# Ultrasonography of the Prenatal Brain

## NOTICE

Medicine is an ever-changing science. As new research and clinical experience broaden our knowledge, changes in treatment and drug therapy are required. The authors and the publisher of this work have checked with sources believed to be reliable in their efforts to provide information that is complete and generally in accord with the standards accepted at the time of publication. However, in view of the possibility of human error or changes in medical sciences, neither the authors nor the publisher nor any other party who has been involved in the preparation or publication of this work warrants that the information contained herein is in every respect accurate or complete, and they disclaim all responsibility for any errors or omissions or for the results obtained from use of the information contained in this work. Readers are encouraged to confirm the information contained herein with other sources. For example and in particular, readers are advised to check the product information sheet included in the package of each drug they plan to administer to be certain that the information contained in this work is accurate and that changes have not been made in the recommended dose or in the contraindications for administration. This recommendation is of particular importance in connection with new or infrequently used drugs.

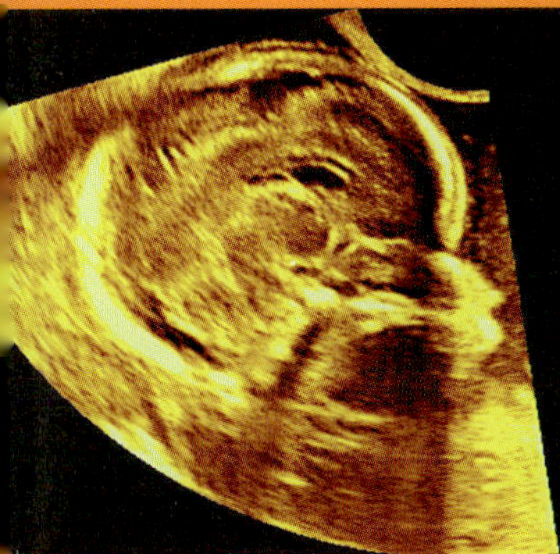

# ULTRASONOGRAPHY OF THE PRENATAL BRAIN

Third Edition

**Ilan E. Timor-Tritsch, MD**
Professor of Obstetrics and Gynecology
Director, Division of Obstetrical and Gynecological Ultrasound
Department of Obstetrics and Gynecology
New York University School of Medicine
New York, New York

**Ana Monteagudo, MD**
Professor of Obstetrics and Gynecology
Director, Bellevue Medical Center Obstetrics and Gynecology, Ultrasound Unit
Fellowship Director
Maternal-Fetal Medicine
Department of Obstetrics and Gynecology
New York University School of Medicine
New York, New York

**Gianluigi Pilu, MD**
Associate Professor of Obstetrics and Gynecology
Department of Obstetrics and Gynecology
University of Bologna, Italy
Bologna, Italy

**Gustavo Malinger, MD**
Associate Clinical Professor of Obstetrics and Gynecology
Director, Division of Prenatal Diagnosis
Co-Director, Fetal Neurology Clinic
Department of Obstetrics and Gynecology
Edith Wolfson Medical Center
Sackler School of Medicine
Tel Aviv University
Holon, Israel

McGraw Hill Medical

New York Chicago San Francisco Lisbon London Madrid Mexico City
Milan New Delhi San Juan Seoul Singapore Sydney Toronto

The McGraw-Hill Companies

**Ultrasonography of the Prenatal Brain, Third Edition**



2 3 4 5 6 7 8 9 0 CTP/CTP 17 16 15 14 13 12

ISBN 978-0-07-161306-4
MHID 0-07-161306-4

This book was set in Warnock Pro by Thomson Digital.
The editor was Alyssa Fried.
The production supervisor was Sherri Souffrance.
Project management was provided by Aakriti Kathuria, Thomson Digital.
The cover designer was Mary McKeon.
China Translation & Printing, Ltd. was printer and binder.

**Library of Congress Cataloging-in-Publication Data**

Ultrasonography of the prenatal brain / [edited by] Ilan E., Timor-Tritsch, Ana Monteagudo, Gianluigi Pilu, Gustavo Malinger. —3rd ed.
p. ; cm.
Includes bibliographical references and index.
ISBN-13: 978-0-07-161306-4 (hardcover : alk. paper)
ISBN-10: 0-07-161306-4 (hardcover : alk. paper)
I. Timor-Tritsch, Ilan E. II. Monteagudo, Ana. III. Pilu, Gianluigi. IV. Malinger, Gustavo.
[DNLM: 1. Fetal Diseases—ultrasonography. 2. Brain—embryology. 3. Brain—growth & development. 4. Echoencephalography. 5. Infant, Newborn, Diseases—ultrasonography. WQ 209]
618.3'207543—dc23
2011035776

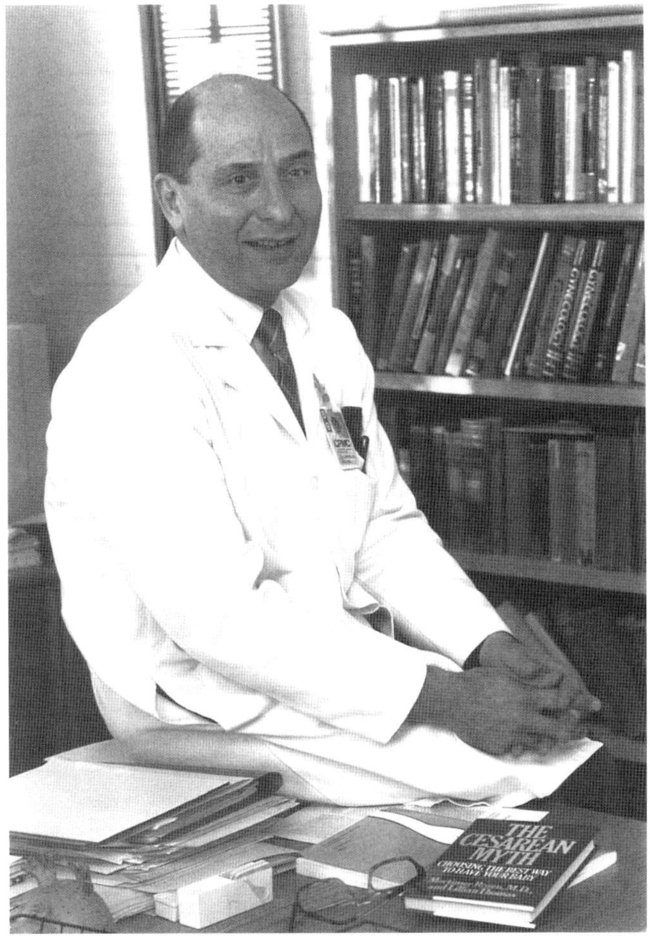

Mortimer G. Rosen, MD
1931–1992

This book is dedicated to Mortimer G. Rosen, friend and mentor, whose early research on the fetal brain was an inspiration to me and many other young researchers struggling to understand the fetal brain. By creating the necessary clinical and scientific environment for such studies, he became very much a part of its "birth." Many years ago, probably at the beginning of his career as a perinatologist, Dr. Rosen recognized the importance of studying the human fetal brain. Surrounded by a growing group of enthusiastic scholars, including residents, maternal-fetal fellows, biomedical engineers, and biochemists, he pursued his research on one of the most difficult subjects: the physiology and the physiopathology of the fetal central nervous system.

Dr. Rosen believed that the then available systems for monitoring fetal health and well-being were inadequate for predicting the intellectual functioning of the neonatal brain. He was always seeking new ways for studying the developing human brain.

When ultrasonography was introduced, Dr. Rosen was among the first to encourage its use in the study of fetal behavioral studies. When he saw the first detailed, crystal clear pictures of the prenatal central nervous system achieved by high frequency transvaginal imaging, he immediately understood the enormous potential of this laboratory technique.

His scientific integrity and skepticism stimulated us to become experts in our field, and furnish objective results to prove the clinical value of high resolution brain scanning of the fetus.

When I presented him with the outline of this book, he was not only supportive, but promised to contribute a special chapter on cerebral palsy, a subject in which he was extremely interested. This is the only time he let us down. The chapter never got further than its introduction. Mort Rosen—my mentor and friend, as well as enthusiastic supporter of our endeavors—passed away in 1992, not living long enough to see the fruits of his labors.

To you, Mort Rosen, in loving memory. I think you would be proud of this work.

Ilan E. Timor-Tritsch, MD

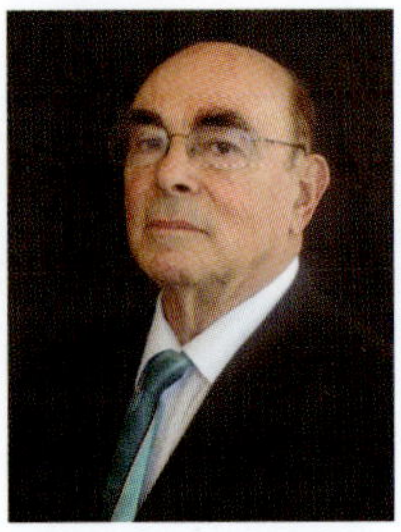

Ilan E. Timor-Tritsch, MD

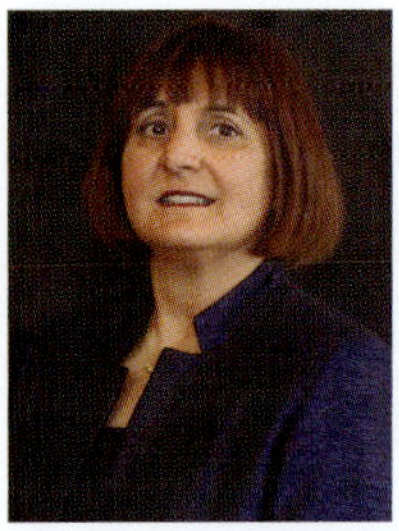

Ana Monteagudo, MD

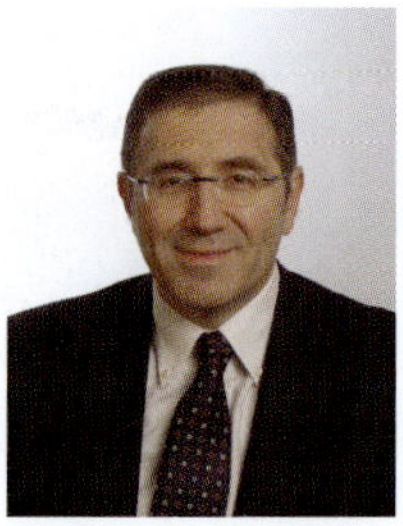

Gianluigi Pilu, MD

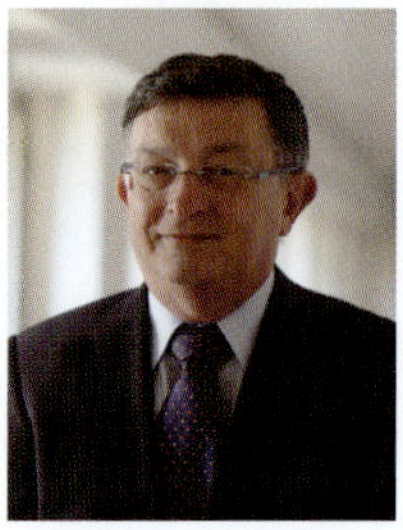

Gustavo Malinger, MD

To my family.

Ilan E. Timor-Tritsch, MD

To my family: my son, Benjamin; my parents, Edith and Miguel; my sister, my niece, and my brother-in-law: Edith A, Carolinna, and Michael who inspired, supported, and encouraged me.

Ana Monteagudo, MD

To my wife and my daughter. Antonella and Isabella, you have all my love.

Gianluigi Pilu, MD

To papá y mamá with love, you will be in my heart forever. To Eyal, Andrés y Nicole, I am very proud of you. To Patricia, you make everything possible.

Gustavo Malinger, MD

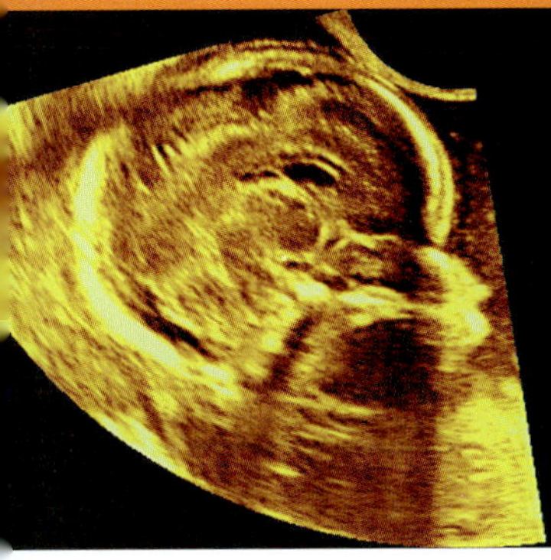

# CONTENTS

# CONTRIBUTORS

**Reuven Achiron, MD**
Professor of Obstetrics and Gynecology
Division of Prenatal Diagnosis
Department of Obstetrics and Gynecology
The Chaim Sheba Medical Center
Tel Hashomer, Israel
(Chapter 17)

**Liat Ben-Sira, MD**
Division of Pediatric Radiology
Department of Radiology
Tel Aviv Medical Center
Sackler School of Medicine
Tel Aviv University
Tel Aviv, Israel
(Chapter 7)

**Zeev Blumenfeld, MD**
Associate Professor
Director, Reproductive Endocrinology
Department of Obstetrics and Gynecology
Rambam Medical Center
Technion-Faculty of Medicine
Haifa, Israel
(Chapter 14)

**Eran Bornstein, MD**
Maternal-Fetal Medicine
Director of Obstetrical Service
Lenox Hill Hospital/North Shore LIJ
New York, New York
(Chapter 11)

**Moshe Bronshtein, MD**
Faculty of Social Welfare & Health Sciences
University of Haifa
AL-KOL Institute of Ultrasound
Haifa, Israel
(Chapter 14)

**Selim Buyukkurt, MD**
Department of Obstetrics and Gynecology
University of Cukurova
School of Medicine
Adana, Turkey
(Chapters 4, 6, 8, 10)

**Shimon Degani, MD**
Professor of Obstetrics and Gynecology
Faculty of Medicine
Technion-Israel Institute of Technology
Director of Ultrasound Unit
Department of Obstetrics and Gynecology
Bnai Zion Medical Center
Haifa, Israel
(Chapter 15)

**Maria Del Rio, MD, PhD**
Department of Obstetrics and Gynecology
Hospital General Hospitalet
Barcelona, Spain
(Chapter 2)

**Tullio Ghi, MD**
Department of Obstetrics and Gynecology
University of Bologna
Bologna, Italy
(Chapter 16)

**Yinon Gilboa, MD**
Department of Obstetrics and Gynecology
The Chaim Sheba Medical Center
Sackler School of Medicine
Tel Aviv University
Tel Aviv, Israel
(Chapter 17)

**Natan Haratz-Rubinstein, MD**
New York Methodist Hospital
Advanced Womens Imaging
Brooklyn, New York
(Chapter 3)

**Ashwin Jadhav, MD, MS**
Assistant Professor
Division of Maternal-Fetal Medicine
Department of Obstetrics and Gynecology
UMDNJ-Robert Wood Johnson Medical School
New Brunswick, New Jersey
(Chapter 10)

**Eldad Katorza, MD**
Department of Obstetrics and Gynecology
The Chaim Sheba Medical Center
Sackler School of Medicine
Tel Aviv University
Tel Aviv, Israel
(Chapter 17)

**Tally Lerman-Sagie, MD**
Associate Clinical Professor
Fetal Neurology Clinic
Division of Pediatric Neurology
Department of Pediatrics
Edith Wolfson Medical Center
Sackler School of Medicine
Tel Aviv University
Holon, Israel
(Chapter 7, 9, 12)

**Gustavo Malinger, MD**
Associate Clinical Professor of Obstetrics and Gynecology
Director, Division of Prenatal Diagnosis
Co-Director, Fetal Neurology Clinic
Department of Obstetrics and Gynecology
Edith Wolfson Medical Center
Sackler School of Medicine
Tel Aviv University
Holon, Israel
(Chapters 4, 6, 7, 8, 9, 10, 12, 16)

**Israel Meizner, MD**
Professor of Obstetrics and Gynecology
Ultrasound Unit
The Helen Schneider Hospital for Women
Rabin Medical Center—Beilinson Campus
Sackler School of Medicine
Tel Aviv University
Tel Aviv, Israel
(Chapter 13)

**Ana Monteagudo, MD**
Professor of Obstetrics and Gynecology
Director, Bellevue Medical Center Obstetrics and Gynecology, Ultrasound Unit
Fellowship Director
Maternal-Fetal Medicine
Department of Obstetrics and Gynecology
New York University School of Medicine
New York, New York
(Chapters 2, 3, 5, 10, 11)

**Fabiola Müller, Dr. habil.rer.nat.**
Professor Emeritus
School of Medicine
University of California, Davis
Davis, California
(Chapter 1)

**Ronan O'Rahilly, MD, DSc**
Professor Emeritus
School of Medicine
University of California, Davis
Davis, California
(Chapter 1)

**Gianluigi Pilu, MD**
Associate Professor of Obstetrics and Gynecology
Department of Obstetrics and Gynecology
University of Bologna, Italy
Bologna, Italy
(Chapters 4, 6, 8, 10, 16)

**Ritsuko K. Pooh, MD, PhD**
Chief Director, Fetal Diagnostic Unit
Clinical Research Institute of Fetal Medicine
Osaka, Japan
(Chapter 15)

**Asuri N. Prasad, MBBS**
Associate Professor of Pediatrics
Section of Clinical Neurosciences
Department of Pediatrics and Child Health
University of Western Ontario, London
Ontario, Canada
(Chapter 12)

**Ilan E. Timor-Tritsch, MD**
Professor of Obstetrics and Gynecology
Director, Division of Obstetrical and Gynecological Ultrasound
Department of Obstetrics and Gynecology
New York University School of Medicine
New York, New York
(Chapters 2, 3, 5, 11)

**Ants Toi, MD, FRCPC, FAIUM**
Professor of Radiology, and of Obstetrics and Gynecology
Associate Professor
University of Toronto
Department of Medical Imaging
Mount Sinai Hospital and University Health Network
Toronto, Canada
(Chapter 7)

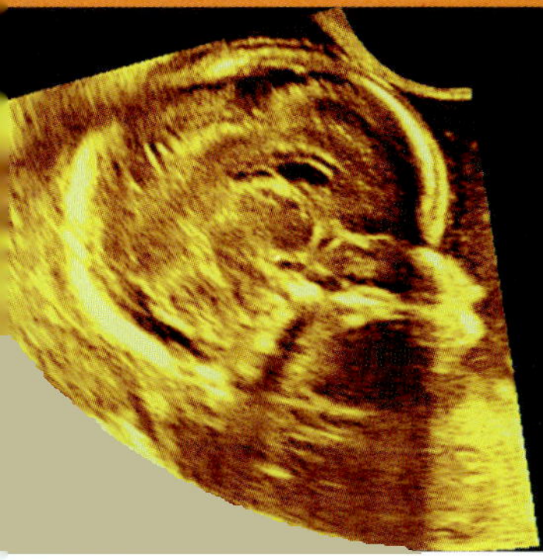

# FOREWORD

Recent advances in imaging of the fetus have furthered our understanding of the neurodevelopment of the fetal brain. This third edition of *Ultrasonography of the Prenatal Brain* has capitalized on incorporating these new technologies in this textbook, to bring to the reader the most advanced information alongside the most impressive images. What Drs. Timor and Monteagudo provided in their first two editions, while nothing short of outstanding, has now been outdone in this third edition. Their choice of Drs. Pilu and Malinger as the additional editors was a work of genius. These two individuals, along with Drs. Timor and Monteagudo, are without a doubt the most talented and knowledgeable in imaging the fetal brain. While expecting excellence from these authors is the norm, the reader will not be disappointed. This text is all you would want and more. In the few chapters in which the editors are not contributors, they have chosen experts who are clearly the most knowledgeable on the specific subjects.

In reading this outstanding text, the reader will quickly marvel at how easily the text flows and is complimented by exquisite companion images. This edition uses advances in MRI fetal imaging to perfection. The just-right use of this modality highlights its most appropriate applications. At the same time the highest quality 2D and 3D images beautifully demonstrate how and why ultrasound remains the frontline modality for prenatal assessment of the fetal brain. The reader can easily follow normal fetal development from the early embryonic period all the way to the third trimester. The authors have created a near-perfect approach that allows the reader to easily recognize even subtle malformations in development. Along with the impeccable images the authors of all chapters have incorporated management recommendations including the appropriate follow-up or use of additional imaging and/or laboratory methods.

This textbook is a major contribution to the literature. It is a must for anyone doing prenatal diagnosis and for every ultrasound laboratory doing any obstetric imaging. Changes made warrant the addition of this text to one's library even if one has the second edition. Whether it is the new information on the molecular diagnosis, metabolic disorders, or infectious or vascular changes, any one of these areas provides enough value in and of itself to warrant ownership of this third edition. In reading this new book I can say that I have been given the advanced privilege of capitalizing on the new information of this edition. I have already translated many of the newly described diagnostic pearls into daily practice. While it was already clear to me before reading this edition that Drs. Timor, Monteagudo, Pilu, and Malinger are the giants of our field and my expectations were high, after reading the text I was not—and you will not be—disappointed. Their prolific writing style, combined with the beautiful diagnostic images and pathological correlation, is impeccable. While many textbooks cannot be easily read in their entirety, this text reads like a novel. The reader gets deeper and deeper involved and cannot put the book down without reading another chapter or two. You learn from every page read. You marvel at the images. Drs. Timor, Monteagudo, Pilu, and Malinger are to be congratulated for bringing us closer to understanding fetal neurodevelopment and anatomy. I am forever humbled by being given this honor to write this foreword.


Lawrence D. Platt, MD
Professor of Obstetrics and Gynecology
David Geffen School of Medicine at UCLA
Director Center for Fetal Medicine
and Women's Ultrasound
Los Angeles, California

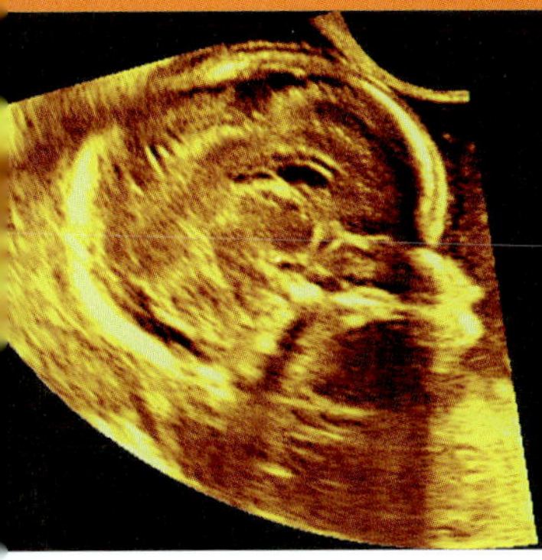

# PREFACE TO THE FIRST EDITION

The concept for this book was born many years ago and was preceded by careful acquisition and selection of representative neurosonograms of normal and abnormal cases. The central nervous system is probably the most elaborate and intricate organ or system in the human body. Minute structural abnormalities can, at times, reflect major functional deficiencies. On the other hand, it would appear that at times major anatomic defects do not seem to be associated with significantly deviant function. It is extremely important to study and understand the normal and abnormal fetal and neonatal central nervous system. The central nervous system is one of the common sites of anatomical malformation in the fetus with chromosomal abnormality. The detection of anomalies within the fetal and neonatal brain is feasible using modern imaging techniques, such as ultrasound, computed tomography, and magnetic resonance imaging.

The aim of prenatal ultrasonography is to be able to reassure the pregnant patient as early as possible that fetal development is normal; or if a malformation is detected to counsel the patient about the nature of the problem. Most anomalies of the central nervous system develop early, and we have the tools to detect these as early as 10 to 16 weeks. Early detection of such central nervous system anomalies is probably the most important advance in modern perinatology. Neonatal ultrasound confirms the prenatal diagnosis. In addition, neonatal neurosonography is a powerful tool in diagnosing central nervous system pathology.

The first chapter deals with the development of the human central nervous system. Its authors are the distinguished professors Ronan O'Rahilly and Fabiola Müller, who have a lifetime of professional experience. Professor O'Rahilly not only took time to write about the embryology of the brain, but also invested valuable time in overseeing the correct anatomical terminology used throughout most of the chapters.

The vast imaging possibilities of ultrasound in general and that of transvaginal sonography in particular regarding the fetal brain, are dealt with at the beginning of our book and lead into the chapters describing the detectable pathology in the fetal and neonatal central nervous system. Because fetal and neonatal neurosonographic scanning is performed using the anterior fontanelle and other calvarial openings, the "classical" axial planes cannot be used to describe the images obtained in the fan-shaped sonographic sections. It was our goal to keep the "classic" planes in use by CT and by MRI imaging of the brain and create a separate and well-defined set of planes and sections for the fetal brain imaging. A new nomenclature regarding the scanning planes of the fetal brain is introduced in Chapters 1, 2, 3, and 4.

We felt that a special and dedicated chapter dealing with biometry of the fetal brain should be included. A large number of tables and graphs as well as measurements of the fetal brain are incorporated for reference.

Because the fetal eye and the fetal face are frequently associated with brain pathology, two special chapters are devoted to these structures. Dr. Israel Meizner and Dr. Moshe Bronshtein's group from Israel have the most imaging experience in these two areas and contributed these two important chapters, which we believe are the most detailed in the literature dealing with those subjects.

Neonatal neurosonology is an established diagnostic entity which has earned its well-deserved place in the armamentarium of the neuroimager since its introduction in 1979. Chapters concerning imaging of the normal and abnormal neonatal brain, and the chapter by Dr. Madhuri Kirpekar dealing with the spine, are included to form a continuum as far as the sonographic neuroimaging work-up of the prenatal and neonatal CNS.

The chapter written by Gianluigi Pilu and Vincenso D'Addario and their co-workers from Italy, made a significant contribution to the book by touching on the subject of the midline brain pathologies and the recently introduced attempts to image the fetal brain using MRI.

It is hard and labor intensive to study the physiological aspects of the brain. This was successfully done by recognized authors such as Jan Nijhuis who reviewed the fetal behavioral states coordinated by the brain and by Shimon Degani and Reuven Lewinsky summarizing the clinical uses of measuring the blood flow to the central nervous system.

Finally, the ethical aspects of neurosonography are explored by Frank Chervenak, who over the years has become an authority in the field of medical ethics.

This book was written for the perinatologists, neonatologists. perinatal geneticists, as well as the imaging specialists such as radiologists, obstetricians, and sonographers who see the fetus and neonate in their clinical practice. These specialists scan the fetal and neonatal brain themselves or are directly involved with managing pregnancies with structural malformations or anomalies of the central nervous system. Special emphasis was placed on the creation of an objective and exhaustive updated review of the pertinent literature so that the reader would have a wide reference base on each subject. As far as the illustrations are concerned, the authors were encouraged to be liberal about including an unrestricted number of cases and their sonographic manifestations in their respective chapters. This may, therefore, lead to some duplication by presenting the same disease or pathology more than once. However, by allowing some deliberate repetition in depicting various cases, we, hopefully, covered the commonly occurring pathologies. We consider such occasional and repetitive presentations as one of the advantages of the text enabling the reader to be educated by the experiences of the different authors and their various points of view.

One of the particular strengths of presenting the sonograms is that we chose to include small body images so that readers could orient themselves as to how an individual sonographic view was obtained. This will, we hope, enable readers to quickly grasp and understand the actual planes used to generate the pictures.

We suggest that neuroimaging of the fetus be included in the structural evaluation of the fetus at any gestational age. We also believe that practitioners involved in fetal and/or neonatal neuroimaging will benefit from using this carefully prepared text.

Ilan E. Timor-Tritsch, MD
Ana Monteagudo, MD
Harris L. Cohen, MD

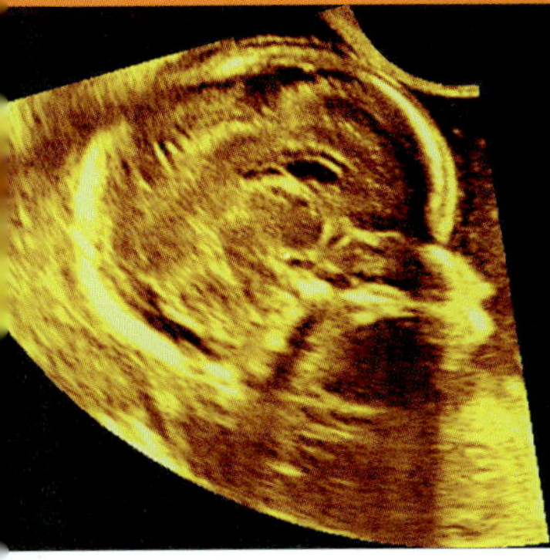

# PREFACE TO THE SECOND EDITION

Responding to the positive feedback to the First Edition of our book we decided to update it and expand its content. An additional reason for this decision was the amount of new and pertinent articles which have accumulated in the last 3–4 years. We wanted to review them and add most of them to the more than 1100 references we used in the First Edition.

As far as the chapters are concerned, every previously written chapter was updated and there are several new chapters. Major changes were made in Chapters 2, 4, 5 and 8 to reflect the new clinical experience in the field of fetal neuroscan and fetal neuro-MRI. New sonographic images of commonly encountered entities were added to the previously published ones. Several rarely seen fetal neuropathologies were also illustrated and were included. All chapters were updated with the newest articles from the literature to justify the term "reference textbook," a term used by many as they mention the First Edition of the book.

Two new chapters (9 and 14) were added dealing with three-dimensional fetal and neonatal neuroscans. Pediatric neurologists and neurosurgeons rely on neonatal CT and MRI images to study the neonatal brain. So far they seemed hesitant to counsel and to plan postnatal (and prenatal) management of pathologies based upon prenatal ultrasound imaging studies. The reason was the prenatal images were obtained at planes unfamiliar to them. They were waiting to see the postnatal imaging studies. Since the introduction of 2D and now 3D transfontanelle fetal neuroimaging by high-frequency, high-resolution ultrasound clear images can be generated in the planes which are familiar to pediatric neurologists and neurosurgeons. The expected result of these images is a better understanding of the pathologies leading to an earlier prenatal counseling and planning for postpartum management before the neonatal studies are available. We predict that the 3D fetal and neonatal brain scan will expand and will be widely employed as effective diagnostic means.

The addition of two new chapters deals with devastating diseases of the fetal brain and attempts for their correction. Chapter 16 summarizes possible causes of cerebral palsy and Chapter 18 is a description of attempts to correct neurological pathologies *in utero*. It seems that after the well-known moratorium to treat diseases of the brain, while the fetus is still in the womb, there may be a place for intrauterine treatment for a well-selected patient population after adequately researched surgical procedures.

The use of the icons at the side of ultrasound images, to indicate the particular plane or section at which the image was generated, was extended to several more chapters. This ensures a better understanding of the anatomy depicted.

We tried (quite successfully) to standardize the anatomic nomenclature throughout the book and based it on the latest issue of the internationally accepted *Nomina Anatomica*. Correctly or incorrectly, some terms are so deeply "embedded" in the daily use, that it may be impossible to constantly correct them. One such example is the word "hydrocephaly" (the accepted, correct way to use it) which over time was changed to "hydrocephalus" and (probably incorrectly) used in many publications. We selected to use the correct term "hydrocephalus" in all chapters.

We hope that the Second Edition of this book will contribute to the understanding and most importantly the earliest possible detection of neurological diseases of the fetus and the newborn.

Ilan E. Timor-Tritsch, MD
Ana Monteagudo, MD
Harris L. Cohen, MD

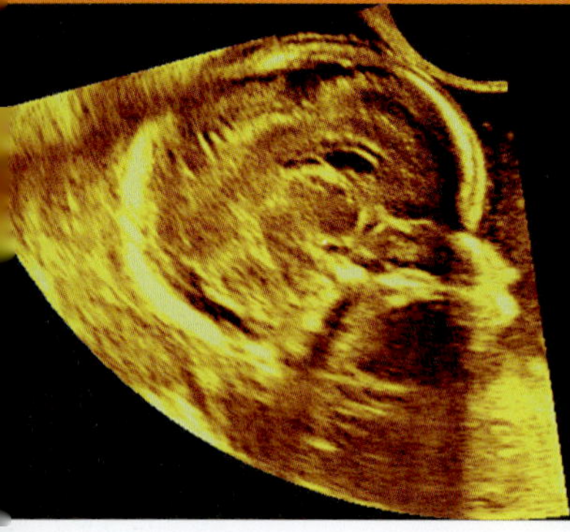

# PREFACE TO THE THIRD EDITION

It is hard to believe, but the first edition of this book saw the light 15 years ago. At the time, it became a useful reference for those who wanted to understand the development, the anatomy, and the pathophysiology of the fetal central nervous system from the viewpoint of ultrasonography.

After a relatively short 5 years—in 2001—the second edition of the book was published. We received encouraging feedback from the ultrasound and the feto-maternal specialists to add the necessary incremental knowledge and include relevant information to publish an updated second edition.

During the time from 2001 to recent days, several things happened that led us to consider the publication of the third edition of the book.

The first compelling reason to update the book was the "outburst" of new clinical research regarding imaging of the fetal brain. The use of high frequency and deep penetrating ultrasound transducer probes yielded increasing resolution, hence more accurate pictures of the fetal brain and spine. These high-resolution pictures found their way into the traditional "printed journals," but even more so into the electronic media. Lectures at courses and webinars, and teaching on CDs and the Internet, spread the understanding and knowledge, requiring an organized way to compile it and reach out to those interested in the subject.

The second impetus to practically rewrite the previous edition was the tremendous improvement and dissemination of three-dimensional ultrasound techniques and magnetic resonance imaging. By resonating to these, we decided to incorporate those two imaging modalities into the individual chapters wherever necessary to enhance understanding, rather than leaving them as stand-alone chapters. In the previous editions, we had placed these two subjects in their separate chapters. Our intention was to emphasize, teach, and incorporate these two important imaging technologies. Now that they are used daily to complement traditional ultrasound imaging of the fetal brain, we incorporated this use as an integral part of the many "older" as well as the new chapters.

The third and not less important reason to redo and rejuvenate the book was the increasing interest in imaging the fetal nervous system as it pertains to imaging the fetal brain. The surging clinical research in Europe, North America, South America, and Israel, to name only a few locations, gave birth to a new generation of young and enthusiastic imagers, maternal–fetal medicine specialists, radiologists, and basic scientists, who literally inundated the field with new observations. As a result of this data surge, conference goers and others kept asking when a new edition of the book would be released.

To answer all three issues and explain the horizons of the new edition, Gustavo Malinger of Israel and Gianluigi Pilu of Italy graciously agreed to serve as co-editors. It was the widening of our perception of teaching that led us to change the format of the chapters completely, making them easier to read and easier to find points of interest. There is no doubt that adding new chapter authors, as well as scores of new 2D and 3D ultrasound images and updated literature were the necessary ingredients to consider this textbook of fetal neuroimaging a relevant reference source.

As to the newly added chapters, we would like to mention them briefly. Ventriculomegaly was given its own importance. It is the most common presenting sonographic sign of brain pathology; therefore, the possible underlying clinico-pathologic reasons for it were "carved out" from the many different sites that were mentioned, creating a dedicated chapter for easy reference.

The different anomalies were reclassified, such as those of the ventral and dorsal induction, and that of cortical development. We tried to pour light upon a diagnostically problematic area of the fetal brain, namely the posterior fossa, focusing on a small but nevertheless important structure, the vermis. Three new chapters dealing with intrauterine insults, intrauterine infections, and metabolic disorders were also added to cover the progress made in those areas that became pertinent to fetal neuroscans.

In short, the newly incorporated chapters, along with those updated and carried over from our last edition, may render this new edition useful for those engaging in the clinical evaluation of the fetal brain.

Ilan E. Timor-Tritsch, MD
Ana Monteagudo, MD
Gianluigi Pilu, MD
Gustavo Malinger, MD

# ACKNOWLEDGMENTS

We thank Ms. Christonia Joseph for her tireless editorial and secretarial work and for coordinating the production of this book. We also thank the editorial team of McGraw-Hill Medical for their work in producing this new edition of our book.

# Ultrasonography of the Prenatal Brain

Chapter 1

# PRENATAL DEVELOPMENT OF THE BRAIN

***Ronan O'Rahilly • Fabiola Müller***

**KEY POINTS**

1. The embryonic period (the first 8 postfertilizational weeks) is subdivided into 23 morphological stages, which, because they are based on internal as well as external criteria, cannot be identified with confidence by ultrasonography.
2. The three major divisions of the brain are found early (stage 9), closure of the neuropores seals the cerebrospinal cavity at 4½ weeks (stage 13), and the five main subdivisions of the brain are visible at 5 weeks (stage 15).
3. The telencephalon is identifiable already at 4 weeks (stage 10) and begins to diverticulate at 5 weeks (during stage 14), but holoprosencephaly is more than a mere failure of diverticulation and may begin as early as 3 weeks (stage 8), as can cyclopia and anencephaly.
4. The appearance of the cortical plate (stage 21) heralds the beginning of lamination of the cerebral cortex, the basal nuclei and internal capsule are progressing, and the brain is developmentally advanced at the end of the embryonic period.
5. Prominent features during the fetal period are the C-shaped structures, including the corpus callosum, and the appearance of sulci and gyri on the cortical surface at the middle of prenatal life.

Prenatal life can be divided conveniently into (1) the embryonic period proper, that is, the first 8 weeks following fertilization, and (2) the fetal period, which extends to birth. The distinction between the embryonic and fetal periods is well founded and has long been established in human embryology. The embryonic period is that time during which new features appear with great rapidity, whereas the fetal period is characterized more by the elaboration of existing structures. Moreover, the vast majority of congenital anomalies appear during the embryonic period. The difference is highlighted by the fact that the embryonic period has been successfully subdivided into morphological stages, whereas the fetal period has so far defied such a procedure.

The embryonic period has been divided into 23 developmental (Carnegie) stages (Table 1-1), which have been listed in detail by O'Rahilly and Müller,[1] in whose monograph the early development of the human embryo has been thoroughly described. Each stage, on average, lasts slightly more than 2 days. The stages are based on both external and internal morphological criteria and depend mainly on features that change rapidly, such as the number of somitic pairs, the early appearance of the eye, and the form of the developing limbs. Although it may sometimes be possible to estimate approximately a given stage on ultrasonography, the staging system is based on having an embryo "in the hand" rather than in utero. Moreover, very early as well as late stages can be identified precisely only by histologic examination.

Although schemes have been devised to subdivide the fetal period according to either measurements or age (one of the simplest, into trimesters, is still very useful), no morphological staging system is available, largely because changes are neither sufficiently rapid nor adequately spectacular.

## TERMINOLOGY

It should be pointed out that, in current usage in anatomy, practically all eponyms (eg, Luschka, Magendie, Monro, Reil, Rolando, and Sylvius) are now obsolete because they convey nothing concerning either the site or the nature of the relevant structure. The addition "of Monro" or "of Sylvius" is superfluous because there is only one interventricular foramen and only one aqueduct in the brain.

## PRENATAL MEASUREMENTS

Several different measurements, such as the biparietal diameter and the ossified femoral length, are very important in later development, but the most useful datum throughout prenatal life is still the greatest length, exclusive of the (flexed) lower limbs.[2] Crown-rump (C-R) length is less satisfactory because point C, which overlies the midbrain, is frequently difficult to locate, and point R is

**Table 1–1. SUMMARY OF DEVELOPMENT OF THE CENTRAL NERVOUS SYSTEM**

| Stage | Greatest Length (mm) | Approximate Age (days) | Key Features |
|---|---|---|---|
| **Embryonic Period** | | | |
| 1–7 | 0.1–0.4 | 1–19 | Very early embryo |
| 8 | 1 | 23 | Neural folds and groove |
| 9 | 2 | 25 | Mesencephalic flexure; rhombencephalon, mesencephalon, prosencephalon; 1–3 S |
| 10 | 3 | 28 | Fusion of neural folds begins; telencephalon and diencephalon distinguishable; optic primordia; 4–12 S |
| 11 | 3.5 | 29 | Rostral neuropore closes; 13–20 S |
| 12 | 4 | 30 | Caudal neuropore closes; secondary neurulation begins; 21–29 S |
| 13 | 5 | 32 | Closed neural tube; primordium of cerebellum; isthmus rhombencephali; 30–? ; Figure 1–2A |
| 14 | 6 | 33 | Pontine flexure; future cerebral hemispheres; all 16 neuromeres present |
| 15 | 8 | 36 | Five subdivisions: medulla, pons, midbrain, diencephalons, telencephalon; Figures 1–2B; 1–3A, B; 1–4 |
| 16 | 10 | 38 | Thalamus; Figure 1–5 |
| 17 | 13 | 41 | Internal and external cerebellar swellings; Figure 1–2C |
| 18 | 15 | 44 | Future corpus striatum; interventricular foramina defined; Figure 1–6 |
| 19 | 17 | 46 | Choroid plexus of fourth ventricle |
| 20 | 20 | 49 | Choroid plexus of lateral ventricles; Figure 1–3C, D |
| 21 | 23 | 51 | Anterior and inferior horns of lateral ventricle; circulus arteriosus complete; Figure 1–2D |
| 22 | 26 | 53 | Internal capsule |
| 23 | 29 | 56 | Caudate nucleus and putamen; anterior commissure begins |
| **Fetal Period** | | | |
| Trimester 1 | | | Cerebellar halves unite, and vermis becomes defined<br>Corpus callosum is still very limited<br>Aqueduct appears narrow<br>Posterior horn of lateral ventricle |
| Trimester 2 | | | Corpus callosum covers roof of third ventricle<br>Sulci and gyri become visible on hemispheric surface<br>Crura cerebri are prominent<br>Hippocampal formation becomes S-shaped<br>Myelinization begins in CNS |
| Trimester 3 | | | Insula buried by opercula |

CNS, central nervous system; S, pairs of somites.

*Note:* The greatest lengths and the postfertizational ages given are approximate only. The latter have been revised to conform to current ultrasonic information.

Data from O'Rahilly and Müller (2001).[15]

imprecise. The greatest length, which is independent of fixed points, is much simpler to ascertain and is in fact what is generally measured.[3,4]

The distinction between stages and measurements should be kept clearly in mind. The "18-mm stage" is incorrect usage, because 18 mm is merely a length, not a stage as the term is used in embryology.

## PRENATAL AGE

Just as postnatal age commences at birth, prenatal age begins at fertilization. Ovulation is sufficiently close, so that the term *postovulatory* has frequently been used to indicate age. Particularly since the advent of in vitro fertilization, however, age is best referred to as postfertilizational.

When a reliable menstrual history is available, or indirectly by the conventional addition of 2 weeks to the age, the duration from the first day of the last menstrual period (LMP) may be used. The duration is expressed in (post) menstrual weeks and days. This is perfectly acceptable provided that the duration is designated as (post)menstrual, and it is not referred to as age. At postmenstrual week 1, an embryo does not even exist.

In summary, two systems of designation are available: (1) age, which is postfertilizational and generally estimated; and (2) (post)menstrual duration, which, although it is not age (and should not be combined with that word), is a useful guide in clinical practice. The type of weeks being used should be specified: postfertilizational weeks or weeks of age, or (post)menstrual weeks. Confusion is thereby eliminated.

It has been shown that the term *gestational age* in the literature is either not defined or is used indiscriminately for postmenstrual weeks and days or for postfertilizational age.[5] The continuing confusion concerning prenatal age is unnecessary and disappears once the ambiguous and superfluous term *gestational age* is abandoned.

The advent of ultrasonography has led to the construction of many elaborate tables of prenatal measurements related to prenatal age, or more generally to intervals since the LMP. Although not all of these tables are in agreement in detail, it would be agreed that at the end of the embryonic period, when the greatest length is ~30 mm, the age is 8 weeks, corresponding to 10 postmenstrual weeks.

## DEVELOPMENT OF THE NERVOUS SYSTEM

The development of the human nervous system is summarized here (Tables 1–1 and 1–2). The most detailed and precise account of the prenatal human brain, with particular emphasis on the embryonic period, is *The Embryonic Human Brain: An Atlas of Developmental Stages*.[6] That study contains a bibliography of 350 entries, and therefore a detailed list of references is not provided here. Some significant features have been summarized recently.[7]

**Table 1–2. FEATURES OF THE BRAIN FOUND BY ULTRASOUND DURING FIRST TRIMESTER**

| Postfertilizational Weeks (Age) | Postmenstrual Weeks | Features |
|---|---|---|
| 5 | 7 | First indication of brain |
| 5–6 | 7–8 | Cerebral hemispheres, lateral ventricles, wide interventricular foramina<br>Future third ventricle<br>Mesencephalon and future aqueduct<br>Rhombencephalon and fourth ventricle |
| 6–7 | 8–9 | Choroid plexuses of lateral ventricle<br>Telencephalon, diencephalon, mesencephalon, metencephalon, myelencephalon<br>Cerebellum, pontine flexure, lateral recesses of fourth ventricle |
| 7–8 | 9–10 | Falx cerebri<br>C-shaped lateral ventricles<br>Narrower third ventricle<br>Isthmus prosencephali (between third ventricle and aqueduct) |
| 8–10 | 10–12 | Growing thalami<br>Cerebellar hemispheres seem to meet<br>Cerebellar peduncles<br>Tentorium cerebelli<br>Fourth ventricle divided by choroid plexus |

Modified from Timor-Tritsch, Blaas. O'Rahilly and Müller, 2006,[6] with permission.

## PRIMARY NEURULATION

The CNS arises mostly from a part of the ectoderm known as the neural plate. The folding of the neural plate to form successively the neural groove and the neural tube is termed *primary neurulation* and is the first visible sign of the nervous system. It begins when the embryo is ~1 mm in length. Closure of the neural groove begins near the junction of the future brain and spinal cord. The still open ends of the developing neural tube are known as the rostral and caudal neuropores, which close successively at about 4 weeks. The closure of the rostral neuropore is bidirectional: rostrocaudal and caudorostral. Although small and variable accessory loci of fusion of the neural folds may sometimes be seen, a specific pattern of multiple sites of fusion, such as has been described in the mouse, does not occur in the human.[8] Moreover, attempts to force the classification of neural tube defects into such a pattern are unconvincing. Primary neurulation is completed by the separation of neural from surface ectoderm by the interposition of mesenchyme.

## SOME EARLY ANOMALIES

In diastematomyelia the spinal cord is partially split longitudinally into right and left halves that are separated by a fibrocartilaginous or bony spur in the vertebral canal. This may be a manifestation of the split notochord syndrome, which is generally attributed to persistence of the neurenteric canal, a temporary communication through the primitive node (at stages 8 through 10).

Anencephaly, a partial absence of the brain and the overlying cranial vault, frequently arises from (1) failure of the rostral neuropore to close, followed by (2) protrusion of the brain (exencephaly), and finally (3) degeneration of the exposed portions.[9] The defect arises early (probably stages 8 and 9), before postfertilizational week 4, and defective production of mesenchyme is considered to be of fundamental importance.[10]

Holoprosencephaly is a variable deficiency in "diverticulation" of the prosencephalon to form the cerebral hemispheres and is usually accompanied by facial malformation. Abnormal induction by an area of the future forebrain near the prechordal plate very early (stages 7 and 8) is believed to be significant.[11] The failure of lateralization may be complete (alobar holoprosencephaly), partial (semilobar), or only rostral (lobar).

Cyclopia is the occurrence within a single orbit of a median eye (sometimes distinguished as synophthalmia) or paired ocular structures.[11,12] The defective lateralization (which is not a fusion) is believed to be caused by the lack of normal inhibition of the median portion of the originally single optic field.[6] Normally, the prechordal plate induces paired optic primordia very early (stages 7 and 8).

Encephalo(meningo)celes are generally in the occipital region. They are covered by skin and hence are believed to arise after closure of the neural tube, probably in the presence of mesenchymal insufficiency. Those situated anteriorly (eg, in the fronto-ethmoidal region) constitute a separate category and are based on a primary disturbance in the separation of neural and surface ectoderm at the site of final closure of the rostral neuropore, resulting secondarily in a mesodermal defect at this site.[13]

## SECONDARY NEURULATION

Secondary neurulation is the continuing formation of the sacrococcygeal part of the spinal cord from the caudal eminence, without direct involvement of the surface ectoderm (neural plate). It begins once the caudal neuropore has closed. The transition from primary to secondary neurulation is at the site of closure of the caudal neuropore. The caudal neuropore closes at the level of somitic pair 31, which corresponds to future vertebral level S2 in the embryo. Because of the ascent of the spinal cord during the fetal period, however, the site of the former caudal neuropore ascends also and corresponds to a higher vertebral level postnatally.

## THE EMBRYONIC BRAIN

### Postmenstrual Weeks 5 to 6 (3 to 4 Weeks of Age)

As the embryo becomes more elongated, the neural groove becomes deeper, and the three major divisions are distinguishable in the folds of the completely open neural groove: the forebrain, the midbrain, and the hindbrain. The site of the midbrain is indicated by the mesencephalic flexure, which remains distinct throughout the embryonic period (Figure 1–1). The neural tube has not yet formed, and the "brain vesicles" are largely a myth. The forebrain soon becomes subdivided (earlier than previously appreciated) into the diencephalon and the telencephalon medium. The embryo is now ~3 mm in length.

### Postmenstrual Weeks 6 to 7 (4 to 5 Weeks of Age)

When both neuropores are closed at 4 to 5 weeks after fertilization, the future ventricular system (Figure 1–2) no longer communicates with the amniotic cavity. At this time, in embryos ~5 mm in length, the first (bilateral) indication of the cerebellum can be discerned.

The cerebral hemispheres (Figure 1–3) become delimited from the telencephalon medium. A bend, the pontine flexure, begins in the hindbrain and allows a subdivision into the metencephalon (the pons and the cerebellum) and the myelencephalon (the medulla oblongata). All five major subdivisions of the brain are then distinguishable: the telencephalon, diencephalon, mesencephalon, metencephalon, and myelencephalon. The initial development of the basal nuclei (a more accurate term than ganglia) now takes place, and the thalami are also discernible (Figures 1–4 and 1–5). The embryo is ~6 mm in length.

In the Arnold-Chiari malformation, a failure of the pontine flexure to form is believed to be important in the abnormal elongation of the hindbrain.

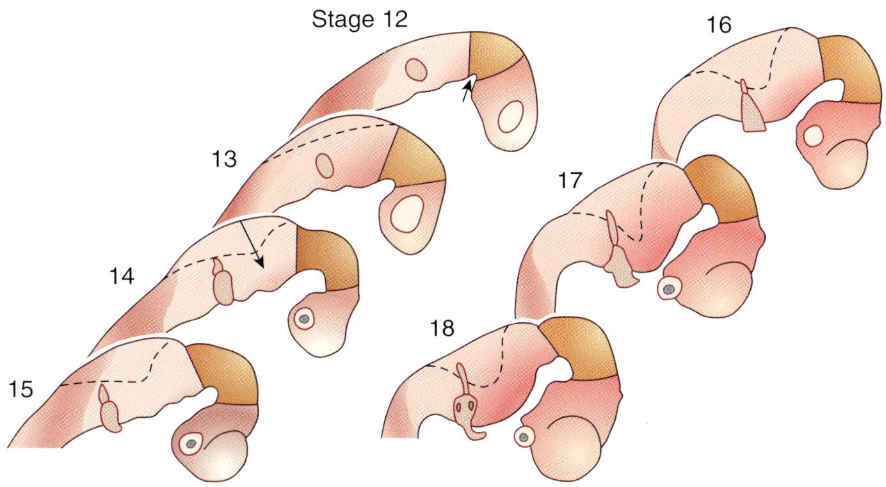


**Figure 1–1.** Right lateral views of the brain at postmenstrual weeks 6 to 8 (4 to 6 weeks of age). The midbrain is shaded, and the mesencephalic flexure (*short arrow*) is evident. The beginning of the pontine flexure can be seen (*larger arrow*). The optic cup and the internal ear are included. (Reproduced from O'Rahilly and Müller, 2006,[6] with permission).

## Postmenstrual Weeks 7 to 8 (5 to 6 Weeks of Age)

The neurohypophysis (Figure 1–3C) begins its evagination, and the longitudinal fissure becomes deeper with continuing growth of the cerebral hemispheres (Figure 1–3D). The basioccipital part of the skull is beginning to chondrify. The embryo is ~12 mm in length.

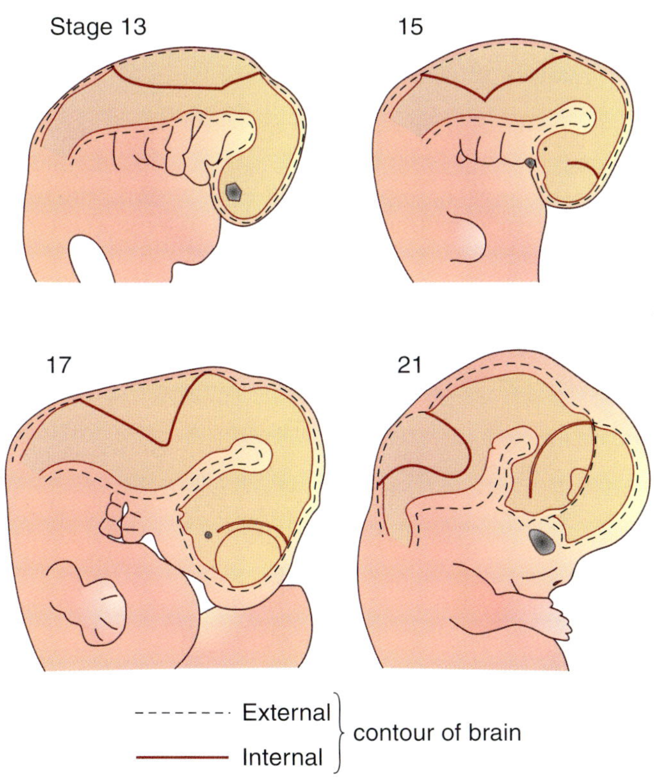


**Figure 1–2.** Right lateral views of the brain in situ to show the ventricular cavities (*shaded*) at postmenstrual weeks 6½ to 9½ (4½ to 7½ weeks of age). The first indication of anterior and inferior horns of the lateral ventricle are visible in the last drawing.

## Postmenstrual Weeks 8 to 9 (6 to 7 Weeks of Age)

A feature that appears very gradually is the flattening of the insular region. The embryo is ~20 mm in length (Figure 1–6).

In the Dandy-Walker syndrome, maldevelopment of the rostral part of the roof of the fourth ventricle is considered to be a significant causative factor.

## Postmenstrual Weeks 9 to 10 (7 to 8 Weeks of Age)

The falx cerebri, indicated initially by a leptomeningeal precursor, is apparent. Ossification is beginning in the occipital region of the skull, and the foramen magnum is definable. The anterior (frontal), posterior (occipital), and inferior (temporal) poles of the cerebral hemispheres, as well as the insula, can be detected, although they are not yet pronounced. The ventricles at this time are shown in Figure 1–7.

Important histologic differentiation takes place in the cerebral cortex, and the internal capsule develops. Numerous nuclei and tracts have been plotted. The anterior and lateral corticospinal tracts are present, and the pyramidal decussation has begun. The spinothalamic tract and thalamocortical fibers (generally considered to be essential for the perception of pain) are appearing. Although the functional significance is far from clear, nociception is present before birth, and it is prudent to assume that pain can be experienced even early in prenatal life.

The embryonic period proper closes at 8 weeks after fertilization, when the greatest length (exclusive of the lower limbs) is ~30 mm. By this time 200 features of the brain have appeared and have been listed.[6]

It is to be stressed that when a structure is first seen in vivo and in utero by current imaging techniques, it should be appreciated that this is usually considerably later than the actual situation elucidated in human embryology.

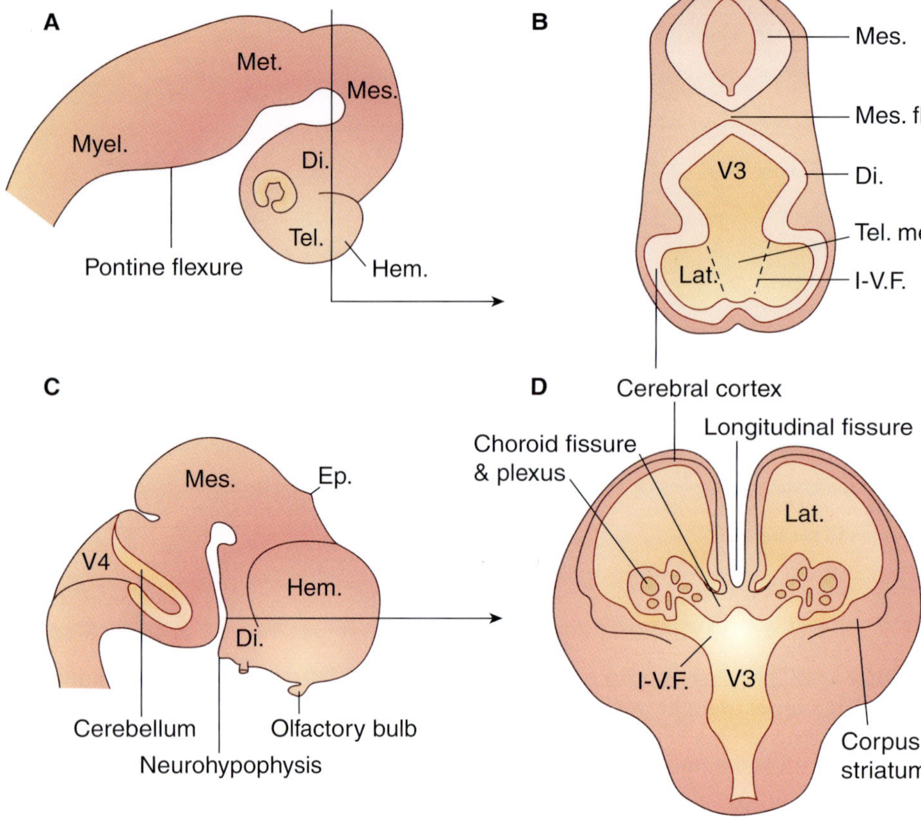


**Figure 1–3.** A and B Postmenstrual week 7 (5 weeks of age). **(A)** The five main subdivisions of the brain (at stage 15). **(B)** The beginning cerebral hemispheres developing from the telencephalon medium. C and D Postmenstrual week 9 (7 weeks of age). **(C)** Typical appearance of the embryonic brain (at stage 20). In **(D)** the wall of each hemisphere has invaginated laterally (at the choroid fissure) into the lateral ventricle to form the choroid plexus. Di., diencephalon; Ep., epiphysis cerebri (pineal gland); Hem., cerebral hemisphere; I-V.F., interventricular foramen; Lat., lateral ventricle; Mes., mesencephalon; Myel., myelencephalon; Tel., telencephalon; Tel. med., telencephalon medium; V3, third ventricle; V4, fourth ventricle.

## VASCULARIZATION

A description of the developing vessels to the brain is available,[14] as are individual details.[6] The internal carotid artery develops early (4 weeks) and is followed by the posterior communicating artery, initially important as the main carotid supply to the hindbrain until the vertebral system is in place and the basilar artery (originally bilateral) becomes dominant. A series of caroticobasilar anastomoses is temporary (4 to 6 weeks), although segments may sometimes persist (eg, a trigeminal artery). With the completion of the anterior communicating artery after the three named cerebral arteries have appeared, the

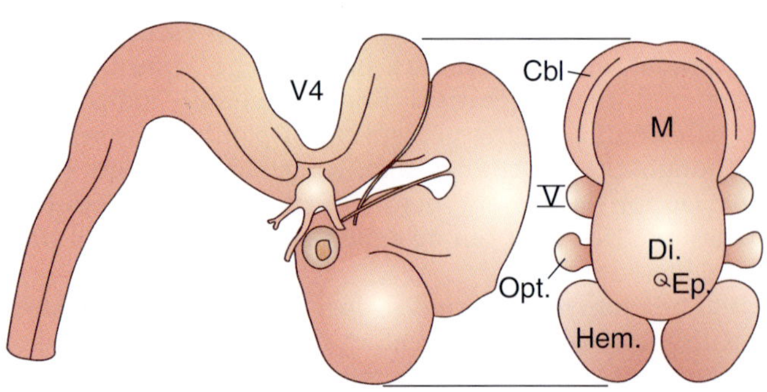


**Figure 1–4.** Right lateral and "end-on" views of the brain at postmenstrual week 8 (6 weeks of age). The pontine and mesencephalic flexures are pronounced (at state 17). The thin roof of the fourth ventricle (V4) is not shown. Included are the optic cup, trigeminal ganglion, and cranial nerves IV and III. Cbl, cerebellum; Di., diencephalon; Ep., epiphysis (pineal); Hem., cerebral hemisphere; Opt., optic cup.

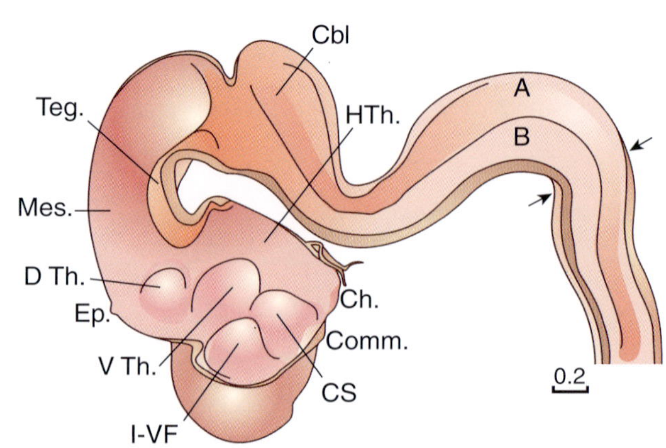


**Figure 1–5.** Medial view at the same stage as the previous figure. The arrows indicate the cerebrospinal junction. A and B, alar and basal laminae; Cbl, cerebellum; Ch., optic chiasma; Comm., commissural plate (future corpus callosum); CS, corpus striatum; DTh., dorsal thalamus; Ep., epiphysis (pineal); HTh., hypothalamus; I-VF, interventricular foramen; Mes., mesencephalon; Teg., tegmentum; VTh., ventral thalamus.

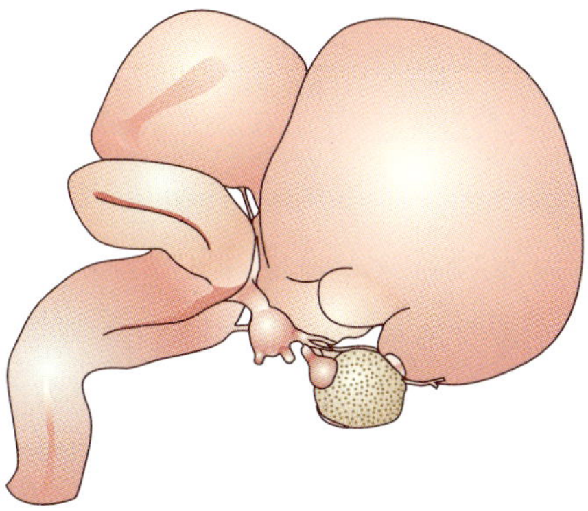

**Figure 1–6.** The brain at the end of the embryonic period (stage 23). The insula is now clearly indented and will later become buried. Most of the diencephalon is by this time covered by the cerebral hemisphere(s). (From O'Rahilly and Müller, 2006,[6] with permission.)

circulus arteriosus (described by Willis) is established by 7 weeks (stage 21).

## SKELETAL SUPPORT[15,16,17]

The skull develops in three overlapping phases: blastemal or membranous (desmocranium), cartilaginous (chondrocranium), and ossific (osteocranium).[18] The inventory of the "membrane bones" is almost complete at the end of the embryonic period, and these components are an important part of the splanchnocranium or viscerocranium, which develops in pharyngeal arches 1 and 2, and uses cartilaginous bars as a template for the mandible and the auditory ossicles. Both endochondral and intramembranous ossification are involved in the skull, which becomes a unity in which the original components are no longer distinct. The spheno-occipital junction is a cartilaginous joint until about puberty, when bony fusion takes place. The much larger portion (neurocranium) of the skull that lies above the orbitomeatal plane protects the brain, which lies in a skeletal bowl from which it is protected by fluid-filled mesenchyme. It is of interest to note that in anencephaly the brain becomes highly differentiated before it begins to disintegrate, but its skeletal base and covering become abnormal early.

The notochord is the distinctive feature of chordates, most of which have a surrounding vertebral column and hence are termed *vertebrates.* The notochord is a complicated "string" that comes to extend from the sphenooccipital junction to the last coccygeal vertebra. It contributes to the nuclei pulposi of the intervertebral discs. Notochordal remains are sometimes found within vertebral bodies, or as a chordoma in the sacrococcygeal or sphenooccipital regions.

The vertebrae (Figure 1–8) arise from sclerotomes derived from somites, which are bilateral mesenchymal segments on each side of the neural tube. The notochord is an axial structure ventral to the tube that eventually

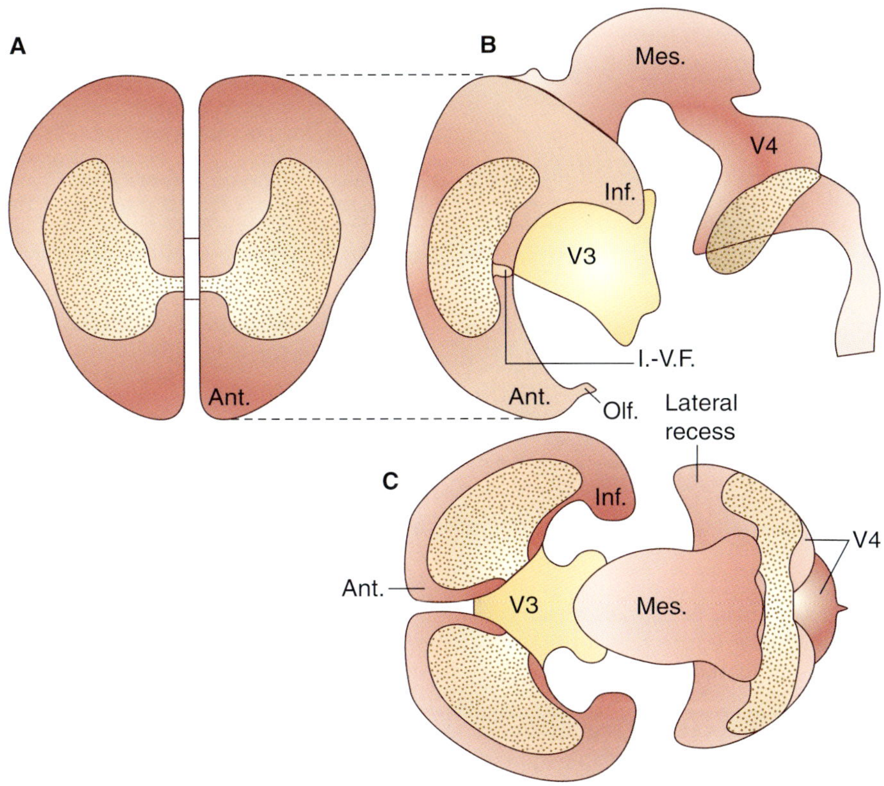


**Figure 1–7.** The ventricular cavities at the end of the embryonic period (stage 23). **(A)** Dorsal view showing the lateral ventricles. **(B)** Left lateral view of the complete ventricular system. **(C)** Dorsal view of the complete ventricular system. In each drawing the choroid plexuses are indicated by stippling. Based on reconstructions by the authors. Ant., anterior or frontal horn; Inf., inferior or temporal horn; I-V.F., interventricular foramen; Mes., mesencephalic ventricle (the future aqueduct); Olf., "olfactory ventricle" (temporary); V3, third ventricle; V4, fourth ventricle.

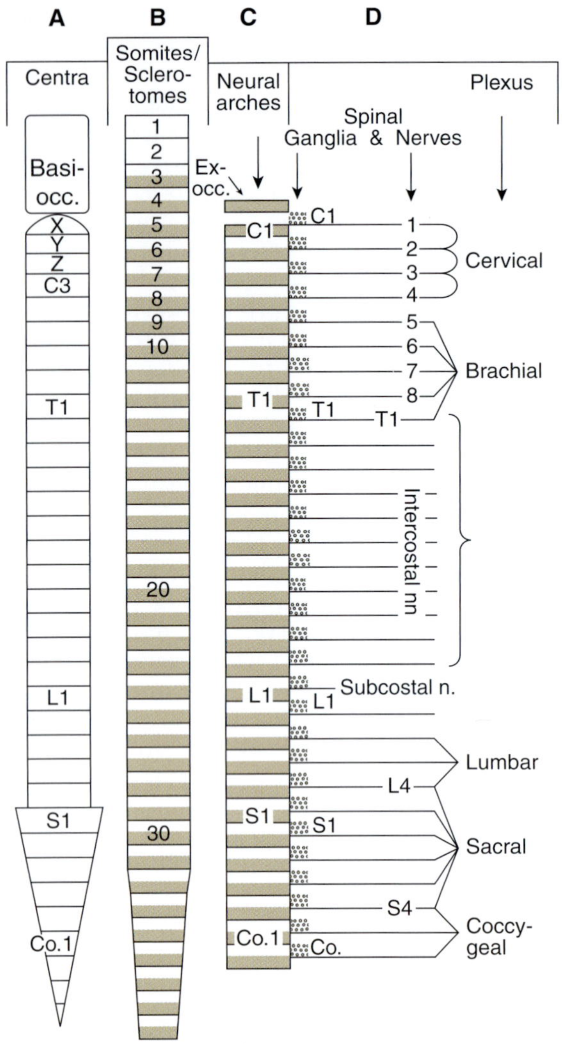


**Figure 1–8.** Early development of the vertebral column. Column **(A)** is the median component: the centra (future bodies). Column **(B)** shows the sclerotomes, which are derived from the somites. Column **(C)** is the lateral component: the neural (future vertebral) arches. The sclerotomes (B) and the neural arches (C) are not in register with the centra (A). Column **(D)** shows the spinal ganglia and nerves. The occipitocervical junction develops between segments 4 and 5 (B, C), whereas the cerebrospinal junction (not shown) occurs between rhombomere 8 and the spinal cord. Sclerotomes 1 to 4 give rise medially (A) to the basioccipital. Sclerotome 4 forms the exoccipital laterally (C). Sclerotome 5 becomes the posterior arch of the atlas, and sclerotome 6 provides the neural arch of the axis. The central pillar of the axis has three components (A): X, the apex of the dens; Y, the base of the dens; and Z, the centrum of the axis. The foramen magnum is between the basioccipital and X in A. Based on reconstructions by the authors. (Reproduced, with permission from, *Journal of Anatomy*, 1994;185:251–258.)

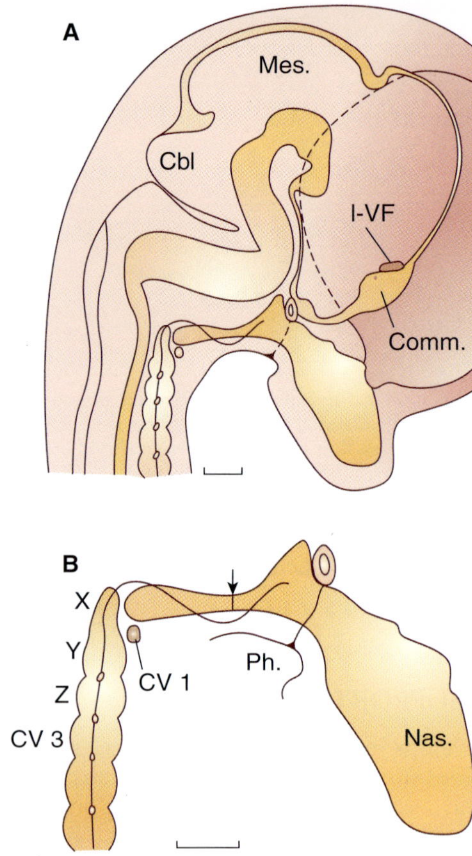


**Figure 1–9.** The brain and cranial base at the end of the embryonic period (stage 23). **(A)** Median section. The left cerebral hemisphere is included. **(B)** The occipitocervical region. The notochord ascends through the tripartite column (Z, Y, X) of the axis, leaves the dens to pass through the foramen magnum, and traverses the basioccipital in the direction of the hypophysis. The arrow represents the approximate position of the sphenooccipital joint. The remains of the stalk from the pharyngeal hypophysis to the adenohypophysis can be detected. Cbl, cerebellum; Comm., commissural plate; CV1, cervical vertebra 1 (anterior arch of the atlas); CV3, cervical vertebra 3; Hyp., adenohypophysis; I-VF, interventricular foramen; Mes, mesencephalon; Nas., nasal septum; Ph., pharynx; X, Y, Z, parts of the axis vertebra. Bars, 1 mm.

becomes embedded in the vertebral bodies and intervertebral discs. An important feature is the development of loose and dense zones in a complicated manner that differs laterally and medially.[15]

The development of the occipitocervical region is very complicated, and the details should be sought in a special account.[19] Medially, a perinotochordal tissue and migrated sclerotomic cells give rise to the basioccipital and to vertebral centra, including a tripartite column that forms the axis vertebra (Figure 1–9). Laterally, sclerotome 4 gives rise to the exoccipital, and sclerotome 5 forms the posterior arch of the atlas.

## SPINA BIFIDA

Spina bifida may be evident (aperta) or concealed (occulta). A cystic mass is generally present in those that are obvious, and these are known as spina bifida cystica. Spinal and cerebral forms of neural tube defects exhibit a close parallelism, as shown in Figure 1–10.

Myelomeningocele (or meningomyelocele), which may arise as a myeloschisis, is usually lumbosacral. Failure of closure of the caudal neuropore is probably a major factor, although the condition is not considered to be a simple failure of neural closure. When the caudal neuropore does not close, fixation between neural and surface ectoderm may hinder the normal ascent of the spinal cord, which becomes tethered. When spina bifida aperta is found in the cervicothoracic region, however, the possibility of reopening of the neural tube needs to be entertained.

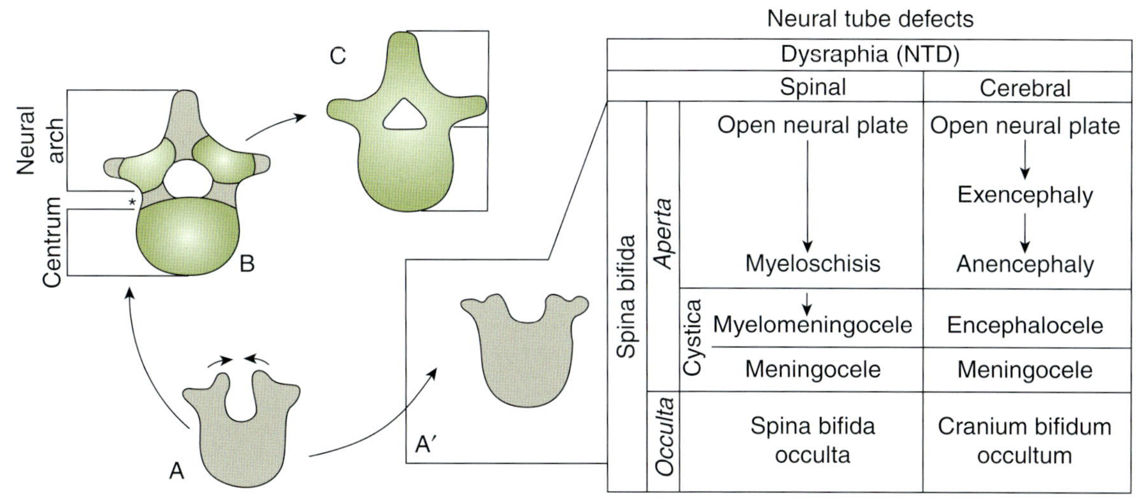


**Figure 1–10.** Neural tube defects. **(A)** The cartilaginous neural processes have not yet united in the embryo. **(B)** Three ossific centers are present in the newborn, providing a radiologic appearance of a normal spina bifida. **(C)** Ossification is complete. The neurocentral joint (asterisk) is a bilateral cartilaginous articulation between the neural arch and the centrum. In A′ a continued lack of closure of a vertebral foramen would constitute a spina bifida.

It is not always appreciated that spina bifida occulta is a normal phase of development. At the end of the embryonic period, the spinal cord and the vertebral column end at the same level. Moreover, ossification has not extended dorsally, so that a total spina bifida occulta exists, and this persists into adulthood in part of the sacral region in about one-fifth of normal persons. During the fetal period, a differential shift in growth occurs whereby the conus medullaris is found at increasingly higher vertebral levels, L3 at birth and L2 or L1 in adulthood.

Spinal meningoceles may arise as herniations in the presence of a mesenchymal deficiency, probably during the time the normal spinal bifida occulta is present. Cerebral meningoceles are rare.

## THE CEREBELLUM

The cerebellum arises as a bilateral organ very early in development (at about 4½ weeks of age). Later in the embryonic period it projects largely into the fourth ventricle in a complicated and temporary manner (Figures 1–4, 1–5, and 1–6). Early in the fetal period, the union of the two halves results in the vermis, which then develops folia and becomes largely obscured by the cerebellar hemispheres. At birth, the form of the cerebellum closely resembles that of the adult.

## THE FETAL BRAIN

The most evident external changes in the fetal period are (1) the union of the cerebellar halves and the definition of the vermis; (2) the increasing concealment of the diencephalon and the mesencephalon, and (later) of part of the cerebellum, by the cerebral hemispheres; (3) further approach of the frontal and temporal poles around the insula, which becomes increasingly buried by opercula; and (4) the appearance of sulci (lateral, central, parieto-occipital, calcarine, etc) on the hemispheric surface at about the middle of prenatal life, at which time the cerebral peduncles become prominent. One of the most noticeable internal changes is the growth of the corpus callosum.

## CORTICAL DEVELOPMENT[6]

The cerebral cortex begins to develop as the cortical plate, lateral to the future corpus striatum (stage 21). The plate divides the cerebral wall into the subpial layer peripherally (future layer 1) and the future white matter centrally. The cortical plate enlarges rapidly and covers most of the lateral part of the cerebral hemispheres at the end of the embryonic period. Cortical layers 2 to 6 develop from the cortical plate during the fetal period. The prefrontal cortex completes its differentiation approximately 6 months after birth. Sulci and gyri begin to appear at about the middle of pregnancy. A vascular network develops within the cortex in trimester 2. The vessels consist of simple epithelial channels at first; a muscularis is acquired only near term.

## C-SHAPED STRUCTURES

Associated with the growth of the relatively fixed corpus striatum and the curved expansion of the cerebral hemispheres to form the temporal lobes, several structures develop in a C-shaped manner: (1) caudate nucleus; (2) choroid plexus and fissure; (3) fornix and fimbria; (4) indusium griseum, hippocampus, and dentate gyrus; (5) corpus callosum (although the splenium does not descend into the temporal lobe); and (6) lateral ventricle.

The commissural plate of the embryo (Figure 1–5) gives rise early in the fetal period to the corpus callosum and the anterior commissure (Figure 1–11A). The corpus callosum, on the median section, is at first merely a compact mass (Figure 1–11B), but its length increases

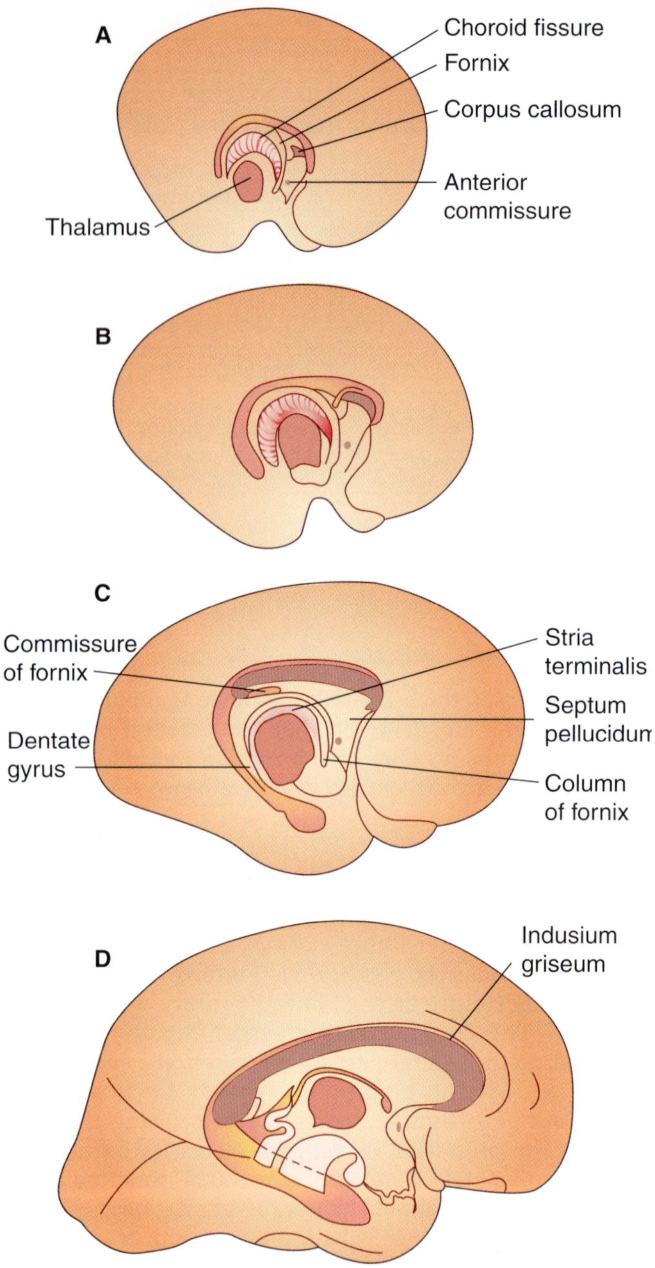


**Figure 1–11.** The development of the corpus callosum (*shown in black*) as seen on the medial surface of the left cerebral hemisphere at postmenstrual weeks 14, 15, 19, and 30. The great increase in its length throughout the fetal period is evident. (Modified from O'Rahilly and Müller, 2006,[6] with permission.)

considerably during the second trimester (Figure 1–11C), and the underlying portion of the commissural plate becomes thinned as the septum pellucidum.

By the middle of prenatal life, the rostrum, genu, central part, and splenium can be distinguished clearly (Figure 1–11D). During the second and third trimesters, the corpus callosum (except in agenesis) gradually forms a solid covering over the roof of the third ventricle. The corpus callosum continues to grow into the third decade of life.

A narrow cavity appears within the septum pellucidum and is known as the cavum septi pellucidi. It has been described by some researchers as arising as a pocket that at first opens into the longitudinal fissure but later becomes sealed by the rostrum of the corpus callosum. According to others, however, the cavum is formed by necrosis within the commissural mass and was never open to the subarachnoid space. The cavum can be identified during the second trimester, after which its posterior portion becomes obliterated before birth, as occurs to its anterior portion usually within a few months after birth. If the posterior portion persists, it is frequently termed the cavum Vergae (see Chapter 2).

The gyrus cinguli, or cingulate gyrus, is so named because it forms a partial girdle around the corpus callosum and follows the callosal curve. It can be distinguished on the medial surface of the cerebral hemisphere during the second trimester. The hippocampal formation (dentate gyrus, hippocampus, subiculum, and parahippocampal gyrus) begins early as bilateral hippocampal thickenings (5 weeks), and its characteristic S-shape becomes clear during the second trimester.

Agenesis of the corpus callosum is assumed to arise already in the commissural plate or field (Figure 1–4), which is a thickening of the embryonic lamina terminalis that appears very early (stage 12).

## THE VENTRICULAR SYSTEM[20]

The ventricles are a significant feature on ultrasonography, and their development is described briefly here. The ventricular system, including the central canal of the medulla and the spinal cord, is derived from the cavity of the neural tube. During the embryonic period and the early portion of the fetal period, the walls of the brain are very thin in most regions; hence, the ventricular system is relatively very large (Figure 1–12A and B). Later, as the walls increase in thickness, the ventricles occupy relatively less of the volume of the brain (Figure 1–12C and D).

In the region of the rhombencephalon, the roof of the brain is already noticeably thin at about 4 to 5 weeks after fertilization, thereby indicating the fourth ventricle (Figure 1–3C), the floor of which has become rhomboid. Extensions of the ventricle that are already detectable early become the lateral recesses (Figure 1–7C) of the fourth ventricle. The median aperture of the fourth ventricle appears, at the earliest, at the end of the embryonic period and is almost constant from early in the fetal period. The lateral apertures appear later, probably during the second trimester.

The cavity of the midbrain (the mesencephalic ventricle) remains relatively wide throughout the embryonic period (Figure 1–5), at the end of which its ends become slightly constricted.[7] It becomes gradually more tubular during the fetal period and would seem to justify the name *aqueduct* at the end of the first trimester.

As the cerebral hemispheres begin to develop, the cavities become the lateral ventricles (Figure 1–3B), and the cavity of the telencephalon medium and the diencephalon becomes delimited as the third ventricle (Figure 1–3B and D). The temporary cavities of the optic

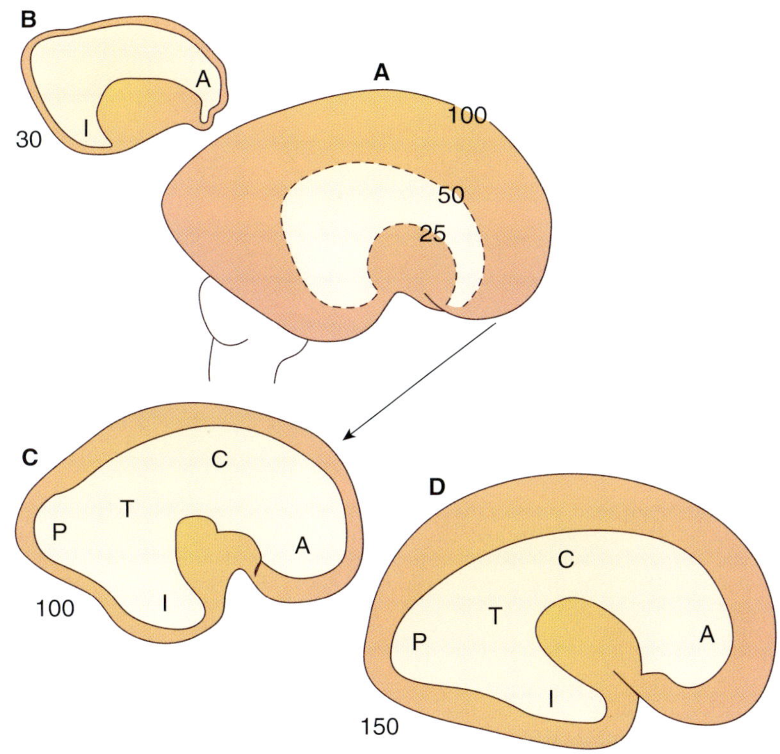


**Figure 1–12.** **(A)** Right lateral outlines of the brain postmenstrual weeks 9½, 12, and 13. **(B)**, **(C)**, and **(D)** Right lateral ventricle at postmenstrual weeks 10, 13, and 19. A comparison of views B, C, and D shows that the wall of the hemisphere (shaded) is becoming thicker; hence, the ventricle appears relatively smaller as age advances. The small evagination from the anterior horn is the temporary "olfactory ventricle." A, anterior horn; C, central part; I, inferior horn; P, posterior horn; T, trigonum. (A is based on Hochstetter,[17] B on O'Rahilly and Müller,[6] and C and D on Westergaard.[22])

cups (the optic ventricles) and their stalks are originally evaginations of the diencephalon. The openings between the third and lateral ventricles become very gradually narrowed (Figure 1–3B and D) to form the interventricular foramina (Figure 1–5).

Growth of the corpus striatum during the last week of the embryonic period further narrows the interventricular foramen (Figure 1–9A) and transforms the formerly spherical lateral ventricle into a characteristic C-shaped cavity (Fig. 1–12B), which extends from anterior (its frontal horn) to inferior (its temporal horn).[6,21,22] The posterior (occipital) horn (Figure 1–12C) develops at about 12 postmenstrual weeks and is very obvious early in the second trimester. The following subdivisions can now be distinguished: the anterior or frontal horn, the central part (which is not really a "body"), and the trigone (frequently referred to as the atrium), from which proceed the posterior or occipital horn and the inferior or temporal horn (Figure 1–12C and D). (Strictly speaking, the collateral trigone is the ventricular floor between the posterior and inferior horns, but the term trigone is commonly used for a portion of the cavity.)

Three different liquids are successively in contact with the developing brain: the amniotic fluid until closure of the neuropores, the ependymal fluid after closure, and the cerebrospinal fluid after the formation of the choroid plexuses.

The choroid plexuses, first that of the fourth ventricle and then those of the lateral ventricles (Figure 1–3D), develop between postmenstrual weeks 8 and 9. The plexuses are noticeably voluminous in the lateral ventricles (Figure 1–7) during the embryonic period and on into fetal life, as is readily seen on ultrasonography. The choroid plexus of the third ventricle develops early in the fetal period, and the interthalamic adhesion (formerly termed the *massa intermedia*) may develop, in some instances, before the middle of prenatal life.

Although indications of the subarachnoid space appear much earlier, the space and most of the cisternae are distinct at the end of the embryonic period, at which time the cerebellomedullary cistern (the cisterna magna) is also discernible.[23]

## MYELINIZATION

Reflexes can occur while nerve fibers are still unmyelinated, and embryonic and fetal movements during the first trimester take place before the onset of myelinization. Myelinization in the CNS begins during the second trimester, although the cerebral hemispheres contain little myelin at birth. Myelin is deposited more rapidly during the first two postnatal years, but the process continues into adulthood.

Fibers associated with related functions tend to become myelinated at the same time, and cortical association fibers are the last to be involved. It is believed that the state of myelinization indicates the functional maturity of the brain and is correlated with psychomotor

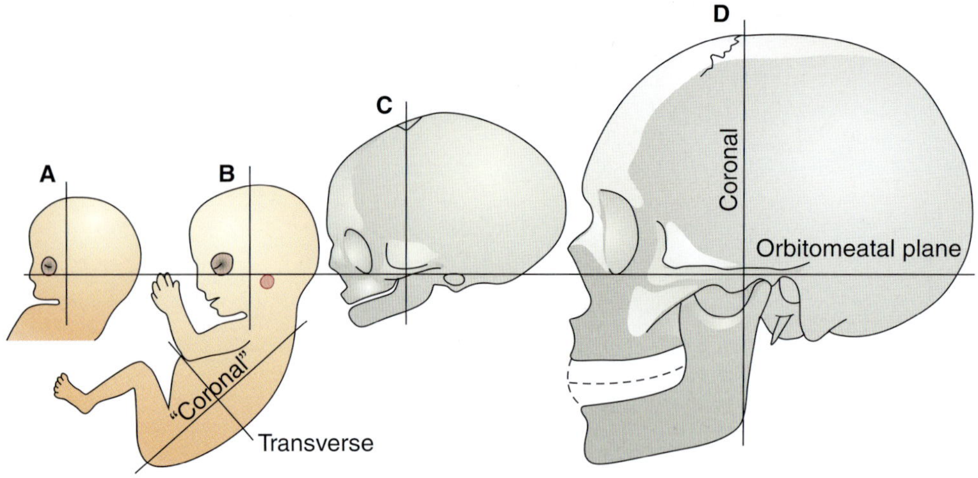


**Figure 1–13.** Left lateral views of the developing head, showing the orbitomeatal plane and examples of the many possible coronal planes. **(A)** End of the embryonic period (stage 23) showing the orbitomeatal plane as determined from graphic reconstructions by the authors. **(B)** A fetus at postmenstrual week 12 illustrating that transverse and "coronal" planes through the trunk differ considerably from horizontal and coronal planes through the head. **(C)** Neonatal skull showing a coronal plane through the anterior fontanelle. **(D)** Adult skull showing a coronal plane through the bregma.

development. Magnetic resonance imaging is particularly suitable for assessing the progress of myelinization.

## PLANES[24]

The three main sets of planes used in anatomy are the horizontal and the two vertical series: coronal and sagittal. One of the sagittal planes is median. There is no limit to the number of sagittal and coronal planes, so that sections are in a, not the, sagittal or coronal plane. Although *frontal* is frequently used as a synonym for *coronal,* in strict usage the term *frontal* should be reserved for the antonym of *occipital.* A particularly important plane in the head is the orbitomeatal (Figure 1–13D), because it is used to ensure that the head is in the standard position. For this purpose, the plane is kept horizontal. In other words, the orbitomeatal and the numerous possible horizontal planes in the adult are all parallel with each other. Strictly coronal planes can be defined as those vertical planes that are at a right angle to the orbitomeatal plane and also at a right angle to the median plane. Strictly coronal planes are necessarily parallel with one another.

It needs to be emphasized that, in anatomy and embryology in general, the unofficial word *midsagittal* should not be used for *median. Coronal* and *sagittal* refer to planes parallel to, but not necessarily through, the coronal and sagittal sutures, respectively. All planes parallel to the median plane are sagittal, so that the unofficial term *parasagittal* is redundant and should be eliminated. If necessary, a plane particularly close to the median could justifiably be termed *paramedian.*

A scheme has been prepared for the embryonic (Figure 1–13A), fetal (Figure 1–13B), and neonatal (Figure 1–13C) heads, positioned in relation to the orbitomeatal plane. The situation is complicated prenatally, however, by the curvature of the body and particularly by the flexion of the head. As a result, a transverse section of the trunk (Figure 1–13B), which would correspond to a horizontal section in the adult, is no longer parallel to the orbitomeatal plane. Similarly, "coronal" planes (of the adult type) in the prenatal trunk differ considerably from those in the head, that is, from vertical planes at a right angle to the orbitomeatal (Figure 1–13B).

The above-mentioned differences are important in discussions of the imaging of the prenatal brain. A further complication arises because many of the planes used in prenatal ultrasonography are oblique, as will be explained in Chapter 2.

## REFERENCES


1. O'Rahilly R, Müller F. *Developmental Stages in Human Embryos, Including a Revision of Streeter's "Horizons" and a Survey of the Carnegie Collection.* Publication 637. Washington, DC: Carnegie Institution of Washington, 1987.
2. O'Rahilly R, Müller F. Embryonic length and cerebral landmarks in staged human embryos. *Anat Rec.* 1984;209:265–271.
3. Böhmer S, Bruhns T, Degenhardt F, et al. Vergleich von vagino- und abdominosonographischen Messergebnissen mit embryologischen Wachstumskurven der Frühschwangerschaft. *Geburtsh Frauenheilk.* 1993;53:792–799.
4. Wisser J, Dirschedl P, Krone S. Estimation of gestational age by transvaginal sonographic measurement of greatest embryonic length in dated human embryos. *Ultrasound Obstet Gynecol.* 1994;4:457–462.
5. O'Rahilly R, Müller F. Prenatal ages and stages: Measures and errors. *Teratology.* 2000;61:382–384.
6. O'Rahilly R, Müller F. *The Embryonic Human Brain: An Atlas of Developmental Stages.* 3rd ed. New York: Wiley-Liss; 2006.
7. O'Rahilly R, Müller F. Significant features in the early prenatal development of the human brain. *Ann Anat.* 2008;105–118.
8. O'Rahilly R, Müller F. The two sites of fusion of the neural folds and the two neuropores in the human embryo. *Teratology.* 2002; 162–170.
9. Müller F, O'Rahilly R. Cerebral dysraphia (future anencephaly) in a human twin embryo at stage 13. *Teratology.* 1984;30:167–177.
10. Müller F, O'Rahilly R. The development of anencephaly and its variants. *Am J Anat.* 1991;190:193–218.

11. Müller F, O'Rahilly R. Mediobasal prosencephalic defects, including holoprosencephaly and cyclopia, in relation to the development of the human forebrain. *Am J Anat.* 1989;185:391–414.
12. O'Rahilly R, Müller F. Interpretation of some median anomalies as illustrated by cyclopia and symmelia. *Teratology.* 1989;40:409–421.
13. Hoving E W. *Frontoethmoidal Encephaloceles.* Groningen: Rijksuniversiteit; 1993.
14. Padget DH. The development of the cranial arteries in the human embryo. *Contr Embryol Carnegie Instn.* 1948;32:205–261.
15. O'Rahilly R, Müller F. *Human Embryology and Teratology.* 3rd ed. New York: Wiley-Liss; 2001.
16. Müller F, O'Rahilly R. The timing and sequence of appearance of neuromeres and their derivatives in staged human embryos. *Acta Anat.* 1997;158:83–99.
17. O'Rahilly R, Müller F. Somites, spinal ganglia, and centra. *Cells Tissues Organs.* 2003;173:75–92.
18. Müller F, O'Rahilly R. The human chondrocranium at the end of the embryonic period proper, with particular reference to the nervous system. *Am J Anat.* 1980;159:33–58.
19. Müller F, O'Rahilly R. Segmentation in staged human embryos: The occipitocervical region revisited. *J Anat.* 2003;203:297–315.
20. O'Rahilly R, Müller F. Ventricular system and choroid plexuses of the human brain during the embryonic period proper. *Am J Anat.* 1990;189:285–302.
21. Hochstetter F. *Beiträge zur Entwicklungsgeschichte des menschlichen Gehirns.* I. Teil. Vienna: Deuticke; 1919.
22. Westergaard E. The lateral cerebral ventricles of human fetuses with a crown rump length of 26–178 mm. *Acta Anat.* 1971;79:409–421.
23. O'Rahilly R, Müller F. The meninges in human development. *J Neuropathol Exp Neurol.* 1986;45:588–608.
24. O'Rahilly R. Making planes plain. *Clin Anat.* 1996;10:128–129.

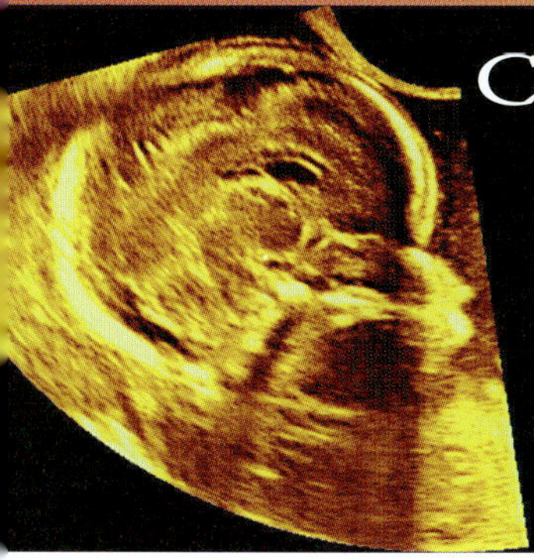

Chapter 2

# NORMAL TWO- AND THREE-DIMENSIONAL NEUROSONOGRAPHY OF THE PRENATAL BRAIN

*Ilan E. Timor-Tritsch • Ana Monteagudo • Maria Del Rio*

**KEY POINTS**

1. Neurosonography of the fetus and the neonate is an informative and noninvasive as well as inexpensive modality that is of great benefit in clinical diagnosis.
2. As technology improves and our understanding of sonoanatomy of the fetal and neonatal brain widens, the distinction between normal and abnormal, as far as anatomy is concerned, becomes increasingly possible.
3. Anomalies and disease of the developing brain area are common. In order to diagnose a deviation from what is normal, it is important to understand and recognize the developmental milestones of the normal brain how it grows, and matures, reaching its almost final anatomy at birth.
4. This chapter presents the sonographic landmarks of developing embryonic and fetal CNS and also suggested new ways to study it systematically.
5. The introduction of TVS in fetal neurosonography adds an additional powerful tool to the diagnostic algorithm, increasing diagnostic precision in patients suspected of an anatomically abnormal fetal CNS.
6. In the future, 2D as well as 3D fetal neurosonography will be used routinely in all pregnant patients to examine the developing brain, the same way we now examine other fetal organs and organ systems.

Problems of the central nervous system (CNS) can range from very simple, that is, merely a variance of the normal, to the most devastating diseases incompatible with life. It is important to recognize these anomalies as the fetus is scanned throughout gestation, starting very early in the first trimester to late in the third.

The prerequisite for differentiating normal from abnormal structures is a thorough knowledge of the CNS anatomy. It is beyond the scope of this and the following chapters to teach the reader advanced neuroanatomy; however, special emphasis is placed on describing basic but sufficiently detailed sonographic neuroanatomy to recognize structures seen by transabdominal (TAS) or transvaginal sonography (TVS). Those interested in scanning the fetal brain to detect deviations from the norm should first refresh their knowledge of neuroanatomy.

It is not sufficient to know only the anatomy of the full-term fetal or neonatal brain. Dealing with the sonographic anatomy and pathology of the fetal brain requires an additional dimension that is of the utmost importance for correctly evaluating the CNS at various prenatal ages of the fetus, that is, knowledge of the evolution of structures from about 6 to 7 postmenstrual weeks to the time of birth. Almost all organs and organ systems are in place by the end of the embryonic period. However, only at approximately 14 to 16 postmenstrual weeks would some of them—the heart and the kidneys, for example—perform almost at the level of perfection in the final month.

All that most organs do during the fetal period is increase in size. The brain, on the other hand, undergoes major developmental changes almost until the last several postmenstrual weeks of intrauterine life. Good examples of this are the changes in the size of the ventricles; the appearance and completion of the development of the corpus callosum; and the deepening, branching, multiplying, and growth of the sulci and the gyri. It is therefore essential to understand the development of various parts of the prenatal brain in order to evaluate it and differentiate abnormal from normal development.

We deal with the prenatal brain in this book. This chapter covers normal anatomy as viewed by sonography, emphasizing the development of the fetal brain from 6 to 7 postmenstrual weeks to term. Of course, the CNS starts to develop at much earlier prenatal ages. However, at these very early prenatal ages, probably up to 7 postmenstrual weeks, the tiny structures still cannot be recognized by presently used ultrasonographic technologies. These methods were dealt with in Chapter 1, on the embryology and development of the early prenatal brain. This chapter therefore will begin with the description of the sonographic appearance of the CNS starting at 6 to 7 postmenstrual weeks.

The reader's expectation for this chapter should be limited to enhancing his or her understanding of the normal prenatal brain anatomy before engaging in the diagnostic process and describing its pathology.

## ULTRASOUND EQUIPMENT

The customary ultrasound (US) equipment is used in imaging the prenatal brain. The two types of US probes employed are the transabdominal and transvaginal US transducer probes. Imaging the fetal brain depends on penetration of the sound waves as well as acoustic impedance of the tissues along the sound path. The acoustic impedances of most biologic tissues are similar. Therefore, only a small fraction of the sound is bounced back at each of these interfaces. The sound is thus successfully transmitted to deeper tissues, which can then be imaged. The soft tissue–bone interface is an exception to this rule. Bone has much higher impedance; thus, at the interface, due to the reflected sound, a very strong echo is produced. The sound energy reflected back is significant, and only a fraction of the attenuated sound waves are transmitted to deeper structures. To illustrate the magnitude of this effect, the acoustic impedance of bone is about 7 times that of water or soft tissues in the fetal body. Imaging of structures behind bone therefore becomes problematic because an acoustic shadow is created. As the fetal skull bones thicken and calcify during the course of gestation, fewer and fewer sound waves penetrate to enable imaging of the brain.

Imaging is also frequency dependent. The higher the frequency is, the better the resolution of the picture. However, the price we pay for increased picture resolution is reduced penetration, or the reduced half-intensity depth. The latter describes the ability of sound to penetrate and is expressed as the thickness of the tissues at which the sound intensity is reduced by half. This half-intensity depth decreases with increased frequency, correlates well with the attainable imaging depth, and is greatly dependent on the medium in which it travels. Excellent through transmission of sound in fluids such as blood or even in body tissue results from their weak sound-absorbing properties. However, bone and air strongly attenuate the intensity of sound. It is clear that the high acoustic impedance of the skull bone, as well as its property to attenuate the intensity of sound, greatly influences the way the brain can be imaged inside its bony case.

It was necessary to find imaginative ways to scan the fetal as well as the neonatal brain. By nature, transabdominal probes use lower frequencies to obtain deeper penetration and greater half-intensity depth. This is one way to penetrate beyond the bony skull. Another way is to scan through "windows" of the skull. These windows are, of course, the fontanelles. The younger the fetus is, the larger the fontanelles and sutures. Because these fontanelles measure ~1 to 2 cm in width, it is natural that sector or curvilinear scanners having a small footprint yield a better picture of the fetal and neonatal brain. These special transducers yield images that are of diagnostic value, even if they are acquired via the transabdominal route using the relatively open sutures, and fontanelles (Figure 2–1A).

Another inventive way to scan the fetal brain is to use extremely high-frequency probes, such as 6.5 to 7.5 or even 9 MHz. Such probes are used in transvaginal gynecologic scanning. If the fetus is in the vertex presentation, it is relatively easy to maneuver the fetal head and the vaginal transducer into a position from which the device can "see" through a fontanelle. If this is successfully achieved, extremely clear pictures of the fetal brain from 13 postmenstrual weeks to term can be obtained.

Since we became aware of the possibility of obtaining limited access to the brain using the transvaginal probe, we have been using it whenever possible (ie, when the fetus is in the vertex presentation). The rather narrow but still open "window" or space between the two parietal bones; namely, the sagittal suture enables by placing the footprint of the vaginal probe over the sagittal suture, a satisfactory picture of the mid-brain structures in the median plane can be obtained. Because of the narrow nature of this space, it is almost impossible to obtain an image of lateral structures.

Transabdominal scanning of the fetal brain using the anterolateral fontanelle or the squamosal suture can, in certain cases, yield clear and clinically diagnostic images. However, the younger the fetus is, or the smaller the structure in question is that must be scrutinized, the more the transabdominal probes will be at handicap as opposed to the higher-resolution transvaginal probes. Under matched conditions the transvaginal probes, which operate at higher frequency, produce better and clinically more useful pictures.[1]

Lately, electronically steered transducers can improve image quality obtained by the abdominal route. This modality employs compound scanning techniques.

Over the last several years, three-dimensional (3D) has become more readily available; therefore, a short explanation of these probes and their use is in place. Both the transabdominal and the transvaginal 3D US probes (at this time) are mechanical transducers. They are controlled by a timing module that determines the number of continuously advancing US pictures acquired and saved into a volume. The acquisition speed ultimately determines the picture resolution and quality. For moving structures (eg, a moving fetal part), high acquisition speed is required; for stationary organs (eg, in gynecology), lower acquisition speed is adequate, which enables obtaining many more sections, hence a higher-resolution end product. In view of the fact that the fetal brain is a stationary organ (except when the fetal head moves), when scanning the fetal brain, one can select a lower acquisition speed. The technique of 3D volume acquisition is relatively simple, and given that an increasing number of new US machines offer 3D technology, it is essential that those readers interested in enhancing their fetal neurosonography skills get acquainted with this powerful scanning technique.

## SCANNING CONCEPT

Fetal brain scanning has emerged from the vast experience gained with neurosonographic imaging of the neonate. The fetal as well as the neonatal head is scanned using the three main body coordinates: the sagittal, coronal (frontal), and horizontal axial planes (Figure 2–1B). Initially, scanning of the neonatal brain was done through the temporal region, obtaining axial

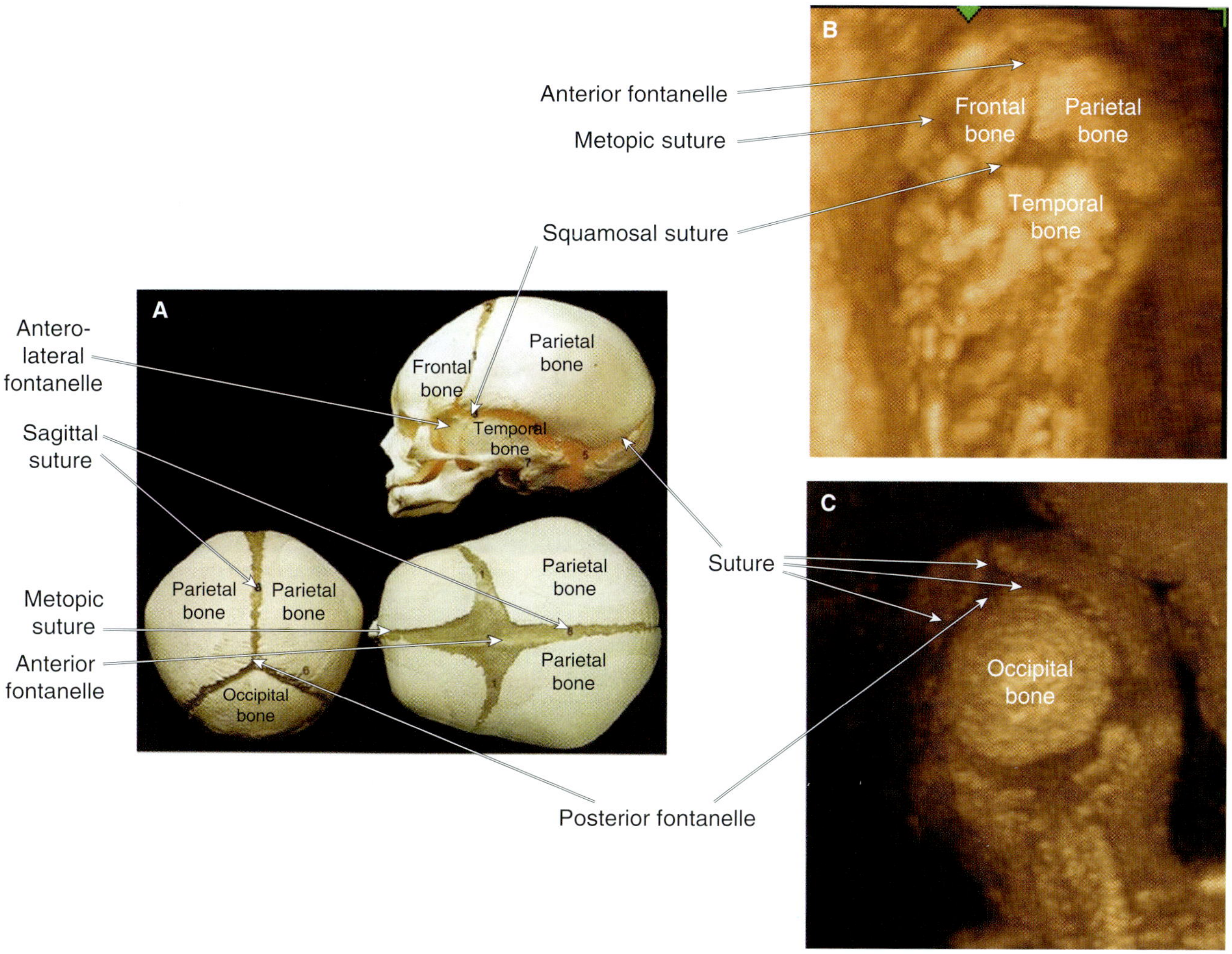


**Figure 2–1A.** Schematic and 3D ultrasound illustration of the fetal skull showing its bones, sutures, and fontanelles. The spaces between the bones can be used as access to the brain. **(A)** Lateral, posterior and superior views (www.uprightdoctor.files.worldpress.com), **(B)** and **(C)** are 3D maximum mode displays of cranial bones and sutures.

sections.[2–9] To achieve this imaging, lower-frequency transducers were used. Two factors contributed significantly to the improved resolution of one neonatal scan: the higher-frequency US transducers (mainly the sector and the small-footprint curvilinear probes) and use of the anterior fontanelle as an acoustic window. The pictures obtained are in the median, paramedian, and different coronal sections, as well as oblique, sections.[10–19] It should be stated at the outset that TAS of the fetal brain usually provides axial and coronal sections. However, it is extremely difficult or almost impossible to obtain sagittal sections (Figure 2–2). At times, though, sagittal sections are needed for imaging of different pathognomonic features and diseases of the brain. Transvaginal scanning through the anterior fontanelle provides us with such median, paramedian, coronal, and oblique sections, much like neonatal scanning (Figure 2–3).[20] Another advantage of scanning the fetal brain using TVS is that the scanning planes obtained are identical and therefore comparable to those performed in the neonate. Continuity of follow-up and comparison between fetal and neonatal scans are then possible by pediatric neurologists and neurosurgeons. The input of these consultants is therefore relevant even in the prenatal period.

An issue of some importance is that fetal neuroimaging requires the use of an end-firing, symmetrical, in-axis (or in-line) vaginal probe. Using an end-firing, off-axis vaginal probe makes symmetrical imaging of the brain and maneuvering of the probe extremely cumbersome (Figure 2–4). The orientation process is also affected, with regard to its speed, simplicity, and teaching. Most off-axis probes require constant use of the left-right orientation key on the control panel to correctly display orientation on the picture.

Blaas et al[21] described the use of the 3D US probe. The development of the three different structures in the brain was defined using this technique. The information obtained by this “spatial scan” was stored in the computer and enabled the user to obtain different pictures, creating not only coronal, sagittal, and axial planes but also selected planes to highlight the spatial embryonic brain anatomy (Figure 2–5) and pathology. Until the 3D technology becomes universally available and widely used, we must

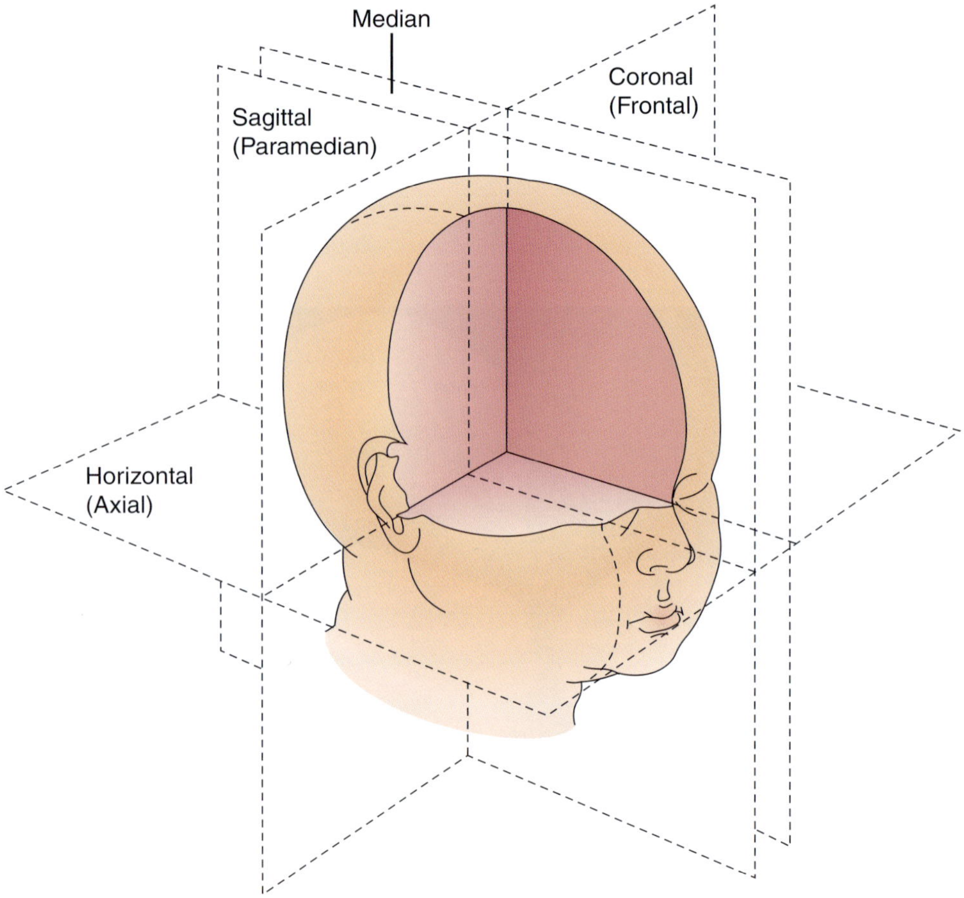


**Figure 2–1B.** The "classical" planes used in the imaging of the fetal brain. The vertical planes are either coronal or sagittal. One of the latter planes is the median plane. There are infinite numbers of coronal and sagittal (paramedian) planes. As far as fetal neurosonography is concerned, the coronal and sagittal planes are reached through the anterior fontanelle in a fetus presenting with the vertex. Several sections through each plane can be generated. The horizontal (axial) planes are achieved classically by a transabdominal 3D scanning.

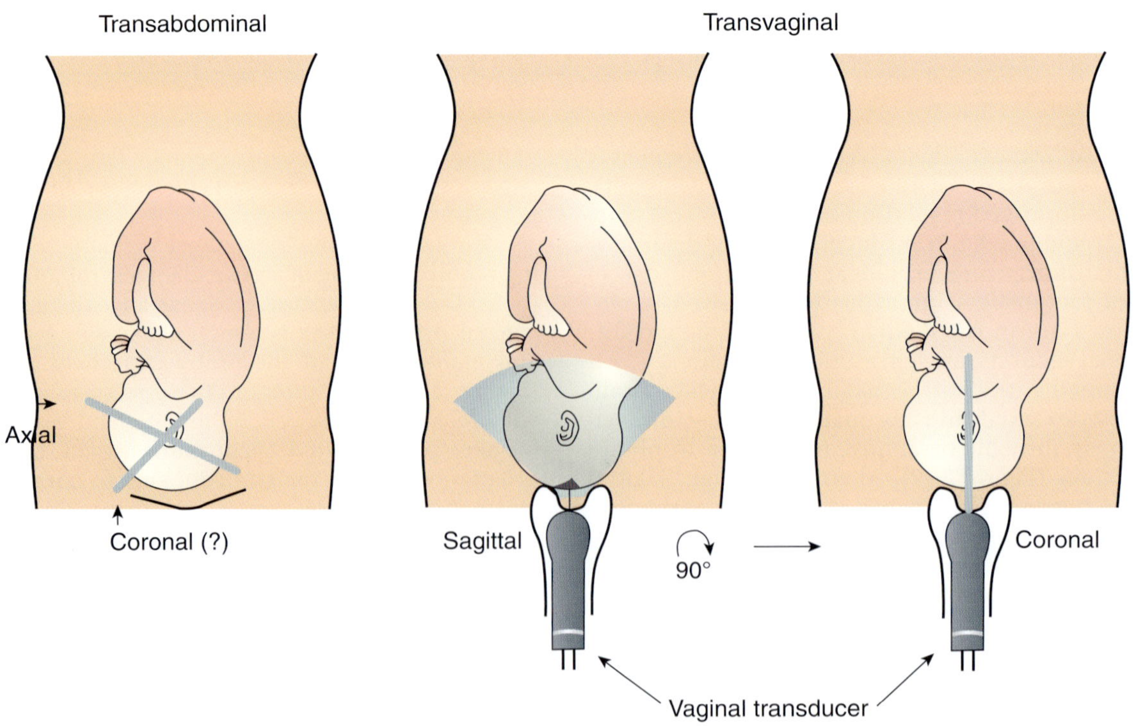


**Figure 2–2.** Schematic illustration of fetal neuroscanning routes. The transabdominal and the 3D routes classically provide axial or coronal views, but rarely sagittal views. The transvaginal approach rarely yields axial views. However, sagittal and coronal planes typically are obtained.

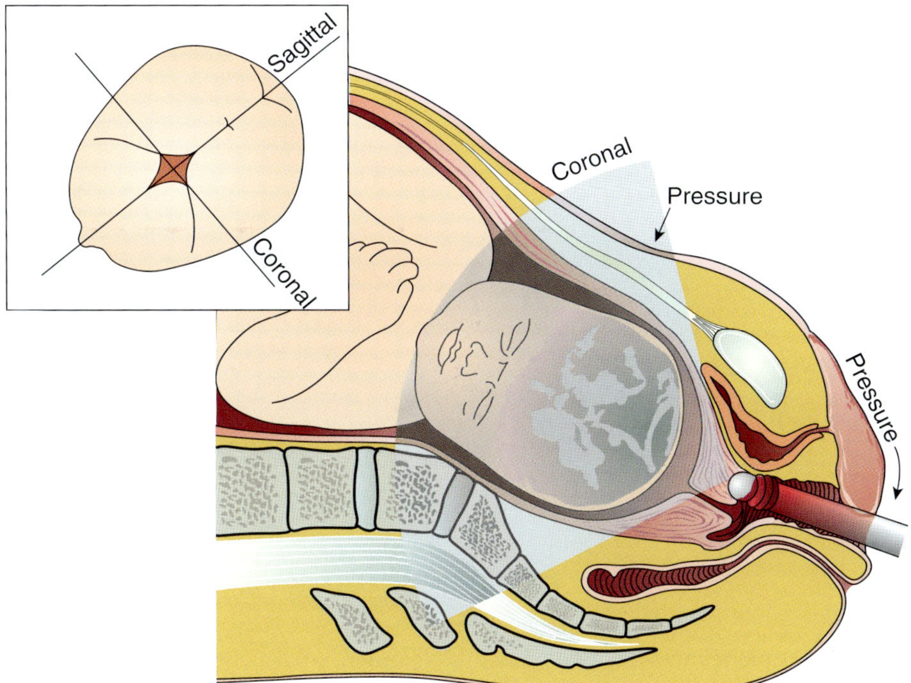


**Figure 2–3.** Schematic drawing depicting the technique of transvaginal sonography during the second and third trimesters. Inset: The relationship of the anterior fontanelle to the transvaginal transducer is demonstrated. (From Monteagudo and colleagues, 1991,[20] with permission.)

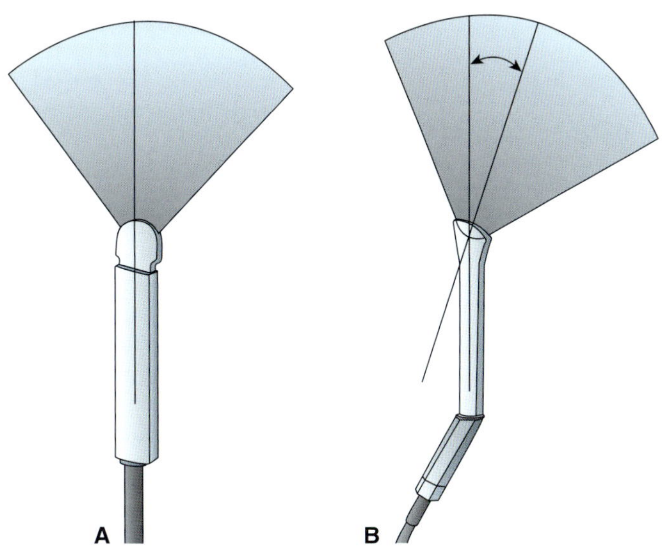


**Figure 2–4.** The different scanning planes of the transvaginal probes most often used. (**A**) Transvaginal fetal neuroscans are imaged best with an end-firing, symmetrical, in-axis probe. (**B**) The tilted, off-axis scanning plane generated by a curvilinear transvaginal probe. In order to scan hemispheres at the same time, the shaft of the probe must be moved from side to side. This may be uncomfortable for the patient, or it may simply be impossible. At times, the probe must be rotated 180° to direct the scanning plane to the other hemisphere.

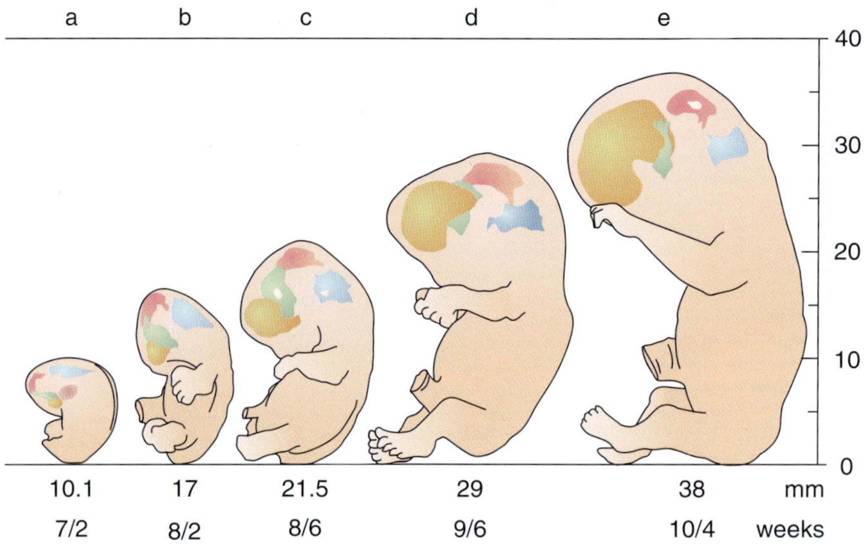


**Figure 2–5.** In vivo 3D ultrasound reconstructions of embryos and early fetuses. (From Blaas HG, 1998,[21] with permission.)

mentally re-create the necessary planes and sections. Thus, knowledge of neuroanatomy remains an important issue.

Another technique that can be used to better describe the anatomy of the fetal brain is color Doppler flow studies. If color flow studies are used, a textbook on neuroanatomy, particularly on the arterial and venous network of the fetal brain, should initially be studied. Color and power Doppler flow studies may become important when anatomical structures such as space-occupying lesions, degenerative changes, or hemorrhages of the brain are examined. Another area still under investigation is the physiology of the blood supply to the brain. This is covered in Chapter 15.

## SCANNING TECHNIQUE

Because TAS is easy to perform and is used routinely by those who engage in ultrasonography of the fetus, it seems redundant to describe its technique. Transvaginal two-dimensional (2D) and 3D scanning of the fetal brain, however, requires more experience and is skill dependent; therefore, we describe it here in detail.

Obviously, due to its small size, the embryonic and early fetal CNS requires the use of a high-resolution transvaginal US probe.[22–30] The CNS structures seen in the first trimester are described later.

Scanning the fetal brain in the second and third trimesters via the vaginal route requires the same safety guidelines used for the customary speculum and palpatory examinations during pregnancy. If these can be performed safely in the second trimester, there is no contraindication to insertion of the vaginal probe for scanning the fetal brain. Of course, as stated before, the fetus must be in the cephalic presentation. At times, when it is of the utmost importance to obtain accurate and more detailed information regarding a disease state, or if an additional sagittal view would significantly contribute to the diagnostic process, it may be important to consider the external cephalic version of the fetus. When a second-trimester fetus is scanned, such a change in the fetal presenting part most of the time can be brought about without effort or can occur spontaneously.

Transvaginal 2D and 3D neuroscanning can be used as early as 10 to 14 postmenstrual weeks. Its technique is relatively simple.[21,24,31,32] The transvaginal probe is prepared in the customary fashion, covering it with a clean condom or one of the digits of a surgical rubber glove after contact gel has been applied to the tip of the probe and, finally, applying some lubricating (K-Y) gel onto the covered tip, making it ready for vaginal insertion. Due to increasing reports of latex allergies in the population, special prelubricated polyvinyl vaginal probe covers are available. The patient should be in the lithotomy position, preferably lying on a gynecologic examination table. Constantly following the image created by the advancing probe on the monitor, the first structure to be viewed (and evaluated as well as measured) is the cervix. The tip of the probe is typically placed on top of the anterior cervical lip. If the patient's bladder is full and displaces the fetal head upward, the patient should be asked to void before the examination proceeds.

To obtain a clear image of the fetal brain, it may be necessary to maneuver the probe and/or the fetal head into the most convenient position. This will be achieved if the axis of the probe and the median plane of the fetal brain (ie, the falx cerebri) are in line (Figure 2–3). Usually, the operator must use both hands to point the probe to the anterior fontanelle or along the metopic and/or sagittal sutures and hold the fetal head in the desired position. Unless skilled help is available to freeze the image and trigger the recording device, a foot pedal is necessary to perform all of the necessary tasks at the same time. An active fetus may be extremely hard to stabilize by the abdominally placed second hand of the operator. To wait for the fetus to enter a quiet sleep state (state 1F) may be a time-consuming option. However, the scanning of an almost motionless fetus in deep sleep does have its dividends.

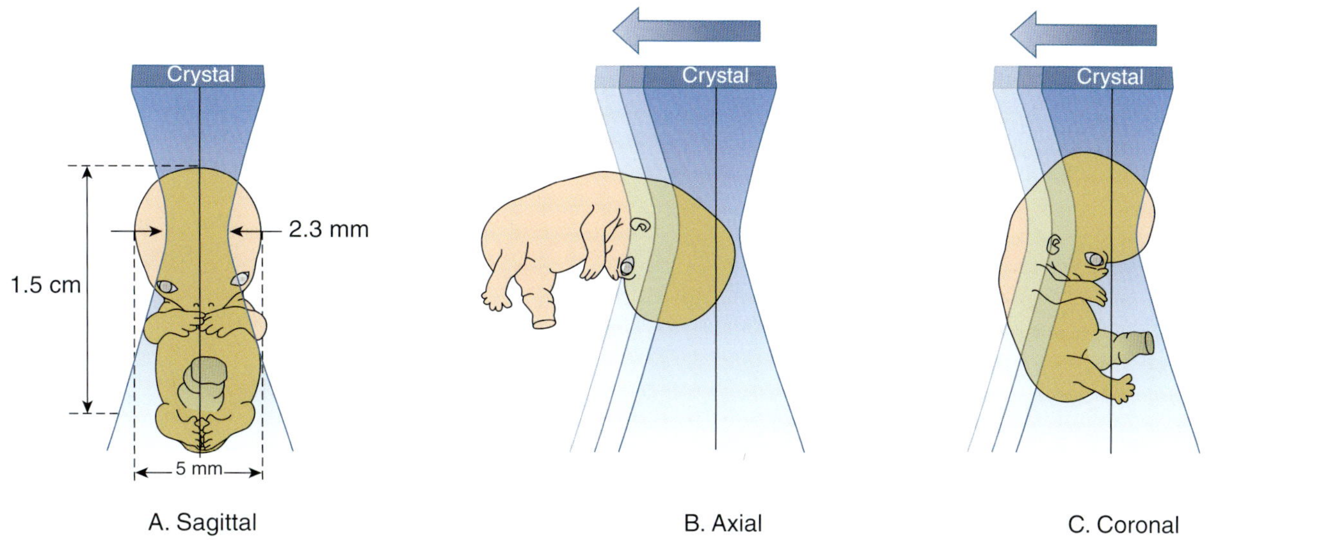


**Figure 2–6.** The effect of slice thickness, or the third dimension of ultrasound imaging, is demonstrated. (**A**) Due to the slice thickness, even at the focal point, a scan in the median plane may include the entire width of the embryonic head. (**B**), (**C**) In axial or coronal planes, two or three sections may be possible. Starting with the fetal period, an increasing number of sections become feasible.

## ORIENTATION AND SCANNING PLANES

In addition to the previously mentioned advantages and disadvantages of TAS and TVS of the fetal CNS, another caveat should be introduced. At times, it is hard or too time-consuming to obtain perfect planes and classical sections of the brain using TVS. This is, of course, a result of the somewhat limited mobility of the vaginal probe and/or the almost constantly moving fetus. Sometimes the fetal head position is such that it prevents the imaging of clear planes. Complementing the scan with an attempt at TAS, rescheduling the scan, or simply allowing the patient to walk for some time may improve the results.

Figure 2–1B depicts the three well-known classical planes of the body, in terms of its planes and sections. These are described below. Additional terms used in the orientation process are *rostral* or *anterior* (toward the face); *occipital, posterior,* or *nuchal* (toward the back); *left lateral* or *right temporal* (toward the respective ear); *caudal, basal,* or *inferior* (toward the base of the skull); and *medial* (toward the middle). It should be noted that the sagittal plane traversing the middle of the body is termed the median (do not use "midsagittal") plane (see Chapter 1).

### Scanning before 12 Postmenstrual Weeks

Ultrasonographic images of the embryonic (up to 9 postmenstrual weeks) or fetal (at and after 9 postmenstrual weeks) period is heavily dependent on several factors. The first factor is the resolution, which, in turn, is a function of the frequency at which the crystals operate. The frequency and, in some ways, the diameter of the piezoelectric crystal determine the slice thickness. The thicker the slice that is insonated and imaged, the more information is "collapsed" into the 2D picture seen on the screen. This slice thickness may, in many cases, be several millimeters. In the case of an embryonic brain at 7 or 8 postmenstrual weeks, the median imaging plane may include the entire width of the head due to the relatively thick imaging slice (Figure 2–6A). This is true even for a high-frequency transvaginal transducer; in the axial or coronal planes, it may be possible to obtain several sections due to the somewhat larger size of the growing embryo (Figure 2–6B and C).

Controlling the thickness of the slice becomes important in postprocessing of 3D US pictures derived from the volume scan. Using the software of several 3D US machines, it is possible to select the desired slice thickness, thus enhancing the displayed image clarity.

Around 9 postmenstrual weeks the size of the embryonic head becomes large enough to yield several sections in each of the three cardinal planes. Because of the small head size, the sections can be obtained in almost a perfect parallel fashion. This becomes increasingly difficult later in pregnancy, as discussed in subsequent sections.

It should also be clear that the terms *axial* (*horizontal*) and *coronal* (*frontal*) *planes* refer to the trunk and become somewhat unclear if applied to the anteflexed embryonic head. Therefore, a coronal plane of the trunk would be axial of the flexed head. It is our understanding, therefore, that the term *axial* in an embryo at 8 to 10 postmenstrual weeks is in a plane parallel with the base of the skull or the orbitomeatal plane (see Chapter 1). A coronal plane of the same fetus is one at 90° to the axial plane (Figure 2–7).

If for any reason (eg, research or clinical observation) it is necessary to image the brain in the first trimester, the observer should place the region of interest rigorously into the exact focal point of the transducer. Thus, it is essential to be knowledgeable about the respective transducer specifications in order to generate high-quality images.

### Scanning after 12 Postmenstrual Weeks

With its increasing size, the developing fetal brain becomes progressively available for high-frequency 5 to 12 MHz

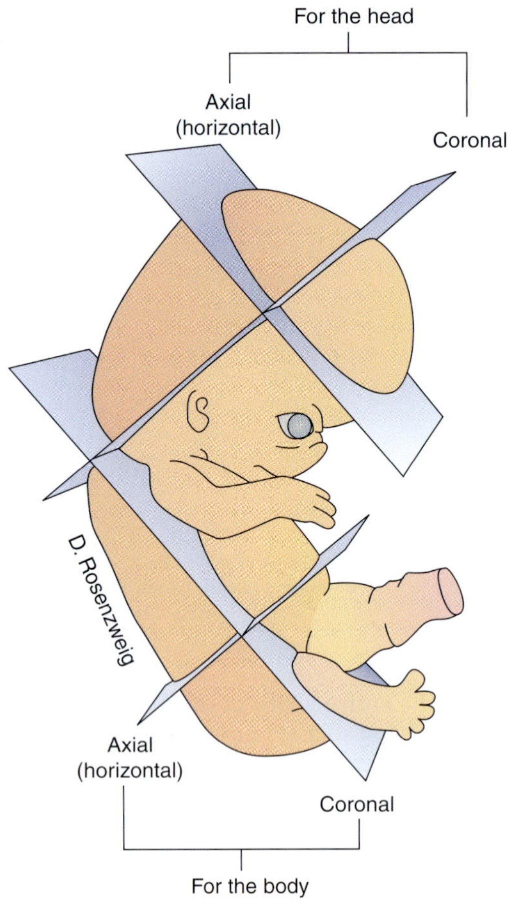


**Figure 2–7.** Due to the flexed posture of the embryonic or early fetal head, the plane that is coronal as far as the trunk is concerned becomes an axial plane when applied to the brain. In the same way, if an axial or transverse section of the trunk is applied to the head, it generates a coronal section of the brain.

TVS. The pictures obtained in the different scanning planes are thus of diagnostic quality. In other words, major diseases of the CNS can be diagnosed, starting at 9 to 11 postmenstrual weeks.

With regard to scanning the fetal brain after 12 weeks, especially after weeks 14 to 15, it is at this point that the thickening skull bones attenuate the high-frequency sound waves of the vaginal probe to a very low level, making imaging from any randomly selected direction increasingly impossible. This is the time at which the window to the fetal brain (ie, the fontanelle) becomes important. This relatively narrow gateway for the sound waves forces certain restrictions on the sonologist or sonographer. First, the tip of the transducer must be kept over the fontanelles or the sagittal (or metopic) suture, to achieve the full scanning potential of the sound output. Second, the different scanning sections in the sagittal, coronal, and oblique planes should be generated by tilting the transducer back and forth (Figure 2–8). Because of the reasons mentioned, these successive sections are not parallel to each other in any given plane, as, for example, with the shifting but always parallel planes of computed tomography (CT) and magnetic resonance imaging (MRI).

This transfontanelle scanning by TVS, common to prenatal and neonatal brain scanning, is really performed in a "radial" fashion. Some of the sagittal and coronal sections are therefore oblique-sagittal and oblique-coronal sections. In the sagittal plane, then, left and right oblique sections are generated; in the coronal plane, occipital and frontal oblique sections are generated (Figure 2–8).

However, as we will see later, if a 3D brain volume is acquired, regardless of the transducer or the scanning route used, the final display will use perfectly parallel planes and sections, as in MRI and CT.

It is important to understand that in order to scan the fetus presenting with the vertex, the free motion of the vaginal probe is restricted by the anatomical limits of the vagina. Only a few "classical" or "pure" planes can therefore be achieved: the median and one coronal plane. In the sagittal planes (to use the best approximation), because of the fan-shaped, radial scanning sections, several left and right oblique sections can be generated on each side of the median plane (Figure 2–8). This is partially overcome by using 3D US. In front of or behind the coronal plane (once again, to use the best approximation), several frontal and occipital oblique sections can be generated (Figure 2–8).

If several sections are created, the 3D anatomy should be re-created mentally by the observer. This "mental processing" will be less and less necessary by the introduction of 3D multiplanar imaging. Three-dimensional imaging of the fetal brain will also eliminate the "radiating" planes, as all planes will be parallel with each other.

If the second- or third-trimester fetus assumes an asynclitic head position, it is sometimes possible to obtain axial planes. The same is true if the head assumes a flexed occipitoanterior position. A detailed study of the posterior fossa should be performed as soon as this presentation is detected. After some time, due to fetal movement, this presenting anatomy may shift away, not to return for the duration of the examination.

As the examination proceeds, we have observed certain conventions in orientation. This serves to introduce a systematic way of displaying the images.

In the sagittal planes the fetal face or the frontal direction should be almost uniformly oriented to the left of the picture. This will orient the posterior fossa and the occipital structures toward the right side of the screen. Likewise, if the lateral ventricles are imaged using these planes, the anterior horn should point toward the left and the posterior horn toward the right side of the monitor.

In the coronal planes the pictures should be taken in such a manner that the fetus should face, or look right at, the examiner. This means that by convention—as is customary in imaging laboratories—the right side of the brain will appear on the left side of the screen, whereas the left side of the prenatal brain will point toward the right of the picture. If no annotation is to be seen on a hard copy, it is assumed that the above-described orientations of the prenatal brain sections in the coronal planes were observed. It seems best, however, to indicate the orientation of the left or right side on at least one of the images. This annotation of the left or right side becomes crucial if an asymmetrical or unilateral lesion is detected.

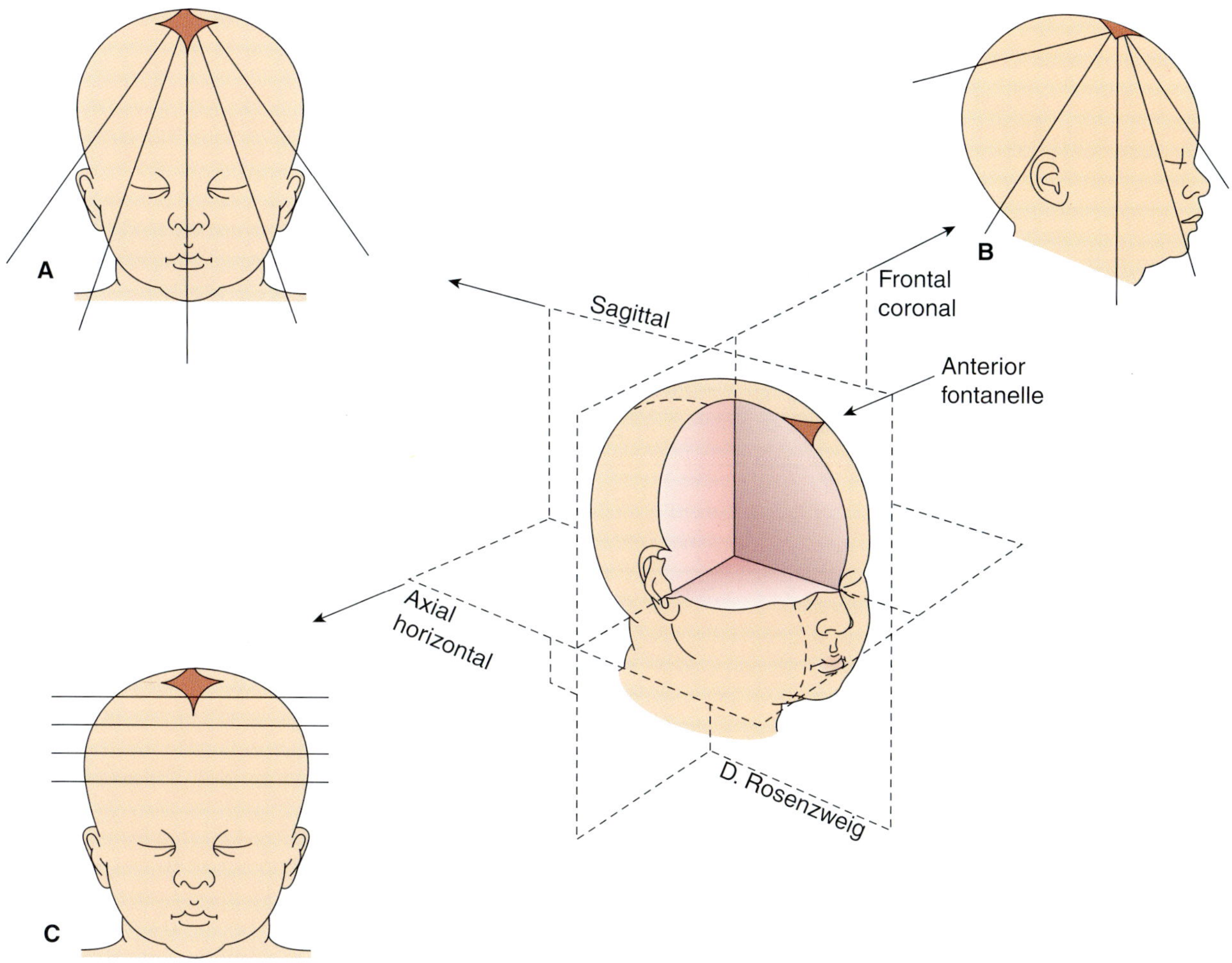


**Figure 2–8.** Scan through the anterior fontanelle. (**A**) The limited motion of the probe within the vagina allows the median plane to be visualized, whereas on each side of it, the planes are oblique and not parallel, and therefore cannot be regarded as strictly sagittal. (**B**) Similarly, a coronal plane can be obtained, whereas those in front of and behind it are oblique planes, not subsequent coronal planes. (**C**) The horizontal planes can be achieved using the transabdominal approach.

If 3D US is used, one should be acquainted with the initial display of the orthogonal planes inherent to the different manufacturers' systems. These orthogonal planes are the customary initial planes appearing on the screen after the acquisition of the volume is completed. Determining the correct side is essential when unilateral brain pathology is encountered.

## BRAIN DEVELOPMENT AND SONOANATOMY FROM 6 POSTMENSTRUAL WEEKS TO TERM

This section deals with the sonoembryology and sonoanatomy of the prenatal brain as it appears and as a continuous function of structural development. It should be clear that parts of the prenatal brain exist and are in different developmental stages even before they can be imaged by ultrasonography. This is particularly true for brain structures revealed by a scan performed during the first 12 to 14 postmenstrual weeks of pregnancy. The structure may well be in place, but due to its size and location, the angle of insonation may not be obvious to the observer. Other structures develop later as a normal process, and because of this they are not seen on early scans.

We present here the normal embryonic and fetal neurosonology in two sections. The first subsection deals with the period up to 9 postmenstrual weeks. The second section comprises the weeks following the ninth postmenstrual week. This is an entirely arbitrary partition. Starting from the 13th postmenstrual week, some of the structures imaged by high-frequency transvaginal transducers are of clinically usable quality. This is also the time after which multiple and clearly discernible brain sections can be obtained using the standard planes.[23]

### Scanning the Embryonic Central Nervous System (6 to 9 Postmenstrual Weeks)

To better understand the development of the embryonic brain, the reader is referred to Chapter 1. After reading that chapter, a clearer perception of the sonographically visualized structures will be possible.

As concerns the age of the embryos and fetuses, the arguments and debates are well known and well

**Table 2–1. CONVERSION TABLE FOR EMBRYONIC AND FETAL AGE AND SIZE**

| Postmenstrual Week | Time From LMP (Weeks and Days) | Time From Fertilization (Weeks and Days) | Days From Fertilization | Crown–Rump Length (cm)[a] | EES (mm) |
|---|---|---|---|---|---|
| 7th | 6 + 0 to 6 + 6 | 4 + 0 to 4 + 6 | ~28–34 | 0.42–0.81 | 1–6 |
| 8th | 7 + 0 to 7 + 6 | 5 + 0 to 5 + 6 | ~35–41 | 0.89–1.38 | 7–13 |
| 9th | 8 + 0 to 8 + 6 | 6 + 0 to 6 + 6 | ~42–48 | 1.47–2.08 | 14–20 |
| 10th | 9 + 0 to 9 + 6 | 7 + 0 to 7 + 6 | ~49–55 | 2.19–2.92 | [b] |
| 11th | 10 + 0 to 10 + 6 | 8 + 0 to 8 + 6 | ~56–62 | 3.05–3.89 | [b] |
| 12th | 11 + 0 to 11 + 6 | 9 + 0 to 9 + 6 | ~63–69 | 4.04–5.00 | [b] |
| 13th | 12 + 0 to 12 + 6 | 10 + 0 to 10 + 6 | ~70–76 | 5.17–6.25 | [b] |
| 14th | 13 + 0 to 13 + 6 | 11 + 0 to 11 + 6 | ~77–83 | 6.43–7.63 | [b] |

LMP, Last menstrual period; EES, early embryonic size.[35]

[a]After Robinson, 1973.[33]

[b]EES measurements of embryonic length are used up to 25 mm or 68 ± 3 base from LMP.

documented. Chapter 1 provides the tools to understand the different views. Table 2–1 contains the embryonic and fetal age conversions, which will allow quick reference for those who would like to rely on the date of the last menstrual period (LMP) to calculate age, as well as for those who are used to expressing age in terms of weeks or days from fertilization (if such a date is known).[33] O'Rahilly and Müller[34] indicated that points C and R of the crown-rump length (CRL, Figure 2–9) are imprecise and frequently are difficult to determine. They emphasized that the best single measurement is the greatest length (GL), exclusive of the lower limbs, and its determination is practicable in both the embryonic and fetal periods. Subsequently, Goldstein[35] expressed concern about measuring the longest diameter of the developing embryo sonographically, calling it the CRL. His measurement, according to the study, does not follow the curvature of the curled-up embryonic body. Therefore, it actually measures the longest diameter (ie, the GL of O'Rahilly and Müller[34]) or the size of the embryo. Goldstein[35] proposed the term *early embryonic size* (EES) for the sonographic measurement. Table 2–1 also contains the EES measurements and their conversions to embryonic age.

Returning to the work of O'Rahilly and Müller,[34] it is clear that the C point (the crown), which, in stages 13 to 20 (6w0d-9w1d from the LMP), is at the point where an imaginary line drawn along the mesencephalic flexure would touch the surface of the embryo, just above the middle of the midbrain (see Figure 2–9), is hard to find sonographically. Even if it can be determined, the CRL would yield a smaller length than the GL or the EES of Goldstein.[35] Figure 2–9 depicts how the C point changes location throughout development from stage 13 to stage 20. Only at stage 23 (10w1d postmenstrual weeks) do the CRL and GL (or EES) become identical as clinically used measurements.

Using currently available US machines, the earliest scan to depict any brain structure can be performed at 7 postmenstrual weeks (5 weeks, or 35 days, from fertilization). At this age one or several sonolucent areas can be detected in the rostral and cephalic pole of the embryo. The detail of the image depends on the resolution of the equipment used.

If attempts are made to image details of the CNS before this embryonic age, a clear fetal pole, at times adjacent to the yolk sac, can be seen (Figures 2–10, 2–11 and 2–12A and B).[36] However, sagittal as well as coronal sections do not yield distinct structures. At times, a tiny sonolucency is seen in the rostral part of the embryo. The nature of this structure is unknown. The parallel lines of the somites (from which the vertebrae are derived) are discernible at or slightly before 7 postmenstrual weeks (Figures 2–12C).

Blaas and colleagues[29,30] studied the brain structures, starting with an embryo with a CRL of 12 mm (7 weeks, 3 days from the LMP). They described the possibility of imaging the cerebral hemispheres (telencephalic vesicles), rhombencephalon, and diencephalons (Figure 2–13). In embryos with a CRL of 16 mm (8 weeks from the LMP), these structures become better defined. Thus, the interventricular foramina (Monro) can be seen (Figure 2–14).

Our group has scanned well-dated embryos from 7 to 10 weeks from the LMP and evaluated the structures imaged. A 6.12 MHz mechanical 3D transvaginal transducer was used. At 8 weeks, 1 day (from the LMP) in the sagittal and axial/coronal planes, we could see all the primitive ventricular suctum (Figure 2–15A, B, and C). Figure 1–4 in Chapter 1 represents a sagittal section of the embryonic brain at a comparable age.

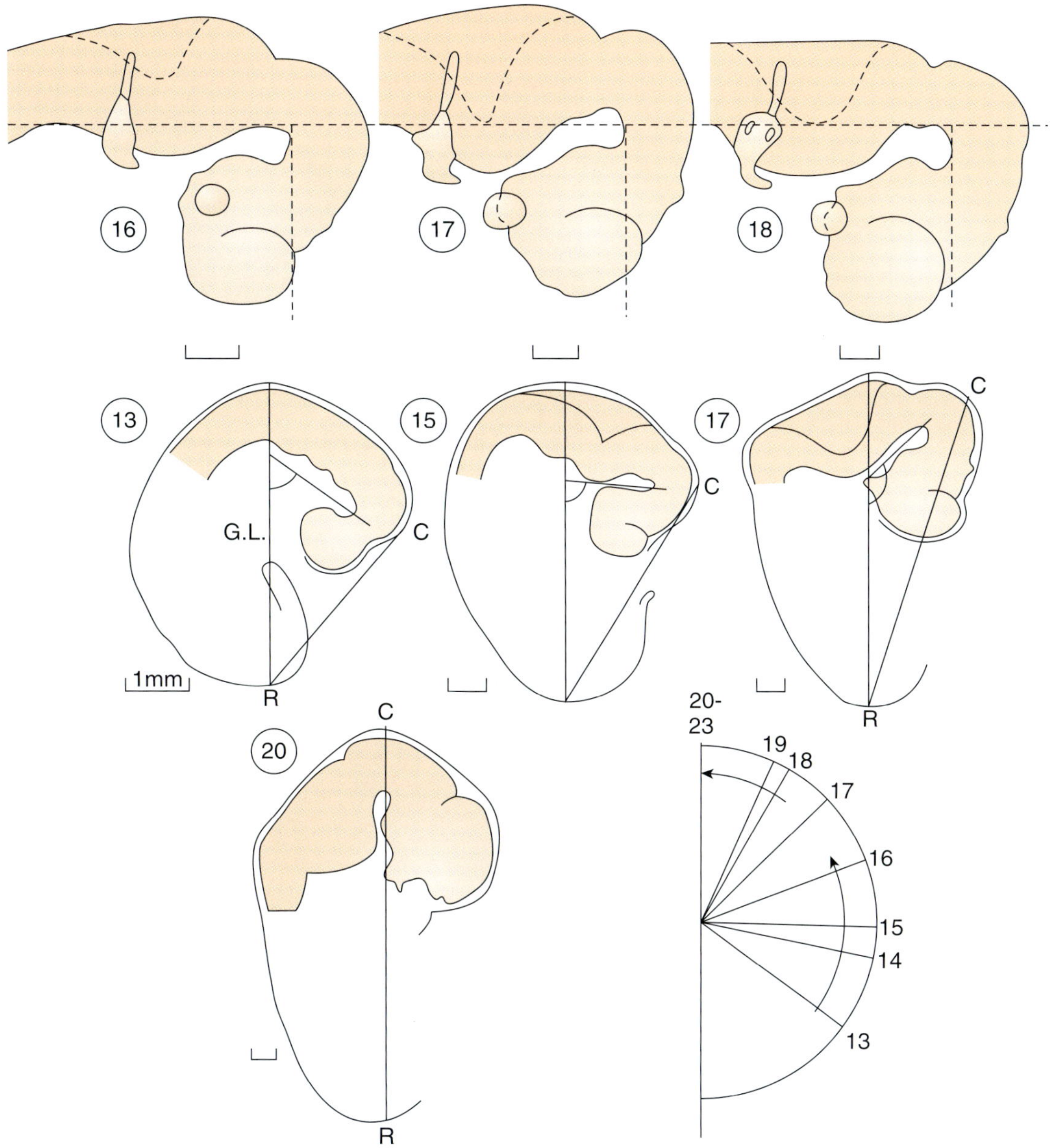


**Figure 2–9.** The outlines of four embryos (right lateral views) with the brain superimposed. The embryos are shown at stages 13, 15, 17, and 20, respectively, and are at 6w1d, 6w5d, 7w5d, 9w1d postmenstrual weeks. In the first three examples, the greatest length (GL) is larger than the crown-rump (C–R) length, whereas the two measurements coincide in the fourth. The last drawing (stages 13 to 23) is a scheme to summarize the "ascent" of point C until the C–R length comes to equal the GL. (From O'Rahilly and Müller, 1984,[34] with permission.)

At 8 weeks, 1 day and 8 weeks, 3 days from the LMP (Figure 2–15), the structures appear clearer, and flexures of the brain, such as the mesencephalic and pontine flexures, were located. The coronal sections revealed the rhombencephalon with regard to the major divisions. Figure 1–4 in Chapter 1 depicts a median section of the brain at 8 weeks, 3 days after the LMP. The subdivisions of the brain (Figure 2–16) could not yet be sufficiently discerned by TVS.[37]

At 8 weeks, 5 days from the LMP (Figure 2–17), the embryo starts to "unfold."[23] The mesencephalic flexure is almost in line with the longitudinal body axis. The cavities of the ventricular system are clearly identifiable. Subdivisions such as the telencephalon, diencephalons, metencephalon, and myelencephalon are seen sonographically not only on sagittal but also on coronal sections.

Observations by Blaas and associates[29,30] are consistent with those described above.

In addition to the already described structures, the choroids fold and slightly later, at 8 weeks, 5 days from LMP, the first sighting of the choroid plexus was reported. Only days later, at 9 weeks, 3 days from the LMP (with a CRL of 25 mm), a better image of the choroid plexus and the cerebellum was seen (Figure 2–18).

From about 9 weeks from the LMP, there is a significant change in the TVS evaluation of the fetus as a whole, particularly of the CNS. Because of their gradual development and increase in size, more structures are

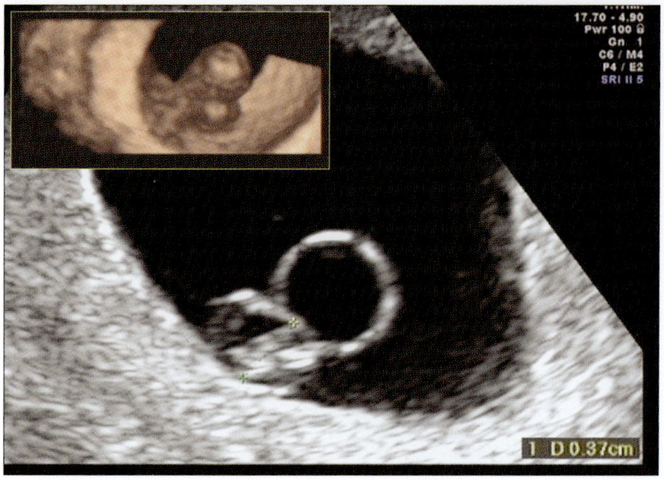


**Figure 2–10.** Pregnancy of 6 weeks 2 days (postmenstrual). The chorionic sac contains the yolk sac and the embryo measuring 3.7 mm. Inlay: 3D rendering of the yolk sac/embryo complex.

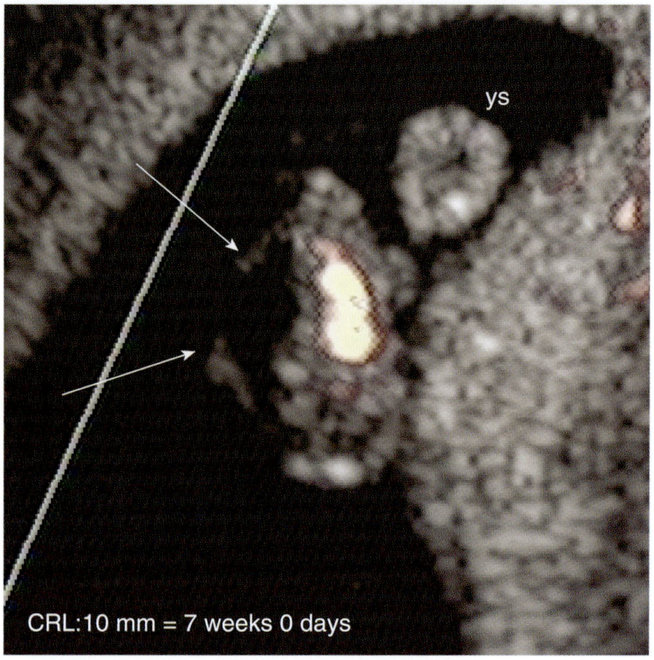


**Figure 2–11.** An embryo at 7 weeks 0 days (postmenstrual). The CR is 10 mm. The amnion (arrows) starts to be seen "separately" the first time by TVS (ys = yolk sac).

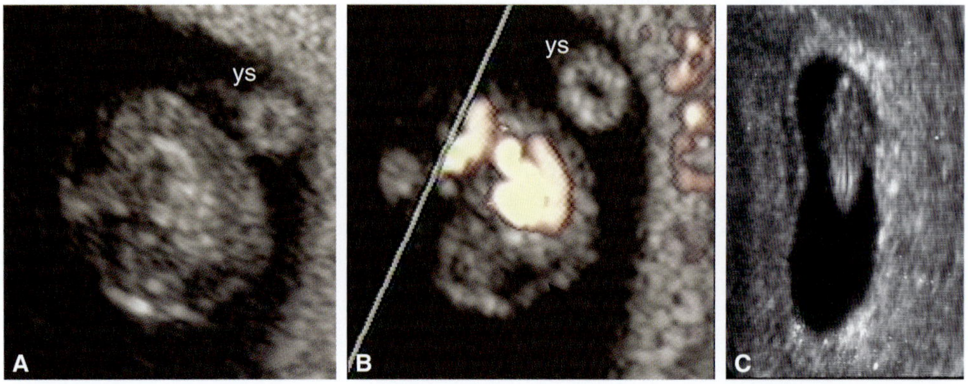


**Figure 2–12.** An embryo at 7 weeks and 2 days (postmenopausal). The CRL is 12 to 13 mm. By the Carnegie classification, this corresponds to a stage 16 embryo at 37th day postfertilization. The arrows point to the rhombencephalon. (**A**) Sagittal image. (**B**) Sagittal image highlighting the heart and umbilical flow. (The patient was scheduled for a termination of the pregnancy.) (**C**) The parallel lines of the spinal structures are evident (ys = yolk sac).

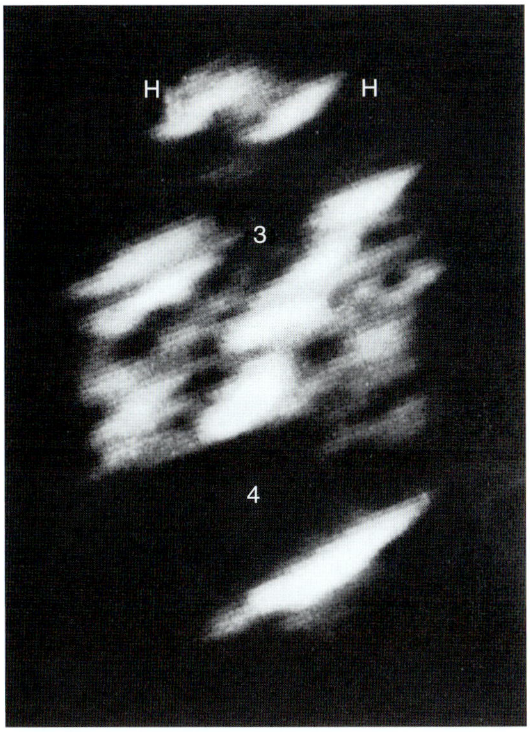


**Figure 2–13.** Transverse/oblique section through the rhombencephalon (4), diencephalon (3), and cerebral hemispheres (H) of an embryo (crown-rump length of 12 mm at 7 postmenstrual weeks 3 days). The bilateral evaginations of the hemispheres are clearly seen. There is still a wide opening to the third ventricle. (From Blaas and colleagues, 1994,[29] with permission.)

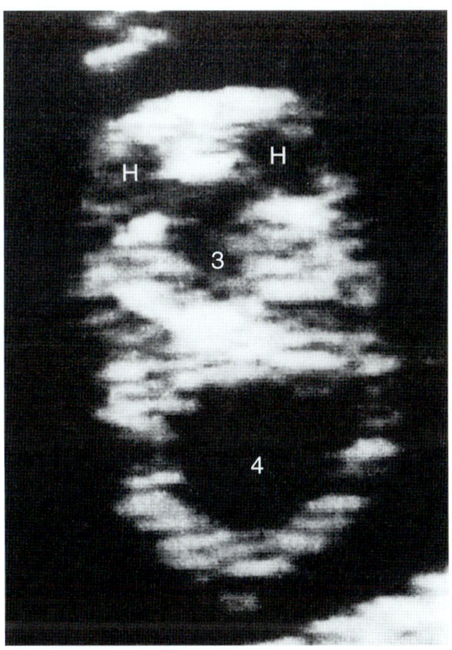


**Figure 2–14.** Transverse/oblique section through the rhombencephalon (4), diencephalon (3), and cerebral hemispheres (H) of an embryo (crown-rump length of 16 mm at 8 postmenstrual weeks 0 days). The borders between the cerebral hemisphere and the third ventricle (3) remain relatively small and start to develop into the interventricular foramina. (From Blaas and colleagues, 1994,[29] with permission.)

better seen. The development of the tortuous, fluid-filled ventricular system is readily imaged in the median plane (Figure 2–19). The subdivisions, as well as the serially connected cavities, appear on both the sagittal and coronal planes. Suddenly, it seems that many more sections can be generated in almost each of the three cardinal planes (Figure 2–19A).[23]

The different parts of the ventricular system are visible at this time. A study of the median section of the embryo at 9 weeks, 5 days from the LMP is depicted in Figure 2–19B. The sonolucent chain of the ventricular system winds itself around the two most prominent solid structures: the echogenic pontine flexure and the mesencephalic flexure. This age marks the stage (Carnegie stage 23) at which the latter points at the "crown" of the head and the true CRL can be measured reliably.[34,35] The first rostral sonolucent structure on this image is the diencephalon. Following the diencephalon, in the caudal direction, are the mesencephalon, the metencephalon, the myelencephalon, and the part of the medulla that contains the central canal. On a paramedian section, the relatively large choroid plexus in the lateral ventricle is depicted. At this age the choroid plexus fills the entire lateral (telencephalic) ventricle. On coronal and axial sections, the falx is seen as an echogenic structure. If the choroid plexus and the falx are imaged by TVS, the age of the embryo must be at least 9 postmenstrual weeks. A reasonably high-quality, high-frequency vaginal probe is necessary to detect the falx, the different ventricles, and the choroid plexuses at or around 9 to 9½ postmenstrual weeks.

## The Developing and Maturing Fetal Brain

The development of the embryonic brain was previously described. As detailed in Chapter 1, the embryonic period lasts up to 8 weeks from fertilization, or roughly 10 postmenstrual weeks. Following this, the fetal period starts; this lasts until delivery takes place. From a sonographic standpoint, there is definitely no visible quantitative reason for this qualitative change. An increasing number of detectable structures are seen from 8 postmenstrual weeks on, without any significant increase at or around the cutoff age at which the designation changes from embryo to fetus.

From 10 postmenstrual weeks on, three axial, three sagittal, and three or four coronal sections in each of the cardinal planes of the fetal head can be obtained.[31]

A 3D model created by computer and based on serial 2D slice scans of fetuses at 8 to 10 postmenstrual weeks is depicted in Figure 2–20. The Norwegian group from Trondheim produced such computer-generated "casts" of the well-delineated ventricular system, which enabled a close study of this system as it changed shape between 8 and 12 postmenstrual weeks.[38] Until a US system becomes widely available to re-create the different brain structures in a 3D fashion, we will have to rely on our own mental re-creation of fetal structures in general, and the brain in particular. To perform such a complex task in our own brain, serial sections of the structure in question must be generated and examined during every scanning session. A similar series of horizontal (axial) slices is depicted in

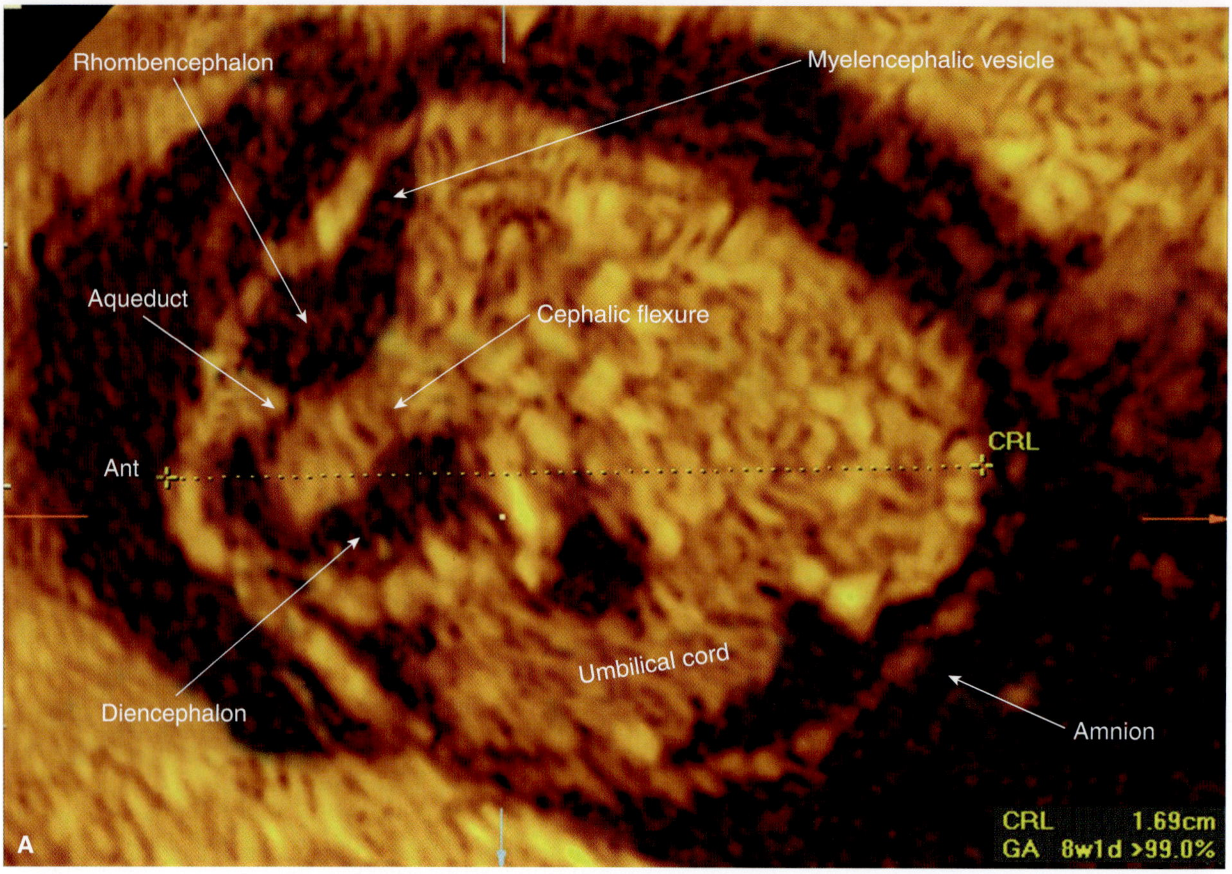


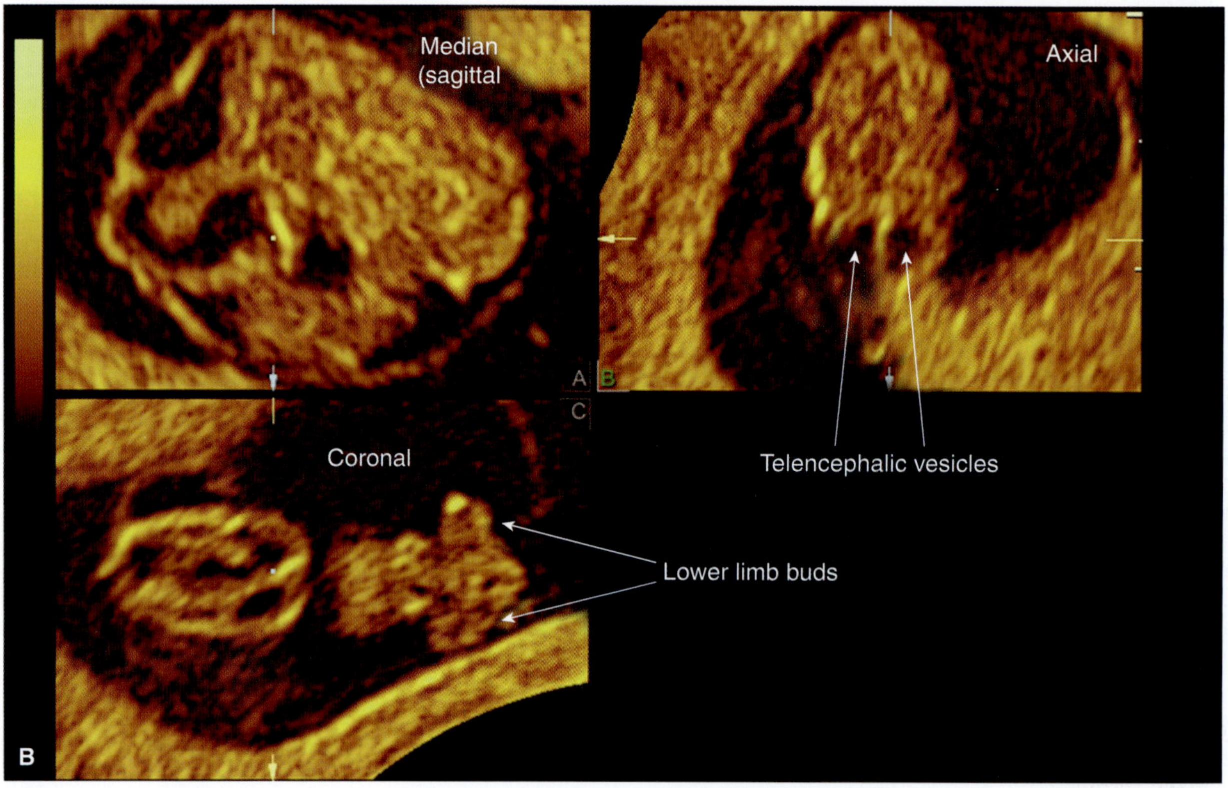


**Figure 2–15.** An 8 weeks and 1 day (postmenopausal) embryo with the crown-rump length of 16.9 mm. By the Carnegie classification, this corresponds to a stage 18 embryo at 43 days postfertilization. (**A**) Median picture showing parts of the anechoic ventricular system. (**B**) The orthogonal planes; the median axial and coronal planes. The lower limb buds and the telencephalic vesicles are highlighted by the arrows.

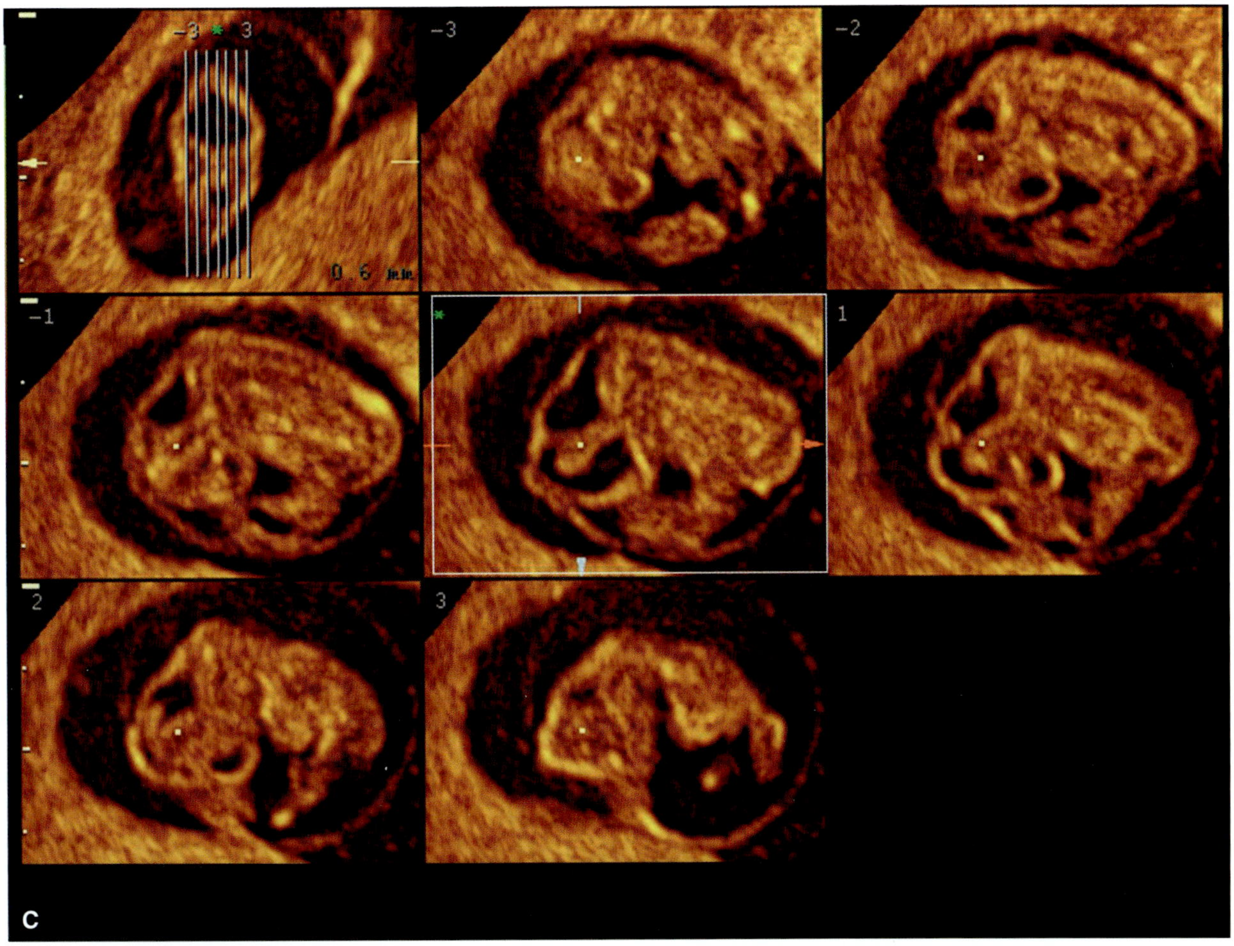

**Figure 2–15.** (*continued*) (**C**) Tomographic, consecutive sagittal sections along the lines shown in the upper left image square. The picture with the white frame is the median plane of the embryo.

Figure 2–21. From these images it is obvious that the choroid plexus of the fetus at 11 to 11½ postmenstrual weeks almost fills the available space within the lateral ventricle. If the gain control is increased, the high brightness of the choroid enables the detection of cysts as small as 2 to 3 mm, should they exist. The falx is sufficiently echoreflective and therefore easily seen. In addition, the third ventricle, the tentorium, the posterior fossa, and the cerebellum and its peduncles leading to the midbrain can be imaged (Figures 2–21 and 2–22). On a very low axial section the foramen magnum can also be seen (Figure 2–21C).

It seems that the presence of the third ventricle can clearly be seen on axial scans at 11, 12, and even 13 postmenstrual weeks (Figures 2–21, 2–22, and 2–23). However, on serial scans at 14 and 16 postmenstrual weeks (Figure 2–30), the space is progressively taken up by the expanding thalamus.

### Three-Dimensional Inversion Rendering of the Developing Ventricular System in the First Trimester

We saw previously the 3D rendering of some brain structures obtained by segmentation techniques by the Trondheim group.[38] Since then, thanks to 3D software developments, new tools are available to study the early fetal brain. One of these methods is the 3D inversion rendering of fluid-filled spaces utilized by our group.[39]

The steps of 3D inversion rendering are the following. First, the volume is obtained, in this case using an ultra-high-frequency transvaginal probe, and stored. Then an inversion algorithm (in our case, the GE-Kretz (GE Healthcare, Milwaukee, WI) 4D view laptop-based software is applied, which inverts the anechoic spaces (fluid) into white echoes. At the conclusion of this process, the fluid-filled ventricular system appears as a cast.

This technique allows the primitive, developing embryonic/fetal ventricular system to be displayed. By performing this display sequence, applying it to the brain of fetuses with increasing gestational ages, we can follow the development of the ventricular system and the brain containing it.

Figures 2–28, 2–30, 2–31, 2–32, 2–33, 2–34 and 2–38 contain the orthogonal display and/or the tomographic (sequential) images of entry of fetuses of increasing gestational ages. The anatomical structures pertaining to each gestational age are indicated with arrows. Similar 3D inversion rendering techniques were also used by Kim et al.[40]

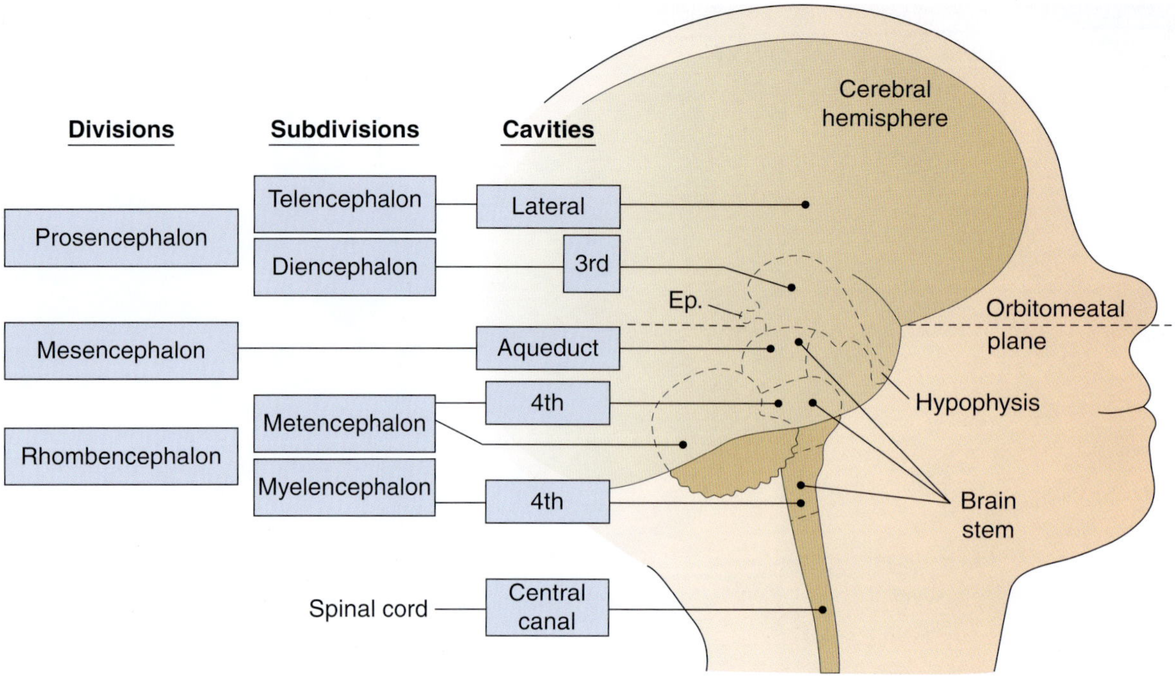


**Figure 2–16.** The divisions, subdivisions, and brain cavities seen in an infant's brain. The metencephalon consists of the cerebellum and the pons. The myelencephalon is the medulla oblongata. The brain stem comprises the midbrain, pons, and medulla. The third ventricle is mainly diencephalic, but it is partly telencephalic. The central canal is mainly in the spinal cord, but it is partly in the medulla. All of these parts are present by 5 postfertilizational (7 postmenstrual) weeks. The subdivisions and the cavities can be detected by high-frequency transvaginal sonography, but only from about 8 to 8½ postmenstrual weeks. (From O'Rahilly and Müller, 2001,[37] with permission.)

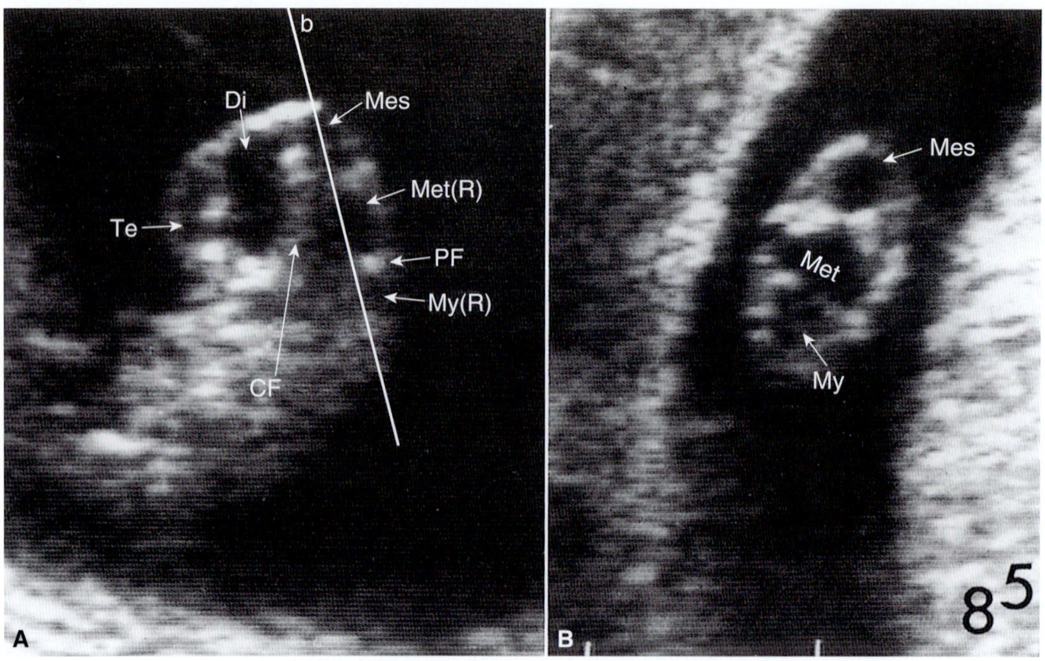


**Figure 2–17.** Median and coronal (posterior oblique) sections of an embryo at 8 postmenstrual weeks and 5 days (crown-rump length, 20 mm). (**A**) Median section showing the following structures: telencephalon (Te), diencephalon (Di), and mesencephalon (Mes). The metencephalon (Met) and myelencephalon (My) are parts of the rhombencephalon (R). The two main flexures, pontine (PF) and mesencephalic (CF), are also seen. (**B**) Coronal oblique section through line b. (Modified from Timor-Tritsch and colleagues, 1991,[23] with permission.)

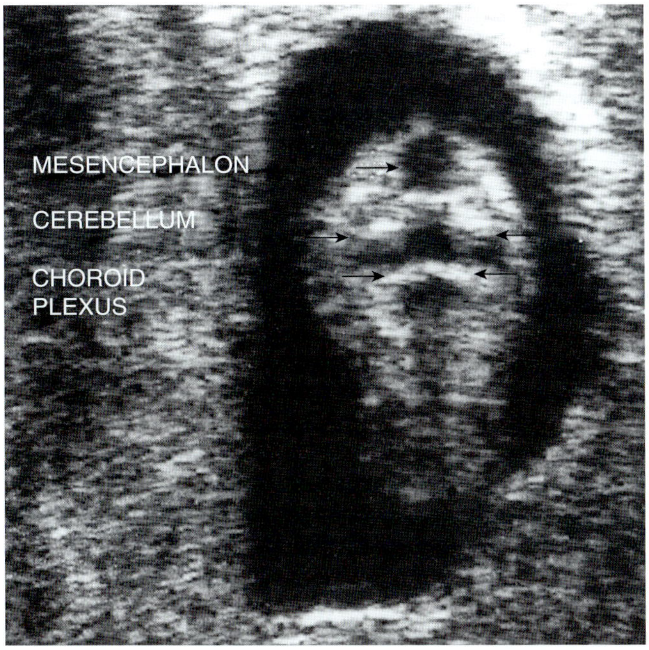


**Figure 2–18.** Coronal section at 9 postmenstrual weeks and 3 days, showing the rhombencephalon (crown-rump length, 25 mm). The mesencephalon, cerebellum, and choroid plexus are marked. (Courtesy of Blaas, Department of Obstetrics and Gynecology, National Center for Fetal Medicine, Trondheim University Hospital, Trondheim, Norway.)

In general terms it is clear that at very early ages (7 to 8 postmenstrual weeks) the rhombencephalon is the dominant structure. Toward the 12th postmenstrual week, the rhombencephalon appears to be small in comparison to the telencephalon and the hemispheres containing the choroid plexus, which at 7 to 8 weeks are relatively small.

The composite picture at the end of the series (Figure 2–29) allows viewers to clearly follow the changes in size of each ventricle (and thus the surrounding brain tissue) and their relationships. It is also evident in the composite that the choroid plexuses of the lateral ventricles become increasingly large, occupying a larger proportion of the lateral ventricles.

A significant change first noted at the 11th to 12th postmenstrual week is the relative increase of the anterior tip of the anterior horns of the lateral ventricles. Note the anterior sonolucent area in front of the choroid plexuses (Figure 2–23) in a fetus at 12 postmenstrual weeks. This is the anterior horn of the lateral ventricle, and it is difficult to overlook. For the next 2 to 3 weeks, it will remain relatively large (Figures 2–34, 2–35, and 2–36). Two simultaneous processes occur from 11 to 16 to 18 postmenstrual week: the choroid plexuses of the lateral ventricles "move back" on top of the thalamus into its final place—the body and the atrium of the lateral ventricle—and progressive growth of the cerebral cortex slowly decreases the size of the horn. Indeed, toward term the anterior horns become slitlike.

At around 14 to 16 postmenstrual weeks, the slowly but constantly growing and thickening skull bones present an increasing obstacle for the high-frequency sound waves that, until this age, have created images of the fetal CNS in a rather unrestricted fashion. The solution to this problem is to use the anterior fontanelle (Figure 2–37) as an acoustic window to continue scanning of the fetal brain. As mentioned previously, scans obtained via the anterior fontanelle do not provide parallel sections in the coronal or sagittal plane. These sections are generated radiating in an oblique fashion with their apex at the fontanelle, as shown in Figure 2–8.

## Coronal Planes

Using the anterior fontanelle as a sonic window, a few perfect midcoronal and a series of oblique coronal sections, from anterior to posterior, can be obtained.

For easier understanding, but even more so for clearer clinical use, three main groups of sections through the above-mentioned planes are described. The three main groups are the frontal, midcoronal, and occipital sections (Table 2–2).[41,42] Each of these may have two or three possible subsections. Their importance is discussed later.

### Sonographic Anatomical Landmarks

Because of extensive changes in the size and location of several anatomical landmarks that are well seen sonographically, it is practical to clearly separate two age groups. One is the age group from 12 to 18 postmenstrual weeks; the second is above at least 18 but clearly above 20 weeks. The groups require partitioning because before 18 postmenstrual weeks, the frontal horn extends frontally and is evident on any of the anterior (frontal) coronal sections.

The sonographically identifiable anatomical landmarks in the coronal sections group are listed in Table 2–2. These landmarks are listed as subdivisions of the following structures: skull, brain, ventricles, cavities, choroid plexus, midbrain, cerebellum, and meninges. Their presence on all of these sections is indicated.[41]

There are several cardinal landmarks, that, if present on a specific plane, are clear markers of the plane in question. Such anatomical markers are the orbits, the passage of the choroid plexus into the third ventricle through the interventricular foramina (Monro), and the posterior horns. The presence of these structures indicates unequivocally that the section was taken at the frontal–2, midcoronal–2, and occipital–1 sections, respectively. These cardinal landmarks are highlighted in Table 2–2 for easier understanding.

There is also a typical and unique clustering of several structures throughout each of the sections. Such a clustering indicates that the section was obtained at a specific and well-defined section. For example, if on a coronal section the orbits and the anterior horns are seen (without the choroid plexus), this can exclusively apply to the Frontal–2 section. On the other hand, if one seeks out the midcoronal–2 section, one would search for an image containing the cross section of the corpus callosum, the choroid plexus containing lateral ventricles, the cavum septi pellucidi, the thalami, and the falx, all seen at the same time. Only this one specific section is consistent

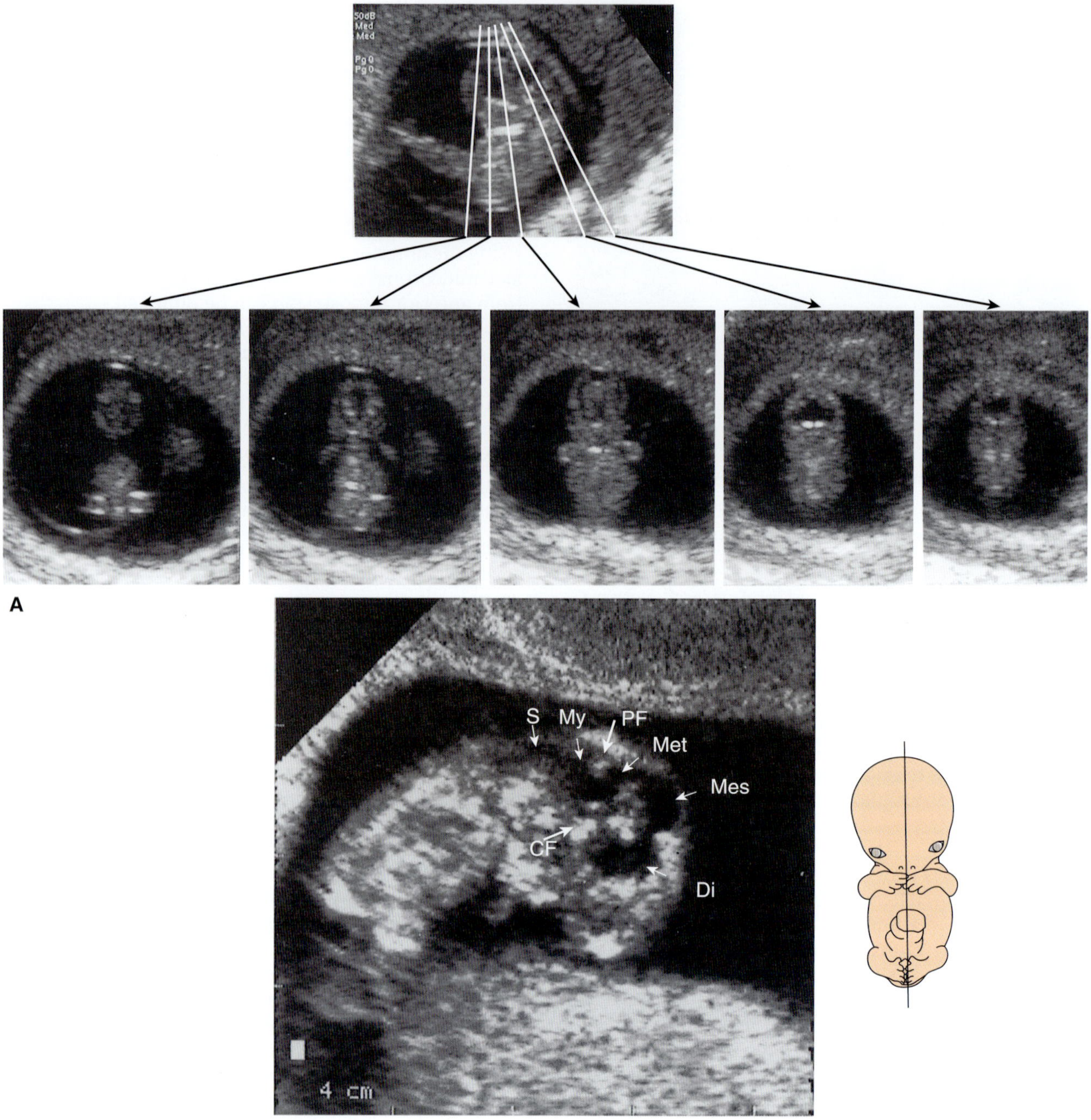


**Figure 2–19.** (**A**) At 9 postmenstrual weeks and 1 day, it is possible to acquire multiple sections in the clanical planes. This picture illustrates five coronal sections obtained using a high frequency transvaginal probe at this age. (**B**) Median section at 9 postmenstrual weeks and 5 days (crown-rump length, 28 mm). The sonolucent and progressively tortuous ventricular system is imaged. Di, diencephalon; Mes, mesencephalon; Met, metencephalon; My, myelencephalon; S, the entrance to the central canal; CF, mesencephalic flexure; PF, pontine flexure. (Modified from Timor-Tritsch and colleagues, 1991,[23] with permission.)

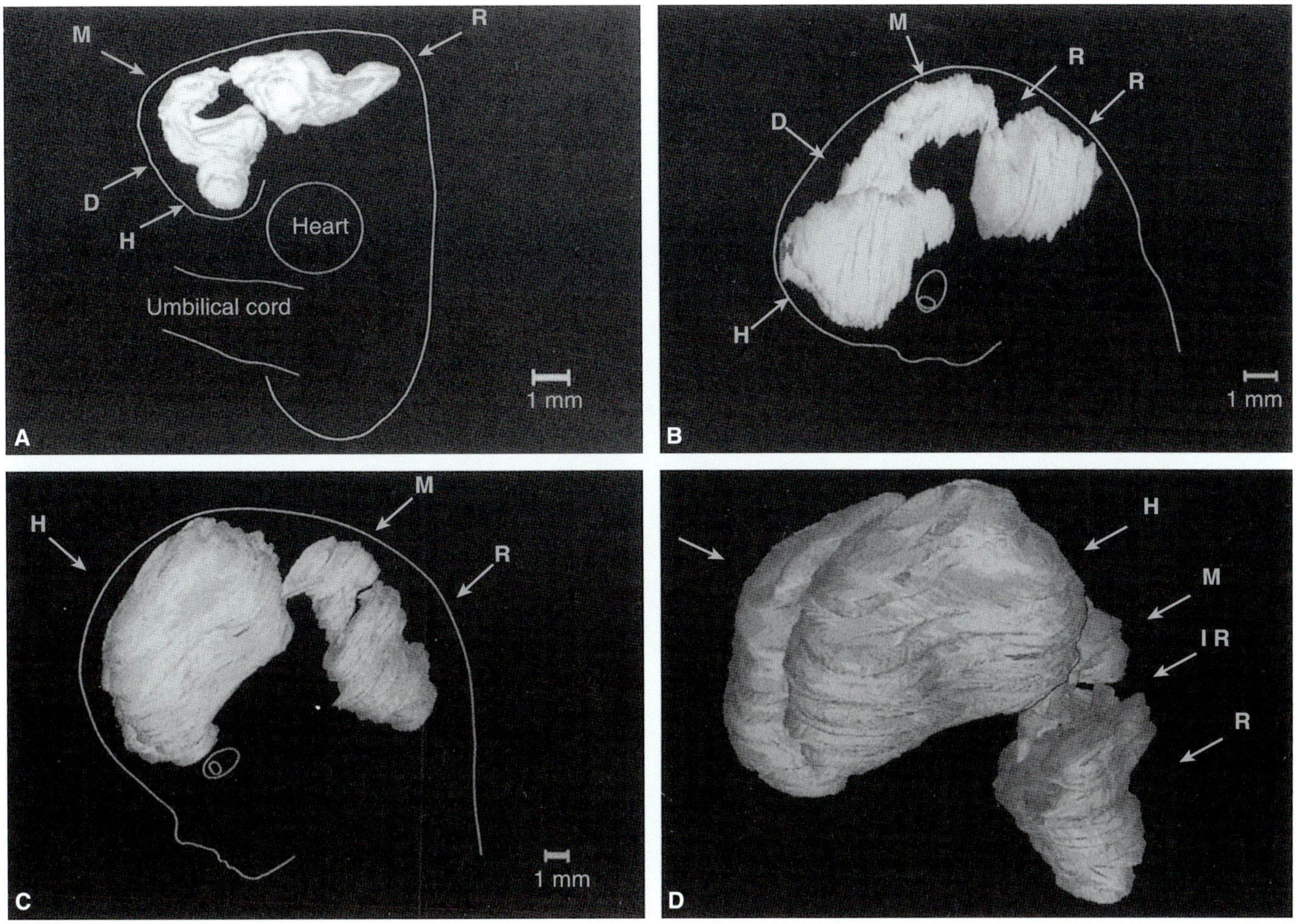


**Figure 2–20.** Three-dimensional representation of the embryonic and fetal ventricular systems. (**A**) Lateral view of the brain cavities in an embryo of 13-mm crown-rump length (CRL). The outline shows the embryonic shape, with head and the umbilical cord. (**B**) Lateral view of the brain cavities in an embryo of 24-mm CRL. The outline shows the embryonic head and eye. (**C**) Lateral view of the brain cavities in a fetus of 40-mm CRL. The outline shows the fetal head and eye. (**D**) Oblique view of the brain cavities in a fetus of 40-mm CRL. H, cerebral hemisphere; D, diencephalon; M, mesencephalon; R, rhombencephalon; IR, isthmus rhombencephali. (From Blaas and colleagues, 1995,[38] with permission.)

with the midcoronal–2 section. This concept holds true for all the specific and unique sections obtained in the two general planes.[38]

Based on these easily recognized sonographic landmarks and the typical picture generated, we refer to the frontal–2 section as the "steer's head" configuration (Figures 2–38A-O1, 2–38C and 2–39E, and 2–39A). The occipital–1 section resembles the "owl's eye" configuration (Figures 2–38A, 2–39E, 2–40B, and 2–41D).

### Structures Seen on Coronal Sections

1. FRONTAL SECTIONS: At 12 to 18 postmenstrual weeks, both frontal–1 and –2 images reveal the widely open anterior horns of the lateral ventricles. The frontal–2 section contains the orbits (steer's head configuration). Later during gestation, the frontal–1 (more anterior frontal) section "cuts" through the white matter only. The longitudinal fissure and the subarachnoid space containing the superior sagittal sinus are present (Figure 2–38A–C).

   Frontal–2 is the typical steer's head configuration and should show only continuous white matter with the anterior horns. The longitudinal fissure is seen (Figures 2–39A–E and 2–41A–D).
2. MIDCORONAL SECTIONS: Three distinct midcoronal sections can be separated. The common denominator of all three is that the anterior horn, with or without the choroid plexus, and the corpus callosum are seen on all three. These are almost true coronal sections because they are close to each other and are generated by a very slight tilt of the probe from the classical coronal plane.

   Structures seen in the midcoronal–1 plane are the laterally and upward slanted frontal horn of the lateral ventricle, the corpus callosum, the interventricular septum, and the cavum septi pellucidi between the heads of the caudate nuclei (Figures 2–39B–C, 2–41B, 2–47 and 2–53A–B).

   Structures seen in the midcoronal–2 plane are the lateral ventricles (body) containing the echogenic choroid plexuses, their extension through the

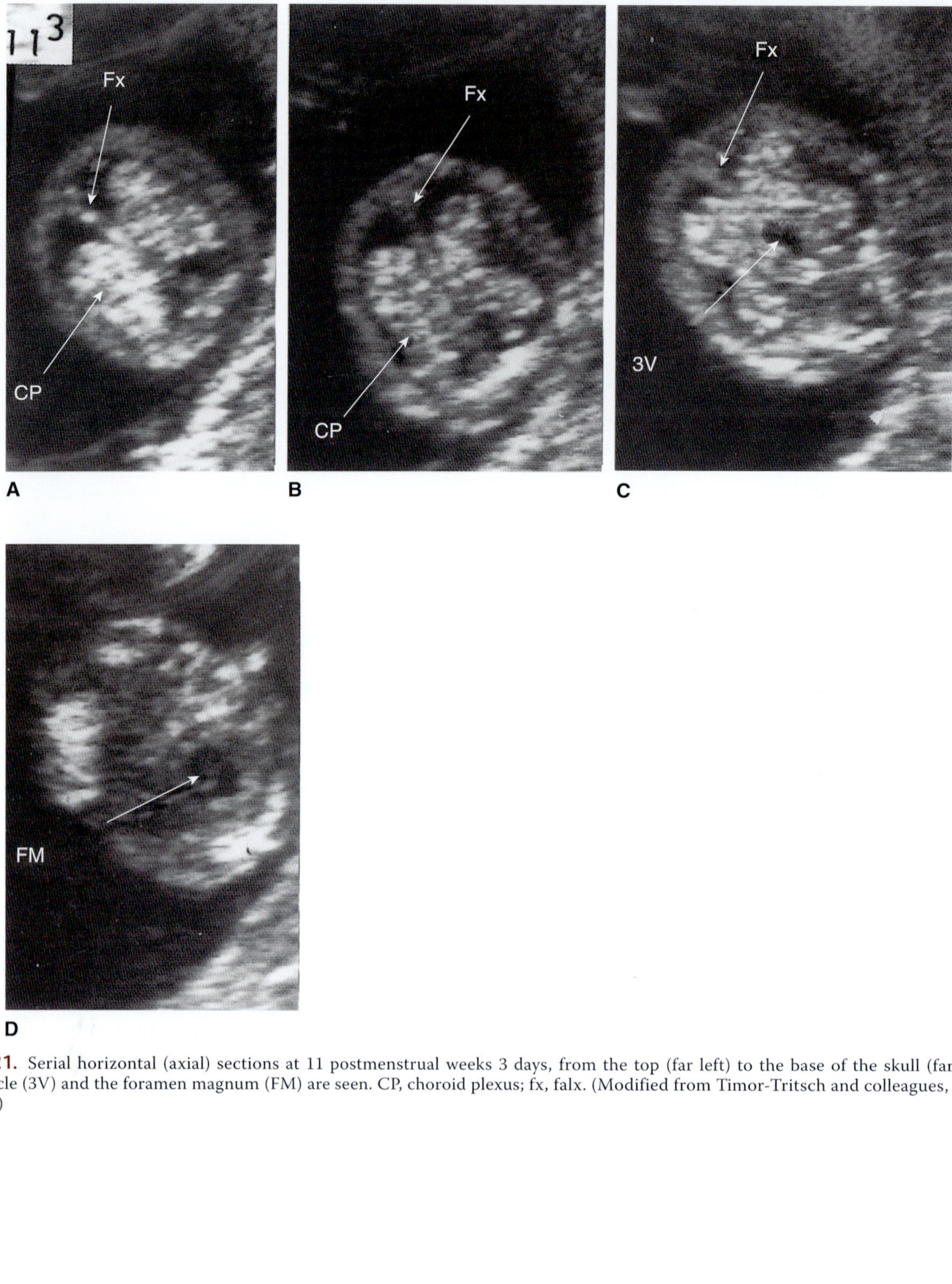


**Figure 2–21.** Serial horizontal (axial) sections at 11 postmenstrual weeks 3 days, from the top (far left) to the base of the skull (far right). The third ventricle (3V) and the foramen magnum (FM) are seen. CP, choroid plexus; fx, falx. (Modified from Timor-Tritsch and colleagues, 1991,[36] with permission.)

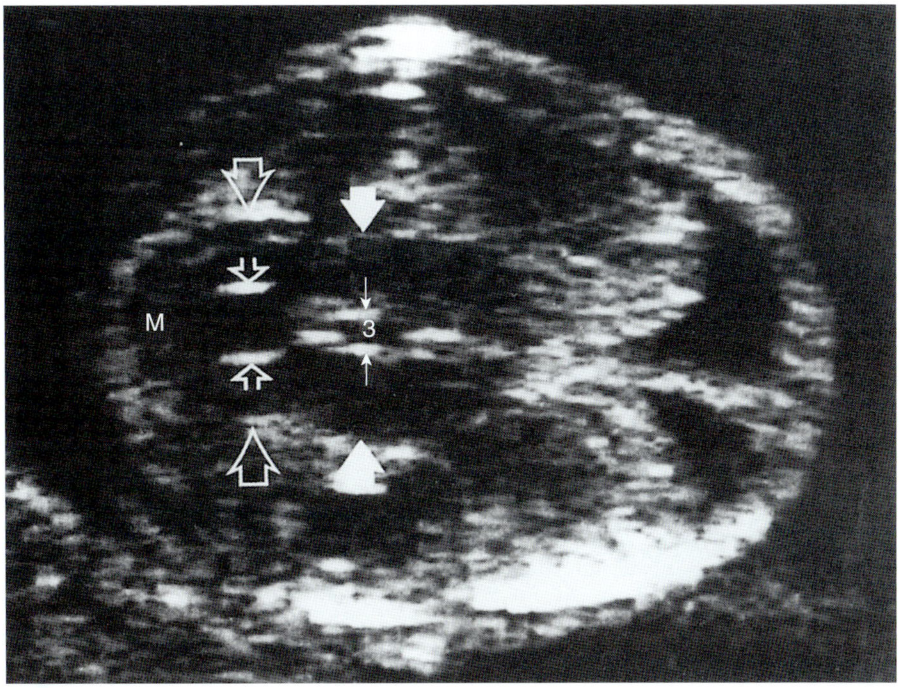


**Figure 2–22.** Horizontal (axial) section through the head of a fetus at 11 postmenstrual weeks and 6 days (crown-rump length, 49 mm). The view is of the diencephalon (bold arrows) and its narrow third ventricle (3), and through the mesencephalon (large open arrows; M), with its wie cavity (small open arrows). AH, anterior horns. (From Blaas and colleagues, 1984,[29] with permission.)

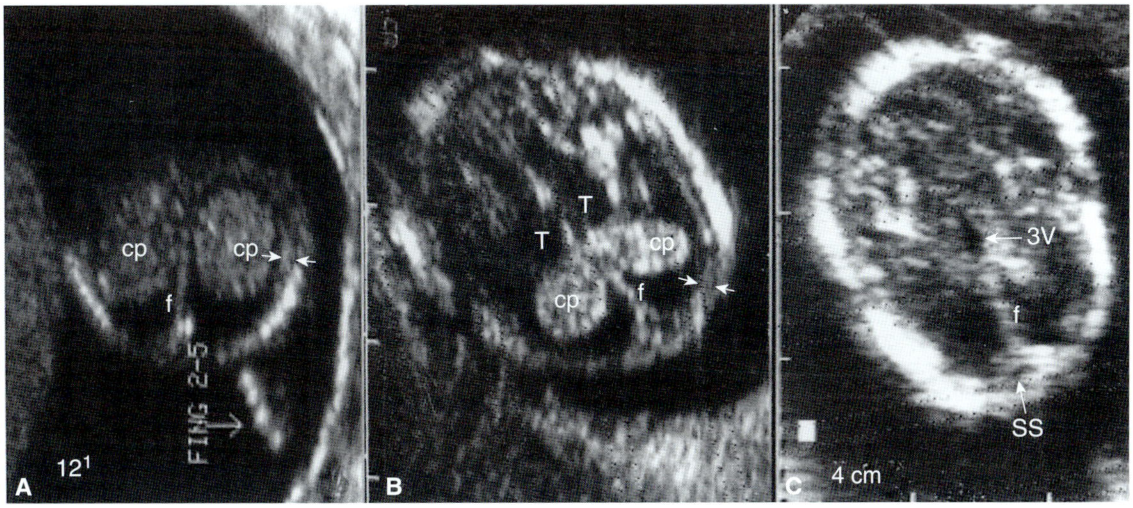


**Figure 2–23.** At 12 postmenstrual weeks 1 day, a frontal oblique section (**A**) shows the falx and the choroid plexus. Axial sections (**B**, **C**) reveal the hyperechoic choroid plexus (cp) on top of the thalamus (T) in the lateral ventricles. Only a thin cerebral cortex mantle is still seen between the small arrows. The third ventricle (3v), the falx (f), and the frontal part of the sagittal sinus (SS) are also seen. (Modified from Timor-Tritsch and colleagues, 1991,[23] with permission.)

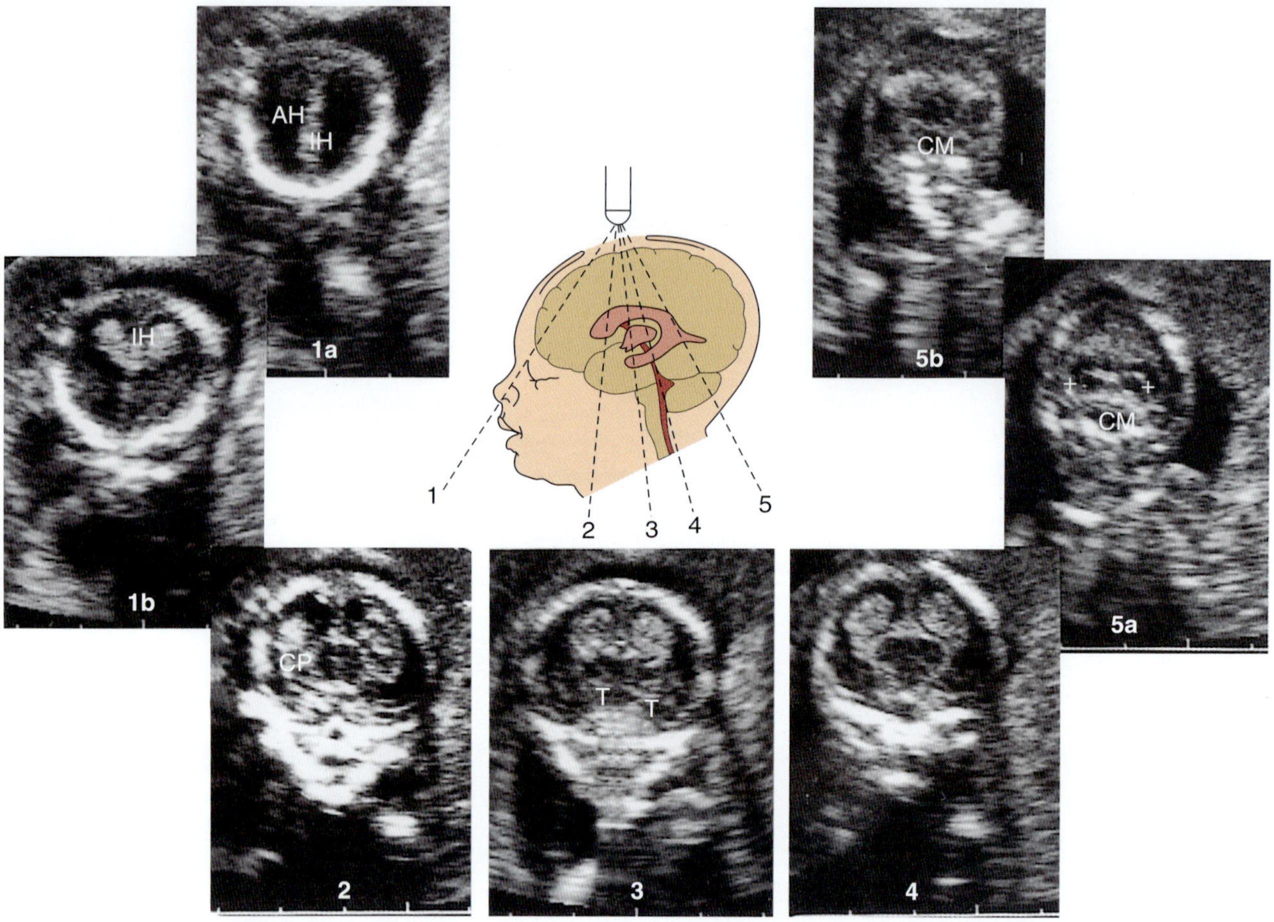


**Figure 2–24.** Serial brain sections at 14 postmenstrual weeks. 1A, 1B. Frontal oblique sections, showing the longitudinal fissure (IH) and the anterior horns (AH). Somewhat more posteriorly (1B), the choroid plexus appears (C). In sections 2 through 4 (midcoronal sections) the changing relationship of the choroid plexus (C) to the thalamus (T) can be seen. 5A and 5B are more posterior occipital oblique sections showing the cisterna magna (CM) and a bicerebellar diameter measurement of the cerebellum. (From Timor-Tritsch and Monteagudo 1991,[24] with permission.)

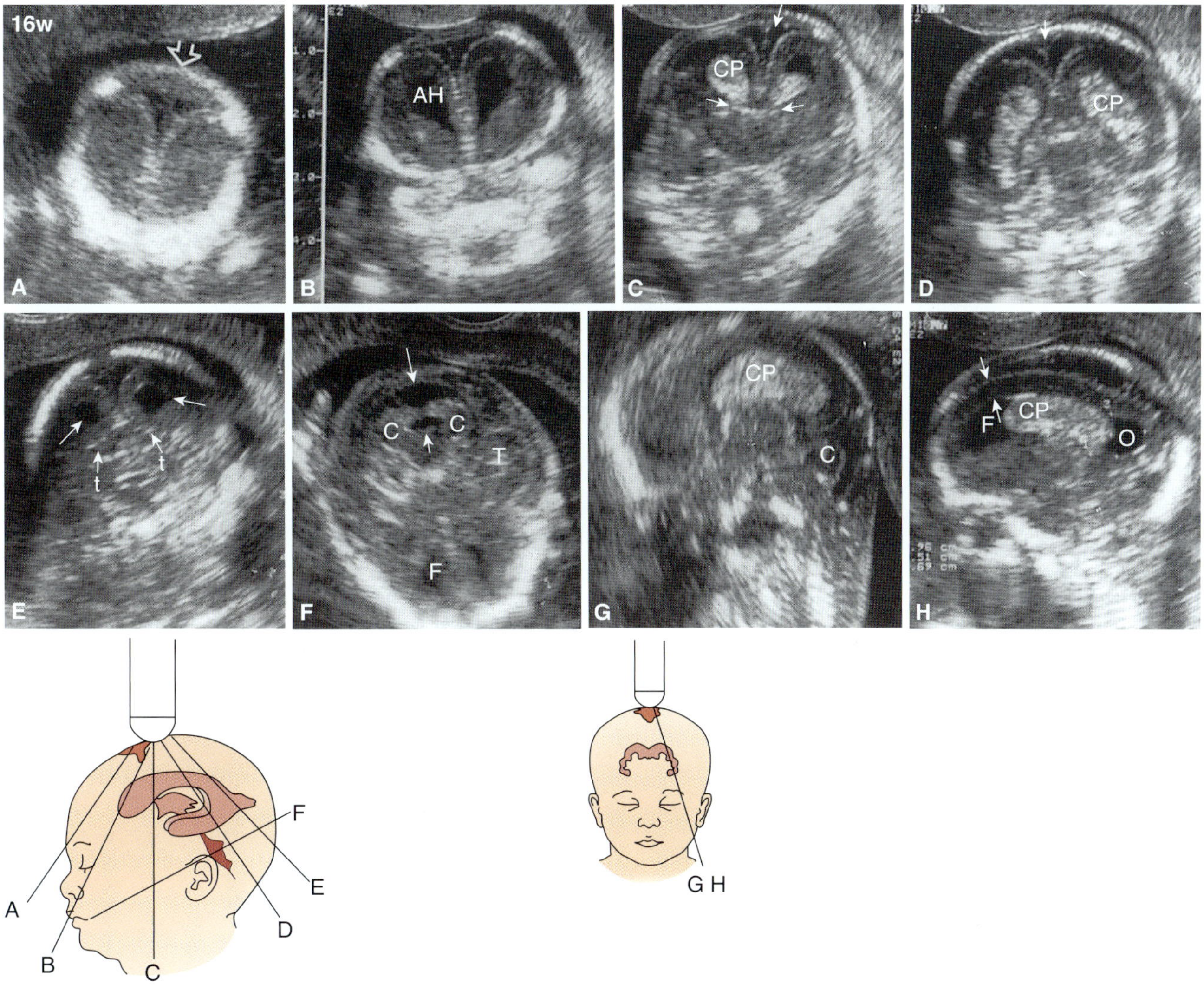


**Figure 2–25.** Serial scans of the fetal brain at 16 postmenstrual weeks. (**A**) An extreme anterior frontal–1 section (see Table 2–2) almost tangential to the fetal skull, showing the wide opening of the anterior fontanelle) (open arrow). (**B**) Frontal–2 section. The cortex and the white matter around the anterior horns are becoming progressively thicker. The sonolucency of the anterior horn (AH) is outstanding. The subarachnoid space is marked by the white arrow. (**C**) Midcoronal section. The choroid plexus (CP) and its connection through the interventricular foramina (small white arrows) are shown. The midline arrow indicates the falx. (**D**) Midcoronal–3 section through the antrum of the lateral ventricles, which are filled entirely by the choroid plexus (CP). The arrow indicates the falx. (**E**) Occipital–1 section. The posterior horns are marked by the small white arrows. The tentorium (t) is also indicated. (**F**) Horizontal section. The sonolucent cisterna magna is highlighted by the large white arrow. The cerebellum (C) and the fourth ventricle (small white arrow) are shown. The anterior horns (F) and the inferior horns (T) are visible using this section. (**G**) An oblique section highlighting the choroid plexus (C) and one of the cerebellar hemispheres (C) (**H**) Right oblique–1 section with the anterior horn (F), posterior horn (O), and choroid plexus (C) situated above the thalamus (T). The thick mass of the brain tissue is indicated by the two small arrows.

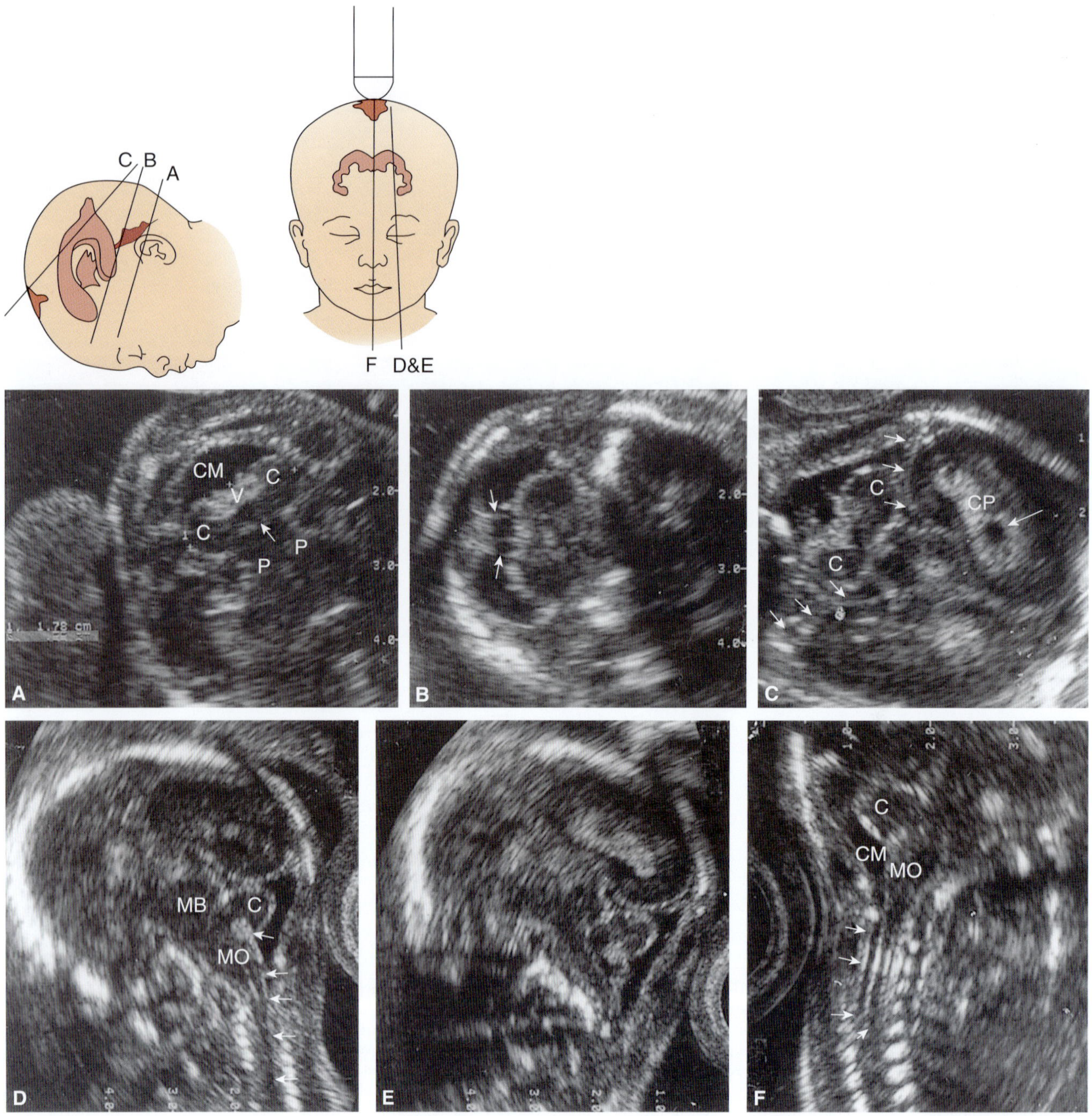


**Figure 2–26.** These series of horizontal and sagittal sections are part of the workup of the posterior fossa in a normal fetus at 16 postmenstrual weeks. (**A**) "Low" horizontal section. The cerebellum (C) measures 1.78 cm, and the cisterna magna measures 0.66 cm. Note the inferior pedunculi (P), the hyperechoic lower portion of the vermis (V), and the fourth ventricle (small arrow). (**B**) The somewhat higher horizontal section of the posterior fossa, highlighting the small, threadlike structures of the arachnoid membrane (small arrows). (**C**) This is a higher, composite horizontal/coronal section that shows the tentorium (small arrows). The cerebellum (C) and the choroid plexus (C), and the choroid plexus (C) with a tiny choroid plexus cyst (small white arrow). (**D**) Almost median section showing the midbrain (MB), medulla oblongata (MO), hyperechoic vermis (small single arrow), and cerebellum (C). The tiny arrow points toward the medulla. This section clearly shows the upper portion of the medulla (multiple small arrows). (**E**) Paramedian section. The structures are similar to those indicated in D. (**F**) Median section of the suboccipital region, highlighting the cerebellum (C), cisterna magna (CM), medulla oblongata (MO), and spinal cord (small arrows).

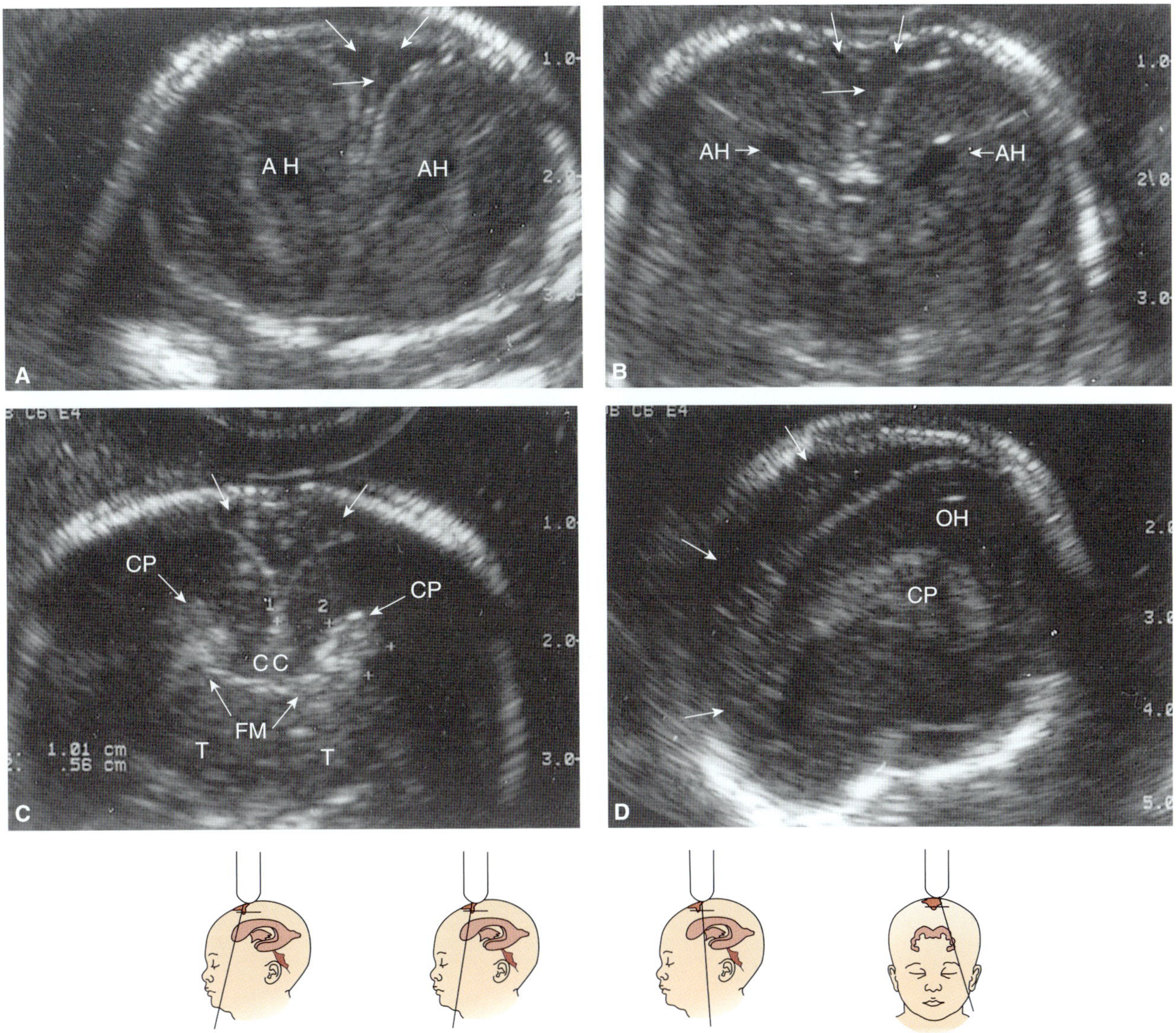


**Figure 2–27.** Additional views of the same fetus imaged in Figure 2–25. In addition, all of these images highlight the subarachnoid space. (**A**) Frontal–2. (**B**) Midcoronal–1 section. (**C**) Midcoronal–2 section. (**D**) Left oblique–1 section. The subarachnoid space is highlighted by small white arrows in all of these sections. AH, Anterior horn; F, falx; CC, corpus callosum; FM, interventricular foramina; CP, Choroid plexus; T, thalamus; OH, posterior horn. The two measurements in C are the distance from the midline to the tip of the anterior horn (1) and the depth of the anterior horn (2). These are normal for this age.

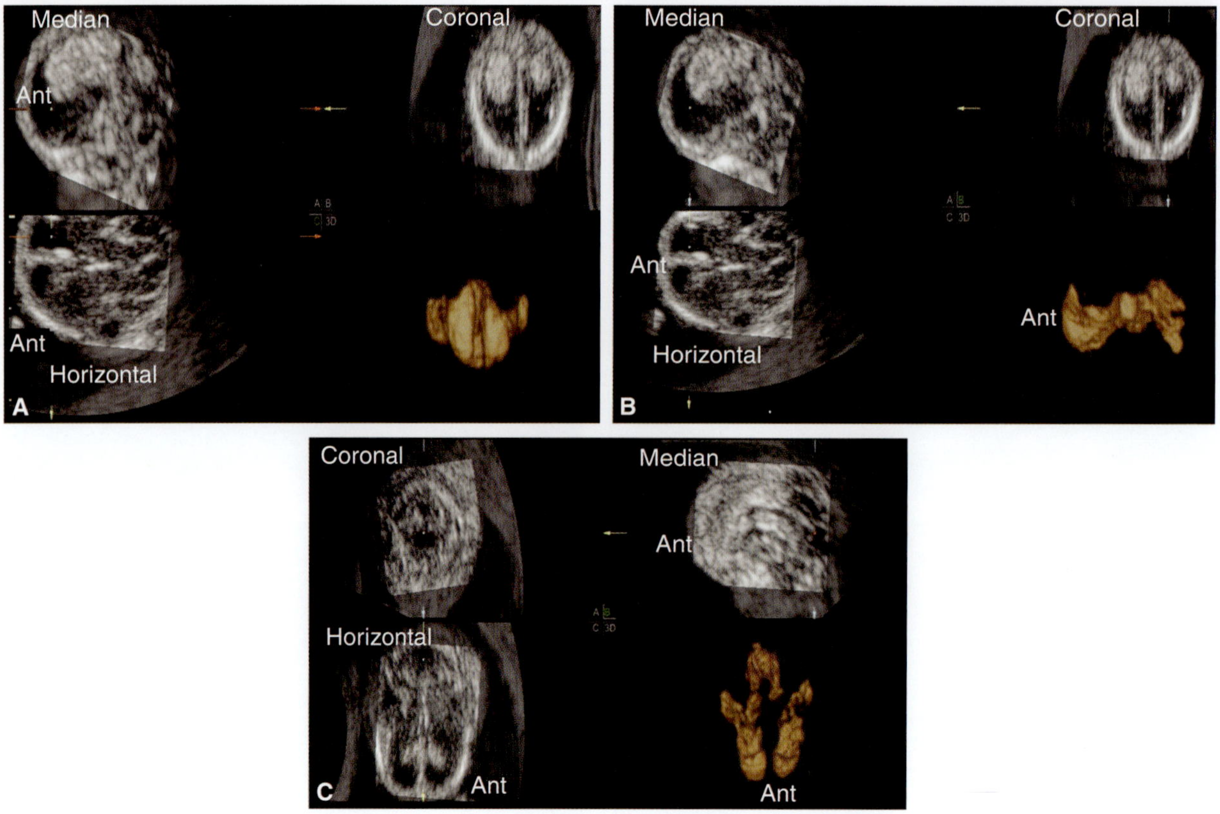


**Figure 2–28.** Structural evaluation of the fetal brain at 15 postmenstrual weeks. Systematic scanning of the lateral ventricles and the choroid plexus can be performed using several horizontal or oblique planes. **(A)** Frontal view of the inversion rendered ventricles. **(B)** Lateral view of the inversion rendered ventricles. **(C)** Superior view of the inversion rendered ventricles. (From Timor-Tritsch and colleagues, 1995,[42] with permission.)

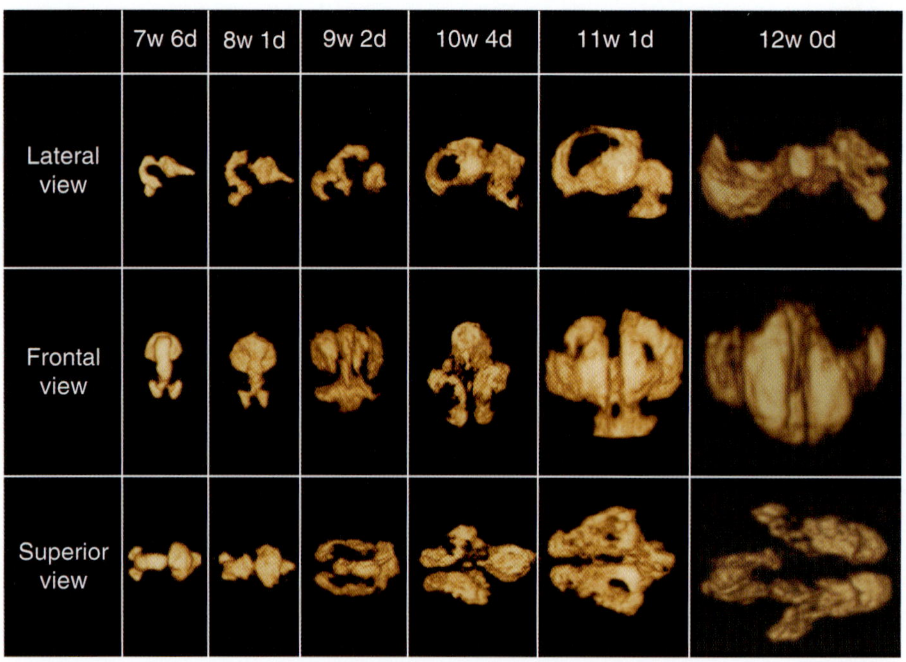


**Figure 2–29.** Composite picture of the 3D inversion renderings of the developing ventricular system from 7 to 12 postmenstrual weeks showing the lateral, frontal, and the superior views. Note the changing relations of size between the anterior horns and the rhombencephilon (fourth ventricle). (From Timor-Tritsch IE et al, 2008,[39] by permission.)

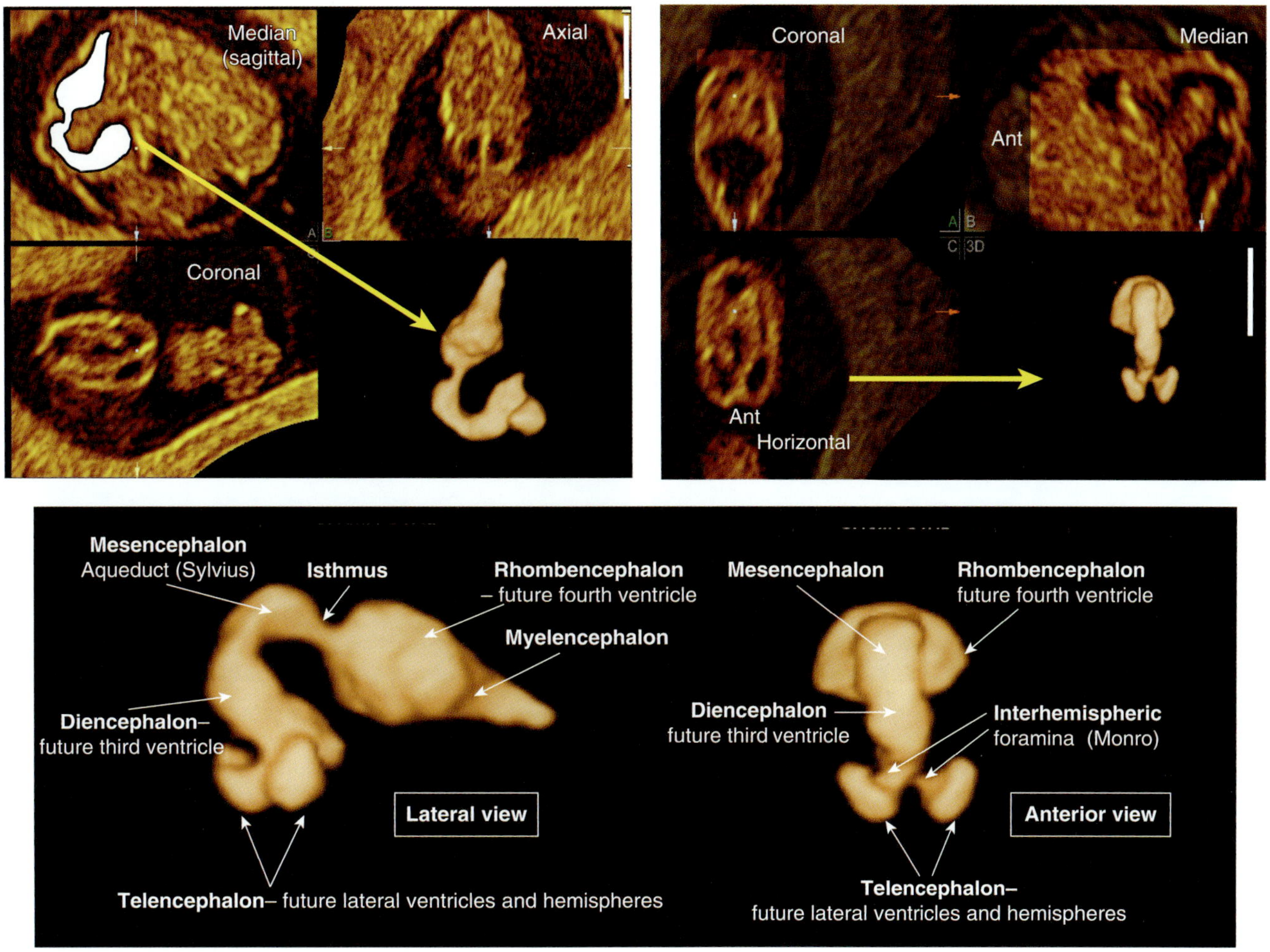


**Figure 2–30.** Inversion rendering of brain ventricles at 8 postmenstrual weeks and 1 day. The upper left and right pictures are orthogonal displays and the resulting 3D inversion renderings offering a lateral (upper left) and an anterior (upper right) view of the cast-like appearance of the ventricles. The two lower pictures detail the anatomic structures seen on the lateral and the anterior views of the 3D inversion renderings. (From Timor-Tritsch IE et al, 2008,[39] by permission.)

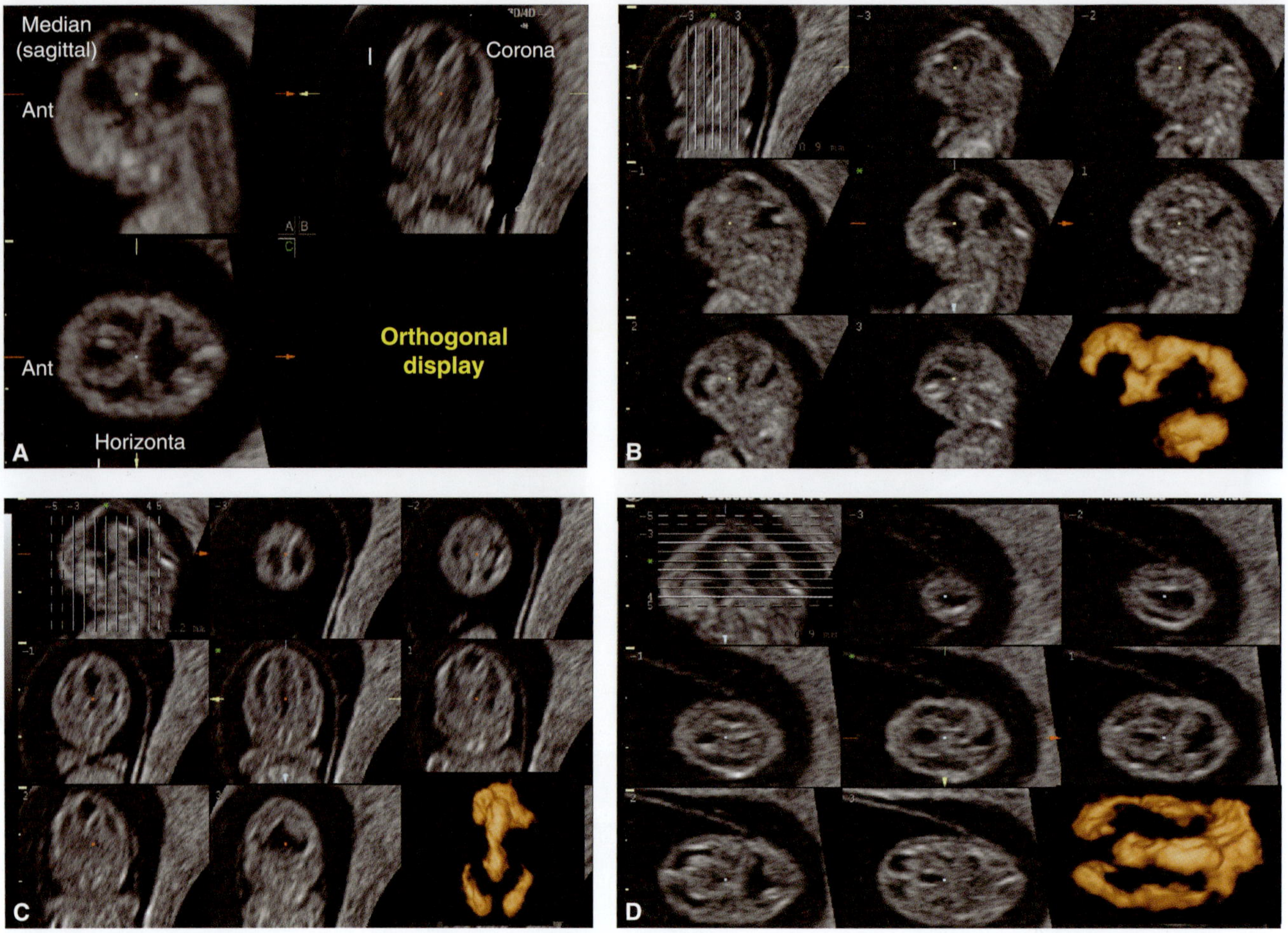


**Figure 2–31.** Inversion rendering of brain ventricles at 9 postmenstrual weeks and 2 days. (**A**) Orthogonal display. (**B**) Tomographic display: sagittal sections with lateral view of 3D inversion rendering. (**C**) Tomographic display: coronal sections with frontal view of 3D inversion rendering. (**D**) Tomograpich display: horizontal sections with superior view of 3D inversion rendering. (From Timor-Tritsch IE et al, 2008,[39] by permission.)

interventricular foramina (Monro) into the space between the thalami (virtual space of the third ventricle), the cavum septi pellucidi below the corpus callosum, the longitudinal fissure, the budding (at 28 postmenstrual weeks) or the developed (after 31 to 32 postmenstrual weeks) cingulate gyrus and sulcus, as well as the triangular subarachnoid space containing the superior sinus (Figures 2–38A–C, 2–39A–E, 2–40B and 2–41A–D).

Structures seen in the midcoronal–3 plane are the lateral ventricles (body) containing the choroid plexuses; at times, the slightly echogenic choroid plexus of the third ventricle between the thalami; the corpus callosum; the longitudinal fissure; and the cingulate gyrus and sulcus. Also, toward term, the secondary and tertiary branches of the cingulate sulcus can be imaged (Figures 2–38A and C, and 2–39D).

3. OCCIPITAL SECTIONS: The occipital oblique sections may be the hardest to obtain.[20,23,32,41,42] If circumstances permit, two distinct sections can be obtained. The occipital–1 section displays the typical owl's eye configuration because the cortical and white matter is seen in a symmetrical fashion surrounding the sonolucent and almost perfectly round posterior horns, above the V-shaped subarachnoid space and below the tentorium and the hemispheres of the cerebellum. At times, the fourth ventricle and the hyperechoic vermis are seen (Figures 2–38C, 2–39E, and 2–41D).

The occipital–2 section is the most posterior one. Rarely seen, however, it contains the tip (smallest sonolucent circle) of the posterior horn and the tentorium, below which the cerebellar hemispheres, vermis, and cerebellomedullary cistern (the cisterna magna) are seen (Figure 2–30).

A faster way to scan the fetal brain in the coronal plane is to use one each of the frontal, midcoronal, and occipital sections. On the frontal–1 section, besides its symmetrical picture, one should not see the anterior horns (these are seen on this section in the case of ventriculomegaly). The midcoronal–2 section should contain the corpus callosum and the left and right thalami, and the choroid plexus should fill the

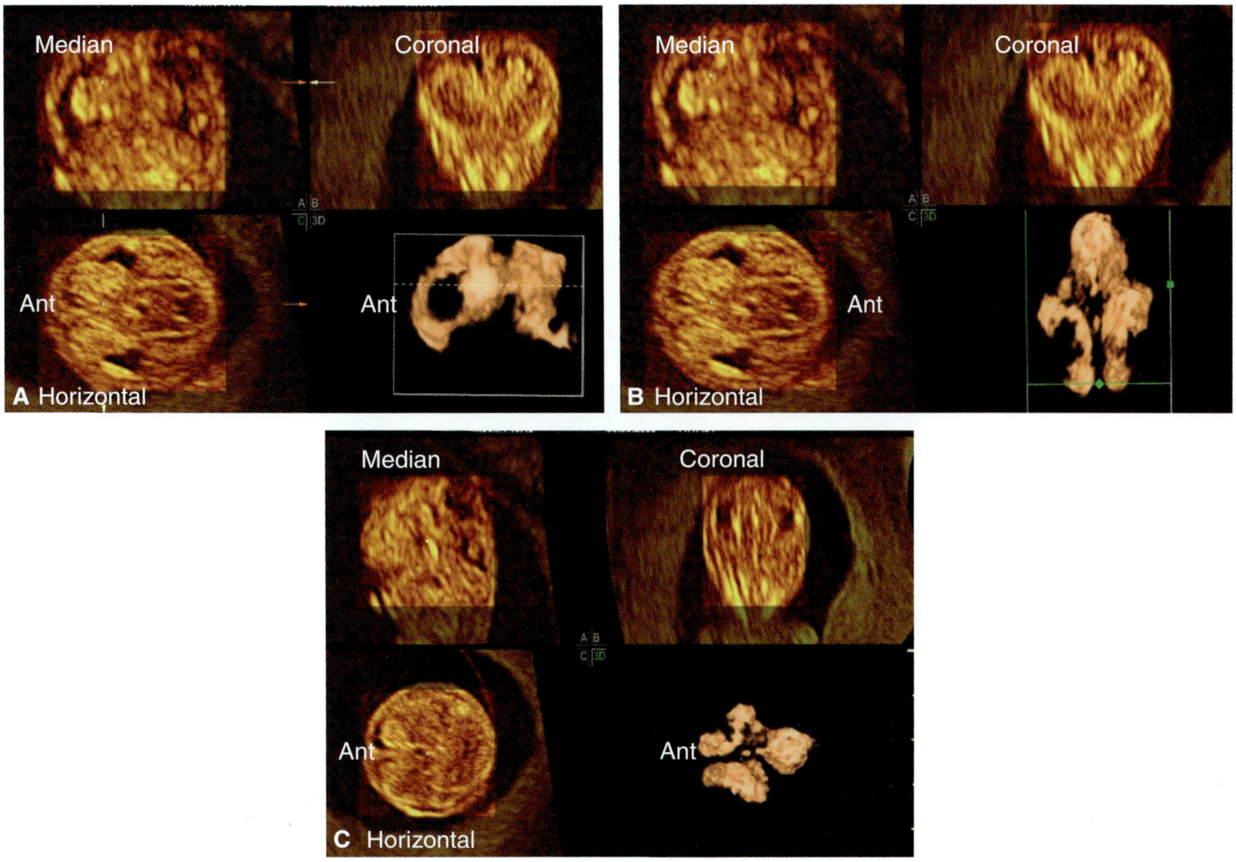


**Figure 2–32.** Inversion rendering of brain ventricles at 10 postmenstrual weeks and 4 days. (**A**) Orthogonal planes and lateral view of 3D inversion rendering. (**B**) Orthogonal planes and anterior view of 3D inversion rendering. (**C**) Orthogonal planes and superior view of 3D inversion rendering. (From Timor-Tritsch IE et al, 2008,[39] by permission.)

body of the lateral ventricle, proceeding through the interventricular foramina. The occipital–1 section should show the normal-size posterior horn (see its normal measurements in Chapter 3), and the tentorium and the cerebellum should fill the posterior fossa. This abbreviated scanning algorithm should not take more than several minutes.

### Structures Seen on Sagittal Sections

Unlike the coronal section, in which the right and left hemispheres are scrutinized simultaneously, sagittal sections are different, since after the image in the median plane is obtained, the right and left hemispheres have to be scanned separately using right and left paramedian or oblique sections.

Table 2–3 contains the pertinent images seen with each of the following structures.

1. MEDIAN SECTION: The hallmark of the median section are the corpus callosum and, below it, the sonolucent cavum septi pellucidi. In addition, the thalamus, the head of the caudate nucleus, their thin-covering tela choroidea, parts of the midbrain, and posteriorly, the hyperechoic vermis are depicted (Figures 2–42, 2–43A, 2–44, and 2–45). Recognition of these structures on this section at 14 postmenstrual weeks is dependent on the quality and resolution of the transducer (Figure 2–34).

   The appearance of the corpus callosum is age dependent and is discussed below. As an example, at 16 postmenstrual weeks (Figure 2–38B), the corpus callosum is not yet evident.

   At times, as a function of the transducer (age dependent) or the depth at which it is situated, the fourth ventricle and the cerebellomedullary cistern become visible (Figures 2–43A and 2–45).
2. OBLIQUE–1 (RIGHT AND LEFT) SECTIONS: The oblique–1 sections should be obtained on the right as well as the left side. Although the sizes of the ventricles in both hemispheres should be the same, slight discrepancies are common. These sagittal sections are of importance and should never be overlooked. Lately, using 3D fetal neuroscanning techniques, we have named such oblique planes the three-horn views because they enable the viewer to evaluate the anterior, posterior, and inferior horns on the same section (see Chapter 9).

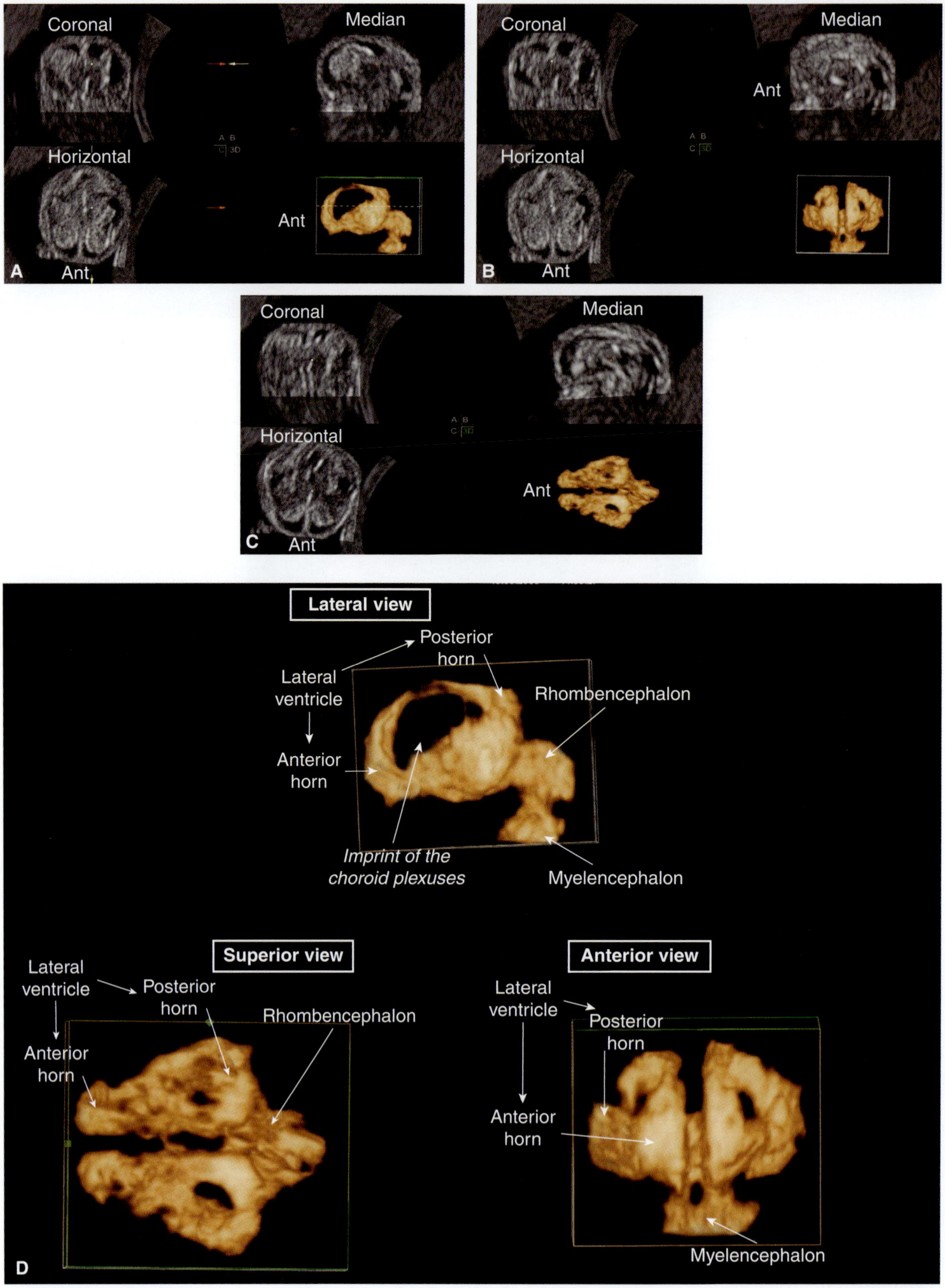


**Figure 2–33.** Inversion rendering of brain ventricles at 11 postmenstrual weeks and 1 day. (**A**) Orthogonal planes and lateral view of 3D inversion rendering. (**B**) Orthogonal planes and anterior view of 3D inversion rendering. (**C**) Orthogonal planes and superior view of 3D inversion rendering. (**D**) Anatomic structures seen on the lateral superior and anterior views of the 3D inversion renderings. Observe the "imprint" of the choroid plexus. (From Timor-Tritsch IE et al, 2008,[39] by permission.)

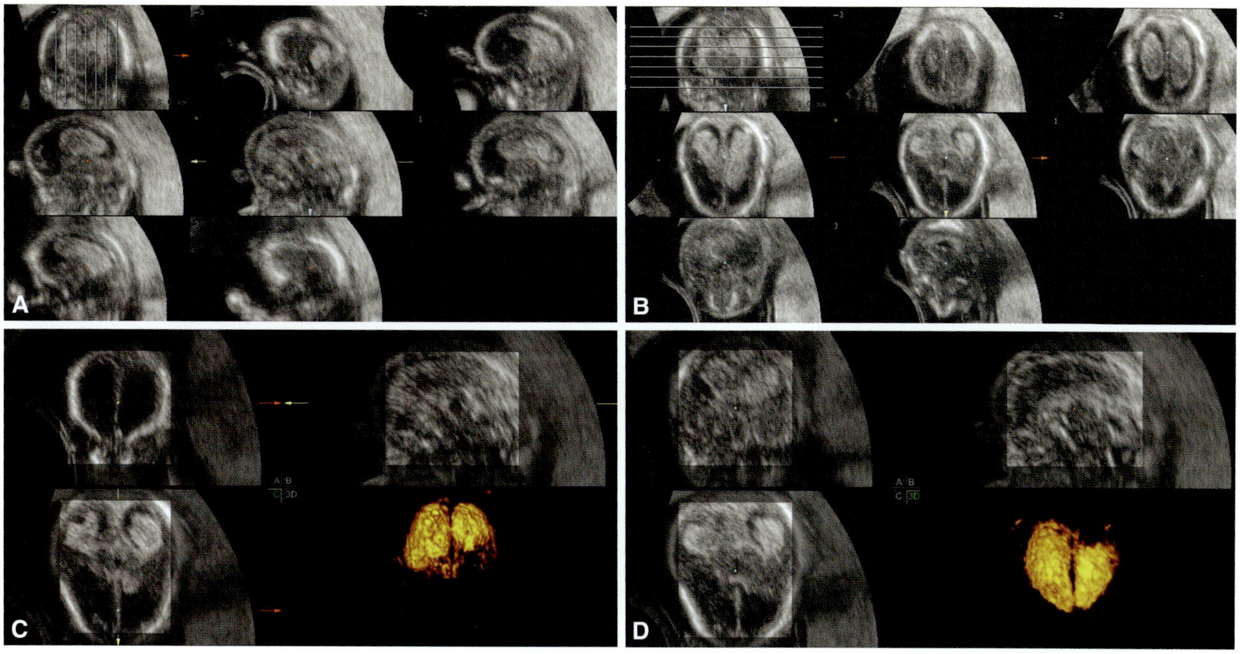


**Figure 2–34.** Fetal brain scan at 12 postmenstrual weeks. **(A)** Sagittal serial tomographic images. **(B)** Axial serial tomographic images. **(C)** Orthogonal plane with an inversion rendering of the relatively large (but normal) anterior horns of the lateral ventricles viewed from the front. **(D)** Orthogonal plane with an inversion rendering of the relatively large (but normal) anterior horns of the lateral ventricles viewed from above.

At 14 postmenstrual weeks the anterior horn is relatively large, and the posterior horn is barely developed and difficult to image (Figures 2–34, 2–35A, B, and 2–38B). At times, the inferior horn is visible in normal fetuses at this age (Figure 2–42). Later, these sections should not contain the inferior horn of the lateral ventricle (Figure 2–31D) because this horn is barely open in a normal brain.

At or after 18 postmenstrual weeks, the anterior horn progressively decreases in size. Toward term it may not be visible at all. The choroid plexus fills the entire antrum above the thalamus. The posterior horn increases its relative size and is easily imaged (Figures 2–40A and 2–43B).

3. OBLIQUE–2 (RIGHT AND LEFT) SECTIONS: If, after scanning through the sagittal planes, the scanning plane of the transducer is further tilted toward the fetal ears, almost tangential scans of the cerebral hemispheric surfaces are obtained. Typical on this section is the still widely gaping lateral sulcus (Sylvius), which appears as if the capital letter V were lying on its side. The apex of the V points toward the occiput (Figure 2–43C). The more advanced the age, the more closed the lateral fissure becomes. Between the two "legs" of the letter V, the tangentially "touched" insula is imaged. The upper lip of the V-shaped edges of the fissure is called the *parietal operculum*; the lower lip is the *temporal operculum*.

## Horizontal (Axial) Planes

At times in the early second trimester the fetus turns conveniently into a position in which an axial view is most revealing. The bone of the skull is still thin enough to enable meaningful TVS scrutiny of the brain.

The horizontal planes allow the gathering of information on two important aspects of brain anatomy. The first is the examination of the entire choroid plexus of the lateral ventricles (Figure 2–34) using different ascending sections. The second is a careful look at the posterior fossa using a posteriorly tilted axial plane (Figures 2–53, 2–59, and 2–60). The images of the posterior fossa are discussed subsequently.

Having pioneered the fetal transfontanelle neuroscan using the high-frequency transvaginal US probe, we are aware of the following.

1. The sections and/or planes obtained through the anterior fontanelle using conventional 2D transvaginal neurosonography were adopted emulating the neonatal transfontanelle approach. All sections are obtained by placing the footprint of the vaginal probe on the anterior fontanelle; the sections therefore "radiate" from one point: the fontanelle. Almost every plane, except the median and one coronal plane, is angled or is oblique and are therefore not parallel to each other. Moving the probe in a fanlike manner from anterior to posterior to obtain the coronal sections and from side to side

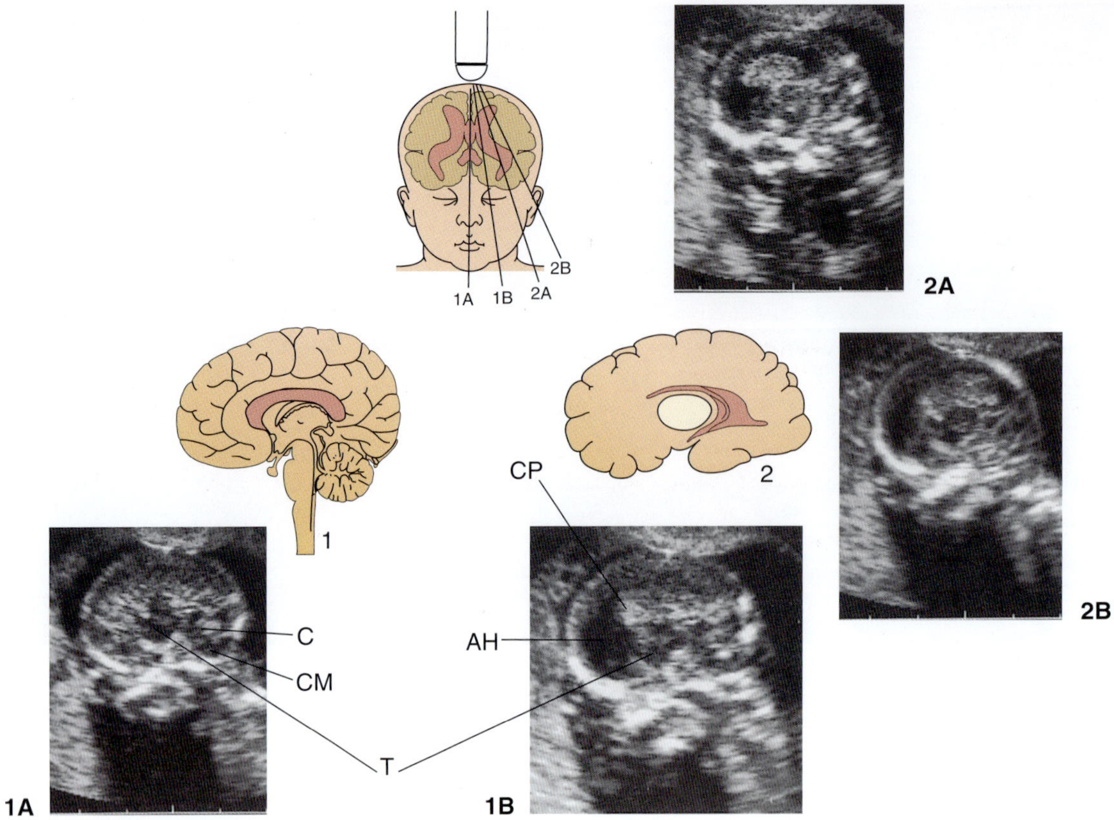


**Figure 2–35.** Median, paramedian, and left oblique sections at 14 postmenstrual weeks. 1A. Median section showing the thalamus (T), the hypoechoic cerebellum (C), and the posterior cisterna magna (CM). 1B. Slightly more lateral paramedian sagittal section showing the relationship between the anterior horn (AH) and the choroid plexus (C) and the thalamus (T). 2A, 2B. Left oblique views also depicting the posterior horn (OH). (From Timor-Tritsch and Monteagudo, 1991,[24] with permission.)

to obtain the sagittal sections results in the desired planes.

2. In contrast to the 2D technique, when a volume of the fetal brain is obtained using the 3D transvaginal US probes through the anterior fontanelle, the volume of the fetal brain can be sequentially sectioned at demand in all three classical orthogonal planes. These planes are parallel to each other and are therefore comparable to those sections obtained using serial tomograms by CT or MRI.
3. Using 3D volume scans, it is easy to render scanning planes that are almost impossible to obtain as a routine procedure. An example is the rendering of axial sections.

Although we use the 2D fetal transfontanelle neuroscan initiated by us,[20,23,24,41] we are increasingly aware of the new, more advanced 3D technique to examine the fetal brain, which will be demonstrated later in this chapter.

## Basic and Targeted Fetal Neurosonogram

The International Society of Ultrasound in Obstetrics and Gynecology (ISUOG) attempted to standardize fetal neurosonography. Guidelines to perform a basic sonographic examination of the fetal CNS were published in *Ultrasound in Obstetrics and Gynecology*.[43] This examination employs only transabdominal US, and its objective is to evaluate the fetal brain only in the general axial (horizontal) planes. It includes three planes: transventricular, transthalamic, and trancerebellar planes, as seen in Figure 2–46. In contrast, the targeted or more detailed fetal neurosonogram contains other planes and sections, such as coronal planes (Figure 2–47) and sagittal planes (Figure 2–48).

## Ventricular System

The embryology of the cerebral ventricles was touched on in Chapter 1, as well as in this chapter. The fetal cerebral ventricular system, as far as ultrasonography is concerned, consists of the following interconnecting structures and their parts (Figure 2–49): the lateral ventricles—anterior (frontal) horn, body, atrium, posterior (occipital) horn, and inferior (temporal) horn—and the interventricular foramina (Monro)—third ventricle, cerebral aqueduct (Sylvius), fourth ventricle, median aperture (Magendie), and lateral apertures (of Luschka).

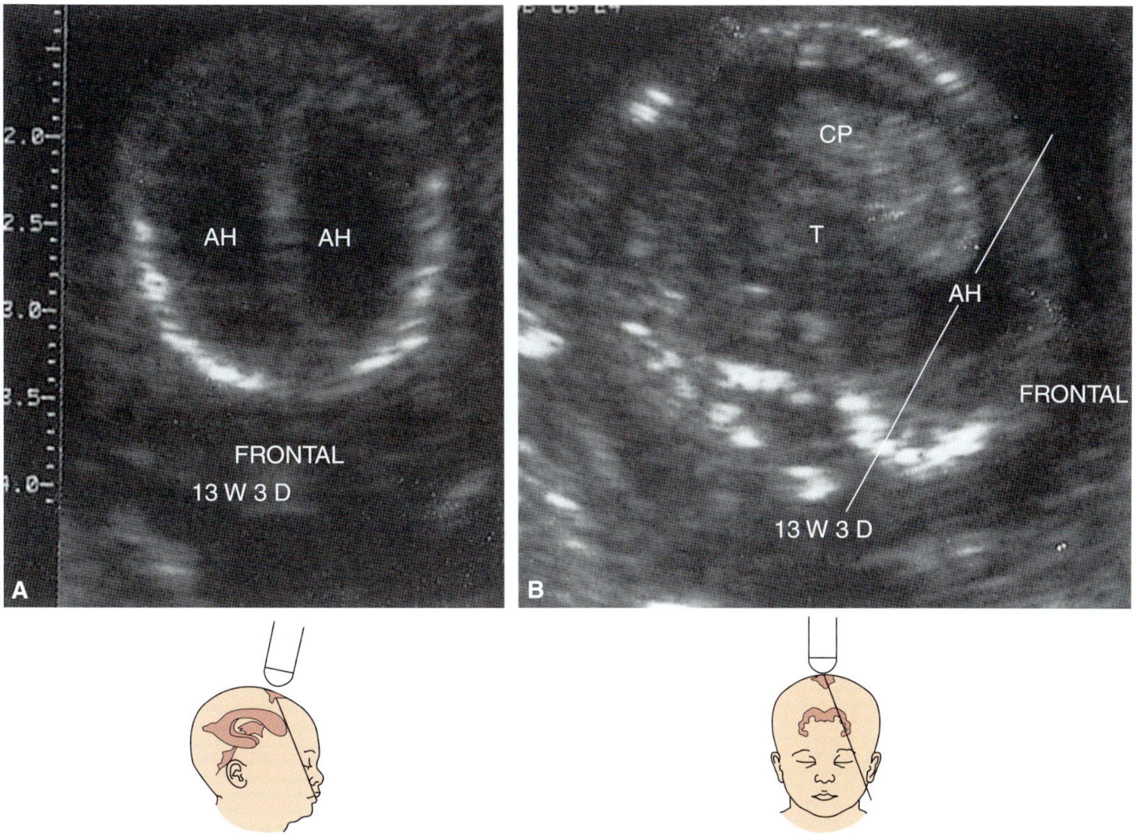


**Figure 2–36.** This image depicts the anterior part of the fetal brain at 13 weeks and 3 days from the last menstrual period. The importance of this image is to show the relatively large and sonolucent anterior horns (AH). (**A**) Frontal slightly slanted section taken at the plane shown by the white line in (**B**) Left oblique section showing the thalamus (T), on top of which the hyperechoic choroid plexus (CP) is seen. Note the ample free space, which is normal at this age.

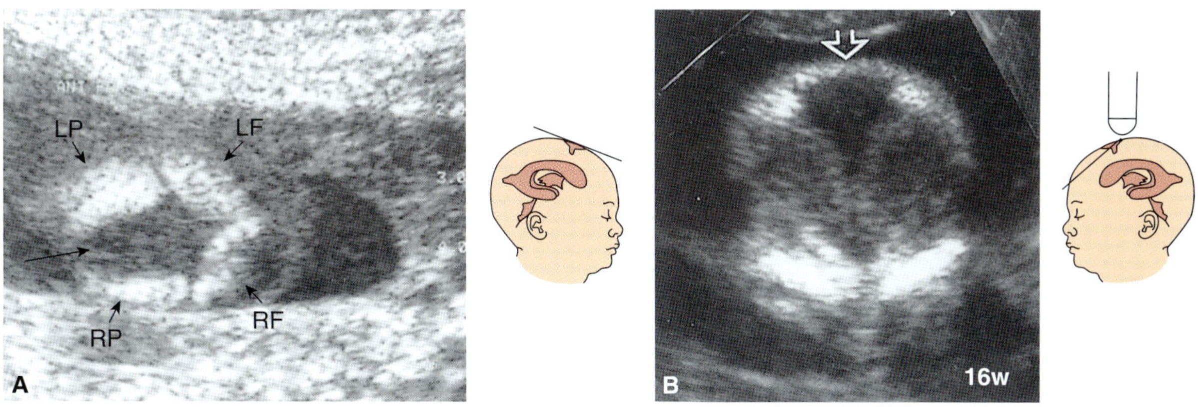


**Figure 2–37.** Images of the fetal skull bones, the fontanelles, and sutures at approximately 16 and at 20 [KT1]postmenstrual weeks. (**A**) Tangential view of the main fontanelle (arrow) through which transvaginal scanning of the fetal brain is performed (ie, the anterior fontanelle). The left and right frontal and parietal bones are also seen (LF, RF, LP, and RP, respectively). (**B**) An anterior coronal (almost tangential) section of the fetal skull showing the anterior fontanelle (arrow).

**Table 2–2. THE CORONAL PLANES**

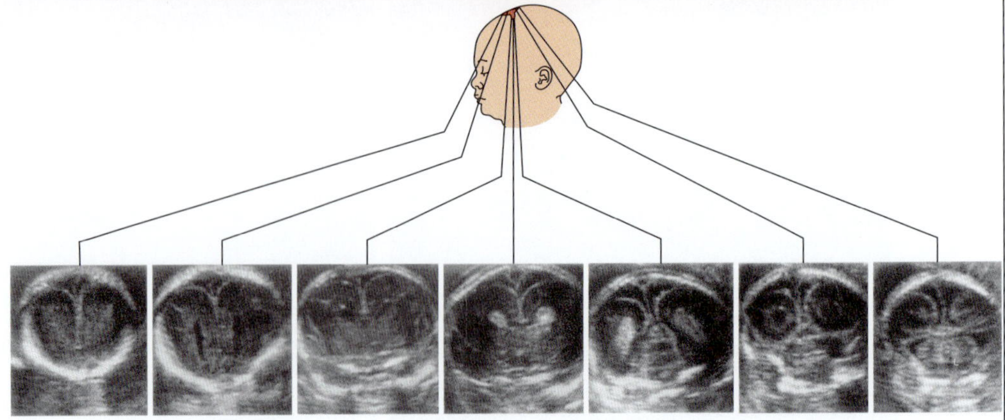

| Anatomical Structures | | FRONTAL GROUP | | MID-CORONAL GROUP | | | OCCIPITAL GROUP | |
|---|---|---|---|---|---|---|---|---|
| | | 1 | 2 | 1 | 2 | 3 | 1 | 2 |
| Skull | | | Orbit | | | | | |
| Ventricles & Connections | Lateral | Only at <16w | Ant. horn | Body | Body<br>Choroid plexus | Atrium<br>Choroid plexus | Post. horn | |
| | Intraventricular foramen | | | | With choroid plexus | | | |
| | Third | | | | (Virtual space) Tela choroidea | | | |
| Cavum septi pellucidi | | | | Cavum septi pellucidi | | | | |
| Midbrain | Corp. callosum | | | Genu | Trunk | Splenium | | |
| | Head of caudate nucleus | | | Caudate nucleus | | | | |
| | Thalamus | | | | Thalamus | | | |
| Cerebellum | Hemisphere | | | | | | Hemispheres | |
| | Vermis | | | | | | | Vermis |
| | 4th Ventricle | | | | | | 4th Ventricle (at times) | |
| Meninges | Falx | F A L X | | | | | | |
| | Tentorium | | | | | | Tentorium | |
| Cisterna magna | | | | | | | | Cisterna magna |

This table summarizes the brain structures imaged on each of the consecutive frontal, midcoronal, and occipital sections.

Reproduced Timor-Tritsch et al, 1996,[41] with permission.

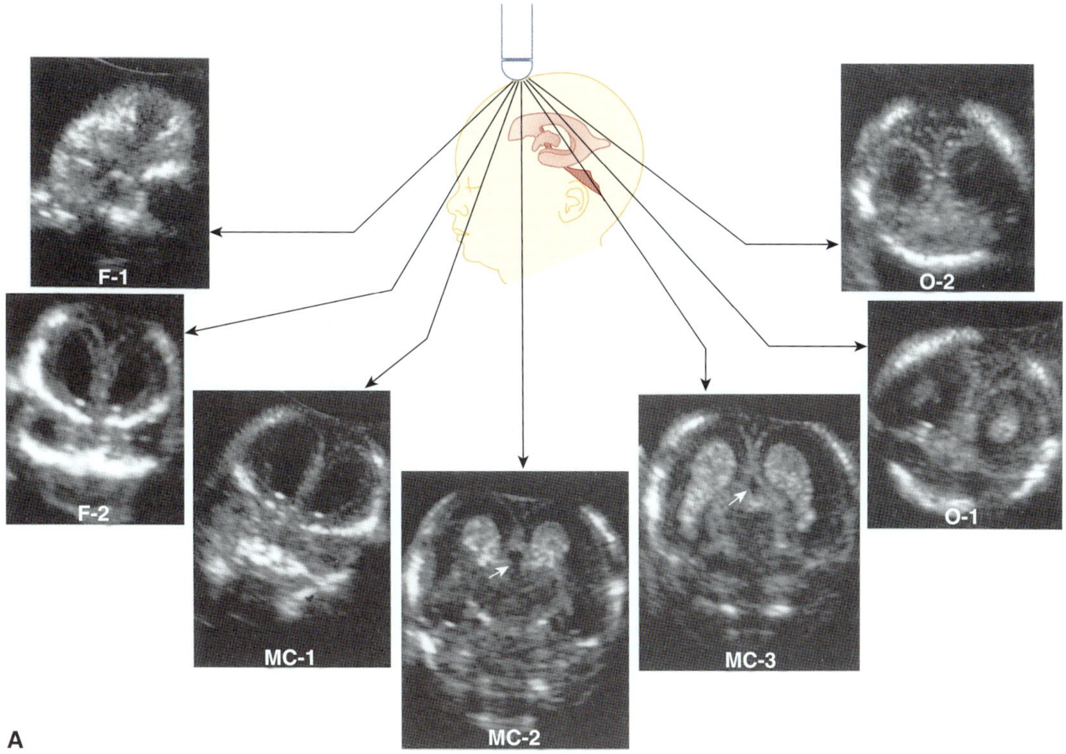


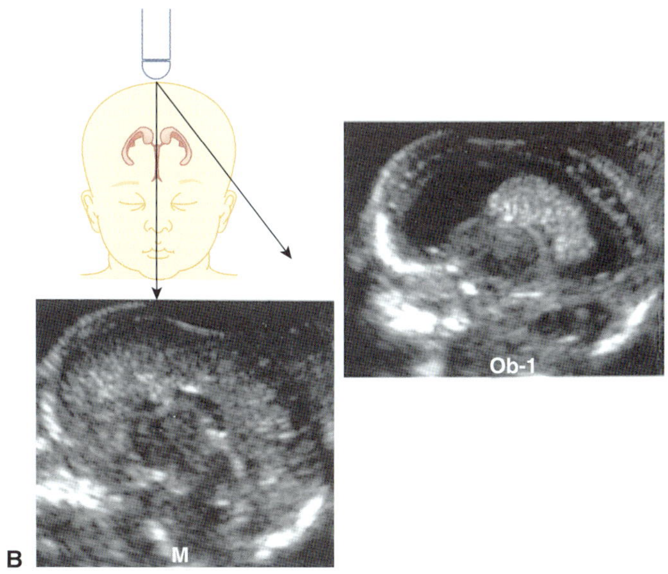


**Figure 2–38.** (**A**) Serial "coronal" sections at 16 postmenstrual weeks from frontal to occipital. Note the anterior fontanelle on F–1, the wide-open anterior horns on F–2 and on MC–1. The incipient cavum septi pellucidi (arrows) are seen on MC–2 and on MC–3. F, Frontal; MC, midcoronal; O, occipital. (**B**) The Median (M) and Oblique–1 (OB–1) sagittal sections of the same fetus at 16 postmenstrual weeks. Note that the corpus callosum is not yet developed and that the lateral ventricles are relatively large on the OB–1 section.

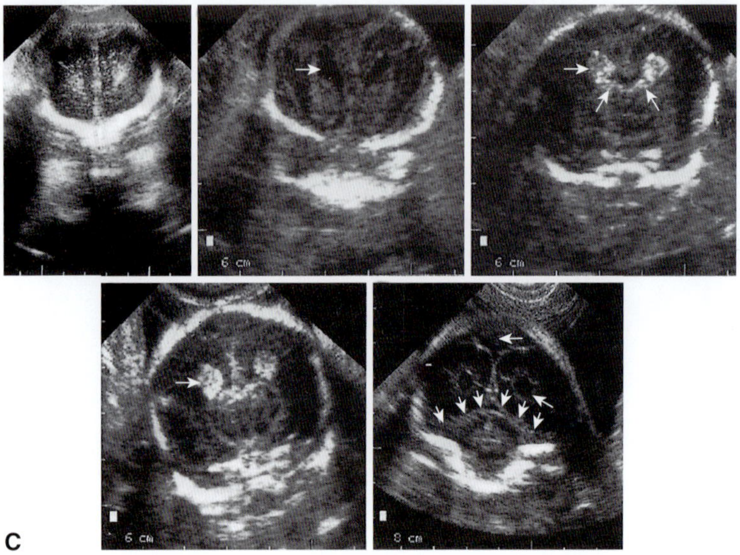

C

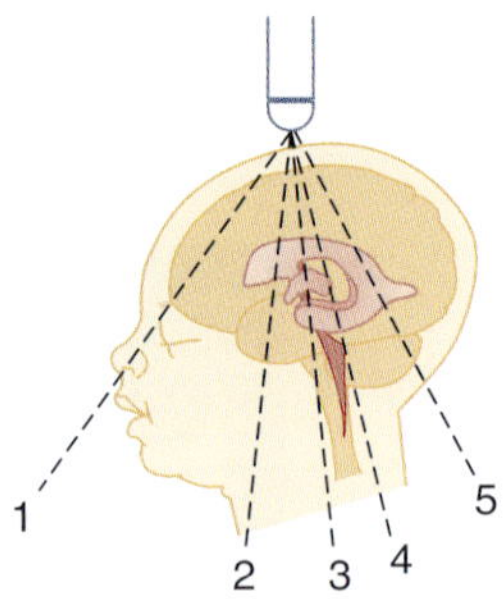


**Figure 2–38.** (*continued*) (**C**) Serial "coronal" brain sections at 18 postmenstrual weeks. (1) Frontal–1 section through the white matter. (2) Frontal–2 section through the anterior horns (AH). (3) Midcoronal–2 section through the choroid plexus (CP) and the interventricular foramina (two small arrows), and the thalamus (T). (4) Midcoronal–3 section through the choroid plexus (C) and the thalamus (T). (5) Occipital–1 section through the posterior (occipital) horn (OH). The arrows indicate the tentorium. C, Cerebellum; f, falx. (Modified from Timor-Tritsch, Monteagudo, 1991,[24] with permission.)

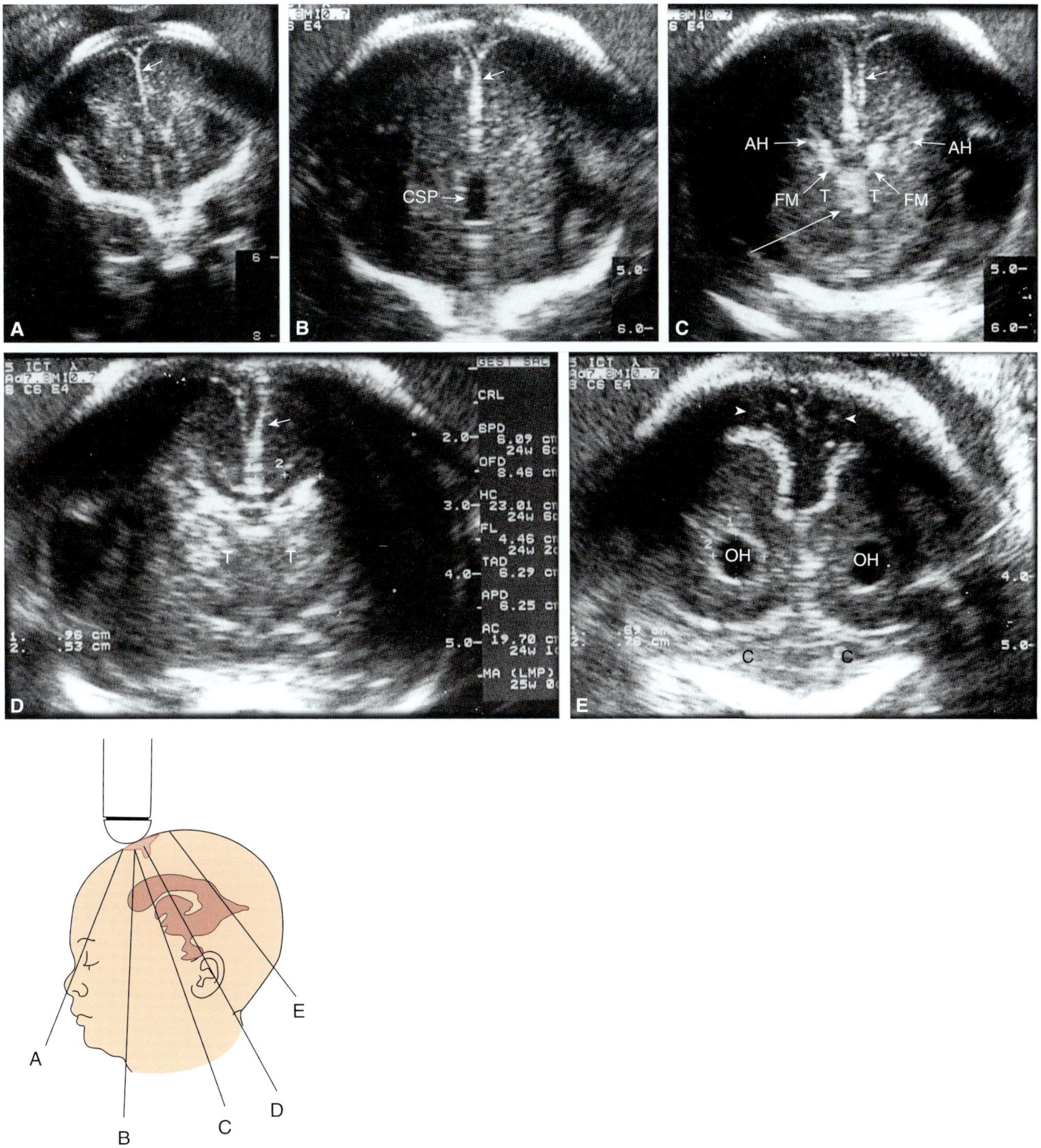


**Figure 2–39.** Serial transvaginal coronal sections at 25 postmenstrual weeks: (**A**) Frontal–1, (**B**) Frontal–2, (**C**) Midcoronal–2, (**D**) Midcoronal–3, and (**E**) Occipital–1. The longitudinal fissure is indicated by small arrows. CSP, cavum septi pellucidi; AH, anterior horn; T, thalamus; FM, interventricular foramina; OH, posterior horn; C, cerebellum. The long arrow in C indicates the choroid plexus within the third ventricle between the thalami; the arrowheads point to the subarachnoid space.

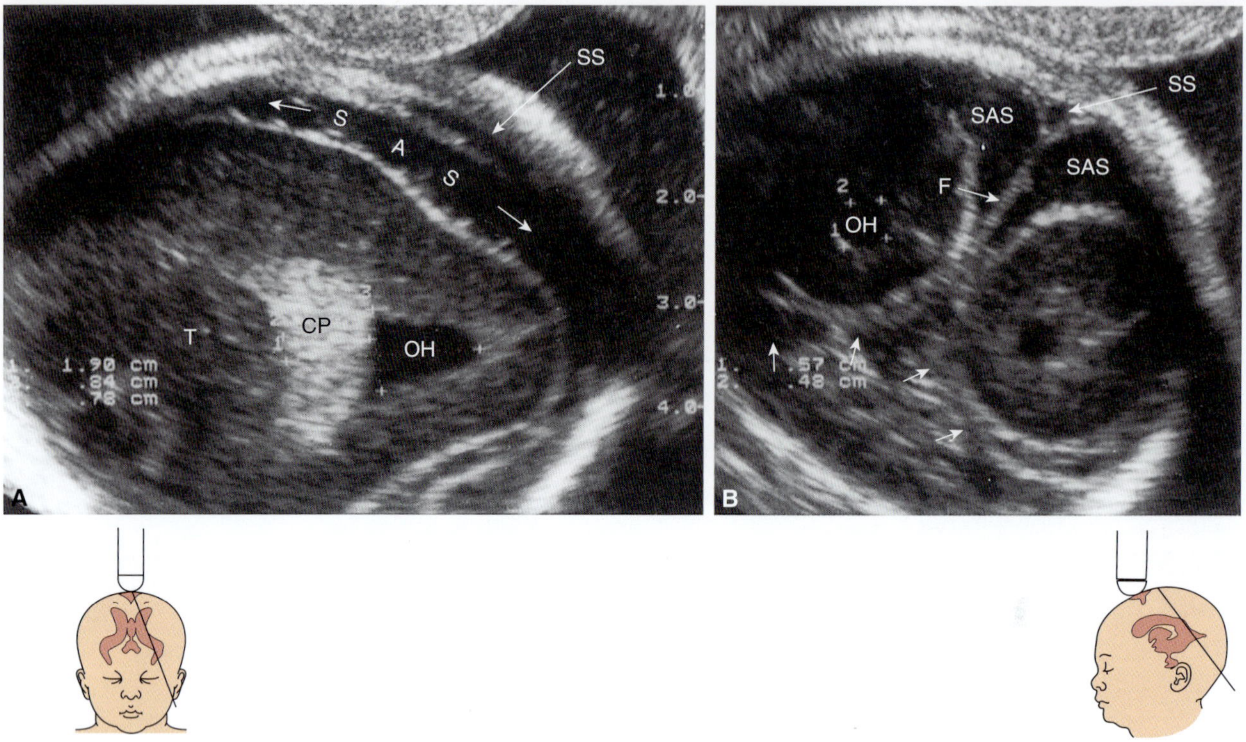


**Figure 2–40.** At 18 postmenstrual weeks, this brain was scanned in (**A**) the left Oblique–1 and (**B**) Occipital–1 planes. The conventional measurements that can be taken of the lateral ventricle and the posterior horn are shown. These measurements are within the normal range. T, Thalamus; CP, choroid plexus; OH, posterior (occipital) horn; SAS, subarachnoid space; F, falx; SS, sagittal sinus. The small arrows indicate the tentorium.

The lateral ventricles are situated in parallel fashion within both cerebral hemispheres. They have three horns (anterior, posterior, and inferior), a body, and a triangular atrium. Even though this is the correct nomenclature of the three horns of the lateral ventricles, on some images the old nomenclature (frontal, occipital, and temporal horns) may still appear. The lateral ventricles are the most obvious when ultrasonography of the fetal brain is undertaken.

The different parts of the lateral ventricles undergo extensive change in their shape and size. The lateral ventricles are at first relatively very large (Figure 1–7 in Chapter 1) and gradually become more slender during the fetal period. The posterior horn is the last to appear (Figure 1–7 in Chapter 1) and is the most variable. Examples of casts by Day[44] of fetal lateral ventricles are shown in Figure 2–50. They are from fetuses at 12, 18, and 32 weeks, respectively. It seems that they match, in general, the sonographic evaluation of the lateral ventricles performed with high-frequency transvaginal transducers. The conclusions of Day's study were (1) the posterior horn develops late in relation to the anterior and inferior horns, (2) the lateral ventricles become progressively more slender in proportion, and (3) the difference in size between homologous ventricles is not as great in the fetus as in the adult, especially in the posterior horn. As the largest of all ventricles, they were readily seen by the relatively low-frequency transabdominal probes. The diagnosis of ventriculomegaly and hydrocephaly was established by measuring the size of the body of the lateral ventricle on the axial transabdominal picture. The term *lateral ventricle–hemisphere width ratio* was coined to refer to objective measurement of ventricular size. The change in this ratio throughout normal gestation was followed up and reported.[45–53] By looking at the published graphs, it is obvious that the relative size of the lateral ventricular width decreases rapidly from ~70% at 18 postmenstrual weeks to 30% at around 28 weeks and stays constant at this level thereafter.

On an axial (horizontal) plane, the normal lateral ventricle should not measure >9 mm. The correct measurements should be taken at a place that contains the choroid plexus.[54]

One of the problems of ventricular measurements by TAS is the lack of standardization. "Obviously normal" and "clearly abnormal" lateral ventricles do not seem to require measurements. However, borderline cases would probably benefit from a quantitative determination of size. Continuous follow-up of a case with suspected ventriculomegaly would also require the values to be put on a conventional graph. There is, however, another pitfall, namely, that different authors measure distances from and to different echogenic "lines" within the head.

The last and probably most important drawback of conventional transabdominal imaging of the fetal brain is the problem of ineffective imaging of the hemisphere close to the transducer (Figure 2–51). This incomplete picture is the reason for a large number of referrals to imaging centers.

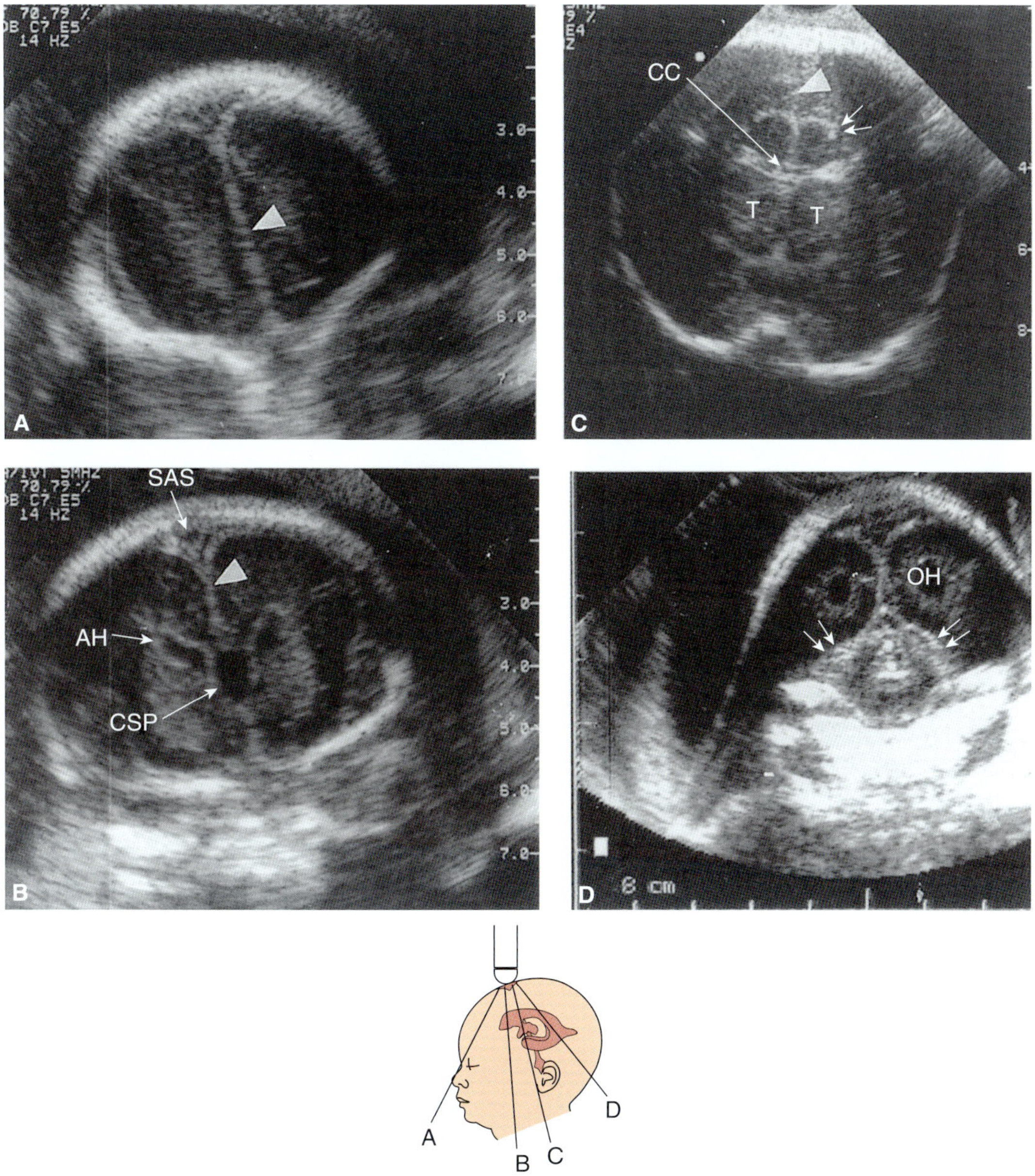


**Figure 2–41.** At 32 postmenstrual weeks: (**A**) Frontal Oblique–1, (**B**) Midcoronal–1, (**C**) Midcoronal–2, and (**D**) Occipital Oblique–1 sections are shown. Note that the longitudinal fissure (arrowheads) in C displays the branching of the cingulate gyrus (two arrows). In D, the tentorium is highlighted with small double arrows. SAS, subarachnoid space containing the superior sagittal sinus, CSP, cavum septi pellucidi; AH, anterior horn; T, Thalamus; CC, corpus callosum; OH, posterior (occipital) horn.

**Table 2–3. SUMMARY OF THE BRAIN STRUCTURES IMAGED ON EACH OF THE CONSECUTIVE MEDIAN, OBLIQUE–1, AND OBLIQUE–2 SECTIONS**

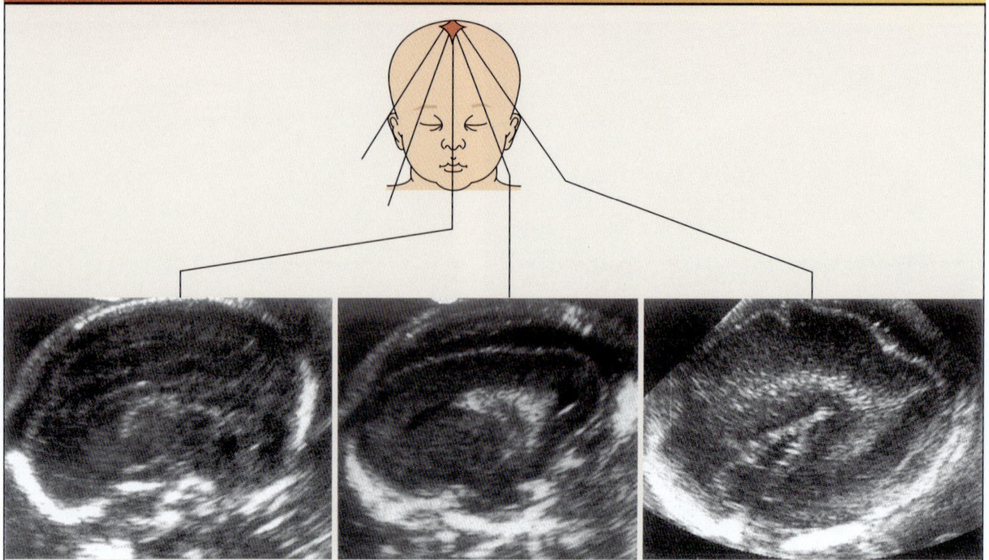

| MEDIAN | OBLIQUE-1 | OBLIQUE-2 |
|---|---|---|
| Corpus callosum | Lateral ventricle | Insula |
| Cavum septi pellucidi | Anterior horn | Parietal operculum |
| Caudate nucleus | Posterior horn | Temporal operculum |
| Thalamus | Atrium | Lateral sulcus |
| Tela choroidea | Choroid plexus | |
| Tectum | Thalami | |
| Corpora quadrigemina | | |
| Vermis | | |
| 4th ventricle | | |
| Cisterna magna | | |

From Timor-Tritsch, et al, 1996,[41] with permission.

If more sophisticated and better US machines are used (eg, compound scanning transducers) and operated by knowledgeable examiners, the transabdominal images have the capability to produce pictures of the fetal brain with a high degree of resolution (Figure 2–52).

Hertzberg and colleagues[55] questioned the validity of these echogenic "lines" mentioned above, postulating that they do not correspond to the walls of the lateral ventricles. In a more recent article, the same author suggests that for a correct measurement of the lateral ventricle on an axial view, the examiner should make "a direct attempt to find the medial wall of the ventricle."[56]

Cardoza and coworkers[48] tried to measure selectively the width of the lateral ventricular atrium according to increasing fetal age. These measurements remained relatively constant throughout gestation (Table 2–4), at a value of 7.6 ± 0.6 mm. This group suggested that atrial diameters >10 mm (>4 standard deviations) should raise suspicion of ventriculomegaly. Other graphs, tables, and nonograms to measure distances from the lateral and medial walls of the lateral ventricles are now available[57–60] (see also Chapter 5). All of these, however, still use the axial views of the head obtained by TAS. Indeed, newer equipment has helped in identifying the above-mentioned components of the lateral ventricles to serve as reproducible landmarks for the measurements. Reece and Goldstein[62] tried to standardize the axial planes obtained by TAS by introducing three successive scanning planes (levels I, II, and III) at the intersection of different intracranial brain structures. Unfortunately (as in the case of all transabdominal scanning approaches), abdominal thickness of the patient, mounting bone thickness, and low transducer frequencies will almost always yield less resolution, hence, a relatively poor fetal neuroscan as opposed to TVS of the brain. However, once the technique of transvaginal neurosonography is observed and mastered, there is no doubt that it will be increasingly used until it almost entirely replaces the transabdominal route, provided that the fetus is in the vertex presentation.[20,23,24,31,32]

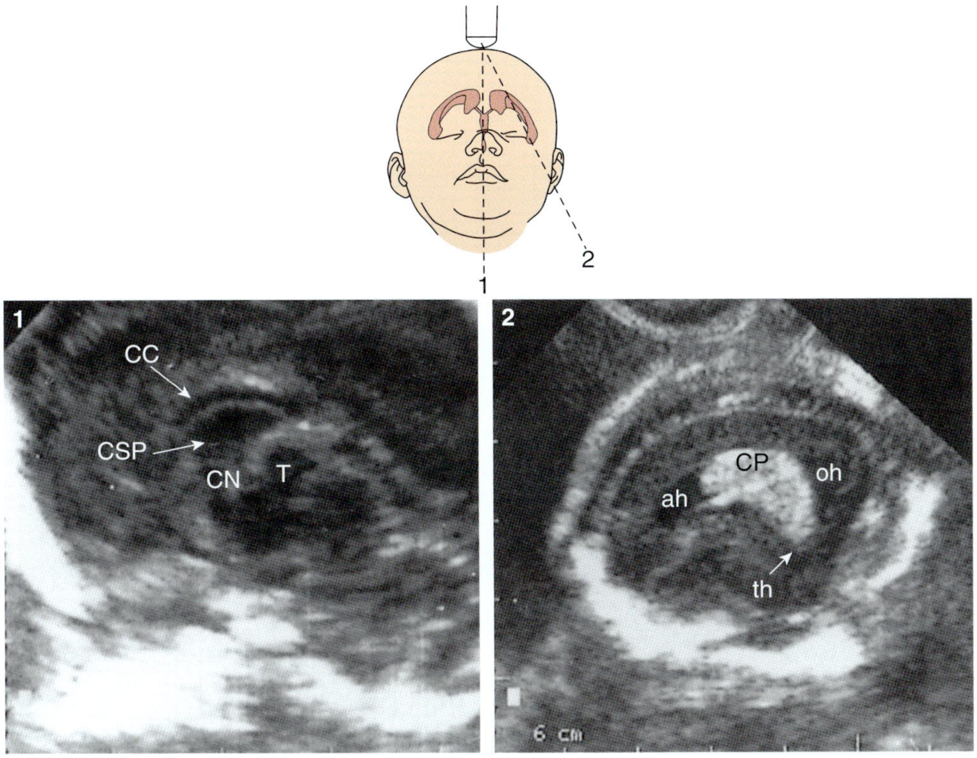


**Figure 2–42.** (1) Median and (2) left Oblique–1 sections at 18 postmenstrual weeks. CC, Corpus callosum; CSP, cavum septi pellucidi; CN, caudate nucleus; T, thalamus; ah, anterior horn; CP, choroid plexus; oh, posterior (occipital) horn; lh, lateral horn. (Modified from Timor-Tritsch and Monteagudo, 1991,[24] with permission.)

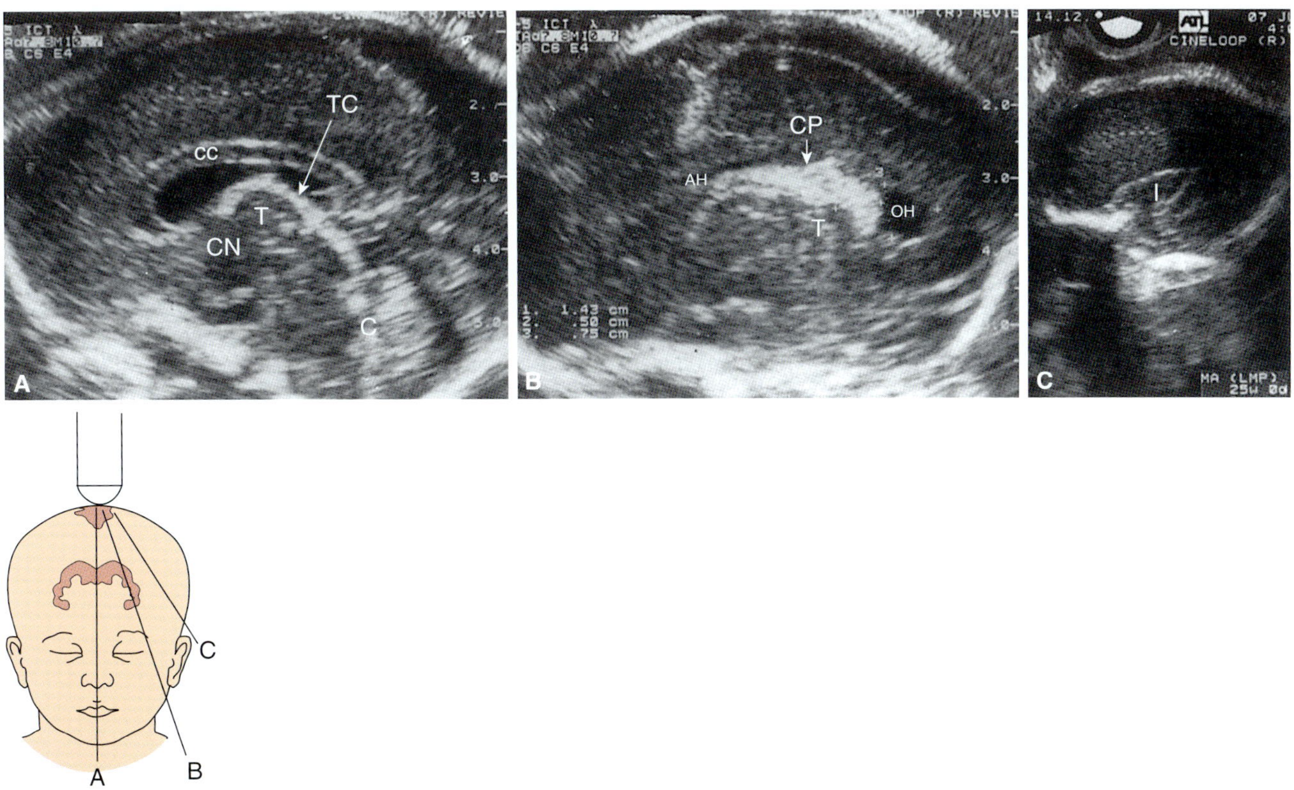


**Figure 2–43.** Serial transvaginal "sagittal" sections at 25 postmenstrual weeks. (**A**) Median section. (**B**) Left Oblique–1 section. (**C**) Left Oblique –2 and extremely lateral section through the still-gaping lateral sulcus, showing the insula. CC, corpus callosum; CN, caudate nucleus; TC, tela choroidea; T, thalamus; C, vermis of the cerebellum; C, choroid plexus; AH, anterior horn; OH, posterior horn; I, insula.

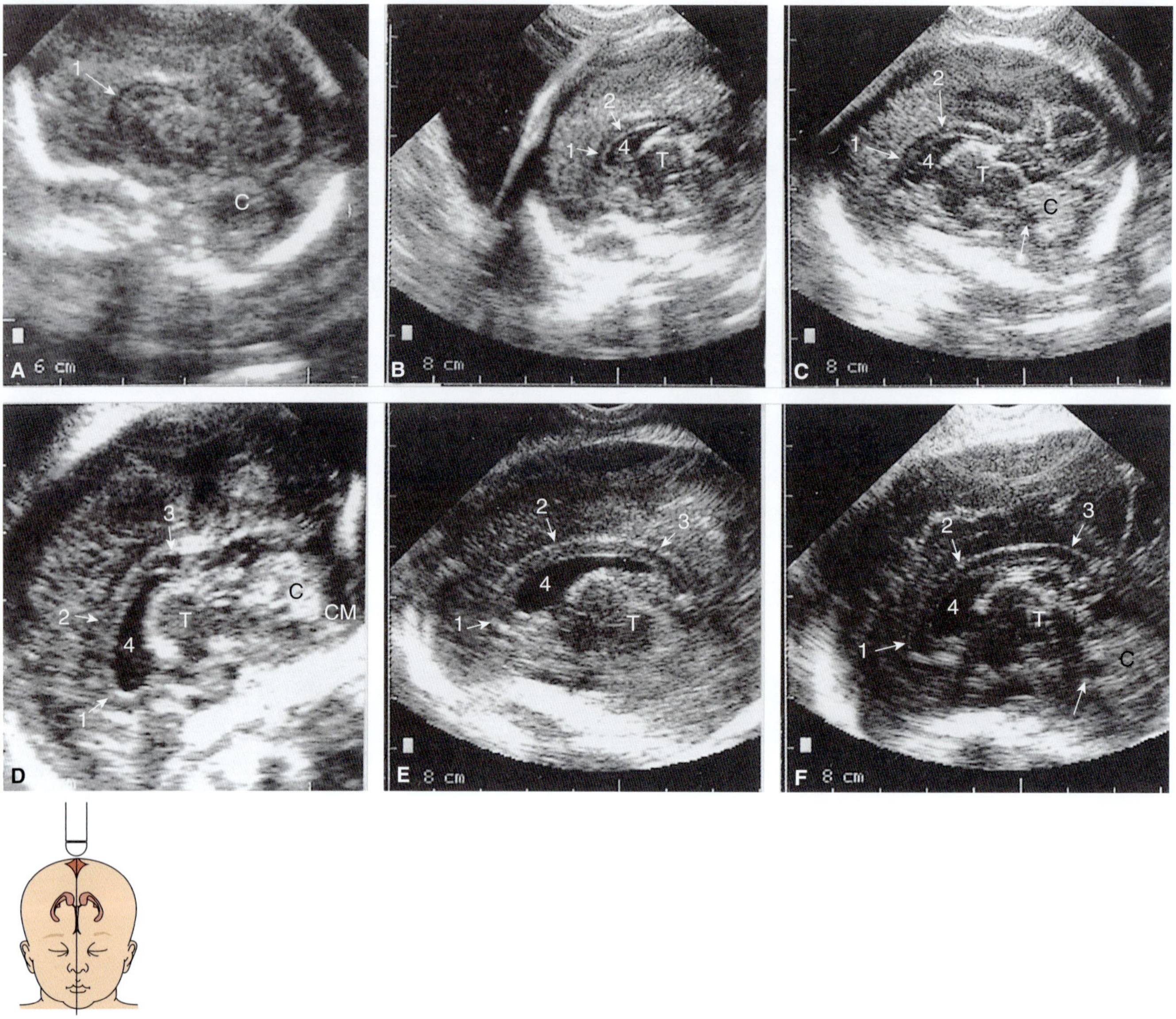


**Figure 2–44.** Transvaginal median images depicting the development of the corpus callosum at (**A**) 18, (**B**, **C**) 22, (**D**) 23, and (**E**, **F**) 28 postmenstrual weeks. C, cerebellum; 1, genu of the corpus callosum; 2, central part (trunk) of the corpus callosum; 3, splenium of the corpus callosum; 4, cavum septi pellucidi; 5, cavum Vergae; T, thalamus; CM, cisterna magna. The white arrows in C and F indicate the fourth ventricle. (Modified from Timor-Tritsch and Monteagudo, 1991,[24] with permission.)

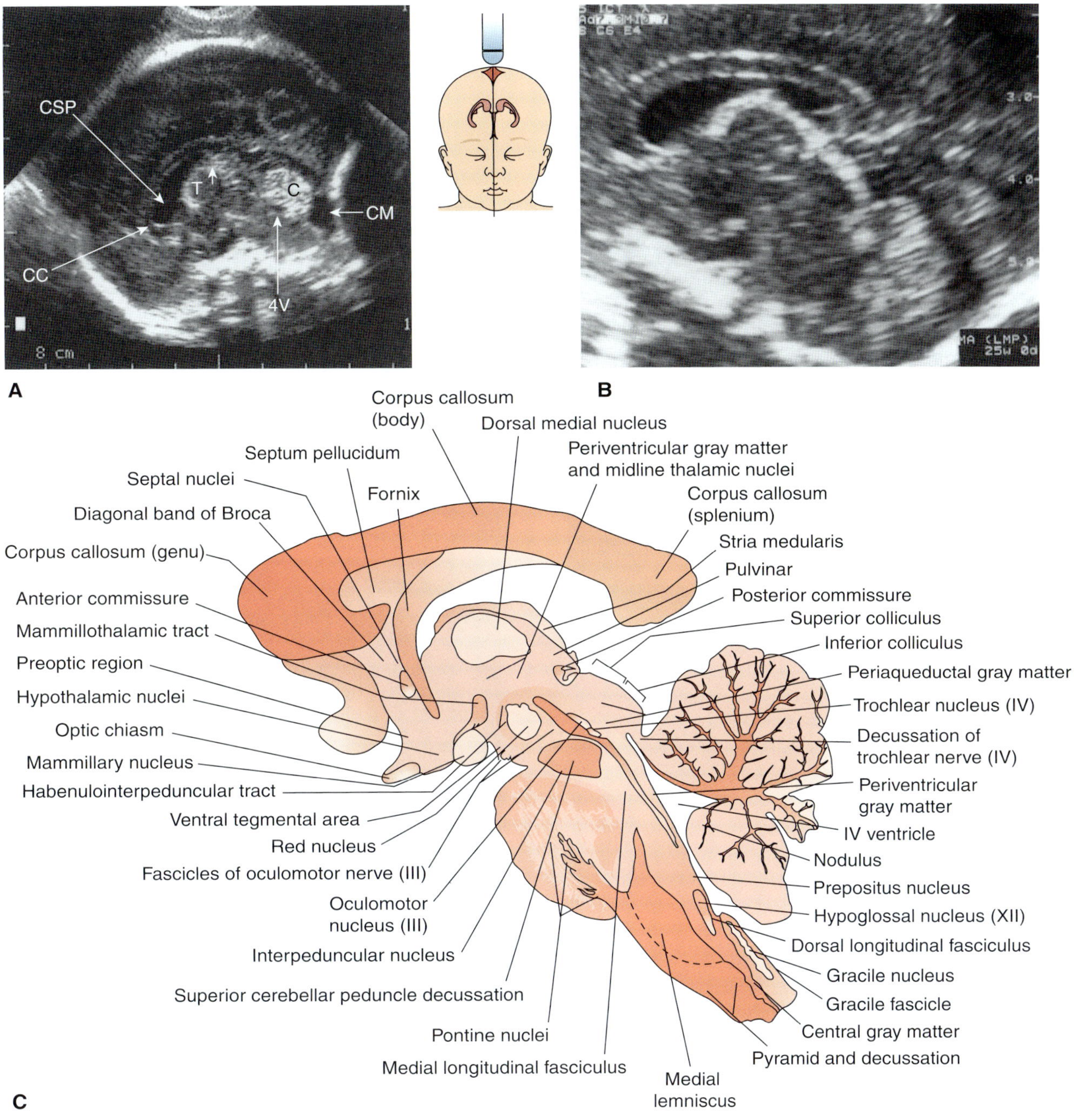


**Figure 2–45.** Sonographically identifiable central structures of the fetal brain at 25 and 28 postmenstrual weeks. (**A**) This transvaginal median section shows the fully developed corpus callosum (CC), the cavum septi pellucidi (CSP), the thalamus (T), the tela choroidea of the third ventricle (small arrow), the vermis of the cerebellum (c), the fourth ventricle (4V), and the cisterna magna (CM) at 28 postmenstrual weeks' gestation. (**B**) Focused median section of the fetal brain at 25 postmenstrual weeks. No annotations were made to identify structures. The image is presented for comparison with the drawing and properly annotated picture in C. (**C**) The anatomic structures of the midbrain. (From Martin, 2003,[61] with permission.)

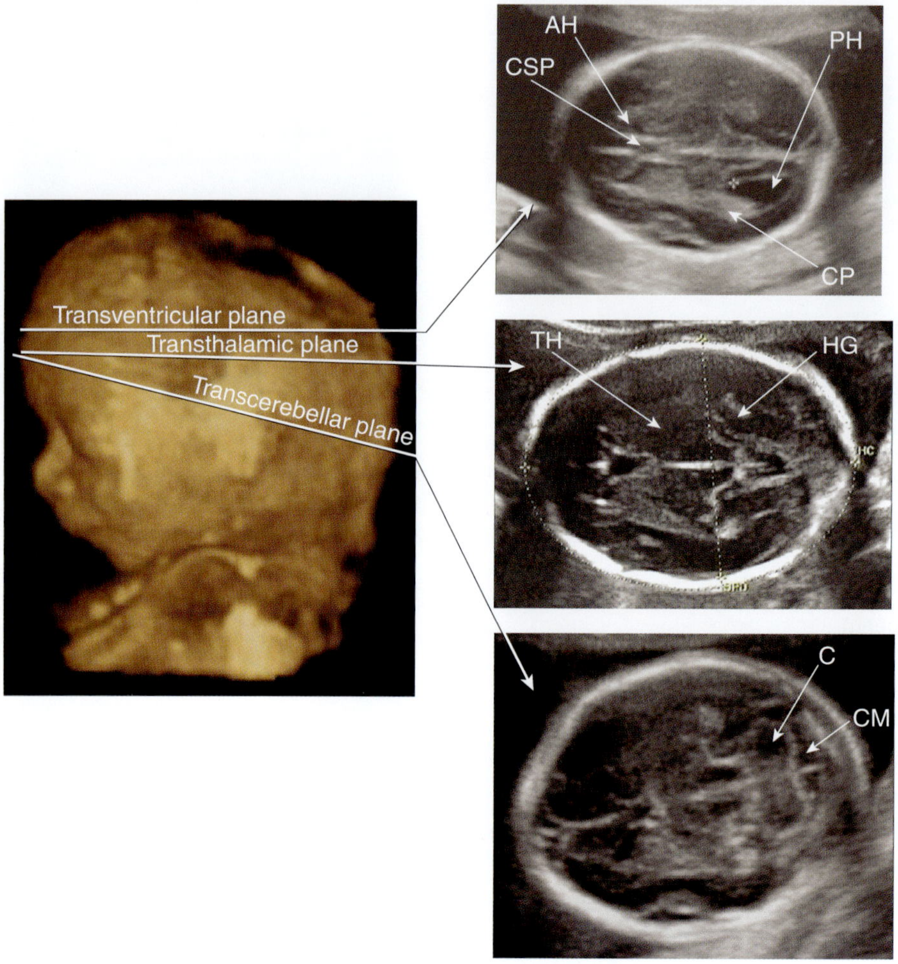


**Figure 2–46.** The basic brain scan is performed by transabdominal sonography and its objective is to evaluate the fetal brain only in the general axial (horizontal) planes. It includes three planes: transventricular, transthalamic, and trancerebellar.

At times, it may become important to perform a cephalic version of a fetus presenting with breech presentation for more accurate studies.

Measurements of the anterior horn–hemispheric width ratio were reported by Campbell in 1979.[63] This ratio decreases from 60% at week 14 to 40% at 21 postmenstrual weeks. Another ratio—that of the frontal horn to the hemispheric width—was measured by Goldstein and collaborators.[58] This ratio diminishes from 50 to 28% from 15 postmenstrual weeks to term. In addition, the size of the frontal lobe can be measured on the TAS picture. Because this measurement correlates with fetal size, it was used to detect microcephaly.[64]

The atrium of the lateral ventricles has also been the subject of numerous studies and serial measurements by various authors. Sonographically, it is easy to recognize the atrium because it contains a large part of the choroid plexus present in the lateral ventricular system. The distance, measured typically on an axial plane, is that from the falx to the lateral wall of the atrium.[59] The ratio between this distance and the hemispheric width was proposed as a sensitive indicator of abnormality. This ratio decreases from 60 to 30% from 15 postmenstrual weeks to 24 weeks.[65] From 27 postmenstrual weeks to term, the same ratio remains fairly constant, at values of 0.56 to 0.51.[48] Pilu and associates[59] suggested that the size of the atrium remains relatively constant across gestation, at about 7 ± 1.3 mm, due to the thickening of the parenchyma. According to this group, this increase in the brain mass is expressed by the slow but constantly increasing distance between the falx and the lateral atrial wall.

The posterior horn is an extremely important structure. It is considered to be the most sensitive indicator of incipient ventriculomegaly. This horn of the lateral ventricle is somewhat neglected in the literature. The reason may be that it is hard to obtain a consistently good-quality image of the posterior horn for purposes of measurement. It is interesting that in a study concentrating

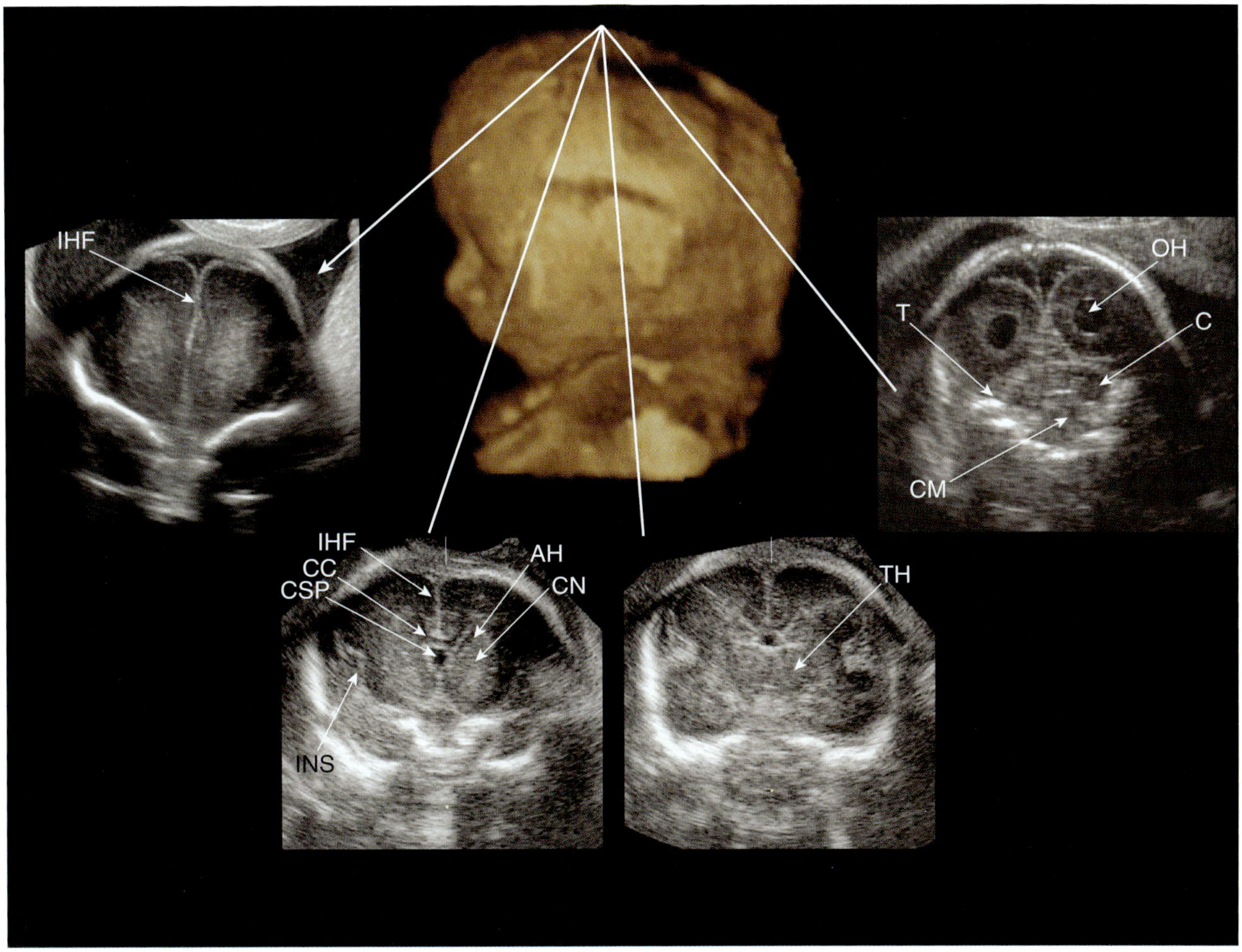


**Figure 2–47.** The targeted or more detailed fetal neurosonogram contains other planes and sections; the coronal planes are displayed in this figure.

on several measurements of the lateral cerebral ventricles to detect impending poor fetal outcome, the most significant increase in size was that of the posterior horn. However, this was not given great importance.[66] Chapter 3 discusses the importance of measuring the size of the posterior horn as well as two ratios in which the size of the posterior horn is compared with the thickness of the choroid plexus within the atria.

The inferior horn extends from the atrium into the temporal lobe. After emerging from the atrium, the horn turns slightly toward the inferior and lateral direction, ending in the center of the temporal lobe (Figure 2–49). The lateral position of this horn is less obvious before 14 to 16 postmenstrual weeks, when the oblique–1 section may include all three horns (ie, anterior, posterior, and inferior). After 16 postmenstrual weeks, the oblique-1 section "cuts" through the anterior and occipital horns but definitely does not include the inferior horn, which is slightly lateral to this plane. Based on our experience, if after 16 postmenstrual weeks all three horns are clearly imaged on the paramedian sagittal section, ventriculomegaly should be seriously considered.

The third ventricle is well imaged in the first and early second trimesters (Figures 2–21, 2–22, and 2–23). However, as gestation progresses, it becomes filled with the choroid plexus (tela choroidea) of the third ventricle and is considered a virtual space. The two contralateral thalami touch each other at the point of the interthalamic adhesion (massa intermedia). Denkhaus and Winsberg[45] claimed to be able to measure the width of the third ventricle on axial TAS images. They suggested a table that lists the width of this ventricle at 2.5 mm as a biparietal diameter of 2.3 cm, increasing to 8.2 mm at term. It is unclear from this report whether or not they saw the choroid plexus within the third ventricle. They also attributed no importance to the clinical value of a change in the size of this ventricle with respect to the diagnosis of antenatal hydrocephaly. Our observation is to the contrary; this is touched on in Chapter 4.

The fourth ventricle can easily be seen on a median plane or an axial section using the occipital approach (Figures 2–44 and 2–45).

## Foramina and the Aqueduct

A pair of narrow interventricular foramina connects the body of the lateral ventricles with the third ventricle. These tiny connections would certainly elude the

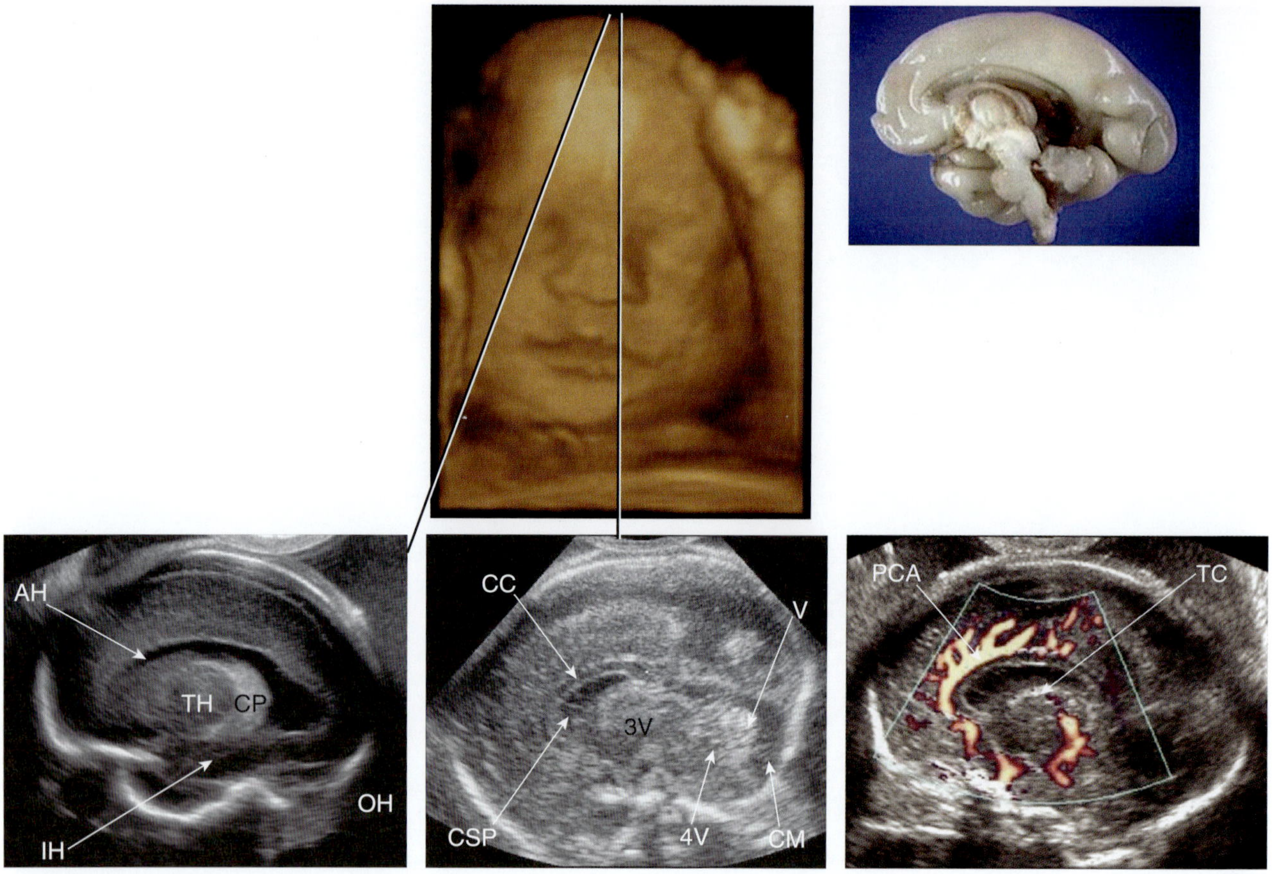


**Figure 2–48.** The targeted or more detailed fetal neurosonogram contains other planes and sections; the sagittal planes are displayed in this figure. The brain specimen supports the ultrasound image.

scanning sound waves if an extremely echogenic structure, namely, the choroid plexus, did not highlight them. These connections were reportedly detected as early as 8½ postmenstrual weeks by the Trondheim group.[29] The interventricular foramina (Monro) are clearly visible from 14 to 16 postmenstrual weeks on and mark the most typical coronal (midcoronal–2) section of the fetal brain (Figures 2–38C and 2–39C).

The cerebral aqueduct (Sylvius), the connection between the third and fourth ventricles, was not reported to be detected by ultrasonography of the normal fetal brain. This may soon change using 3D imaging when a special plane to detect and study this extremely thin structure can be created by the multiplanar capability of this technique.

Using a posterior (occipital) axial or median approach, the median aperture (Magendie) can be seen (Figure 2–44). This aperture is wide open before 16 postmenstrual weeks and is more easily detected before 20 postmenstrual weeks than after. This aperture becomes wide open in cases of abnormal dilations of the cerebellomedullary cistern (the cisterna magna) and the fourth ventricle (see Chapter 4).

## Choroid Plexuses

An integral part of the ventricular system is a complex tissue dedicated to the production of cerebrospinal fluid (CSF): the choroid plexuses. These structures are found in all lateral ventricles.

The choroid plexuses consist of villi in large numbers, the outer (ventricular) surface of which is covered by a single-layered, modified cuboidal epithelium (ependyma). The inner layer is a stromal core derived from the pia. The capillaries found in each of these villi are the major source of CSF production.

Embryologically, the choroid plexuses develop from the anteriorly located ventricles, more precisely, from their medial and upper wall. The stroma and the covering pia are derived from the mesenchyme. Even though the choroid plexuses are present from 6 to 7 postmenstrual weeks on, it takes several weeks until it becomes large and echogenic enough to be detected by a high-frequency transvaginal probe. At 8 to 8½ postmenstrual weeks, it is small in size and already significantly echogenic (Figure 2–18). Starting from the ninth postmenstrual week, it is consistently seen on the two sides of the falx within the lateral ventricles. It can be said that it is the most striking sonographic intracranial structure well beyond the end of the first trimester. At 9 to 11 postmenstrual weeks, the choroid plexuses fill both lateral ventricles (Figures 2–21, and 2–23). As pregnancy progresses, their relative size compared with the lateral ventricular size decreases. They "move" posteriorly and assume their permanent anatomical site within the atrium, "hugging" the thalami

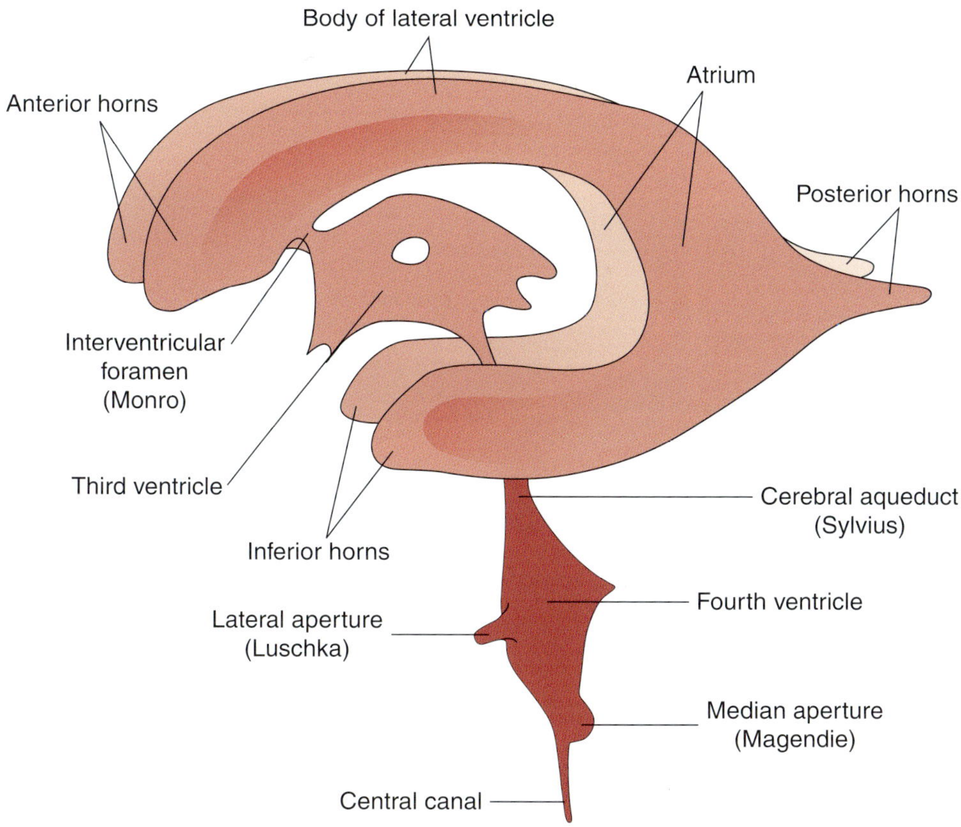


**Figure 2–49.** The ventricular system of the brain, seen from the left side.

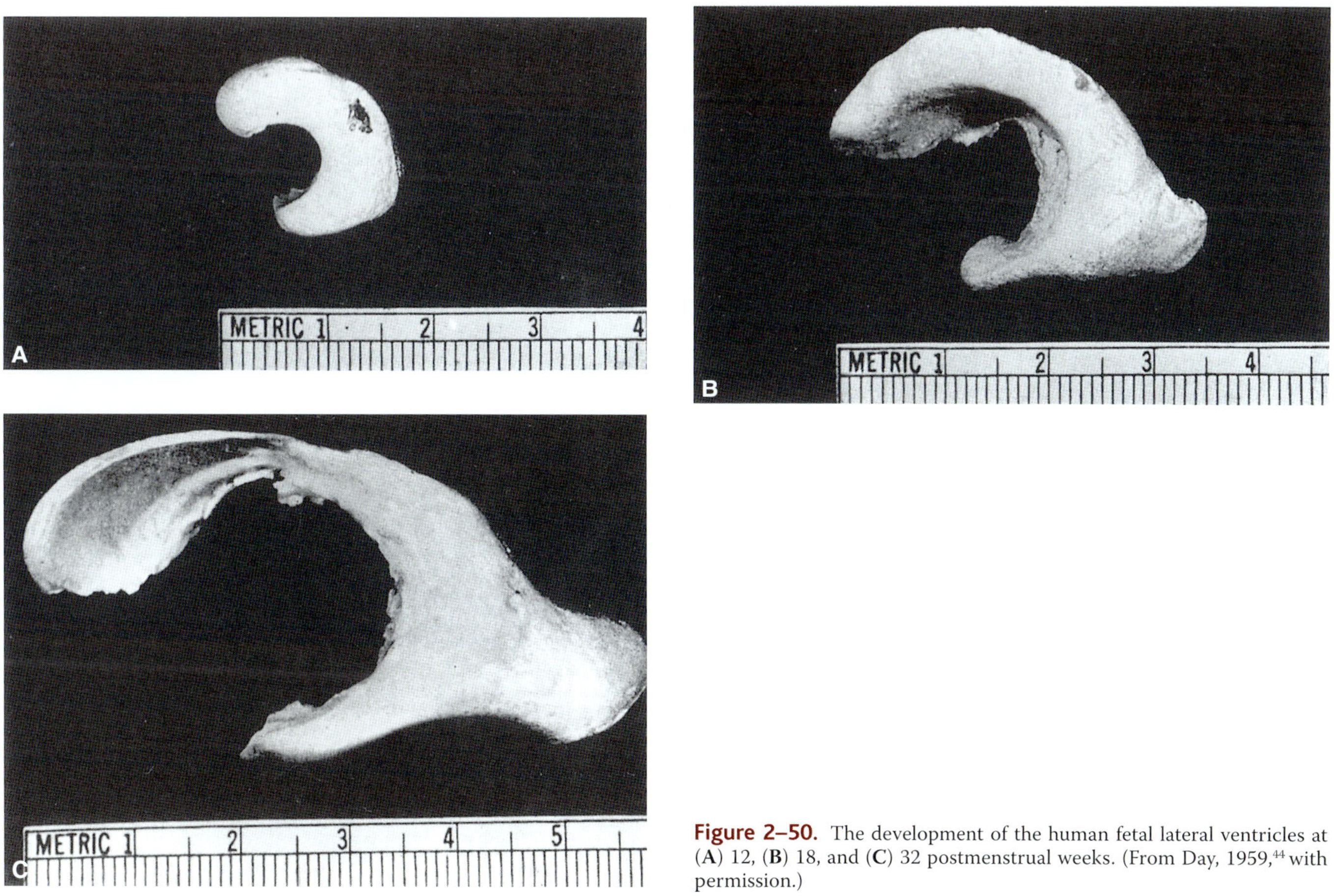


**Figure 2–50.** The development of the human fetal lateral ventricles at (**A**) 12, (**B**) 18, and (**C**) 32 postmenstrual weeks. (From Day, 1959,[44] with permission.)

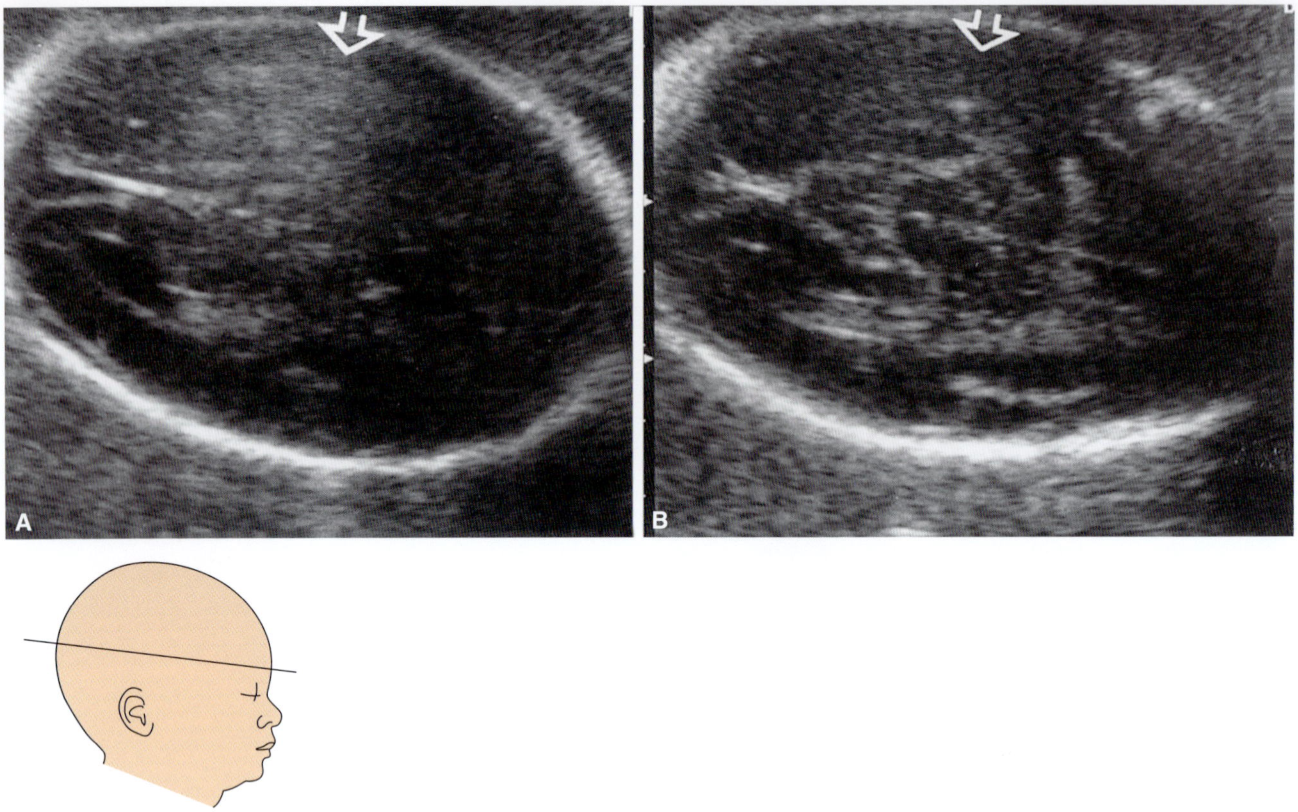


**Figure 2–51.** (**A**, **B**) Two axial sections of the brain at 26 postmenstrual weeks, showing the obscured near field due to ineffective transabdominal imaging of the hemisphere close to the transducer (open arrows).

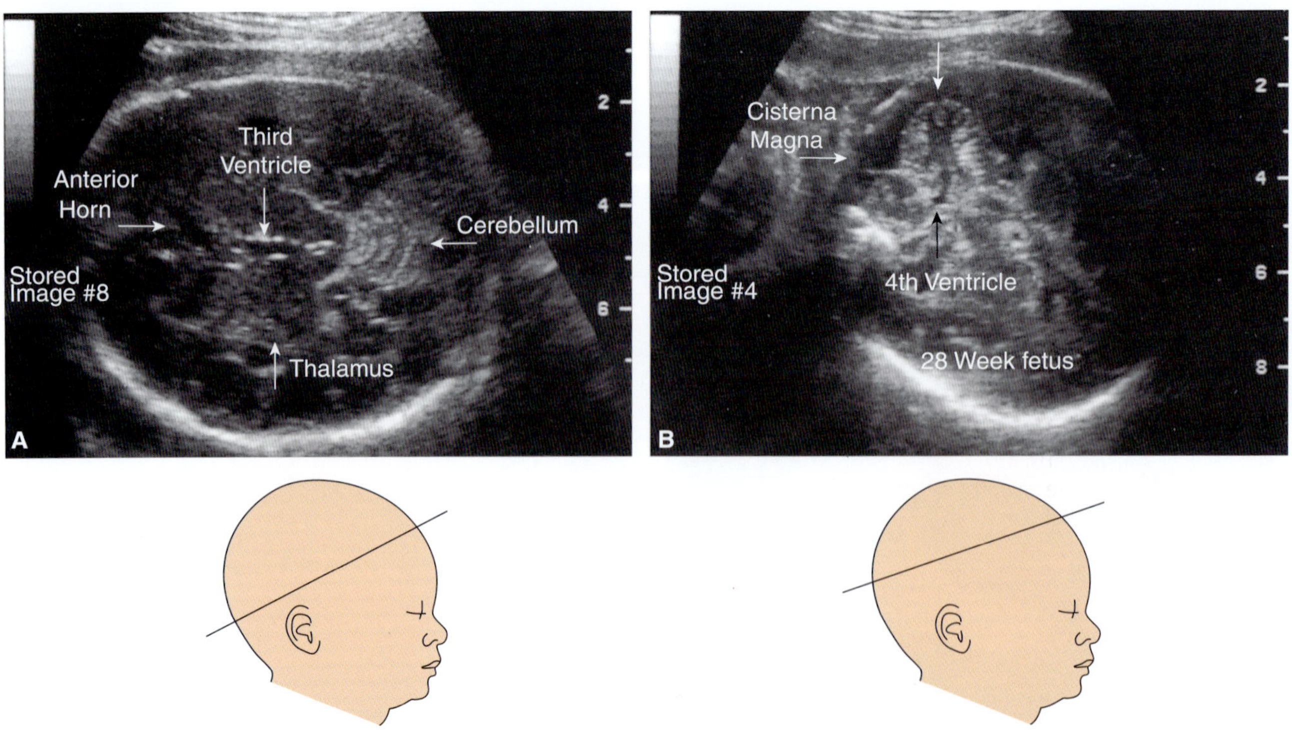


**Figure 2–52.** The more advanced technology of the transabdominal transducer allows visualization of very fine detail of the cerebellum as well as the fourth and third ventricles at 28 postmenstrual weeks. **A** and **B** axial sections tilted slightly backward.

**Table 2–4. DIAMETER OF THE NORMAL LATERAL VENTRICULAR ATRIUM AS A FUNCTION OF POSTMENSTRUAL AGE**

| Postmenstrual Weeks | Mean ± SD (mm) | Range (mm) |
|---|---|---|
| 14–20 | 7.6 ± 0.7 | 6.0–9.0 |
| 21–25 | 7.7 ± 0.5 | 7.0–9.0 |
| 26–30 | 7.5 ± 0.7 | 6.5–9.0 |
| 31–38 | 7.6 ± 0.5 | 7.0–8.5 |

Modified from Cardoza and colleagues, 1988,[51] with permission.

from posterior and above (Figure 2–35). Their posterior contour is smooth. If they lose their regular contour, one should suspect an adjacent intraventricular hemorrhage. An obviously thin or dangling choroid plexus should arouse suspicion of ventriculomegaly or hydrocephaly. The tela choroidea is the thin choroid plexus layer covering the thalami, extending into the third ventricle (Figures 2–39C and 2–43). The choroid plexus of the fourth ventricle is extremely difficult to image. Therefore, to our knowledge, it is not mentioned in the pertinent literature.

It should be emphasized that the choroid plexus may give rise to tumors, such as choroid plexus papilloma and carcinoma.

## THE CAVA

The cavum septi pellucidi and its posterior part, the cavum Vergae, are not strictly part of the ventricular system; if found at autopsies of infants and adults, they are generally considered insignificant. The cavum septi pellucidi and the cavum Vergae are, in fact, the same structure, the former located anteriorly and the latter positioned posteriorly to a vertical plane formed by the columns of the fornix. The two usually communicate with each other (Figure 2–53A and B). The presence or absence of the cavum septi pellucidi as a function of age was studied by Shaw and Alvord.[67] Dissecting the brains of 374 normal subjects, they found that 100% of the premature infants had a cavum septi pellucidi wider than 1 mm. The cavum Vergae closes first, well before term, and the cavum septi pellucidi starts to close just before term. Table 2–5 also shows that at 6 months of age only 12% of the brains had a recognizable cavum. This group did not report on the age of the premature infants.

Jou et al[68] measured the width of the cavum septi pellucidi from 19 to 42 weeks in 608 fetuses. They found that this measurement increased gradually to 27 weeks when it plateaued until term.

Larroche and Bandey[69] noted that the cavum Vergae is typically absent at birth. This was observed following pneumoencephalographic studies in neonates.

The cava forms simultaneously with the corpus callosum. The appearance of the cava on ultrasonographic images is also limited to the first detection of the corpus callosum, that is, about 17 to 18 postmenstrual weeks. At term these spaces become almost obliterated.

Even though it will be discussed in detail later in this chapter when we describe the arteries of the brain, we have to mention here the pericallosal artery. This artery closely follows the corpus callosum. As a matter of fact, three structures and their development are closely interrelated: the corpus callosum; above it, the pericallosal artery; and below it, the cavum septi pellucidi. This parallel development becomes important when deviant development of the corpus callosum is discussed.

The cavum septi pellucidi is best imaged on the median (Figures 2–42, 2–43, 2–44, 2–45) and the midcoronal–1 and –2 (Figures 2–39 and 2–41B) sections. Two lateral walls separate this structure from the anterior horns of the lateral ventricles (Figure 2–41B). Failing to detect these lateral walls should arouse suspicion of disease, such as agenesis of the corpus callosum, septo-optic dysplasia, schizencephaly, hydrocephaly, and porencephaly.[70]

### Corpus Callosum

The corpus callosum is one of the important structures of the brain, connecting the right and left hemispheres. In fact, it is the largest interconnecting structure and consists of myelin-coated nerve fibers that cross the median plane. It forms the roof of the cavum septi pellucidi and the cavum Vergae. The development of these structures (ie, the corpus callosum and the cava) is closely linked. Because the roof of the cavum septi pellucidi is the corpus callosum itself, it is clear that if there is no roof, there is no cavum.

If the corpus callosum is scanned through the anterior fontanelle, the sound waves meet this structure at almost a right angle. The sonographic picture in the median plane of the developed corpus callosum is that of two parallel echogenic lines with a sonolucent strip of ~3 to 5 mm between them. The upper line is generated by the deepest points of the longitudinal fissure. The lower echogenic line is the roof of the cavum septi pellucidi and the cavum Vergae. The pericallosal artery closely follows the upper boundary of the corpus callosum. The midcoronal–1 and –2 sections depict this commissural structure as semilunar.

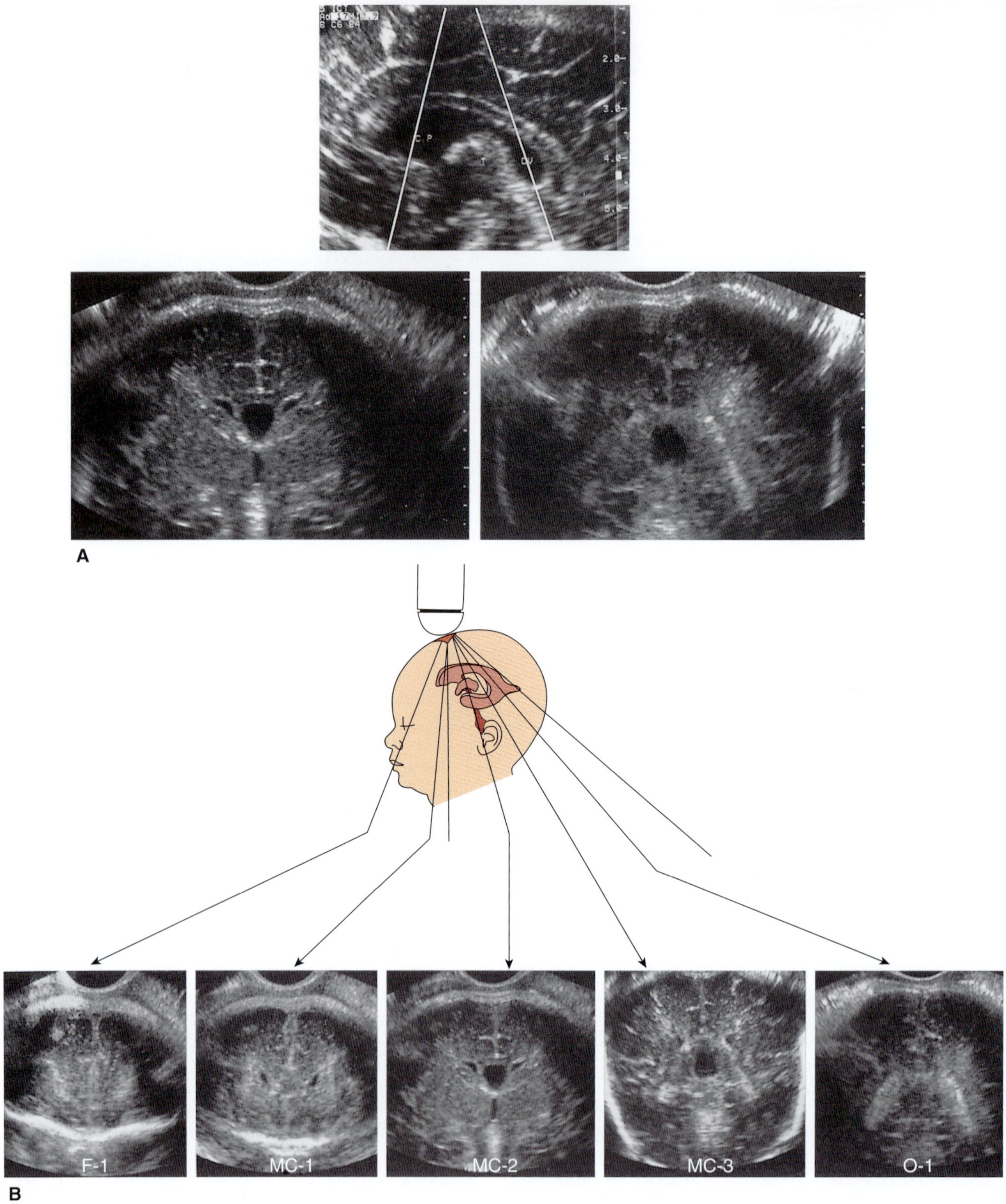


**Figure 2–53.** The cavum Vergae in the brain of this normal 28-week old fetus is the posterior part of the cavum septi pellucidi. (**A**) The two lower images were generated along the white lines seen on the median plane. The anterior section "cuts" through the cavum septi pellucidi (CP). The posterior coronal section highlights the cavum Vergae (CV). (**B**) The systematic scanning using the transfontanelle approach reveals the normal cavum septi pellucidi on the MC–2 plane and the still open cavum Vergae on the MC–3 plane. This study uses the sequential "coronal" planes.

**Table 2–5. INCIDENCE OF OPEN CAVUM SEPTI PELLUCIDI AS A FUNCTION OF AGE**

| Age | Percentage Present |
|---|---|
| Premature | 100 |
| Full term to 7 days | 97 |
| 8 days to 1 month | 85 |
| 6 month to 16 years | 12 |

Modified from Shaw and Alvord, 1969,[67] with permission.

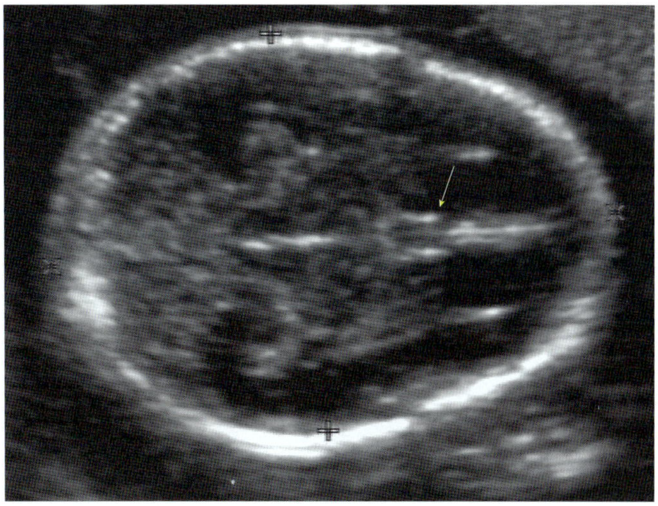

**Figure 2–54.** The columns of the fornix (arrow) appear as parallel echogenic lines in the "BPD plane" but slightly inferior.

After understanding the anatomy and the sonographic presentation of the corpus callosum in the various scanning planes, its development should be discussed. The corpus callosum is a relatively late-developing structure reported to develop between the 12th and 18th postmenstrual weeks.[71,72] It is also known that it develops in an anterior-to-posterior direction,[69] but this development can be followed sonographically.[20,24,72–74] (See Chapter 1.)

In Figure 2–35, which represent coronal and sagittal sections of fetuses at 14 postmenstrual weeks, it is not yet possible to discern the corpus callosum. At 16 postmenstrual weeks, the first hint of its sonographic appearance is present (Figure 2–38). At 18 postmenstrual weeks (Figures 2–38 and 2–42), the anterior portion of the genu and almost all of the central part are seen. Figure 2–44 depicts images of the corpus callosum from 18 to 28 postmenstrual weeks.

At 22 to 23 postmenstrual weeks, the median section shows the totally formed corpus callosum (Figure 2–45). This structure has four parts, from anterior to posterior: the rostrum, the genu (knee), the trunk, and the splenium (see Figure 2–45C).

The importance of knowing this pattern is because, at times and for various reasons, the development of the corpus callosum is incomplete.[72,73,75] Such a partial agenesis of the corpus callosum appears on the sonographic image as if it had been "caught" at an early stage of development. The lack of development of this structure is discussed in Chapter 5.

Normative measurements of the length as well as the thickness of the corpus callosum were published.[76]

We have to mention here that on some of axial sections there is a structure that can be mistaken for the cavum septi pellucidi. These structures are the columns of the fornix (Figure 2–54). These are seen as parallel echogenic lines that appear if the BPD plane is slightly shifted (in a parallel fashion) toward the base of the skull. In a retrospective study of 20 consecutive sonograms on pregnant patients between 18 and 24 postmenstrual weeks, the columns of the fornix could be identified in all fetuses. To mistake the columns of the fornix in a case of agenesis of the corpus callosum may lead to misdiagnosis of this entity.[77]

## Subarachnoid Spaces and Cisterns

In scanning the normal fetal brain, spaces of different shapes and sizes can be seen between the cortex and the bony skull or between structures of the brain itself. Fine cords of the arachnoid, delicate blood vessels, and probably arachnoid granulations produce a variety of echoes within this space (Figures 2–39B–E, 2–55, and 2–56). Figures 2–55 and 2–56 show an ultrasonographic image and a drawing of the subarachnoid space.

Early in pregnancy, it is rare to detect subarachnoid spaces. However, around 14 to 16 postmenstrual weeks, they can be revealed using high-frequency TVS (Figures 2–40, 2–55, and 2–57). The relative sizes of these spaces decrease as pregnancy advances. In a study by Laing and colleagues,[78] 122 fetuses from 21 to 40 postmenstrual weeks were scanned transabdominally. A subdural space was sought on a transaxial scan. Eighty-three percent of the fetuses with this subdural space were less than 30 postmenstrual weeks, whereas 77% lacking this sign were older than 30 weeks. All of the fetuses were normal at birth. These investigators concluded that if a wide subarachnoid space is seen in late pregnancy, it should be investigated following birth, as a prominent space may predispose a neonate to subdural hematoma.[79]

It is possible that Laing's group[78] studied the space immediately adjacent to the lateral sulcus (of Sylvius). This fluid-filled space was also studied by Jeanty and collaborators.[80] The latter came to the conclusion that the structure (ie, the cortex) below the internal table of the bone overlapping this area in which the pulsations of the middle cerebral artery is seen should be termed the *insula* and not the *sylvian fissure*. Such an area is shown in Figure 2–58.

The subarachnoid space overlying the insula is also shown in the subsection dealing with the sulci, fissures, and gyri in this chapter.

It is worth discussing the echoes appearing within the subarachnoid space seen in Figure 2–55. These may be

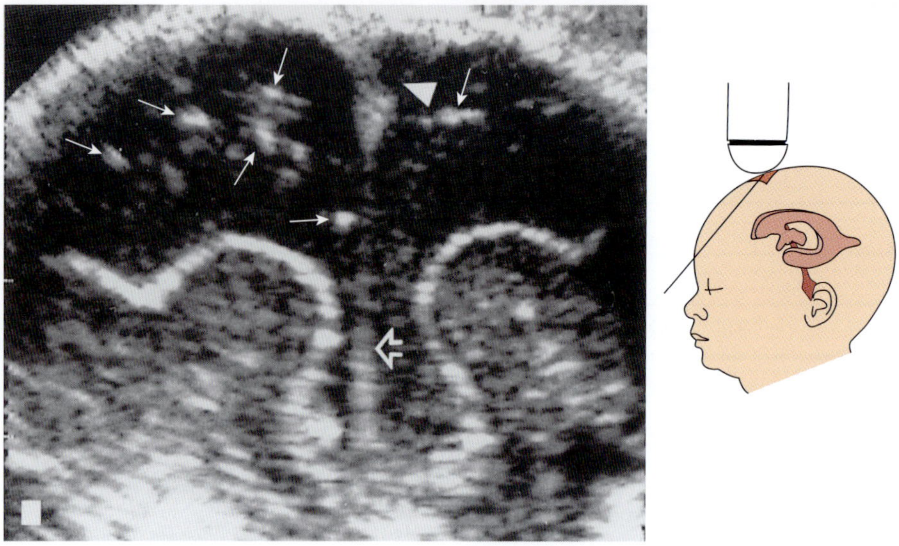

**Figure 2–55.** The subarachnoid space is shown on this Frontal–1 section. The small arrows indicate the hyperechoic structures thought to represent cross-sections of blood vessels or arachnoid granulations in the subarachnoid space. The open arrow indicates the falx; the arrowhead marks the sagittal sinus.

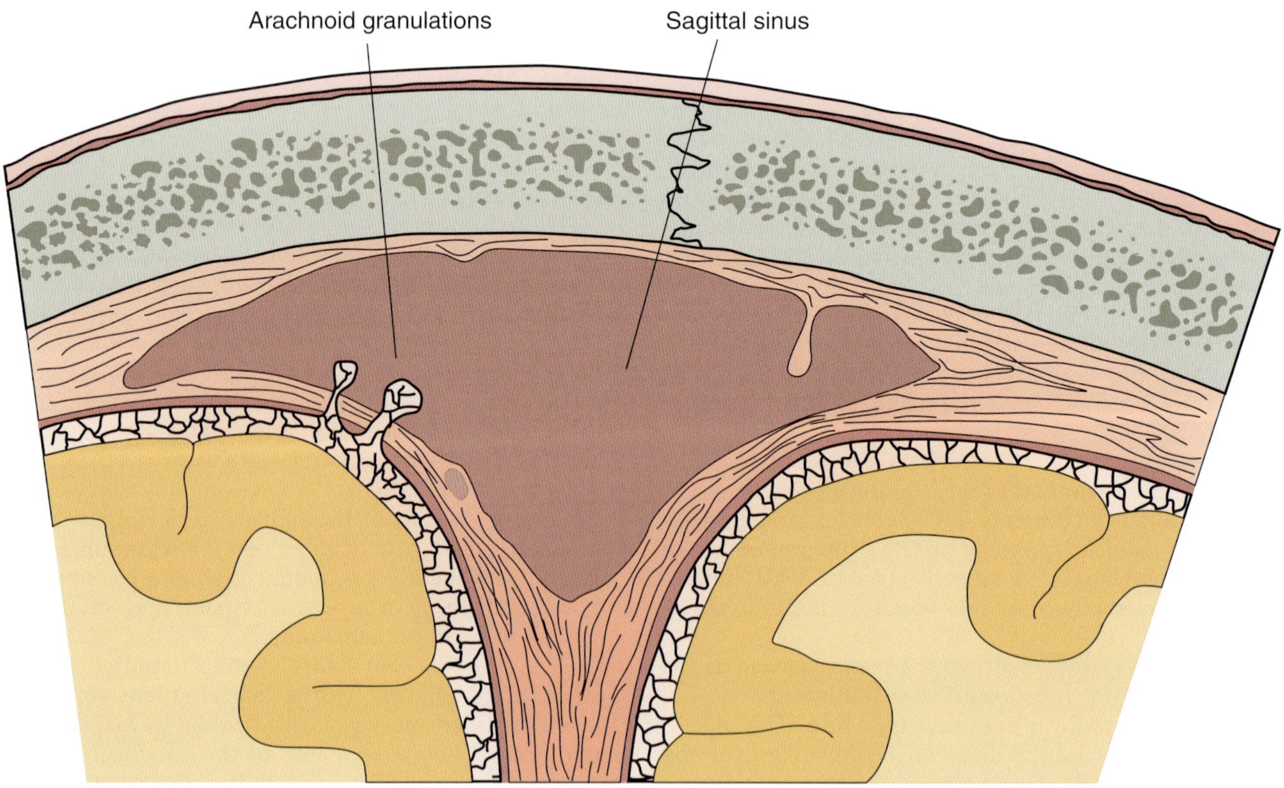


**Figure 2–56.** Schematic drawing of a similar section depicted in Figure 2–55, showing the subarachnoid space and the arachnoid granulations bulging into the areas supplied by blood and which drain the cerebrospinal fluid.

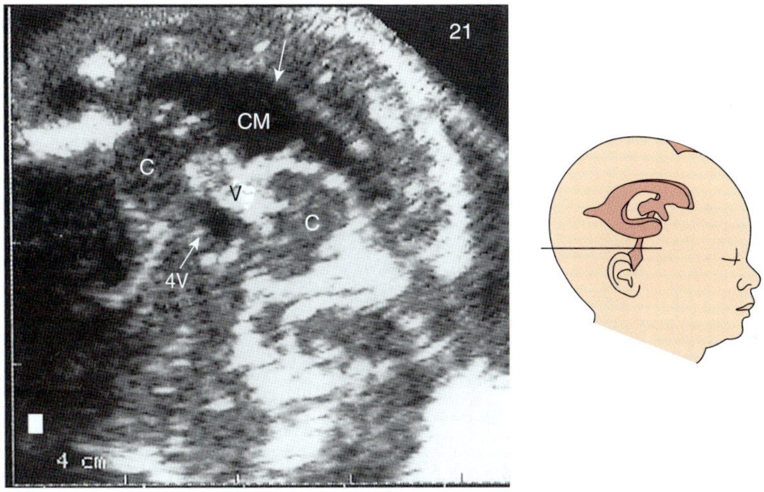


**Figure 2–57.** Axial section of the posterior fossa in a normal fetus at 21 postmenstrual weeks. CM, cisterna magna; C, cerebellum; V, vermis; 4V, fourth ventricle.

cross sections of vessels; however, on color Doppler and power Doppler scans, these do not demonstrate flow. An additional hypothesis is that they may represent cross sections of arachnoid granulations (Figure 2–56).

Several cisterns in the subarachnoid space can be seen by neurosonography of the fetal brain. The cisterns are scattered around as well as within the folds of the brain. We could not detect cisterns such as that of the lamina terminalis or the chiasmatic, interpeduncular, and pontine cisterns (cisterna magna); at times, the superior (interpeduncular) cistern below the cerebellum and the quadrigeminal cistern and the bilateral cisterna ambiens above the cerebellum have been imaged by ultrasonography.[81]

The cisterna magna has been seen as early as 12 to 14 postmenstrual weeks (Figures 2–36, and 2–57). From

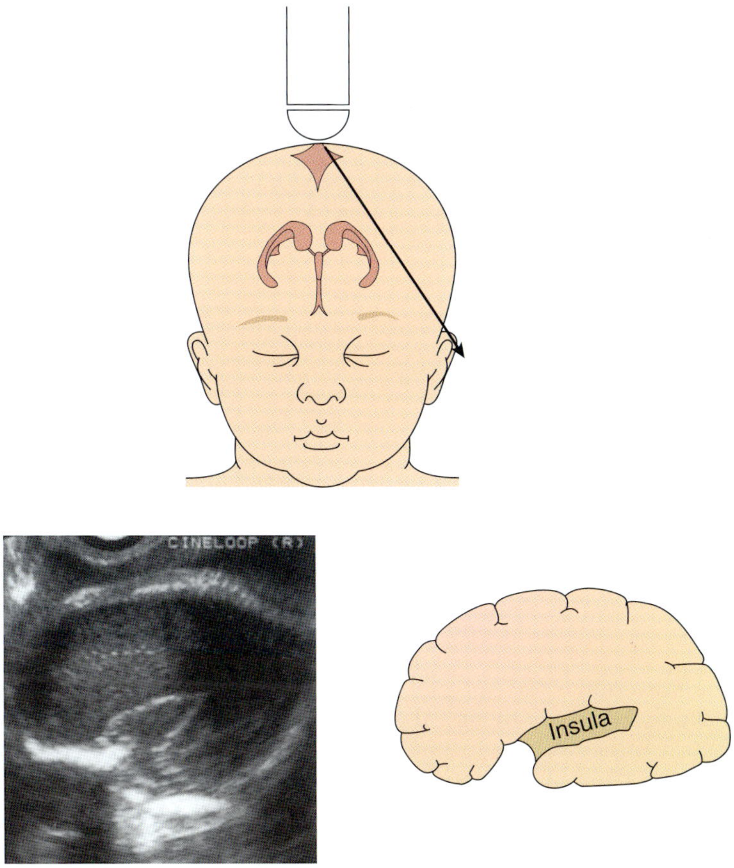


**Figure 2–58.** Left Oblique-2 section through the insula. Pulsations of the middle cerebral artery may be detected scanning through this view.

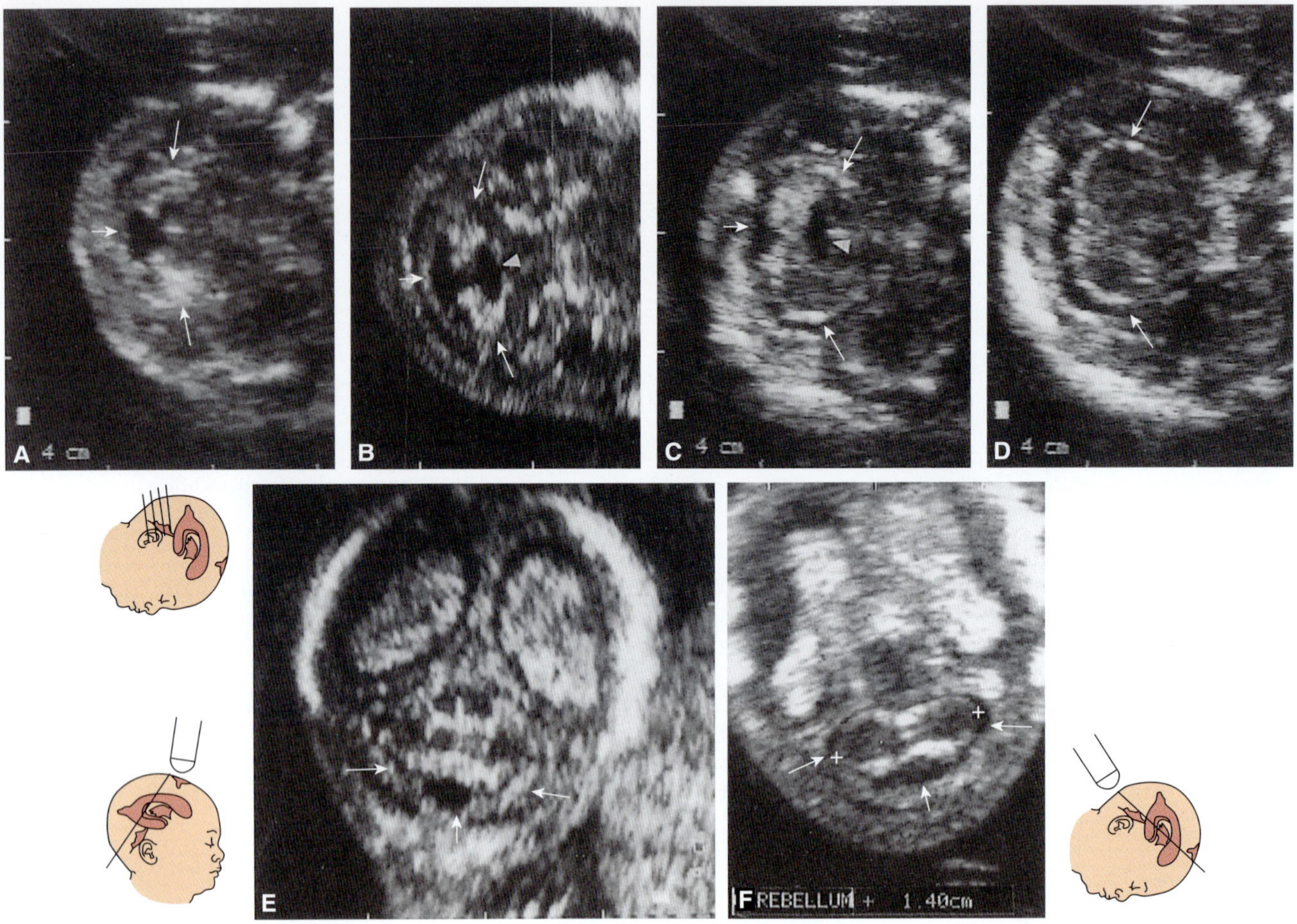


**Figure 2–59.** Structural evaluation of the brain at 15 postmenstrual weeks. The posterior fossa and the cerebellum are studied on these serial sections. The two slanted arrows on both sides of the cerebellum throughout the six images point to the two cerebral hemispheres. (**A**) Low axial section depicting the cisterna magna (small arrow). (**B**) The higher axial plane reveals the widening cisterna magna (small arrow) and the lower pole of the fourth ventricle (arrowhead). (**C**) A somewhat "higher" axial section shows the hemispheres and the fourth ventricle (arrowhead). (**D**) This is the highest of axial sections depicting the cerebellum at the level where the bicerebellar diameter measurement is usually taken. Note the hyperechoic cortex surrounded by sonolucent cerebrospinal fluid and the low echogenicity of the medulla. (**E**) Coronal section showing the cisterna magna (small white arrow in the median plane), the inverted-funnel-shaped tentorium (two black arrows), and the choroid plexus (cp). (**F**) A combined oblique axial-coronal section showing the bicerebellar diameter, which measures 1.4 cm. The small arrow in the midline indicates the cisterna magna. (From Timor-Tritsch and colleagues, 1995,[42] with permission.)

14 postmenstrual weeks on, it is easy to visualize this relatively large sonolucent structure in the posterior fossa (2–45, 2–51, and 2–57).

As mentioned before, using a posterior (occipital) approach and a transvaginal probe, some of the fine details of the posterior fossa and the cisterna magna, as well as the quadrigeminal cistern, can be revealed (Figure 2–59). The connection between the fourth ventricle and the cisterna magna through the median aperture can also be seen if the correct section and plane are applied (Figures 2–60, 2–61, 2–62, 2–63, and 2–64).

The exact anatomy of the posterior fossa, but more so the connections between the fourth ventricle and the cisterns around the cerebellum (eg, the cisterna magna), should be well known to those engaging in neurosonography of the fetal posterior fossa. Variations in the size of these CSF-filled spaces are not uncommon. The size of the cisterna magna in normal neonates was measured and ranges between 3 and 8 mm, with a mean value of 4.5 mm.[78] As opposed to an increase in the size of this space due to disease, there is also restriction of this cistern due to pathology (Arnold-Chiari type II malformation). It is therefore of the utmost importance that this space be examined in the context of the entire CNS.

The use of high-frequency (possibly through the transvaginal route) transducers is probably warranted, along with sound knowledge of the anatomy and neuropathology of this region.

At times, only TAS of the ventricular system is feasible (eg, with breech or transverse positions of the fetus). In such cases one should be familiar with nomograms developed for atrial measurements. One of these nomograms was suggested by Pilu and coworkers.[59] After conducting a prospective study of 171 normal pregnancies from 15 postmenstrual weeks to term, the following were found: (1) the atrial width remained fairly constant during pregnancy (0.69 ± 0.13 cm = 2 standard deviations); and (2) significant relationships were found between the cerebroatrial

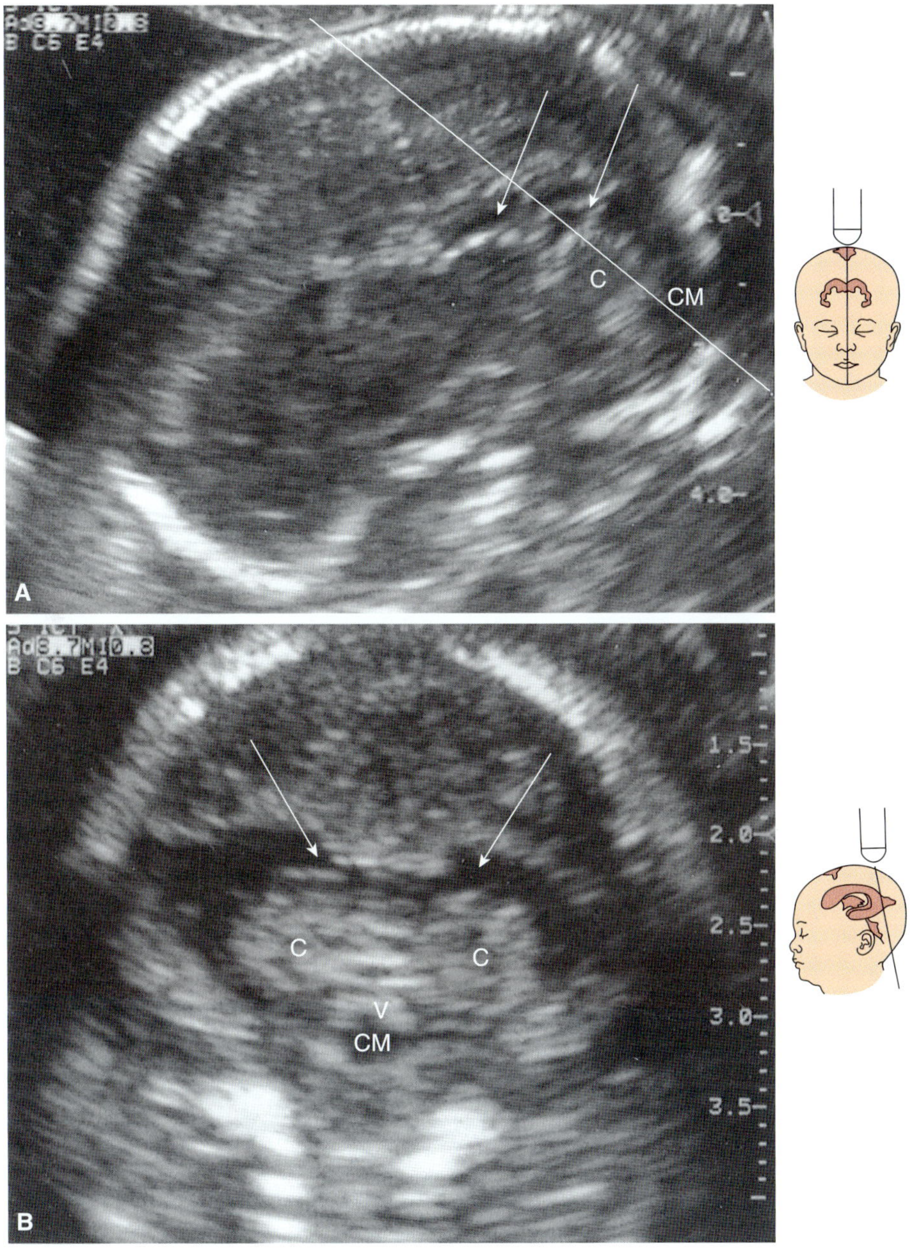


**Figure 2–60.** The cisterns around the cerebellum in a normal fetus at 17 postmenstrual weeks. (**A**) Median section. The two arrows indicate the quadrigeminal cisterns. C, cerebellum; CM, cisterna magna. (**B**) Coronal view obtained along the white line in A. The two arrows point to the cisterna ambiens above the cerebellar hemispheres. Note the generous amount of cerebrospinal fluid around the cerebellar hemispheres (**C**). A small segment of the cisterna magna (CM) is also shown below the vermis (V).

distance (Figure 2–65) and age ($R^2$ = 0.936; $P$ = 0.0001) and between the cerebroatrial distance and the biparietal diameter, as well as between the atrial width–cerebroatrial distance ratio and age.

It is hard to compare ventricular measurements taken on axial sections using TAS with those obtained on paramedian sagittal sections using TVS. In spite of this, it seems that the general trend, for example, the very slow increase of fetal atrial size seen using the two methods, is comparable.[52]

## Posterior Fossa and Upper Spinal Cord

Transvaginal sonographic examination of the posterior fossa is feasible using a variety of approaches and scanning planes. All of them are useful and informative.

After 10 to 12 postmenstrual weeks, several larger structures of this anatomical area, such as the cerebellar hemispheres and the cisterna magna, are discernible (Figures 2–35A, 1B, 2A, 2B). At 16 to 18 postmenstrual weeks, the posterior fossa lends itself to excellent imaging.

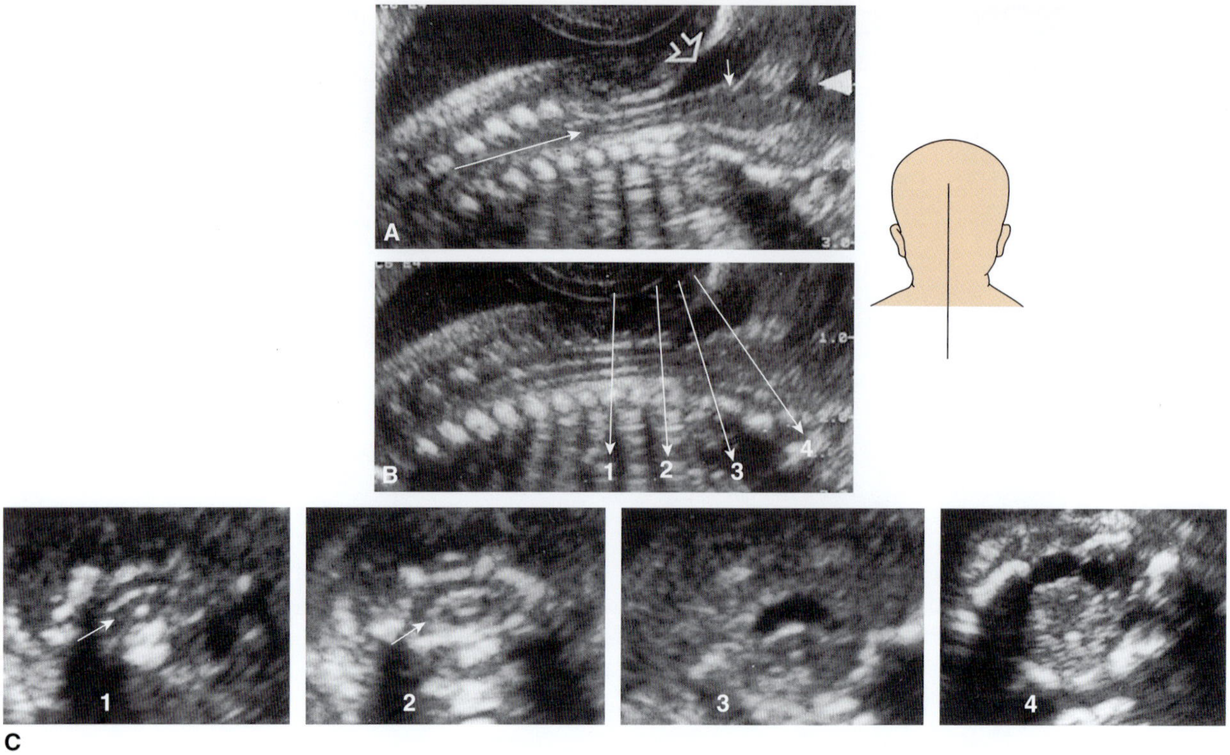


**Figure 2–61.** (**A**, **B**) Median sections through the posterior fossa and the upper portion of the spinal cord. The open arrow indicates the cisterna magna; the small arrow, the medulla oblongata; and the arrowhead, the fourth ventricle (at 17 postmenstrual weeks). B is similar to A, the arrows and the numbers showing the levels at which the cross-sections shown in **C** were taken. (1, 2) These sections were taken at the cervical level. The arrow indicates the spinal cord. (3, 4) These sections were obtained at the level of the medulla oblongata.

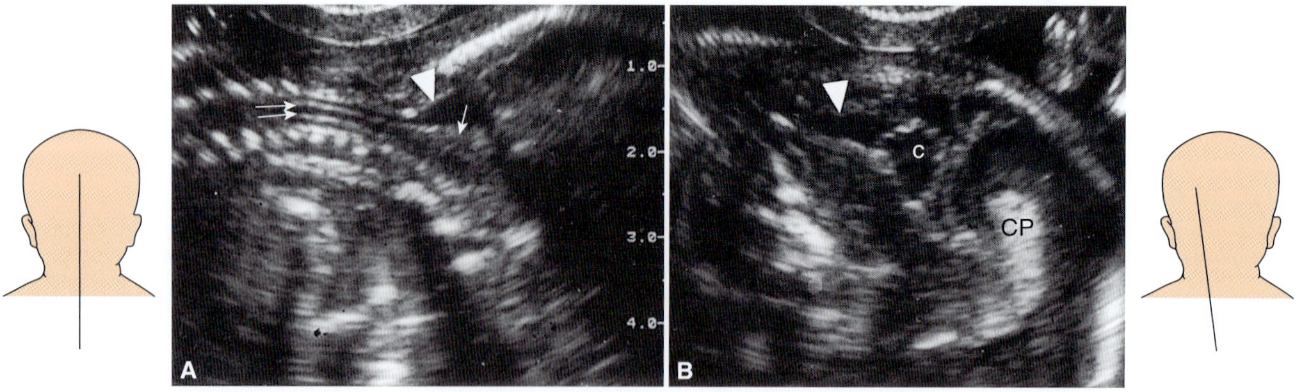


**Figure 2–62.** Imaging the upper spinal cord and the posterior fossa at 18 postmenstrual weeks. (**A**) Median section. The small arrow indicates the medulla oblongata; the arrowhead, the cisterna magna; the double arrow, the spinal cord. (**B**) Paramedian section through the cerebellar hemisphere (C) and the posterior horn of the lateral ventricle with the choroid plexus (CP).

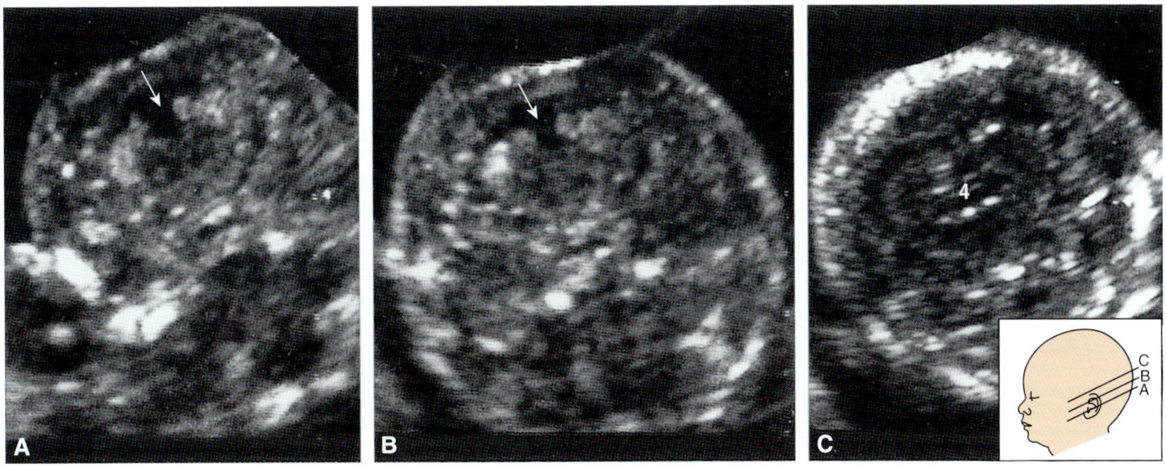


**Figure 2–63.** Anatomy of the cerebellum and the vermis in the posterior fossa at 15 to 16 postmenstrual weeks. (**A**) A low almost-axial section reveals the open communication (Magendie) between the cerebello medullary cistern (cisterna magna) and the fourth ventricle (arrow). (**B**) A somewhat higher section still shows the communication. (**C**) The highest of the three sections demonstrates that the vermis at this level is already present.

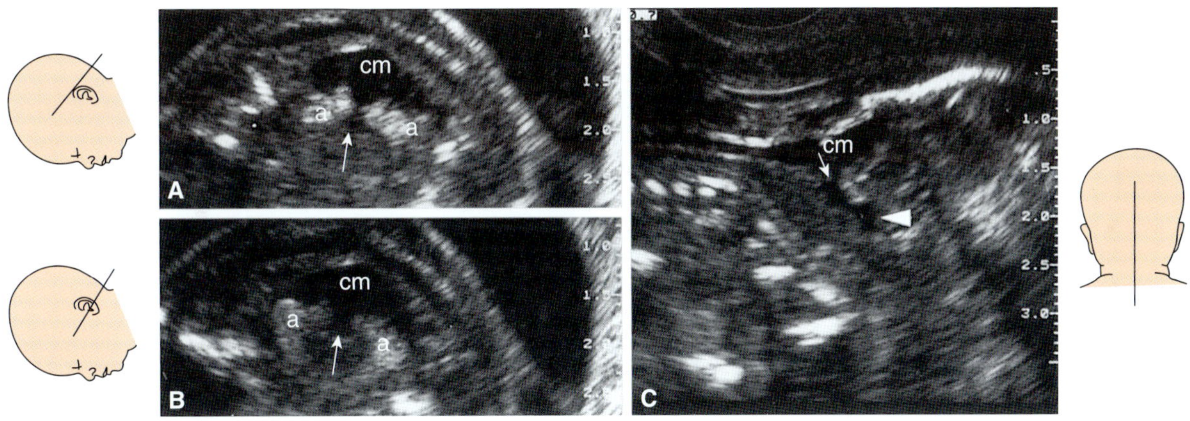


**Figure 2–64.** Anatomy of the posterior fossa at 19 postmenstrual weeks and 4 days. **A, B.** Two parallel axial sections demonstrating the still partially open connection between the cisterna magna (cm) and the median aperture of the fourth ventricle (small arrows). The slightly more echogenic lowermost portions of the two cerebellar hemispheres are evident. The arrowhead indicates the fourth ventricle. a, Amygdala. **C.** Median section. The white line is the plane along which the two axial sections in A and B were taken. p, pons; c, cerebellum. The arrowhead marks the fourth ventricle.

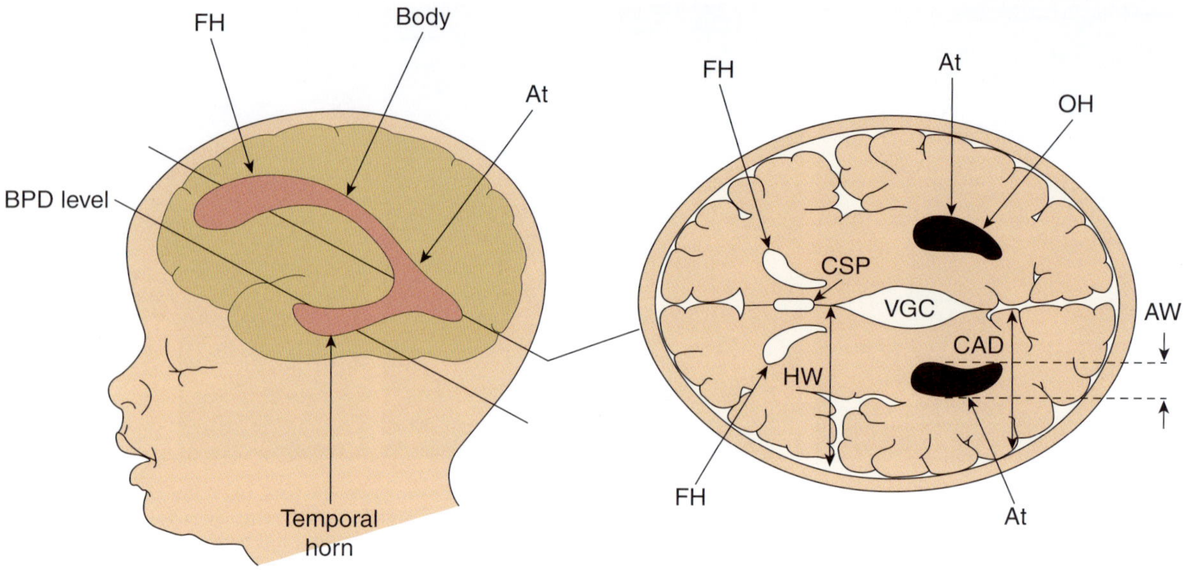


**Figure 2–65.** Schematic representation of a sagittal view of the fetal ventricular system at a level slightly above that normally used for obtaining the biparietal diameter. FH, Frontal horn; At, atrium; OH, occipital horn; CSP, cavum septi pellucidi; HW, hemispheric width; CAD, cerebroatrial distance; VGC, cerebral vein of Galen; AW, atrial width. (From Pilu and colleagues, 1989,[59] with permission.)

Studying the infratentorial region reveals the following structures: the cisterna magna, with fine, linear echoes of the arachnoid; the hemispheres, with their hyperechoic cortex; the extremely hyperechoic vermis; the pons; the fourth ventricle; and, on a median section, the connection between the fourth ventricle and the cisterna magna, that is, the median aperture (Magendie).

The late closure of the cerebellar vermis, toward the 18th postmenstrual week, was documented by Bromley et al[82] using transabdominal scanning. Using the transfontanelle approach, we have noted several fetuses with even later "closure" of the vermis, with normal neonatal outcome.

For easier orientation the posterior fossa is depicted in the following figures: horizontal (axial) sections—Figures 2–52; 2–59; 2–61; and 2–64A and B; coronal sections—Figures 2–38-5, and 2–59; and median and sagittal sections—Figures 2–43A, 2–45, 2–59A and B, 2–60A and B, and 2–64C.

Figures 2–61A, B and 2–62A, depict the upper spinal cord. To achieve a good view of the posterior fossa and the upper spinal cord, the transducer should ideally be over the nuchal area of the fetus. It is obvious that such views are not always possible. Gentle manipulation of the fetal position using the abdominally placed second hand of the scanning person, in combination with equally gentle touching with the tip of the vaginal probe, may ease the fetus into the desired position.

By knowing the normal anatomy of the posterior fossa, early detection of pathology (eg, Dandy-Walker malformation, atrophy of the vermis, and posterior cephalocele) is feasible as early as 10 to 11 postmenstrual weeks.

Because the size of the cerebellum is easy to image on axial as well as coronal sections, this structure has been discussed in detail by various authors. The bicerebellar (lateral edge-to-lateral edge) measurement has been plotted and published by several centers.[83,84]

## Sulci, Fissures, and Gyri

Examination of the sulci, fissures, and gyri is one of the many instances when fetal neuroimaging is fashioned after that of the neonatal brain scanning by ultrasonography.

Neuropathologists and pediatric neurologists use sequential sulcal and gyral developments as a clinical estimate of fetal age, particularly between 22 and 34 postmenstrual weeks.[85–90] Deformities or delayed development of the cingulate gyrus may predict disease in the immediate neighborhood of this structure.[91]

In spite of the fact that rather crude timing of the fetal age is possible, based on the developmental stages of the gyri and the sulci, it seems that perinatologists may never have to rely on these markers to determine age. However, it may at times be important to assess cortical maturation and development, as well as diseases that affect formation of the cerebral cortex.

Performing antenatal neurosonography enables us to evaluate some of the sulci, fissures, and gyri of the developing fetal brain. Before these structures are shown as they progressively appear on the US screen, a list of the major sulci, fissures, and gyri of the mature human brain is shown in Figures 2–66 through 2–70. These images depict the mature brain in normal neonates. The next step is to examine the sequential appearance of the sulci, fissures, and gyri as a function of increasing fetal age, expressed in weeks from the LMP. Tables 2–6 and 2–7 were compiled using data from Chi and associates.[92] This group examined photographs of 507 brains and serial sections of 209 brains

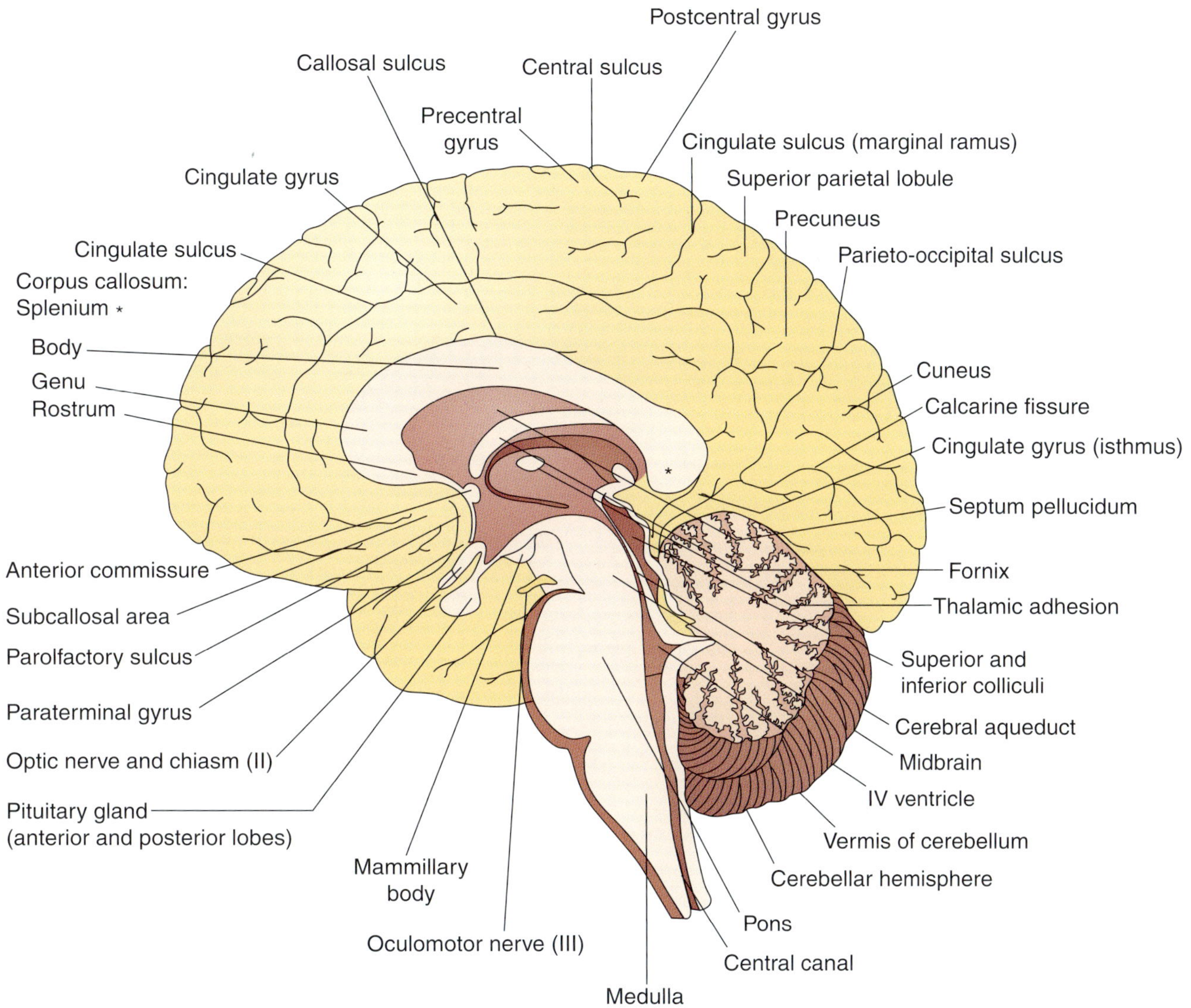


**Figure 2–66.** Medial surface of the cerebral hemisphere and median section through the diencephalon, brain stem, cerebellum, and rostral spinal cord of a mature brain. The sulci, the gyri, and other major structures of the medial cerebral surface are shown. (From Martin, 2003,[61] with permission.)

from pathologic specimens of fetuses 10 to 44 weeks from the LMP. They concluded that many gyri become well defined within a short period (between 26 and 28 postmenstrual weeks). Thereafter, only a few gyri develop. During the last trimester, the gyri and the sulci become more prominent and deep, giving rise to secondary and tertiary gyri.

In 1977 a study examining 80 brains ranging in age from 22 postmenstrual weeks to 1 month of postnatal life was published by Dorovini-Zis and Dolman.[93] They concluded that at 22 postmenstrual weeks, the cerebral hemispheres are smooth, and the lateral sulci on both sides are wide open. The parieto-occipital and calcarine fissures are present on the medial surface. By 24 postmenstrual weeks, the central sulcus begins to form, and the cingulate sulcus is seen. By 26 postmenstrual weeks, deepening of these fissures and sulci occurs. A great growth spurt takes place between 28 and 30 postmenstrual weeks. The sulci and the gyri deepen and become more branched. Figure 2–66 depicts the development of the sulci and the gyri as described in the work of Dorovini-Zis and Dolman.[93]

Slagle's group[91] studied the development of the cingulate sulcus in preterm infants by performing cranial ultrasonographic scans. Two hundred eleven infants from 24 to 40 postmenstrual weeks were studied on their third prenatal day of life. These investigators identified five patterns: (1) a discontinuous line of the sulcus appears; (2) a continuous line appears; (3) first branches of the primary sulcus appear (marginal ramus); (4) multiple branches of the primary sulcus appear; and (5) multiple branches appear and merge with other sulci, giving the surface a "cobblestone" appearance.

Figure 2–71 depicts the sequential appearance of these five patterns. The first pattern appeared at

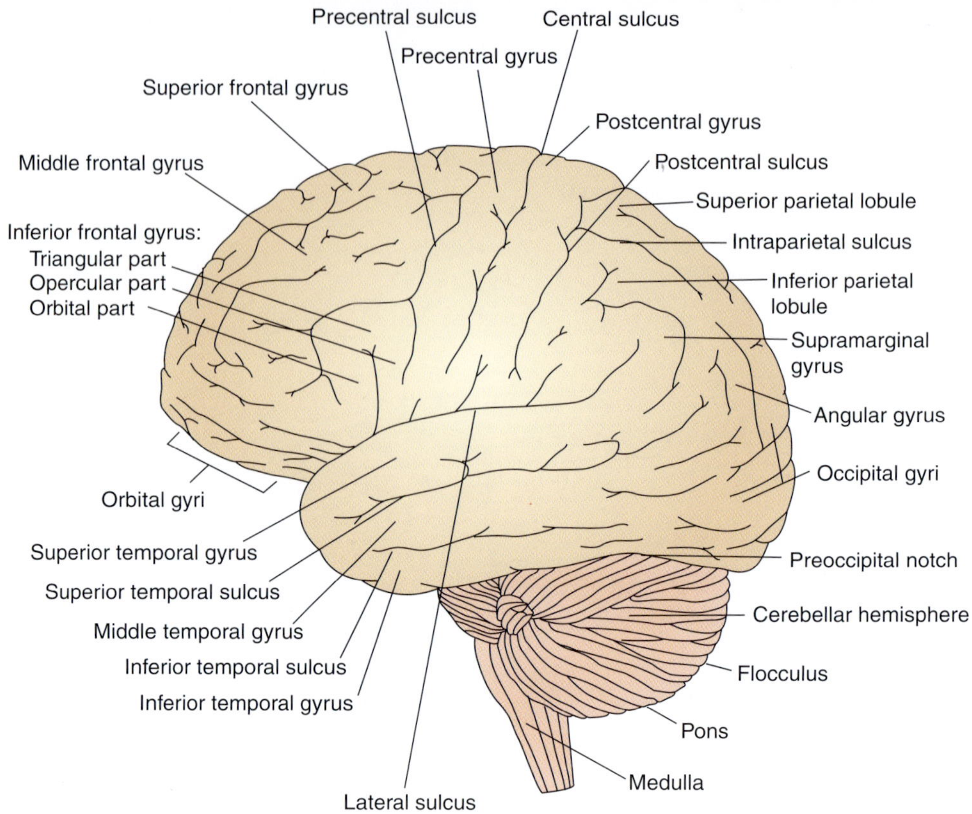


**Figure 2–67.** Lateral surface of the cerebral hemisphere, emphasizing the gyri and the sulci of a mature brain. (From Martin, 2003,[61] with permission.)

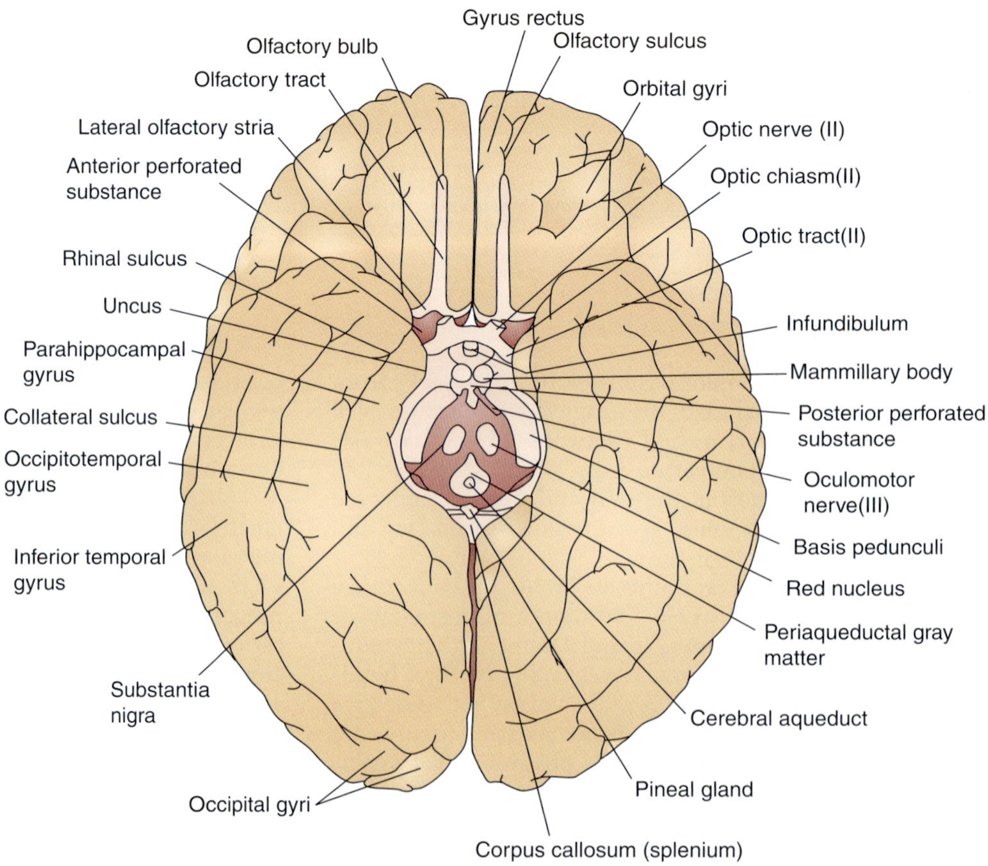


**Figure 2–68.** Inferior surface of the cerebral hemispheres and the diencephalon. The gyri and the sulci are marked. The brain stem is transected at the rostral midbrain. (From Martin, 2003,[61] with permission.)

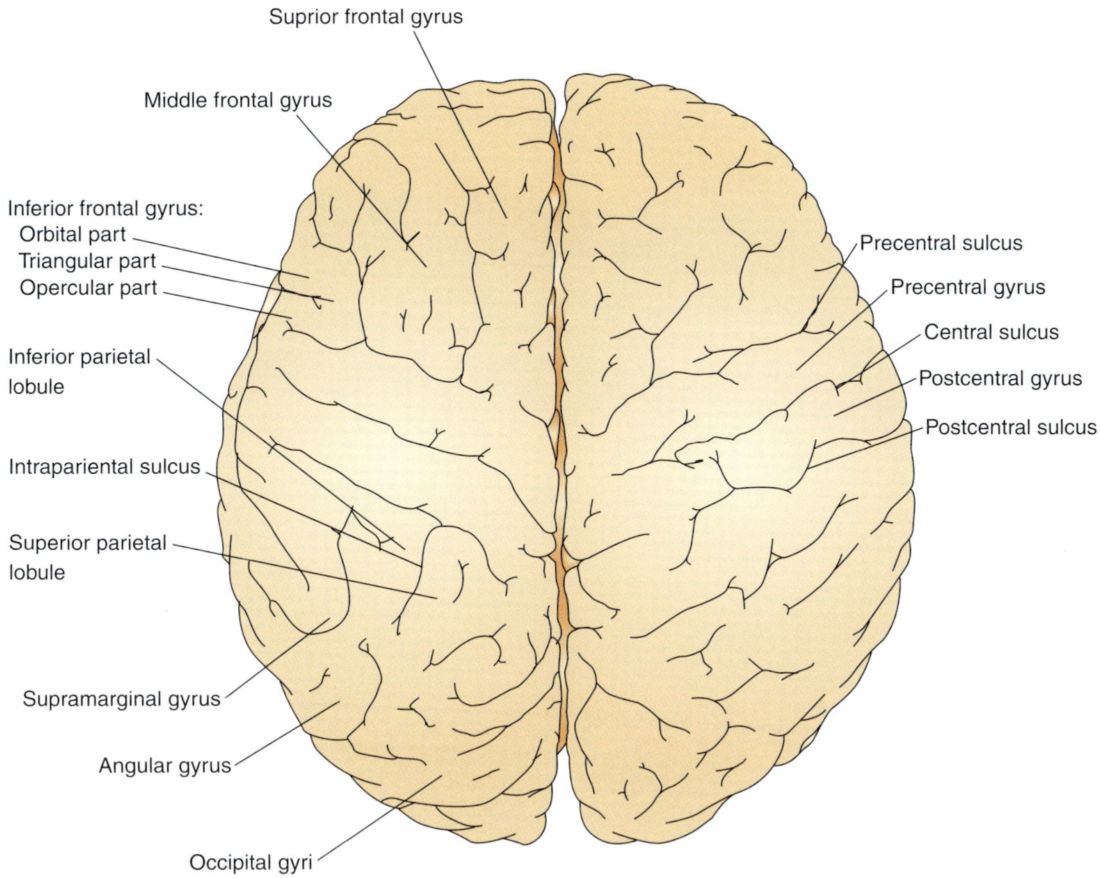


**Figure 2–69.** Gyri and sulci of the superior surface of the cerebral hemisphere. (From Martin, 2003,[61] with permission.)

24 postmenstrual weeks, the first line was seen at 26 ± 2 postmenstrual weeks, first branching appeared at 32 ± 3 postmenstrual weeks, multiple branches occurred at 34 ± 3 postmenstrual weeks, and the cobblestone pattern appeared after 38 postmenstrual weeks. This study suggested that cingulate sulcus maturation occurs in a predictable pattern (Figure 2–72). Slagle and colleagues[91] also studied 30 infants with evidence of brain damage. These infants showed significant delay in the postnatal development of the cingulate sulcus.

Our observations of the developing cortex using transvaginal ultrasonography focused on three readily available planes. The first is the median plane, which touches the medial aspect of the cerebral hemisphere and scans along the longitudinal fissure. The second available plane is a midcoronal plane at the level of the anterior horns. The third is an extreme lateral right or left oblique plane "touching" almost tangentially the upper surface of the cerebral hemispheres, emphasizing the lateral sulcus and the insula.[94]

We focused on the following sulci and fissures: on the median plane the cingulate sulcus with its marginal ramus, the posterior occipital sulcus, and the calcarine sulcus; and on the coronal plane the longitudinal fissure, with its progressive branching of the cingulate sulcus. Finally, on the lateral sagittal section we examined the shape of the lateral sulcus and the underlying insula. Figures 2–73, 2–74, and 2–75 clearly show progressive deepening and branching as well as curving of the different fissures and sulci and the appearance of the insula, respectively. Relative flatness of the cortex is present until 24 to 25 postmenstrual weeks, with widely gaping longitudinal fissures, calcarine, posterior occipital fissures, and lateral sulcus (insula). At 28 to 30 postmenstrual weeks, significant depth and branching of the sulci and fissures occur. Between 30 and 60 postmenstrual weeks, more secondary branching develops, and at 38 postmenstrual weeks, the tertiary branching is seen.[94]

The clinical significance of these observations is still not clear. It may be possible to establish whether the cortex progresses along a well-defined and age-dependent pattern. It may also be feasible to detect diseases of the fetal brain that are expressed by a delayed or nonexistent maturational process.

The sonographic appearance of the sulci and the fissures is dependent on the higher-echogenicity pia mater (pachymeninx) and the pia-arachnoid complex, also called the "soft brain covering," or the leptomeninx. Note that the high echogenicity of the choroid plexus is due to the highly vascular and abundant presence of the pia mater. The highly echogenic leptomeninx or the choroid plexus in close proximity to the CSF generates a

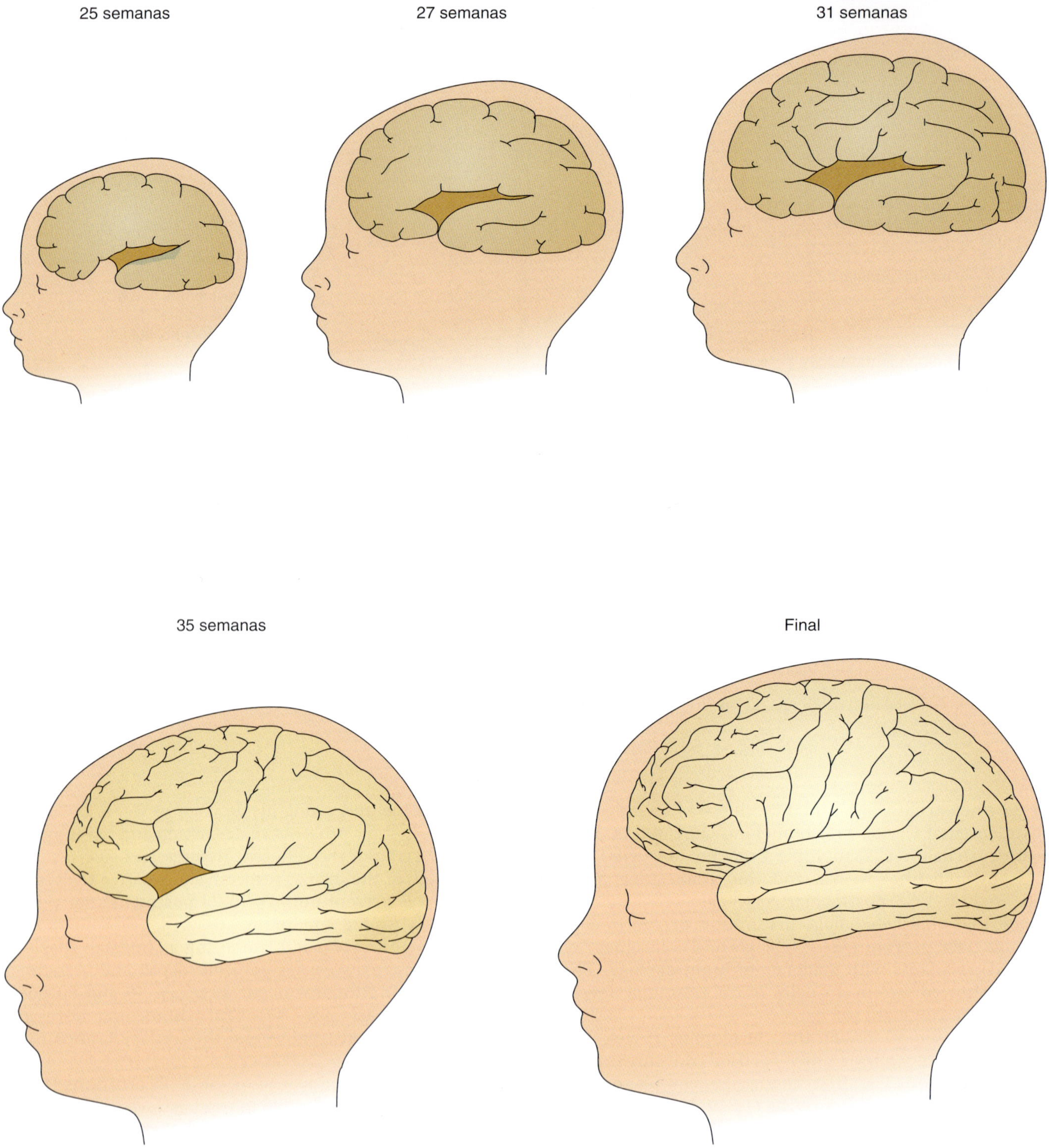


**Figure 2–70.** The surface of the fetal brain is relatively smooth in the first 20 weeks after which the sulci, gyri, and fissures develop. This image demonstrates the concept of the gradual changes in the surface of the fetal brain throughout the pregnancy. (Reproduced, with permission, from Dr P. Jeanty, Editor www.Thefetus.net. *Magnetic Resonance in the Fetus,* Part 1. H. Werner, et al. Thefetusnet.net, 2005.)

**Table 2–6. TEMPORAL DEVELOPMENT OF THE CEREBRAL HEMISPHERES**

| Gestational Age* (No. Examined) | Sulci and Fissures | Gyri |
|---|---|---|
| 10–15 weeks (n = 6) | Interhemispheric fissure, sylvian fissure, transverse cerebral fissure, callosal sulcus | — |
| 16–19 weeks (n = 13) | Parieto-occipital fissure, olfactory sulcus, circular sulcus, cingulate sulcus, calcarine fissure | Gyrus rectus, insula, cingulate gyrus |
| 20–23 weeks (n = 41) | Rolandic sulcus, collateral sulcus, superior temporal sulcus | Parahippocampal gyrus, superior temporal gyrus |
| 24–27 weeks (n = 46) | Prerolandic sulcus, middle temporal sulcus, postrolandic sulcus, interparietal sulcus, superior frontal sulcus, lateral occipital sulcus | Prerolandic gyrus, middle temporal gyrus, postrolandic gyrus, superior and inferior parietal lobules, superior and middle frontal gyri, superior and inferior occipital gyrus, cuneus and lingual gyrus, fusiform gyrus |
| 28–31 weeks (n = 36) | Inferior temporal sulcus, inferior frontal sulcus | Inferior temporal gyrus, triangular gyrus, medial and lateral orbital gyrus, callosomarginal gyrus, transverse temporal gyrus, angular and supramarginal gyrus, external occipitotemporal gyrus |
| 32–35 weeks (n = 29) | Marginal sulcus<br>Secondary superior, middle, and inferior frontal; superior and middle temporal; superior and inferior parietal; prerolandic and postrolandic, superior and inferior occipital sulci and gyri; insular gyri | Paracentral gyrus |
| 36–39 weeks (n = 31) | Secondary transverse and inferior temporal and cingulate sulci and gyri; tertiary superior, middle, and inferior frontal and superior and inferior parietal sulci and gyri | Anterior and posterior orbital gyri |
| 40–44 weeks (n = 29) | Secondary orbital, callosomarginal, and insular sulci and gyri; tertiary inferior temporal and superior and inferior occipital gyri and sulci | |

From Chi and colleagues, 1977,[92] with permission.

*Postmenstrual weeks.

highly visible interface, which appears as bright echoes. The dura is prominent in those places where it protrudes into the brain to separate structures. These two dura-containing places are the falx (Figures 2–21, 2–38, 2–39, 2–41, 2–53, and 2–59) and the tentorium (Figures 2–31, 2–38, 2–40, and 2–41). The pia closely follows the surface of the cortex. Wherever a fissure or a sulcus is present, the pia (and, at times, the arachnoid) closely follows, making this a sonographically easily recognized structure. In the case of the cerebellar cortex, and even more so the vermis of the cerebellum, which have extremely abundant and tightly folded gyri and sulci, the sonographic image shows extremely bright echoes. The sonographic hallmark of the vermis is its easily recognizable high echogenicity, due to the repeatedly infolded double layers of leptomeninges (Figures, 2–44, 2–45, 2–51, 2–57, 2–63, and 2–64).

It is hard to image sonographically the convexity of the cerebral hemisphere. Thus, it is rare to see a small area of the tangential picture of the gyri and the sulci. However, the medial surface of the cerebral hemisphere along the longitudinal fissure is easily imaged by the ultrasonographic techniques. It is this flat surface where good images of the cortex are obtained.

Fetal and neonatal sulcal examination by ultrasonography is a noninvasive and convenient method to assess cerebral maturation. This cerebral maturation has so far been proven only in neonates. However, if the proper methodology is developed for use in fetal neurosonology, it may prove to be useful.

**Table 2–7. REGIONAL DEVELOPMENT OF THE CEREBRAL HEMISPHERES**

| Lobe | Fissures and Sulci | Weeks* | Gyri | Weeks |
|---|---|---|---|---|
| Frontal | Interhemispheric fissure | 10 | Gyrus rectus | 16 |
| | Transverse cerebral fissure | 10 | Insula | 18 |
| | Callosal sulcus | 14 | Cingulate gyrus | 18 |
| | Sylvian fissure | 14 | Prerolandic gyrus | 24 |
| | Olfactory sulcus | 16 | Superior frontal gyrus | 25 |
| | Circular sulcus | 18 | Middle frontal gyrus | 27 |
| | Cingulate sulcus | 18 | Triangular gyrus | 28 |
| | Rolandic sulcus | 20 | Medial and lateral orbital gyrus | 28 |
| | Prerolandic sulcus | 24 | Callosomarginal gyrus | 28 |
| | Superior frontal sulcus | 25 | Anterior and posterior orbital gyrus | 36 |
| | Inferior frontal sulcus | 28 | | |
| Parietal | Interhemispheric fissure | 10 | Cingulate gyrus | 18 |
| | Transverse cerebral fissure | 10 | Postrolandic gyrus | 25 |
| | Sylvian fissure | 14 | Superior parietal lobule | 26 |
| | Parieto-occipital fissure | 16 | Inferior parietal lobule | 26 |
| | Rolandic sulcus | 20 | Angular gyrus | 28 |
| | Postrolandic sulcus | 25 | Supramarginal gyrus | 28 |
| | Interparietal sulcus | 26 | Paracentral gyri | 35 |
| Temporal | Sylvian fissure | 14 | Superior temporal gyrus | 23 |
| | Superior temporal sulcus | 23 | Parahippocampal gyrus | 23 |
| | Collateral sulcus | 23 | Middle temporal gyrus | 26 |
| | Middle temporal sulcus | 26 | Fusiform gyrus | 27 |
| | Inferior temporal sulcus | 30 | Inferior temporal gyrus | 30 |
| | | | External occipitotemporal gyrus | 30 |
| | | | Transverse temporal gyrus | 31 |
| Occipital | Interhemispheric fissure | 10 | Superior occipital gyri | 27 |
| | Calcarine fissure | 16 | Inferior occipital gyri | 27 |
| | Parieto-occipital sulcus | 16 | Cuneus | 27 |
| | Collateral sulcus | 23 | Lingual gyrus | 27 |
| | Lateral occipital sulcus | 27 | External occipitotemporal gyrus | 30 |

After Chi and colleagues, 1977,[92] with permission.

*Postmenstrual weeks.

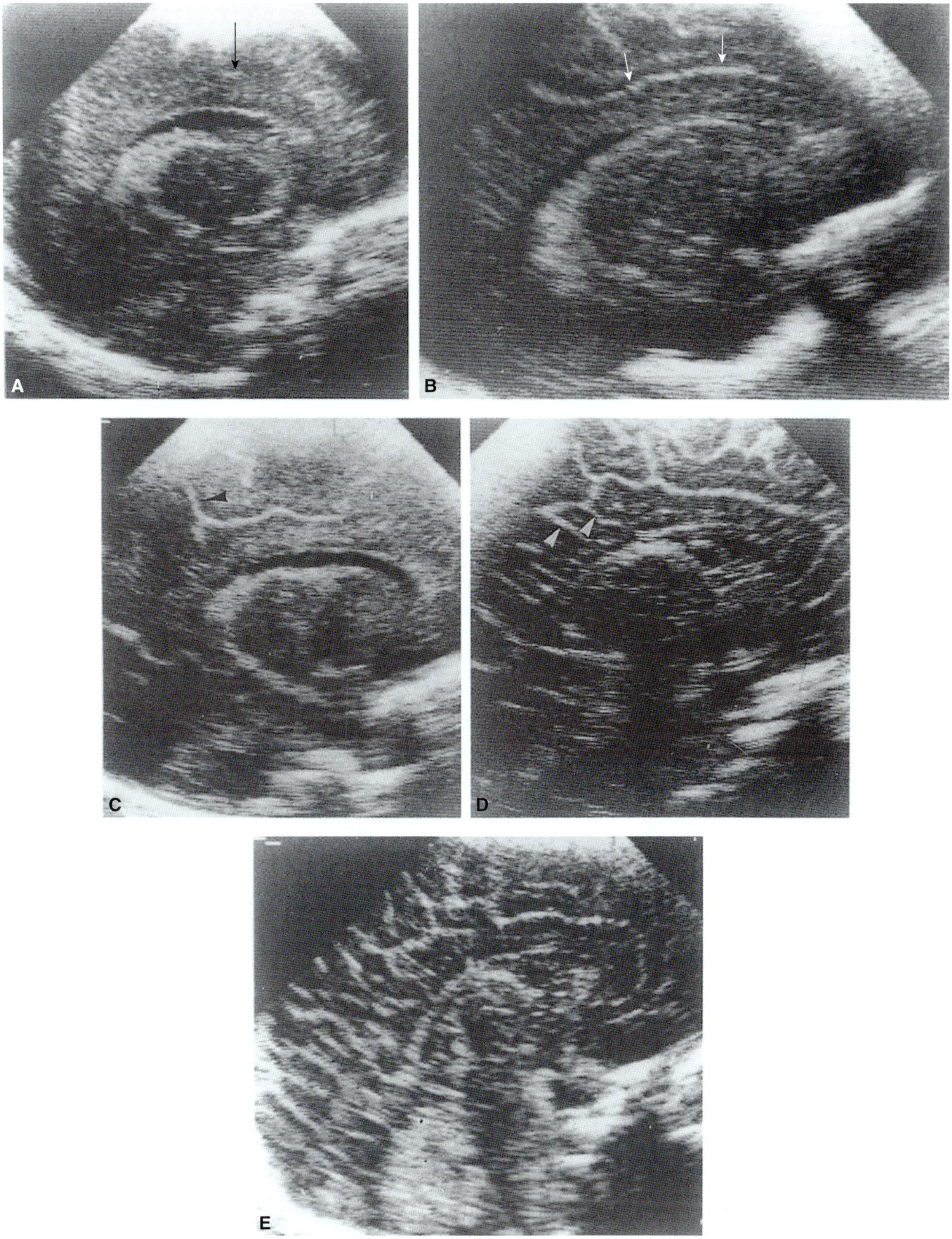


**Figure 2–71.** Developmental stages of the cingulate sulcus. Paramedian sonograms demonstrating five developmental stages: (**A**) The presence of one or more discontinuous linear echoes (arrow); (**B**) Continuity—a single continuous linear echo (arrows); (**C**) First branch—perpendicular echo of the primary sulcus (arrowhead); (**D**) Multiple branches—additional branches off the primary sulcus (arrowheads); and (**E**) "Cobblestone" pattern branches from the cingulate sulcus, merging with other cortical sulci. (From Slagle and colleagues, 1989,[91] with permission.)

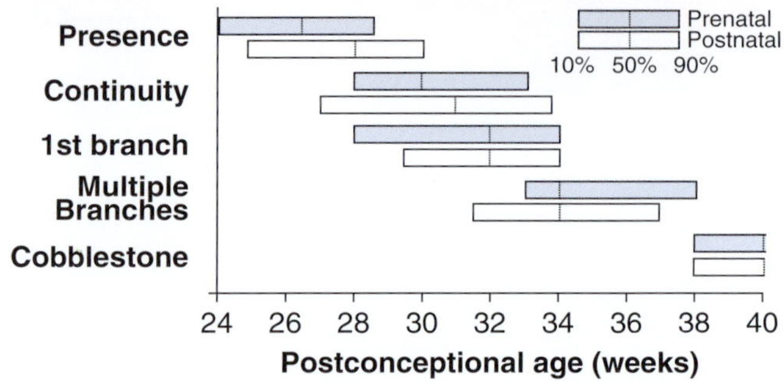


**Figure 2–72.** Developmental sequence of the cingulate sulcus. Shown is a comparison of the 10%, 50%, and 90% levels of prenatal (stippled bars) and postnatal (open bars) development of the cingulate sulcus. There was no difference in cingulate sulcus landmark timing between prenatal (determined on initial sonograms of 211 infants of 24 to 40 postmenstrual weeks' gestational age) and postnatal development (determined on serial ultrasound examinations from week 1 of age to 40 weeks' postconceptual age in the 144 infants born at less than 32 weeks' postmenstrual age). (From Slagle and colleagues, 1989,[91] with permission.)

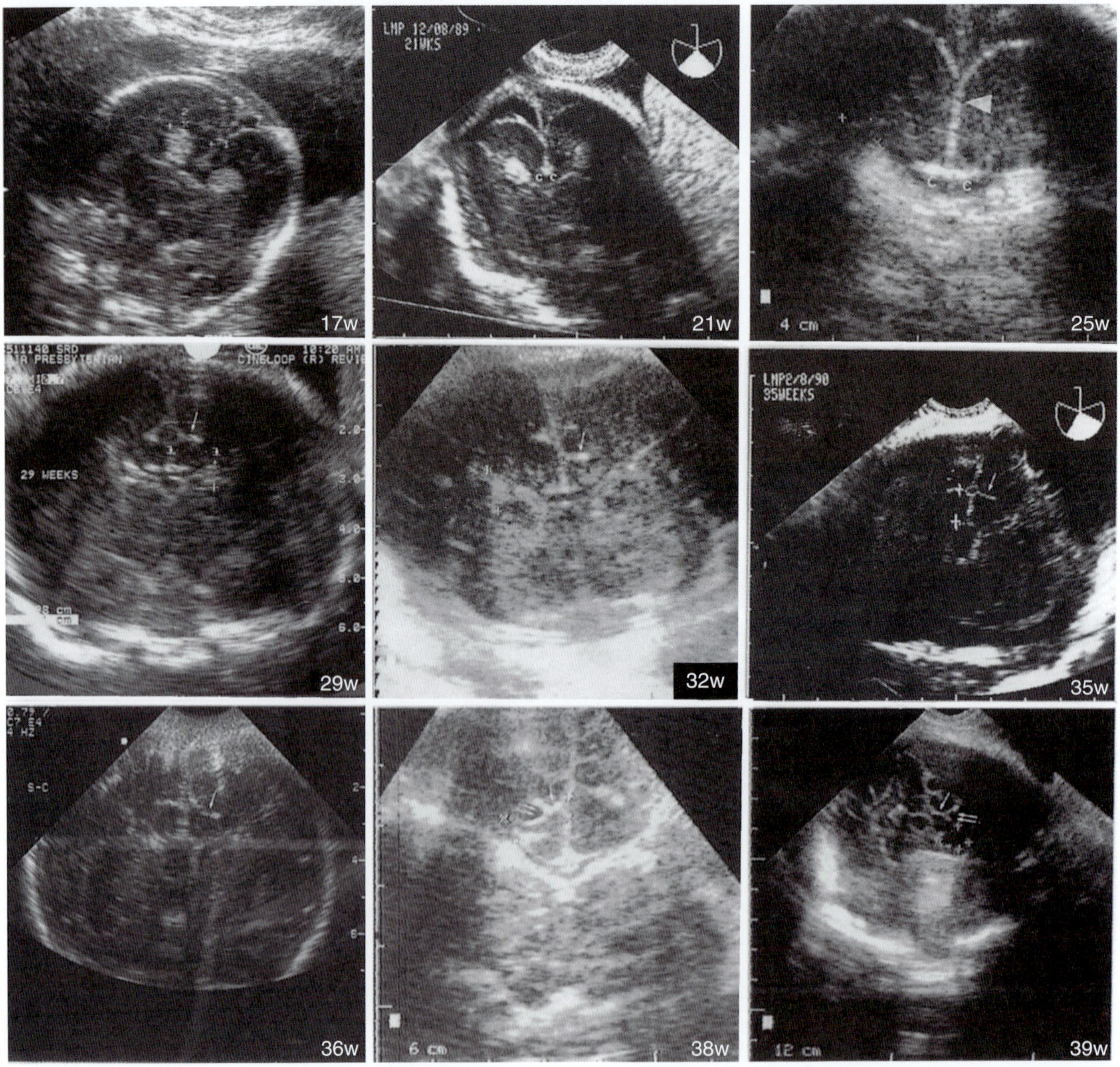


**Figure 2–73.** Development of the sulci and the gyri. Coronal sections (usually midcoronal–2) from 17 to 39 postmenstrual weeks are depicted. Note that at first the straight line of the longitudinal fissure (arrowhead shown at 25 postmenstrual weeks). At 25 to 28 postmenstrual weeks (not shown), the first indentation of the cingulate sulcus (small single arrow) appears and remains evident up to 36 weeks. At 37 to 38 postmenstrual weeks, secondary and, finally, tertiary branches appear (small double arrows). CC, corpus callosum; CG, cingulate gyrus. (From Monteagudo et al, 1997,[94] with permission.)

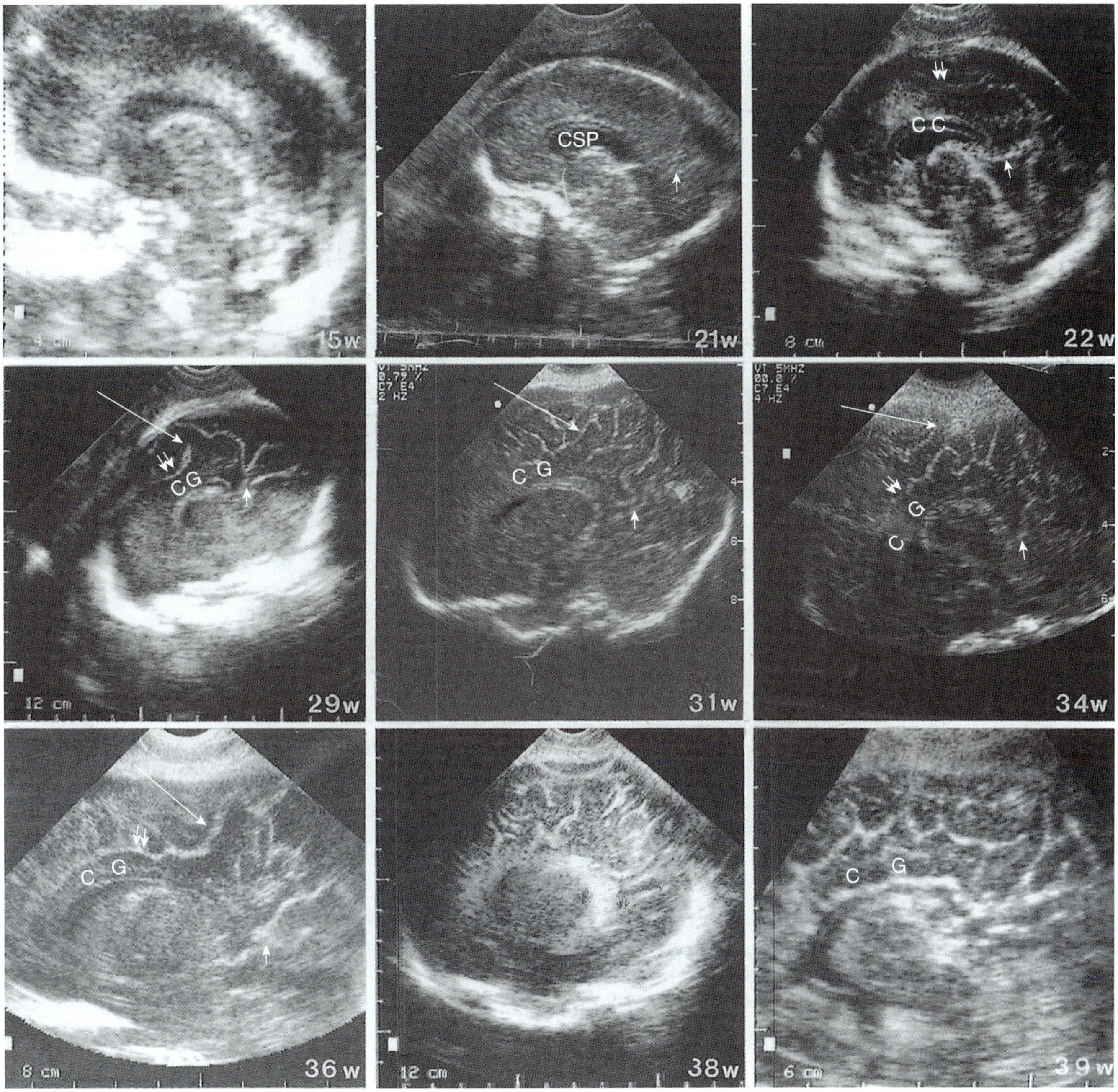


**Figure 2–74.** Development of the fissures, sulci, and gyri. The median sections from 15 to 39 postmenstrual weeks show the first appearance of the cingulate gyrus (CG), the cingulate sulcus (small double arrow) at 22 postmenstrual weeks, and the calcarine fissure and the parieto-occipital sulcus (arrow) at 21 postmenstrual weeks. Note the progressive appearance of the "cobblestone" gyral pattern, fully recognizable at 38 to 39 postmenstrual weeks. The long arrow points to the callosomarginal sulcus. CC, corpus callosum; CG, cingulate gyrus. (From Monteagudo et al, 1997,[94] with permission.)

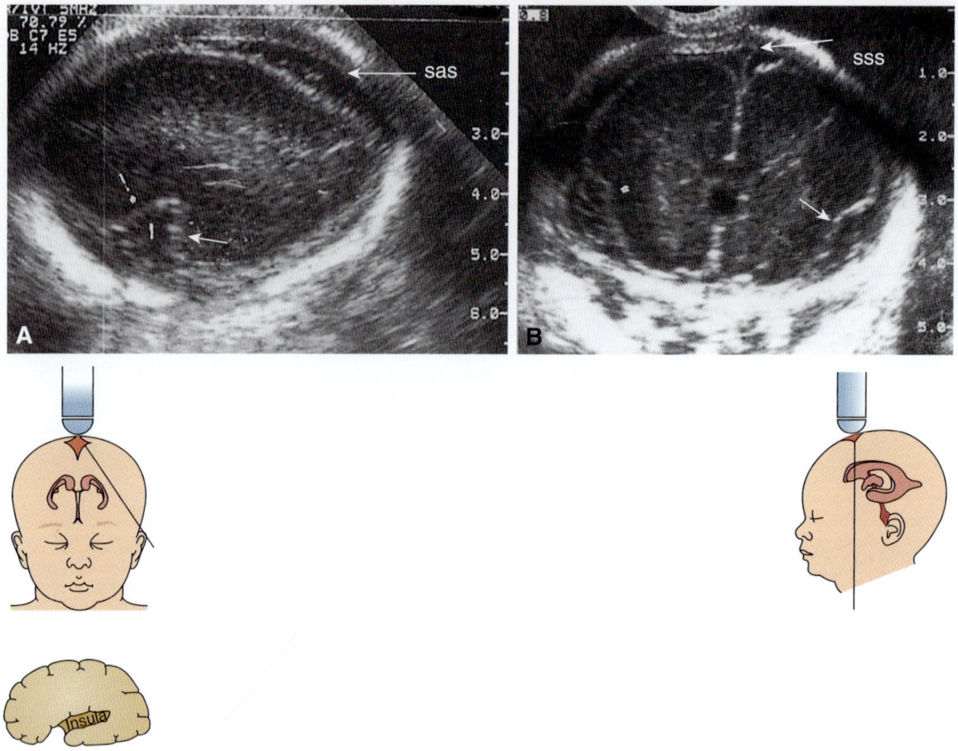


**Figure 2–75.** The insula, lateral sulcus, and subarachnoid space at 25 postmenstrual weeks. (**A**) On the left Oblique–2 extremely lateral sagittal section of the subarachnoid space (sas), the operculum (arrows), and the insula are shown. (**B**) On the Midcoronal–1 plane, the subarachnoid space surrounding the superior sagittal sinus (sss) and the insula (arrows) are depicted.

## THREE-DIMENSIONAL FETAL NEUROSCAN

A thorough description of 3D US equipment and its functioning, including the explanation of the physics behind the different types of display modalities, is beyond the scope of this chapter. However, for those readers who are interested, we refer them to several texts and articles available in the literature.[95,96]

We will focus on the three basic steps in performing a 3D US study: acquisition, storage, and display. This section will review these three main components of 3D US and explain how to "manipulate" the acquired volumes. In this volume, this manipulation is also referred as "navigating" or "scrolling."

Before performing volume imaging of the fetal brain, a dedicated fetal neurosonography should be performed using the transabdominal and/or the transvaginal 2D scanning approach. Normal 2D US appearance of the fetal CNS has been described in depth in this chapter.

### Volume Acquisition

A well-planned and well-executed volume acquisition is the most important first step in the process of creating good-quality 3D US images. The volume can be obtained using a manual sweep with the probe, across the volume of interest, or automatically, with mechanical transducers enabling fast acquisition of data without movement of the probe itself. The US industry is slowly phasing out manual acquisition, favoring automated acquisition for many valid reasons. At present, volume US (3D sonography) can be performed using transabdominal or transvaginal scan heads.

Initiating a 3D US examination is similar to that of a 2D US. Once the targeted brain structures of interest are clearly seen on the monitor, the region of interest is selected by using the volume box on the 2D image. Then the special transabdominal or transvaginal 3D transducer is activated. To obtain the volume, the 3D probe creates an extremely rapid sequence of images that are automatically stored into a single volume. Every subsequent activation of the transducer creates a new and separate volume that can be accessed later as needed. The volume acquisition results in a single 3D static data set that consists of numerous successive 2D sectional images. As a result, it becomes possible to re-create any desired image by slicing through the volume in any of the three classical planes (coronal, sagittal, and axial), as well as any other plane referred to as "anyplane." We recommend capturing several volumes of the same structure in different planes.

The first display of images, usually the multiplanar orthogonal planes, appears automatically on the screen. At this point the quality of the picture is examined. If the quality of the displayed images, hence the acquired volume, seems acceptable, the volume can be stored.

Acquisition of good-quality 3D volume is the basis of any 3D analysis. Most factors that determine the acquisition quality can be controlled and varied by the operator, such as grayscale settings, acquisition speed, frame rate, and acoustic shadowing. However, fetal position, fetal movement, maternal obesity, and fluid–tissue interface may challenge 3D assessment, just as in 2D US. When volume acquisition takes place, the following factors need to be considered.

1. GRAYSCALE SETTINGS: Because poor-quality 2D images will create poor-quality 3D images, it is mandatory to optimize the grayscale 2D image prior to volume acquisition. The machine settings applied to a good 2D US image should be those applied to a diagnostic-quality 3D US image. We should therefore pay special attention to use the best settings, as the quality of the acquired volume will determine the success in effectively "reading" the 3D images.
2. ACQUISITION TIME AND ANGLE OF ROTATION: These are two of the main features defining volume quality. Angle of rotation determines the number of sections obtained during acquisition. The wider the angle of rotation, the bigger the volume that is acquired and the longer the acquisition time that is required. The longer the acquisition time, the clearer the image will be. However, the probability of movement artifacts increases. Thus, because acquisition speed is inversely correlated with resolution, care should be taken to adjust acquisition time as well as the size of the volume containing the structure to be evaluated. When acquiring a volume of the fetal brain in the sagittal or coronal plane, an angle of rotation of 60 to 80° is suggested, whereas when an axial approach is used, a 45 to 60° angle should be used.
3. ACOUSTIC SHADOWING: As discussed earlier, after 15 to 16 weeks' gestation, mounting bone thickness may preclude an adequate evaluation of 3D images, as any shadowing on the 2D image will be embedded in the 3D volume. Therefore, an attempt to acquire the volume through an acoustic window, just as with 2D US, is highly recommended.

   When the volumes are acquired transvaginally, two volumes should be taken. One should be acquired on the sagittal plane obtained by aligning the US plane with the longitudinal axis of the fetal brain using any of the fontanelles or sagittal suture as an acoustic window. The bregmatic fontanelle offers the largest acoustic window in the anterior portion of the brain. The second volume should be acquired on the coronal plane, which is achieved by rotating the probe 90° from the previous scanning plane. Most of the time both approaches are possible. The examiner can always help obtain the desired plane by applying gentle external manipulation of the fetal head with a free hand.

   In scanning transabdominally, the 3D volume is generally obtained using an axial approach. We recommend using two perpendicular planes: an axial plane that can be obtained through the squamosal suture and a sagittal plane through the metopic suture; the latter is sometimes hard to obtain, but it yields excellent quality volumes. However, acquisition in any plane may be feasible; in that case, on-screen or off-line rotation of the brain into the customary classic planes is possible.

   The advantages of the 2D transvaginal transfontanelle approach compared with conventional transabdominal scanning of the fetal brain have been described previously in this chapter, as well as in the literature.[41] However, two distinct advantages are added to 2D transvaginal imaging when using 3D transvaginal US.

   First, the axial section, which is rarely seen with 2D transvaginal transfontanelle imaging, can be reconstructed on the orthogonal sections, although this reconstructed image will be of lesser quality compared with that of the sagittal and coronal planes. Second, the 2D sections obtained from "slicing" the 3D volume are parallel to each other, whereas, when using 2D transvaginal transfontanelle neurosongraphy, the planes obtained radiate from a single point, usually from the anterior fontanelle, and are oblique to one another (Figure 2–76). This may present a real advantage when pictures are presented to neurology or neurosurgeon consultants because they are generally more familiar with the parallel tomographic images of MRI or CT scans.

   The most commonly used scanning approach is clearly the transabdominal 2D scan. It is therefore natural that most will use 3D scanning of the fetal brain by transabdominal volume acquisition. It should be remembered, however, that when using the transabdominal route, good-quality images may not be feasible at all times. We strongly recommend performing a transvaginal acquisition whenever possible. Furthermore, in those fetuses with suspicion of brain anomaly or when it is impossible to obtain a view in order to correctly assess normal brain anatomy, an external version of the fetus into the vertex presentation is warranted. This procedure should be tried before one decides to obtain an MRI of the fetal brain, as a good-quality transvaginally obtained volume is superior to most MRI images.
4. FETAL MOVEMENT: Fetal movements during the volume acquisition are the main cause of motion artifacts and are demonstrated by the presence of wavelike stripes on images on almost all planes (Figure 2–77). In order to minimize movement artifacts, if possible, the acquisition should be performed during fetal rest or between periods of fetal movements. The choice of longer acquisition times is best for a quiet fetus, whereas faster speeds should be applied for an active fetus. In addition, the patient can be asked to hold her breath during the acquisition time (this will not influence artifacts created by the fetus).
5. FETAL POSITION: Other factors that can compromise image quality are position of the fetal head, a fetal hand above the face or if the face is targeted, a fetal face too close to the uterine wall or an anterior placenta. As mentioned before, sometimes the fetal head may need to be manipulated by the nonscanning

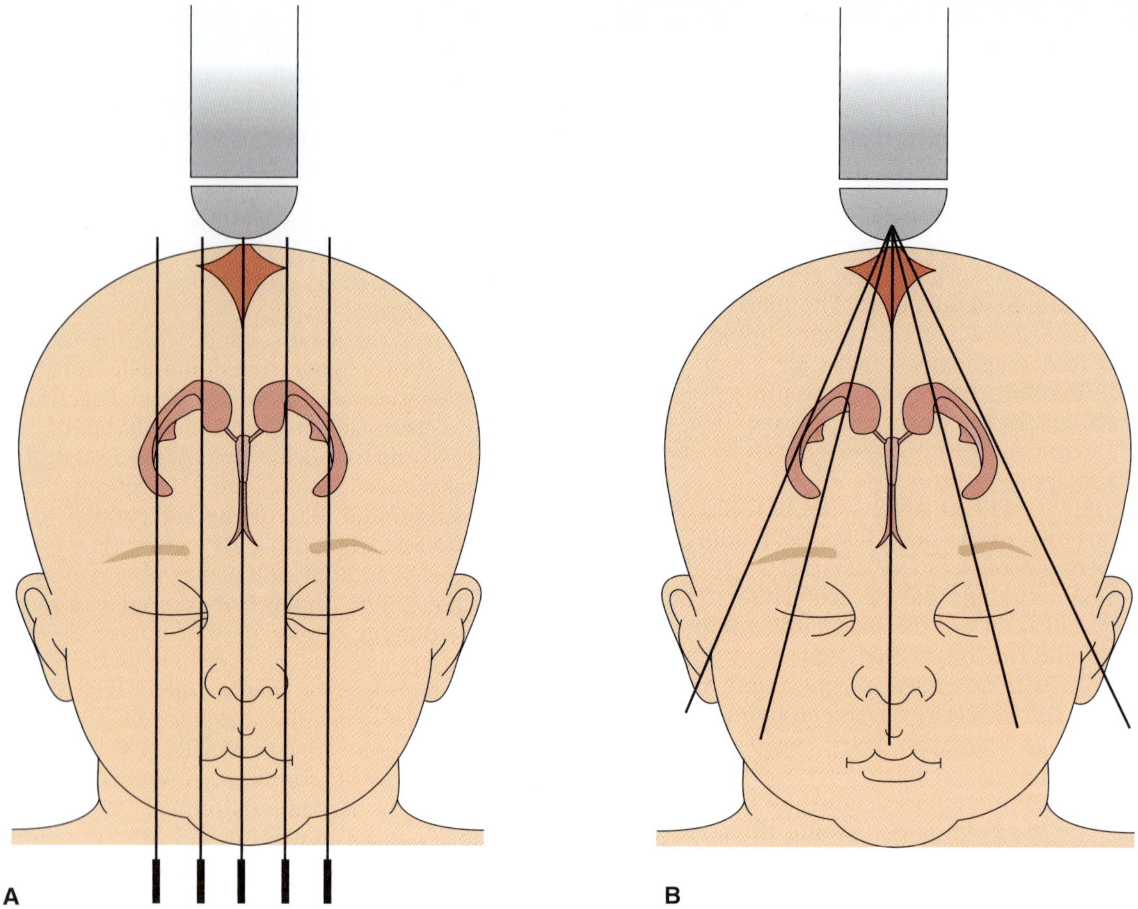


**Figure 2–76.** The diagrams demonstrate the different angles in which the coronal and sagittal views are obtained with 3D (**A**) and 2D (**B**) transvaginal ultrasound. The sections recreated from the 3D volume are parallel to each other, similar to those obtained when using a CT or an MRI (**A**). When scanning with conventional 2D ultrasound through the anterior fontanelle, the planes arise from a single point (fontanelle) and fan-out laterally (**B**).

hand to allow access to fontanelles, which serve as an acoustic window.

6. FLUID–TISSUE INTERFACE: Among the factors that may interfere with good-quality surface-rendering imaging is oligohydramnios, the absence of or low amount of amniotic fluid around the region of interest.

Luckily, if the fetus is in the vertex presentation, many of the above hindrances are avoided, enabling the examiner to concentrate only on positioning the fontanelles and/or sutures vis-à-vis the footprint of the probe.

We should bear in mind that the acquisition plane provides the best image, thus the best information, whereas images on the reconstructed planes are of lesser quality. This limitation of 3D US is important when evaluating targeted structures that are better evaluated in a specific plane. Thus, spending the time necessary to obtain the adequate acquisition plane is warranted. As the technology (ie, the number of acquired slices) increases and resolution improves, the quality of the reconstructed planes is expected to improve, too.

## Data Storage

Once the volume has been acquired, it can be processed directly on the US system at the time of acquisition, or the stored digital volumes can be saved to the computer's hard disk. Transferring the data onto a CD or a smaller storage device allows the volume to be analyzed off-line using manipulation and postprocessing proprietary and brand-specific software. Different manufacturers have their own software to analyze 3D US volumes, including 4DView (GE Healthcare www.volusonclub.net/emea/4DView), QLAB (Koninklijke Philips Electronics www.healthcare.philips.com), SonoView Pro (Samsung Medison America, Cypress, CA www.samsungmedisonusa.com.), and Inspace interactive 3D viewer (Siemens). Unfortunately, they are not interchangable.

## Display Modalities

Multiple displays are available for the analysis of 3D volumes. These have been extensively described in the literature.[97–100] Of all the available displays, the primary modes most used for the purposes of a fetal neuroscan

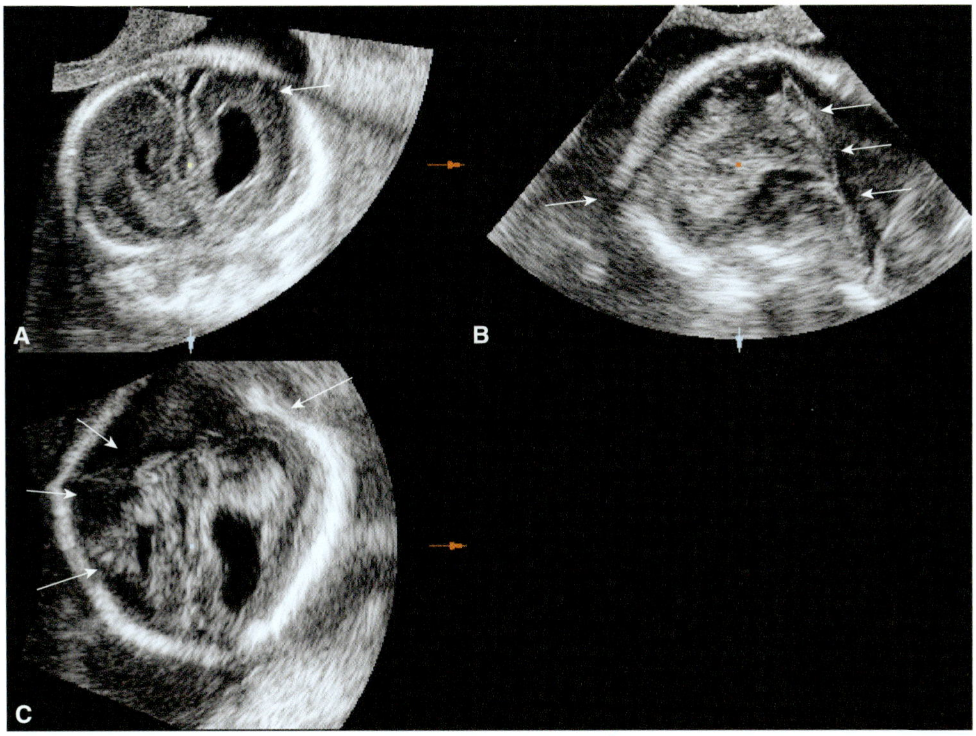


**Figure 2–77.** Multiplanar display mode of the fetal brain. After a brain volume has been acquired, the three orthogonal planes are displayed on the screen and volume quality can be assessed. Box A shows a coronal plane through the anterior horns of the lateral ventricles, box B a sagittal view, and box C an axial plane. No alignment of the different planes has been performed; therefore, the views shown in the three planes are asymmetrical. Note in this case how motion during volume acquisition has led to the presence of artifacts, which are demonstrated as wave-like stripes in all three orthogonal planes (arrows).

are the multiplanar mode, the tomographic display, and the inversion mode. However, the other less used modes will be described here, as they have shown potential in improving visualization of different fetal CNS structures.

### Multiplanar Imaging (Orthogonal Planes)

This image modality is the first type of display that we use and the one that in our experience is the mainstay of 3D US evaluation of the fetal brain. It allows simultaneous display of an image in the three classical anatomical planes (coronal, sagittal, and axial). The three boxes containing the orthogonal displays are called box A (upper left), which contains the plane parallel to the acquisition plane or starting plane, and box B (upper right) and box C (lower left), which contain the reconstructed planes. This allows simultaneous visualization of all three mutually perpendicular sectional planes. A fourth box may appear on the display screen if the rendering mode is activated; this is called box D (lower right), which contains the rendered image. This screen display corresponds to that seen when using the GE 4DView (www.volusoncub.net/emea/4DView) software (Figures 2–78 and 2–79).

An important tool available in the orthogonal display mode is the marker dot. The place of the marker dot indicates the same anatomical location on all three orthogonal planes, as at this very point the three planes meet (Figures 2–78 and 2–79). Thus, the relationships between different anatomical structures can readily and easily be assessed by moving this dot in one of the planes and evaluating the corresponding structure on the other two planes. Once we realize this, we are in possession of a powerful tool to localize anatomy and pathology.

A major advantage of using the multiplanar mode is that views that are not easily accessible by customary 2D transabdominal or even transvaginal US such, as the sagittal plane, can be obtained by scrolling or navigating in the volume in a continuous fashion at will.[101] Because one can move freely in the saved brain volume in all three planes, virtually any desired diagnostic plane can be achieved.

Because spatial orientation when scrolling in the volume may appear difficult for inexperienced sonographers, a standardization of transabdominal and transvaginal 3D images is strongly recommended. This will in turn avoid erroneous topographical interpretations. We refer the reader to the literature[102] for a thorough description of standardization of 3D images. Still, different operators and centers may have their preferred way to display the "starting" orthogonal display. However, our group usually displays the orthogonal planes on the screen as follows: in box A, regardless of the acquisition plane, the coronal section of the head; in box B, the median section with the fetal face facing box A (this allows the right and left sides to

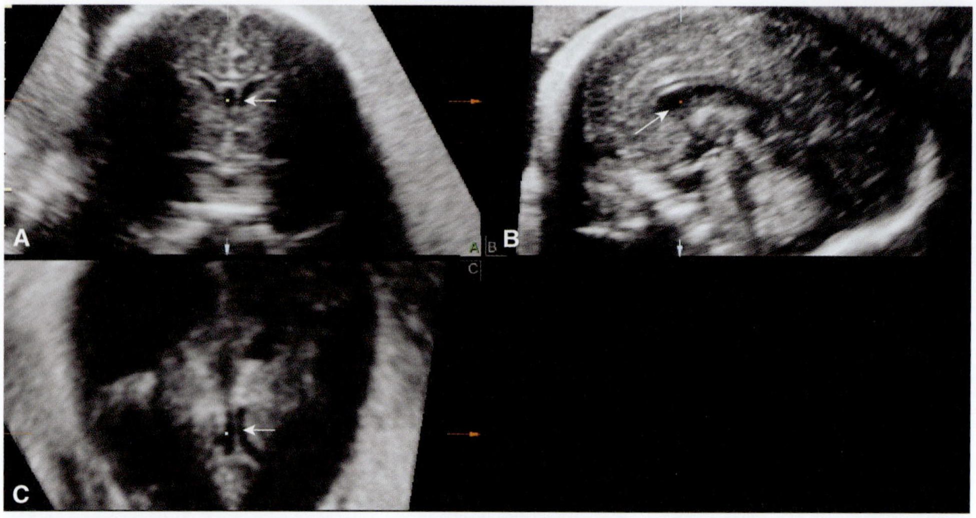


**Figure 2–78.** Multiplanar display of the fetal brain at 22 weeks' gestation in the three orthogonal planes: the coronal plane in box A, the median plane in box B, and the axial plane in box C. Note the "marker dot" representing the intersection of the three orthogonal planes (arrows), which is placed in this image in the cavum septi pellucidi.

be displayed as in traditional imaging); in box C, the axial section with the forehead facing inferior on the screen (Figure 2–80). Other groups using different US equipment might display the three planes of the volume in a different manner, with box C demonstrating the sagittal section of the fetal head. There is one advantage to leaving the display unaltered without any rotation: one can realize in which plane the volume was acquired.

Once the volume is orientated as desired, one can start navigating or scrolling in the volume. Each box can be "activated" so that all the functions selected will pertain to that box only. A systematic scrolling protocol is suggested to perform a complete sweep in each of the three orthogonal planes in order to include all the recommended planes for dedicated neurosonography. Using five to seven continuous coronal, three sagittal, and three axial sections will allow a detailed evaluation of the fetal brain anatomy. In addition, other sections and planes can be generated at will.

### Multiplanar Mode and Evaluation of Midline Structures

Although 3D US has not been proven to be superior to 2D US in the evaluation of the intracranial anatomy, the use of 3D reconstruction of sagittal planes has been proposed in the literature as an adjunct to traditional 2D neurosonography for evaluating midline structures.[103–106]

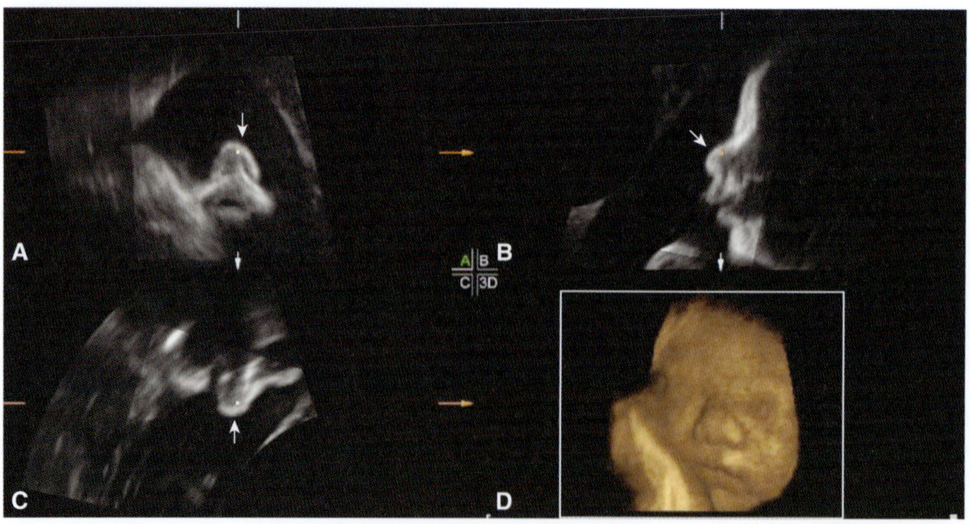


**Figure 2–79.** Multiplanar display of a fetal face at 32 weeks' gestation in the three orthogonal planes: the coronal plane in box A, the median plane in box B, the axial plane in box C, and a rendered image showing the fetal face in box D are presented. Note how both imaging modalities, the multiplanar display and the surface rendering mode, can be used to complement each other. The "marker dot" is placed in this image on the tip of the nose and one can evaluate the integrity of the upper lip on the coronal plane of the multiplanar display and on the rendered image.

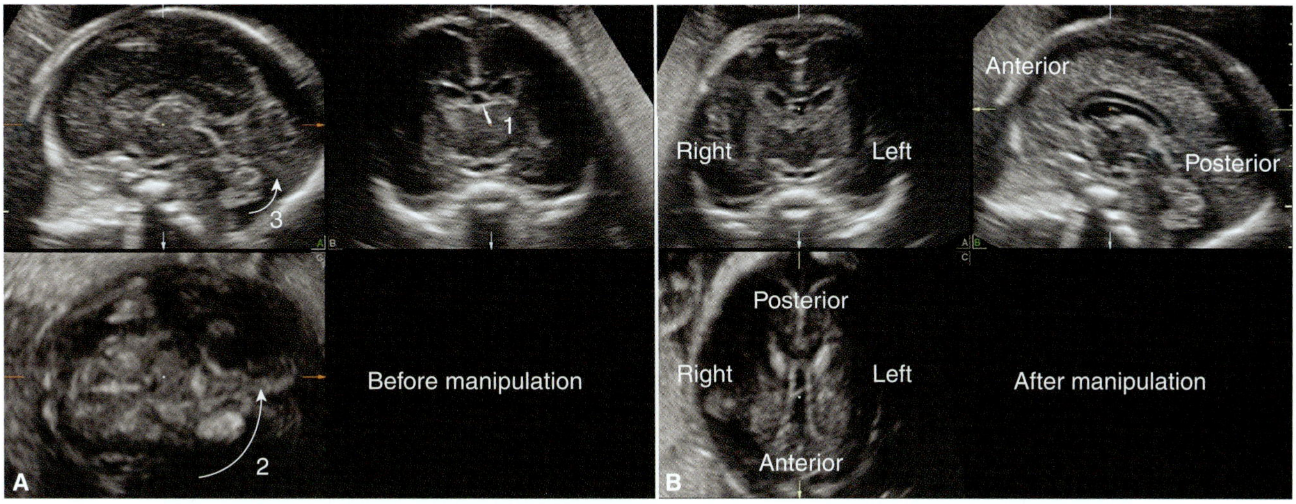


**Figure 2–80.** Multiplanar image of the fetal brain before and after manipulation of the volume in order to display the three orthogonal planes as desired. (**A**) Before manipulation the following steps were performed: 1) the marker dot in box B was placed in the cavum septi pelucidi; 2) 90° Z axis rotation of the axial image in box C was performed so that the front of the fetal head faces downwards; 3) "fine-tune" into the perfect orientation of the three orthogonal planes in order to achieve a perfect alignment in all planes was performed. (**B**) After manipulation, the orthogonal planes are displayed as follows: in box A, the coronal section of the head, in box B, the sagittal section with the fetus facing the left side of the screen, and in box C, the axial section with the forehead facing inferior on the screen.

This is especially useful when a median plane is difficult to obtain due to unfavorable fetal position or when examiners do not use a transvaginal approach. In such cases, 3D US imaging enables a rapid and easy mode to obtain the median plane by scrolling in the volume, as described previously.

A good correlation has been demonstrated between the median plane obtained directly by 2D US and those reconstructed with 3D US.[103] Recent studies, including our experience, have shown improved visualization of midline structures, such as the corpus callosum, the brainstem, and the vermis, with 3D US.[104–106] Because direct visualization of the corpus callosum using standard axial planes is not feasible due to its arched shape, coronal and median planes have to be obtained using a 2D transvaginal or transabdominal approach. However, a 3D reconstructed sagittal plane may be obtained from an axial or coronal approach, allowing rapid and easy evaluation of the midline structures. Most authors demonstrated that this technique enables adequate evaluation of the corpus callosum through the transabdominal scanning route.[100–103] However, the following aspects specific to visualization of the corpus callosum and structures of the posterior fossa have to be considered.

The appearance of the reconstructed image will depend on the plane of the volume acquisition. When a 3D transabdominal scanning is performed, and a median plane approach is used, the corpus callosum appears as a thin sonolucent stripe with well-defined echogenic contours (Figure 2–81A) On a reconstructed image from an axial plane, some authors suggest that the corpus callosum is depicted as a comma-shaped echogenic structure overlying the cavum septi pellucidi (CSP);[104–105] others that the corpus callosum may not be differentiated clearly from the CSP,[106–108] and a single anechoic comma-shaped image on top of the third ventricle is seen instead (Figure 2–81B). Interestingly, other authors believe that this echogenic structure overlying the CSP corresponds instead to the interface of the cingulate gyrus, the cingulate sulcus, the CSF, and the blood flow of the callosal arteries.[109] Therefore, because these may be only indirect signs of callosal integrity, when brain pathology is suspected, a median plane approach is highly recommended in order to visualize directly the corpus callosum.

### Multiplanar Mode and Evaluation of the Posterior Fossa

One of the main advantages of using the multiplanar mode to evaluate the posterior fossa is that it enables simultaneous visualization of the three orthogonal planes of the cerebellum (Figure 2–82). This allows an easier and more rapid assessment of the integrity of the vermis, along with its size and position. However, at times, when evaluating the posterior fossa with 3D US, a suboptimal quality image is obtained, and the infratentorial structures, such as the cerebellum, the vermis, the fourth ventricle, and the cistern magna, are blurred. This is due to acoustic shadowing of the petrous ridges of the bony base of the skull. When an axial approach is used, this shadowing can be minimized by keeping an angle of ~45° between the incident US beam and the midline, as suggested by Pilu et al.[108] When the sagittal or coronal plane of acquisition is used in scanning through the posterior fontanelle, image quality can be improved. Other experts suggest the use of a transabdominal transfontanellar approach to improve visualization of the cerebellar structures, as well as the corpus callosum.[108]

### Multiplanar Mode and the Three-Horn View

Evaluation of the lateral ventricles is part of fetal neurosonography. This includes the measurement of the

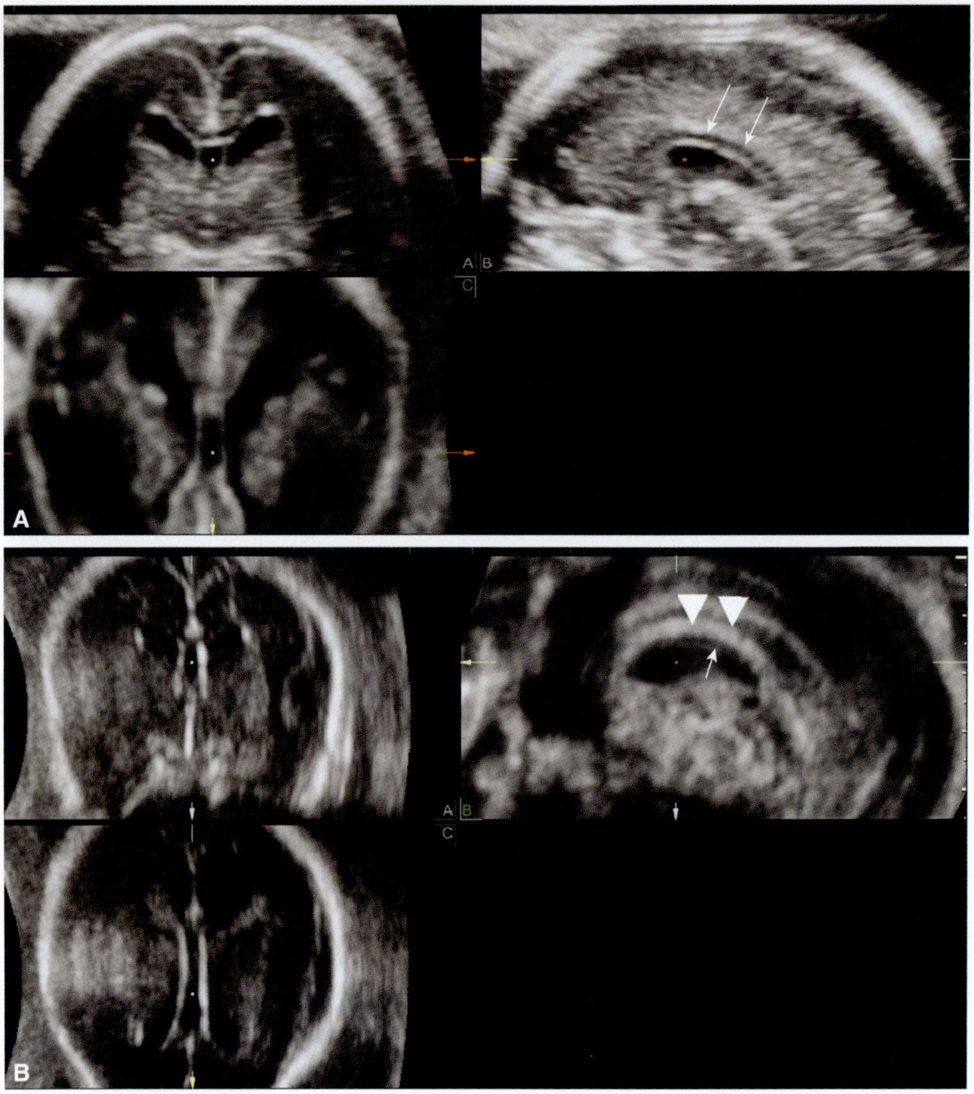


**Figure 2–81.** Multiplanar analysis of an ultrasound volume of the fetal head obtained by transabdominal scanning: (**A**) volume acquired using a sagittal plane and (**B**) volume acquired using an axial plane. Note the difference of resolution of the CC. When a sagittal plane is used, the CC appears as a thin sonolucent stripe with well-defined echogenic contours (arrows). When an axial plane is used, the CC is not easily differentiated from the cavum septi pellucidi. Sometimes a thin echogenic contour that separates it from the underlying CSP (thin arrow) and a comma-shaped echogenic structure overlying both the CC and CSP (arrow head) are seen, as demonstrated in this case.

atrium of the lateral ventricle in the axial plane.[110,111] Other measurements of the ventricular system using transabdominal and transvaginal transfontanelle US have been previously published.[32,112,113] However, our observations led us to believe that the "classical" measurement of the lateral ventricles in the axial plane does not truly represent the dynamic and progressive change in shape and size that takes place in all three horns. We therefore looked for a single scanning plane that reveals all three horns (anterior, posterior, and inferior) simultaneously. We termed this plane the "three-horn view."[114] This scanning plane can be visualized with 2D transvaginal transfontanelle sonography when an oblique section of the brain is obtained; this section is lateral to the median section of the brain. However, using 3D US is an easier way to obtain the three-horn view, regardless of the acquisition plane. After obtaining the proper volume of the fetal brain, it takes only few minutes to manipulate the volume in order to accomplish the three-horn view, as described elsewhere (Figure 2–83). This view can be used to compare the appearance of the ventricular horns and their sizes, providing diagnostic and clinically useful information.

## Tomographic Display

This mode allows a successive and sequential display in which multiple images parallel to each other are displayed at the same time. It is one of the most useful static display modalities used during fetal neuroscan because it enables the visualization of serial sections similar to those used by CT and MRI. One can alternate and create tomographic series using all three orthogonal planes (Figures 2–84,

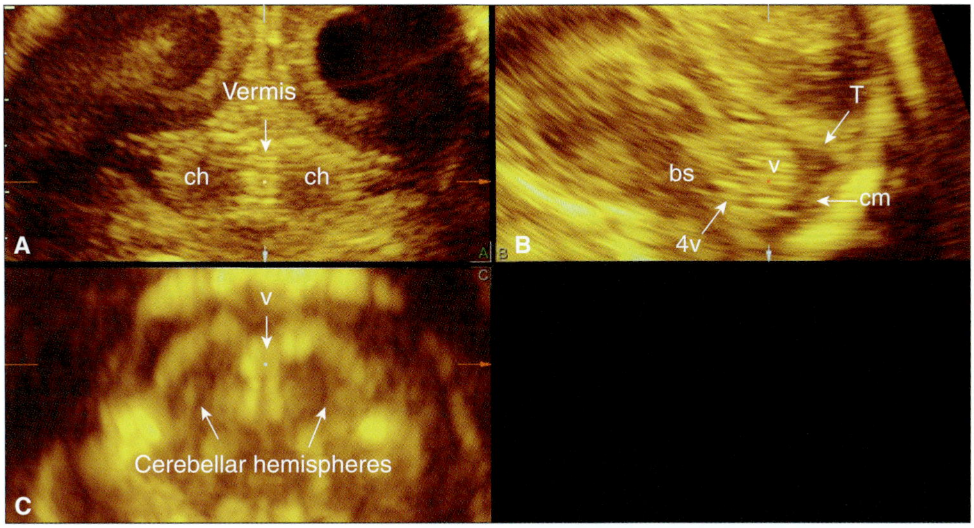


**Figure 2–82.** Multiplanar analysis of an ultrasound volume depicting the posterior fossa of a normal fetal brain at 22 weeks acquired by transabdominal ultrasound using the sagittal fontanelle as an acoustic window. This mode allows simultaneous visualization of the three orthogonal planes of the cerebellum and the main landmarks in order to assess the integrity of the vermis. In the coronal (**A**) and the axial plane (**C**) the cerebellar vermis (v) is shown as an echogenic structure in between the two cerebellar hemispheres (ch), which are less echogenic. In the median plane (**B**), the vermis together with other structures seen on that view such as the tentorium (T), the fourth ventricle (4v), the cistern magna (cm), and the brainstem (bs) are presented. Note that the "marker dot" is placed on the vermis.

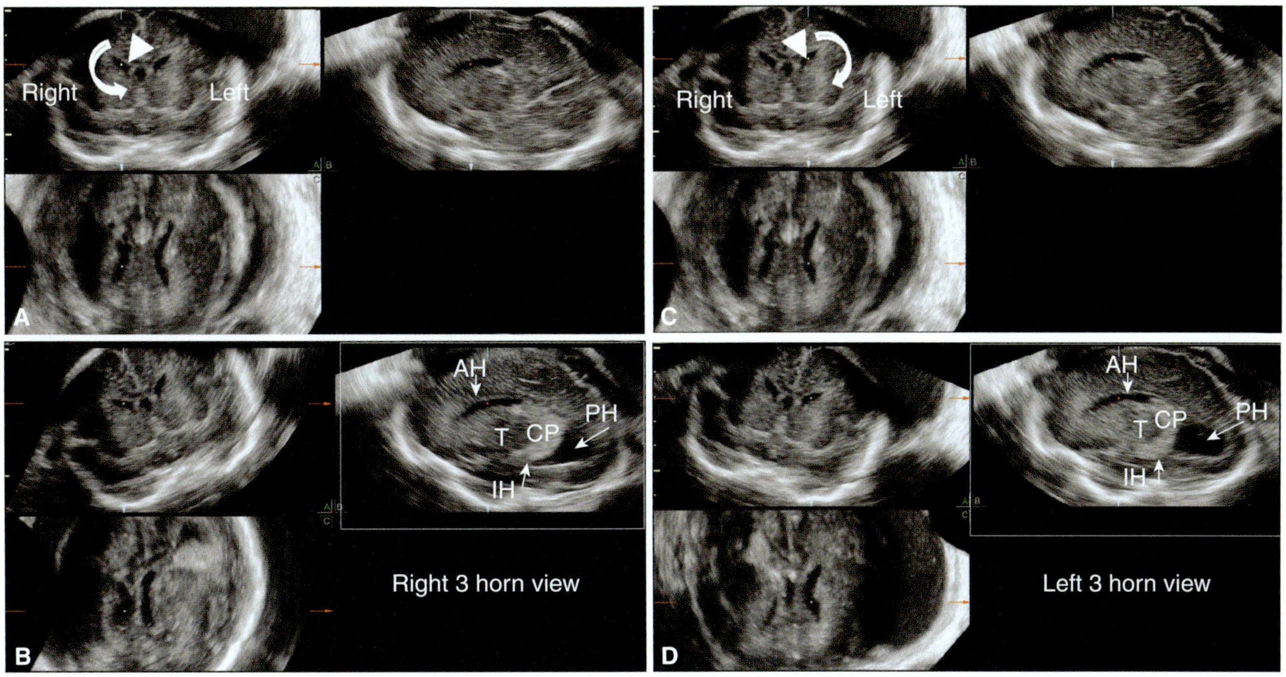


**Figure 2–83.** The "three-horn views" of a normal fetal brain at 22 weeks. In order to generate the right 3HV, first the desired coronal plane is selected and aligned with the other two orthogonal planes. Then the marker dot (arrowhead) is placed in the right lateral ventricle and the mid-coronal plane is rotated to the right as shown in image a. The result is the 3HV shown in a parasagittal view (highlighted in a box) as presented in image b. To obtain the left 3HV, the first step is identical to that of obtaining the right 3HV. The only difference is that the mid-coronal plane is rotated to the left as shown in image c. The result is the 3HV shown in a parasagittal view (highlighted in a box) presented in image d. Note in both lateral ventricles the thin anterior horn (AH), the posterior horn (PH) of normal size, and the closed inferior horn (IH). Other structures seen on that view are the choroid plexus (CP) and the thalamus (T).

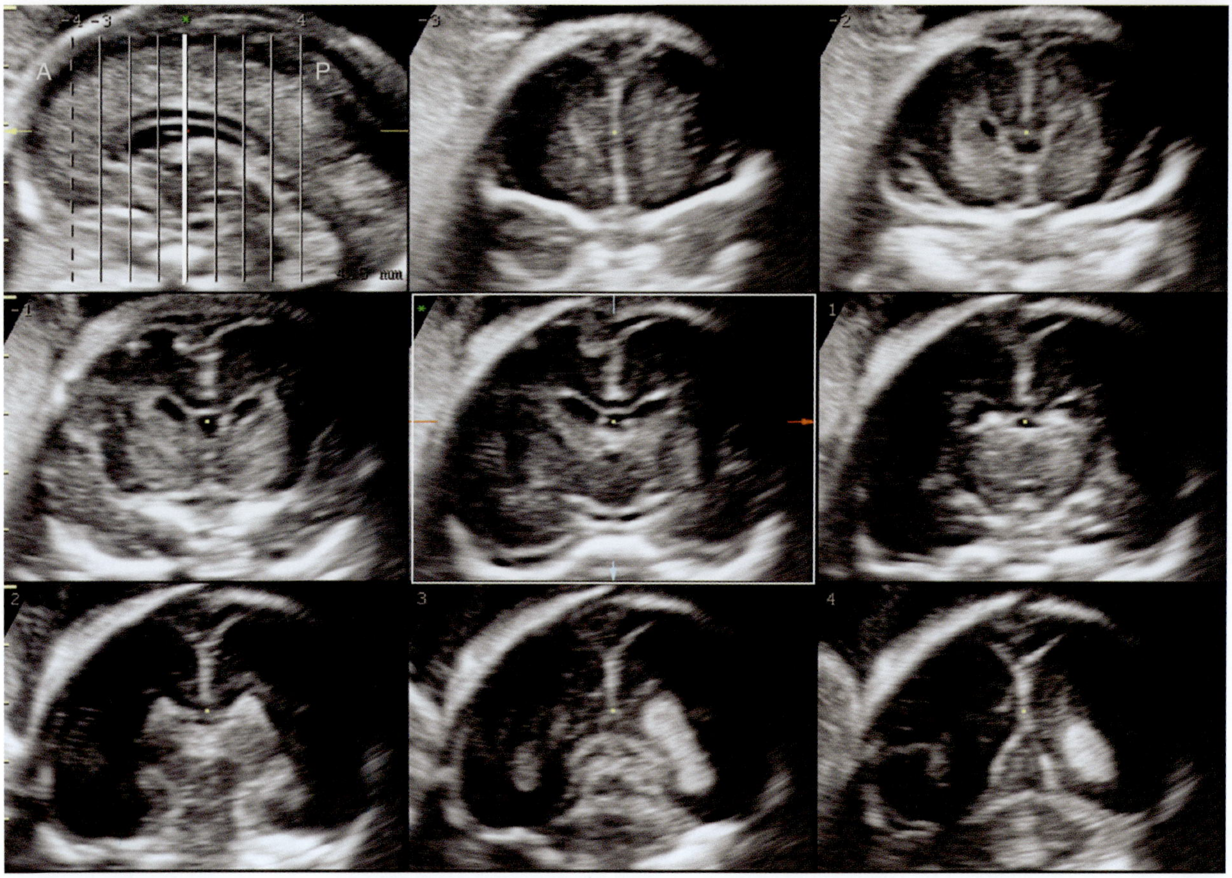

**Figure 2–84.** Tomographic ultrasound image obtained on a normal fetal brain at 22 weeks' gestation demonstrating successive coronal sections displayed from anterior (A) to posterior (P). The coronal planes correspond to the planes that are marked crossing the brain on the sagittal image. The slice interval is 4.5 mm and the "marker dot" is seen in the midline on the cavum septi pellucidi.

2–85, and 2–86). Usually a reference image is shown in the upper left side of the picture, with the parallel lines representing the pertinent picture in a string of consecutive sections displayed sequentially. The examiner can define the distance between the slices usually ranging from 2 to 5 mm. The same display format can be applied to grayscale, Doppler, or power Doppler containing volumes.

### Volume Rendering

Rendering displays includes a variety of modes. The most commonly used are the surface and the inversion rendering modes. Advantages of the rendering modes include the use of different lighting, filtering, and transparency levels, which allows better visualization and perception of certain structures.

### Thick-Slice Rendering

In this mode, a number of successive slices are "collapsed" into one single rendered 2D picture or plane, which enhances edges, improves contrast detection, and gives more depth to the image. If rendering boxes are placed on the orthogonal planes, then on two of the planes the boxes are narrowed to a minimum; thus, the picture in the rendering box represents the thick-slice image of many collapsed 2D images (Figure 2–87). It is useful to study structures requiring better definition, such as the vermis, the spine, and the lateral ventricles. This method of obtaining the thick-slice display was lately replaced by the one-step volume contrast imaging (VCI) display mode 4D View (GE Healthcare).

### Static Volume Contrast Imaging

This software application is essentially the same as the thick-slice rendering, but instead of manipulating the volume as described above using the thick-slice mode, the same process is achieved by touching only one simple control. By controlling the slice thickness to be between 2 and 5 mm, thus defining the number of tissue layers, US artifacts, such as speckles and noise pixels, are decreased so that anatomical edges are enhanced. This process results in an image with improved tissue contrast[115] (Figures 2–88 and 2–89). Improved resolution and contrast using volume contrast imaging was compared to those of 2D US images by different authors studying the posterior fossa.

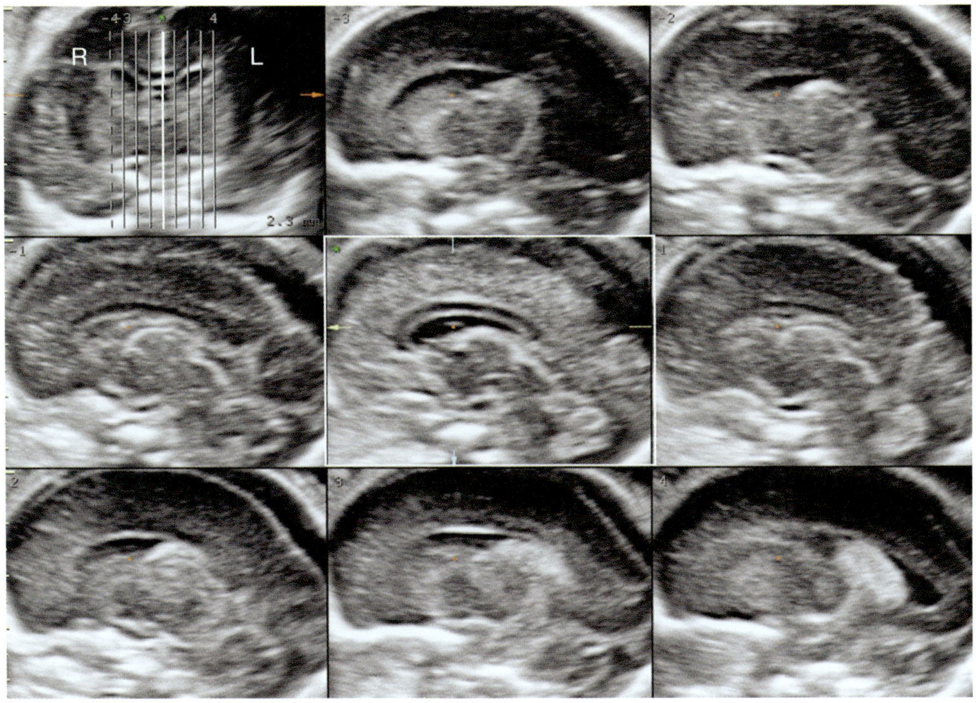


**Figure 2–85.** Tomographic ultrasound image obtained on a normal fetal brain at 22 weeks' gestation showing successive sagittal sections displayed from left to right. The sagittal planes correspond to the planes that are marked crossing the brain on the coronal image. The slice interval is 2.3 mm and the marker dot is seen in the midline on the cavum septi pellucidi, therefore both right (R) and left (L) of the median sections are seen.

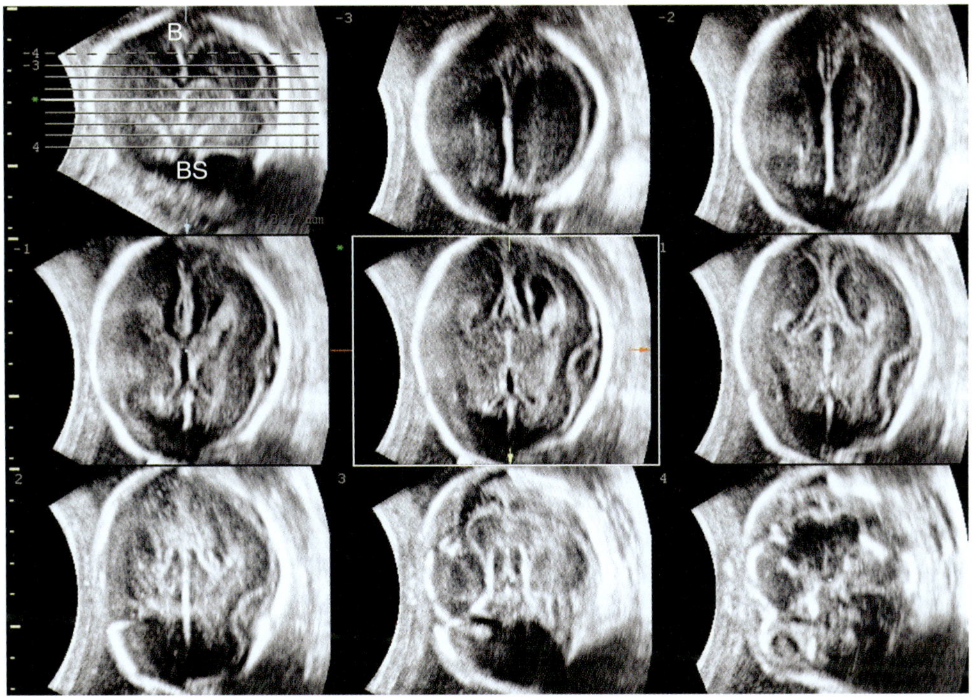


**Figure 2–86.** Tomographic ultrasound image obtained on a normal fetal brain at 22 weeks' gestation demonstrating successive axial planes displayed from the bregma (B) to the base of the skull (BS). The axial planes correspond to the planes that are marked crossing the brain on the coronal image. The slice interval is 3.7 mm and the "marker dot" is seen in the midline on the cavum septi pellucidi.

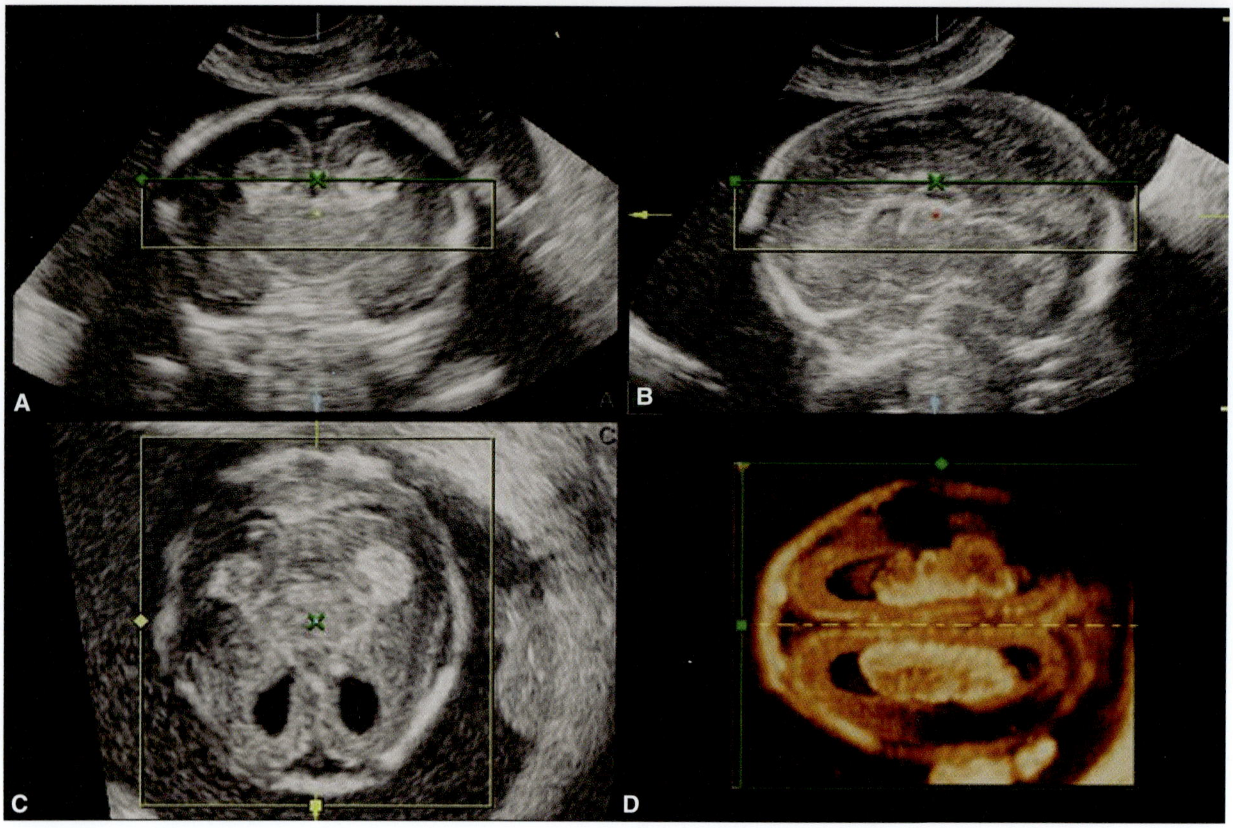


**Figure 2–87.** "The thick slice" mode is demonstrated. Box A shows a fetal brain at 22 weeks in the coronal plane, box B in the median plane, and box C in the axial plane. The box or region of interest shows the selected area of the volume in all three planes that has been "collapsed" into a 2D image enabling enhanced edge detection presented in box D as a "thick slice." Note that the region of interest is placed at a level in which both lateral ventricles are shown.

The application of this filter improved the definition of the landmarks of structures such as the cerebellar vermis and fourth ventricle.[116]

### Surface Rendering

The image rendering of the fetal body surface is the most widely known and most commonly used display modality of 3D. This mode allows reconstruction of surface features of a given structure resembling a photograph (Figure 2–90). The surface effect is achieved by various directional illumination combinations. A selection of lighting, gradient, and opacity levels can enhance the clarity and the desired quality of the surface-rendering effect. It is important to understand that a significant amount of fluid has to be between the transducer and the surface to be rendered. Because certain brain anomalies are associated with facial dysmorphism, this image mode can be very helpful in order to rule out or confirm anomalies involving the face. In addition, the images provided can be of invaluable help for parents as well as for consulting physicians. No detailed neurosonogram is complete without looking at facial structures. This is even more important when CNS anomalies are detected. Several anomalies of the brain have been associated with pathognomonic features. This is why surface rendering of the face and/or the skull is so useful.

### Radiograph, Maximum ("Bone"), or Transparency Mode

This mode allows selective imaging of the bony structures by eliminating weaker echoes originating from the soft tissues of the fetus and prominently displaying strong echoes. This results in a picture similar to a radiograph of the bony structures of the fetus. Therefore, this mode is an ideal tool in the demonstration of the cranial bones, as well as the corresponding sutures[117,118] (Figure 2–1A). This issue was discussed earlier in this chapter. When searching for anomalies of the skull or the fetal skeleton, this proves an invaluable tool.

### 3D Sonoangiography

This mode enables selective imaging of blood vessels after a 3D acquisition of power or color Doppler containing volume.[119,120] The technique of volume acquisition and manipulation is the same as with other 3D US modes. This feature is often used to assess the cerebral blood supply in normal and abnormal conditions. We are

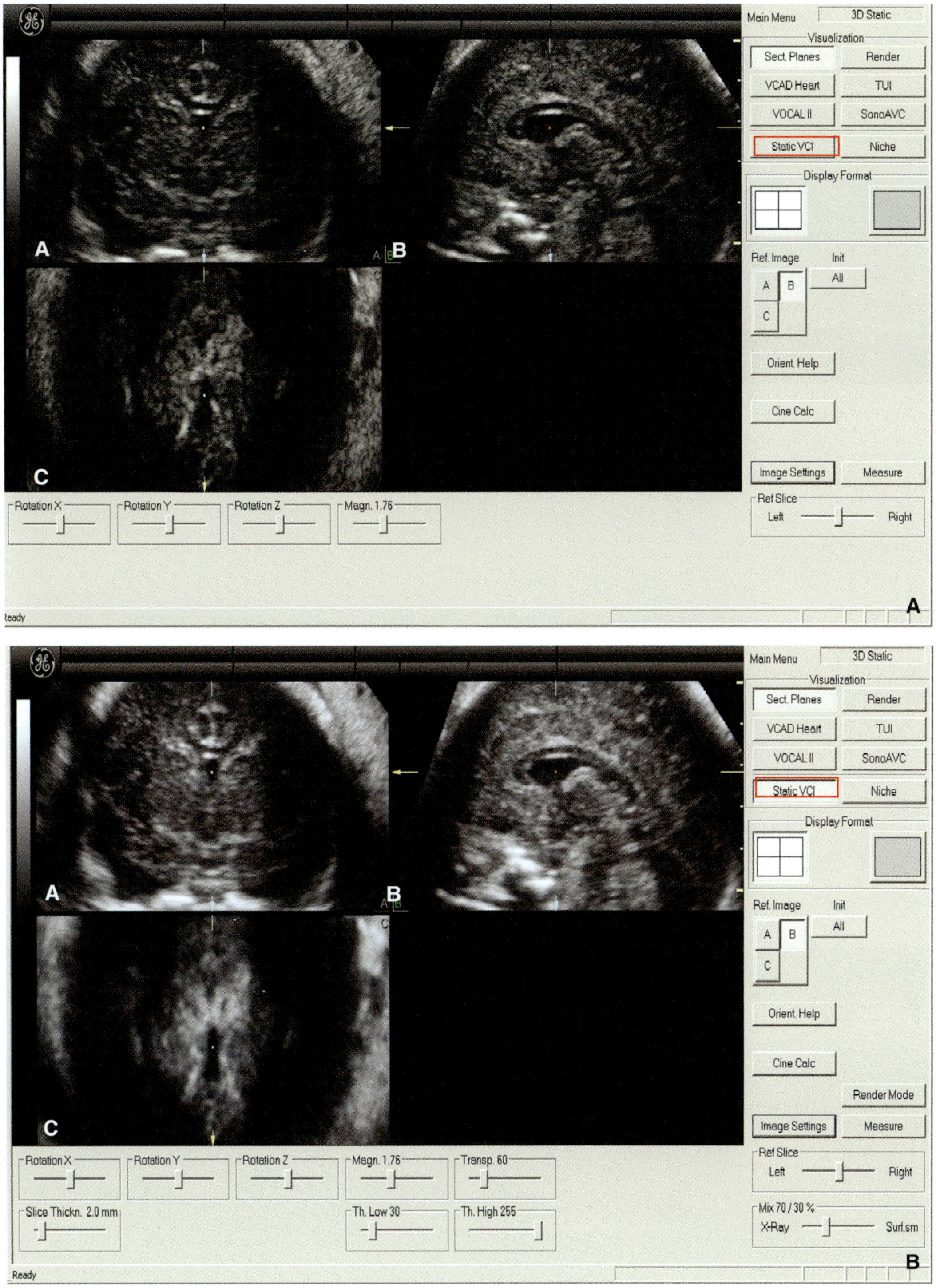


**Figure 2–88.** Multiplanar display of the fetal brain in the three orthogonal planes before (a) and after applying the static volume contrast imaging (b) just by touching one simple control (highlighted) and adjusting the desired slice thickness, in this case set at 2 mm. Note the difference in resolution and contrast of the images. On both images box A shows the coronal plane, box B shows the median plane, and box C shows the axial plane of the fetal head.

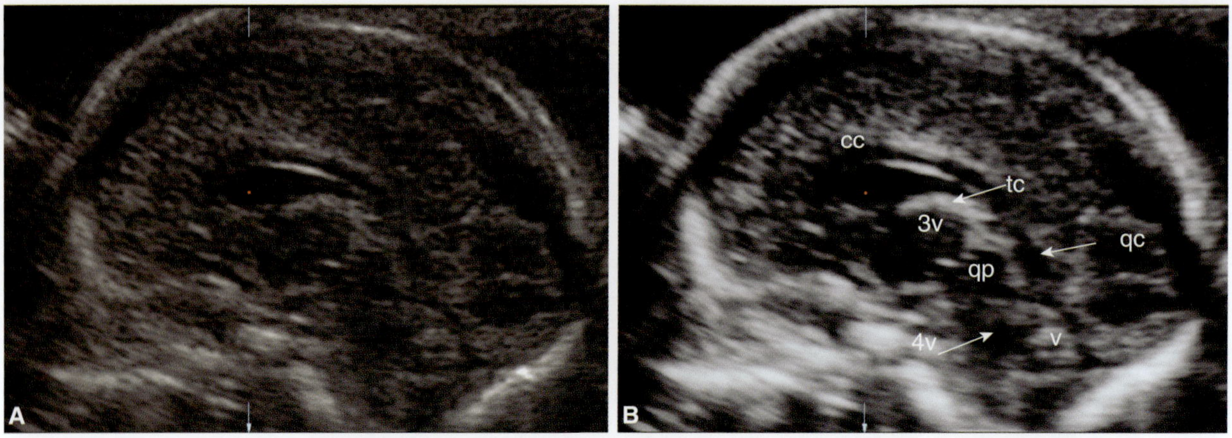


**Figure 2–89.** Sagittal view of the normal fetal head at 22 weeks of gestation. Comparison of two images obtained from the same ultrasound volume, using a standard plane mode (a) and with static volume contrast imaging with a thickness of 3 mm (b). Note the difference in resolution and contrast of the images, which allows better differentiation of different structures such as the corpus callosum (cc), tela choroidea (tc), quadrigeminal plate (qp), quadrigeminal cistern (qc), third ventricle (3v), fourth ventricle (4v), and vermis (v). The structures on (a) are identical to those marked on (b).

mainly interested in the course of the pericallosal branch of the anterior cerebral artery (Figure 2–91), especially in those cases in which agenesis of the corpus callosum is suspected, as the presence of this artery is a useful marker of at least partial callosal integrity. In other cases, such as space-occupying lesions, the anatomy of the vessels may be helpful in determining the size and extent of the lesion. It is true that the course of any main vessel in the brain can be obtained and followed by regular 2D sonoangiography; however, it certainly requires great skill and is sometimes impossible, whereas 3D US allows a median plane to be obtained quite easily just by manipulating the volume and aligning the axial and coronal planes in the right position. Furthermore, a vascular tree of the whole brain corresponding to the brain volume included in the region of interest is displayed in a 3D fashion as a rendered image allowing rotation using the three orthogonal planes and viewing

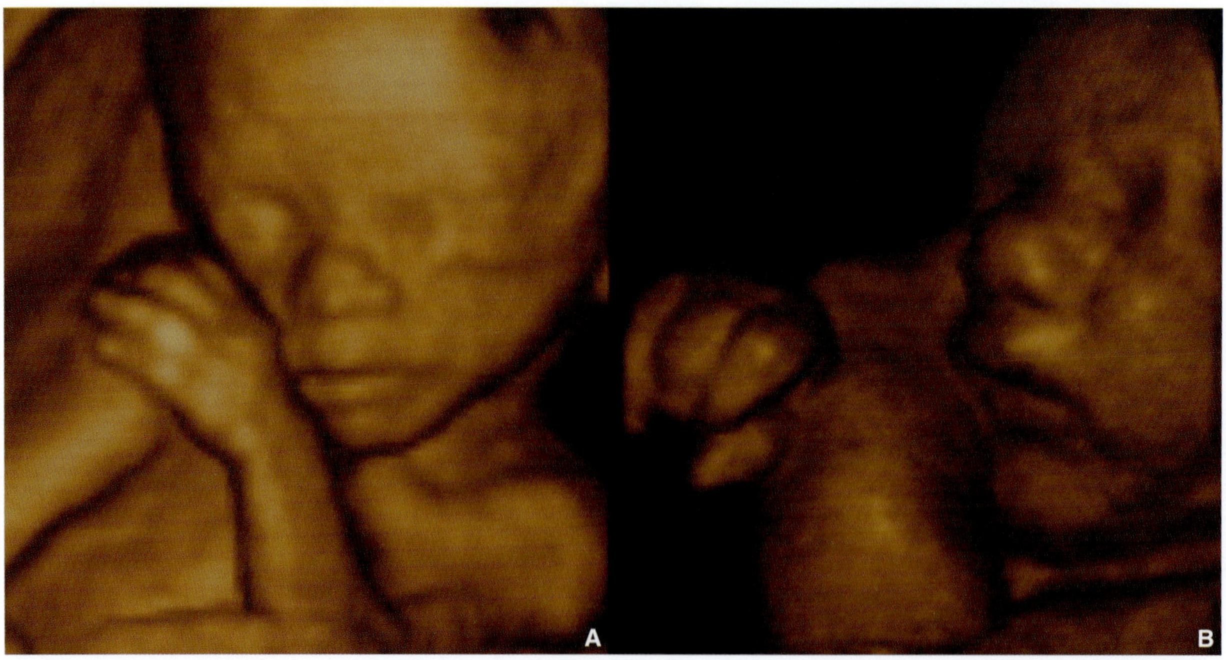


**Figure 2–90.** Surface rendering mode. Normal fetal face at 20 weeks (a) and at 32 weeks (b). Note how the nose and lips can be seen and recognized, resembling a photograph.

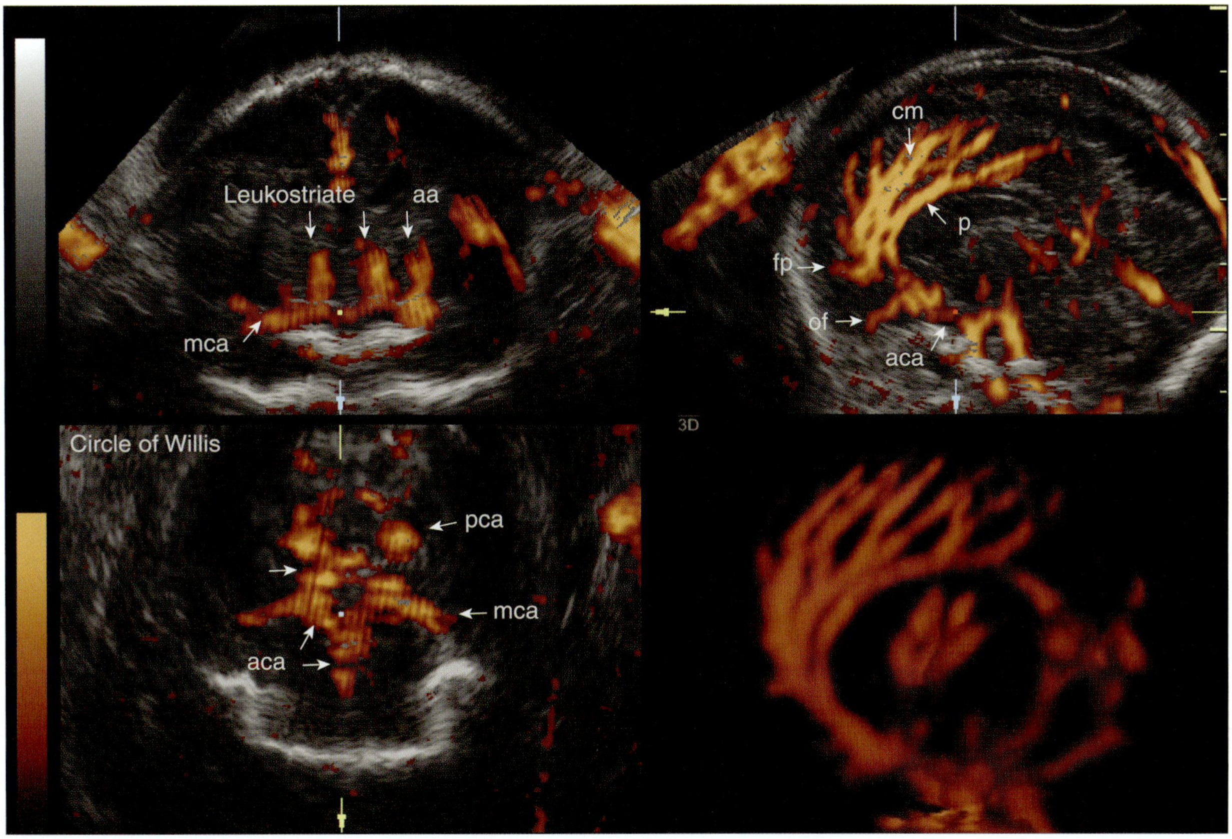


**Figure 2–91.** 3D angiography display mode enables selective imaging of blood flow through vessels after a 3D acquisition of a volume with power Doppler. The anterior cerebral artery (acm), callosomarginal artery (cm), the pericallosal artery (p), orbitofrontal (of), fronto polar artery (fp), middle cerebral atery (mca), posterior cerebral artery (pca), and posterior communicating artery (Post Com) are presented.

the course of the vessels from different angles. In addition, this image modality is an excellent teaching tool for students and residents. For more details see Chapter 15.

### Glass Body Mode

While color Doppler or power Doppler is switched on, it is possible to simultaneously display grayscale and color flow information. When the color rendering is used in conjunction with the transparency mode, a "glass body" mode is achieved (Figure 2–92).

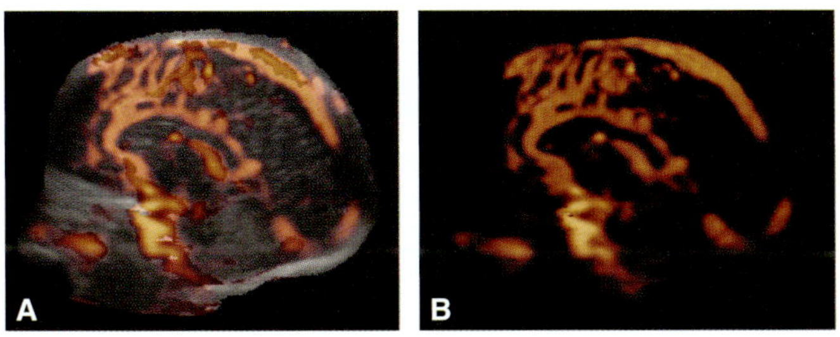


**Figure 2–92.** Glass body display mode. When a volume with grey scale is used in conjunction with the color rendering, the "glass body" display is achieved allowing us to see the brain vessels through the transparent skull at 22 weeks (a). Volume data can also be displayed as color rendering alone (b). The pericallosal artery and branches are demonstrated.

### Inversion Mode

This display mode inverts the anechoic fluid-filled areas of the acquired volume into echogenic structures. Thus, the on-screen appearance is that of a castlike image of the studied structure. This mode can be particularly useful to display the ventricular system or any pathologic fluid-filled space of the fetal brain[39,121] (Figure 2–93). The use of the inversion was demonstrated earlier in this chapter when discussing sonoembryology. At that early stage of fetal brain development, 3D US has made it possible to visualize planes of the embryonic brain not available in 2D US. Furthermore, the inversion rendering mode allows volume estimation of embryonic brains[21,122] and has been shown to be very helpful in understanding normal development of the fetal brain at these early stages by displaying casts of the fluid-filled cavities.[40] Figures 2–18, 2–24, 2–25, 2–26, 2–27, 2–28, and 2–29 show the use of this display pertaining to the normal development of the ventricular system. When using the inversion or the surface-rendering mode, artifacts may result from skull shadowing or from amniotic fluid; these can be eliminated using the electronic scalpel during off-line volume manipulation, as with any of the images obtained by surface rendering. The electronic scalpel and the eraser enable removal of structures that may obliterate or

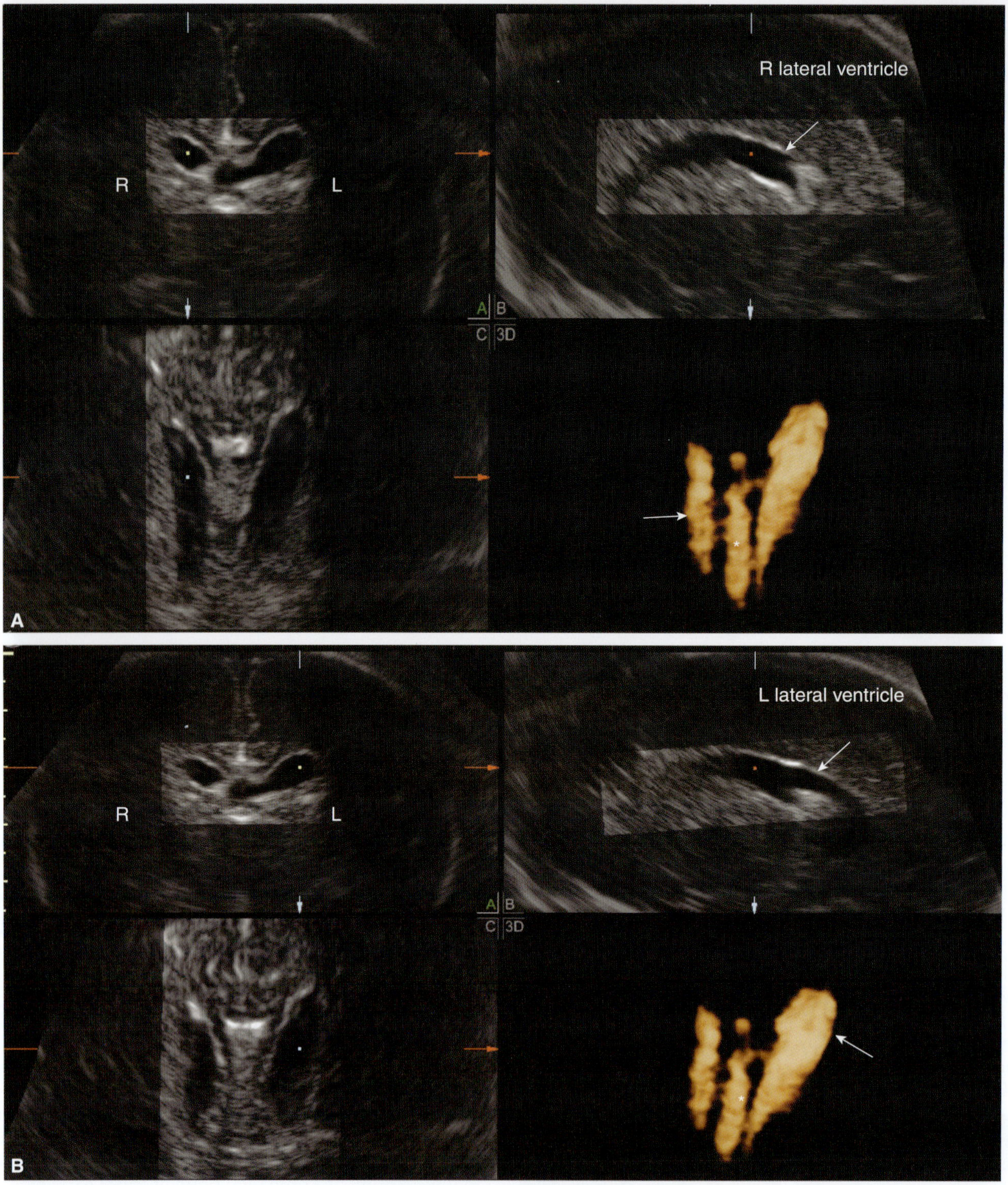


**Figure 2–93.** Multiplanar display of an ultrasound volume of a normal fetal brain at 21 weeks. The three orthogonal planes, coronal, sagittal, and axial planes, of the right and left lateral ventricles are presented in images a and b, respectively. Inversion mode demonstrates the shape of both lateral ventricles (arrows) and the cavum septi pellucidi (asterisk). Note the asymmetry of both ventricles depicted in both imaging modalities.

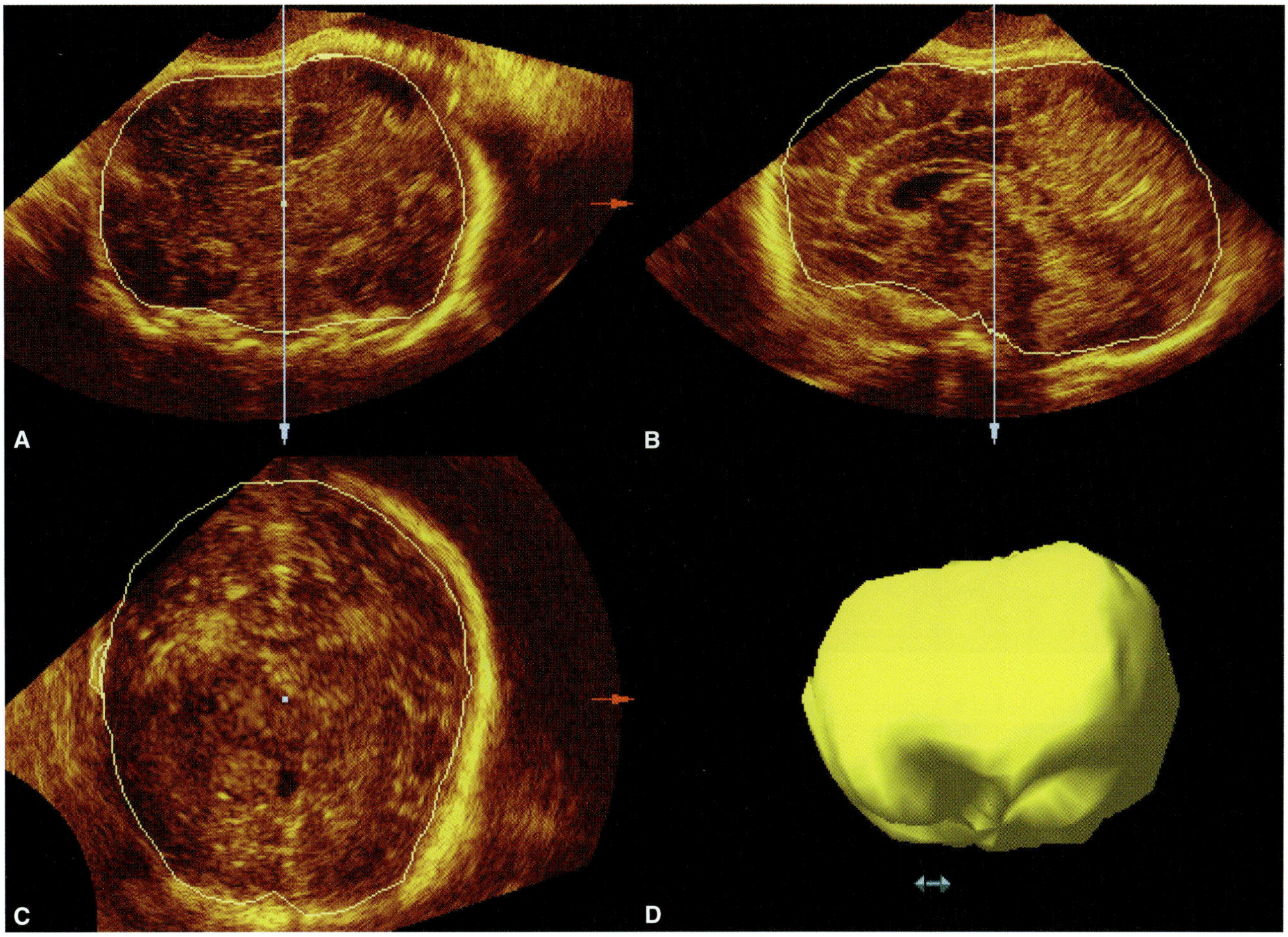


**Figure 2–94.** Measurement of fetal brain volume with 3D ultrasound. With the VOCAL mode, the internal borders of the head are traced manually with stepwise rotation of 30 degrees, taking the skull base as the lower border. First the coronal plane was fixed as the anchor (box A), with the "marker dot" on the midline. Second, the volume was determined by scrolling through the fetal head from one end to the other end and measuring the areas of eight to ten serial coronal cuts. Third, the areas were calculated at the inner edge of the fetal skull bone by manual tracing. The VOCAL mode measures the distance between each coronal cut and adds automatically the slices in between them to obtain the fetal brain volume. Box D shows the final volume reconstruction of the total intracranial region using VOCAL.

obscure the object to be studied, improving evaluation of the targeted object.[123]

One of the most important advantages of using volume scanning in general, more specifically, fetal neuroscanning, is that all of the different displays and rendering modes can be derived from the originally acquired volumes. In addition, any of the volumes displayed can be rotated around all three orthogonal planes to achieve the right plane.

### Volume Calculation: Virtual Organ Computer-Aided Analysis (VOCAL)

The acquisition of a 3D volume allows the reconstruction of a 2D image on which different, commonly used measurements can be performed. Among these are biparietal diameter, head circumference, ventricular dimensions, and different cerebellar measurements. However, the real advantage over 2D images is its potential to calculate the volume of a selected region of interest.

The VOCAL software (GE Healthcare, Kretz-Technik) enables the ultrasonographer to trace on-screen stepwise rotating organs such as the brain and to delineate or "cut out" their actual shapes. After doing this, the volume of the "cut-out" organ can be measured, and its content can be displayed using grayscale, glass body, or angiography display modes (Figure 2–94). Volume measurements can be achieved using either the multiplanar mode or the VOCAL software. If the volume was acquired using color or power Doppler, the vessel arrangement of the organ, as well as quantification of the blood flow containing voxels, can be counted and displayed in a quantitative fashion. This is one of the display modes toward which a significant amount of research activity is directed to evaluate its potential clinical use. Good intra- and interobserver reproducibility of intracranial volume calculation has been reported, as well as a good correlation with biparietal diameter (BPD) and head circumference (HC), by different

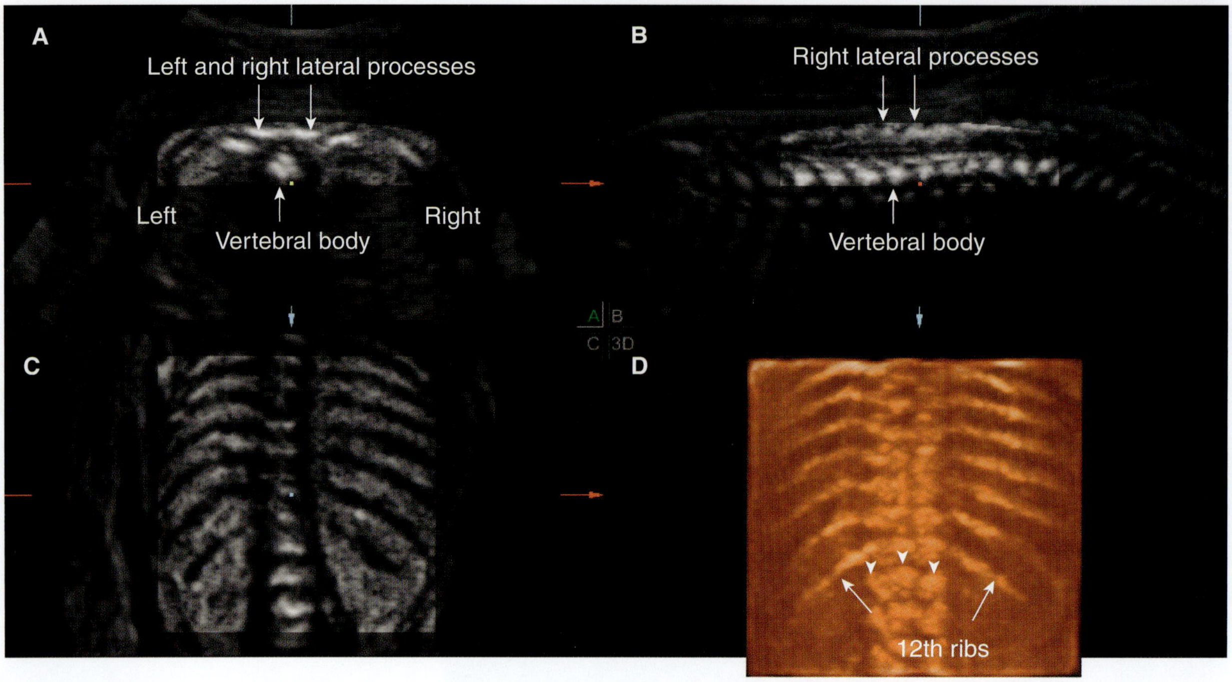


**Figure 2–95.** Multiplanar mode and maximum or x-ray display of the fetal spine and ribs at 20 weeks' gestation. This mode allows simultaneous visualization of the three orthogonal planes of the spine and evaluation of the three ossification centers, the lateral processes, and the bodies of the vertebrae. Axial plane in box A, sagittal plane in box B, and coronal plane in box C. Note that the ribs are not demonstrated in box C, but their shadow is visible, since the marker dot is placed on the body of the vertebrae anterior to the level of the ribs. The maximum mode was applied to obtain the rendered image as demonstrated in box D, which allows the identification of the 12th ribs and visualization of the three ossification centers simultaneously (arrowheads).

authors, making it available for research and eventually for clinical use.[124–126]

## THE FETAL SPINE

Because the spinal cord is part of the CNS and is found within the vertebral canal, it is imperative to evaluate the bony casing of the spinal cord. When evaluating the spine, 3D US appears to be an important adjunct to 2D imaging in arriving at the correct diagnosis when an abnormality is suspected.

### Technique

The choice of which transducer to use to obtain the volume will depend upon the orientation of the spine and its size. As gestation advances, the best way to obtain 3D images of the fetal column is by using the transabdominal US probe. With regards to the plane of acquisition, the best results are obtained by using the sagittal view. It is important to adjust the angle of rotation in order to include the ribs in the volume. Once the volume is acquired, the next step is to rotate the spine to obtain perfect sagittal and coronal planes.

The 3D volume can be evaluated using multiplanar display, volume rendering with the maximum-intensity mode, or a combination of both methods. The major advantage of the use of 3D when evaluating the fetal spine is that this image modality allows simultaneous visualization of the three ossification centers, the lateral processes, and the vertebral bodies of each vertebra[127–130] (Figures 2–95, 2–96, and 2–97). This allows a better understanding of the complex anatomy of the spine compared with 2D US.[132,133] An additional advantage is the possibility of rotating the volume around all three orthogonal planes and visualizing the spine from different angles.[129–132]

Furthermore, in the cases of neural tube defects, 3D US has been shown to be useful in determining the level and extent of the lesion.[127,128,133–135] This can be easily achieved by using the maximum mode in a thin slice, which allows the identification of the 12th rib; thus, the vertebral segments can be counted starting with the one connected to the last identifiable rib (Figure 2–95). However, 3D rendering of the spine may sometimes be inconclusive, especially in cases of small and low defects, as pointed out in a recent review of 3D US examination of the fetal CNS. The authors stated that a normal 3D image of the bony elements of the spine is not reassuring with regard to the presence of spina bifida.[136]

Other applications of 3D US have included the measurement of the size and volume of the thoracolumbar spine,[137] the spinal length,[138] and the size of the lumbar spinal canal,[139] with no clinical use suggested. At times, the surface-rendering mode may be used to demonstrate the cutaneous surface of the spine, which might be clinically useful when evaluating an open spina bifida.

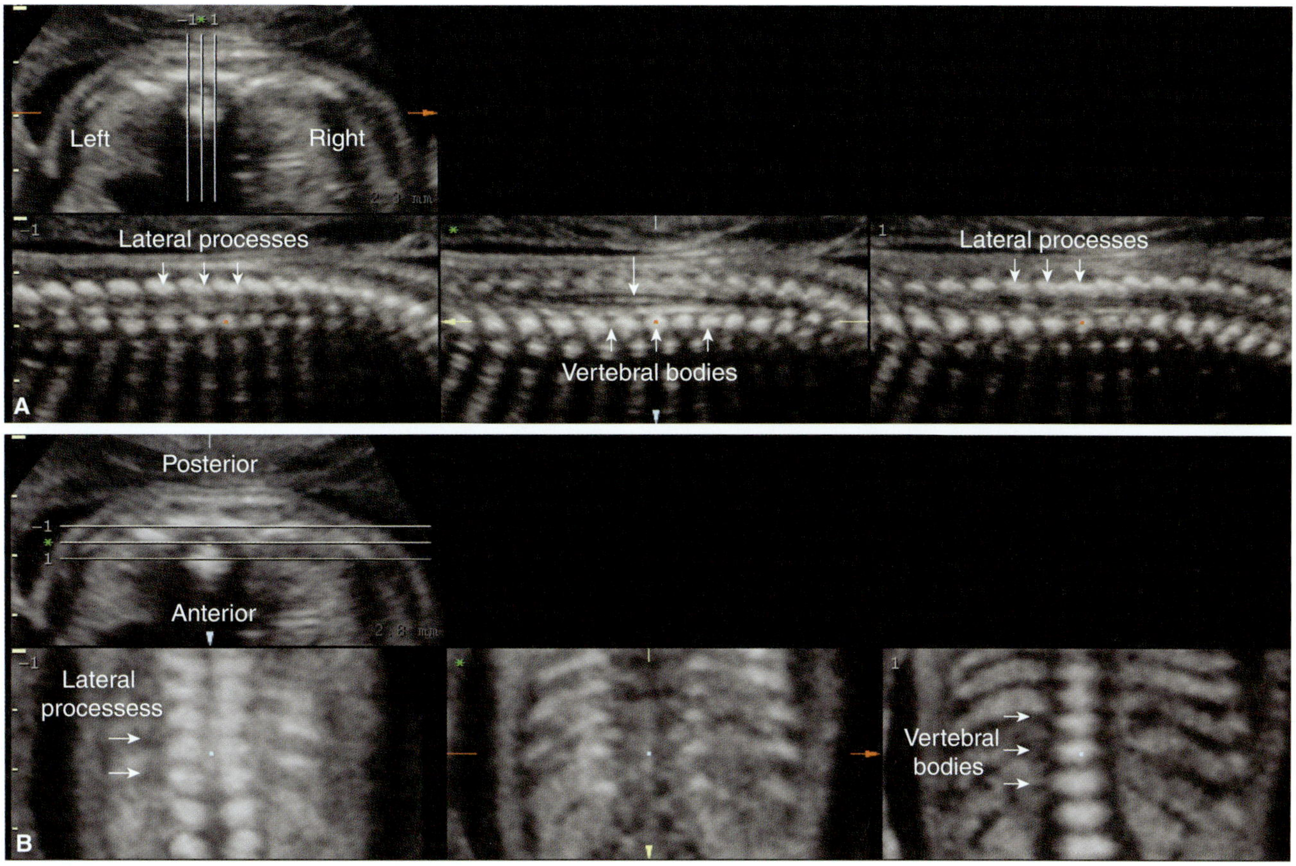


**Figure 2–96.** Tomographic ultrasound images obtained on a normal fetal spine at 24 weeks. (**A**) Sagittal views displayed from left to right. (**B**) Coronal views displayed from posterior to anterior. The body of the vertebrae and the lateral processes from different angles are viewed. Note how the contents of the neural canal are demonstrated in the central image of the sagittal sequence (arrow).

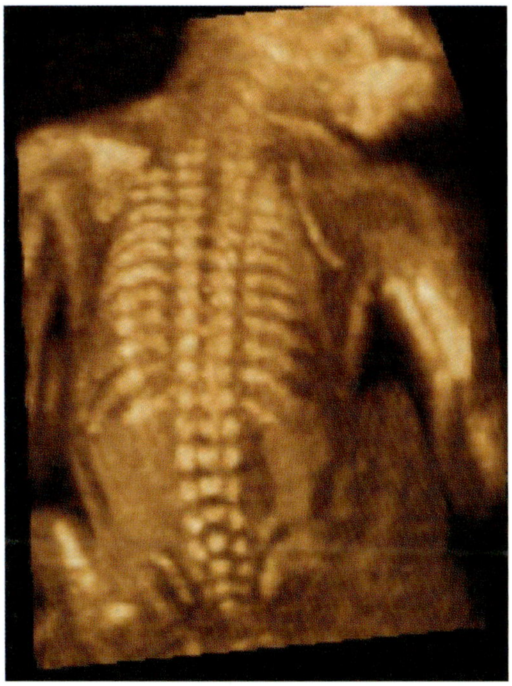

**Figure 2–97.** Rendering image obtained on a normal spine at 20 weeks. Note that depending on the gestational age of the fetus, visualization of the entire spine in a single image can be presented.

## REFERENCES


1. Kossoff G. Griffith KA, Dixon CE. Is the quality of transvaginal images superior to transabdominal ones under matched conditions? *Ultrasound Obstet Gynecol.* 1991;1:29–35.
2. Kossoff G, Garret WJ, Radavaniovich G. Ultrasonic atlas normal brain of infant. *Ultrasound Med Biol.* 1974;1:259–266.
3. Garret WJ, Kossoff G, Jones RF. Ultrasonic cross-sectional visualization of hydrocephalus in infants. *Neuroradiology.* 1975;8:279–288.
4. Lees RF, Harrison RB, Sims TL. Gray scale ultrasonography in the evaluation of hydrocephalus and associated abnormalities in infants. *Am J Dis Child.* 1978;132:376–378.
5. Babcock DS, Han BK, LeQuesne GW. B-mode gray scale ultrasound of the head in the newborn and young infant. *AJR.* 1980;134:457–468.
6. Skolnick ML, Rosenbaum AE, Matzuk T, et al. Detection of dilated cerebral ventricle in infants: A correlative study between ultrasound and computed tomography. *Radiology.* 1979;131:447–451.
7. Haber K, Wachter RD, Christenson PC, et al. Ultrasonic evaluation of intracranial pathology in infants: A new technique. *Radiology.* 1980;134:173–178.
8. Vlieger M. Evaluations of echoencephalography. *J Clin Ultrasound.* 1980;8:38.
9. Johnson ML, Rumack CM. Ultrasonic evaluation of the neonatal brain. *Radiol Clin North Am.* 1980;18:117–131.
10. Ben-Ora A. Eddy L, Hatch G, et al. The anterior fontanelle as an acoustic window to the neonatal ventricular system. *J Clin Ultrasound.* 1980;8:65–67.
11. Dewbury KC, Aluwihare APR. The anterior fontanelle as an ultrasound window for study of the brain: A preliminary report. *Br J Radiol.* 1980;53:81–84.

12. Grant EG, Schellinger D, Borts FT, et al. Real-time sonography of the neonatal and infant head. *AJR.* 1981;136:265–270.
13. Slovis TL, Kuhns LR. Real-time sonography of the brain through the anterior fontanelle. *AJR.* 1981;136:277–286.
14. Edwards MK, Brown DL, Muller J, et al. Cribside neurosonography: Real-time sonography for intracranial investigation of the neonate. *AJR.* 1981;136:271–276.
15. Pigadas A, Thompson JR, Grube GL. Normal infant brain anatomy: Correlated real-time sonograms and brain specimens. *AJNR.* 1981;2:339–344.
16. Harwood-Nash DC, Flodmark O. Diagnostic imaging of the neonatal brain: Review and protocol. AJNR. 1982;3:103–115.
17. Cremin BJ, Chilton SJ, Peacock WJ. Anatomical landmarks in anterior fontanelle ultrasonography . *Br J Radiol.* 1983;56:517.
18. Richardson DJ, Grant EG. Scanning techniques and normal anatomy. In: Grant GE, ed. *Neurosonography of Preterm Neonate.* New York: Springer-Verlag;1986:1–24.
19. Naidich TP, Yousefzadeh DK, Gusnard DA. Sonography of the normal neonatal head. Supratentorial structures: State-of-the-art imaging. *Neuroradiology.* 1986;28:408–427.
20. Monteagudo A, Reuss ML, Timor-Tritsch IE. Imaging the fetal brain in the second and third trimesters using transvaginal sonography. *Obstet Gynecol.* 1991;77:27–32.
21. Blaas HG, Eik-Nes SH, Berg S, Torp H. In vitro three dimensional ultrasound reconstructions of embryos and early fetuses. *Lancet.* 1998;352:1182–1186.
22. Timor-Tritsch IE, Farine D. Rosen MG. A close look at early embryonic development with the high-frequency transvaginal transducer. *Am J Obstet Gynecol.* 1988;159:676–681.
23. Timor-Tritsch IE, Monteagudo A, Warren WB. Transvaginal ultrasonographic definition of the central nervous system in the first and early second trimesters. *Am J Obstet Gynecol.* 1991;164: 497–503.
24. Timor-Tritsch IE, Monteagudo A. Transvaginal sonographic evaluation of the fetal central nervous system. *Obstet Gynecol Clin North Am.* 1991;18:713–748.
25. Warren WB, Timor-Tritsch IE, Peisner DB, et al. Dating the early pregnancy by sequential appearance of embryonic structures. *Am J Obstet Gynecol.* 1989;161:747–753.
26. Timor-Tritsch IE, Peisner DB, Raju S. Sonoembryology: An organ-oriented approach using a high-frequency vaginal probe. *J Clin Ultrasound.* 1990;18:286–298.
27. Achiron R, Achiron A. Transvaginal ultrasonic assessment of the early fetal brain. *Ultrasound Obstet Gynecol.* 1991;1:336–344.
28. Kushnir U, Shalev J, Bronstein M, et al. Fetal intracranial anatomy in the first trimester of pregnancy: Transvaginal ultrasonographic evaluation. *Neuroradiology.* 1989;31:222–225.
29. Blaas HG, Eik-Nes SH, Kiserud T, et al. Early development of the forebrain and midbrain: A longitudinal ultrasound study from 7 to 12 postmenstrual weeks of gestation. *Ultrasound Obstet Gynecol.* 1994;4:183–192.
30. Blaas HG, Eik-Nes SH, Kiserud T, et al. Early development of the hindbrain: A longitudinal ultrasound study from 7 to 12 weeks of gestation. *Ultrasound Obstet Gynecol.* 1995;5:151–160.
31. Monteagudo A, Timor-Tritsch IE, Reuss, ML, et al. Transvaginal sonography of the second- and third-trimester fetal brain. In: Timor-Tritsch IE, Rottem S, eds. *Transvaginal Sonography.* 2nd ed. New York: Chapman & Hall, 1991. pp 393–426.
32. Monteagudo A, Timor-Tritsch IE, Moomjy M. Nomograms of the fetal lateral ventricles using transvaginal sonography. *J Ultrasound Med.* 1993;5:265–269.
33. Robinson HP. Sonar measurements of fetal crown rump length as means of assessing maturity in the first trimester of pregnancy. *Br Med J.* 1973;4:28–31.
34. O'Rahilly R, Müller F. Embryonic length and cerebral landmarks in staged human embryos. *Anat Rec.* 1984;209:265–271.
35. Goldstein SR. Embryonic ultrasonographic measurements: Crown-rump length revisited. *Am J Obstet Gynecol.* 1991;165:497–501.
36. Timor-Tritsch IE, Blumenfeld Z, Rottem S. Sonoembryology. In: Timor-Tritsch IE, Rottem S, eds. *Transvaginal Sonography,* 2nd ed. New York: Chapman & Hall; 1991:275.
37. O'Rahilly R, Müller F. *Human Embryology and Teratology.* 3rd ed. New York: Wiley–Liss; 2001.
38. Blaas HG, Eik-Nes SH, Kiserud T, et al. Three-dimensional imaging of the brain cavities in human embryos. *Ultrasound Obstet Gynecol.* 1995;5:228–232.
39. Timor-Tritsch IE, Monteagudo A, Santos R. Three-dimensional inversion rendering in the first- and early second-trimester fetal brain: Its use in holoprosencephaly. *Ultrasound Obstet Gynecol.* 2008;32(6):744–750.
40. Kim MS, Jeanty P, Turner C, Benoit B. Three-dimensional sonographic evaluation of embryonic brain development. *J Ultrasound Med.* 2008;27:119–124
41. Timor-Tritsch IE, Monteagudo A. Transvaginal fetal neurosonography: Standardization of the planes and sections by anatomic landmarks. *Ultrasound Obstet Gynecol.* 1996;8:42–47.
42. Timor-Tritsch IE, et al. Sonoembryology in the structural evaluation of the fetus from 6 to 16 weeks. In: Reed GB, Claireaux AE, Cockburn F, Eds. *Diseases of* the *Fetus and Newborn.* 2nd ed. London: Chapman & Hall; 1995:897–917.
43. Malinger G, Monteagudo A, Pilu G, Timor-Tritsch IE, Toi A. Sonographic examination of the fetal central nervous system: guidelines for performing the 'basic examination and the fetal neurosonogram.' *Ultrasound Obstet Gynecol.* 2007;29:109–116.
44. Day WR. Casts of foetal lateral ventricles. *Brain.* 1959;82:109–115.
45. Denkhaus H, Winsberg F. Ultrasonic measurement of the fetal ventricular system. *Radiology.* 1979;131:781–787.
46. Johnson ML, Dunne MG, Mack LA, et al. Evaluation of fetal intracranial anatomy by static and realtime ultrasound. *J Clin Ultrasound.* 1980;8:311.
47. Horbar J, Leahy K, Lucey J. Ultrasound identification of lateral ventricular asymmetry in the human neonate. *J Clin Ultrasound.* 1983;11:67.
48. Hadlock FP, Deter RL, Park SK. Real-time sonography: Ventricular and vascular anatomy of the fetal brain in utero. *AJR.* 1981;136: 133–137.
49. Jeanty P, Dramaix-Wilmet M, Delbeke D, et al. Ultrasonic evaluation of fetal ventricular growth. *Neuroradiology.* 1981;21:127–133.
50. Pretorius DH, Rose JA, Manco-Johnson ML. Exclusion of fetal ventriculomegaly with a single measurement of the width of the lateral ventricular atrium. *Radiology.* 1988;169:711.
51. Cardoza JD, Goldstein RB, Filly RA. Exclusion of fetal ventriculomegaly with a single measurement of the width of the lateral ventricular atrium. *Radiology.* 1988;169:711.
52. Chinn DH, Callen PW, Filly RA. The lateral ventricle in early second trimester. *Radiology.* 1983;148:529–531.
53. Lustig-Gillman I, Snyder JR, Silverman F, et al. Sonographic anatomy of the fetal cerebral ventricles, with reference to the early diagnosis of hydrocephaly. *J Perinat Med.* 1984;12:185–191.
54. Filly RA, Cardoza JD, Goldstein R, Barkovich AJ. Detection of fetal central nervous system anomalies: a practice level of effort for a routine sonogram. *Radiology.* 1989;172:403–408.
55. Hertzberg BS, Sowie JD, Burder PC, et al. The three lines: Origin of a sonographic landmark in the fetal head. *AJR.* 1987;149:1009–1012.
56. Hertzberg BS, Kliewer MA, Bovie JD: Fetal cerebral ventriculomegaly: Misidentification of the true medial boundary of the ventricle at US. *Radiology.* 1997;205:813–816.
57. Siedler DE, Filly RA. Relative growth of the higher brain structures. *J Ultrasound Med.* 1987;6:573–576.
58. Goldstein I, Reece EA, Pilu G, et al. Sonographic evaluation of the normal developmental anatomy of fetal cerebral ventricles. 1: The frontal horn. *Obstet Gynecol.* 1988;72:588–592.
59. Pilu G, Reece EA, Goldstein I, et al. Sonographic evaluation of normal developmental anatomy of the fetal cerebral ventricles. 2: The atria. *Obstet Gynecol.* 1989;73:250–256.
60. Goldstein I, Reece EA, Pilu G, et al. Sonographic evaluation of the normal developmental anatomy of the fetal cerebral ventricles. 4: The posterior horn. *Am J Perinatol.* 1990;7:79–83.
61. Martin JH, ed. *Neuroanatomy: Text and Atlas.* 3rd ed. New York: McGraw-Hill; 2003.
62. Reece EB, Goldstein I. Three-level view of fetal brain imaging in the prenatal diagnosis of congenital anomalies. *Matern Fetal Med.* 1999:8:249–252.
63. Campbell S. Diagnosis of fetal abnormalities by ultrasound. In: Milunsky A, ed. *Genetic Disorders and the Fetus.* New York: Plenum; 1979:431–467.

64. Goldstein I, Reece EA, Pilu G, et al. Sonographic assessment of the fetal frontal lobe: A potential tool for the prenatal diagnosis of microcephaly. *Am J Obstet Gynecol.* 1988;158:1057–1062.
65. Campbell S, Pearce JM. Ultrasound visualization of congenital malformations. *Br Med Bull.* 1983;39:322–331.
66. Mahony BS, Nyberg DA, Hirsch JH, et al. Mild idiopathic lateral cerebral ventricular dilation in utero: Sonographic evaluation. *Radiology.* 1988;169:715–721.
67. Shaw CM, Alvord EC. Cava septi pellucidi and vergae: Their normal and pathological states. *Brain.* 1969;92:213–224.
68. Jou HJ, Shyu MK, Wu SC, et al. Ultrasound measurement of the fetal cavum septi pellucidi. *Ultrasound Obstet Gynecol.* 1998;12: 419–421.
69. Larroche JC, Bandey J. Cavum septi lucidi, cavum vergae, cavum veli interpositi: Cavités de la ligne médiane. Etude anatomique et pneumoencéphalographique dans la période néo-natale. *Biol Neonat.* 1961;3:193–236.
70. Kostovic I, Lukinovic N, Judas M, et al. Structural basis of the developmental plasticity in the human cerebral cortex: The role of the transient subplate zone. *Metab Brain Dis.* 1989;4:17–23.
71. Lemire RJ, Loeser JD, Leech RW, et al. *Normal and Abnormal Development of the Human Nervous System.* New York: Harper & Row; 1975;260–277.
72. Pilu G, Sandri F, Perolo A, et al. Sonography of fetal agenesis of the corpus callosum: A survey of 35 cases. *Ultrasound Obstet Gynecol.* 1993;3:318–329.
73. Comstock CH, Culp D, Gonzales J. Agenesis of the corpus callosum in the fetus: Its evolution and significance. *J Ultrasound Med.* 1985;4:613–616.
74. Malinger G, Zakut H. The corpus callosum: Normal fetal development as shown by transvaginal sonography. *AJR.* 1993;161: 1041–1043.
75. Guibert-Tranier F, Piton J, Billerey L, et al. Agenesis of the corpus callosum. *J Neuroradiol.* 1982;9:135–160.
76. Achiron R, Achiron A. Development of the human corpus callosum: a high resolution, cross sectional sonographic study. *Ultrasound Obstet Gynecol.* 2001;18:343–347.
77. Callen PW, Callen AL, Glenn OA, Toi A. Columns of the fornix, not to be mistaken for the cavum septi pellucidi on prenatal sonography. *J Ultrasound Med.* 2008;27(1):25–31.
78. Laing FC, Stamler CE, Jeffrey BR. Ultrasonography of the fetal subarachnoid space. *J Ultrasound Med.* 1983;2:29–32.
79. Kapila A, Trice J Spies WG, et al. Enlarged cerebrospinal fluid in infants with subdural hematoma. *Radiology.* 1982;142:669–672.
80. Jeanty P, Chervenak FA, Romero R, et al. The sylvian fissure: A commonly mislabeled cranial landmark. *J Ultrasound Med.* 1984;3:15–18.
81. Mahony BS, Callen PW, Tilly RA. The fetal cisterna magna. *Radiology.* 1984;153:73–76.
82. Bromley B, Nadel AS, Parker S, Estroff JA, Benacerraf BR. Closure of the cerebellar vermis: Evaluation with second trimester US. *Radiology.* 1994;193:761–763.
83. Goldstein I, Reece EA, Pilu G, et al. Cerebellar measurements with ultrasonography in the evaluation of fetal growth and development. *Am J Obstet Gynecol.* 1987;156:1065–1069.
84. Hill LM, Quzick D, Fried J, et al. The transverse cerebellar diameter in estimating gestational age in the large-for-gestational-age fetus. *Obstet Gynecol.* 1990;75:983–992.
85. Turner OA. Growth and development of the cerebral cortical pattern in man. *Arch Neurol Psychol.* 1948;59:1–12.
86. Dooling EC, Chi JG Gilles FH. Telencephalic development, changing gyral patterns. In: Gilles FH, ed. *The Developing Human Brain.* Boston: Wright-PSG; 1983:94–96.
87. Worthen NJ, Gilbertson V, Lau C. Cortical sulcal development seen on sonography: Relationship to gestational parameters. *J Ultrasound Med.* 1986:5:153–156.
88. Salamon G, Raynaud C, Reis J, et al. *Magnetic Resonance Imaging of the Pediatric Brain: An Anatomical Atlas.* New York; Raven; 1990.
89. Hansen PE, Ballesteros MC, Soila K, et al. MR imaging of the developing human brain, part 1. Prenatal development. *Radiographics.* 1993:13:21–36.
90. Naidich TP, Grant JL, Altman N, et al. The developing cerebral surface: Preliminary report on the patterns of sulcal and gyral maturation—Anatomy, ultrasound, and magnetic resonance imaging. *Neuroimaging Clin North Am.* 1994;4:201–240.
91. Slagle TA, Oliphant M, Gross SJ. Cingulate sulcus development in preterm infants. *Pediatr Res.* 1989;26:598–602.
92. Chi JG, Dooling EC, Gilles FH. Gyral development of the human brain. *Ann Neurol.* 1977;1:86–93.
93. Dorovini-Zis K, Dolman CL. Gestational development of the brain. *Arch Pathol Lab Med.* 1977;101:192–195.
94. Monteagudo A, Timor-Tritsch IE. Development of fetal gyri and sulci: a transvaginal sonographic study. *Ultrasound Obstet Gynecol.* 1997;9:222–228.
95. Baba K, Jurkovic D. Three-dimensional ultrasound in obstetrics and gynecology. The Parthenon Publishing Group: 1997.
96. Nelson TR, Downey DB, Pretorius DH, et al. Three-dimensional ultrasound. Philadelphia: Loppincott, Williams & Wilkins: 1999.
97. Blaas HG, Eik-Nes SH, Berg S. Three-dimensional fetal ultrasound. *Baillieries Best Pract Res Clin Obstet Gynecol.* 2000;14:611–627.
98. Timor-Tritsch IE, Monteagudo A. Three and four-dimensional ultrasound in obstetrics and gynecology. *Curr Opin Obstet Gynecol.* 2007;19:157–175.
99. Abuhamad AZ. Standarization of 3-dimensional volumes in obstetric sonography: A required step for training and automation. *J Ultrasound Med.* 2005;24:397–401.
100. Gonçalves LF, Lee W, Espinoza J, Romero R. Three and 4-dimensional ultrasound in obstetric practice: Does it help? *J Ultrasound Med.* 2005:24:1599–1624.
101. Monteagudo A, Timor-Tritsch IE, Mayberry P. Three dimensional transvaginal neurosonography of the fetal brain: "Navigating" in the volume scan. *Ultrasound Obstet Gynecol.* 2000;16:307–313.
102. Merz E, Benoit B, Blaas HG, et al. Standarization of three-dimensional images in obstetrics and gynecology: Consensus statement. *Ultrasound Obstet Gynecol.* 2007;29:697–703.
103. Pilu G, Segata M, Ghi T, et al. Diagnosis of midline anomalies of the fetal brain with the three-dimensional median view. *Ultrasound Obstet Gynecol.* 2006;27:522–529.
104. Correa F, Lara C, Bellver J, Remohi J, Pellicer A, Serra V. Examination of the fetal brain by transabdominal three dimensional ultrasound: potential for routine neurosonographic studies. Ultrasound Obstet Gynecol 2006;27:503–508.
105. Plasencia W, Dagklis T, Borenstein M, Csapo B, Nicolaides KH. Assessment of the corpus callosum at 20–24 weeks' gestation by three-dimensional ultrasound exaination. *Ultrasound Obstet Gynecol.* 2007;30:169–172.
106. Viñals F, Muñoz M, Naveas R, Giuliano A. Transfrontal three dimensional visualization of the midline cerebral structures. *Ultrasound Obstet Gynecol.* 2007;30:162–168.
107. Bornstein E, Monteagudo A, Santos R, Keeler SM, Timor-Tritsch IE. A systematic technique using 3-dimensional ultrasound provides a simple and reproducible mode to evaluate the corpus callosum. *Am J Obstet Gynecol.* 2010;202(2):201.e1–5.
108. Pilu G, Ghi T, Carletti A, Segata M, Perolo A, Rizzo N. Three-dimensional ultrasound examination of the fetal central nervous system. *Ultrasound Obstet Gynecol.* 2007;30:233–245.
109. Malinger G, Lerman-Sagie T, Viñals F. Three-dimensional sagittal reconstruction of the corpus callosum: fact or artifact? *Ultrasound Obstet Gynecol.* 2006;28:742–743.
110. Denkhaus H, Winsberg F. Ultrasonic measurement of the fetal ventricular system. *Radiology.* 1979;131:781–787.
111. Cardoza JD, Goldstein RB, Filly RA. Exclusion of fetal ventriculomegaly with a single measurement: The width of the lateral ventricular atrium. *Radiology.* 1988;169:711–714.
112. Goldstein I, Reece EA, Pilu G, et al. Sonographic evaluation of the normal developmental anatomy of the fetal cerebral ventricles. 1: The frontal horn. *Obstet Gynecol.* 1988;72:588–592.
113. Goldstein I, Reece EA, Pilu G, et al. Sonographic evaluation of the normal developmental anatomy of the fetal cerebral ventricles. 4: The posterior horn. *Am J Perinatol.* 1990;7:79–83.
114. Timor-Tritsch I.E, Monteagudo A, Mayberry P. Three-dimensional ultrasound evaluation of the fetal brain: the three horn view. *Ultrasound Obstet Gynecol.* 2000;16:302–306.
115. Ruano R, Benachi A, Aubry M, Dumez Y, Dommergues M. Volume contrast imaging: A new approach to identify fetal thoracic structures. *J Ultrasound Med.* 2004;23:403–408.

116. Viñals F, Munoz M, Naveas R, Schalper J, Giuliano S. The fetal cerebellar vermis: anatomy and biometry assessment using 4D volume contrast imaging in the C-plane (VCI-C). *Ultrasound Obstet Gynecol.* 2005;26:622–627.
117. Pretorius DH, Nelson TR. Prenatal visualization of cranial sutures and fontanelles with three-dimensional ultrasonography. *J Ultrasound Med.* 1994;13:871–876.
118. Dikkeboom CM, Roelfsema NM, Van Adrichem LN, Wladimiroff JW. The role of three-dimensional ultrasound in visualizing the fetal cranial sutures and fontanels during the second half of pregnancy. *Ultrasound Obstet Gynecol.* 2004;24:134–140.
119. Chang CH, Yu CH, Ko HC. Three-dimensional power Doppler ultrasound for the assessment of the fetal brain blood flow in normal gestation. *Ultrasound Med Biol.* 2003;29:1273–1279.
120. Pooh RK, Pooh KH. The assessment of fetal brain morphology and circulation by transvaginal 3D sonography power Doppler. *J Perinat Med.* 2002;30:48–56.
121. Benacerraf BR. Inversion mode display of 3D sonography: Applications in obstetrics and gynecology imaging. *Am J Roentgenol.* 2006;187:965–997.
122. Blaas H-GK, Eik-Nes SH. The description of the early development of the human central nervous system using two- and three dimensional ultrasound. In: Hanson M, Lagercrantz H (eds). *The Newborn Brain—Neuroscience and Clinical Applications.* Cambridge: Cambridge University Press: 2002:278–288.
123. Merz E, Miric-Tesanic, Welter C. Value of the electronic scalpel (cut mode) in the evaluation of the fetal face. *Ultrasound Obstet Gynecol.* 2000;16:564–568.
124. Endres LK, Cohen L. Reliability and validity of 3D fetal brain volumes. *JUM.* 2001;20:1265–1269.
125. Chang CH, Yu CH, Chang FM, Ko HC, Chen HY. The assessment of normal fetal brain volume by 3-D ultrasound. *Ultrasound Med Biol.* 2003;29:1267–1272.
126. Roelfsema NM. 3D sonographic measurement of normal fetal brain volume during the second half of pregnancy. *AJOG.* 2004;190(1): 275–280.
127. Johnson DD, Pretorius DH, Riccabona M, Budorick NE, Nelson TR. Three-dimensional ultrasound of the fetal spine. *Obstet Gynecol.* 1997;89:434–438.
128. Mueller GM, Weiner CP, Yankowitz J. Three-dimensional ultrasound in the evaluation of fetal head and spine anomalies. *Obstet Gynecol.* 1996;88:372–378.
129. Budorick NE, Pretorius DH, Nelson TR. Sonography of the fetal spine: technique, imaging findings, and clinical implications. *AJR Am J Roentgenol.* 1995;164:421–428.
130. Riccabona M, Johnson D, Pretorius DH, Nelson TR. Three dimensional ultrasound: Display modalities in the fetal spine and thorax. *Eur J Radiol.* 1996;22:141–145.
131. Yanagihara T, Hata T. Three-dimensional sonographic visualization of fetal skeleton in the second trimester of pregnancy. *Gynecol Obstet Invest.* 2000;49:12–16.
132. Nelson TR, Pretorius DH. Visualization of the fetal thoracic skeleton with three-dimensional sonography: A preliminary report. *AJR Am J Roentgenol.* 1995;164:1485–1488.
133. Lee W, Chaiworapongsa T, Romero R, et al. A diagnostic approach for the evaluation of spina bifida by three-dimensional ultrasonography. *J Ultrasound Med.* 2002;21:619–626.
134. Bonilla-Musoles F, Machado LE, Osborne NG, et al. Two- and three-dimensional ultrasound in malformations of the medullary canal: Report of four cases. *Prenat Diagn.* 2001;21:622–626.
135. Lazebnik N, Bornstein E, Timor-Tritsch IE. The utility of volume sonography for the detection of fetal spine abnormalities. *Ultrasound Clin.* 2008;3(4):517–528.
136. Pilu G, Ghi T, Carletti A, Segata M, Perolo A, Rizzo N. Three-dimensional ultrasound examination of the fetal central nervous system. *Ultrasound Obstet Gynecol.* 2007;30(2):233–245.
137. Schild RL, Wallny T, Fimmers R, Hansmann M. The size of the fetal thoraco lumbar spine: A three-dimensional ultrasound study. *Ultrasound Obstet Gynecol.* 2000;16:468–472.
138. Ulm MR, Kratochwil A, Oberhuemer U, et al. Ultrasound evaluation of fetal spine length between 14 and 24 weeks' gestation. *Prenat Diagn.* 1999;19:637–641.
139. Wallny T, Schild RL, Fimmers R, Hansmann ME. Three dimensional sonographic evaluation of the fetal lumbar spinal canal. *J Anat.* 2002;200:439–443.

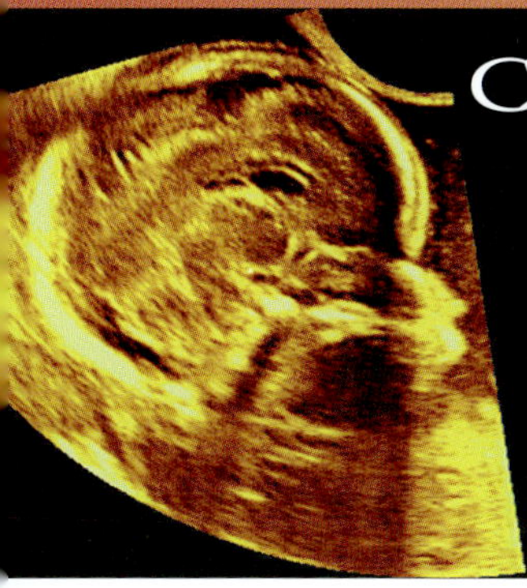

Chapter 3

# BIOMETRY OF THE FETAL BRAIN

*Natan Haratz-Rubinstein • Ana Monteagudo • Ilan E. Timor-Tritsch*

## INTRODUCTION

Prenatal diagnosis should be instituted accurately and early enough to achieve an excellent level of care of the obstetric patient. Ultrasonography, with its increasingly better resolution and image quality, is making it easier for health care providers to make appropriate management decisions. Assessing whether a structure is normal or abnormal may not always be feasible, but if doubt exists regarding its normalcy, it must be carefully and diligently pursued. In addition, several measurements, such as the biparietal diameter (BPD) and the head circumference (HC), can be used to determine the gestational age of a fetus, especially during the first half of pregnancy. Correct estimation of gestational age is of paramount importance because adequate management of both low- and high-risk obstetric populations relies heavily on knowing the precise gestational age.

The tables in this chapter have been compiled from the literature for the sole purpose of serving as an easy reference against which measurements can be compared. An attempt has been made to include as many tables of different parameters as possible. These tables, assembled in a single chapter, will allow the sonographer or sonologist to more easily make the differentiation between normal and abnormal measurements, without having to search different textbooks and articles for a particular measurement.

This chapter is divided into four main sections. The first, crown-rump length (CRL), although not a brain or head measurement, is included to provide a means of predicting embryonic or fetal age. This parameter is of obvious importance and eliminates the need to turn to another source.

The second section, dealing with head measurements, can be used not only to date the pregnancy but also to aid in the diagnosis of microcephaly and alterations in fetal head shape. This section also includes measurements of orbital diameters, which can be of help in the diagnosis of eye pathology.

The third section provides a variety of tables concerning the different portions of the fetal ventricular system, mainly for the purpose of making early diagnosis of ventriculomegaly possible. Congenital hydrocephaly is one of the most frequently described anomalies, with an incidence of 0.3 to 1.5 per 1000 births. The importance of in utero detection of this anomaly cannot be overemphasized. This section also includes tables that we have generated using the transvaginal-transfontanelle approach to the fetal brain using 5 to 7.5 MHz transvaginal probes. These tables enhance and complement the widely accepted transabdominally generated tables, thereby advancing the field of fetal neurosonography and giving new meaning to the term *early diagnosis*.

The fourth and final section includes measurements of other intracranial structures, such as the thalami, basal nuclei, cerebellum, and cerebellomedullary cistern. These can assist the sonographer or sonologist in the diagnosis of pathologies such as Dandy-Walker and Arnold-Chiari malformations.

This chapter attempts to provide the reader with a unique reference guide to fetal brain measurements.

## CROWN-RUMP LENGTH

### Definition

The CRL represents the longest measurable length of the embryo or fetus, excluding the inferior limbs or the yolk sac.[1,2]

### How to Measure It (Figure 3–1)

In a longitudinal scan, the CRL is measured from a point immediately over the middle of the midbrain (crown) to the embryonic or fetal rump. O'Rahilly and Müller[1] suggested that from 28 to 44 postovulatory days (6.0 to 8.5 postmenstrual weeks,* or Carnegie stages 13 to 18), the maximum longitudinal length of the embryo is not truly represented by the CRL, but by what they called the greatest length. This is explained by the fact that during these stages, the normal flexion of the embryonic head locates the middle of the midbrain below the highest point of the head. As pregnancy advances, the head extends, making

* Fetal and embryonic age is described here in reference to postmenstrual weeks. Postovulatory age is approximately 2 weeks less than postmenstrual age.

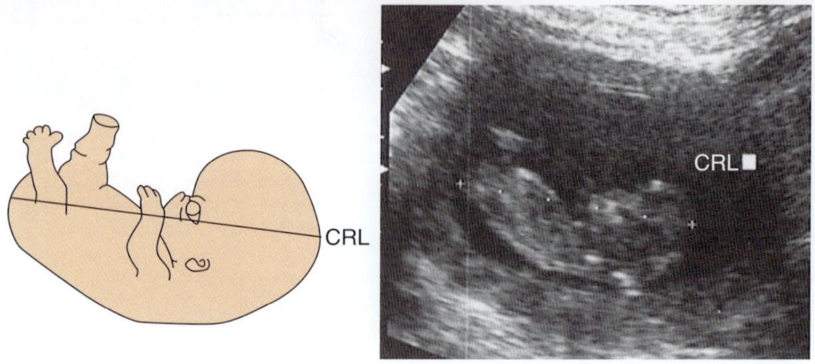


Figure 3–1.

the middle of the midbrain match the highest point of the head and thus becoming a true "crown" reference point (see Chapters 1 and 2).

### Comments

Although the CRL is obviously not a measurement of the brain, it will be included in this chapter as a reference for the assessment of estimated age, a parameter of utmost importance when evaluating the embryo and the fetus, and one against which most biometry tables are plotted. The validity of this parameter for determination of age in the first trimester has been widely reported in the literature.[2–4] The average of three measurements should be used to diminish random errors in the technique. The variability in predicting postmenstrual age with the CRL changes over time, with a reported range of error of ± 8% of the estimate.[2] Possible factors contributing to this range are (1) normal biologic variation in fetal size, (2) variation in the times of ovulation and fertilization, and (3) errors attributed to the measurement technique.[3] Nevertheless, the CRL remains the gold standard measurement for dating pregnancy in the first trimester, with the exception of in vitro fertilization cases (Tables 3–1 and 3–2).

Blaas and colleagues[5] described the use of three-dimensional (3D) transvaginal sonography to outline in detail the outer contours of embryos at 7 to 10 weeks of gestation. Using this technique, they were able to describe the contours of the brain cavities, as well as calculate volumes that corresponded well with the descriptions from classic human embryology.

## HEAD MEASUREMENTS

### Biparietal Diameter

#### Definition

The BPD represents the widest transverse dimension of the fetal head.

#### How to Measure It (Figure 3–2)

The fetal head should be imaged in a horizontal (axial) plane. The transducer should be tilted to match the angle of inclination of the head in the vertical axis of the fetus so that a horizontal section can be obtained. This is recognized by the appearance of the midline echo and the widest fetal head diameter at right angles with it. The transducer should then be rotated (following the position of the fetal spine) until the head appears as an ovoid and a small anechoic area is detected in the midline, one-third of the distance from the sinciput.[6] According to Hadlock and colleagues,[7] this plane represents a section along the sub-occipital-bregmatic axis, angled ~40°, to the canthomeatal line. Intracranial landmarks that should be recognized in an anterior-to-posterior fashion are (see Figure 3–2 for abbreviations) the falx cerebri (F); the cavum septi pellucidi (CSP), which corresponds to the midline anechoic area described by Campbell and Thoms;[6] the cerebral peduncles (P); and again, the falx cerebri in the midline. Laterally, one should be able to recognize, depending on the age of the fetus, the anterior horns (AH) of the lateral ventricles, the hypoechoic thalami (T), and the choroid plexus (CP) in the atrium (A) of each lateral ventricle. Halfway between the thalami and the calvarium, a linear echo corresponding to the insula (I) can be seen, with the pulsating middle cerebral artery within. Once the correct plane has been identified, the calipers should be placed at the outer surface of the skull table nearest the transducer and at the inner margin of the opposite skull table, with gain settings adjusted so that the width of the skull table nearer the transducer is 3 to 5 mm.

#### Comments

The BPD was one of the first sonographic parameters used to estimate fetal age.[8] It has been shown to be a reliable predictor of menstrual age in the first half of pregnancy, being the most accurate between 12 and 18 (± 1.2) weeks. As pregnancy progresses, the BPD loses its power to correctly predict gestational age, with a margin of error of ± 3.2 weeks at 36 to 42 weeks (Tables 3–3 and 3–4).[9]

The observed variation in the third trimester has been related to (1) technical errors in imaging, (2) genetic variations in head size in fetuses of equal age, and (3) differences in the times of ovulation and fertilization during the menstrual period.

Sonographic measurement of the BPD may be misleading if the fetal head shape is abnormal. It has been postulated that extrinsic factors such as breech presentation

**Table 3–1. NOMOGRAM OF THE SONOGRAPHICALLY DETERMINED CROWN-RUMP LENGTH AS A FUNCTION OF GESTATIONAL AGE**

| Postmenstrual Gestational Age (weeks + days) | CRL (mm) | | Postmenstrual Gestational Age (weeks + days) | CRL (mm) | |
|---|---|---|---|---|---|
| | Mean | SD | | Mean | SD |
| 6 + 2 | 6.7 | 2.9 | 10 + 2 | 35.5 | 6.9 |
| 6 + 3 | 7.4 | 3.1 | 10 + 3 | 36.9 | 7.0 |
| 6 + 4 | 8.0 | 3.2 | 10 + 4 | 38.4 | 7.2 |
| 6 + 5 | 8.7 | 3.4 | 10 + 5 | 39.9 | 7.3 |
| 6 + 6 | 9.5 | 3.5 | 10 + 6 | 41.4 | 7.4 |
| 7 + 0 | 10.2 | 3.7 | 11 + 0 | 43.0 | 7.6 |
| 7 + 1 | 11.0 | 3.8 | 11 + 1 | 44.6 | 7.7 |
| 7 + 2 | 11.8 | 3.9 | 11 + 2 | 46.2 | 7.9 |
| 7 + 3 | 12.6 | 4.1 | 11 + 3 | 47.8 | 8.0 |
| 7 + 4 | 13.5 | 4.2 | 11 + 4 | 49.5 | 8.1 |
| 7 + 5 | 14.4 | 4.4 | 11 + 5 | 51.2 | 8.3 |
| 7 + 6 | 15.3 | 4.5 | 11 + 6 | 52.9 | 8.4 |
| 8 + 0 | 16.3 | 4.6 | 12 + 0 | 54.7 | 8.6 |
| 8 + 1 | 17.3 | 4.8 | 12 + 1 | 56.5 | 8.7 |
| 8 + 2 | 18.3 | 4.9 | 12 + 2 | 58.3 | 8.8 |
| 8 + 3 | 19.3 | 5.1 | 12 + 3 | 60.1 | 9.0 |
| 8 + 4 | 20.4 | 5.2 | 12 + 4 | 62.0 | 9.1 |
| 8 + 5 | 21.5 | 5.3 | 12 + 5 | 63.9 | 9.3 |
| 8 + 6 | 22.6 | 5.5 | 12 + 6 | 65.9 | 9.4 |
| 9 + 0 | 23.8 | 5.6 | 13 + 0 | 67.8 | 9.5 |
| 9 + 1 | 25.0 | 5.8 | 13 + 1 | 69.8 | 9.7 |
| 9 + 2 | 26.2 | 5.9 | 13 + 2 | 71.8 | 9.8 |
| 9 + 3 | 27.4 | 6.0 | 13 + 3 | 73.9 | 10.0 |
| 9 + 4 | 28.7 | 6.2 | 13 + 4 | 76.0 | 10.1 |
| 9 + 5 | 30.0 | 6.3 | 13 + 5 | 78.1 | 10.2 |
| 9 + 6 | 31.3 | 6.5 | 13 + 6 | 80.2 | 10.4 |
| 10 + 0 | 32.7 | 6.6 | 14 + 0 | 82.4 | 10.5 |
| 10 + 1 | 34.0 | 6.7 | | | |

CRL, crown-rump length; SD, standard deviation.

Reproduced, with permission, from Robinson HP, 1975.[3]

**Table 3–2. PREDICTED MENSTRUAL AGE FROM CROWN-RUMP LENGTH MEASUREMENTS**

| CRL (cm) | MA (weeks) | CRL (cm) | MA (weeks) | CRL (cm) | MA (weeks) |
|---|---|---|---|---|---|
| 0.2 | 5.7 | 4.2 | 11.1 | 8.2 | 14.2 |
| 0.3 | 5.9 | 4.3 | 11.2 | 8.3 | 14.2 |
| 0.4 | 6.1 | 4.4 | 11.2 | 8.4 | 14.3 |
| 0.5 | 6.2 | 4.5 | 11.3 | 8.5 | 14.4 |
| 0.6 | 6.4 | 4.6 | 11.4 | 8.6 | 14.5 |
| 0.7 | 6.6 | 4.7 | 11.5 | 8.7 | 14.6 |
| 0.8 | 6.7 | 4.8 | 11.6 | 8.8 | 14.7 |
| 0.9 | 6.9 | 4.9 | 11.7 | 8.9 | 14.8 |
| 1.0 | 7.2 | 5.0 | 11.7 | 9.0 | 14.9 |
| 1.1 | 7.2 | 5.1 | 11.8 | 9.1 | 15.0 |
| 1.2 | 7.4 | 5.2 | 11.9 | 9.2 | 15.1 |
| 1.3 | 7.5 | 5.3 | 12.0 | 9.3 | 15.2 |
| 1.4 | 7.7 | 5.4 | 12.0 | 9.4 | 15.3 |
| 1.5 | 7.9 | 5.5 | 12.1 | 9.5 | 15.3 |
| 1.6 | 8.0 | 5.6 | 12.2 | 9.6 | 15.4 |
| 1.7 | 8.1 | 5.7 | 12.3 | 9.7 | 15.5 |
| 1.8 | 8.3 | 5.8 | 12.3 | 9.8 | 15.6 |
| 1.9 | 8.4 | 5.9 | 12.4 | 9.9 | 15.7 |
| 2.0 | 8.6 | 6.0 | 12.5 | 10.0 | 15.9 |
| 2.1 | 8.7 | 6.1 | 12.6 | 10.1 | 16.0 |
| 2.2 | 8.9 | 6.2 | 12.6 | 10.2 | 16.1 |
| 2.3 | 9.0 | 6.3 | 12.7 | 10.3 | 16.2 |
| 2.4 | 9.1 | 6.4 | 12.8 | 10.4 | 16.3 |
| 2.5 | 9.2 | 6.5 | 12.8 | 10.5 | 16.4 |
| 2.6 | 9.4 | 6.6 | 12.9 | 10.6 | 16.5 |
| 2.7 | 9.5 | 6.7 | 13.0 | 10.7 | 16.6 |
| 2.8 | 9.6 | 6.8 | 13.1 | 10.8 | 16.7 |
| 2.9 | 9.7 | 6.9 | 13.1 | 10.9 | 16.8 |
| 3.0 | 9.9 | 7.0 | 13.2 | 11.0 | 16.9 |
| 3.1 | 10.0 | 7.1 | 13.3 | 11.1 | 17.0 |
| 3.2 | 10.1 | 7.2 | 13.4 | 11.2 | 17.1 |
| 3.3 | 10.2 | 7.3 | 13.4 | 11.3 | 17.2 |
| 3.4 | 10.3 | 7.4 | 13.5 | 11.4 | 17.3 |

*(continued)*

**Table 3–2. PREDICTED MENSTRUAL AGE FROM CROWN-RUMP LENGTH MEASUREMENTS (CONTINUED)**

| CRL (cm) | MA (weeks) | CRL (cm) | MA (weeks) | CRL (cm) | MA (weeks) |
|---|---|---|---|---|---|
| 3.5 | 10.4 | 7.5 | 13.6 | 11.5 | 17.4 |
| 3.6 | 10.5 | 7.6 | 13.7 | 11.6 | 17.5 |
| 3.7 | 10.6 | 7.7 | 13.8 | 11.7 | 17.6 |
| 3.8 | 10.7 | 7.8 | 13.8 | 11.8 | 17.7 |
| 3.9 | 10.8 | 7.9 | 13.9 | 11.9 | 17.8 |
| 4.0 | 10.9 | 8.0 | 14.0 | 12.0 | 17.9 |
| 4.1 | 11.0 | 8.1 | 14.1 | 12.1 | 18.0 |

CRL, Crown-rump length; MA, menstrual age.

Modified, with permission, from Hadlock FP, Shah YP, Kanon DJ, Lindsey JV. Fetal crown-rump length: Reevaluation of relation to menstrual age (5–18 weeks) with high-resolution real time US. *Radiology*. 1992;182:501–505.

and oligohydramnios can alter fetal head shape.[10,11] In an attempt to identify variations in the shape of the fetal skull that might adversely affect the potential of the BPD in estimating age, Hadlock and associates[12] developed the so-called cephalic index (CI). When this parameter is abnormal, other measurements, such as the HC, abdominal circumference, or femur length, should be used to predict fetal age.

## CEPHALIC INDEX

### Definition

The CI is the relationship between the short and long axes of the fetal skull, measured at the level of the BPD.

### How to Measure It

The widest transverse and longitudinal (occipitofrontal diameter [OFD]) dimensions of the fetal skull at the level of the BPD are measured from outer margin to outer margin. The CI can then be calculated using the following simple equation:

$$\text{CI} = \text{short axis (transverse)}/\text{long axis (OFD)} \times 100$$

### Comments

The clinical application of the CI lies in its property to discriminate between the normal fetal head shape and the head that is abnormal enough to alter fetal age estimation based on the BPD. Thus, in situations that may modify

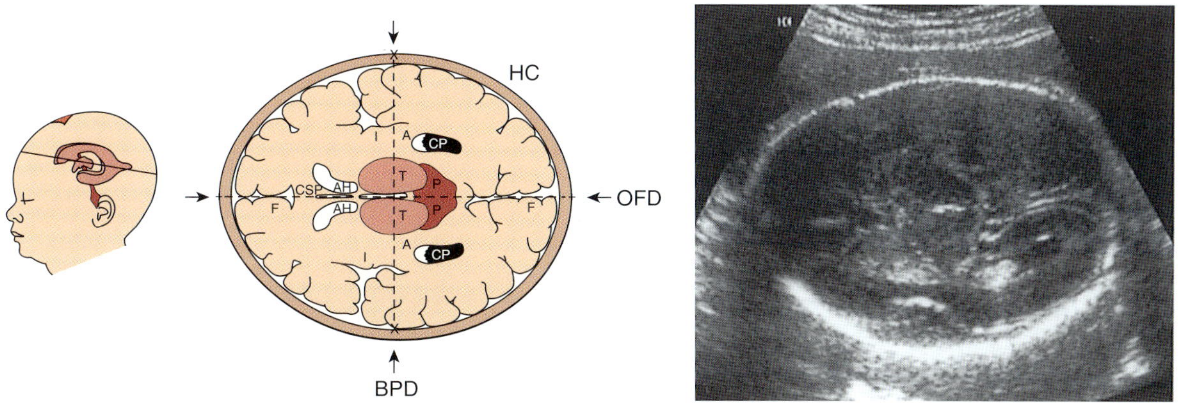


**Figure 3–2.**

**Table 3–3. PREDICTED FETAL BIPARIETAL DIAMETER AT SPECIFIC MENSTRUAL AGES**

| Menstrual Age (weeks) | Biparietal Diameter (cm) | Menstrual Age (weeks) | Biparietal Diameter (cm) |
|---|---|---|---|
| 12.0 | 1.7 | 26.0 | 6.5 |
| 12.5 | 1.9 | 26.5 | 6.7 |
| 13.0 | 2.1 | 27.0 | 6.8 |
| 13.5 | 2.3 | 27.5 | 6.9 |
| 14.0 | 2.5 | 28.0 | 7.1 |
| 14.5 | 2.7 | 28.5 | 7.2 |
| 15.0 | 2.9 | 29.0 | 7.3 |
| | | 29.5 | 7.5 |
| 15.5 | 3.1 | 30.0 | 7.6 |
| 16.0 | 3.2 | 30.5 | 7.7 |
| 16.5 | 3.4 | 31.0 | 7.8 |
| 17.0 | 3.6 | 31.5 | 7.9 |
| 17.5 | 3.8 | 32.0 | 8.1 |
| 18.0 | 3.9 | 32.5 | 8.2 |
| 18.5 | 4.1 | 33.0 | 8.3 |
| 19.0 | 4.3 | 33.5 | 8.4 |
| 19.5 | 4.5 | 34.0 | 8.5 |
| 20.0 | 4.6 | 34.5 | 8.6 |
| 20.5 | 4.8 | 35.0 | 8.7 |
| 21.0 | 5.0 | 35.5 | 8.8 |
| 21.5 | 5.1 | 36.0 | 8.9 |
| 22.0 | 5.3 | 36.5 | 8.9 |
| 22.5 | 5.5 | 37.0 | 9.0 |
| 23.0 | 5.6 | 37.5 | 9.1 |
| 23.5 | 5.8 | 38.0 | 9.2 |
| 24.0 | 5.9 | 38.5 | 9.2 |
| 24.5 | 6.1 | 39.0 | 9.3 |
| 25.0 | 6.2 | 39.5 | 9.4 |
| 25.5 | 6.4 | 40.0 | 9.4 |

Reproduced, with permission, from Hadlock and colleagues, 1984.[9]

**Table 3–4. ASSESSMENT OF GESTATIONAL AGE FROM THE BIPARIETAL DIAMETER**

| | Gestational Age (weeks + days) | | |
|---|---|---|---|
| Biparietal Diameter (mm) | 5th Percentile | 50th Percentile | 95th Percentile |
| 10 | 7 + 0 | 10 + 1 | 13 + 1 |
| 11 | 7 + 2 | 10 + 2 | 13 + 3 |
| 12 | 7 + 3 | 10 + 4 | 13 + 4 |
| 13 | 7 + 5 | 10 + 5 | 13 + 5 |
| 14 | 7 + 6 | 10 + 6 | 14 + 0 |
| 15 | 8 + 1 | 11 + 1 | 14 + 1 |
| 16 | 8 + 2 | 11 + 2 | 14 + 3 |
| 17 | 8 + 4 | 11 + 4 | 14 + 4 |
| 18 | 8 + 5 | 11 + 5 | 14 + 6 |
| 19 | 9 + 0 | 12 + 0 | 15 + 0 |
| 20 | 9 + 1 | 12 + 2 | 15 + 2 |
| 21 | 9 + 3 | 12 + 3 | 15 + 3 |
| 22 | 9 + 4 | 12 + 5 | 15 + 5 |
| 23 | 9 + 6 | 12 + 6 | 16 + 0 |
| 24 | 10 + 1 | 13 + 1 | 16 + 1 |
| 25 | 10 + 2 | 13 + 3 | 16 + 3 |
| 26 | 10 + 4 | 13 + 4 | 16 + 5 |
| 27 | 10 + 6 | 13 + 6 | 17 + 0 |
| 28 | 11 + 0 | 14 + 1 | 17 + 1 |
| 29 | 11 + 2 | 14 + 3 | 17 + 3 |
| 30 | 11 + 4 | 14 + 4 | 17 + 5 |
| 31 | 11 + 6 | 14 + 6 | 18 + 0 |
| 32 | 12 + 1 | 15 + 1 | 18 + 1 |
| 33 | 12 + 3 | 15 + 3 | 18 + 3 |
| 34 | 12 + 4 | 15 + 5 | 18 + 5 |
| 35 | 12 + 6 | 16 + 0 | 19 + 0 |
| 36 | 13 + 1 | 16 + 2 | 19 + 2 |
| 37 | 13 + 3 | 16 + 4 | 19 + 4 |
| 38 | 13 + 5 | 16 + 6 | 19 + 6 |
| 39 | 14 + 0 | 17 + 1 | 20 + 1 |
| 40 | 14 + 2 | 17 + 3 | 20 + 3 |
| 41 | 14 + 4 | 17 + 5 | 20 + 5 |

*(continued)*

**Table 3–4. ASSESSMENT OF GESTATIONAL AGE FROM THE BIPARIETAL DIAMETER (CONTINUED)**

| | Gestational Age (weeks + days) | | |
|---|---|---|---|
| **Biparietal Diameter (mm)** | **5th Percentile** | **50th Percentile** | **95th Percentile** |
| 42 | 14 + 6 | 18 + 0 | 21 + 0 |
| 43 | 15 + 1 | 18 + 2 | 21 + 2 |
| 44 | 15 + 3 | 18 + 4 | 21 + 4 |
| 45 | 15 + 6 | 18 + 6 | 21 + 6 |
| 46 | 16 + 1 | 19 + 1 | 22 + 1 |
| 47 | 16 + 3 | 19 + 3 | 22 + 4 |
| 48 | 16 + 5 | 19 + 5 | 22 + 6 |
| 49 | 17 + 0 | 20 + 1 | 23 + 1 |
| 50 | 17 + 3 | 20 + 3 | 23 + 3 |
| 51 | 17 + 5 | 20 + 5 | 23 + 6 |
| 52 | 18 + 0 | 21 + 0 | 24 + 1 |
| 53 | 18 + 2 | 21 + 3 | 24 + 3 |
| 54 | 18 + 5 | 21 + 5 | 24 + 5 |
| 55 | 19 + 0 | 22 + 0 | 25 + 1 |
| 56 | 19 + 2 | 22 + 3 | 25 + 3 |
| 57 | 19 + 5 | 22 + 5 | 25 + 6 |
| 58 | 20 + 0 | 23 + 1 | 26 + 1 |
| 59 | 20 + 3 | 23 + 3 | 26 + 3 |
| 60 | 20 + 5 | 23 + 6 | 26 + 6 |
| 61 | 21 + 1 | 24 + 1 | 27 + 1 |
| 62 | 21 + 3 | 24 + 4 | 27 + 4 |
| 63 | 21 + 6 | 24 + 6 | 27 + 6 |
| 64 | 22 + 1 | 25 + 2 | 28 + 2 |
| 65 | 22 + 4 | 25 + 4 | 28 + 5 |
| 66 | 22 + 6 | 26 + 0 | 29 + 0 |
| 67 | 23 + 2 | 26 + 2 | 29 + 3 |
| 68 | 23 + 5 | 26 + 5 | 29 + 5 |
| 69 | 24 + 0 | 27 + 1 | 30 + 1 |
| 70 | 24 + 3 | 27 + 3 | 30 + 4 |
| 71 | 24 + 6 | 27 + 6 | 30 + 6 |
| 72 | 25 + 1 | 28 + 2 | 31 + 2 |
| 73 | 25 + 4 | 28 + 5 | 31 + 5 |

*(continued)*

**Table 3–4. ASSESSMENT OF GESTATIONAL AGE FROM THE BIPARIETAL DIAMETER (CONTINUED)**

| Biparietal Diameter (mm) | Gestational Age (weeks + days) | | |
|---|---|---|---|
| | 5th Percentile | 50th Percentile | 95th Percentile |
| 74 | 26 + 0 | 29 + 0 | 32 + 1 |
| 75 | 26 + 3 | 29 + 3 | 32 + 4 |
| 76 | 26 + 6 | 29 + 6 | 32 + 6 |
| 77 | 27 + 1 | 30 + 2 | 33 + 2 |
| 78 | 27 + 4 | 30 + 5 | 33 + 5 |
| 79 | 28 + 0 | 31 + 1 | 34 + 1 |
| 80 | 28 + 3 | 31 + 3 | 34 + 4 |
| 81 | 28 + 6 | 31 + 6 | 35 + 0 |
| 82 | 29 + 2 | 32 + 2 | 35 + 3 |
| 83 | 29 + 5 | 32 + 5 | 35 + 6 |
| 84 | 30 + 1 | 33 + 1 | 36 + 2 |
| 85 | 30 + 4 | 33 + 4 | 36 + 5 |
| 86 | 31 + 0 | 34 + 0 | 37 + 1 |
| 87 | 31 + 3 | 34 + 3 | 37 + 4 |
| 88 | 31 + 6 | 35 + 0 | 38 + 0 |
| 89 | 32 + 2 | 35 + 3 | 38 + 3 |
| 90 | 32 + 5 | 35 + 6 | 38 + 6 |
| 91 | 33 + 2 | 36 + 2 | 39 + 2 |
| 92 | 33 + 5 | 36 + 5 | 39 + 6 |
| 93 | 34 + 1 | 37 + 1 | 40 + 2 |
| 94 | 34 + 4 | 37 + 5 | 40 + 5 |
| 95 | 35 + 0 | 38 + 1 | 41 + 1 |
| 96 | 35 + 4 | 38 + 4 | 41 + 4 |
| 97 | 36 + 0 | 39 + 0 | 42 + 1 |
| 98 | 36 + 3 | 39 + 4 | 42 + 4 |
| 99 | 37 + 0 | 40 + 0 | 43 + 0 |

From Jeanty P. Fetal biometry. In Fleischer AC, Romero R, et al. *The Principles and Practice of Ultrasonography in Obstetrics and Gynecology*. 4th ed. East Norwalk, CT: Appleton & Lange; 1991:100, with permission.

the fetal head shape, (eg, oligohydramnios and breech presentation[13,14]), other parameters, such as the HC, should be used.

Hadlock and coworkers[12] suggested that the CI is constant throughout gestation, with a mean value of 78.3 and a standard deviation (SD) of 4.4. A CI $>1$ SD from the mean ($<74$ or $>83$) was found to be associated with a significant change in the BPD measurement expected for any given age. Using the CI, certain variations in the shape of the fetal skull, such as dolichocephaly (CI $<74$) and brachycephaly (CI $>84$), have been described.[12]

Gray and collaborators[10] proposed that the CI varies with advancing age (Table 3–5). These authors also suggested that the normal CI range is within 1 SD of the mean, with a sensitivity of 84% and a false-positive rate of 35% for detection of a misleading BPD value.

The head/abdominal circumference ratio was used to determine growth restriction in fetuses.[15]

**Table 3–5. CEPHALIC INDEX: MEAN AND NORMAL RANGE**

| Week | Mean Cephalic Index | −1 SD | +1 SD |
|---|---|---|---|
| 14 | 81.5 | 77.8 | 85.3 |
| 15 | 81.0 | 77.3 | 84.8 |
| 16 | 80.5 | 76.8 | 84.3 |
| 17 | 80.1 | 76.4 | 83.9 |
| 18 | 79.7 | 76.0 | 83.5 |
| 19 | 79.4 | 75.7 | 83.2 |
| 20 | 79.1 | 75.4 | 82.9 |
| 21 | 78.8 | 75.1 | 82.6 |
| 22 | 78.6 | 74.9 | 82.4 |
| 23 | 78.4 | 74.7 | 82.2 |
| 24 | 78.3 | 74.6 | 82.0 |
| 25 | 78.1 | 74.4 | 81.9 |
| 26 | 78.0 | 74.3 | 81.8 |
| 27 | 78.0 | 74.3 | 81.8 |
| 28 | 78.0 | 74.3 | 81.8 |
| 29 | 78.0 | 74.3 | 81.8 |
| 30 | 78.1 | 74.4 | 81.9 |
| 31 | 78.2 | 74.5 | 82.0 |
| 32 | 78.3 | 74.6 | 82.1 |
| 33 | 78.5 | 74.8 | 82.3 |
| 34 | 78.7 | 75.0 | 82.5 |
| 35 | 78.9 | 75.2 | 82.7 |
| 36 | 79.2 | 75.5 | 83.0 |
| 37 | 79.5 | 75.8 | 83.3 |
| 38 | 79.9 | 76.2 | 83.7 |
| 39 | 80.3 | 76.6 | 84.1 |
| 40 | 80.7 | 77.0 | 84.5 |

From Gray and colleagues, 1989,[10] with permission.

## HEAD CIRCUMFERENCE

### Definition

The HC represents the outer perimeter of the fetal calvarium measured at the level of the BPD.

### How to Measure It

The correct anatomical plane that should be used to measure the HC corresponds to the axial plane described by Campbell and Thoms,[6] previously delineated in the section on BPD. Ideally, the formula for the circumference of an ellipse should be used.[16]

$$HC = \sqrt{(\text{transverse diameter})^2 + (\text{longitudinal diameter})^2/2} \times \pi$$

Both transverse and longitudinal diameters should be outer-to-outer distances (as for the CI). Adequate calculation of the HC can also be made using the formula[17]

$$[D1 + D2] \times 1.57$$

The HC can also be measured along the outer perimeter of the calvarium, using a map measurer or electronic digitizer, as originally described by Hadlock's group.[17,18] The calculation of a circumference from two diameters is equivalent to the electronically digitized perimeter measurement, although the probability of technical errors between these techniques exists.

### Comments

The HC was originally described as a useful index to estimate fetal age in cases in which variations in head shape (eg, dolichocephaly or brachycephaly) adversely affected the accuracy of the BPD.[19] Several authors have demonstrated that the HC is a better predictor of fetal age than the BPD.[20–22] This is because the HC is more shape independent, and thus is less prone to be affected by molding of the fetal head (Tables 3–6 and 3–7).

As with other parameters, such as the BPD, the variability for estimation of age via the HC progressively increases with advancing menstrual age, ranging from ±1.19 at the 12- to 18-week interval to ±2.70 at the 36- to 42-week interval (Table 3–8).[9]

The HC has also been used in equations developed to estimate fetal weight,[23] to monitor normal fetal growth as well as intrauterine growth restriction,[24,25] and for the diagnosis of microcephaly (Table 3–9). Microcephaly is a clinical syndrome characterized by an abnormally small head. Most authors agree that the diagnosis of microcephaly should be suspected when the HC is 3 SD below the mean for a given gestational age.[26–28] Nevertheless, the antenatal accuracy for the diagnosis of microcephaly using this parameter has been reported to be as low as 56.2%.[28] To overcome this low performance, other measurements, such as the frontal lobe distance and the thalamic frontal lobe distance, have been proposed.[29] Other typical features of microcephalic fetuses, such as a cone-shaped head, a large face, large ears, and a sloping forehead ("birdhead"),[29] as well as associated

**Table 3–6. PREDICTED HEAD CIRCUMFERENCE AT SPECIFIC MENSTRUAL AGES**

| Menstrual Age (weeks) | Head Circumference (cm) | Menstrual Age (weeks) | Head Circumference (cm) |
|---|---|---|---|
| 12.0 | 6.8 | 26.5 | 25.1 |
| 12.5 | 7.5 | 27.0 | 25.6 |
| 13.0 | 8.2 | 27.5 | 26.1 |
| 13.5 | 8.9 | 28.0 | 26.6 |
| 14.0 | 9.7 | 28.5 | 27.1 |
| 14.5 | 10.4 | 29.0 | 27.5 |
| 15.0 | 11.0 | 29.5 | 28.0 |
| 15.5 | 11.7 | 30.0 | 28.4 |
| 16.0 | 12.4 | 30.5 | 28.8 |
| 16.5 | 13.1 | 31.0 | 29.3 |
| 17.0 | 13.8 | 31.5 | 29.7 |
| 17.5 | 14.4 | 32.0 | 30.1 |
| 18.0 | 15.1 | 32.5 | 30.4 |
| 18.5 | 15.8 | 33.0 | 30.8 |
| 19.0 | 16.4 | 33.5 | 31.2 |
| 19.5 | 17.0 | 34.0 | 31.5 |
| 20.0 | 17.7 | 34.5 | 31.8 |
| 20.5 | 18.3 | 35.0 | 32.2 |
| 21.0 | 18.9 | 35.5 | 32.5 |
| 21.5 | 19.5 | 36.0 | 32.8 |
| 22.0 | 20.1 | 36.5 | 33.0 |
| 22.5 | 20.7 | 37.0 | 33.3 |
| 23.0 | 21.3 | 37.5 | 33.5 |
| 23.5 | 21.9 | 38.0 | 33.8 |
| 24.0 | 22.4 | 38.5 | 34.0 |
| 24.5 | 23.0 | 39.0 | 34.2 |
| 25.0 | 23.5 | 39.5 | 34.4 |
| 25.5 | 24.1 | 40.0 | 34.6 |
| 26.0 | 24.6 | | |

After Hadlock and colleagues, 1984,[9] with permission.

Table 3–7. ASSESSMENT OF GESTATIONAL AGE FROM THE HEAD CIRCUMFERENCE

| Head Perimeter (mm) | Gestational Age (weeks + days) | | |
|---|---|---|---|
| | 5th Percentile | 50th Percentile | 95th Percentile |
| 80 | 10 + 5 | 12 + 4 | 14 + 2 |
| 84 | 11 + 0 | 12 + 5 | 14 + 4 |
| 88 | 11 + 2 | 13 + 0 | 14 + 6 |
| 92 | 11 + 4 | 13 + 2 | 15 + 0 |
| 96 | 11 + 6 | 13 + 4 | 15 + 2 |
| 100 | 12 + 1 | 13 + 6 | 15 + 4 |
| 104 | 12 + 3 | 14 + 1 | 15 + 6 |
| 108 | 12 + 5 | 14 + 3 | 16 + 1 |
| 112 | 13 + 0 | 14 + 5 | 16 + 3 |
| 116 | 13 + 2 | 15 + 0 | 16 + 5 |
| 120 | 13 + 4 | 15 + 2 | 17 + 0 |
| 124 | 13 + 6 | 15 + 4 | 17 + 2 |
| 128 | 14 + 1 | 15 + 6 | 17 + 5 |
| 132 | 14 + 3 | 16 + 1 | 18 + 0 |
| 136 | 14 + 5 | 16 + 4 | 18 + 2 |
| 140 | 15 + 0 | 16 + 6 | 18 + 4 |
| 144 | 15 + 3 | 17 + 1 | 18 + 6 |
| 148 | 15 + 5 | 17 + 3 | 19 + 2 |
| 152 | 16 + 0 | 17 + 6 | 19 + 4 |
| 156 | 16 + 3 | 18 + 1 | 19 + 6 |
| 160 | 16 + 5 | 18 + 3 | 20 + 1 |
| 164 | 17 + 0 | 18 + 6 | 20 + 4 |
| 168 | 17 + 3 | 19 + 1 | 20 + 6 |
| 172 | 17 + 5 | 19 + 3 | 21 + 2 |
| 176 | 18 + 0 | 19 + 6 | 21 + 4 |
| 180 | 18 + 3 | 20 + 1 | 21 + 6 |
| 184 | 18 + 5 | 20 + 4 | 22 + 2 |
| 188 | 19 + 1 | 20 + 6 | 22 + 4 |
| 192 | 19 + 3 | 21 + 2 | 23 + 0 |
| 196 | 19 + 6 | 21 + 4 | 23 + 3 |
| 200 | 20 + 2 | 22 + 0 | 23 + 5 |
| 204 | 20 + 4 | 22 + 2 | 24 + 1 |

*(continued)*

Table 3–7. ASSESSMENT OF GESTATIONAL AGE FROM THE HEAD CIRCUMFERENCE (CONTINUED)

| | Gestational Age (weeks + days) | | |
|---|---|---|---|
| Head Perimeter (mm) | 5th Percentile | 50th Percentile | 95th Percentile |
| 208 | 21 + 0 | 22 + 5 | 24 + 3 |
| 212 | 21 + 2 | 23 + 1 | 24 + 6 |
| 216 | 21 + 5 | 23 + 3 | 25 + 2 |
| 220 | 22 + 1 | 23 + 6 | 25 + 4 |
| 224 | 22 + 4 | 24 + 2 | 26 + 0 |
| 228 | 22 + 6 | 24 + 5 | 26 + 3 |
| 232 | 23 + 2 | 25 + 0 | 26 + 6 |
| 236 | 23 + 5 | 25 + 3 | 27 + 2 |
| 240 | 24 + 1 | 25 + 6 | 27 + 4 |
| 244 | 24 + 4 | 26 + 2 | 28 + 0 |
| 248 | 25 + 0 | 26 + 5 | 28 + 3 |
| 252 | 25 + 3 | 27 + 1 | 28 + 6 |
| 256 | 25 + 6 | 27 + 4 | 29 + 2 |
| 260 | 26 + 1 | 28 + 0 | 29 + 5 |
| 264 | 26 + 4 | 28 + 3 | 30 + 1 |
| 268 | 27 + 1 | 28 + 6 | 30 + 4 |
| 272 | 27 + 4 | 29 + 2 | 31 + 0 |
| 276 | 28 + 0 | 29 + 5 | 31 + 3 |
| 280 | 28 + 3 | 30 + 1 | 31 + 6 |
| 284 | 28 + 6 | 30 + 4 | 32 + 2 |
| 288 | 29 + 2 | 31 + 0 | 32 + 6 |
| 292 | 29 + 5 | 31 + 4 | 33 + 2 |
| 296 | 30 + 1 | 32 + 0 | 33 + 5 |
| 300 | 30 + 5 | 32 + 3 | 34 + 1 |
| 304 | 31 + 1 | 32 + 6 | 34 + 5 |
| 308 | 31 + 4 | 33 + 3 | 35 + 1 |
| 312 | 32 + 1 | 33 + 6 | 35 + 4 |
| 316 | 32 + 4 | 34 + 2 | 36 + 0 |
| 320 | 33 + 0 | 34 + 6 | 36 + 4 |
| 324 | 33 + 4 | 35 + 2 | 37 + 0 |
| 328 | 34 + 0 | 35 + 5 | 37 + 4 |
| 332 | 34 + 4 | 36 + 2 | 38 + 0 |

*(continued)*

**Table 3–7. ASSESSMENT OF GESTATIONAL AGE FROM THE HEAD CIRCUMFERENCE (CONTINUED)**

| | Gestational Age (weeks + days) | | |
|---|---|---|---|
| **Head Perimeter (mm)** | **5th Percentile** | **50th Percentile** | **95th Percentile** |
| 336 | 35 + 0 | 36 + 5 | 38 + 4 |
| 340 | 35 + 3 | 37 + 2 | 39 + 0 |
| 344 | 36 + 0 | 37 + 5 | 39 + 4 |
| 348 | 36 + 4 | 38 + 2 | 40 + 0 |
| 352 | 37 + 0 | 38 + 5 | 40 + 4 |
| 356 | 37 + 4 | 39 + 2 | 41 + 0 |
| 360 | 38 + 0 | 39 + 6 | 41 + 4 |
| 364 | 38 + 4 | 40 + 2 | 42 + 1 |

From Jeanty P. Fetal biometry. In Fleischer AC, Romero R, Manning FA, Jeanty P, James AE. *The Principles and Practice of Ultrasonography in Obstetrics and Gynecology*. 4th ed. East Norwalk, CT: Appleton & Lange; 1991:102, with permission.

anomalies such as ventricular enlargement, porencephaly, and cephaloceles,[28] should be carefully searched. Some investigators have postulated that a reduction in blood supply to the underdeveloped cerebral hemispheres in fetuses with microcephaly could be detected with color Doppler and power Doppler imaging.[30]

As the nomograms for HC require knowledge of the accurate fetal age, and this information is not always available, the use of ratios such as the HC-to-femur length ratios has the advantage of reducing dependence on reliable age evaluation (Table 3–10).[28] This ratio assumes that limb growth is not affected in fetuses with microcephaly, which might not always be the case.

## ORBITAL DIAMETERS: INNER ORBITAL DIAMETER, OUTER ORBITAL DIAMETER, AND OCULAR DIAMETER

### Definition

The inner orbital, or interorbital, diameter (IOD) is defined as the distance between the medial border of one orbit and the medial border of the opposite orbit. The outer orbital, or biorbital, diameter (OOD) is defined as the distance between the lateral border of one orbit and the lateral border of the opposite orbit.[31] The ocular diameter corresponds to the distance between the medial border and the lateral border of a single orbit.

**Table 3–8. VARIABILITY IN PREDICTING MENSTRUAL AGE USING THE BIPARIETAL DIAMETER AND THE HEAD CIRCUMFERENCE**

| | Subgroup Variability (± 2 SD) in Weeks | | | | |
|---|---|---|---|---|---|
| **Fetal Parameters** | **12–18 Weeks** | **18–24 Weeks** | **24–30 Weeks** | **30–36 Weeks** | **36–42 Weeks** |
| Biparietal diameter | ±1.19 | ±1.73 | ±2.18 | ±3.08 | ±3.20 |
| Head circumference | ±1.19 | ±1.48 | ±2.06 | ±2.98 | ±2.70 |

Modified from Hadlock and colleagues, 1984,[9] with permission.

**Table 3–9. MEANS AND STANDARD DEVIATIONS OF THE HEAD CIRCUMFERENCE AS A FUNCTION OF GESTATIONAL AGE**

| | | Head Circumference (mm): SD Below Mean | | | | |
|---|---|---|---|---|---|---|
| **Week** | **Mean** | **−1** | **−2** | **−3** | **−4** | **−5** |
| 20 | 175 | 160 | 145 | 131 | 116 | 101 |
| 21 | 187 | 172 | 157 | 143 | 128 | 113 |
| 22 | 198 | 184 | 169 | 154 | 140 | 125 |
| 23 | 210 | 195 | 180 | 166 | 151 | 136 |
| 24 | 221 | 206 | 191 | 177 | 162 | 147 |
| 25 | 232 | 217 | 202 | 188 | 173 | 158 |
| 26 | 242 | 227 | 213 | 198 | 183 | 169 |
| 27 | 252 | 238 | 223 | 208 | 194 | 179 |
| 28 | 262 | 247 | 233 | 218 | 203 | 189 |
| 29 | 271 | 257 | 242 | 227 | 213 | 198 |
| 30 | 281 | 266 | 251 | 236 | 222 | 207 |
| 31 | 289 | 274 | 260 | 245 | 230 | 216 |
| 32 | 297 | 283 | 268 | 253 | 239 | 224 |
| 33 | 305 | 290 | 276 | 261 | 246 | 232 |
| 34 | 312 | 297 | 283 | 268 | 253 | 239 |
| 35 | 319 | 304 | 289 | 275 | 260 | 245 |
| 36 | 325 | 310 | 295 | 281 | 266 | 251 |
| 37 | 330 | 316 | 301 | 286 | 272 | 257 |
| 38 | 335 | 320 | 306 | 291 | 276 | 262 |
| 39 | 339 | 325 | 310 | 295 | 281 | 266 |
| 40 | 343 | 328 | 314 | 299 | 284 | 270 |
| 41 | 346 | 331 | 316 | 302 | 287 | 272 |
| 42 | 348 | 333 | 319 | 304 | 289 | 275 |

SD, standard deviation.

From Chervenak and colleagues, 1984,[28] with permission.

## How to Measure It (Figure 3–3)

To measure the orbital diameters, an axial plane slightly caudad to the BPD is commonly used. The criteria used for this section are (1) a symmetrical section, (2) both eyes imaged and of equal diameter, and (3) the largest possible diameter of the eyes.[32] Measurements of orbital diameters can also be accomplished using a coronal plane, ~2 cm posterior to the glabella-alveolar line.[31]

## Comments

The study of the orbital diameters should help in the diagnosis of hypotelorism, hypertelorism, and microphthalmos. Trout and colleagues[33] have found that in cases of hypotelorism, both the IOD and the OOD clearly fall below 2 SD of the mean. In cases of hypertelorism, the IOD fell above the 95th percentile, whereas the OOD measurement fell within normal limits but near the 95th

**Table 3–10. MEANS AND STANDARD DEVIATIONS OF THE FEMUR LENGTH: HEAD CIRCUMFERENCE RATIOS AS A FUNCTION OF GESTATIONAL AGE**

| | | SD Below Mean | | | | |
|---|---|---|---|---|---|---|
| **Week** | **Mean** | **−5** | **−4** | **−3** | **−2** | **−1** |
| 20 | 0.180 | 0.107 | 0.122 | 0.137 | 0.152 | 0.167 |
| 21 | 0.190 | 0.111 | 0.126 | 0.141 | 0.156 | 0.171 |
| 22 | 0.190 | 0.115 | 0.130 | 0.145 | 0.160 | 0.175 |
| 23 | 0.190 | 0.118 | 0.133 | 0.148 | 0.163 | 0.178 |
| 24 | 0.200 | 0.121 | 0.136 | 0.151 | 0.166 | 0.181 |
| 25 | 0.200 | 0.123 | 0.138 | 0.153 | 0.168 | 0.183 |
| 26 | 0.200 | 0.125 | 0.140 | 0.155 | 0.170 | 0.185 |
| 27 | 0.200 | 0.127 | 0.142 | 0.157 | 0.172 | 0.187 |
| 28 | 0.200 | 0.129 | 0.144 | 0.159 | 0.174 | 0.189 |
| 29 | 0.200 | 0.130 | 0.145 | 0.160 | 0.175 | 0.190 |
| 30 | 0.210 | 0.131 | 0.146 | 0.161 | 0.176 | 0.191 |
| 31 | 0.210 | 0.132 | 0.147 | 0.162 | 0.177 | 0.192 |
| 32 | 0.210 | 0.134 | 0.149 | 0.164 | 0.179 | 0.194 |
| 33 | 0.210 | 0.135 | 0.150 | 0.165 | 0.180 | 0.195 |
| 34 | 0.210 | 0.136 | 0.151 | 0.166 | 0.181 | 0.196 |
| 35 | 0.210 | 0.138 | 0.153 | 0.168 | 0.183 | 0.198 |
| 36 | 0.210 | 0.140 | 0.155 | 0.170 | 0.185 | 0.200 |
| 37 | 0.220 | 0.142 | 0.157 | 0.172 | 0.187 | 0.202 |
| 38 | 0.220 | 0.144 | 0.159 | 0.174 | 0.189 | 0.204 |
| 39 | 0.220 | 0.147 | 0.162 | 0.177 | 0.192 | 0.207 |
| 40 | 0.230 | 0.151 | 0.166 | 0.181 | 0.196 | 0.211 |
| 41 | 0.230 | 0.155 | 0.170 | 0.185 | 0.200 | 0.215 |
| 42 | 0.230 | 0.160 | 0.175 | 0.190 | 0.205 | 0.220 |

SD, standard deviation.

From Chervenak and colleagues, 1984,[28] with permission.

percentile. Hypotelorism has been associated with chromosomal anomalies (trisomy 13, trisomy 21, 18p−, 5p−, and 14q +), holoprosencephaly, Meckel-Gruber syndrome, microcephaly, maternal phenylketonuria, and others.[32–34] Hypertelorism can occur as an isolated defect but has also been associated with a long list of malformations and syndromes, such as frontal, ethmoidal, or sphenoidal meningoencephalocele; median cleft syndrome; and craniosynostosis.[34]

Mayden and associates[31] developed nomograms of orbital measurements as a function of the BPD, which are taken as a classical reference to which newer data are compared (Table 3–11). Nomograms for orbital diameters as a function of age have been published because the

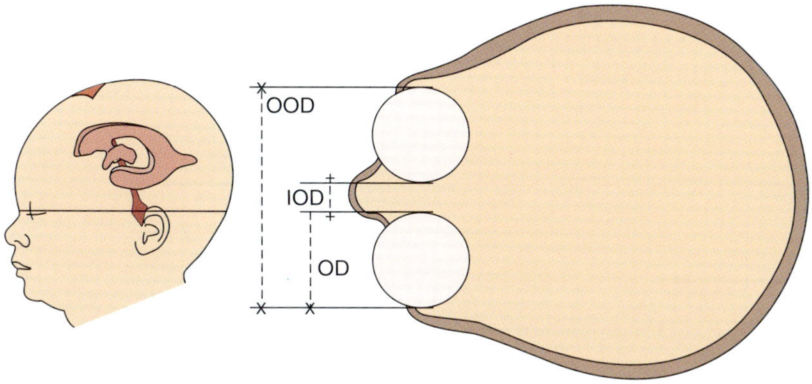


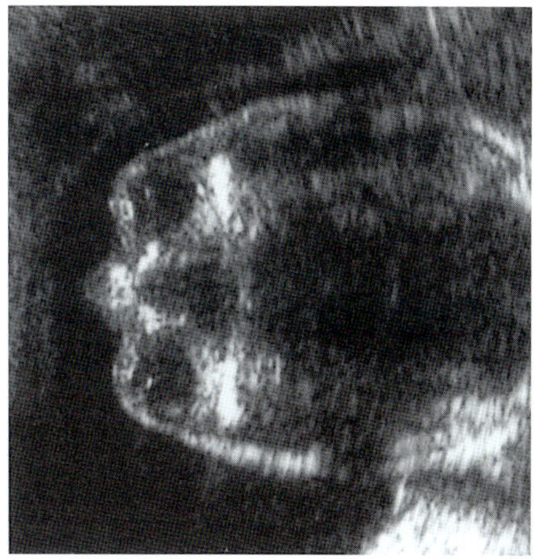

Figure 3–3.

**Table 3–11. NOMOGRAM FOR EVALUATION OF THE INNER AND OUTER ORBITAL DIAMETERS IN THE FETUS VERSUS BIPARIETAL DIAMETER**

| Biparietal Diameter (cm) | Inner Orbital Diameter (cm) | Outer Orbital Diameter (cm) |
|---|---|---|
| 1.9 | 0.5 | 1.3 |
| 2.0 | 0.5 | 1.4 |
| 2.1 | 0.6 | 1.5 |
| 2.2 | 0.6 | 1.6 |
| 2.3 | 0.6 | 1.7 |
| 2.4 | 0.7 | 1.7 |
| 2.5 | 0.7 | 1.8 |
| 2.6 | 0.7 | 1.9 |
| 2.7 | 0.8 | 2.0 |
| 2.8 | 0.8 | 2.1 |
| 2.9 | 0.8 | 2.1 |
| 3.0 | 0.9 | 2.2 |
| 3.1 | 0.9 | 2.3 |
| 3.2 | 0.9 | 2.4 |
| 3.3 | 1.0 | 2.5 |
| 3.4 | 1.0 | 2.5 |
| 3.5 | 1.0 | 2.6 |
| 3.6 | 1.0 | 2.7 |
| 3.7 | 1.1 | 2.7 |
| 3.8 | 1.1 | 2.8 |

*(continued)*

**Table 3–11. NOMOGRAM FOR EVALUATION OF THE INNER AND OUTER ORBITAL DIAMETERS IN THE FETUS VERSUS BIPARIETAL DIAMETER (CONTINUED)**

| Biparietal Diameter (cm) | Inner Orbital Diameter (cm) | Outer Orbital Diameter (cm) |
|---|---|---|
| 4.0 | 1.2 | 3.0 |
| 4.2 | 1.2 | 3.1 |
| 4.3 | 1.2 | 3.2 |
| 4.4 | 1.3 | 3.2 |
| 4.5 | 1.3 | 3.3 |
| 4.6 | 1.3 | 3.4 |
| 4.7 | 1.3 | 3.4 |
| 4.8 | 1.4 | 3.5 |
| 4.9 | 1.4 | 3.6 |
| 5.0 | 1.4 | 3.6 |
| 5.1 | 1.4 | 3.7 |
| 5.2 | 1.4 | 3.8 |
| 5.3 | 1.5 | 3.8 |
| 5.4 | 1.5 | 3.9 |
| 5.5 | 1.5 | 4.0 |
| 5.6 | 1.5 | 4.0 |
| 5.7 | 1.5 | 4.1 |
| 5.8 | 1.6 | 4.1 |
| 5.9 | 1.6 | 4.2 |
| 6.0 | 1.6 | 4.3 |
| 6.1 | 1.6 | 4.3 |
| 6.2 | 1.6 | 4.4 |
| 6.3 | 1.7 | 4.4 |
| 6.4 | 1.7 | 4.5 |
| 6.5 | 1.7 | 4.5 |
| 6.6 | 1.7 | 4.6 |
| 6.7 | 1.7 | 4.6 |
| 6.8 | 1.7 | 4.7 |
| 6.9 | 1.7 | 4.7 |
| 7.0 | 1.8 | 4.8 |

*(continued)*

**Table 3–11. NOMOGRAM FOR EVALUATION OF THE INNER AND OUTER ORBITAL DIAMETERS IN THE FETUS VERSUS BIPARIETAL DIAMETER (CONTINUED)**

| Biparietal Diameter (cm) | Inner Orbital Diameter (cm) | Outer Orbital Diameter (cm) |
|---|---|---|
| 7.1 | 1.8 | 4.8 |
| 7.3 | 1.8 | 4.9 |
| 7.4 | 1.8 | 5.0 |
| 7.5 | 1.8 | 5.0 |
| 7.6 | 1.8 | 5.1 |
| 7.7 | 1.8 | 5.1 |
| 7.8 | 1.8 | 5.2 |
| 7.9 | 1.9 | 5.2 |
| 8.0 | 1.9 | 5.3 |
| 8.2 | 1.9 | 5.4 |
| 8.3 | 1.9 | 5.4 |
| 8.4 | 1.9 | 5.4 |
| 8.5 | 1.9 | 5.5 |
| 8.6 | 1.9 | 5.5 |
| 8.8 | 1.9 | 5.6 |
| 8.9 | 1.9 | 5.6 |
| 9.0 | 1.9 | 5.7 |
| 9.1 | 1.9 | 5.7 |
| 9.2 | 1.9 | 5.8 |
| 9.3 | 1.9 | 5.8 |
| 9.4 | 1.9 | 5.8 |
| 9.6 | 1.9 | 5.9 |
| 9.7 | 1.9 | 5.9 |

From Mayden and colleagues, 1982,[31] with permission.

**Table 3–12. NOMOGRAM FOR EVALUATION OF THE INNER AND OUTER ORBITAL DIAMETERS IN THE FETUS VERSUS GESTATIONAL AGE**

| | Inner Orbital Diameter (mm) | | | Outer Orbital Diameter (mm) | | |
|---|---|---|---|---|---|---|
| Gestational Age (weeks) | 5th Percentile | 50th Percentile | 95th Percentile | 5th Percentile | 50th Percentile | 95th Percentile |
| 13 | 4 | 7 | 10 | 12 | 16 | 20 |
| 14 | 5 | 8 | 11 | 14 | 18 | 22 |
| 15 | 5 | 8 | 11 | 17 | 21 | 25 |
| 16 | 6 | 9 | 12 | 19 | 23 | 27 |
| 17 | 7 | 10 | 13 | 21 | 25 | 29 |
| 18 | 8 | 11 | 14 | 24 | 27 | 31 |
| 19 | 8 | 11 | 14 | 26 | 30 | 34 |
| 20 | 9 | 12 | 15 | 28 | 32 | 36 |
| 21 | 10 | 13 | 16 | 30 | 34 | 38 |
| 22 | 10 | 13 | 16 | 32 | 36 | 40 |
| 23 | 11 | 14 | 17 | 33 | 37 | 41 |
| 24 | 12 | 14 | 17 | 35 | 39 | 43 |
| 25 | 12 | 15 | 18 | 37 | 41 | 45 |
| 26 | 13 | 16 | 19 | 39 | 43 | 47 |
| 27 | 13 | 16 | 19 | 40 | 44 | 48 |
| 28 | 14 | 17 | 20 | 42 | 46 | 50 |
| 29 | 14 | 17 | 20 | 43 | 47 | 51 |
| 30 | 15 | 18 | 21 | 45 | 49 | 52 |
| 31 | 15 | 18 | 21 | 46 | 50 | 54 |
| 32 | 16 | 19 | 22 | 47 | 51 | 55 |
| 33 | 17 | 20 | 23 | 48 | 52 | 56 |
| 34 | 17 | 20 | 23 | 49 | 53 | 57 |
| 35 | 18 | 21 | 24 | 50 | 54 | 58 |

From Trout and colleagues, 1994,[33] with permission.

authors[33] felt that some patients could have pathologic intracranial conditions that might alter the BPD, making this measurement less reliable (Table 3–12).

Microphthalmos can be suspected when the orbital diameter falls below the fifth percentile for age (Table 3–13). Because this is a statistical definition, careful examination of the intraorbital anatomy, as well as detection of associated anomalies, is warranted. Conditions associated with microphthalmos include chromosomal (trisomies 13 and 18 and trisomy 9 mosaic), environmental (fetal toxoplasmosis, rubella, varicella, and alcohol syndrome and maternal phenylketonuria), and multiple syndromes (eg, frontonasal dysplasia, Fraser syndrome, Lenz syndrome, and Fanconi syndrome).[35]

**Table 3–13. NOMOGRAM FOR EVALUATION OF THE OCULAR DIAMETER VERSUS GESTATIONAL AGE**

| | Ocular Diameter (mm) | | |
|---|---|---|---|
| Gestational Age (weeks) | 5th Percentile | 50th Percentile | 95th Percentile |
| 11 | — | — | — |
| 12 | 1 | 3 | 6 |
| 13 | 2 | 4 | 7 |
| 14 | 3 | 5 | 8 |
| 15 | 4 | 6 | 9 |
| 16 | 5 | 7 | 9 |
| 17 | 5 | 8 | 10 |
| 18 | 6 | 9 | 11 |
| 19 | 7 | 9 | 12 |
| 20 | 8 | 10 | 13 |
| 21 | 8 | 11 | 13 |
| 22 | 9 | 12 | 14 |
| 23 | 10 | 12 | 15 |
| 24 | 10 | 13 | 15 |
| 25 | 11 | 13 | 16 |
| 26 | 12 | 14 | 16 |
| 27 | 12 | 14 | 17 |
| 28 | 13 | 15 | 17 |
| 29 | 13 | 15 | 18 |
| 30 | 14 | 16 | 18 |
| 31 | 14 | 16 | 19 |
| 32 | 14 | 17 | 19 |
| 33 | 15 | 17 | 19 |
| 34 | 15 | 17 | 20 |
| 35 | 15 | 18 | 20 |
| 36 | 16 | 18 | 20 |
| 37 | 16 | 18 | 21 |
| 38 | 16 | 18 | 21 |
| 39 | 16 | 19 | 21 |
| 40 | 16 | 19 | 21 |

Adapted from Romero and colleagues, 1988,[34] with permission.

## THE VENTRICULAR SYSTEM

For practical purposes, we have divided the analysis of the ventricular system depending on the sonographic modality used, transabdominal or transvaginal.

## TRANSABDOMINAL SONOGRAPHY

### Lateral Ventricular Width–Hemispheric Width Ratio

#### Definition

The lateral ventricular width–hemispheric width (LVW/HW) ratio represents the percentage of the whole cerebral hemisphere that corresponds to the lateral ventricle, measured in an axial plane.

#### How to Measure It (Figure 3–4)

The widths of the lateral ventricles and the hemispheres are measured in a plane parallel to the BPD, but slightly closer to the top of the head. In this section, the lateral ventricles (LVs) appear as two linear echoes, roughly parallel to the midline. The LVW is then measured as the distance from the midline to the first echoes of the LVs. This measurement is thus slightly greater than that of the actual LV, because it does not use its medial wall as the internal landmark. The HW is the largest distance between the midline and the inner edge of the skull, measured perpendicular to the midline. To avoid tilting errors, one should be able to recognize both LVs as being equal in size.[36]

#### Comments

The normal LVW/HW ratio at 15 weeks can be as high as 71%, with a mean of 56% and a range of 40% to 71%. By 37 postmenstrual weeks, the mean is 29%, with a range of 24% to 34% (Table 3–14). These data reflect the rapid growth of the cerebral hemispheres as pregnancy progresses, making the LVW/HW decrease with advancing age.[37]

The LVW/HW ratio was developed to monitor ventricular growth in an attempt to provide an early diagnosis of hydrocephaly at a time when the classical diagnosis of intrauterine hydrocephaly relied on the finding of a BPD > 11 cm or a head-to-abdomen ratio > 2.[38] Although this ratio provided a way to diagnose hydrocephaly up to 2 months before the BPD was pathologically enlarged,[36] other parameters, such as the width of the lateral ventricular atrium were able to do that too.[37] Transvaginal neurosonography can evaluate the fetal ventricular system in a much more accurate way and somewhat earlier.

One of the major drawbacks of the LVW/HW ratio is that echogenic "lines" previously used to delineate the ventricular walls are instead reflections from small venous structures deep in the fetal white matter.[39] Also, the wide SD of this ratio renders it ineffective for detecting early ventricular dilation.[40]

## ANTERIOR (FRONTAL) HORN OF THE LATERAL VENTRICLES AND CAVUM SEPTI PELLUCIDI

#### Definition

The anterior horn corresponds to the portion of the lateral ventricles anterior to the interventricular foramen.

The cavum septi pellucidi (CSP) is a closed cavity in the brain, located on the midline of the transverse plane between the two leaves of septum pellucidum, which separate the lateral ventricles.

#### How to Measure It (Figure 3–5)

To allow proper visualization of the anterior horn with transabdominal sonography, a horizontal (axial) scanning plane parallel and slightly anterior to that for the BPD should be used. In this section one should be able to recognize, in an anterior-to-posterior fashion, the anterior horns (AHs), the CSP, and the atria of the lateral ventricles (A). The cerebrofrontal horn distance (CFHD) can then be measured from the midline echo to the lateral wall of the anterior horn distal to the transducer. It should be kept in mind that from about 30 postmenstrual weeks on, the lumen of the anterior horns is very hard to visualize, and only its lateral aspect is defined. The frontal HW is measured from the leading edge of the midline echo

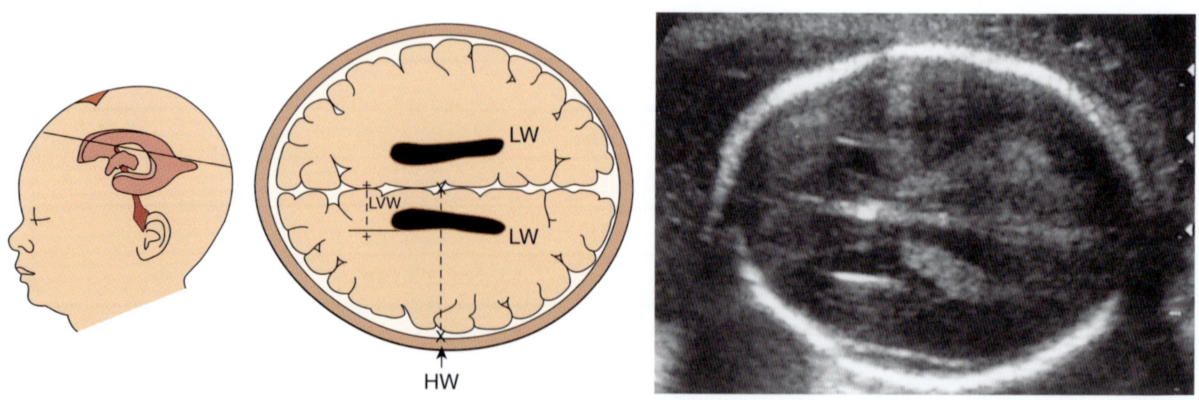


**Figure 3–4.**

**Table 3–14. NOMOGRAM FOR EVALUATION OF THE LATERAL VENTRICULAR WIDTH–HEMISPHERIC WIDTH RATIO**

| Menstrual Age (weeks) | Lateral Ventricular Width (LVW) (cm) | Hemispheric Width (HW) (cm) | Ratio LVW/HW (% ± 2 SD) |
|---|---|---|---|
| 15 | 0.75 | 1.4 | 56 (40–71) |
| 16 | 0.86 | 1.5 | 57 (45–69) |
| 17 | 0.85 | 1.5 | 52 (42–62) |
| 18 | 0.83 | 1.8 | 46 (40–52) |
| 19 | — | — | — |
| 20 | 0.82 | 1.9 | 43 (29–57) |
| 21 | 0.76 | 2.2 | 35 (27–43) |
| 22 | 0.82 | 2.6 | 32 (26–38) |
| 23 | 0.83 | 2.5 | 33 (24–42) |
| 24 | 0.83 | 2.7 | 31 (23–39) |
| 25 | 1.1 | 3.0 | 34 (26–42) |
| 26 | 0.9 | 3.0 | 30 (24–36) |
| 27 | 0.9 | 3.0 | 28 (23–34) |
| 28 | 1.1 | 3.3 | 31 (18–45) |
| 29 | 1.0 | 3.4 | 29 (22–37) |
| 30 | 1.0 | 3.4 | 30 (26–34) |
| 31 | 1.0 | 3.4 | 29 (23–36) |
| 32 | 1.1 | 3.6 | 31 (26–36) |
| 33 | 1.1 | 3.4 | 31 (25–37) |
| 34 | 1.1 | 3.8 | 28 (23–33) |
| 35 | 1.1 | 3.8 | 29 (26–31) |
| 36 | 1.1 | 3.9 | 28 (23–34) |
| 37 | 1.2 | 4.1 | 29 (24–34) |
| Term | 1.2 | 4.3 | 28 (22–33) |

From Johnson and colleagues, 1980,[37] with permission.

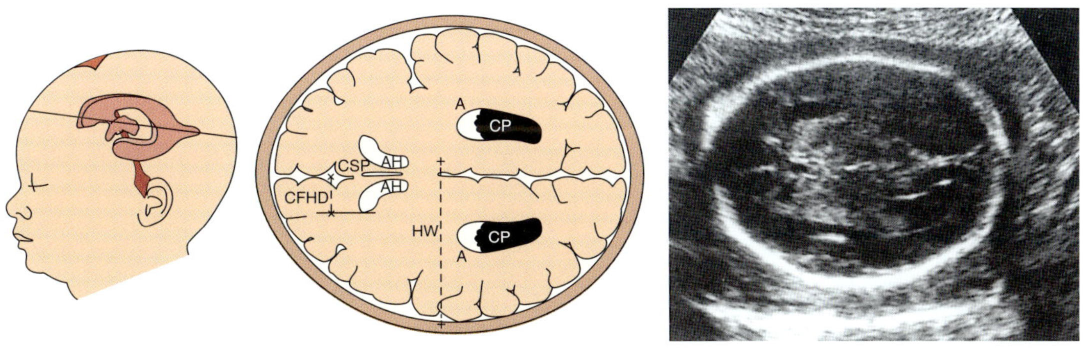


**Figure 3–5.**

**Table 3–15. NOMOGRAM OF THE CEREBROFRONTAL HORN DISTANCE THROUGHOUT PREGNANCY (IN CENTIMETERS)**

| Gestational Age (weeks) | Mean ± 2 SD | Percentile 10th | Percentile 50th | Percentile 90th |
|---|---|---|---|---|
| 15 | 0.7 ± 0.10 | 0.6 | 0.7 | 0.9 |
| 16 | 0.8 ± 0.12 | 0.5 | 0.8 | 1.0 |
| 17 | 0.9 ± 0.16 | 0.7 | 0.9 | 1.2 |
| 18 | 0.8 ± 0.05 | 0.8 | 0.9 | 0.9 |
| 19 | 0.8 ± 0.10 | 0.7 | 0.8 | 0.9 |
| 20 | 0.8 ± 0.10 | 0.7 | 0.8 | 1.0 |
| 21 | 0.8 ± 0.08 | 0.7 | 0.8 | 0.9 |
| 22 | 0.8 ± 0.07 | 0.7 | 0.8 | 0.9 |
| 23 | 0.9 ± 0.10 | 0.7 | 0.8 | 1.0 |
| 24 | 0.8 ± 0.07 | 0.7 | 0.9 | 0.9 |
| 25 | 0.8 ± 0.05 | 0.7 | 0.8 | 0.8 |
| 26 | 0.9 ± 0.11 | 0.8 | 1.0 | 1.1 |
| 27 | 1.0 ± 0.17 | 0.8 | 1.0 | 1.2 |
| 28 | 0.9 ± 0.13 | 0.8 | 0.9 | 1.1 |
| 29 | 1.0 ± 0.09 | 0.9 | 1.0 | 1.1 |
| 30 | 1.0 ± 0.12 | 0.8 | 1.0 | 1.2 |
| 31 | 1.0 ± 0.16 | 0.8 | 1.0 | 1.3 |
| 32 | 1.1 ± 0.08 | 1.0 | 1.1 | 1.2 |
| 33 | 1.1 ± 0.12 | 0.9 | 1.1 | 1.2 |
| 34 | 1.1 ± 0.13 | 0.9 | 1.0 | 1.2 |
| 35 | 1.2 ± 0.15 | 1.0 | 1.1 | 1.4 |
| 36 | 1.2 ± 0.10 | 1.1 | 1.2 | 1.3 |
| 37 | 1.1 ± 0.00 | 1.1 | 1.1 | 1.1 |
| 38 | 1.2 ± 0.06 | 1.2 | 1.2 | 1.3 |
| 39 | 1.3 ± 0.19 | 1.0 | 1.3 | 1.4 |
| 40 | 1.2 ± 0.00 | 1.2 | 1.2 | 1.2 |

From Goldstein and colleagues, 1988,[41] with permission.

to the inner aspect of the fetal calvarium at the point of maximal HW.[41]

## Comments

The relative size of the anterior horns decreases with advancing gestational age. This was demonstrated by Goldstein and coworkers,[41] who found that, in spite of an increasing CFHD throughout pregnancy, the CFHD/HW ratio decreases throughout gestation, from 50% at 15 menstrual weeks to 28% at term (Tables 3–15 and 3–16). These findings correlate with previous reports[42] and are related to the fact that the internal lumina of the ventricles are progressively reduced and molded by the growth of

**Table 3–16. NOMOGRAM OF THE FRONTAL HEMISPHERIC WIDTH THROUGHOUT PREGNANCY**

| | | Percentile | | |
|---|---|---|---|---|
| Gestational Age (weeks) | Mean ± 2 SD (cm) | 10th | 50th | 90th |
| 15 | 1.5 ± 0.11 | 1.3 | 1.5 | 1.6 |
| 16 | 1.6 ± 0.12 | 1.5 | 1.7 | 1.8 |
| 17 | 1.7 ± 0.10 | 1.6 | 1.8 | 1.9 |
| 18 | 2.0 ± 0.07 | 1.9 | 2.0 | 2.1 |
| 19 | 2.1 ± 0.09 | 2.0 | 2.1 | 2.2 |
| 20 | 2.2 ± 0.10 | 2.1 | 2.3 | 2.3 |
| 21 | 2.3 ± 0.09 | 2.2 | 2.3 | 2.5 |
| 22 | 2.5 ± 0.07 | 2.4 | 2.5 | 2.6 |
| 23 | 2.7 ± 0.13 | 2.5 | 2.7 | 2.9 |
| 24 | 2.8 ± 0.10 | 2.6 | 2.9 | 2.9 |
| 25 | 3.0 ± 0.04 | 3.0 | 3.0 | 3.1 |
| 26 | 3.1 ± 0.11 | 3.0 | 3.3 | 3.4 |
| 27 | 3.3 ± 0.12 | 3.1 | 3.3 | 3.4 |
| 28 | 3.4 ± 0.09 | 3.3 | 3.5 | 3.5 |
| 29 | 3.6 ± 0.15 | 3.4 | 3.6 | 3.8 |
| 30 | 3.7 ± 0.20 | 3.4 | 3.8 | 3.9 |
| 31 | 3.9 ± 0.19 | 3.6 | 3.9 | 4.2 |
| 32 | 3.9 ± 0.17 | 3.5 | 3.9 | 4.1 |
| 33 | 4.0 ± 0.10 | 3.8 | 4.0 | 4.1 |
| 34 | 4.1 ± 0.18 | 3.8 | 4.2 | 4.2 |
| 35 | 4.4 ± 0.34 | 3.9 | 4.4 | 4.8 |
| 36 | 4.4 ± 0.13 | 4.2 | 4.4 | 4.5 |
| 37 | 4.4 ± 0.00 | 4.4 | 4.4 | 4.4 |
| 38 | 4.3 ± 0.22 | 4.1 | 4.3 | 4.6 |
| 39 | 4.6 ± 0.14 | 4.5 | 4.5 | 4.8 |
| 40 | 4.4 ± 0.00 | 4.4 | 4.4 | 4.4 |

From Goldstein and colleagues, 1988,[41] with permission.

the basal nuclei, the corpus striatum, and the knee of the corpus callosum.

The septi pellucidi are two thin, translucent leaves that extend from the anterior part of the body, the genu, and the rostrum of the corpus callosum to the superior surface of the fornix. They begin to develop at 10 to 12 weeks of gestation and reach an adult form by the 17th week of gestation (Table 3–17).[43] They are also part of the limbic system and are important relay stations, which are linked with the main hippocampus and hypothalamus. For a more extensive review of the sonographic diagnosis of CSP abnormalities, see Chapter 5.

**Table 3–17. MEAN WIDTH AND STANDARD DEVIATION OF THE CAVUM SEPTI PELLUCIDI AT VARIOUS GESTATIONAL AGES IN 608 FETUSES**

| Gestational Age (weeks) | −2 SD | −1 SD | Mean Width (mm) | +1 SD | +2 SD | *n* |
|---|---|---|---|---|---|---|
| 19–20 | 2.08 | 2.74 | 3.40 | 4.06 | 4.7 | 43 |
| 21–22 | 2.60 | 3.33 | 4.06 | 4.81 | 5.52 | 104 |
| 23–24 | 3.02 | 3.88 | 4.74 | 5.60 | 6.46 | 92 |
| 25–26 | 3.96 | 4.76 | 5.56 | 6.36 | 7.16 | 36 |
| 27–28 | 4.12 | 5.27 | 6.42 | 7.57 | 8.72 | 18 |
| 29–30 | 4.37 | 5.29 | 6.11 | 7.13 | 8.05 | 24 |
| 31–32 | 4.43 | 5.47 | 6.51 | 7.55 | 8.59 | 77 |
| 33–34 | 4.04 | 5.26 | 6.48 | 7.70 | 8.92 | 116 |
| 35–36 | 4.37 | 5.41 | 6.45 | 7.49 | 8.53 | 55 |
| 37–38 | 3.81 | 5.09 | 6.37 | 7.65 | 8.93 | 27 |
| 39–40 | 4.64 | 5.47 | 6.30 | 7.13 | 7.96 | 10 |
| 41–42 | 3.62 | 4.55 | 5.48 | 6.41 | 7.34 | 6 |

CSP, cavum septi pellucidi; SD, standard deviation.

From Jou and colleagues, 1998,[43] with permission.

## ATRIUM OF THE LATERAL VENTRICLES

### Definition

The atrium, or the trigone, is the triangular portion of the lateral ventricle that is connected anteriorly to the body, posteriorly to the posterior horn, and inferiorly to the inferior horn. The lateral ventricular atrium width (LVAW) is the widest dimension of the atrium of the lateral ventricles that can be measured in an axial plane.

### How to Measure It (Figure 3–6)

The atrium (A) of the lateral ventricles can be measured near the axial plane previously described for the BPD.[39] It can be easily recognized by the presence of the highly echogenic choroid plexus (CP) within it, marking the lateral wall of the ventricle farther from the transducer. The electronic calipers are then placed using an outer-to-inner (leading edge-to-leading edge) technique. Other

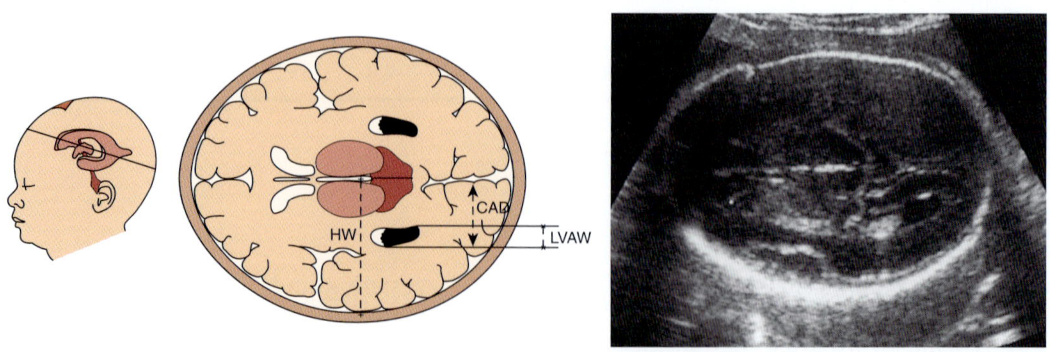


**Figure 3–6.**

**Table 3–18. DIAMETER OF THE LATERAL VENTRICULAR ATRIUM ACCORDING TO GESTATIONAL AGE**

| Gestational Age (weeks) | Lateral Ventricular Atrium Diameter (mm) | |
|---|---|---|
| | Mean ± SD | Range |
| 14–20 | 7.6 ± 0.7 | 6.0–9.0 |
| 21–25 | 7.7 ± 0.5 | 7.0–9.0 |
| 26–30 | 7.5 ± 0.7 | 6.5–9.0 |
| 31–38 | 7.6 ± 0.5 | 7.0–8.5 |
| All | 7.6 ± 0.6 | 6.0–9.0 |

SD, standard deviation.

Modified from Cardoza and colleagues, 1988,[39] with permission.

parameters that can be used to evaluate the ventricular atrium are the cerebroatrial distance (CAD), atrial width/HW ratio, atrial width/CAD ratio, and CAD/HW ratio. The CAD is measured in the same plane as the distance between the midline and the outer border of the atrial lumen. The HW corresponds to the distance between the midline and the inner border of the calvarium.

## Comments

It is important to place the calipers across the ventricle that contains the choroid plexus just across the indentation of the cortex marking the parietooccipital fissure. This anatomic landmark becomes increasingly evidence and marked as the gestational age increases.

The ventricular atrium is a structure easily recognized due to the presence within it of the choroid plexus, which is among the most noticeable intracranial landmarks. During the second and third trimesters, the choroid plexus normally fills the atrium of the lateral ventricles, touching the lateral ventricular walls. Ventricular enlargement can thus be suspected when a separation ≥3 mm can be measured between the ventricular surface of the choroid plexus and the adjacent ventricular wall.[44]

The LVAW is an excellent measurement for verifying the state of the ventricular system. It is age independent, with a mean of 7.6 mm, which remains stable with little change (SD 0.6 mm) throughout gestation, certainly a very useful feature for any parameter used to evaluate a normal fetal structure (Table 3–18). For practical purposes, a normal upper limit of 10 mm for atrial width has been established.[45,46] Another advantage of this measurement is its low reported intra- and interobserver variability.[39] Other authors[47] prefer morphological criteria, such as the shrunken appearance of the choroid plexus in hydrocephaly, rather than absolute measurements for estimation of the cerebral ventricles.

Typically, a reverberation artifact from the fetal calvarium obscures the ventricle closest to the transducer, but variations in the angle of the beam and maternal position can make visualization of this ventricle possible.[44] Both atria should be visualized if the uncommon but reported[48] possibility of unilateral ventriculomegaly is to be ruled out in the atria closest to the transducer.

The CAD increases as pregnancy progresses, reflecting the steady growth of the cerebral hemispheres (Table 3–19). The decreasing atrial width/HW, atrial width/CAD, and CAD/HW ratios (Tables 3–20, 3–21,

**Table 3–19. NOMOGRAM OF THE CEREBROATRIAL DISTANCE THROUGHOUT PREGNANCY**

| Gestational Age (weeks) | Mean ± SD (cm) |
|---|---|
| 15–17 | 1.16 ± 0.08 |
| 18–20 | 1.35 ± 0.09 |
| 21–23 | 1.45 ± 0.10 |
| 24–26 | 1.59 ± 0.13 |
| 27–29 | 1.81 ± 0.14 |
| 30–32 | 1.96 ± 0.17 |
| 33–35 | 2.04 ± 0.15 |
| 36–38 | 2.15 ± 0.21 |
| 39–40 | 2.36 ± 0.15 |

From Pilu and colleagues, 1989,[49] with permission.

**Table 3–20. NOMOGRAM OF THE ATRIAL WIDTH–HEMISPHERIC WIDTH RATIO VERSUS GESTATIONAL AGE**

| Gestational Age (weeks) | Mean ± 2 SD (%) |
|---|---|
| 15 | 49 ± 10 |
| 16 | 47 ± 9 |
| 17 | 46 ± 6 |
| 18 | 42 ± 8 |
| 19 | 35 ± 8 |
| 20 | 20 ± 8 |
| 21 | 33 ± 6 |
| 22 | 27 ± 6 |
| 23 | 23 ± 8 |
| 24 | 22 ± 8 |
| 25 | 20 ± 4 |
| 26 | 21 ± 4 |
| 27 | 19 ± 6 |
| 28 | 18 ± 6 |
| 29 | 16 ± 2 |
| 30 | 14 ± 2 |
| 31 | 17 ± 4 |
| 32 | 15 ± 6 |
| 33 | 17 ± 4 |
| 34 | 15 ± 4 |
| 35 | 17 ± 6 |
| 36 | 13 ± 4 |
| 37 | 13 ± 4 |
| 38 | 13 ± 4 |
| 39 | 14 ± 2 |
| 40 | 14 ± 2 |

From Pilu and colleagues, 1989,[49] with permission.

and 3–22) indicate that the relative size of the atrium decreases with brain growth, probably due not to an actual decrease in its size, which is relatively constant, but to growth of brain tissue throughout fetal life.[49]

## POSTERIOR (OCCIPITAL) HORN OF THE LATERAL VENTRICLES

### Definition

The posterior or occipital horn of the lateral ventricles represents the posterior continuation of the atria of the lateral ventricles.

### How to Measure It (Figure 3–7)

The posterior horns (PHs) are better imaged in a horizontal plane at a level slightly above that normally used for the BPD. They appear sonographically as a sonolucent area in continuation with the atria, located at the posterior lobe of the fetal head. To measure them, the electronic calipers are placed in the echo-dense medial and lateral walls (PHW). The cerebroposterior horn distance (CPHD) is measured between the falx cerebri and the lateral wall of the posterior horn.[50]

### Comments

As reported by Goldstein's group,[50] the width of the posterior horn of the lateral ventricles ranges between 5 and 9 mm, with a mean value of 7.06 mm and an SD of ± 1.36 mm throughout pregnancy. The CPHD increases with advancing gestational age, and the posterior horn width/CPHD ratio decreases as pregnancy progresses (Tables 3–23 and 3–24). These findings are consonant with those reported by Siedler and Filly,[51] who demonstrated that throughout pregnancy, the telencephalic structures grow at a much faster rate than the diencephalon and the lateral ventricles.

Callen and associates[52] evaluated the cerebral cortical mantle thickness in fetuses with hydrocephaly. The sonographic images suggested that the posterior horn appears to dilate first and more severely than the rest of the ventricular system. Thus, the evaluation of the posterior horn probably leads to an early diagnosis of this pathology.

## TRANSVAGINAL SONOGRAPHY

### First Trimester

### Definition

A detailed definition of the development of the embryonic and fetal human brain is given in Chapter 1. Reading that chapter first will aid in understanding the development of the structures we describe here using sonography.

### How to Measure It (Figures 3–8, 3–9, 3–10, 3–11, and 3–12)

In the extensive work of Blaas and collaborators,[53,54] transvaginal sonographic evaluation during the first trimester

**Table 3–21. NOMOGRAM OF THE ATRIAL WIDTH–CEREBROATRIAL DISTANCE RATIO THROUGHOUT PREGNANCY**

| | | Percentile | | |
|---|---|---|---|---|
| Gestational Age (weeks) | Mean ± 2 SD (cm) | 10th | 50th | 90th |
| 15 | 0.59 ± 0.086 | 0.50 | 0.60 | 0.70 |
| 16 | 0.70 ± 0.060 | 0.58 | 0.72 | 0.75 |
| 17 | 0.67 ± 0.101 | 0.53 | 0.66 | 0.81 |
| 18 | 0.63 ± 0.058 | 0.57 | 0.61 | 0.71 |
| 19 | 0.56 ± 0.071 | 0.50 | 0.53 | 0.69 |
| 20 | 0.54 ± 0.766 | 0.42 | 0.53 | 0.64 |
| 21 | 0.54 ± 0.043 | 0.50 | 0.53 | 0.62 |
| 22 | 0.48 ± 0.048 | 0.40 | 0.50 | 0.54 |
| 23 | 0.44 ± 0.079 | 0.31 | 0.43 | 0.56 |
| 24 | 0.43 ± 0.094 | 0.27 | 0.46 | 0.57 |
| 25 | 0.37 ± 0.388 | 0.31 | 0.39 | 0.41 |
| 26 | 0.39 ± 0.380 | 0.35 | 0.41 | 0.44 |
| 27 | 0.36 ± 0.067 | 0.28 | 0.35 | 0.44 |
| 28 | 0.37 ± 0.095 | 0.26 | 0.35 | 0.50 |
| 29 | 0.31 ± 0.063 | 0.20 | 0.32 | 0.41 |
| 30 | 0.29 ± 0.046 | 0.21 | 0.28 | 0.35 |
| 31 | 0.34 ± 0.059 | 0.24 | 0.37 | 0.40 |
| 32 | 0.30 ± 0.064 | 0.17 | 0.32 | 0.40 |
| 33 | 0.36 ± 0.070 | 0.27 | 0.35 | 0.44 |
| 34 | 0.30 ± 0.600 | 0.24 | 0.27 | 0.39 |
| 35 | 0.36 ± 0.072 | 0.29 | 0.33 | 0.47 |
| 36 | 0.28 ± 0.043 | 0.23 | 0.29 | 0.33 |
| 37 | 0.25 ± 0.043 | 0.25 | 0.25 | 0.25 |
| 38 | 0.29 ± 0.038 | 0.27 | 0.28 | 0.35 |
| 39 | 0.28 ± 0.034 | 0.25 | 0.27 | 0.32 |
| 40 | 0.33 ± 0.330 | 0.33 | 0.33 | 0.33 |

From Pilu and colleagues, 1989,[49] with permission.

**Table 3–22. NOMOGRAM OF THE CEREBROATRIAL DISTANCE–HEMISPHERIC WIDTH RATIO THROUGHOUT PREGNANCY**

| | | Percentile | | |
|---|---|---|---|---|
| **Gestational Age (weeks)** | **Mean ± 2 SD (cm)** | **10th** | **50th** | **90th** |
| 15 | 0.82 ± 0.090 | 0.71 | 0.80 | 1.00 |
| 16 | 0.73 ± 0.069 | 0.64 | 0.71 | 0.86 |
| 17 | 0.70 ± 0.062 | 0.61 | 0.70 | 0.76 |
| 18 | 0.70 ± 0.055 | 0.60 | 0.72 | 0.75 |
| 19 | 0.65 ± 0.014 | 0.63 | 0.65 | 0.67 |
| 20 | 0.63 ± 0.610 | 0.55 | 0.62 | 0.75 |
| 21 | 0.66 ± 0.046 | 0.60 | 0.67 | 0.73 |
| 22 | 0.60 ± 0.044 | 0.52 | 0.61 | 0.65 |
| 23 | 0.58 ± 0.050 | 0.54 | 0.56 | 0.67 |
| 24 | 0.54 ± 0.040 | 0.46 | 0.54 | 0.59 |
| 25 | 0.58 ± 0.033 | 0.55 | 0.57 | 0.62 |
| 26 | 0.57 ± 0.033 | 0.53 | 0.57 | 0.63 |
| 27 | 0.57 ± 0.025 | 0.53 | 0.57 | 0.60 |
| 28 | 0.51 ± 0.054 | 0.44 | 0.49 | 0.57 |
| 29 | 0.55 ± 0.040 | 0.51 | 0.54 | 0.62 |
| 30 | 0.51 ± 0.050 | 0.46 | 0.50 | 0.61 |
| 31 | 0.53 ± 0.050 | 0.46 | 0.53 | 0.60 |
| 32 | 0.54 ± 0.056 | 0.46 | 0.52 | 0.60 |
| 33 | 0.52 ± 0.042 | 0.45 | 0.53 | 0.58 |
| 34 | 0.30 ± 0.060 | 0.24 | 0.27 | 0.39 |
| 35 | 0.52 ± 0.034 | 0.48 | 0.53 | 0.57 |
| 36 | 0.49 ± 0.024 | 0.46 | 0.49 | 0.52 |
| 37 | 0.57 ± 0.024 | 0.57 | 0.57 | 0.57 |
| 38 | 0.53 ± 0.038 | 0.48 | 0.53 | 0.59 |
| 39 | 0.54 ± 0.026 | 0.52 | 0.53 | 0.57 |
| 40 | 0.50 ± 0.026 | 0.50 | 0.50 | 0.50 |

From Pilu and colleagues, 1989,[49] with permission.

was accomplished using a high-frequency (7.5 MHz) transducer. The prosencephalon (forebrain) and the mesencephalon (midbrain) were defined using median, oblique, and horizontal planes. In the median plane, the length and height of the cavities of the mesencephalon (ML-MH) and the diencephalon (DL-DH) can be obtained. In the horizontal plane, the widths of the mesencephalon (MW) and diencephalon cavities (DW), the hemispheres (HW), and the choroid plexus (CPW) of the lateral ventricles are measured. In the oblique plane, the length of the hemisphere (HL) can be measured as the longest possible distance from the anterior to the posterior border of the cortex. The height of the hemisphere (HH) is measured over the frontal horn, not including the basal nuclei.

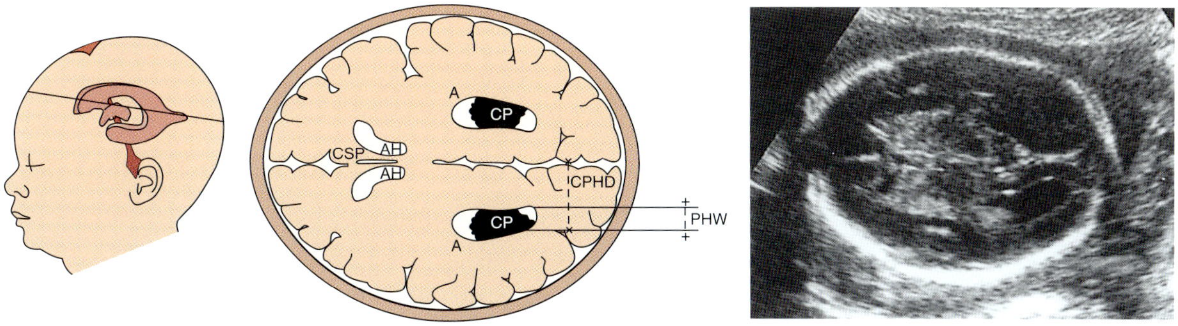


Figure 3–7.

To evaluate the rhombencephalon (hindbrain), the scanning plane follows the neuroaxis as it bends. During week 7, the plane is horizontal (the depth [-RD-] and the height [-RH-] are measured), gradually tilting to a coronal plane at the end of the embryonic period. In coronal planes, the width and height of the cerebellum (CW-CH), the choroid plexuses (CPW-CPH), and the rhombencephalic cavity (RW—RH) are measured.

## Comments

Several studies have demonstrated that sonographic evaluation of the embryonic central nervous system (CNS) is possible.[53–56] A detailed biometric analysis has been presented by Blaas and coworkers,[53,54] showing an increase in the measurements of all evaluated structures with advancing gestational age, with the exception of the width of the diencephalon, which decreases slowly during the first trimester, probably due to diencephalic wall growth (Figures 3–13, 3–14, 3–15, and 3–16; Tables 3–25 and 3–26).

The expanding field of neurosonoembryology not only has the potential to evaluate growth but also can help in diagnosing conditions, such as exencephaly, holoprosencephaly, cephalocele, craniorachischisis, and Dandy-Walker malformation,[53,54] at a much earlier stage than was

**Table 3–23. NOMOGRAM OF THE CEREBROPOSTERIOR HORN DISTANCE THROUGHOUT PREGNANCY**

| Gestational Age (weeks) | Mean ± 2 SD (mm) | Percentile | | |
|---|---|---|---|---|
| | | 10th | 50th | 90th |
| 15–16 | 9.2 ± 0.83 | 8.0 | 9.0 | 10.0 |
| 17–18 | 11.36 ± 1.41 | 9.0 | 11.0 | 13.0 |
| 19–20 | 11.0 ± 1.52 | 9.0 | 11.0 | 13.8 |
| 21–22 | 12.4 ± 1.55 | 11.0 | 12.0 | 15.2 |
| 23–24 | 14.0 ± 1.22 | 12.0 | 14.0 | 15.0 |
| 25–26 | 14.8 ± 1.39 | 12.0 | 15.0 | 16.0 |
| 27–28 | 16.18 ± 2.13 | 13.0 | 16.5 | 19.0 |
| 29–30 | 18.0 ± 2.37 | 15.2 | 17.0 | 22.0 |
| 31–32 | 22.7 ± 2.08 | 21.0 | 22.0 | 25.0 |
| 33–34 | 19.7 ± 3.28 | 15.0 | 19.5 | 25.0 |
| 35–36 | 22.6 ± 3.71 | 17.0 | 23.0 | 27.0 |
| 37–38 | 20.3 ± 3.14 | 16.0 | 20.5 | 25.0 |
| 39–40 | 20.2 ± 2.77 | 17.0 | 20.0 | 23.0 |

From Goldstein and colleagues, 1990,[50] with permission.

**Table 3–24. NOMOGRAM OF THE POSTERIOR HORN WIDTH–CEREBROPOSTERIOR HORN DISTANCE RATIO THROUGHOUT GESTATION**

| Gestational Age (weeks) | Mean ± SD (mm) |
|---|---|
| 15–16 | 0.67 ± 0.071 |
| 17–18 | 0.60 ± 0.87 |
| 19–20 | 0.60 ± 0.76 |
| 21–22 | 0.51 ± 0.05 |
| 23–24 | 0.46 ± 0.03 |
| 25–26 | 0.49 ± 0.05 |
| 27–28 | 0.42 ± 0.06 |
| 29–30 | 0.43 ± 0.06 |
| 31–32 | 0.37 ± 0.01 |
| 33–34 | 0.41 ± 0.10 |
| 35–36 | 0.41 ± 0.08 |
| 37–38 | 0.39 ± 0.06 |
| 39–40 | 0.47 ± 0.05 |

From Goldstein and colleagues, 1990,[50] with permission.

previously done with conventional transabdominal scans, permitting the appropriate management to be carried out in a timely fashion.

## SECOND AND THIRD TRIMESTERS

### Definition

Because the evaluated structures are the same as with transabdominal sonography, there is no need to redefine them here (see Chapter 2).

### How to Measure It (Figures 3–17, 3–18, and 3–19)

In fetuses in the vertex presentation, transvaginal evaluation of the brain during the second and third trimesters can be accomplished by aligning the ultrasound beam of the transducer with the longitudinal axis of the fetal head through the anterior fontanelle.[57] To allow proper alignment, the fetal head can be gently manipulated by the free hand of the examiner. If the fetus is in a nonvertex presentation, and the transabdominal scan is suboptimal, an external cephalic version may be considered in selected cases. Usually, end-firing probes with frequencies of 5 or 7.5 MHz are used.[57,58] Oblique and coronal planes can be used to measure the cerebral ventricles in the following fashion.[57,58] (See description of measurement in oblique and coronal planes.)

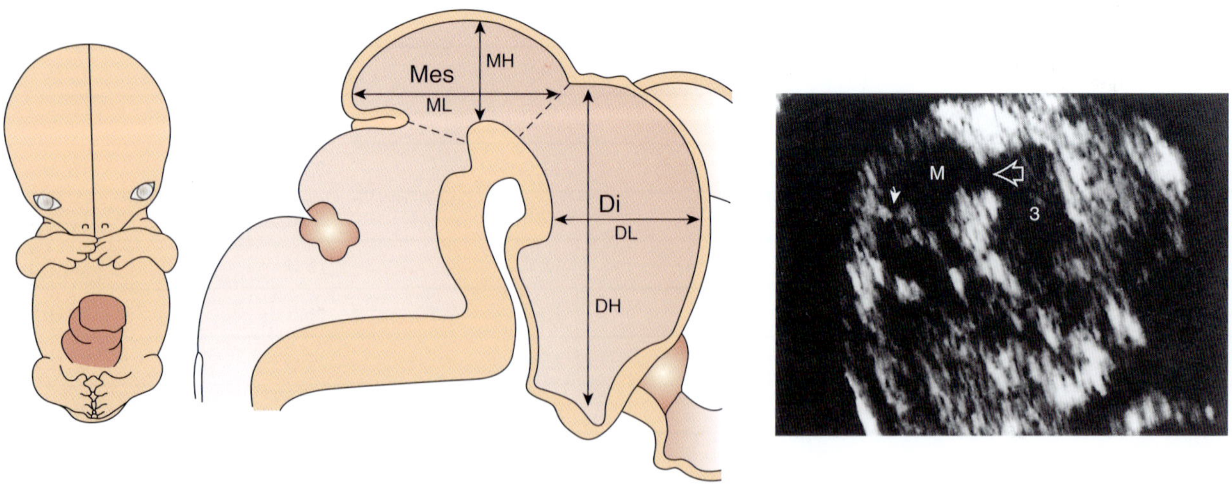


**Figure 3–8.** M, Mesencephalon; 3, diencephalon.

**DESCRIPTION OF MEASUREMENTS IN OBLIQUE AND CORONAL PLANES**[57,58]

| Number | Plane | Measurement |
|---|---|---|
| 1 | Oblique– 1 (Figure 3–17) | Thalamus–choroid plexus interface to the tip of the posterior (occipital) horn (TCP-TOH) |
| 2 | | Choroid plexus thickness (CPT) |
| 3 | | Posterior (occipital) horn height (OHH) |
| 4 | Midcoronal–2 (Figure 3–18) | Midline to the upper edge of the lateral ventricle (MUELV) |
| 5 | | Depth of the lateral ventricle (DLV) |
| 6 | Occipital–1 (posterior coronal) (Figure 3–19) | Width of the posterior (occipital) horn (WOH) |
| 7 | | Height of the posterior (occipital) horn (HOH) |
| Ratio | | Thalamus to tip of posterior horn (TCP-TOH)/choroid plexus thickness (CPT) |
| Ratio | | Posterior horn height (oblique plane) (OHH)/choroid plexus thickness (CPT) |

## Comments

In 1989 Kushnir and colleagues[59] proposed the use of transvaginal sonography to examine certain biometric parameters (CRL, BPD, HC, LVW, and HW) in a group of 50 patients whose pregnancies were between 12 and 14 gestational weeks. In 1991 our group[57] described for the first time the feasibility of the routine transvaginal sonographic evaluation of the fetal brain during the second half of pregnancy. With this approach, using the anterior fontanelle, images of diagnostic quality of the intracranial anatomy can be obtained. The differentiation between normal and pathologic brain structures is easier and avoids the disadvantages of the transabdominal route. Such disadvantages may be (1) the inadequate visualization of the cerebral hemispheres due to reverberation artifacts, a deeply engaged fetal head, or maternal obesity and abdominal scarring; and (2) the presence of pseudohydrocephalus, unilateral hydrocephaly, and pseudoepidural artifact, which are detected using conventional axial planes.[60]

Using this technique, nine nomograms of the fetal lateral ventricles were developed and evaluated using the

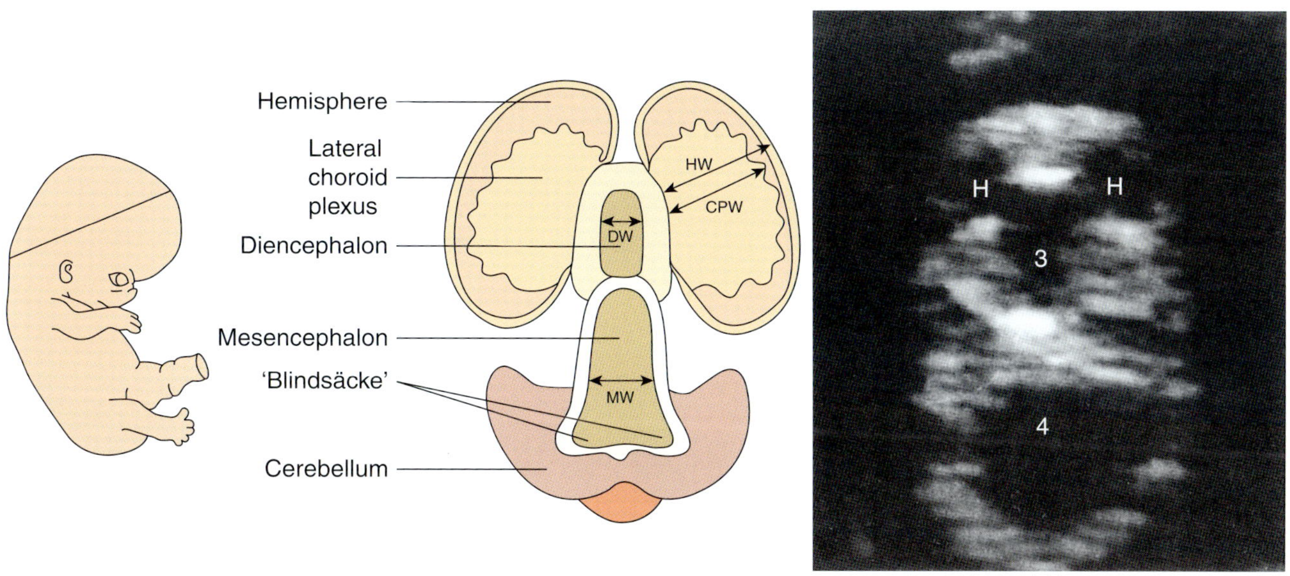


**Figure 3–9.** H, Hemisphere; 3, diencephalon; 4, rhombencephalon. (From Blaas HG and colleagues, 1995 with permission.)

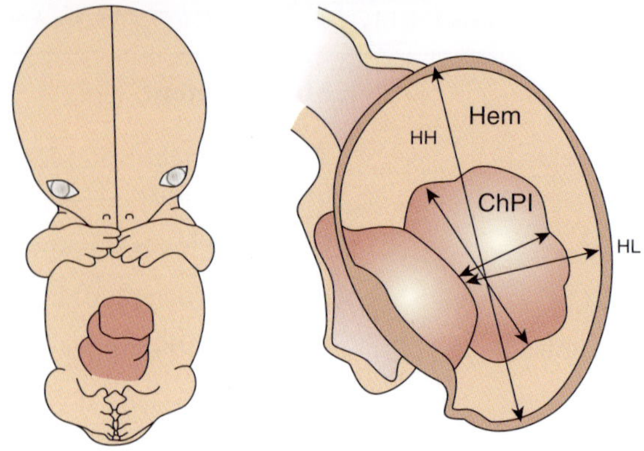


**Figure 3–10.**

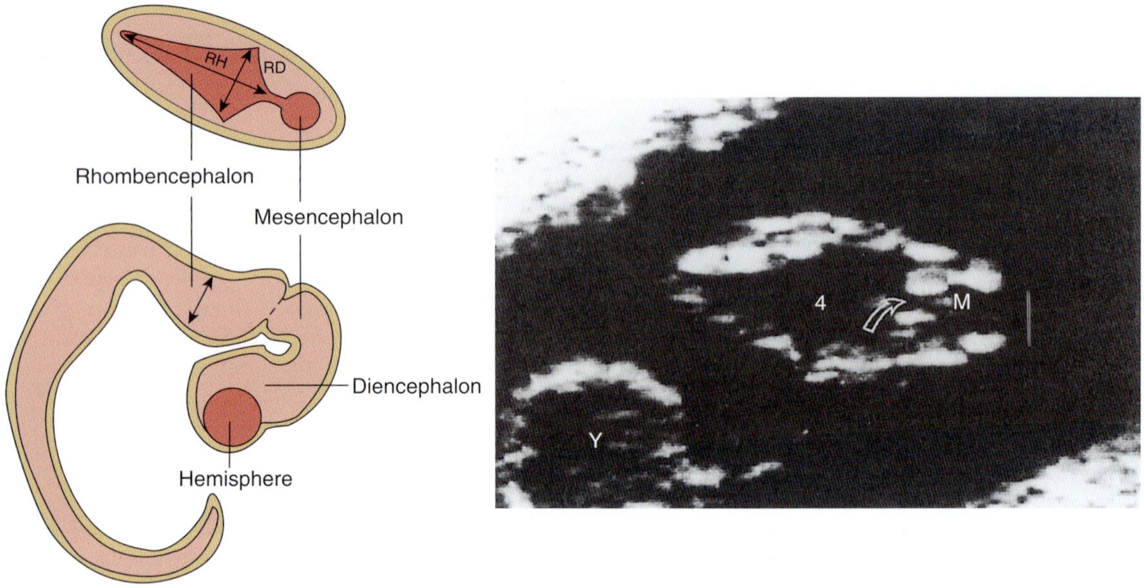


**Figure 3–11.** M, Mesencephalon; 4, rhombencephalon. (From Blaas HG and colleagues, 1995 with permission.)

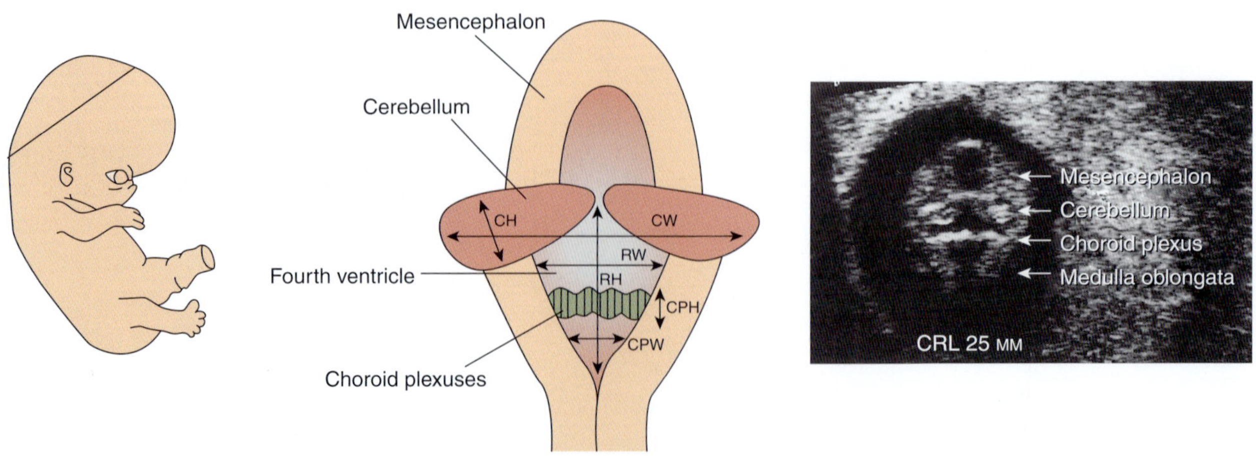


**Figure 3–12.** (From Blaas HG and colleagues, 1995 with permission.)

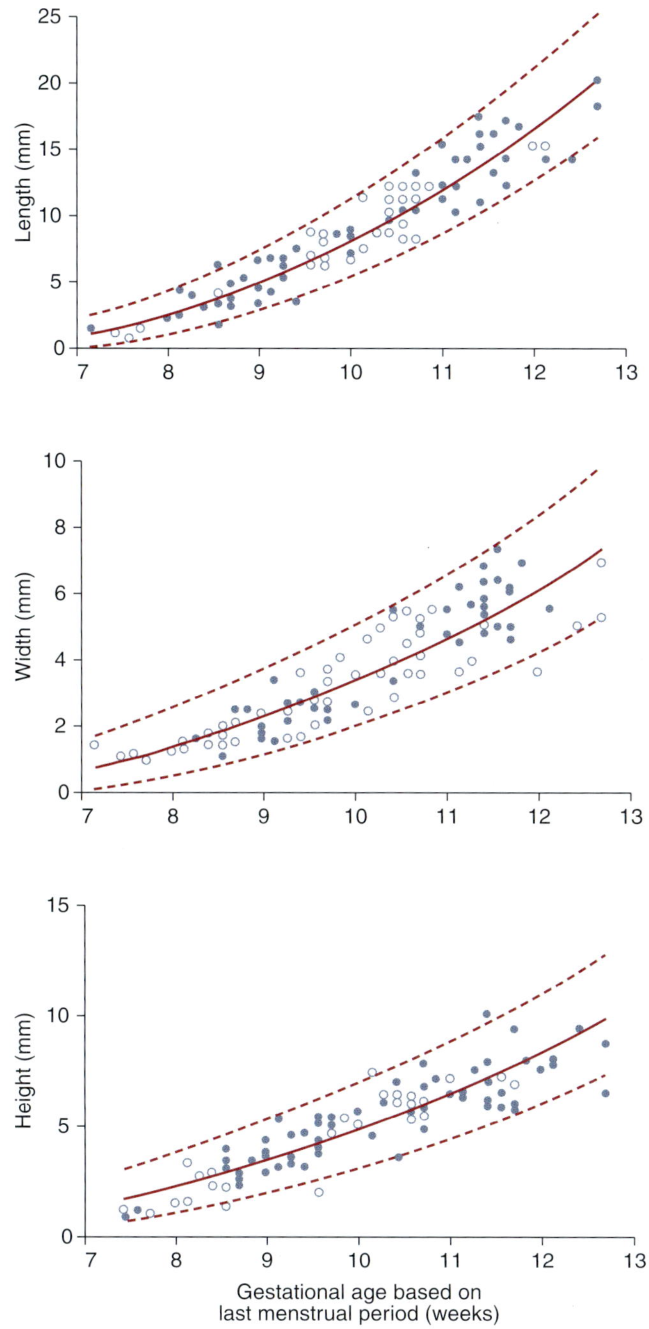


**Figure 3–13.** Hemispheres. (From Blaas and colleagues, 1994 and 1995, with permission.)

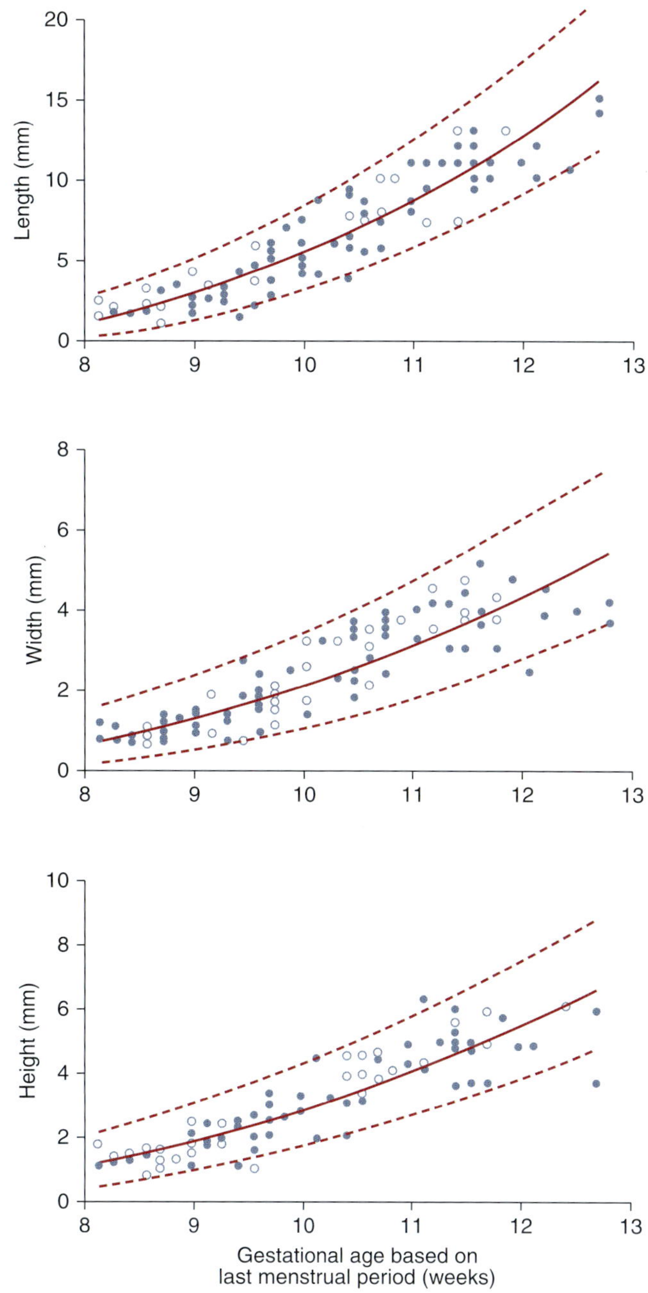


**Figure 3–14.** Choroid plexus of the lateral ventricle. (From Blaas and colleagues, 1994 and 1995, with permission.)

sagittal and coronal planes (Tables 3–26 through 3–36). The occipital plane is usually the hardest to image due to maternal discomfort while maneuvering the probe. Measurements such as the TCP-TOH, OHH, and MUELV increased in a linear fashion as pregnancy advanced. Measurements such as the CPT, DLV, WOH, HOH, and the ratios TCP-TOH/CPT and OHH/CPT demonstrated little, if any, association with gestational age.[60]

One of the major applications of these nomograms is the early diagnosis of hydrocephaly. Two early changes have been described. The first is the dilation of the posterior horn in an up-and-down fashion, where the resistance to the cerebrospinal fluid (CSF) pressure is least,[61,62] and the second is the squeezed appearance of the choroid plexus, probably as a result of the increasing CSF pressure.[63] In our experience,[58] measurement of the choroid plexus alone was not discriminatory, but when its thickness was used as a denominator in the two ratios, it became a very sensitive measurement. We propose that although all seven measurements may add important clinical information, evaluation of the OHH (number 3) in the oblique–1 plane and measurements of the lateral ventricle

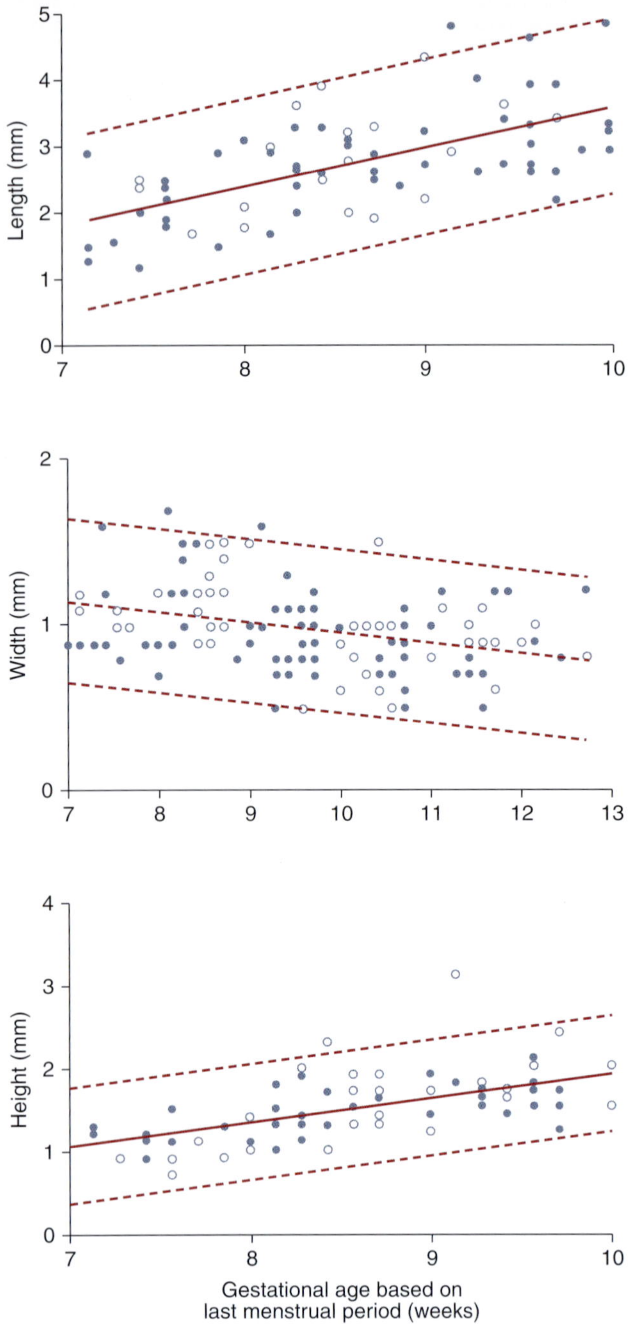


**Figure 3–15.** Diencephalon. (From Blaas and colleagues, 1994 and 1995, with permission.)

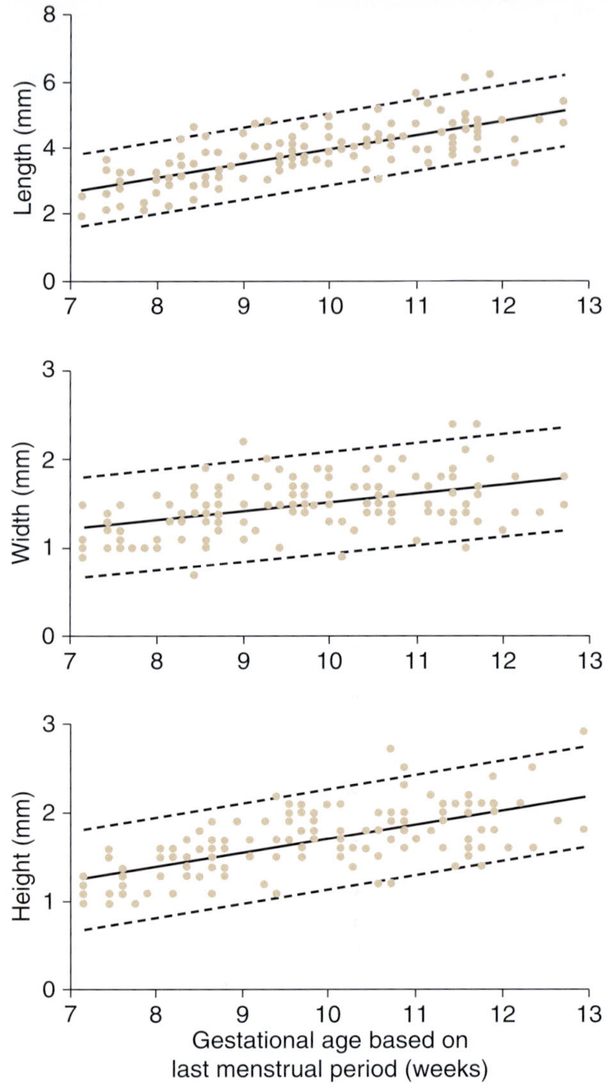


**Figure 3–16.** Mesencephalon. (From Blaas and colleagues, 1994 and 1995, with permission.)

and the HOH (numbers 5 and 7) in the midcoronal–2 and occipital–1 planes are the best markers of early ventricular dilation. If a single plane had to be chosen as the first-line indicator of ventriculomegaly with the transvaginal route, the oblique–1 plane should be selected because in this plane the OHH can be obtained, and the two ratios can be calculated.[58]

Transvaginal neurosonography not only has a place in the diagnosis of ventricular dilation, but also can be of invaluable help in diagnosing almost any type of congenital CNS anomaly.[64] The sonographic planes described can also be used for evaluating the appearance and development of the corpus callosum. By 18 weeks of gestation, all the components of the corpus callosum are present and can be visualized on transvaginal sonography in ~95% of cases (Table 3–27).[65] Transvaginal sonography provides an excellent method for direct examination of this structure, allowing for the diagnosis of anomalies such as agenesis and hypogenesis, as well as more subtle findings associated with "callosal thinning," particularly in cases of infection, periventricular leukomalacia, inborn errors of the metabolism, and anomalies of neuronal migration.

**Table 3–25. EQUATIONS OF THE REGRESSIONS, INCLUDING THE 95% PREDICTION INTERVALS**

| Independent Variable | Dependent Variable | Equations |
|---|---|---|
| Hemispheres | | |
| Gestational age | Length | $y = (-3.34 + 0.62x \pm 1.96 \times 0.26)^2$ |
| Gestational age | Width | $y = (-1.45 + 0.33x \pm 1.96 \times 0.21)^2$ |
| Gestational age | Depth | $y = (-1.25 + 0.34x \pm 1.96 \times 0.22)^2$ |
| Choroid plexus of the lateral ventricles | | |
| Gestational age | Length | $y = (-3.99 + 0.63x \pm 1.96 \times 0.29)^2$ |
| Gestational age | Width | $y = (-1.71 + 0.32x \pm 1.96 \times 0.21)^2$ |
| Gestational age | Height | $y = (-1.55 + 0.32x \pm 1.96 \times 0.19)^2$ |
| Diencephalon | | |
| Gestational age | Length | $y = -2.15 + 0.575x \pm 1.96 \times 0.63$ |
| Gestational age | Width | $y = 1.63 - 0.07x \pm 1.96 \times 0.24$ |
| Gestational age | Height | $y = -0.87 + 0.28x \pm 1.96 \times 0.34$ |
| Mesencephalon | | |
| Gestational age | Length | $y = -0.32 + 0.42x \pm 1.96 \times 0.54$ |
| Gestational age | Width | $y = 0.54 + 0.1x \pm 1.96 \times 0.28$ |
| Gestational age | Height | $y = 0.01 + 0.16x \pm 1.96 \times 0.28$ |

The gestational age is based on the date of the last menstrual period.
From Blaas and colleagues, 1995,[54] with permission.

**Table 3–26. MEAN SIZE AND 95% PREDICTION INTERVALS OF THE RHOMBENCEPHALIC STRUCTURES**

| Gestational Age (weeks + days) | Rhombencephalon (mm) | | | Cerebellum (mm) | | Chorold Plexus (mm) | |
|---|---|---|---|---|---|---|---|
| | Length | Width | Depth | Width | Height | Width | Height |
| 7 + 0 | 3.8 (2.2–5.3) | 2.1 (0.6–3.7) | 1.5 (0.4–2.6) | | | | |
| 8 + 0 | 3.9 (2.3–5.4) | 3.1 (1.5–4.7) | 2.1 (1.0–3.2) | | | | |
| 9 + 0 | 4.0 (2.5–5.6) | 3.8 (2.2–5.4) | 2.5 (1.5–3.6) | 4.8 (3.0–7.1) | 1.4 (0.7–2.1) | 3.2 (1.8–4.6) | 1.1 (0.6–1.6) |
| 10 + 0 | 4.1 (2.6–5.7) | 4.3 (2.7–5.8) | 2.9 (1.8–3.9) | 5.8 (3.8–8.3) | 1.7 (1.0–2.4) | 3.5 (2.1–4.9) | 1.1 (0.6–1.6) |
| 11 + 0 | 4.3 (2.7–5.8) | 4.5 (2.9–6.1) | 3.1 (2.0–4.2) | 6.9 (4.7–9.6) | 2.1 (1.4–2.8) | 3.8 (2.4–5.2) | 1.2 (0.7–1.7) |
| 12 + 0 | 4.4 (2.8–5.9) | 4.5 (2.9–6.1) | 3.2 (2.2–4.3) | 8.1 (5.7–11.0) | 2.5 (1.8–3.2) | 4.1 (2.7–5.6) | 1.3 (0.8–1.8) |

From Blaas and colleagues, 1995,[54] with permission.

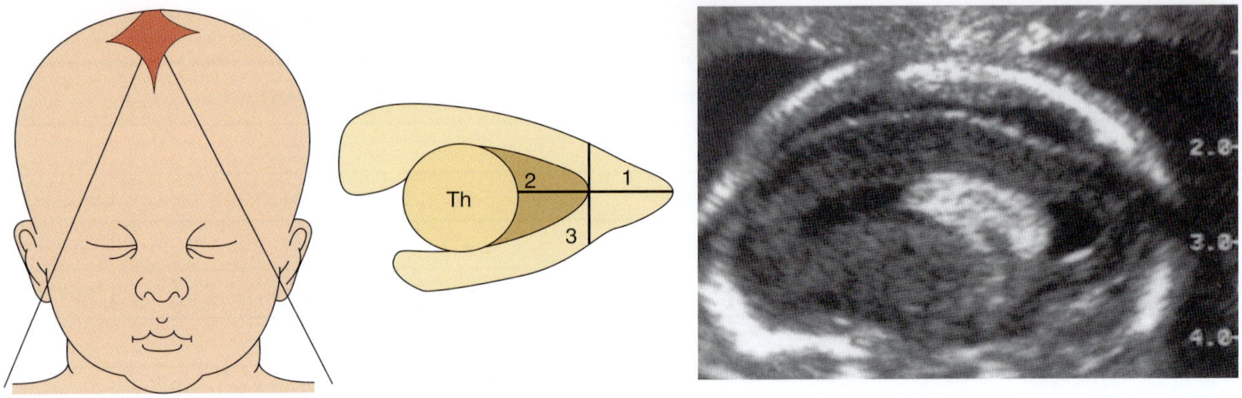


**Figure 3–17.** Measurement of the Thaamus-to-tip of the posterior horn (1), choroid plexus thickness (2) and posterior horn height (3).

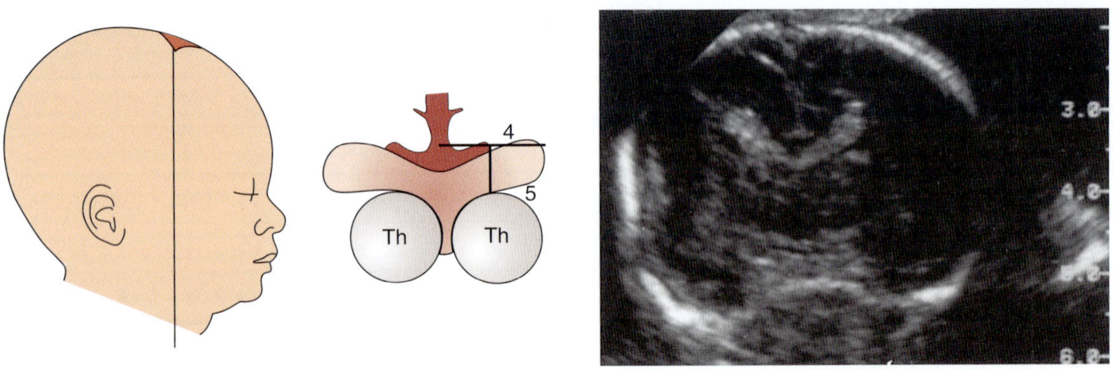


**Figure 3–18.** Measurement of the Midline-to-upper edge of the lateral ventricle (4) and depth of the lateral ventricle (5).

## OTHER INTRACRANIAL STRUCTURES

### Thalamus, Basal Nuclei–Insula, and Temporal Operculum

#### Definitions

The thalamus is a diencephalic structure separated from the epithalamus by the epithalamic sulcus and from the hypothalamus by the hypothalamic sulcus. It develops rapidly on each side and bulges into the cavity of the third ventricle, molding and reducing its size. In most brains (70%) the thalami fuse in the midline, forming a bridge of gray matter called the massa intermedia.[66]

The basal nuclei are an arbitrary group that includes the corpus striatum, the amygdaloid body, and the claustrum. The corpus striatum and the claustrum are telencephalic structures, whereas the amygdaloid body is of diencephalic origin. From a clinical point of view, the subthalamic nucleus and the substantia nigra are added, to complete the basal structures affected pathologically in the so-called extrapyramidal motor diseases.[67]

The temporal operculum corresponds to the caudal end of the temporal lobe, growing forward and downward to form the posterocaudal edge of the lateral sulcus. The insula is a portion of the cerebral cortex buried by the folds of frontal, parietal, and temporal cortices that form the walls of the lateral sulcus.[68]

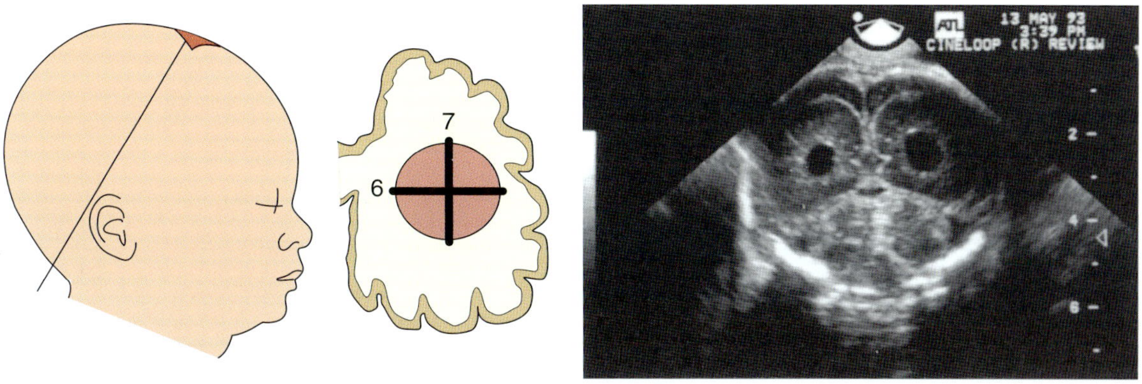


**Figure 3–19.** Measurement of the width (6) and weight (7) of the posterior horn.

**Table 3–27. BIOMETRY OF THE CORPUS CALLOSUM**

| | | Thickness (mm) | | |
|---|---|---|---|---|
| Gestational Age (weeks) | Length (mm) | Genu | Body | Splenlum |
| 18–19 | 16.9 ± 2.4 | 2.2 ± 0.5 | 1.3 ± 0.1 | 2.1 ± 0.1 |
| 20–21 | 20.6 ± 4.4 | 2.3 ± 0.6 | 1.6 ± 0.1 | 2.1 ± 0.1 |
| 22–23 | 23.3 ± 3.0 | 2.7 ± 0.6 | 1.7 ± 0.2 | 3.1 ± 0.2 |
| 24–25 | 29.8 ± 2.3 | 3.0 ± 0.6 | 1.9 ± 0.3 | 3.0 ± 0.3 |
| 26–27 | 33.7 ± 2.4 | 3.5 ± 0.6 | 2.0 ± 0.2 | 3.3 ± 0.6 |
| 28–29 | 25.8 ± 2.8 | 4.0 ± 0.7 | 2.0 ± 0.4 | 4.0 ± 0.8 |
| 30–31 | 36.8 ± 1.4 | 4.2 ± 0.5 | 2.1 ± 0.4 | 4.1 ± 0.7 |
| 32–33 | 39.1 ± 4.3 | 4.5 ± 1.2 | 2.5 ± 0.6 | 4.2 ± 0.8 |
| 34–35 | 40.6 ± 6.4 | 4.6 ± 0.5 | 2.5 ± 0.5 | 4.4 ± 0.8 |
| 36–37 | 41.9 ± 3.5 | 5.0 ± 0.4 | 2.5 ± 0.4 | 4.4 ± 1.3 |
| 38–39 | 43.0 ± 4.2 | 4.8 ± 0.7 | 2.6 ± 0.5 | 4.4 ± 0.6 |
| 40–42 | 44.0 ± 3.8 | 4.8 ± 0.4 | 2.6 ± 0.5 | 4.4 ± 0.7 |

From Malinger and colleauges, 1993,[65] with permission.

**Table 3–28. THALAMUS TO THE TIP OF THE POSTERIOR HORN**

| Estimated Gestational Age (weeks) | 5th Percentile (mm) | 50th Percentile (mm) | Percentile 95th (mm) |
|---|---|---|---|
| 14 | 6.06 | 13.34 | 20.62 |
| 15 | 6.47 | 13.75 | 21.03 |
| 16 | 6.87 | 14.15 | 21.43 |
| 17 | 7.27 | 14.55 | 21.83 |
| 18 | 7.68 | 14.96 | 22.24 |
| 19 | 8.08 | 15.36 | 22.64 |
| 20 | 8.49 | 15.77 | 23.05 |
| 21 | 8.89 | 16.17 | 23.45 |
| 22 | 9.29 | 16.57 | 23.85 |
| 23 | 9.70 | 16.98 | 24.26 |
| 24 | 10.10 | 17.38 | 24.66 |
| 25 | 10.51 | 17.79 | 25.07 |
| 26 | 10.91 | 18.19 | 25.47 |
| 27 | 11.31 | 18.60 | 25.88 |
| 28 | 11.72 | 19.00 | 26.28 |
| 29 | 12.12 | 19.40 | 26.68 |
| 30 | 12.53 | 19.81 | 27.09 |
| 31 | 12.93 | 20.21 | 27.49 |
| 32 | 13.34 | 20.62 | 27.90 |
| 33 | 13.74 | 21.01 | 28.30 |
| 34 | 14.14 | 21.42 | 28.70 |
| 35 | 14.55 | 21.83 | 29.11 |
| 36 | 14.95 | 22.23 | 29.51 |
| 37 | 15.36 | 22.64 | 29.92 |
| 38 | 15.76 | 23.04 | 30.32 |
| 39 | 16.16 | 23.44 | 30.72 |
| 40 | 16.57 | 23.85 | 31.13 |

From Monteagudo et al, 1993,[60] by permission.

**Table 3–29. CHOROID PLEXUS THICKNESS**

| Estimated Gestational Age (weeks) | 5th Percentile (mm) | 50th Percentile (mm) | 95th Percentile (mm) |
|---|---|---|---|
| 14 | 4.41 | 8.89 | 13.37 |
| 15 | 4.48 | 8.96 | 13.44 |
| 16 | 4.55 | 9.03 | 13.51 |
| 17 | 4.62 | 9.10 | 13.58 |
| 18 | 4.69 | 9.17 | 13.65 |
| 19 | 4.76 | 9.24 | 13.72 |
| 20 | 4.83 | 9.31 | 13.79 |
| 21 | 4.90 | 9.38 | 13.86 |
| 22 | 4.97 | 9.45 | 13.93 |
| 23 | 5.04 | 9.52 | 14.00 |
| 24 | 5.11 | 9.59 | 14.07 |
| 25 | 5.18 | 9.66 | 14.14 |
| 26 | 5.25 | 9.73 | 14.21 |
| 27 | 5.32 | 9.80 | 14.28 |
| 28 | 5.39 | 9.87 | 14.34 |
| 29 | 5.45 | 9.93 | 14.41 |
| 30 | 5.52 | 10.00 | 14.48 |
| 31 | 5.59 | 10.07 | 14.55 |
| 32 | 5.66 | 10.14 | 14.62 |
| 33 | 5.73 | 10.21 | 14.69 |
| 34 | 5.80 | 10.28 | 14.76 |
| 35 | 5.87 | 10.35 | 14.83 |
| 36 | 5.94 | 10.42 | 14.90 |
| 37 | 6.00 | 10.49 | 14.97 |
| 38 | 6.08 | 10.56 | 15.04 |
| 39 | 6.15 | 10.63 | 15.11 |
| 40 | 6.22 | 10.70 | 15.18 |

From Monteagudo et al, 1993,[60] by permission.

**Table 3–30. POSTERIOR HORN HEIGHT**

| Estimated Gestational Age (weeks) | 5th Percentile (mm) | 50th Percentile (mm) | 95th Percentile (mm) |
|---|---|---|---|
| 14 | 1.97 | 6.91 | 11.85 |
| 15 | 2.20 | 7.14 | 12.08 |
| 16 | 2.42 | 7.36 | 12.30 |
| 17 | 2.64 | 7.58 | 12.53 |
| 18 | 2.87 | 7.81 | 12.75 |
| 19 | 3.09 | 8.03 | 12.97 |
| 20 | 3.32 | 8.26 | 13.20 |
| 21 | 3.54 | 8.48 | 13.42 |
| 22 | 3.76 | 8.70 | 13.64 |
| 23 | 3.99 | 8.93 | 13.87 |
| 24 | 4.21 | 9.15 | 14.09 |
| 25 | 4.43 | 9.37 | 14.31 |
| 26 | 4.66 | 9.60 | 14.54 |
| 27 | 4.88 | 9.82 | 14.76 |
| 28 | 5.11 | 10.05 | 14.98 |
| 29 | 5.33 | 10.27 | 15.21 |
| 30 | 5.55 | 10.49 | 15.43 |
| 31 | 5.78 | 10.72 | 15.66 |
| 32 | 6.00 | 10.94 | 15.88 |
| 33 | 6.22 | 11.16 | 16.10 |
| 34 | 6.45 | 11.39 | 16.33 |
| 35 | 6.67 | 11.61 | 16.55 |
| 36 | 6.90 | 11.84 | 16.78 |
| 37 | 7.12 | 12.06 | 17.00 |
| 38 | 7.34 | 12.28 | 17.22 |
| 39 | 7.57 | 12.51 | 17.45 |
| 40 | 7.79 | 12.73 | 17.67 |

From Monteagudo et al, 1993,[60] by permission.

**Table 3–31. MIDLINE TO THE UPPER EDGE OF THE LATERAL VENTRICLE**

| Estimated Gestational Age (weeks) | 5th Percentile (mm) | 50th Percentile (mm) | 95th Percentile (mm) |
|---|---|---|---|
| 14 | 3.95 | 8.39 | 12.83 |
| 15 | 4.19 | 8.63 | 13.07 |
| 16 | 4.44 | 8.88 | 13.32 |
| 17 | 4.68 | 9.12 | 13.56 |
| 18 | 4.93 | 9.37 | 13.81 |
| 19 | 5.17 | 9.61 | 14.05 |
| 20 | 5.42 | 9.86 | 14.30 |
| 21 | 5.67 | 10.11 | 14.55 |
| 22 | 5.91 | 10.35 | 14.79 |
| 23 | 6.16 | 10.60 | 15.04 |
| 24 | 6.40 | 10.84 | 15.28 |
| 25 | 6.65 | 11.09 | 15.53 |
| 26 | 6.89 | 11.33 | 15.77 |
| 27 | 7.14 | 11.58 | 16.02 |
| 28 | 7.39 | 11.83 | 16.27 |
| 29 | 7.63 | 12.07 | 16.51 |
| 30 | 7.98 | 12.32 | 16.76 |
| 31 | 8.12 | 12.56 | 17.00 |
| 32 | 8.37 | 12.81 | 17.25 |
| 33 | 8.62 | 13.06 | 17.50 |
| 34 | 8.86 | 13.30 | 17.74 |
| 35 | 9.11 | 13.55 | 17.99 |
| 36 | 9.35 | 13.79 | 18.23 |
| 37 | 9.60 | 14.04 | 18.48 |
| 38 | 9.84 | 14.28 | 18.72 |
| 39 | 10.09 | 14.53 | 18.97 |
| 40 | 10.34 | 14.78 | 19.22 |

From Monteagudo et al, 1993,[60] by permission.

**Table 3–32. DEPTH OF THE LATERAL VENTRICLE**

| Estimated Gestational Age (weeks) | 5th Percentile (mm) | 50th Percentile (mm) | 95th Percentile (mm) |
|---|---|---|---|
| 14 | 2.25 | 5.49 | 8.73 |
| 15 | 2.18 | 5.42 | 8.66 |
| 16 | 2.11 | 5.35 | 8.59 |
| 17 | 2.04 | 5.28 | 8.52 |
| 18 | 1.97 | 5.21 | 8.45 |
| 19 | 1.91 | 5.15 | 8.39 |
| 20 | 1.84 | 5.08 | 8.32 |
| 21 | 1.77 | 5.00 | 8.25 |
| 22 | 1.70 | 4.94 | 8.18 |
| 23 | 1.63 | 4.87 | 8.11 |
| 24 | 1.56 | 4.80 | 8.04 |
| 25 | 1.49 | 4.73 | 7.97 |
| 26 | 1.42 | 4.66 | 7.90 |
| 27 | 1.35 | 4.59 | 7.83 |
| 28 | 1.28 | 4.52 | 7.76 |
| 29 | 1.23 | 4.45 | 7.69 |
| 30 | 1.14 | 4.38 | 7.62 |
| 31 | 1.07 | 4.31 | 7.55 |
| 32 | 1.00 | 4.24 | 7.48 |
| 33 | 0.93 | 4.17 | 7.41 |
| 34 | 0.87 | 4.11 | 7.35 |
| 35 | 0.80 | 4.04 | 7.28 |
| 36 | 0.73 | 3.97 | 7.21 |
| 37 | 0.66 | 3.90 | 7.14 |
| 38 | 0.59 | 3.83 | 7.07 |
| 39 | 0.52 | 3.76 | 7.00 |
| 40 | 0.45 | 3.69 | 6.93 |

From Monteagudo et al, 1993,[60] by permission.

**Table 3–33. WIDTH OF THE POSTERIOR HORN**

| Estimated Gestational Age (weeks) | 5th Percentile (mm) | 50th Percentile (mm) | 95th Percentile (mm) |
|---|---|---|---|
| 14 | 1.23 | 5.53 | 9.83 |
| 16 | 1.31 | 5.61 | 9.91 |
| 17 | 1.36 | 5.66 | 9.96 |
| 18 | 1.40 | 5.70 | 10.00 |
| 19 | 1.44 | 5.74 | 10.04 |
| 20 | 1.48 | 5.78 | 10.08 |
| 21 | 1.52 | 5.82 | 10.12 |
| 22 | 1.56 | 5.86 | 10.16 |
| 23 | 1.60 | 5.90 | 10.20 |
| 24 | 1.65 | 5.95 | 10.25 |
| 25 | 1.69 | 6.00 | 10.29 |
| 26 | 1.73 | 6.03 | 10.33 |
| 27 | 1.77 | 6.07 | 10.37 |
| 28 | 1.82 | 6.12 | 10.42 |
| 29 | 1.86 | 6.16 | 10.46 |
| 30 | 1.90 | 6.20 | 10.50 |
| 31 | 1.94 | 6.24 | 10.54 |
| 32 | 1.98 | 6.28 | 10.58 |
| 33 | 2.02 | 6.32 | 10.62 |
| 34 | 2.07 | 6.37 | 10.67 |
| 35 | 2.10 | 6.40 | 10.71 |
| 36 | 2.15 | 6.45 | 10.75 |
| 37 | 2.19 | 6.49 | 10.79 |
| 38 | 2.23 | 6.53 | 10.83 |
| 39 | 2.28 | 6.58 | 10.88 |

From Monteagudo et al, 1993,[60] by permission.

**Table 3–34. HEIGHT OF THE POSTERIOR HORN**

| Estimated Gestational Age (weeks) | 5th Percentile (mm) | 50th Percentile (mm) | 95th Percentile (mm) |
|---|---|---|---|
| 14 | 0.70 | 5.80 | 10.90 |
| 16 | 0.94 | 6.04 | 11.14 |
| 17 | 1.06 | 6.16 | 11.26 |
| 18 | 1.18 | 6.28 | 11.38 |
| 19 | 1.30 | 6.40 | 11.50 |
| 20 | 1.42 | 6.52 | 11.62 |
| 21 | 1.54 | 6.64 | 11.74 |
| 22 | 1.66 | 6.76 | 11.86 |
| 23 | 1.78 | 6.88 | 11.98 |
| 24 | 1.90 | 7.00 | 12.10 |
| 25 | 2.02 | 7.12 | 12.22 |
| 26 | 2.15 | 7.25 | 12.35 |
| 27 | 2.27 | 7.37 | 12.47 |
| 28 | 2.39 | 7.49 | 12.59 |
| 29 | 2.51 | 7.61 | 12.71 |
| 30 | 2.63 | 7.73 | 12.83 |
| 31 | 2.75 | 7.85 | 12.95 |
| 32 | 2.87 | 7.97 | 13.07 |
| 33 | 2.99 | 8.09 | 13.19 |
| 34 | 3.11 | 8.21 | 13.31 |
| 35 | 3.23 | 8.33 | 13.43 |
| 36 | 3.34 | 8.45 | 13.55 |
| 37 | 3.47 | 8.57 | 13.67 |
| 38 | 3.59 | 8.69 | 13.79 |
| 39 | 3.71 | 8.80 | 13.91 |

From Monteagudo et al, 1993,[60] by permission.

**Table 3–35. RATIO OF THE THALAMUS TO THE TIP OF THE OCCIPITAL (POSTERIOR) HORN TO CHOROID PLEXUS THICKNESS**

| Estimated Gestational Age (weeks) | 5th Percentile (mm) | 50th Percentile (mm) | 95th Percentile (mm) | Estimated Gestational Age (weeks) | 5th Percentile (mm) | 50th Percentile (mm) | 95th Percentile (mm) |
|---|---|---|---|---|---|---|---|
| 14 | 0.50 | 1.55 | 2.60 | 28 | 0.95 | 1.99 | 3.05 |
| 15 | 0.54 | 1.59 | 2.64 | 29 | 0.98 | 2.03 | 3.08 |
| 16 | 0.57 | 1.62 | 2.68 | 30 | 1.00 | 2.06 | 3.11 |
| 17 | 0.59 | 1.65 | 2.70 | 31 | 1.04 | 2.09 | 3.14 |
| 18 | 0.63 | 1.68 | 2.73 | 32 | 1.07 | 2.12 | 3.17 |
| 19 | 0.66 | 1.71 | 2.76 | 33 | 1.10 | 2.15 | 3.20 |
| 20 | 0.69 | 1.74 | 2.79 | 34 | 1.14 | 2.19 | 3.24 |
| 21 | 0.73 | 1.78 | 2.83 | 35 | 1.17 | 2.22 | 3.27 |
| 22 | 0.76 | 1.81 | 2.86 | 36 | 1.20 | 2.25 | 3.30 |
| 23 | 0.79 | 1.84 | 2.89 | 37 | 1.23 | 2.28 | 3.33 |
| 24 | 0.82 | 1.87 | 2.92 | 38 | 1.26 | 2.31 | 3.36 |
| 25 | 0.85 | 1.90 | 2.95 | 39 | 1.29 | 2.34 | 3.39 |
| 26 | 0.88 | 1.93 | 2.98 | 40 | 1.32 | 2.37 | 3.42 |
| 27 | 0.91 | 1.96 | 3.01 | | | | |

From Monteagudo et al, 1993,[60] by permission.

**Table 3–36. RATIO OF THE OCCIPITAL (POSTERIOR) HORN HEIGHT TO THE CHOROID PLEXUS THICKNESS**

| Estimated Gestational Age (weeks) | 5th Percentile (mm) | 50th Percentile (mm) | 95th Percentile (mm) |
|---|---|---|---|
| 14 | 0.02 | 0.85 | 1.68 |
| 15 | 0.04 | 0.86 | 1.69 |
| 16 | 0.05 | 0.88 | 1.71 |
| 17 | 0.07 | 0.90 | 1.72 |
| 18 | 0.84 | 0.91 | 1.74 |
| 19 | 0.10 | 0.93 | 1.75 |
| 20 | 0.12 | 0.94 | 1.77 |
| 21 | 0.13 | 0.96 | 1.79 |
| 22 | 0.15 | 0.97 | 1.80 |
| 23 | 0.16 | 0.99 | 1.82 |
| 24 | 0.18 | 1.00 | 1.83 |
| 25 | 0.19 | 1.02 | 1.85 |
| 26 | 0.21 | 1.04 | 1.87 |
| 27 | 0.23 | 1.05 | 1.88 |
| 28 | 0.24 | 1.07 | 1.90 |
| 29 | 0.26 | 1.09 | 1.91 |
| 30 | 0.27 | 1.10 | 1.93 |
| 31 | 0.29 | 1.12 | 1.94 |
| 32 | 0.31 | 1.13 | 1.96 |
| 33 | 0.32 | 1.15 | 1.98 |
| 34 | 0.24 | 1.16 | 1.99 |
| 35 | 0.35 | 1.18 | 2.00 |
| 36 | 0.37 | 1.20 | 2.02 |
| 37 | 0.38 | 1.21 | 2.04 |
| 38 | 0.40 | 1.23 | 2.06 |
| 39 | 0.42 | 1.24 | 2.07 |
| 40 | 0.43 | 1.26 | 2.09 |

From Monteagudo et al, 1993,[60] by permission.

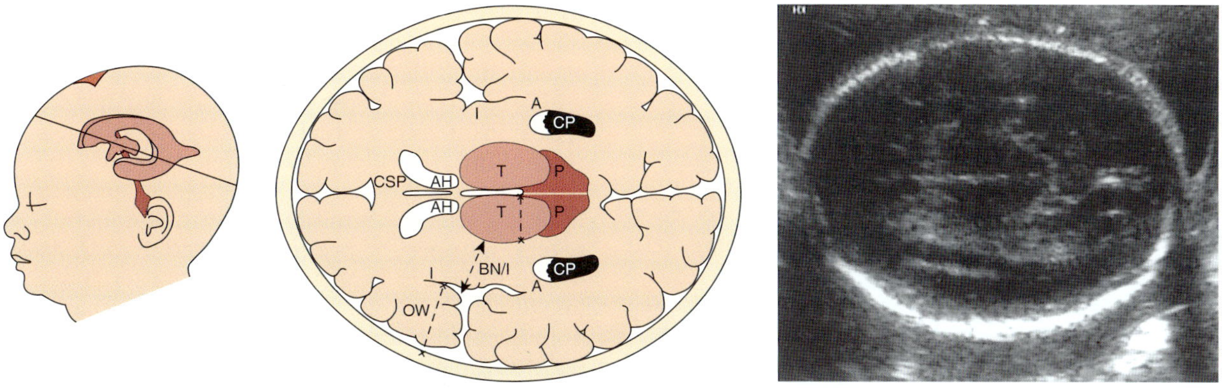


**Figure 3–20.**

## How to Measure It (Figure 3–20)

These structures can be readily outlined in the standard horizontal BPD plane previously described.[5,8] The hypoechoic thalamus (T) is measured at the anterior tip of the ambient cistern. The basal nuclei (BN) and insula (I) can be measured as a whole from the edge of the thalamus to the echo of the cistern of the lateral sulcus. The opercular width (OW) of the temporal lobe corresponds sonographically to the distance between the inner surface of the temporal bone and the cistern of the lateral sulcus at the point of its invagination into the cerebral cortex.[51]

## Comments

The cerebral hemispheres buckle as their growth increases, creating the sulci and the gyri. The largest infolding corresponds to the developing lateral sulcus, where the caudal end of the cerebral hemispheres grows to form the operculum of the temporal lobe. With the described measurement method, the OW is overestimated in the second trimester because the gap that exists between the inner bone surface and the insular cortex is not taken into consideration. On the other hand, in the third trimester this measurement is underestimated because the distance between the cistern of the lateral sulcus and the calvarium does not represent exactly the full width of the developing temporal operculum. Nevertheless, by 35 postmenstrual weeks, the OW has approximately doubled from the time of its first appearance.[51]

By 18 postmenstrual weeks, the basal nuclei and the insular cortex can be identified. Siedler and Filly[51] proposed that with transabdominal sonography, the basal nuclei appear as two zones of different echogenicity: (1) an echogenic curvilinear strip marginating the thalamus and posterolateral to the frontal horns that corresponds to the caudate and lentiform nuclei; and (2) a sonolucent band lateral to the previously described, corresponding to the external capsule, claustrum, and extreme capsule. The insular cortex is included when measuring this hypoechoic band.

The thalami, in the BPD plane, appear sonographically as two hypoechoic oval structures separated in the midline by the third ventricle. Their width increases from 7 ± 0.8 mm at 15 to 20 postmenstrual weeks to 9 ± 0.7 mm at 31 to 35 postmenstrual weeks, undergoing considerably less growth than the temporal operculum and the basal nuclei-insula (Table 3–37).

**Table 3–37. MEASUREMENTS OF FETAL INTRACRANIAL STRUCTURES**

| Gestational Age (weeks) | Thalamus (mm) | | | Basal Nuclel–Insula (mm) | | | Temporal Operculum (mm) | | |
|---|---|---|---|---|---|---|---|---|---|
| | Mean | Range | SD | Mean | Range | SD | Mean | Range | SD |
| 15–20 | 7 | 6–9 | 0.8 | 6 | 5–7 | 0.7 | 6 | 5–7 | 0.9 |
| 21–25 | 8 | 6–9 | 0.7 | 7 | 6–11 | 1.2 | 9 | 7–11 | 1.0 |
| 26–30 | 8 | 8–9 | 0.4 | 9 | 8–12 | 1.2 | 11 | 10–13 | 0.6 |
| 31–35 | 9 | 8–10 | 0.7 | 11 | 9–14 | 1.1 | 13 | 11–15 | 0.7 |

SD, standard deviation.

From Siedler and Filly, 1987,[51] with permission.

## POSTERIOR FOSSA: CEREBELLUM AND CEREBELLOMEDULLARY CISTERN (CISTERNA MAGNA)

### Definitions

The cerebellum is a suprasegmental portion of the brain located within the cranial posterior fossa that receives input from virtually the entire nervous system, playing a key role in movement coordination.[69]

The cerebellomedullary cistern (CMC) corresponds to a portion of the subarachnoid space that bathes the cranial posterior fossa in CSF. It arcs around the cerebellum posteriorly, invaginating in the midline between the cerebellar hemispheres.[70]

### How to Measure It (Figure 3–21)

To evaluate the posterior fossa, a horizontal plane of the fetal head equal to that used for determination of the BPD must be obtained. Once the landmarks of the thalami (T) and the cavum septum pellucidum (CSP) are identified, a slight caudal rotation of the transducer will bring the characteristic butterfly-like appearance of the cerebellum into view. The transverse cerebellar diameter (TCD) can then be measured as the widest diameter across both hemispheres in an outer-to-outer fashion.[71]

The CMC depth is evaluated in the same plane and measured in the median plane from the posterior aspect of the cerebellum to the inner table of the occiput.

### Comments

The fetal cerebellum can be visualized sonographically as early as 10 to 11 postmenstrual weeks. It grows rapidly in the second trimester following a linear relationship with gestational age, so that during this period, measurements in millimeters equal approximately the gestational age in weeks. However, as pregnancy advances, the growth curve of the cerebellum tends to flatten, showing a slower rate of evolution (Tables 3–38 and 3–39).[71]

Because the cerebellum is located inside the posterior fossa and is surrounded by the dense petrous ridges and the occipital bone, it should be able to withstand deformation by extrinsic pressure better than the parietal bone. Keeping this concept in mind, several authors[71–73] proposed that the TCD, as opposed to the BPD, can better predict gestational age in cases in which variations of the fetal head shape, such as dolichocephaly and brachycephaly, have been described (eg, breech presentation, oligohydramnios, twins, and uterine anomalies).

Intrauterine growth retardation remains a major cause of perinatal morbidity and mortality, affecting 4% to 8% of all deliveries in so-called developed countries.[74] In order to better evaluate fetal biometry, when intrauterine growth retardation is suspected, the TCD should also be used. Cabbad and associates[75] found that 22 out of 23 asymmetrically growth-impaired fetuses had a TCD lower than expected but within the normal range, suggesting that this measurement could be used to help estimate gestational age in these cases. On the other hand, Hill and colleagues[76] found in a group of 116 diabetic and nondiabetic singleton gestations with an estimated fetal weight at or above the 90th percentile that the TCD did not overestimate gestational age in the nondiabetic group and overestimated age in the diabetic group by only 0.5 postmenstrual weeks, rendering it a useful tool for predicting age in this population. The TCD has also been used to evaluate fetal growth in twin gestations.[77] Dilmen and colleagues[78] used the TCD/AC ratio obtained by transabdominal sonography to evaluate fetal growth. Ten of 11 fetuses with TCD/AC ratios exceeding 2 SD (0.1648) were found to have asymmetrical intrauterine growth retardation upon neonatal examination.

Because many congenital alterations of the cranial posterior fossa can modify the normal size of the CMC,

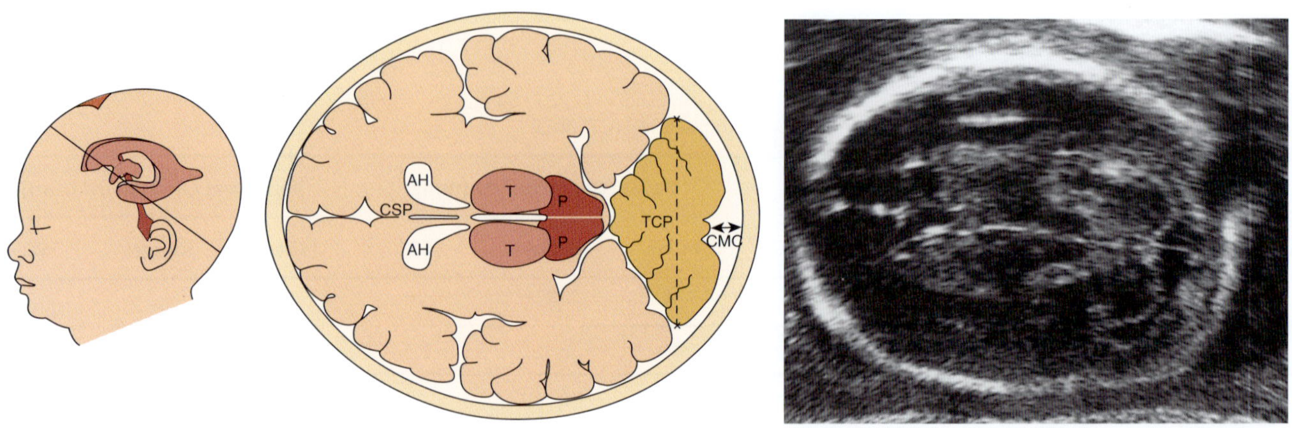


**Figure 3–21.**

**Table 3–38. PREDICTED GESTATIONAL AGES FOR TRANSVERSE CEREBELLAR DIAMETERS OF 14 TO 56 MM**

| Cerebellar Diameter (mm) | Gestational Age (weeks) | Cerebellar Diameter (mm) | Gestational Age (weeks) |
|---|---|---|---|
| 14 | 15.2 | 35 | 29.4 |
| 15 | 15.8 | 36 | 30.0 |
| 16 | 16.5 | 37 | 30.6 |
| 17 | 17.2 | 38 | 31.2 |
| 18 | 17.9 | 39 | 31.8 |
| 19 | 18.6 | 40 | 32.3 |
| 20 | 19.3 | 41 | 32.8 |
| 21 | 20.0 | 42 | 33.4 |
| 22 | 20.7 | 43 | 33.9 |
| 23 | 21.4 | 44 | 34.4 |
| 24 | 22.1 | 45 | 34.8 |
| 25 | 22.8 | 46 | 35.3 |
| 26 | 23.5 | 47 | 35.7 |
| 27 | 24.2 | 48 | 36.1 |
| 28 | 24.9 | 49 | 36.5 |
| 29 | 25.5 | 50 | 36.8 |
| 30 | 26.2 | 51 | 37.2 |
| 31 | 26.9 | 52 | 37.5 |
| 32 | 27.5 | 54 | 38.0 |
| 33 | 28.1 | 55 | 38.3 |
| 34 | 28.8 | 56 | 38.5 |

From Hill and colleagues, 1990,[76] with permission.

its evaluation deserves special consideration when searching for infratentorial anomalies. The mean normal CMC depth has been reported to be 5 mm (range 1 to 10 mm), with an SD of ±3 mm. The CMC can be enlarged in Dandy-Walker malformation, as well as in posterior fossa arachnoid cysts. Joubert syndrome also should be considered in the differential diagnosis of an enlarged CMC. In both conditions, the cerebellar hemispheres and fourth ventricles can be of normal size, the inferior and posterior vermian dysplasia is common to both disorders, and, in both, the CMC communicates with the fourth ventricle. Joubert syndrome, however, is associated with bilaterally enlarged echogenic kidneys, agenesis of the corpus callosum, occipital encephalocele, facial anomalies, and polydactyly.[79] However, it is important to keep in mind that in the absence of other findings (eg, hydrocephaly, shift of the midline, or dysgenesis of the cerebellar vermis), a prominent CMC is unlikely to be of clinical significance. On the contrary, in Arnold-Chiari malformation, the CMC is diminished in size, typically measuring ≤2 mm.[70] In this case, the cerebellum can have a flattened, wedged appearance, giving the impression of the so-called banana sign.[80]

The cerebellar vermis should also be adequately imaged when evaluating the sonographic appearance of the cerebellum. Vermian agenesis is commonly found

**Table 3–39. NOMOGRAM OF THE TRANSVERSE CEREBELLAR DIAMETER ACCORDING TO PERCENTILE DISTRIBUTION**

| | Cerebellar Diameter (mm) | | | | |
|---|---|---|---|---|---|
| Gestational Age (weeks) | 10th Percentile | 25th Percentile | 50th Percentile | 75th Percentile | 90th Percentile |
| 15 | 10 | 12 | 14 | 15 | 16 |
| 16 | 14 | 16 | 16 | 16 | 17 |
| 17 | 16 | 17 | 17 | 18 | 18 |
| 18 | 17 | 18 | 18 | 19 | 19 |
| 19 | 18 | 18 | 19 | 19 | 22 |
| 20 | 18 | 19 | 20 | 20 | 22 |
| 21 | 19 | 20 | 22 | 23 | 24 |
| 22 | 21 | 23 | 23 | 24 | 24 |
| 23 | 22 | 23 | 24 | 25 | 26 |
| 24 | 22 | 24 | 25 | 27 | 28 |
| 25 | 23 | 21.5 | 28 | 28 | 29 |
| 26 | 25 | 28 | 29 | 30 | 32 |
| 27 | 26 | 28.5 | 30 | 31 | 32 |
| 28 | 27 | 30 | 31 | 32 | 34 |
| 29 | 29 | 32 | 34 | 36 | 38 |
| 30 | 31 | 32 | 35 | 37 | 40 |
| 31 | 32 | 35 | 38 | 39 | 43 |
| 32 | 33 | 36 | 38 | 40 | 42 |
| 33 | 32 | 36 | 40 | 43 | 44 |
| 34 | 33 | 38 | 40 | 41 | 44 |
| 35 | 31 | 37 | 40.5 | 43 | 47 |
| 36 | 36 | 29 | 43 | 52 | 55 |
| 37 | 37 | 37 | 45 | 52 | 55 |
| 38 | 40 | 40 | 48.5 | 52 | 55 |
| 39 | 52 | 52 | 52 | 55 | 55 |

Modified from Goldstein and colleagues, 1987,[71] with permission.

with Dandy-Walker malformation and variants, as well as in association with other malformations and syndromes. Although uncommon, agenesis if the cerebellar vermis can be part of the Dandy-Walker malformation or an isolated finding. It may also present as complete or partial agenesis.[81] It is generally accepted that vermian development should be completed by 18 weeks of gestation; however, other authors[82] have suggested that the diagnosis of the different types of vermian hypoplasia should not be performed before 24 weeks of gestation.[85] At this point, the vermis should have completed its development to allow accurate measurements. Vermian

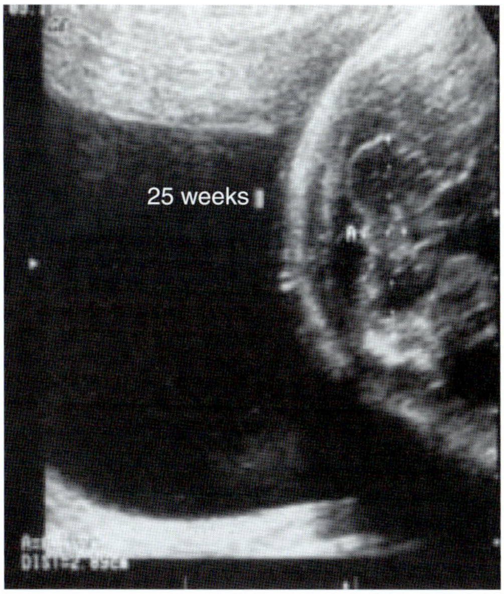


**Figure 3–22.** Transverse (axial) sonogram of the fetal head at the level of the thalamus, showing the width of the cerebellar vermis at 25 week of gestation. (Reproduced, with permission, from *Ultrasound Obstet Gynecol.* 2002;19:136–139. Blackwell Science Ltd. The development of the fetal vermis: an in-utero sonographic evaluation.[84])

width and height are commonly evaluated in the transverse (axial) plane for width and sagittal plane for height (Figure 3–22).

More recently,[88,92] vermian development and anatomy have been described using multiplanar 3D ultrasound. With this technique, the characteristic features of the cystic malformations of the posterior fossa (ie, upward displacement of the tentorium, counterclockwise rotation, and hypoplasia of the cerebellar vermis) can be more easily evaluated (Tables 3–40 through 3–49).

## Frontal Lobe

### Definition

The frontal lobe corresponds to the portion of the cerebral hemisphere anterior to the central sulcus and an imaginary line drawn at the level of the lateral sulcus up to the circular sulcus of the insula.[68]

### How to Measure It (Figure 3–23)

Frontal lobe measurements are accomplished in the plane in which the BPD is measured (eg, the horizontal plane). The frontal lobe distance (FLD) is measured between the anterior margin of the medial wall of the frontal horn of the lateral ventricles and the middle hyperechogenic frontal bone. The thalamic frontal lobe distance (TFD) is measured from the most posterior landmark of the thalami to the middle hyperechogenic frontal bone.

### Comments

Frontal lobe measurements (ie, FLD and TFD) (Tables 3–50 and 3–51) can be used as an adjunct for the diagnosis of microcephaly, as several investigators agree that this entity is associated with a decreased size of the frontal fossa and flattening of the frontal bone, with other lobes of the brain remaining unchanged.[81–83] Goldstein and coworkers[29] reported on three cases of postnatally confirmed microcephaly in which the FLD and the TFD were below the 10th percentile. Although this is a small series, measuring the frontal lobe seems to be a logical suggestion in cases where microcephaly is suspected, as it adds only a few seconds to the scanning session. Frontal lobe measurements (especially the TFD) have also been used to aid in the antenatal midtrimester diagnosis of Down syndrome. Bahado-Singh and collaborators[83] found that among 19 fetuses with Down syndrome, 10 (52%) had a TFD below the 10th percentile for gestational age. It

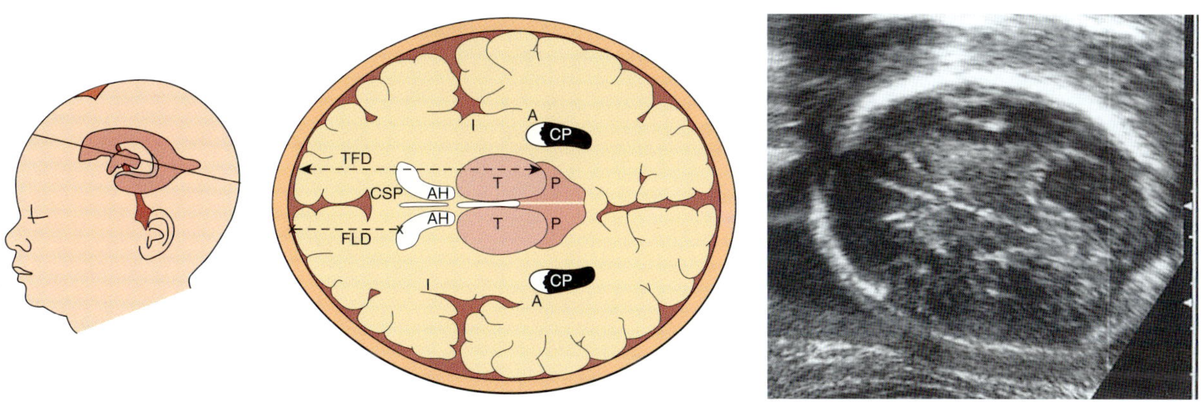


**Figure 3–23.**

**Table 3–40. VERMIS SIZE (WIDTH AND HEIGHT) ACCORDING TO GESTATIONAL AGE (MEAN ± SD)**

| Gestational Week | Number of Patients | Vermis Width (mean, mm, (SD)) | Vermis Height (mean, mm, (SD)) |
|---|---|---|---|
| 18–20 | 8 | 5 (0.76) | 5.88 (0.85) |
| 21 | 17 | 5.76 (0.83) | 6.47 (0.94) |
| 22 | 17 | 6.24 (0.66) | 6.88 (0.60) |
| 23 | 31 | 6.90 (0.54) | 7.71 (0.90) |
| 24 | 25 | 8.12 (0.67) | 8.44 (0.71) |
| 25 | 26 | 8.58 (0.81) | 8.62 (0.75) |
| 26 | 18 | 9.11 (0.96) | 9.17 (0.71) |
| 27 | 18 | 9.78 (0.81) | 10.00 (0.91) |
| 28–29 | 17 | 10.4 (1.17) | 10.5 (0.87) |
| 30–31 | 12 | 11.3 (1.22) | 11.6 (0.79) |
| 32 | 14 | 12.3 (1.54) | 12.1 (1.27) |
| 33 | 16 | 11.8 (1.29) | 12.2 (1.11) |
| 34 | 10 | 13.0 (1.05) | 13.0 (0.94) |
| 35–36 | 18 | 14.2 (1.25) | 14.2 (1.20) |
| 37–38 | 9 | 15.4 (1.01) | 15.3 (0.87) |
| Total | 256 | | |

SD, standard deviation.

After Zalel et al, 2002,[84] with permission.

**Table 3–41. CORRELATION OF VERMIS HEIGHT AND GESTATIONAL AGE ($r = 0.937$)**

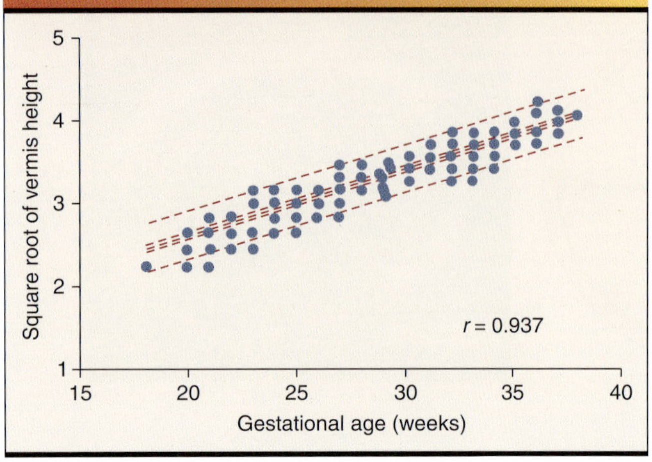


Reproduced from Zalel et al, 2002,[84] with permission.

**Table 3–42. CORRELATION OF VERMIS WIDTH AND GESTATIONAL AGE ($r = 0.934$)**

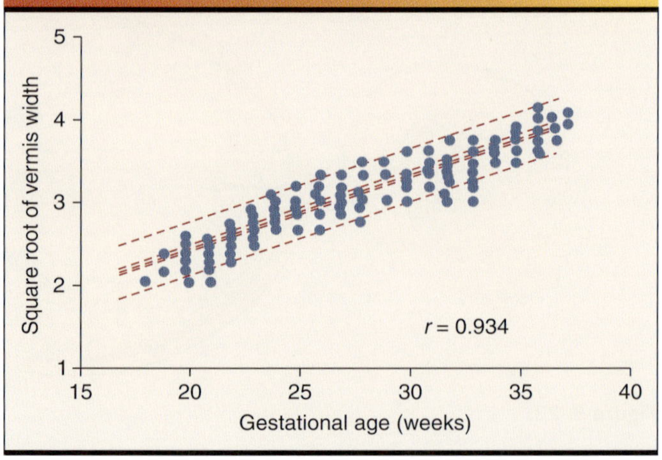


Reproduced from Zalel et al, 2002,[84] with permission.

**Table 3–43. CORRELATION OF VERMIS HEIGHT AND BIPARIETAL DIAMETER ($r$ = 0.937)**

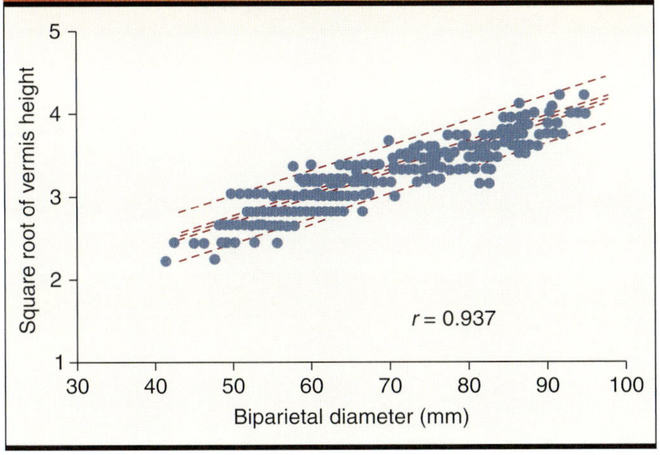


Reproduced from Zalel et al, 2002,[84] with permission.

**Table 3–44. CORRELATION OF VERMIS WIDTH AND BIPARIETAL DIAMETER ($r$ = 0.936)**

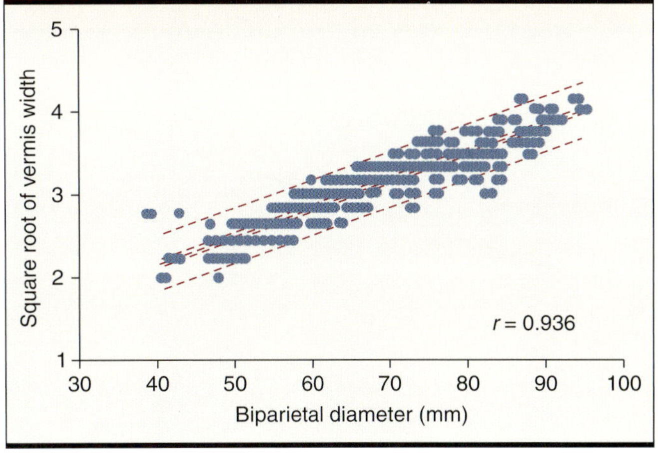


Reproduced from Zalel et al, 2002,[84] with permission.

**Table 3–45. MEAN ± SD MEASUREMENTS OBTAINED BY VOLUME CONTRAST IMAGING IN THE CORONAL PLANE OF THE CEREBELLAR VERMIS IN 203 NORMAL FETUSES**

| Gestational Age (weeks) | Patients ($n$) | Carniocaudal Diameter (mm) | Anteroposterior Diameter (mm) | Surface Area ($cm^2$) |
|---|---|---|---|---|
| 18–19 | 10 | 10.5 ± 1.3 | 8.3 ± 0.8 | 0.6 ± 0.05 |
| 20–21 | 19 | 12.7 ± 1.4 | 9.1 ± 1.6 | 0.7 ± 0.3 |
| 22–23 | 46 | 14.2 ± 1.6 | 10.5 ± 1.7 | 1.2 ± 0.2 |
| 24–25 | 45 | 15.8 ± 1.6 | 12 ± 1.4 | 1.5 ± 0.3 |
| 26–27 | 28 | 17.6 ± 1.7 | 13.5 ± 1.8 | 1.7 ± 0.3 |
| 28–29 | 19 | 19.6 ± 1.7 | 13.9 ± 1.1 | 2.1 ± 0.2 |
| 30–31 | 16 | 20.9 ± 1.5 | 15.5 ± 1.6 | 2.4 ± 0.06 |
| 32–33 | 20 | 22.8 ± 1.6 | 18.2 ± 1.7 | 3.4 ± 0.2 |

From Vinals et al, 2005,[94] with permission.

**Table 3–46. CORRELATION BETWEEN VERMIS SUPEROINFERIOR DIAMETER AND GESTATIONAL AGE**

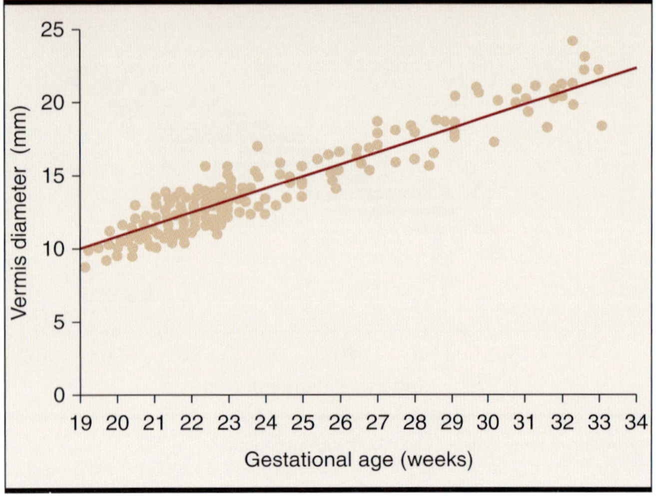


From Achiron et al, 2004,[93] with permission.

**Table 3–47. CORRELATION OF CEREBELLAR VERMIS CRANIOCAUDAL (CC) DIAMETER WITH GESTATIONAL AGE (GA)**

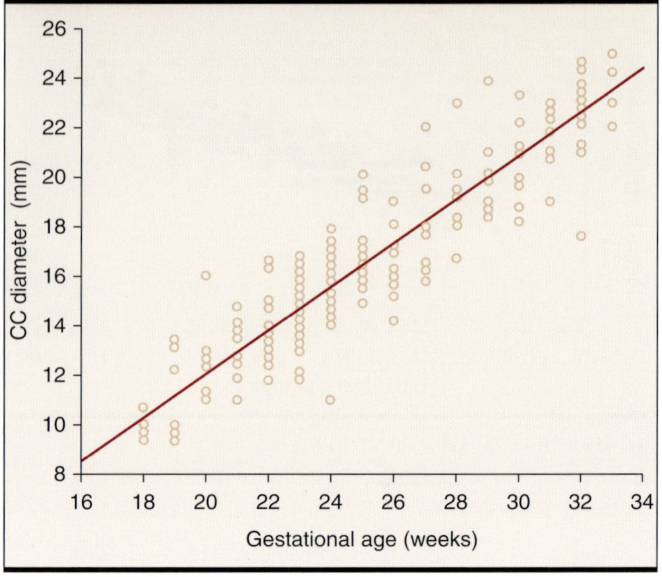


From Vinals et al, 2005),[94] with permission.

**Table 3–48. CORRELATION OF CEREBELLAR VERMIS ANTEROPOSTERIOR (AP) DIAMETER WITH GESTATIONAL AGE (GA)**

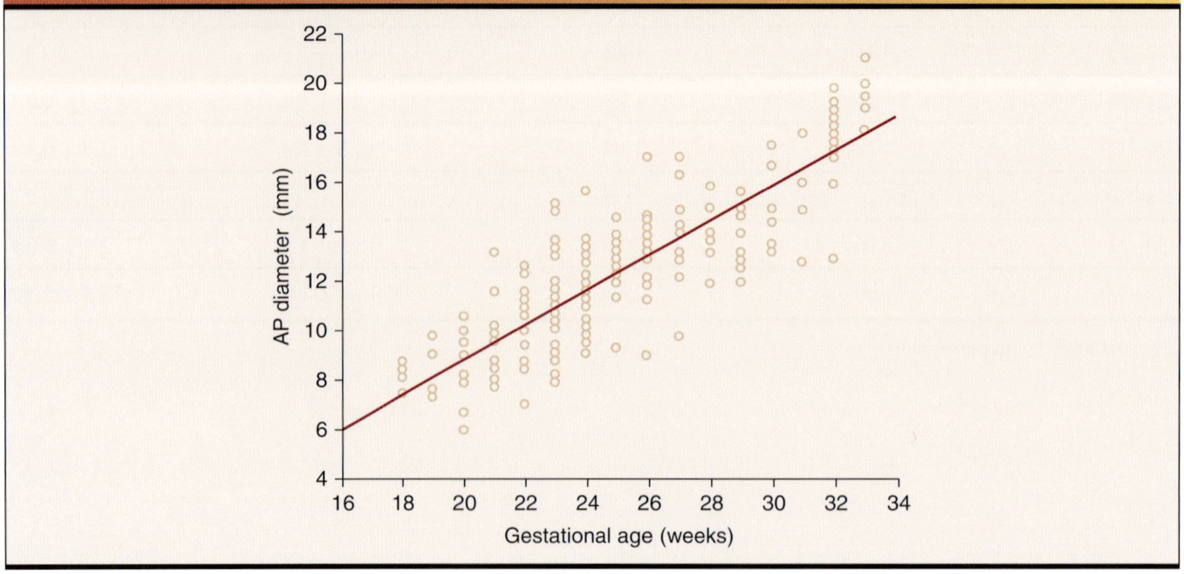


From Vinals et al, 2005,[94] with permission.

**Table 3–49. PERCENTILE MEASUREMENTS CEREBELLAR VERMIS (SUPEROINFERIOR DIAMETER) ACCORDING TO GESTATIONAL AGE**

| | | Superoinferior Diameter (mm) | | | | |
|---|---|---|---|---|---|---|
| GA (weeks) | *n* | 5th | 25th | 50th | 75th | 95th |
| 19–20 | 18 | 6.5 | 9.1 | 9.5 | 10 | 11.1 |
| 21–22 | 114 | 10.1 | 10.9 | 11.7 | 12.1 | 13.2 |
| 23-24 | 82 | 11.4 | 12.3 | 13 | 13.6 | 15.2 |
| 25–26 | 20 | 13.1 | 14.3 | 14.8 | 15.4 | 16.4 |
| 27–28 | 15 | 15.3 | 16 | 16.8 | 17.9 | 18.6 |
| 29–30 | 11 | 15.6 | 17.5 | 18.5 | 20.3 | 20.9 |
| 31–32 | 13 | 17.2 | 19.6 | 20.1 | 20.7 | 21 |
| 33–34 | 14 | 18.3 | 20.6 | 21.5 | 22.8 | 24 |

GA, gestational age.

From Achiron et al, 2004,[84] with permission.

is possible that the combination of these measurements with other reported signs (eg, enlarged nuchal fold, cardiovascular anomalies, hyperechogenic bowel, and hydronephrosis) could further enhance the ability of ultrasonography to diagnose this condition in utero.

## CORPUS CALLOSUM

### Definition

The corpus callosum is a brain commissure composed of fibers that connect the cerebral hemispheres with each other.[87–92]

### How to Measure It

The corpus callosum can be evaluated in both the midsagittal and coronal planes, where it can be found between the cingulate gyrus above and the cavum septi pellucidi below. The length of the corpus callosum is measured from the most anterior aspect of the genu to the most posterior aspect of the splenium along a straight rostrocaudal line.[87,95]

Tables 3–52 to 3–53 Measurements of the normal fetal corpus callosum by gestational age

### Comments

The corpus callosum is a telencephalic structure that connects the left and right cerebral hemispheres. It is the largest white matter structure in the brain, consisting of 200 million to 250 million axonal projections. Much of the interhemispheric communication in the brain is conducted across the corpus callosum. The fetal corpus callosum can be used as a marker for normal brain development and maturation. During the prenatal period, changes in the length of the corpus callosum could be used as an indicator of abnormal development[86,88–91] (Tables 3–52, 3–53, 3–54, and 3–55; Figures 3–24, 3–25, 3–26, 3–27, 3–28, and 3–29).

The corpus callosum is composed of four parts (from front to back): rostrum, genu, body, and splenium (Figure 3–24). The formation of the corpus callosum starts with the development of the genu; the body and splenium develop at a later stage. If the normal developmental process is disturbed, the corpus callosum may be completely or partially absent.[89] Given the anteroposterior fashion of its development, it is usually the posterior body and splenium that get affected. Prenatal evaluation of the corpus callosum can be accomplished via the transvaginal-transfontanellar approach (in the fetus in the vertex presentation) or transabdominally when the fetal presentation is breech.[90,91] Adequate evaluation of the corpus callosum requires its visualization both in the median and coronal planes, which are easily obtainable using the transvaginal-transfontanellar route.[88] More recently, the use of the 3D multiplanar technique has been proposed[92] for the evaluation of the fetal brain. The corpus callosum can be fully evaluated in the fetus from the 18th gestational week onward, reaching its final adultlike configuration closer to the 28th week of gestation. A full discussion of corpus callosum abnormalities is beyond the scope of this chapter and will be discussed further in this book.

Table 3–50. MEASUREMENTS OF THE FRONTAL LOBE DISTANCE

| Gestational Age (weeks) | Mean ± 2 SD (cm) | Percentile | | | | |
|---|---|---|---|---|---|---|
| | | 10th | 25th | 50th | 75th | 90th |
| 16 | 1.4 ± 0.4 | 1.0 | 1.4 | 1.5 | 1.6 | 1.8 |
| 17 | 1.6 ± 0.2 | 1.5 | 1.6 | 1.6 | 1.8 | 1.8 |
| 18 | 1.6 ± 0.2 | 1.4 | 1.4 | 1.7 | 1.7 | 1.8 |
| 19 | 1.7 ± 0.2 | 1.4 | 1.5 | 1.8 | 1.9 | 1.9 |
| 20 | 1.7 ± 0.2 | 1.7 | 1.7 | 1.9 | 1.8 | 1.9 |
| 21 | 1.8 ± 0.4 | 1.4 | 1.5 | 2.0 | 2.0 | 2.1 |
| 22 | 1.8 ± 0.4 | 2.3 | 2.3 | 2.3 | 2.3 | 2.3 |
| 23 | 1.8 ± 0.4 | 1.8 | 1.9 | 2.1 | 2.2 | 2.3 |
| 24 | 1.9 ± 0.2 | 2.0 | 2.0 | 2.0 | 2.0 | 2.0 |
| 25 | 2.2 ± 0.4 | 2.0 | 2.0 | 2.3 | 2.4 | 2.5 |
| 26 | 2.3 ± 0.4 | 2.0 | 2.1 | 2.3 | 2.4 | 2.5 |
| 27 | 2.5 ± 0.6 | 2.5 | 2.5 | 2.7 | 3.1 | 3.2 |
| 28 | 2.8 ± 0.2 | 2.4 | 2.5 | 2.6 | 2.6 | 2.7 |
| 29 | 2.7 ± 0.2 | 2.7 | 2.7 | 2.8 | 2.8 | 2.8 |
| 30 | 2.8 ± 0.6 | 2.6 | 2.6 | 2.7 | 3.2 | 3.4 |
| 31 | 2.9 ± 0.4 | 2.7 | 2.7 | 2.8 | 3.0 | 3.0 |
| 32 | 3.0 ± 0.6 | 3.0 | 3.0 | 3.3 | 3.6 | 3.8 |
| 33 | 3.1 ± 0.6 | 2.5 | 2.6 | 3.2 | 3.4 | 3.4 |
| 34 | 3.2 ± 0.2 | 2.9 | 3.0 | 3.1 | 3.2 | 3.3 |
| 35 | 3.2 ± 0.4 | 3.2 | 3.4 | 3.5 | 3.7 | 4.0 |
| 36 | 3.2 ± 0.4 | 2.9 | 2.9 | 3.2 | 3.4 | 3.4 |
| 37 | 3.4 ± 0.4 | 3.1 | 3.2 | 3.4 | 3.6 | 3.8 |
| 38 | 3.5 ± 0.4 | 3.2 | 3.2 | 3.5 | 3.9 | 4.0 |
| 39 | 3.7 ± 0.6 | 3.5 | 3.5 | 3.7 | 4.2 | 4.3 |
| 40 | 4.0 ± 0.6 | 3.8 | 3.8 | 3.9 | 4.5 | 4.5 |

SD, standard deviation

From Goldstein and colleagues, 1988,[29] with permission.

**Table 3–51. MEASUREMENTS OF THALAMIC FRONTAL LOBE DISTANCE**

| Gestational Age (weeks) | Mean ± 2 SD (cm) | Percentile | | | | |
|---|---|---|---|---|---|---|
| | | 10th | 25th | 50th | 75th | 90th |
| 15 | 3.2 ± 0.4 | 3.2 | 3.2 | 3.2 | 3.2 | 3.2 |
| 16 | 3.2 ± 0.4 | 2.9 | 3.1 | 3.2 | 3.4 | 3.5 |
| 17 | 3.6 ± 0.6 | 3.2 | 3.4 | 3.5 | 3.8 | 4.5 |
| 18 | 3.7 ± 0.6 | 3.3 | 3.3 | 3.7 | 3.9 | 3.9 |
| 19 | 3.8 ± 0.4 | 3.5 | 3.5 | 3.7 | 3.9 | 4.0 |
| 20 | 4.1 ± 0.4 | 4.0 | 4.0 | 4.0 | 4.3 | 4.4 |
| 21 | 4.1 ± 0.4 | 3.9 | 3.9 | 4.1 | 4.4 | 4.5 |
| 22 | 4.6 ± 0.4 | 4.6 | 4.6 | 4.6 | 4.6 | 4.6 |
| 23 | 4.6 ± 0.4 | 4.6 | 4.6 | 4.6 | 4.6 | 4.6 |
| 24 | 4.7 ± 0.4 | 4.6 | 4.6 | 4.6 | 4.9 | 4.9 |
| 25 | 5.1 ± 0.6 | 4.7 | 4.8 | 5.2 | 5.3 | 5.4 |
| 26 | 5.2 ± 0.6 | 4.8 | 5.0 | 5.3 | 5.4 | 5.5 |
| 27 | 5.6 ± 0.8 | 5.3 | 5.6 | 5.6 | 6.8 | 7.2 |
| 28 | 5.7 ± 0.4 | 5.5 | 5.6 | 5.7 | 6.0 | 6.2 |
| 29 | 6.1 ± 0.4 | 6.0 | 6.0 | 6.1 | 6.4 | 6.4 |
| 30 | 6.2 ± 1.2 | 5.5 | 5.7 | 5.9 | 6.4 | 7.4 |
| 31 | 6.2 ± 0.8 | 6.1 | 6.1 | 6.1 | 6.2 | 6.2 |
| 32 | 6.4 ± 0.8 | 6.2 | 6.2 | 6.4 | 6.9 | 7.1 |
| 33 | 6.5 ± 0.6 | 5.9 | 6.0 | 6.3 | 6.5 | 6.6 |
| 34 | 6.7 ± 0.6 | 6.2 | 6.4 | 6.7 | 7.0 | 7.2 |
| 35 | 6.9 ± 0.6 | 6.6 | 6.7 | 7.1 | 7.2 | 7.3 |
| 36 | 7.0 ± 0.4 | 6.5 | 6.5 | 6.6 | 6.9 | 6.9 |
| 37 | 7.2 ± 0.6 | 6.2 | 6.4 | 6.7 | 7.0 | 7.1 |
| 38 | 7.3 ± 0.8 | 6.5 | 6.6 | 7.2 | 7.3 | 7.4 |
| 39 | 7.5 ± 0.8 | 7.1 | 7.0 | 7.4 | 7.7 | 7.8 |
| 40 | 7.7 ± 0.8 | 7.4 | 7.4 | 7.6 | 8.1 | 8.1 |

SD, standard deviation.

From Goldstein and colleagues, 1988,[29] with permission.

**Table 3–52. WIDTH OF FETAL CORPUS CALLOSUM BY GESTATIONAL AGE**

| Gestational Age (weeks) | Observations (n) | Lower 95% CI | Mean Width (mm) | Upper 95% CI |
|---|---|---|---|---|
| 16 | 4 | 1.61 | 2.38 | 3.14 |
| 17 | 8 | 2.08 | 2.63 | 3.17 |
| 18 | 7 | 2.82 | 3.99 | 5.15 |
| 19 | 18 | 3.80 | 4.18 | 4.55 |
| 20 | 21 | 3.93 | 4.43 | 4.93 |
| 21 | 21 | 4.40 | 5.02 | 5.64 |
| 22 | 18 | 4.56 | 4.99 | 5.43 |
| 23 | 22 | 4.90 | 5.39 | 5.88 |
| 24 | 18 | 5.49 | 6.16 | 6.83 |
| 25 | 23 | 5.26 | 5.68 | 6.11 |
| 26 | 18 | 5.74 | 6.40 | 7.06 |
| 27 | 12 | 5.72 | 6.69 | 7.66 |
| 28 | 9 | 6.50 | 7.19 | 7.88 |
| 29 | 10 | 5.35 | 6.18 | 7.01 |
| 30 | 12 | 6.45 | 7.16 | 7.87 |
| 31 | 10 | 5.92 | 6.63 | 7.34 |
| 32 | 7 | 5.43 | 6.61 | 7.80 |
| 33 | 4 | 4.81 | 6.58 | 8.34 |
| 34 | 6 | 5.90 | 7.32 | 8.73 |
| 35 | 5 | 5.43 | 7.16 | 8.89 |
| 36 | 2 | 5.60 | 8.60 | 8.80 |
| 37 | 3 | 2.98 | 7.67 | 12.36 |

CI, confidence interval.

From Achiron et al, 2001,[95] by permission.

**Table 3–53. THICKNESS OF FETAL CORPUS CALLOSUM BY GESTATIONAL AGE**

| Gestational Age (weeks) | Observations (n) | Lower 95% CI | Mean Thickness (mm) | Upper 95% CI |
|---|---|---|---|---|
| 16 | 4 | 0.42 | 0.75 | 1.08 |
| 17 | 8 | 0.58 | 1.12 | 1.32 |
| 18 | 7 | 1.12 | 1.30 | 1.48 |
| 19 | 18 | 1.03 | 1.13 | 1.24 |
| 20 | 21 | 1.31 | 1.47 | 1.63 |
| 21 | 21 | 1.60 | 1.73 | 1.86 |
| 22 | 18 | 1.82 | 2.00 | 2.18 |
| 23 | 22 | 1.87 | 2.04 | 2.20 |
| 24 | 18 | 1.90 | 2.07 | 2.24 |
| 25 | 23 | 1.89 | 2.11 | 2.34 |
| 26 | 18 | 1.87 | 2.09 | 2.31 |
| 27 | 12 | 1.94 | 2.14 | 2.35 |
| 28 | 9 | 1.66 | 2.14 | 2.63 |
| 29 | 10 | 1.73 | 1.99 | 2.25 |
| 30 | 12 | 2.04 | 2.35 | 2.66 |
| 31 | 10 | 1.93 | 2.37 | 2.81 |
| 32 | 7 | 1.96 | 2.66 | 3.36 |
| 33 | 4 | 2.13 | 2.75 | 3.37 |
| 34 | 6 | 2.20 | 2.62 | 3.03 |
| 35 | 5 | 2.21 | 2.76 | 3.31 |
| 36 | 2 | 2.20 | 2.50 | 3.00 |
| 37 | 3 | 1.98 | 2.27 | 2.55 |

CI, confidence interval.

From Achiron et al, 2001,[95] by permission.

**Table 3–54. LENGTH OF NORMAL FETAL CORPUS CALLOSUM BY GESTATIONAL AGE**

| Gestational Age (weeks) | No. of Observations (n) | Lower Limit 95% CI | Mean Length (mm) | Upper Limit of 95% CI |
|---|---|---|---|---|
| 16 | 14 | 8.0 | 9.4 | 10.7 |
| 17 | 15 | 10.5 | 12.0 | 13.5 |
| 18 | 11 | 12.2 | 14.0 | 15.8 |
| 19 | 18 | 15.7 | 16.6 | 17.5 |
| 20 | 20 | 17.7 | 18.7 | 19.7 |
| 21 | 21 | 21.0 | 22.2 | 23.4 |
| 22 | 26 | 22.8 | 23.9 | 24.9 |
| 23 | 33 | 24.6 | 25.6 | 26.5 |
| 24 | 25 | 25.1 | 26.0 | 26.9 |
| 25 | 30 | 28.1 | 29.0 | 29.9 |
| 26 | 30 | 30.9 | 31.8 | 32.8 |
| 27 | 35 | 32.9 | 33.8 | 34.7 |
| 28 | 25 | 33.3 | 34.6 | 35.8 |
| 29 | 36 | 34.2 | 35.5 | 36.8 |
| 30 | 29 | 36.3 | 37.7 | 39.1 |
| 31 | 17 | 36.0 | 36.5 | 37.0 |
| 32 | 28 | 37.6 | 38.5 | 39.5 |
| 33 | 30 | 37.1 | 38.2 | 39.3 |
| 34 | 12 | 37.8 | 39.8 | 41.9 |
| 35 | 27 | 41.0 | 42.6 | 44.2 |
| 36 | 14 | 42.4 | 44.7 | 47.0 |
| 37 | 12 | 42.4 | 45.0 | 47.6 |
| 38 | 25 | 43.2 | 44.2 | 45.3 |
| 39 | 16 | 41.8 | 43.2 | 44.6 |

CI, confidence interval.

From Hai-chun et al, 2009,[87] by permission.

**Table 3–55. LENGTH OF FETAL CORPUS CALLOSUM BY GESTATIONAL AGE**

| Gestational Age (weeks) | Observations (n) | Lower 95% CI | Mean Length (mm) | Upper 95% CI |
|---|---|---|---|---|
| 16 | 4 | 2.95 | 3.75 | 4.55 |
| 17 | 8 | 4.77 | 6.24 | 7.70 |
| 18 | 7 | 10.04 | 12.51 | 14.99 |
| 19 | 18 | 14.51 | 15.78 | 17.05 |
| 20 | 21 | 18.13 | 18.95 | 19.77 |
| 21 | 21 | 19.54 | 20.38 | 21.23 |
| 22 | 18 | 21.53 | 22.39 | 23.24 |
| 23 | 22 | 23.19 | 24.45 | 25.72 |
| 24 | 18 | 26.32 | 27.61 | 28.90 |
| 25 | 23 | 28.66 | 29.65 | 30.64 |
| 26 | 18 | 29.91 | 31.44 | 32.98 |
| 27 | 12 | 32.75 | 34.33 | 35.92 |
| 28 | 9 | 32.30 | 34.44 | 36.59 |
| 29 | 10 | 34.21 | 36.40 | 38.59 |
| 30 | 12 | 37.14 | 38.33 | 39.52 |
| 31 | 10 | 36.18 | 37.30 | 38.42 |
| 32 | 7 | 38.37 | 40.43 | 42.49 |
| 33 | 4 | 31.44 | 38.50 | 45.56 |
| 34 | 6 | 41.40 | 42.50 | 43.60 |
| 35 | 5 | 40.82 | 45.60 | 50.38 |
| 36 | 2 | 40.00 | 44.00 | 45.00 |
| 37 | 3 | 42.5 | 44.67 | 46.84 |

CI, confidence interval.

From Achiron et al, 2001,[95] by permission.

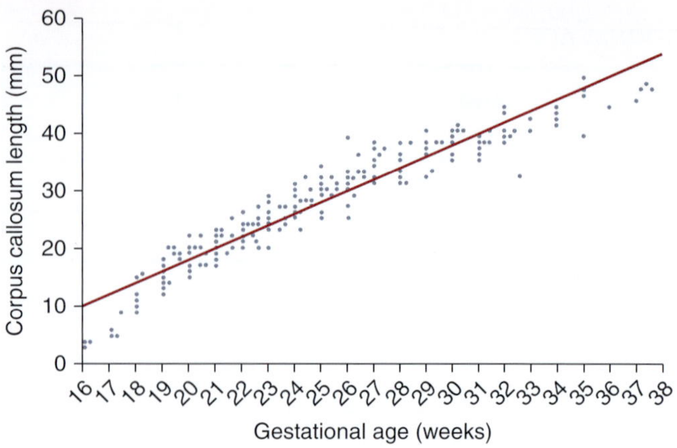


**Figure 3–24.** Individual scatter plot of length of the corpus callosom with gestational age of 258 normal fetuses showing a linear regression ($r$ = 0.779). (Reproduced, with permission, from *Ultrasound Obstet Gynecol.* 2001;18:343–347.[95])

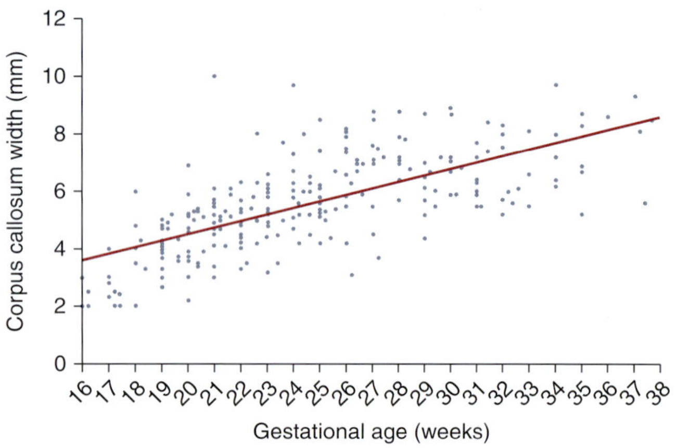


**Figure 3–25.** Individual scatter plot of width of the corpus callosom with gestational age of 258 normal fetuses showing a linear regression ($r$ = 0.676). (Reproduced, with permission, from *Ultrasound Obstet Gynecol.* 2001;18:343–347.[95])

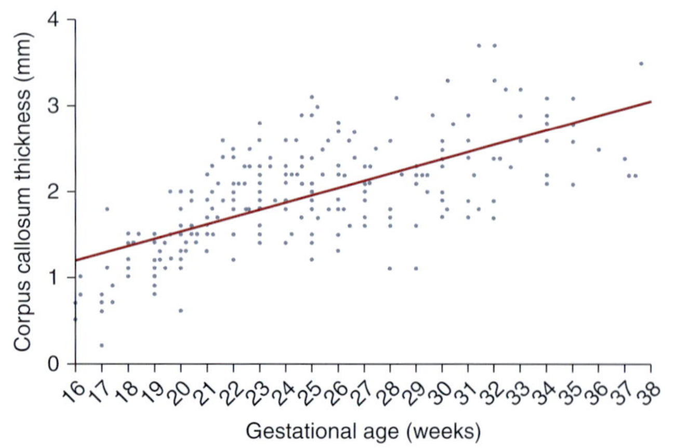


**Figure 3–26.** Individual scatter plot of thickness of the corpus callosom with gestational age of 258 normal fetuses showing a linear regression ($r$ = 0.494). (Reproduced, with permission, from *Ultrasound Obstet Gynecol.* 2001;18:343–347.[95])

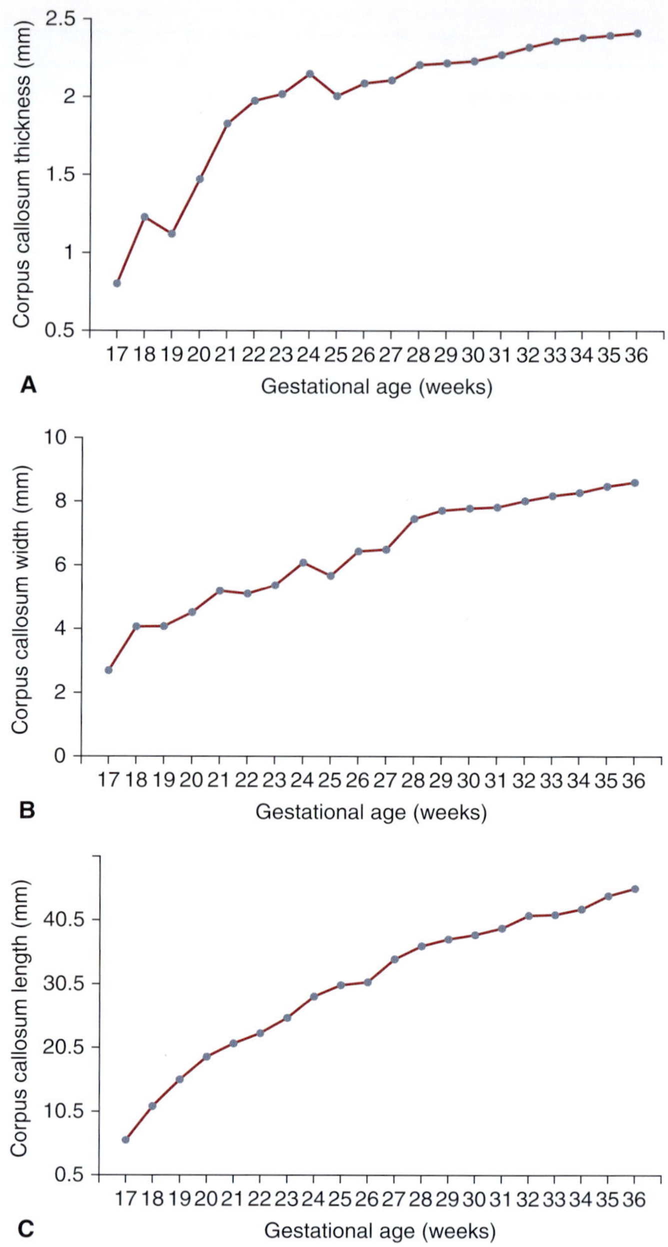


**Figure 3–27.** Maximum growth in thickness **(A)** and width **(B)** of the corpus callosum occurred between 19 and 21 weeks' gestation, while its length **(C)** followed a constant growth rate. (Reproduced, with permission, from *Ultrasound Obstet Gynecol.* 2001;18:343–347.[95])

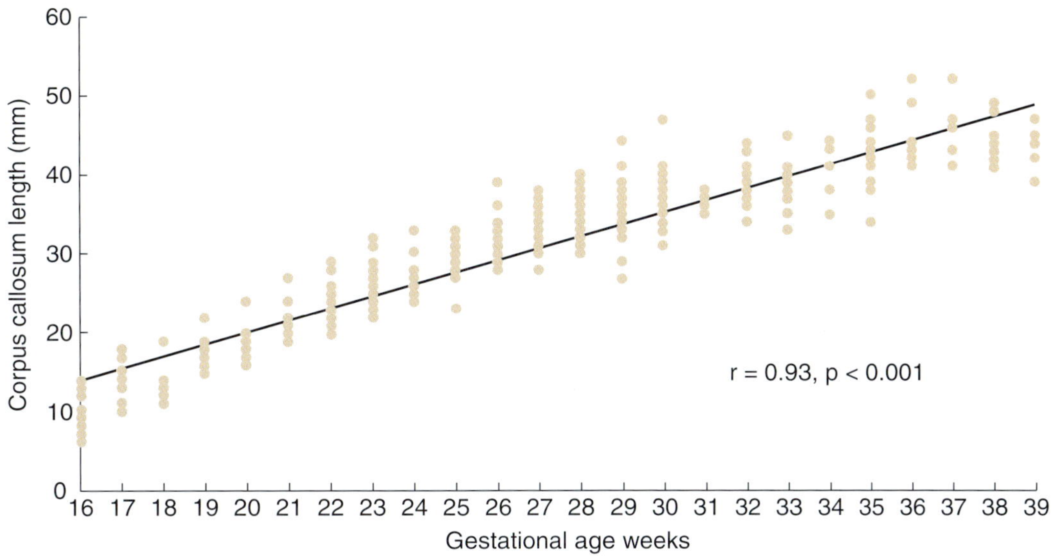


**Figure 3–28.** Scatterplot of the length of the corpus callosum by gestational age in 549 normal fetuses. (Reproduced, with permission, from *JCU*. 2009;37:75–77.[87])

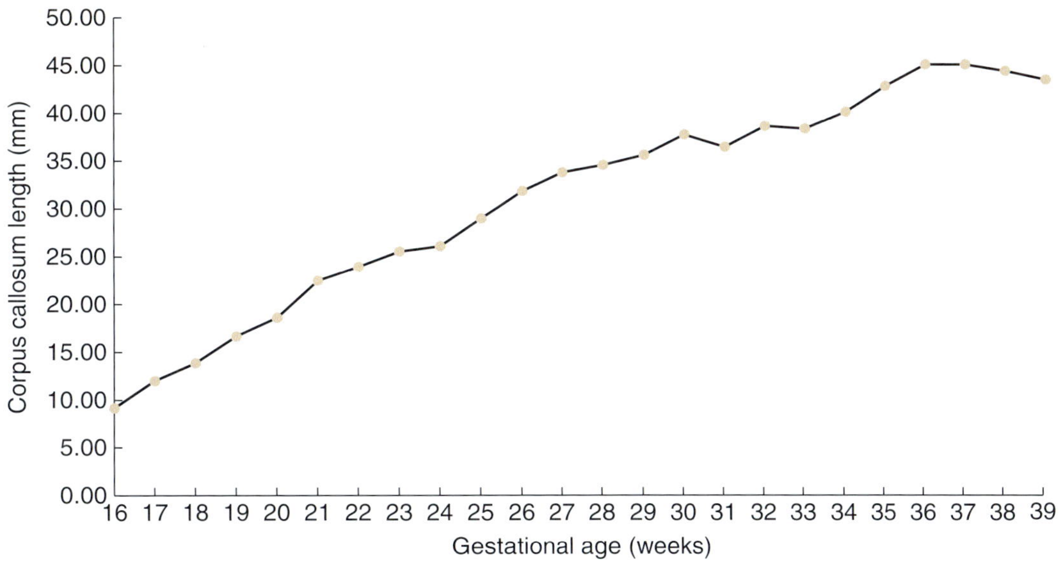


**Figure 3–29.** Relationship between the mean length of the corpus callosum and gestational age. (Reproduced, with permission, from *JCU*. 2009;37:75–77.[87])

## SUMMARY

The numeric information as well as their applications were compiled in this chapter. At places more than one author's metrics are quoted since different ultrasound laboratories or perinatal practitioners have one over another.

Most tables, graphs and the needed informations were updated using the newest publications.

## REFERENCES


1. O'Rahilly R, Müller F. Embryonic length and cerebral landmarks in staged human embryos. *Anat Rec*. 1984;209:265–271.
2. Robinson HP. Sonar measurement of fetal crown–rump length as means of assessing maturity in first trimester of pregnancy. *Br Med J*. 1973;4:28–31.
3. Robinson HO, Fleming JEE. A critical evaluation of sonar "crown–rump" length measurements. *Br J Obstet Gynaecol*. 1975;82: 702–710.
4. Ott WJ. Accurate gestational dating: Revisited. *Am J Perinatol*. 1994;11:404–408.
5. Blaas HG, Eik-Nes SH, Berg S, Torp H. In vivi three-dimensional ultrasound reconstructions of embryos and early fetuses. *Lancet*. 1998;352:1182–1186.
6. Campbell S, Thoms A. Ultrasound measurement of the fetal head to abdomen circumference ratio in the assessment of growth retardation. *Br J Obstet Gynaecol*. 1977;84:165–174.
7. Hadlock FP, Deter RL, Harrist RB, et al. Fetal biparietal diameter: Rational choice of plane section for sonographic measurement. *AJR Am J Roentgenol*. 1982;138:871–874.
8. Campbell S. An improved method of fetal cephalometry. *J Obstet Gynecol Br Commonw*. 1968;75:568–576.
9. Hadlock FP, Deter RL, Harrist RB, et al. Estimating fetal age: Computer assisted analysis of multiple fetal growth parameters. *Radiology*. 1984;152:497–501.
10. Gray DL, Songster GS, Parvin CA, et al. Cephalic index: A gestational age-dependent biometric parameter. *Obstet Gynecol*. 1989;74: 600–603.
11. Wolfson RN, Zador IE, Halvorsen P, et al. Biparietal diameter in premature rupture of membranes: Errors in estimating gestational age. *J Clin Ultrasound*. 1983;11:371–374.
12. Hadlock FP, Deter RL, Carpenter RJ, et al. Estimating fetal age: Effect of head shape on BPD. *AJR Am J Roentgenol*. 1981;137:83–85.
13. Hill LM, Breckle R, Gehrking WC. The variable effects of oligohydramnios on the biparietal diameter and the cephalic index. *J Ultrasound Med*. 1984;3:93–95.
14. Kasby CB, Poll V. The breech head and its ultrasound significance. *Br J Obstet Gynaecol*. 1982;89:106–110.
15. al Ryami N, Walker MG, Proctor LK, Yinon Y, Windrim RC, Kingdom JC. Utility of head/abdomen circumference ratio in the evaluation of severe, early-onset intrauterine growth restriction. *J Obstet Gynecol Can*. 2011;33:715–719.
16. Ott WJ. The use of ultrasonic fetal head circumference for predicting expected date of confinement. *J. Clin Ultrasound*. 1984;12:411–415.
17. Hadlock FP. Ultrasound determination of menstrual age. In: Callen PW, ed. *Ultrasonography in Obstetrics and Gynecology*. Philadelphia: WB Saunders; 1994:94–95.
18. Hadlock FP, Deter RL, Harrist RB, et al. Fetal head circumference: Relation to menstrual age. *AJR Am J Roentgenol*. 1982;138:649–653.
19. Hadlock FP, Deter RL, Carpenter RJ, et al. The effect of head shape on the accuracy in estimating fetal gestational age. *AJR Am J Roentgenol*. 1981;137:83–85.
20. Hadlock FP, Harrist RB, Martinez-Poyer J. How accurate is the second trimester fetal dating? *J Ultrasound Med*. 1991;10:557–561.
21. Benson CB, Doubilet PM. Sonographic prediction of gestational age: Accuracy of second and third trimester fetal measurements. *AJR Am J Roentgenol*. 1991;157:1275–1277.
22. Hill LM, Guzick D, Hixson J, et al. Composite assessment of gestational age: A comparison of institutionally derived and published regression equations. *Am J Obstet Gynecol*. 1992;166:551–555.
23. Hadlock FP, Harrist RB, Carpenter RJ, et al. Sonographic estimation of fetal weight. *Radiology*. 1984;150:535–540.
24. Benson CB, Boswell SB, Brown DL, et al. Improved prediction of intrauterine growth retardation with use of multiple parameters. *Radiology*. 1988;168:7–12.
25. Benson CB, Bellville JS, Lentini JF, et al. Intrauterine growth retardation: Diagnosis based on multiple parameters—A prospective study. *Radiology*. 1990;177:499–502.
26. Romero R, Pilu G, Jeanty P, et al, eds. *Prenatal Diagnosis of Congenital Anomalies*. Norwalk, CT: Appleton & Lange; 1988: 54–59.
27. Kurtz AB, Wapner RJ, Rubin CS, et al. Ultrasound criteria for in utero diagnosis of microcephaly. *J Clin Ultrasound*. 1980;8:11–16.
28. Chervenak FA, Jeanty P, Cantraine F, et al. The diagnosis of fetal microcephaly. *Am J Obstet Gynecol*. 1984;149:512–517.
29. Goldstein I, Reece EA, Pilu G, et al. Sonographic assessment of the fetal frontal lobe: A potential tool for prenatal diagnosis of microcephaly. *Am J Obstet Gynecol*. 1988;158:1057–1062.
30. Pilu G, Falco P, Milano V, Perolo A, Bovicelli L. Prenatal diagnosis of microcephaly assisted by vaginal sonography and power Doppler ultrasound. *Obstet Gynecol*. 1998;11:357–360.
31. Mayden KL, Tortora M, Berkowitz RL, et al. Orbital diameters: A new parameter for prenatal diagnosis and dating. *Am J Obstet Gynecol*. 1982;144:289–297.
32. Jeanty P, Dramaix-Wilmet M, Van Gansbeke D, et al. Fetal ocular biometry by ultrasound. *Radiology*. 1982;143:513–516.
33. Trout T, Budorick NE, Pretorius DH, et al. Significance of orbital measurements in the fetus. *J Ultrasound Med*. 1994;13:937–943.
34. Romero R, Pilu G, Jeanty P, et al, eds. *Prenatal Diagnosis of Congenital Anomalies*. Norwalk, CT: Appleton & Lange; 1988: 81–97.
35. Birnholz JC. Ultrasonic fetal ophthalmology. *Early Hum Dev*. 1985;12:199–209.
36. Jeanty P, Dramaix-Wilmet M, Delbeke D, et al. Ultrasonic evaluation of fetal ventricular growth. *Neuroradiology*. 1981;21:127–131.
37. Johnson ML, Dunne MG, Mack LA, et al. Evaluation of fetal intracranial anatomy by static and real time ultrasound. *J Clin Ultrasound*. 1980;8:311–318.
38. Kurjak A. Ultrasound diagnosis of congenital malformations. In: de Viegler, ed. *Handbook of Clinical Ultrasound*. New York: Wiley; 1988:189–202.
39. Cardoza JD, Goldstein RB, Filly RA. Exclusion of fetal ventriculomegaly with a single measurement: The width of the lateral ventricular atrium. *Radiology*. 1988;169:711–714.
40. Hadlock FP, Deter RL, Park SK. Real-time sonography: Ventricular and vascular anatomy of the fetal brain in utero. *AJR Am J Roentgenol*. 1981;136:133–137.
41. Goldstein I, Reece EA, Pilu G, et al. Sonographic evaluation of the normal developmental anatomy of the fetal cerebral ventricles: 1. The frontal horn. *Obstet Gynecol*. 1988;72:588–592.
42. Denkhaus H, Winsberg F. Ultrasonic measurement of the fetal ventricular system. *Radiology*. 1979;131:781–787.
43. Jou HJ, Shyu MK, Wu SC, Chen SM, Su CH, Hsieh FJ. Ultrasound measurement of the fetal cavum septi pellucidi. *Ultrasound Obstet Gynecol*. 1998;12:419–421.
44. Mahony BS, Nyberg DA, Hirsch JH, et al. Mild idiopathic cerebral ventricular dilatation in utero: Sonographic evaluation. *Radiology*. 1988;169:715–721.
45. Filly RA, Cardoza JD, Goldstein RB, et al. Detection of fetal central nervous system anomalies: A practical level of effort for a routine sonogram. *Radiology*. 1989;172:403–408.
46. Farrell TA, Hertzberg BS, Kliewer MA, et al. Fetal lateral ventricles: Reassessment of normal values for atrial diameter at US. *Radiology*. 1994;193:409–411.
47. Chinn DH, Callen PW, Filly RA. The lateral cerebral ventricle in early second trimester. *Radiology*. 1983;148:529–531.
48. Hartung RW, Yiu-Chiu V. Demonstration of unilateral hydrocephalus in utero. *J Ultrasound Med*. 1983;2:369–371.
49. Pilu G, Reece EA, Goldstein I, et al. Sonographic evaluation of the normal developmental anatomy of the fetal cerebral ventricles: 2. The atria. *Obstet Gynecol*. 1989;73:250–255.
50. Goldstein I, Reece EA, Pilu G, et al. Sonographic evaluation of the normal developmental anatomy of the fetal cerebral ventricles: 4. The posterior horn. *Am J Perinatol*. 1990;7:79–83.

51. Siedler DE, Filly RA. Relative growth of the higher fetal brain structures. *J Ultrasound Med.* 1987;6:573–576.
52. Callen PW, Hashimoto BE, Newton TH. Sonographic evaluation of cerebral cortical mantle thickness in the fetus and neonate with hydrocephalus. *J Ultrasound Med.* 1986;5:251–255.
53. Blaas HG, Eik-Nes SH, Kiserud T, et al. Early development of the forebrain and midbrain: A longitudinal study from 7 to 12 weeks of gestation. *Ultrasound Obstet Gynecol.* 1994;4:183–192.
54. Blaas HG, Eik-Nes SH, Kiserud T, et al. Early development of the hindbrain: A longitudinal ultrasound study from 7 to 12 weeks of gestation. *Ultrasound Obstet Gynecol.* 1995;5:151–160.
55. Achiron R, Achiron A. Transvaginal ultrasound assessment of the early fetal brain. *Ultrasound Obstet Gynecol.* 1991;164:497–503.
56. Timor-Tritsch IE, Monteagudo A, Warren WB. Transvaginal ultrasonographic definition of the central nervous system in the first and early second trimesters. *Am J Obstet Gynecol.* 1991;164:497–503.
57. Monteagudo A, Reuss ML, Timor-Tritsch IE. Imaging the fetal brain in the second and third trimesters using transvaginal sonography. *Obstet Gynecol.* 1991;77:27–32.
58. Monteagudo A, Timor-Tritsch IE, Moomjy M. In utero detection of ventriculomegaly during the second and third trimesters by transvaginal sonography. *Ultrasound Obstet Gynecol.* 1994;4:193–198.
59. Kushnir U, Shalev J, Bronshtein M, et al. Fetal intracranial anatomy in the first trimester of pregnancy: Transvaginal ultrasonographic evaluation. *Neuroradiology.* 1989;31:222–225.
60. Monteagudo A, Timor-Tritsch IE, Moomjy M. Nomograms of the fetal lateral ventricles using transvaginal sonography. *J Ultrasound Med.* 1993;5:265–269.
61. Poland RL, Slovis TL, Sharankaran S. Normal values for ventricular size determined by real time sonographic techniques. *Pediatr Radiol.* 1985;15:12–14.
62. Sauerbrei EE, Digney M, Harrison PB, et al. Ultrasonic evaluation of neonatal intracranial hemorrhage and its complications. *Radiology.* 1981;130:677–685.
63. Chin DH, Callen PW, Filly RA. The lateral cerebral ventricle in early second trimester. *Radiology.* 1983;148:529–531.
64. Monteagudo A, Tharakan T, Timor-Tritsch IE. Sonographic neuroembryology of the central nervous system. *J Assoc Acad Minority Physicians.* 1995;6:34–37.
65. Mallinger G, Zakut H. The corpus callosum: Normal fetal development as shown by transvaginal sonography. *AJR Am J Roentgenol.* 1993;161:1041–1043.
66. Moore KL. ed. *The Developing Human: Clinically Oriented Embryology*. 4th ed. Philadelphia: WB Saunders; 1988:364–401.
67. O'Rahilly R, Múller F, eds. *The Embryonic Human Brain: An Atlas of Developmental Stages.* New York: Wiley-Liss; 1994:15–25.
68. Crosby EC, Humphrey T, Lauer EW, eds. *Correlative Anatomy of the Nervous System.* New York: Macmillan; 1962:343–345.
69. Martin JH. ed. *Neuroanatomy: Text and Atlas.* New York: Elsevier; 1989:240–266.
70. Mahony BS, Callen PW, Filly RA, et al. The fetal cisterna magna. *Radiology.* 1984;153:773–776.
71. Goldstein I, Reece EA, Pilu G, et al. Cerebellar measurements with ultrasonography in the evaluation of fetal growth and development. *Am J Obstet Gynecol.* 1987;156:1065–1069.
72. McLeary RD, Kuhns LR, Barr M. Ultrasonography of the fetal cerebellum. *Radiology.* 1984;151:439–442.
73. Hata K, Hata T, Daisaku S, et al. Ultrasonographic measurement of the fetal transverse cerebellum in utero. *Gynecol Obstet Invest.* 1989;28:111–112.
74. Creasy RK, Resnick R, eds. *Maternal—Fetal Medicine: Principles and Practice.* Philadelphia: WB Saunders; 1994:558–560.
75. Cabbad M, Kofinas A, Simin N, et al. Fetal weight-cerebellar diameter discordance as an indicator of asymmetrical fetal growth impairment. *J Reprod Med.* 1992;37:794–798.
76. Hill LM, Guzick D, Fries J, et al. The transverse cerebellar diameter in estimating gestational age in the large for gestational age fetus. *Obstet Gynecol.* 1990;75:981–985.
77. Shimizu T, Gaudette S, Nimrod C. Transverse cerebellar diameter in twin gestations. *Am J Obstet Gynecol.* 1992;167:1004–1008.
78. Dilmen G, Toppane MF, Turban NO, Ozturk M, Isik S. Tranverse cerebellar diameter/abdominal circumference index for assessing fetal growth. *Fetal Diagn Ther.* 1996;11(1):50–56.
79. Scanaill SN, Crowley P, Hogan M, Stuart B. Abnormal prenatal sonographic findings in the posterior cranial fossa: A case of Joubert's syndrome. *Ultrasound Obstet Gynecol.* 1999;13:71–74.
80. Nicolaides KH, Campbell S, Gabbe SG, et al. Ultrasound screening for spina bifida: Cranial and cerebellar signs. *Lancet.* 1986;2:72–74.
81. Devies H, Kizman BH. Microcephaly. *Arch Dis Child.* 1972;123:204–206.
82. Martin HP. Microcephaly and mental retardation. *Am J Dis Child.* 1970;119:129–131.
83. Bahado-Singh RO, Wyse L, Dorr MA, et al. Fetuses with Down syndrome have disproportionately shortened frontal lobe dimensions on ultrasonographic examination. *Am J Obstet Gynecol.* 1992;167:1009–1014.
84. Zalel Y, Seidman DS, Brandt N, Lipitz S, Achiron R. The development of the fetal vermis: An in-utero sonographic evaluation. *Ultrasound Obstet Gynecol.* 2002;19:136–139.
85. Malinger G, Lev D, Lerman-Sagie T. The fetal cerebellum: Pitfalls in diagnosis and management. *Prenat Diagn.* 2009;29:372–380.
86. Paladini D, Volpe P. Posterior fossa and vermian morphometry in the characterization of the fetal cerebellar abnormalities: A prospective three-dimensional ultrasound study. *Ultrasound Obstet Gynecol.* 2006;27:482–489.
87. Hai-chun Zhang, Jie Yang, Zhong-ping Chen, Xiao-yan Ma. Sonographic study of the development of fetal corpus callosum in a Chinese population. *J Clin Ultrasound.* 2009;37:75–77.
88. Monteagudo A, Timor-Tritsch IE. Normal sonographic development of the central nervous system from the second trimester onwards using 2D, 3D and transvaginal sonography. *Prenat Diagn.* 2009;29:326–339.
89. Volpe P, Campobasso G, De Robertis V, Rembouskos G. Disorders of prosencephalic development. *Prenat Diagn.* 2009;29:340–354.
90. Monteagudo A, Reuss ML, Timor-Tritsch IE. 1991. Imaging the fetal brain in the second and third trimesters using transvaginal sonography. *Obstet Gynecol.* 77:127–132.
91. Malinger G, Zakut H. 1993. The corpus callosum: Normal fetal development as shown by transvaginal sonography. *AJR Am J Roentgenol.* 1993;161:1041–1043.
92. Pilu G, Segata M, Ghi T, *et al.* 2006. Diagnosis of midline anomalies of the fetal brain with the three dimensional median view. *Ultrasound Obstet Gynecol.* 2006;27:522–529.
93. Achiron R, Kivilevich Z, Lipitz S, Gamzu R, Almog B, Zalel Y Development of the fetal pons: In-utero ultrasonographic study. *Ultrasound Obstet Gynecol.* 2004;24:506–510.
94. Vinals F, Munoz M, Naveas R, Shalper J, Giuliano A. The fetal cerebellar vermis: anatomy and biometric assessment using volume contrast imaging in the C-plane (VCI-C). *Ultrasound Obstet Gynecol.* 2005;26(6):622–627.
95. Achiron R, Achiron A. Development of the human fetal corpus callosum: A high resolution, cross sectional sonographic study. *Ultrasound Obstet Gynecol.* 2001;18:343–347.

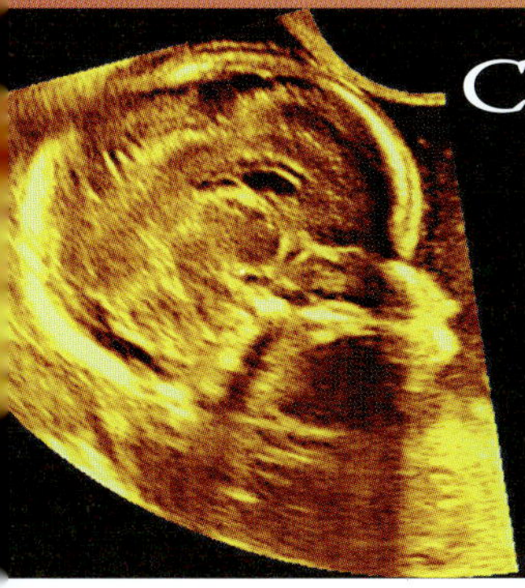

# Chapter 4

# VENTRICULOMEGALY

*Gianluigi Pilu • Gustavo Malinger • Selim Buyukkurt*

### KEY POINTS

1. Ventriculomegaly is not a diagnosis. It is a sign. The search for all underlying causes should be immediately undertaken.
2. Ventriculomegaly is frequently associated with a large number of intra- and extracranial chromosomal as well as nonchromosomal anomalies.
3. For measuring the lateral ventricle it is recommended to use an axial view of the brain and to place the clipers at the level of the parieto-occipital fissure that is usually well demonstrated from 20 weeks' gestation.
4. Congenital ventriculomegaly has a increased recurrence rate and after the birth of an affected infant a targeted neurscan is recommended in a subsequent pregnancy.

*Ventriculomegaly,* a term commonly employed to indicate the enlargement of the lateral cerebral ventricles, is found in ~1% of fetuses at midgestation and is the most common abnormal fetal cerebral diagnosis.

Although the enlargement of the lateral ventricles encompasses a wide spectrum of severity, at present a width of the atrium <10 mm is considered normal, 10 to 15 mm indicates mild ventriculomegaly, and >15 mm represents severe ventriculomegaly. This categorization has prognostic implications. Fetuses with normal ventricles have an exceedingly low risk of cerebral anomalies. Fetuses with mild ventriculomegaly in the majority of cases are normal at birth but have an increased risk of an abnormal outcome. Fetuses with severe ventriculomegaly have a very high probability of an abnormal outcome.

Enlargement of the cerebral lateral ventricles is not an anomaly per se. The clinical significance of this finding is that it signals to the possibility of associated anomalies of the brain or other organs. The final prognosis depends more on such anomalies than on the degree of ventricular dilation.

Fetuses with mild ventriculomegaly in particular have an increased risk of chromosomal aberrations.

## MILD LATERAL CEREBRAL VENTRICULOMEGALY

### Synonyms

Mild hydrocephaly, borderline ventriculomegaly

### Definition and Diagnosis

The widely accepted definition of mild cerebral lateral ventriculomegaly is an atrial width of 10 to 15 mm on the transverse plane (Figure 4–1)[1–3]

### Prevalence

Seen in 1% of fetuses[4]

### Pathogenesis and Pathology

In many cases, it probably represents a normal variant. In other cases, mild enlargement of the lateral ventricles may be the only obvious epiphenomenon of heterogeneous cerebral anomalies.

### Differential Diagnosis

Isolated mild ventriculomegaly should be differentiated from more complex abnormalities of the fetal brain that frequently have a different prognosis (eg, agenesis of the corpus callosum and cortical malformations). Several reports suggest that magnetic resonance imaging (MRI) may be a useful adjunct to sonography, particularly in late gestation.[5,6]

### Implications for Targeted Examination

The main problem in cases that are referred with mild dilatation of the lateral ventricles is to exclude other neural and extraneural malformations. We recommend careful multiplanar examination of the fetal brain, performed if possible with a high-resolution vaginal probe, and a detailed evaluation of the spine. Both lateral ventricles should be visualized and assessed, as this condition can be

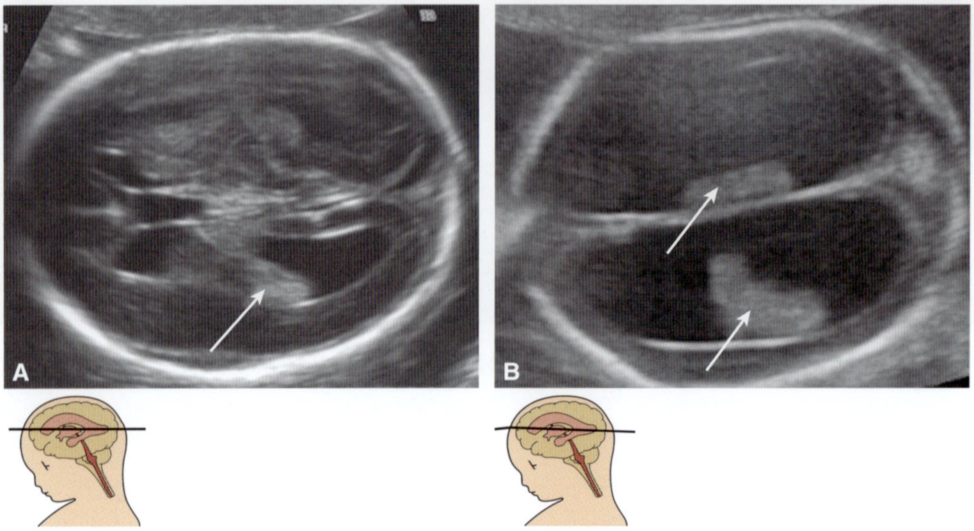


**Figure 4–1.** Mild **(A)** and severe **(B)** ventriculomegaly in midtrimester fetuses. Atrial width is 10 and 16 mm, respectively. Arrows indicate the dangling choroid plexuses.

unilateral (Figure 4–2). A stepwise ultrasound (US) evaluation of the fetal brain should be performed in order to exclude associated anomalies (Figure 4–3). Although the use of MRI has also been advocated,[5,6] we believe that when following the protocol suggested in Figure 4–3, the role of fetal MRI remains limited to those cases in which technical issues impairs US visualization. A detailed evaluation of the entire fetal anatomy, including fetal echocardiography, should also be performed. These examinations may be incomplete or limited during the third trimester.

## Implications for Sonographic Screening

In all standard sonographic examinations, a view of the lateral ventricles should be obtained, and at least one of the atria should be visualized and assessed. A qualitative evaluation is acceptable, and the presence of the choroid plexus filling the cavity of the atrium, being closely apposed to both the medial and lateral walls of the ventricle, is indicative of normalcy. A quantitative approach, however, is favored, and a measurement <10 mm is considered normal between 15 and 40 weeks.[7] Congenital

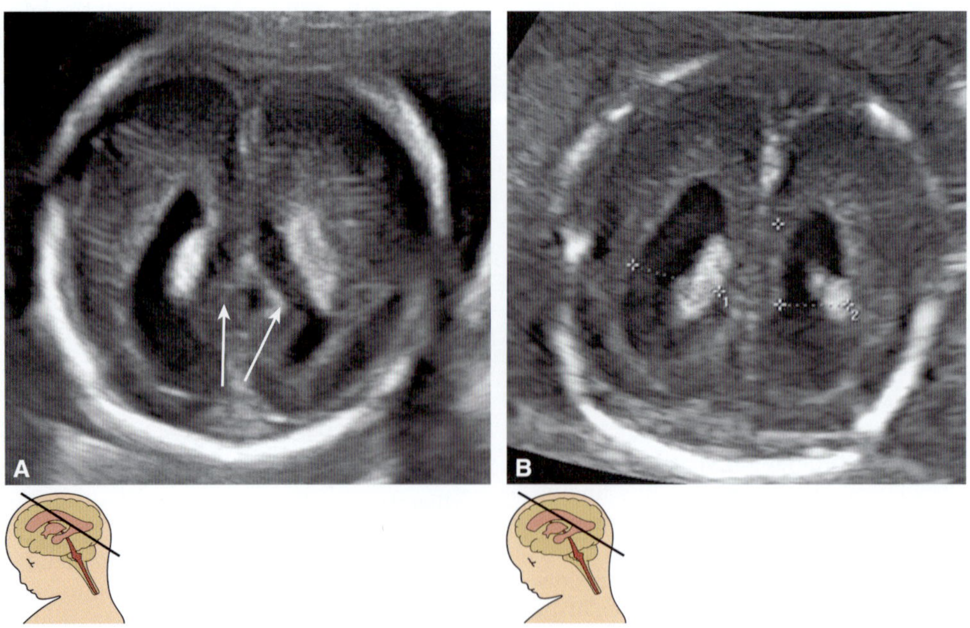


**Figure 4–2.** **(A)** Unilateral ventriculomegaly. The calcarine fissure (*arrows*) is significantly less pronounced in the ventriculomegalic hemisphere than in the controlateral one. **(B)** Bilateral ventriculomegaly. The calcarine fissure is not seen in this image, even though it was obtained at 21 weeks. A delayed cortical maturation is frequently encountered with ventriculomegaly. The clinical significance of such finding is uncertain. Both of these fetuses had a completely normal outcome and normal neurologic development at long-term follow-up.

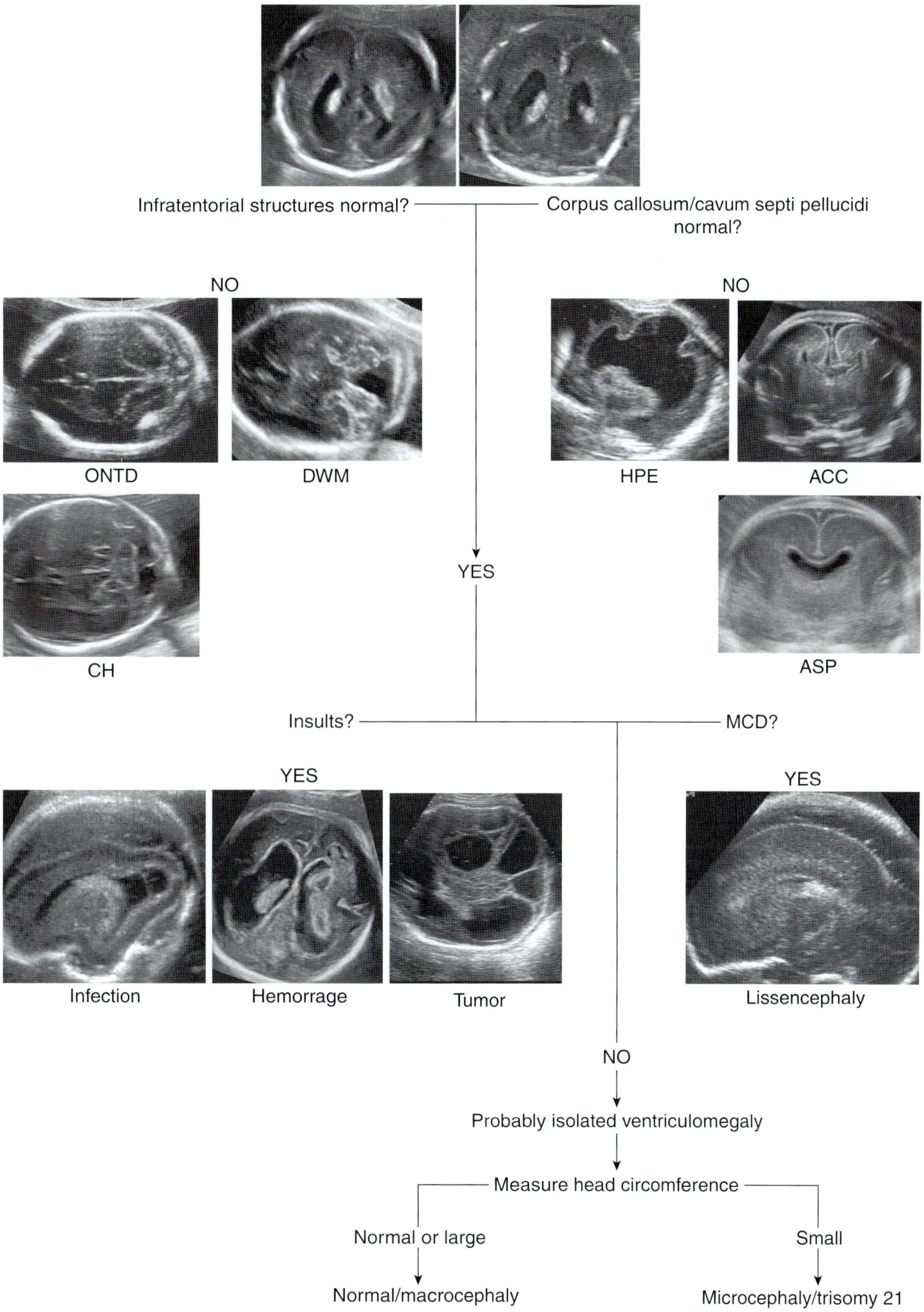


**Figure 4–3.** Flowchart for the investigation of fetuses with mild bilateral ventriculomegaly. Ventriculomegaly may be present with any congenital or acquired brain anomaly. Isolated mild ventriculomegaly may be diagnosed only after exclusion of these central nervous system anomalies. ONTD, open neural tube defects (Chapter 5); DWC, Dandy-Walker complex (Chapter 8); HPE, holoprosencephaly (Chapter 6); ACC, agenesis of the corpus callosum (Chapter 6); MCD, malformations of cortical development (Chapter 7); IVH, intraventricular hemorrhage (Chapter 12); HC, head circumference.

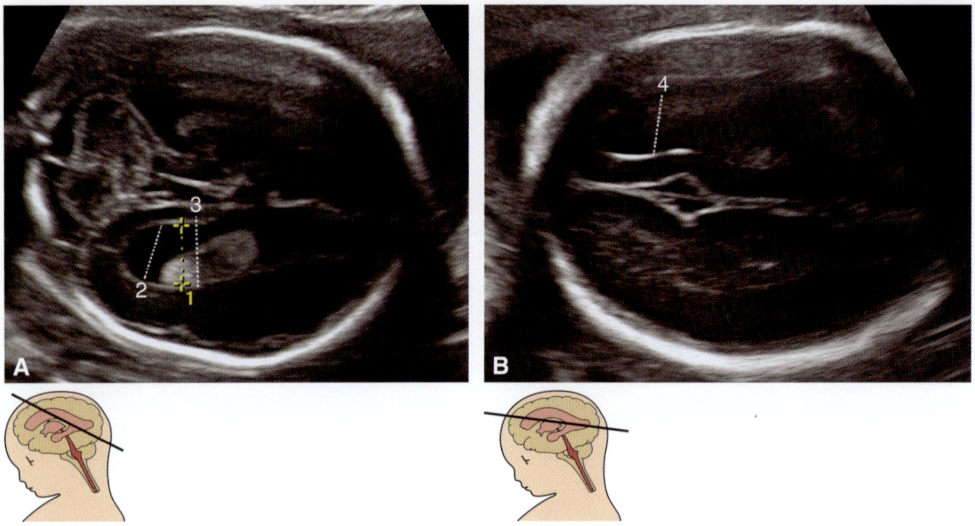


**Figure 4–4.** Pitfalls in the measurement of the lateral ventricle. **(A)** Axial plane. The correct measurement of the lateral ventricular width (LVW) is numbered 1. The measurements depicted as 2 and 3 are wrong; 2 is positioned in the occipital horn, and 3 measures not only the ventricles but also part of the brain parenchyma. **(B)** This image shows a common error in measuring the proximal lateral ventricle. The proximal ventricle is difficult to visualize in a true axial plane, and the operator tilted the transducer to reach access to show the proximal ventricle. This plane shows a poorly visualized ventricle in an oblique plane, and measurement 4 overestimates the LVW.

ventriculomegaly may develop late in gestation, and a normal midtrimester exam does not exclude this condition. The correct measurement of the lateral ventricles is important to avoid false-positive diagnoses of ventriculomegaly. Common errors in measurement include placing the calipers in the brain parenchyma instead of at the inner border of the ventricular wall, measuring the ventricle not perpendicular to their walls, measuring the occipital horn, or measuring the lateral ventricle not in a truly axial plane. A specific approach has been described that proposes **placing the calipers at the level of the parietooccipital fissure, an easily recognizable landmark beginning around 20 weeks' gestation**[8] (Figure 4–4).

### Prognosis

Fetal mild cerebral ventriculomegaly is an elusive entity. It is frequently seen without consequences. However, most of the available studies are consistent in indicating an increased risk of abnormal outcomes.[2,3] The likelihood of trisomy 21 is increased 9-fold over the general population.[2] Despite careful antenatal assessment, anomalies will be present at birth in ~13% of cases.[2] Most of these anomalies are mild and of little consequence, but developmental malformations of the cerebrum, including progressive hypertensive hydrocephaly, cystic brain lesions, and abnormal cortical development, have been documented in up to 4% of cases.[2] The rate of neurodevelopmental delay in infants with a prenatal diagnosis of isolated mild ventriculomegaly is ~11%, and it is unclear whether this is increased or not over the general population. The most important prognostic factor is the association with other abnormalities undetected at the time of the first diagnosis (~13% of cases) and progression of the ventricular dilation (~16% of cases).[2]

### Obstetric Management

Mild lateral cerebral ventriculomegaly is frequently associated with neural and extraneural anomalies; therefore, a careful evaluation of the fetal anatomy should be carried out using expert US examination and, if possible, transvaginalneurosonography. Where available, fetal MRI may be indicated, although there is no consensus on the optimal time for this examination. The likelihood ratio for trisomy 21 is about 9, and invasive testing for chromosomal analysis should be offered. Maternal serum cytomegalovirus (CMV) and *Toxoplasma* studies should be considered. Follow-up sonograms and/or MRI in the third trimester should be considered.[2]

## SEVERE CEREBRAL LATERAL VENTRICULOMEGALY

### Synonym

Hydrocephaly

### Definition and diagnosis

Overt enlargement of the lateral ventricles (atrial width >15 mm) in the absence of other sonographically demonstrable central nervous system anomalies[2,3]

### Prevalence

The incidence of hydrocephaly, a condition that overlaps with severe ventriculomegaly, ranges between 0.3 and 1.5 in 1000 births in different series.[9] In many fetuses, associated anomalies are present, but isolated ventriculomegaly accounts for 10% to 60% of cases in different series.[10–12]

## Pathogenesis

In the majority of cases, cerebral lateral ventriculomegaly is the consequence of associated cerebral abnormalities. Isolated severe ventriculomegaly is usually the consequence of an obstruction along the normal pathway of the cerebrospinal fluid. When this is associated with intracranial hypertension, the term *obstructive hydrocephaly* is commonly used.[10]

## Etiology

Congenital severe ventriculomegaly is a heterogeneous disease for which genetic, infectious, teratogenetic, and neoplastic causes have been implicated. X-linked hydrocephaly accounts for ~5% of all cases. This condition is caused by mutations in the gene at Xq28 encoding for L1, a neural cell adhesion molecule (*L1CAM*). Mutations in this gene are also responsible for other syndromes with clinical overlap; these are frequently referred to as the X-linked hydrocephaly spectrum, or L1 spectrum, and include MASA (mental retardation, aphasias, shuffling gait, and adducted thumbs), complicated X-linked spastic paraplegia (SP 1), X-linked mental retardation–clasped thumb (MR-CT) syndrome, and some forms of X-linked agenesis of the corpus callosum.[13–16] A multifactorial pattern of inheritance is probably responsible for most other cases of congenital hydrocephaly.[14] Infections implicated in the determination of congenital ventriculomegaly include toxoplasmosis, syphilis, CMV, mumps, and influenza virus.

## Pathology

Severe lateral ventriculomegaly (Figures 4–1 and 4–5) can result from different pathologic entities. In our experience, fetuses with this finding usually have other neural and extraneural malformations. Even those with presumably isolated ventricular dilation were found in the majority of cases to have complex abnormalities. In a large series, only 10% of fetuses with severe ventricular dilation were found not to have associated malformations.[12] Only a small proportion of fetuses are found to have isolated obstructive hydrocephaly, either aqueductal stenosis or communicating hydrocephaly. In these cases, the degree of ventricular enlargement is variable. Knowledge about the pathogenesis of congenital ventriculomegaly is largely incomplete. Thinning of the cortex, macrocrania, and symptoms of intracranial hypertension are frequently found. Studies performed in experimental animals and based on biopsies of brain tissue obtained in children at the time of shunting seem to demonstrate the following sequence of events: Initially, there is disruption of the ependymal lining, followed by edema of the white matter and proliferation of astrocytes and fibrosis of the cortex.

## Recurrence Risk

Apart from X-linked hydrocephaly (recurrence risk 50% of males), isolated congenital ventriculomegaly is mostly multifactorially determined. Couples with a previously affected child have a recurrence risk of 4%.[17]

## Associated Anomalies

Extracranial abnormalities occur in 30% to 60% of cases.[10,12] Chromosomal aberrations are found in 11% of cases (6% of fetuses with ventriculomegaly as the only antenatal finding, 25% of cases with multiple anomalies).[18] The X-linked hydrocephaly spectrum is frequently associated with abduction of the thumbs, abnormal facies, and absence or dehiscence of the septum pellucidum (Figure 4–5).[19]

## Diagnosis

Overt lateral cerebral ventriculomegaly is defined as a measurement >15 mm (Figures 4–2 and 4–3).[3,20]

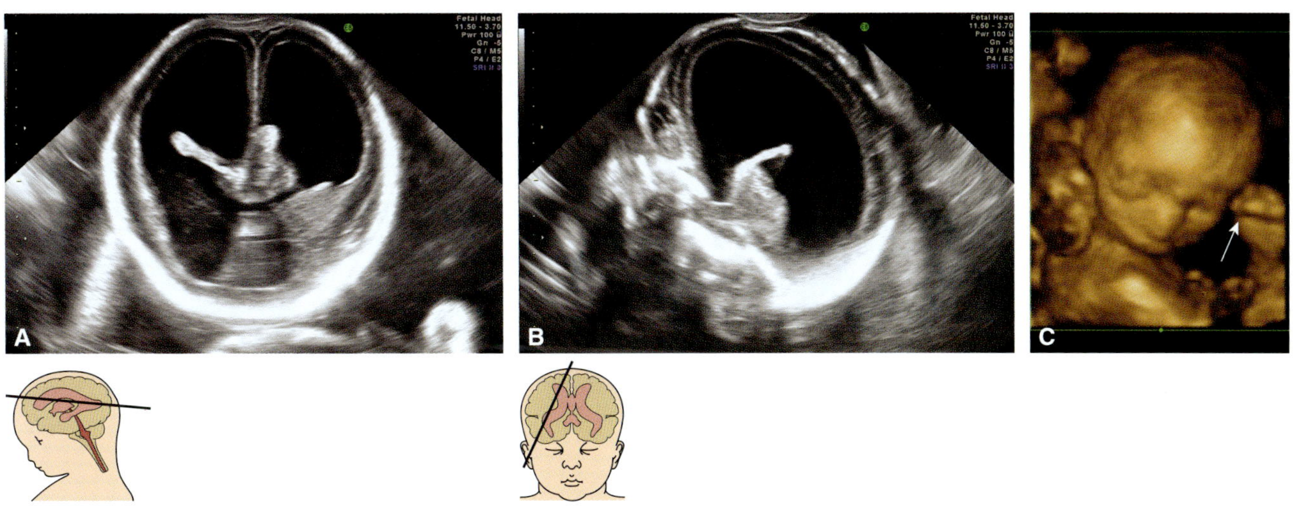


**Figure 4–5.** Severe ventriculomegaly in a fetus with X-linked hydrocephaly. **(A)** Axial plane. **(B)** Coronal plane. **(C)** Three-dimensional ultrasonography reconstruction of the body surface shows the adducted thumb (*arrow*).

## Differential Diagnosis

The main problem is distinguishing isolated ventriculomegaly from more complex abnormalities of the fetal brain that frequently have a different prognosis, including intracranial hemorrhage,[21] cortical malformations,[22] Walker-Warburg syndrome,[23] or X-linked hydrocephaly spectrum.[19] Identifying such conditions is usually a major challenge. When severe isolated ventriculomegaly is identified, genetic analysis for X-linked hydrocephaly should be offered. Ventriculomegaly may be associated with cortical malformations, and the diagnosis of these conditions is often difficult or impossible. In particular, it has been recently demonstrated that ventriculomegalic brains have delayed cortical maturation (Figure 4–2); it is unclear whether this has an impact on the final outcome or not.[24] Several authors have suggested that MRI can be helpful in the assessment of ventriculomegalic fetuses, particularly in advanced gestation.[5,6]

## Implications for Targeted Examinations

For patients at risk for fetal cerebral ventriculomegaly (eg, because of a previously affected child or because of TORCH [toxoplasmosis, other infections, rubella, CMV, herpes simplex virus] infection), we recommend careful multiplanar examination of the fetal brain, performed if possible with a high-resolution vaginal probe, including visualization and assessment of both lateral ventricles. It has been our experience, and it has been reported in a handful of cases, that ventriculomegaly may develop only in late gestation or after birth, particularly with the X-linked hydrocephaly spectrum.[14] The patients at risk should be informed that a normal midtrimester sonogram does not rule out this condition. Couples with a previously affected child should receive genetic counseling, because sometimes a generic diagnosis of congenital hydrocephaly may hinder a more complex anomaly with significant genetic implications. For example, patients at risk for X-linked hydrocephaly spectrum should be offered DNA analysis, as the recurrence rate is high, and midtrimester-sonography is frequently unsuccessful.[13]

## Implications for Sonographic Screening

In all standard sonographic examinations, a view of the lateral ventricles should be obtained, and at least one of the atria should be visualized and assessed. A qualitative evaluation is acceptable, and the presence of the choroid plexus filling the cavity of the atrium, being closely apposed to both the medial and lateral walls of the ventricle, is indicative of normalcy. A quantitative approach, however, is favored, and a measurement <10 mm is considered normal between 15 and 40 weeks.[7] Congenital ventriculomegaly may develop late in gestation, and a normal midtrimester exam does not exclude this condition.

## Prognosis

In a review, isolated ventriculomegaly diagnosed in utero was associated with a postnatal survival rate of 70%, and 59% of the survivors had a normal developmental quotient at follow-up.[11] In most, though not all cases with isolated progressive ventriculomegaly, intracranial hypertension develops after birth, and a shunting procedure is necessary. In a large pediatric series (excluding cases with X-linked hydrocephaly and congenital infections), the survival rate was 62% at 10 years, and 50% of survivors had a low developmental quotient (<60). Only 29% of infants attending school reached a normal academic level. Macrocrania at birth, ventricular size, and age at surgery had no influence on the outcome.[25] The X-linked hydrocephaly spectrum carries a severe prognosis, being usually associated with severe neurologic deficits and premature death.[13,15,16]

## Obstetric Management

A search for associated congenital anomalies, including fetal karyotyping and a workup for congenital infections associated with hydrocephaly (ie, toxoplasmosis, CMV, and rubella), is indicated. Before viability, the option of pregnancy termination should be offered to the parents. Little data exist to support any specific management plan in continuing pregnancies. There is no evidence that anticipation of delivery is beneficial. Most infants with ventriculomegaly do not have macrocrania; therefore, a trial of labor is indicated in the vertex presentation. Cesarean section should be reserved for standard obstetrical indications. Whether cephalocentesis should be offered in cases with macrocrania to overcome cephalopelvic disproportion is debated. In one series cephalocentesis resulted in perinatal mortality in >90% of cases.[26] Careful aspiration with fine needles guided with high-resolution US equipment, trying to limit as much as possible damage to brain parenchyma and cerebral vessels, may cause much less harm than these rather old data indicate.

Intrauterine treatment consisting of the implantation of a ventricular-amniotic shunt for the relief of intracranial pressure during gestation has been attempted.Although preliminary experience in animal models was encouraging, the clinical application of these procedures remains undetermined. In a group of 39 treated fetuses, the perinatal mortality rate was 18%, and 66% of the survivors were affected by moderate to severe handicaps.[27] However, the new fetal endoscopic technique may provide a different approach to the problem in the future.[28]

## REFERENCES


1. Cardoza JD, Goldstein RB, Filly RA. Exclusion of fetal ventriculomegaly with a single measurement: The width of the lateral ventricular atrium. *Radiology.* 1988;169(3):711–714.
2. Melchiorre K, Bhide A, Gika AD, Pilu G, Papageorghiou AT. Counseling in isolated mild fetal ventriculomegaly. *Ultrasound Obstet Gynecol.* 2009;34(2):212–224.
3. Patel MD, Filly AL, Hersh DR, Goldstein RB. Isolated mild fetal cerebral ventriculomegaly: Clinical course and outcome. *Radiology.* 1994;192(3):759–764.
4. Salomon LJ, Bernard JP, Ville Y. Reference ranges for fetal ventricular width: a non-normal approach. *Ultrasound Obstet Gynecol.* 2007;30(1):61–66.
5. Benacerraf BR, Shipp TD, Bromley B, Levine D. What does magnetic resonance imaging add to the prenatal sonographic diagnosis of ventriculomegaly? *J Ultrasound Med.* 2007;26(11):1513–1522.

6. Salomon LJ, Ouahba J, Delezoide AL, et al. Third-trimester fetal MRI in isolated 10- to 12-mm ventriculomegaly: Is it worth it? *BJOG.* 2006;113(8):942–947.
7. ISUOG. Sonographic examination of the fetal central nervous system: Guidelines for performing the basic examination and the fetal neurosonogram. *Ultrasound Obstet Gynecol.* 2007;29(1):109–116.
8. Guibaud L. Fetal cerebral ventricular measurement and ventriculomegaly: Time for procedure standardization. *Ultrasound Obstet Gynecol.* 2009;34(2):127–130.
9. Myrianthopoulos NC. Epidemiology of central nervous system malformations. In: Vinken PJ, Bruyn GW, eds. *Handbook of Clinical Neurology.* Amsterdam: Elsevier; 1977:139–171.
10. Chervenak FA, Berkowitz RL, Romero R, et al. The diagnosis of fetal hydrocephalus. *Am J Obstet Gynecol.* 1983;147(6):703–716.
11. Gupta JK, Bryce FC, Lilford RJ. Management of apparently isolated fetal ventriculomegaly. *Obstet Gynecol Surv.* 1994;49(10):716–721.
12. Nyberg DA, Mack LA, Hirsch J, Pagon RO, Shepard TH. Fetal hydrocephalus: sonographic detection and clinical significance of associated anomalies. *Radiology.* 1987;163(1):187–191.
13. Fransen E, Vits L, Van Camp G, Willems PJ. The clinical spectrum of mutations in L1, a neuronal cell adhesion molecule. *Am J Med Genet.* 1996;64(1):73–77.
14. Schrander-Stumpel C, Fryns JP. Congenital hydrocephalus: Nosology and guidelines for clinical approach and genetic counselling. *Eur J Pediatr.* 1998;157(5):355–362.
15. Schrander-Stumpel C, Howeler C, Jones M, et al. Spectrum of X-linked hydrocephalus (HSAS), MASA syndrome, and complicated spastic paraplegia (SPG1): Clinical review with six additional families. *Am JMed Genet.* 1995;57(1):107–116.
16. Varadi V, Csecsei K, Szeifert GT, Toth Z, Papp Z. Prenatal diagnosis of X linked hydrocephalus without aqueductal stenosis. *J Med Genet.* 1987;24(4):207–209.
17. Varadi V, Toth Z, Torok O, Papp Z. Heterogeneity and recurrence risk for congenital hydrocephalus (ventriculomegaly): A prospective study. *Am J Med Genet.* 1988;29(2):305–310.
18. Schwanitz G, Schuler H, Gembruch U, Zerres K. Chromosomal findings in fetuses with ultrasonographically diagnosed ventriculomegaly. *Ann Genet.* 1993;36(3):150–153.
19. Timor-Tritsch IE, Monteagudo A, Haratz-Rubinstein N, Levine RU. Transvaginal sonographic detection of adducted thumbs, hydrocephalus, and agenesis of the corpus callosum at 22 postmenstrual weeks: The MASA spectrum or L1 spectrum. A case report and review of the literature. *Prenat Diagn.* 1996;16(6):543–548.
20. Goldstein RB, La Pidus AS, Filly RA, Cardoza J. Mild lateral cerebral ventricular dilatation in utero: Clinical significance and prognosis. *Radiology.* 1990;176(1):237–242.
21. Ghi T, Simonazzi G, Perolo A, et al. Outcome of antenatally diagnosed intracranial hemorrhage: Case series and review of the literature. *Ultrasound Obstet Gynecol.* 2003;22(2):121–130.
22. Malinger G, Kidron D, Schreiber L, et al. Prenatal diagnosis of malformations of cortical development by dedicated neurosonography. *Ultrasound Obstet Gynecol.* 2007;29(2):178–191.
23. Strigini F, Valleriani A, Cecchi M, et al. Prenatal ultrasound and magnetic resonance imaging features in a fetus with Walker-Warburg syndrome. *Ultrasound Obstet Gynecol.* 2009;33(3):363–365.
24. Levine D, Barnes PD. Cortical maturation in normal and abnormal fetuses as assessed with prenatal MR imaging. *Radiology.* 1999;210(3):751–758.
25. Renier D, Sainte-Rose C, Pierre-Kahn A, Hirsch JF. Prenatal hydrocephalus: Outcome and prognosis. *Childs Nerv Syst.* 1988;4(4):213–222.
26. Chervenak FA, Berkowitz RL, Tortora M, Hobbins JC. The management of fetal hydrocephalus. *Am J Obstet Gynecol.* 1985;151(7):933–942.
27. Manning FA, Harrison MR, Rodeck C. Catheter shunts for fetal hydronephrosis and hydrocephalus: Report of the International Fetal Surgery Registry. *N Engl J Med.* 1986;315(5):336–340.
28. von Koch CS, Gupta N, Sutton LN, Sun PP. In utero surgery for hydrocephalus. *Childs Nerv Syst.* 2003;19(7–8):574–586.

# Chapter 5

# ANOMALIES OF DORSAL INDUCTION

*Ana Monteagudo • Ilan E. Timor-Tritsch*

**KEY POINTS**

1. Failure of closure of the neural tube during neurulation results in neural tube defects. Neurulation, both primary and secondary, are completed by approximately 32 post-ovulatory days.
2. Not all cases of neural tube defects are open lesions. Approximately 20% of spina bifida and 80% of cephaloceles are closed lesions. In this scenario the MSAFP is normal and the diagnosis is made at the time of the ultrasound examination.
3. Approximately 80 to 90% of children with Chiari II will develop hydrocephaly.
4. During the second and third trimesters the "classic" sonographic findings that aid in the diagnosis of spina bifida are the lemon and banana signs. Recently, three additional findings have been described: pointed lateral ventricles, beaked tectum, and interhemispheric cyst. In the first trimester, the newly proposed "intracranial translucency" may become an early sign of open spina bifida.

Anomalies of dorsal induction are those that result from failure or abnormal closure of the neural tube. Essentially these anomalies are better known as neural tube defects (NTDs). NTDs result from failure of the neural tube to close during primary neurulation. They are characterized by the presence of a cerebral, spinal, or combined cerebral/spinal defect or dysraphia.

The normal appearance of the fetal central nervous system (CNS) results from primary neurulation or dorsal induction; this in turn results in the formation of the brain and spinal cord exclusive of those segments caudal to the lumbar area. During primary neurulation, fusion of the neural fold occurs first in the dorsal region of the lower medulla at approximately 22 days after conception. Fusion does not proceed continuously in a caudal to rostral fashion as previously believed (the "zipper" theory).[1] There are two fusion sites, and closure occurs bidirectional with the anterior neuropore closing before the rostral neuropore.[2,3] Secondary neurulation, or caudal neural tube formation, occurs approximately between 26 and 32 postovulatory days and results in the formation of the lower sacral and coccygeal segments.[4] It is during secondary neurulation that canalization occurs (see Chapter 1). Table 5–1 lists the defects that arise as a result of abnormal primary neurulation in decreasing order of severity.

In the United States, all pregnant women are routinely offered screening with maternal serum alpha-fetoprotein (MSAFP) for neural tube defects at 15 to 18 postmenstrual weeks. MSAFP is one of the components of the quad screen (alpha-fetoprotein, human chorionic gonadotropin, estriol, and inhibin-A), which is commonly used at present for screening of Down syndrome and open NTDs. Among low-risk women, MSAFP screening results in the detection of 80% to 90% of cases of fetal open NTDs.[5] Limb et al[6] published a study on the changes in prenatal detection and birth status of anencephaly between 1972 and 1990 in the Malformations Surveillance program of Brigham and Women's Hospital in Boston. In the 1970s, half of the infants with anencephaly were born alive at an average gestational age of 35.6 weeks, and few were diagnosed prenatally; between 1988 and 1990, however, all affected fetuses were diagnosed either by prenatal ultrasonography or as a result of MSAFP, and the average age at delivery was 18 weeks.

MSAFP levels are expressed as multiples of the median (MoMs). An abnormal value is one that exceeds 2.5 MoMs. Elevated MSAFP levels are associated with NTDs, as well as a variety of other conditions (Table 5–2). In a retrospective study of 773 cases with elevated MSAFP, Reichler et al[7] evaluated the percentage of fetal anomalies detected. They found that there was a progressive increase in the incidence of fetal anomalies as a direct function of the level of the MSAFP (Figure 5–1).

NTDs can be categorized as open or closed, depending on whether or not they are covered by skin[8] (Table 5–3). In an open NTD, the neural tissue is exposed or covered only by the thinnest of membranes; therefore, the lesion is directly in contact with the amniotic fluid. In these cases, the alpha-fetoprotein (AFP) molecule freely diffuses across the lesion, which results in an abnormally increased level in the amniotic fluid, hence in the maternal serum. Not all cases of NTDs are open lesions. For example, whereas all anencephaly are open defects, only 80% of spina bifida and 18% of cephaloceles are open NTDs.[8] In a closed neural tube lesion, the defect is covered by skin or a thick membrane. In these cases, AFP cannot freely diffuse across the lesion into the amniotic fluid; therefore, the MSAFP

**Table 5–1. NEURAL TUBE DEFECTS: DEFECTS OF PRIMARY NEURULATION**

| |
|---|
| Craniorachischisis totalis |
| Anencephaly |
| Myeloschisis |
| Encephalocele |
| Myelomeningocele, Arnold-Chiari malformation |

Modified, with permission, from Volpe JJ. *Neurology of the Newborn.* 5th ed. Philadelphia: WB Saunders; 2008:3–50.

level will be within the normal limits. Prenatal diagnosis in these cases will not be made on the basis of the serum or amniotic fluid AFP. An ultrasound (US) examination must therefore be performed in a timely fashion.

Acetylcholinesterase (AchE), unlike AFP, is not a normal component of the amniotic fluid. It is derived from neural tissue and is always seen in the amniotic fluid in the presence of an open NTD. Also, AchE may be present in cases of abdominal wall defects in which a nerve plexus is exposed to the amniotic fluid. It is essential to know that AchE is normally found in fetal blood and may therefore be found in amniotic fluid that at the time of amniocentesis has been contaminated with fetal blood.[9,10]

The occult dysraphic conditions affect the lower sacral and coccygeal areas of the spine. These lesions are covered by skin and may go on undetected, even after the birth of the infant. The important issue is that 4.1% of siblings of patients with these occult dysraphic conditions exhibit disorders of primary neurulation, such as meningocele and anencephaly.[11,12]

**Table 5–2. NON–NEURAL TUBE MALFORMATIONS ASSOCIATED WITH ELEVATED MSAFP**

| |
|---|
| **Fetal Conditions** |
| Multiple pregnancy |
| Intrauterine fetal demise |
| Wrong dates (i.e. pregnancy more advanced) |
| Ventral wall defects: omphalocele, gastroschisis |
| Renal: congenital nephrosis, bilateral renal agenesis, polycystic kidney or infantile |
| Intestinal atresia |
| Triploidy |
| Congenital skin disorders: epidermolysis bullosa or aplasia cutis |
| Teratoma: sacrococcygeal, pharyngeal |
| Congenital cystic adenomatoid malformation (congenital cystic adenomatoid malformation type III) |
| Turner syndrome with cystic hygroma |
| Oligohydramnios |
| **Placental conditions** |
| Hemangioma |
| **Maternal Conditions** |
| Maternal infection: parvovirus, cytomegalovirus, hepatitis |
| Maternal malignancy: hepatoma, ovarian teratoma |
| Abdominal pregnancy |
| Fetomaternal hemorrhage |

## EXENCEPHALY–ANENCEPHALY SEQUENCE

### Synonyms

Anencephaly, exencephaly, acrania

### Definition

Exencephaly is the absence of the calvarium and skin resulting in exposure of the brain. It appears to be the embryologic predecessor of anencephaly. Anencephaly is the complete absence of the calvarium, skin, meninges, and forebrain.

### Incidence

The reported incidence of NTDs of which anencephaly is the most common is about 1 case per 1000 live births worldwide.[6,13–15] However, the incidence of NTDs is different among different patient populations. In the United States, the prevalence of NTDs is higher among Hispanic women than among non-Hispanic white or non-Hispanic black women.[16,17] For example, in Puerto Rico, where most residents are Hispanic, the prevalence of NTDs is 8.68 per 10,000 live births, which is higher than in the mainland United States, which is 5.59 per 10,000.[17]

### Pathogenesis

Anencephaly and related disorders are no longer theorized to be simple NTDs, but are complex developmental malformations that primarily affect the production of mesenchyme. This results in skeletal defects and imperfect fusion of the neural folds.[18,19]

The developmental sequence of events leading to anencephaly was first elucidated in experimental animals exposed to high doses of vitamin A. Subsequent studies in the human embryo have suggested that in humans it progresses in a similar fashion.[19–22] The three phases in the development of anencephaly are (1) dysraphia or a failure of the neural groove to close in the rostral region (new evidence has suggested that the defect may occur as early as 18 to 20 postovulatory days, as a mesenchymal defect, far earlier than previously believed); (2) exencephaly, or

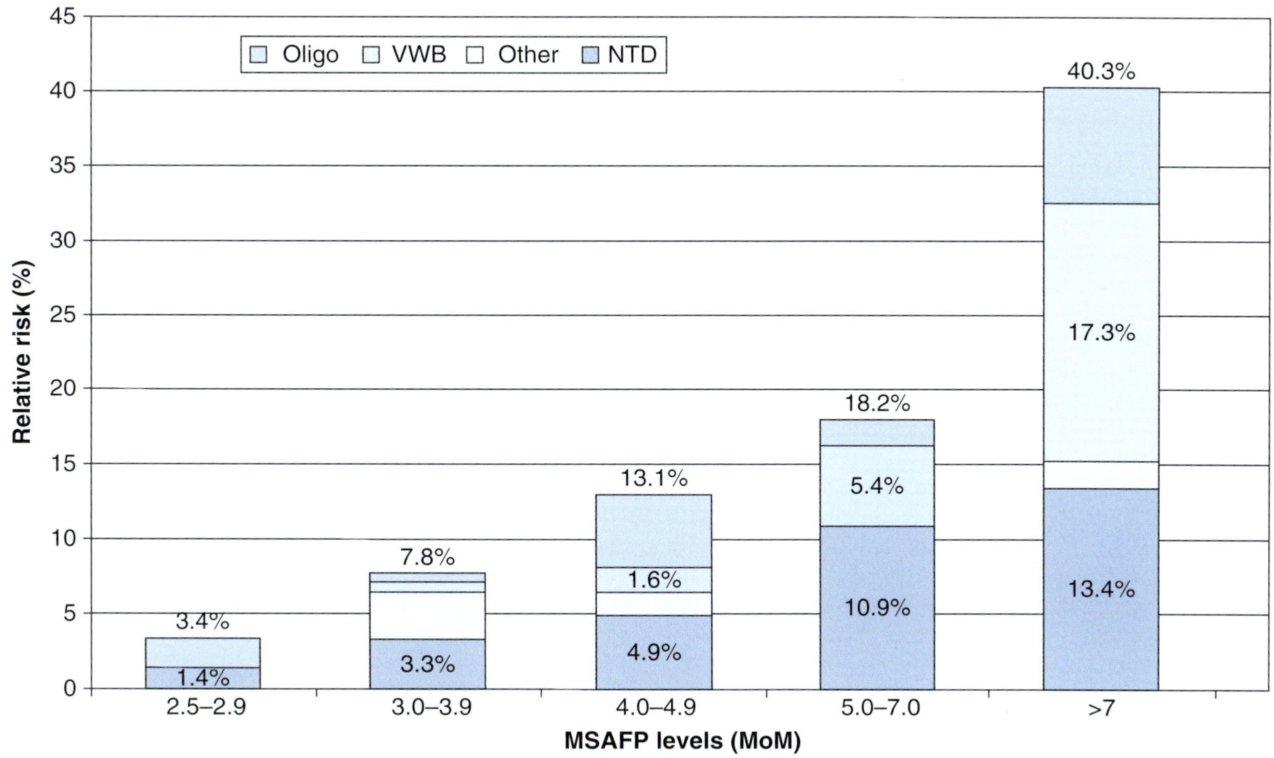


**Figure 5–1.** Anomalies and oligohydramnios distribution as a function of elevated maternal serum alpha-fetoprotein (MSAFP). Other, subchorionic bleeding, intra-abdominal echogenicity, hydronephrosis, echogenic bowel, dilated kidney, heart defect; NTD, neural tube defect; VWD, ventral wall defect; Oligo, oligohydramnios; MoM, multiple of the median. (Reproduced, with permission, from Reichler et al. AJOG 1994;1071:1052.)[7]

exposure of a well-developed and differentiated brain outside the skull during the embryonic period; and (3) disintegration of the exposed brain during the fetal period, resulting in anencephaly[4,18,20,21] (Table 5–4). It appears that early on during development the generation of the brain and the skull is relatively independent of each other and that the brain of anencephalic fetuses attains a high degree of differentiation before it disintegrates.[21] Using prenatal sonography, the development of anencephaly from exencephaly has been observed and reported.[23] This breakdown of the brain tissue has been corroborated by findings of primitive neuronal cells in the amniotic fluid.[24]

**Table 5–3. CLASSIFICATION OF NEURAL TUBE DEFECTS**

| Location of Defect | Open | Closed |
|---|---|---|
| Cranial | Anencephaly | Cephalocele |
| Craniospinal | Craniorachischisis | Iniencephaly |
| Spinal | Meningomyelocele | Lumbosacral lesions |

Modified, with permission, from Lemire RJ. Anencephaly. In: Myrianthopoulos NC. Handbook of Clinical Neurology Malformations. Vol 6. Amsterdam: Elsevier; 1987.

## Etiology

Exencephaly/anencephaly, as well as other NTDs, can be isolated or can be part of a malformation syndrome. Isolated NTDs, which account for the majority of cases, have a multifactorial origin involving both genetic and environmental factors.[25] In these cases, one of the most important factors is the maternal serum folic acid levels. Maternal serum levels $<200$ μg/L have been associated with a significant risk of NTDs. Syndromes associated with NTDs can be the result of a chromosomal abnormality (eg, trisomy 13, 18, or 21) or a single gene disorder (eg, Meckel-Gruber syndrome).[26] Teratogenic exposure results in a small number of cases of anencephaly and spina bifida.[26] Maternal diabetes (pregestational) is associated with a 2- to 10-fold increase in malformations (eg, NTDs), and exposure to valproic acid and/or carbamazepine is associated with a 1% to 2% risk of spina bifida but not necessarily anencephaly.[26] Other factors associated with NTDs are maternal obesity (patients with a body mass index [BMI]

**Table 5–4. THREE PHASES IN THE DEVELOPMENT OF ANENCEPHALY**

| |
|---|
| Dysraphia |
| Exencephaly |
| Anencephaly |

>29 kg/m$^2$ having a 1.5- to 3.5-fold increase in risk) and hyperthermia (2-fold increase).[26]

## Associated Anomalies

Other malformations can also be seen in anencephalic fetuses. However, due to the severity and lethality of this malformation, searching for other malformations does not alter the management or the prognosis for the fetus. Among the other associated malformations are hypoplastic or anomalous folding of the ears; subcutaneous clefts of the nose, cleft lip, and/or palate; diaphragmatic hernia; omphalocele; limb and cardiac malformations; and hydronephrosis.[27] Joo et al[28] reported that in a series of 743 cases of NTDs, 385 had anencephaly, 307 had spina bifida, and 51 had encephalocele. They found that the most commonly associated anomaly with anencephaly is spina bifida (24%), a CNS anomaly; it can also be seen with cephaloceles (10%). Non-CNS malformations seen with anencephaly run the gamut of almost all organ systems, such as congenital heart defects in 6.5% (eg, atrial septal defect [ASD], ventricular septal defect [VSD], coarctation of the aorta, and univentriculat heart), gastrointestinal anomalies in 5.2% (eg, esophageal atresia, jejunal atresia, and intestinal malformation), urogenital anomalies in 3.1% (eg, hydronephrosis and polycystic kidneys), facial malformations in 19.2% (eg, hypo- and hypertelorism, proboscis, and cleft palate), limb anomalies in 4.1% (eg, clubfoot), and abdominal wall defects in 7.5% (eg, omphalocele, diaphragmatic hernia, and costal anomalies).[28] Among 77 anencephalic fetuses who underwent karyotype, 97.4% had normal chromosomes, with one case each of trisomy 18 and 21.

Craniorachischisis refers to a defect in which the open cranial defect (anencephaly) is in continuity with the completely open spine (spinal dysraphism). In this defect total failure of neurulation has occurred and is believed to arise no later than 20 to 22 days after conception. Most of the fetuses affected with this extensive malformation are spontaneously aborted early in pregnancy.[11] Craniorachischisisis presents in up to 10% of anencephalic fetuses.[29] Sonography demonstrates the anencephaly and the extensive spinal dysraphism (Figure 5–2).

Polyhydramnios complicates up to 50% of anencephalic pregnancies, which usually develops during the second half of gestation. It is theorized that polyhydramnios results from decreased fetal swallowing.[29–32]

## Risk of Recurrence

Anencephaly, like most NTDs, has a polygenic inheritance. In addition, several other factors, such as ethnicity, geographic location, and nutritional deficiency (eg, folate), may play significant roles in the occurrence of NTDs. The risk of an NTD increases significantly if there is a family history of an NTD. Deak et al[15] reported on a data set of more than 1000 families affected by NTDs. They found both sex-influenced and maternal (imprinting) effects in the etiology of NTDs. Other factors associated with increased risk of NTDs are diabetes and exposure to valproic acid, thalidomide, and alcohol, as well as exposure to hyperthermia.[33]

Recurrence risk for NTDs is related to the family's history. If one of the parents has an NTD, the risk to the offspring is as high as 4.5%.[34] If a previous full sibling is affected, the recurrence risk is 4%; if two previous siblings are affected, this risk increases to as high as 10%. The recurrence risk among half-siblings is ~0.5% to 0.8%.[15] The risk for second-degree relatives (eg, grandparents and grandchildren, uncles and aunts, nephews and nieces) is 0.5%, and for third degree (eg, first cousins), it is similar to that of the general population.[15] In monozygotic twins, the concordance rate for NTDs is 7.7%; for dizygotic twins, it is 4%[15] (Figure 5–3).

Folic acid can help prevent 50% to 70% of the cases of NTDs. Most studies suggest that folic acid works by correcting a nutritional deficiency of folic acid; however, exactly how it works is not known. Folates have two main physiologic effects: as a cofactor for the enzymes that synthesize DNA and RNA and for the conversion of homocysteine to methionine. The gene for 5, 10-methylenehydrofolate (MTHFR) catalyzes the conversion of MTHFR into 5-methyl-tetrahydrofolate, which is the major circulating form of folate. There are two mutations in the MTHFR gene that are associated with NTDs: the C677T and the A1298C mutations. Specifically, C677T has been linked to an increased risk of spina bifida and anencephaly. This mutation causes a mild enzymatic dysfunction that results in mild hemocystenemia in persons whose folate status is not optimal. Lower vitamin $B_{12}$ levels during pregnancy have also been associated with increased risk of NTDs.[1,35,36]

A decrease in folate intake has been shown to be associated with an increased risk of NTDs.[37–39] In view of this association, the U.S. Centers for Disease Control and Prevention (CDC) recommends that all women of childbearing age should consume 400 µg of folic acid per day for prevention of NTDs.[40] However, public health campaigns have not had a significant impact on the prevalence of NTDs.[26] Approximately 40% of women of childbearing age report taking folic acid, although racial and ethnic differences are noted, with Hispanic women who have the highest rate of NTDs reporting the lowest rate of consumption of folic acid.[41] In 1998 the U.S. Food and Drug Administration (FDA) mandated that folic acid should be added to all grain products in the United States; since that time, many other countries have followed suit. Over the last 10 years since the fortification of cereal grain products was mandated, there has been a 26% decrease in NTDs in the United States.[41] On the other hand, the amount of folic acid in these foods is small, and women of childbearing age still need to continue to supplement their diet with folic acid. Worldwide, as reported in 2007 by the CDC, the percentage of wheat flour fortification increased from 18% in 2004 to 27% in 2007.[42] More recently, Bell and Oakley[43] reported that the Flour Fortification Initiative now includes 67 countries that fortify wheat flour and 6 countries that fortify both wheat and maize (corn) flour; this has resulted globally in a 9% decrease of folic acid–preventable NTDs.

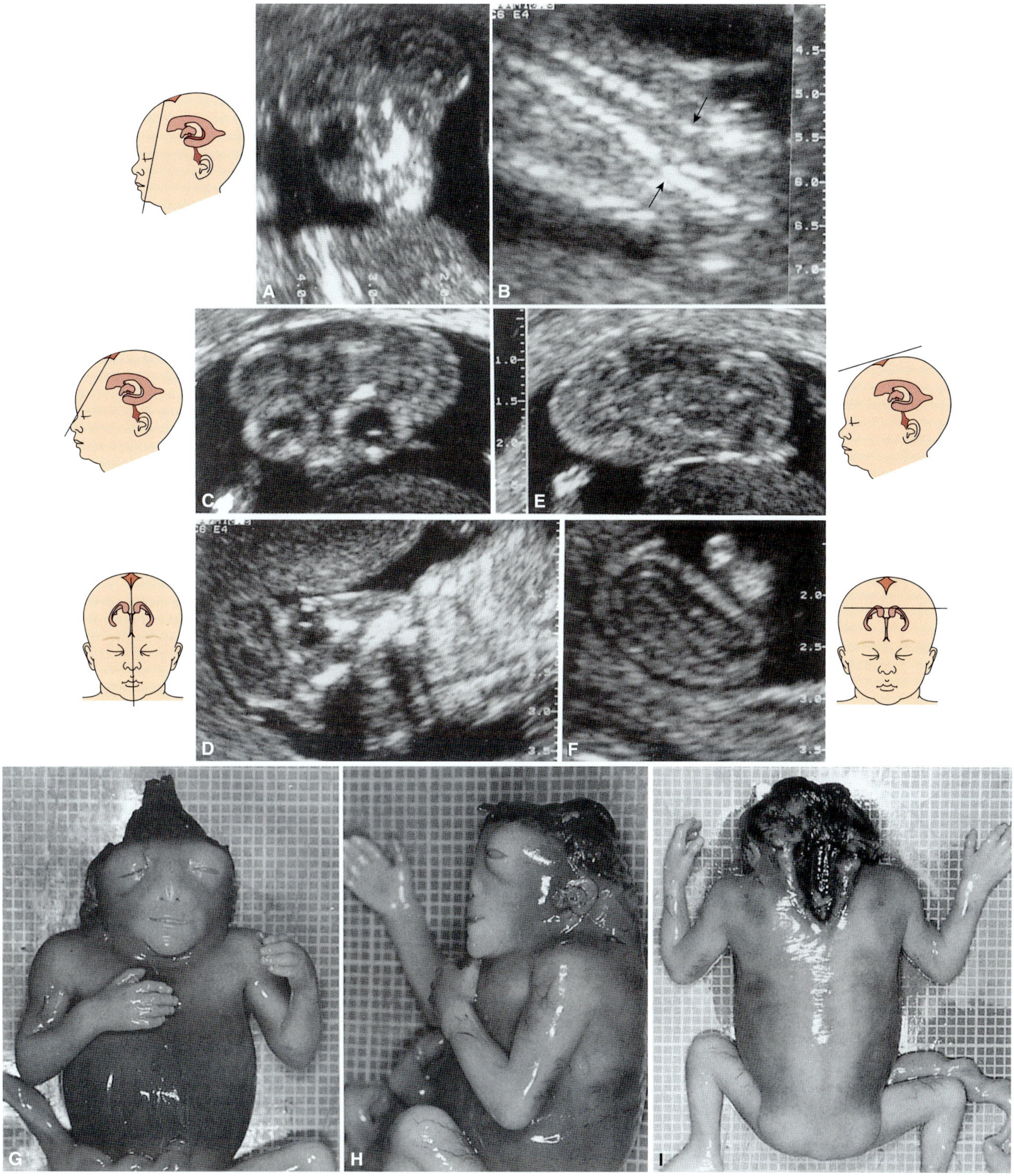


**Figure 5–2.** Exencephaly at 17 postmenstrual weeks. **(A)** Coronal section demonstrating the eyes (lens) showing strabismus and the brain tissue without the calvarium. **(B)** The splayed upper part of the spinal column (*arrow*). **(C)** Coronal section highlighting the orbit with the lens pointing downward (strabismus). **(D)** A median section showing the flat profile (*arrow*). **(E)** and **(F)** Horizontal sections of the brain. No hyperechoic bony structure surrounding the brain tissue is seen. **(G), (H),** and **(I)** Pictures of the aborted specimen from the front, side, and back, respectively. Note the resemblance of the specimen to the respective sonographic pictures.

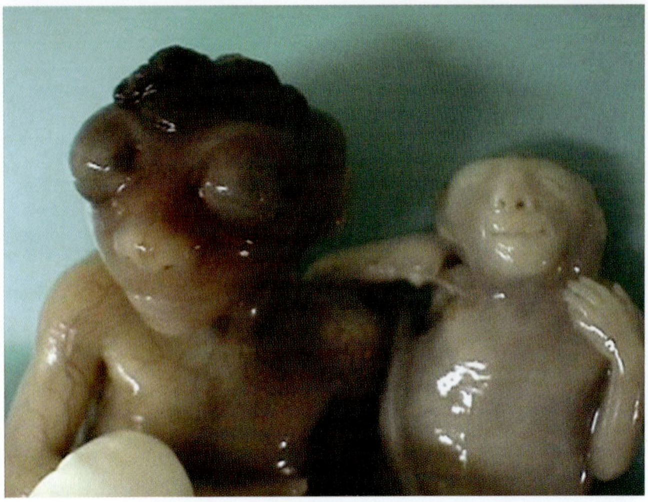

**Figure 5–3.** Discordant dizygotic twins concordant for anencephaly. Pregnancy following invitro fertilization and intracytoplasmic sperm injection. (Courtesy of Gustavo Malinger.)

Recurrence risk can be significantly decreased with the use of periconceptional folic acid. For women who have had a prior child with an NTD, the recommended dose of folic acid is 4 mg daily started at least 1 month before conception and to be continued for the first 12 weeks of pregnancy.[40] Doses of folic acid >1 mg must be taken under the supervision of a physician in order not to mask an underlying condition, such as pernicious anemia (vitamin $B_{12}$ deficiency).

## Sonographic Diagnosis

Anencephaly is a historically important malformation in the field of US, as it was the first malformation reported using transabdominal sonography in a fetus at 17 postmenstrual weeks.[44] Almost 20 years later, it became the first malformation reported using transvaginal sonography (TVS) in a fetus at 11 weeks, 5 days (postmenstrual).[45]

Using TVS, the integrity of the cranium can be assessed as early as the first trimester of pregnancy. This is because ossification of the fetal cranium begins and subsequently accelerates after 9 postmenstrual weeks.[46,47] Abnormal mineralization of the cranial bones can be sonographically determined by the early second trimester by assessing the degree of echogenicity of the bone.[48] Well-mineralized bone is highly echogenic. Absence of an echogenic outer border surrounding the fetal brain must raise the suspicion of the presence of exencephaly-anencephaly sequence (Figures 5–4 and 5–5). The visualization of echogenic "milky" amniotic fluid during the first or early second trimester is considered diagnostic for the presence of anencephaly (Figures 5–6 and 5–7).

Exencephaly refers to a "transient" malformation in which the brain is exposed to the amniotic fluid. It is the second stage of the development of the clinically apparent anencephaly in humans.[31,48–53] In exencephaly a relatively large amount of well-developed brain is present in the absence of a fetal cranium, with significant portions of the cranium missing, but there is preservation of the face and bones of the base of the skull. Preservation of the bones of the face and skull is also seen in anencephaly, although during the

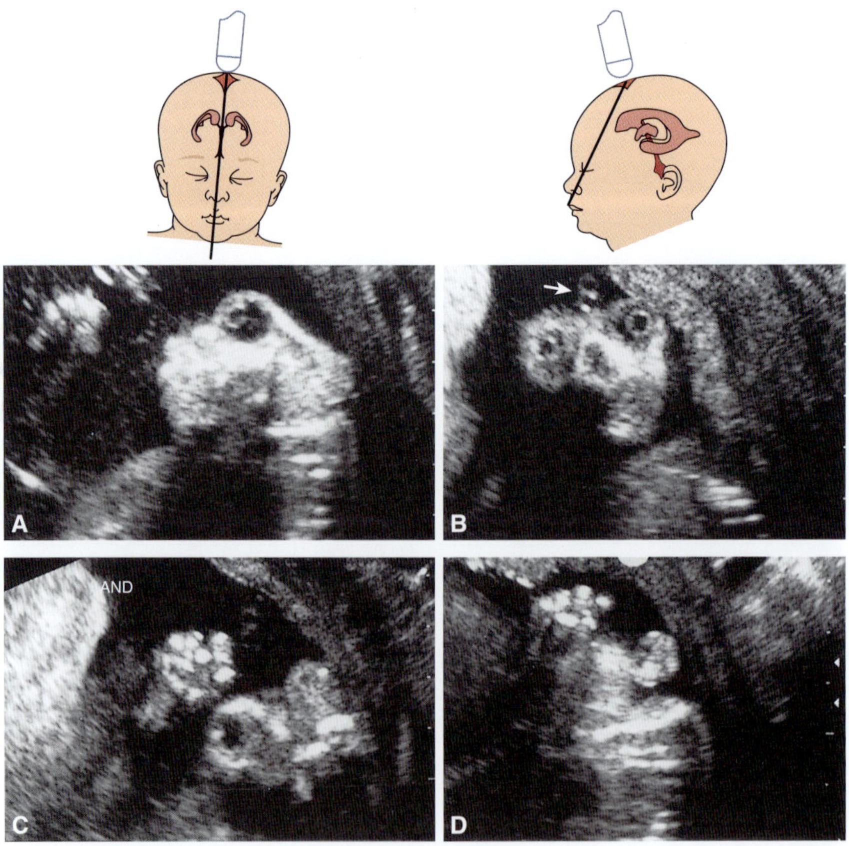


**Figure 5–4.** Anencephaly at 20 postmenstrual weeks. **(A)** Median section depicting a relatively normal profile of the fetal head. However, the skull is totally missing. **(B)** A coronal section of the face showing the fetal orbits with the lenses within. The arrow points to the two-vessel cord present in this fetus. **(C)** and **(D)** are two views of the hands of the fetus. Note that the hands are clenched with overlapping digits.

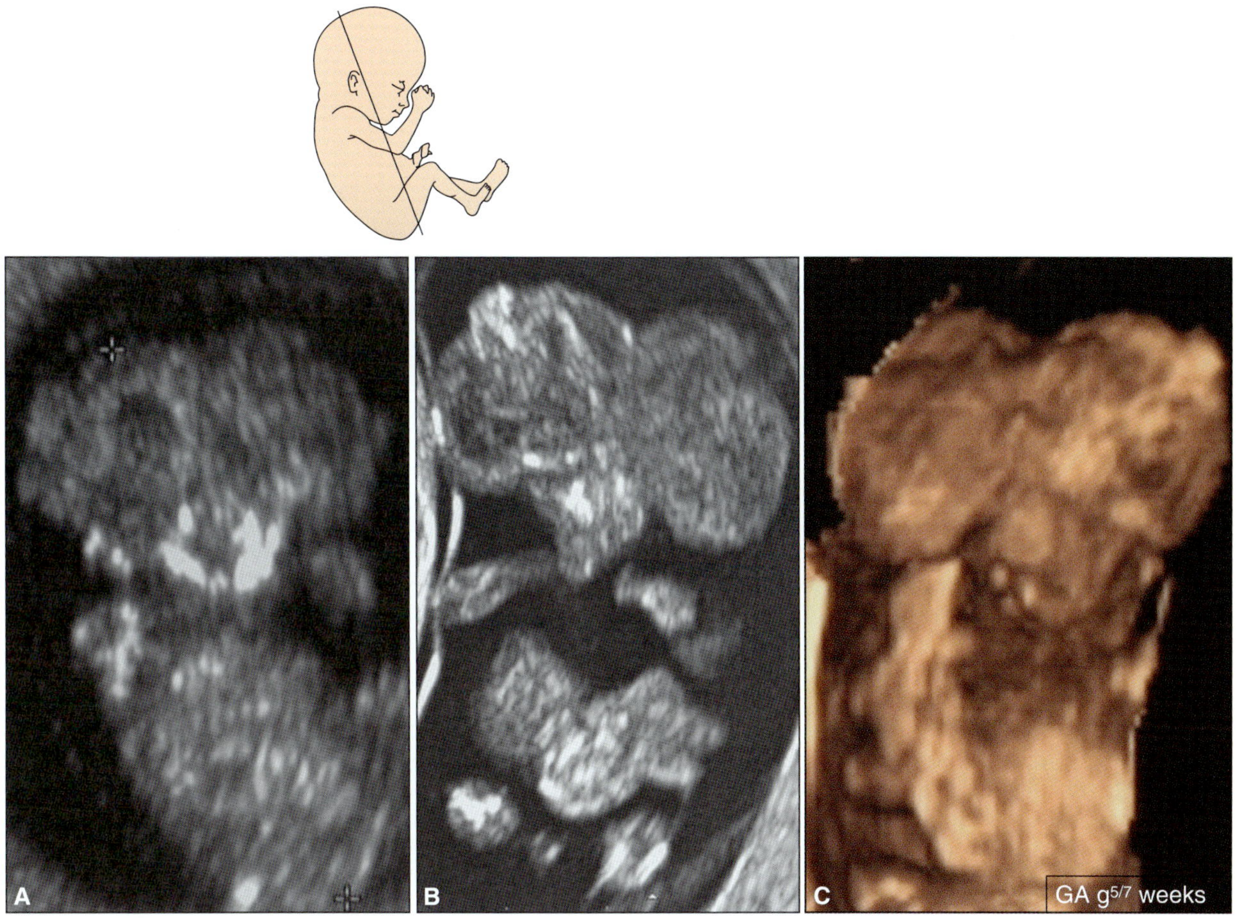


**Figure 5–5.** The fetal head is seen in three different views in this fetus with exencephaly at 9 weeks, 5 days. **(A), (B)** Using two-dimensional (2D) sonography, the exposed brain is shown as disorganized and lacking any of the anatomical landmarks usually seen at this gestational age. **(C)** Three-dimensional (3D) reconstruction of this pathology. The typical appearance of the "Mickey Mouse"–shaped head is evident.

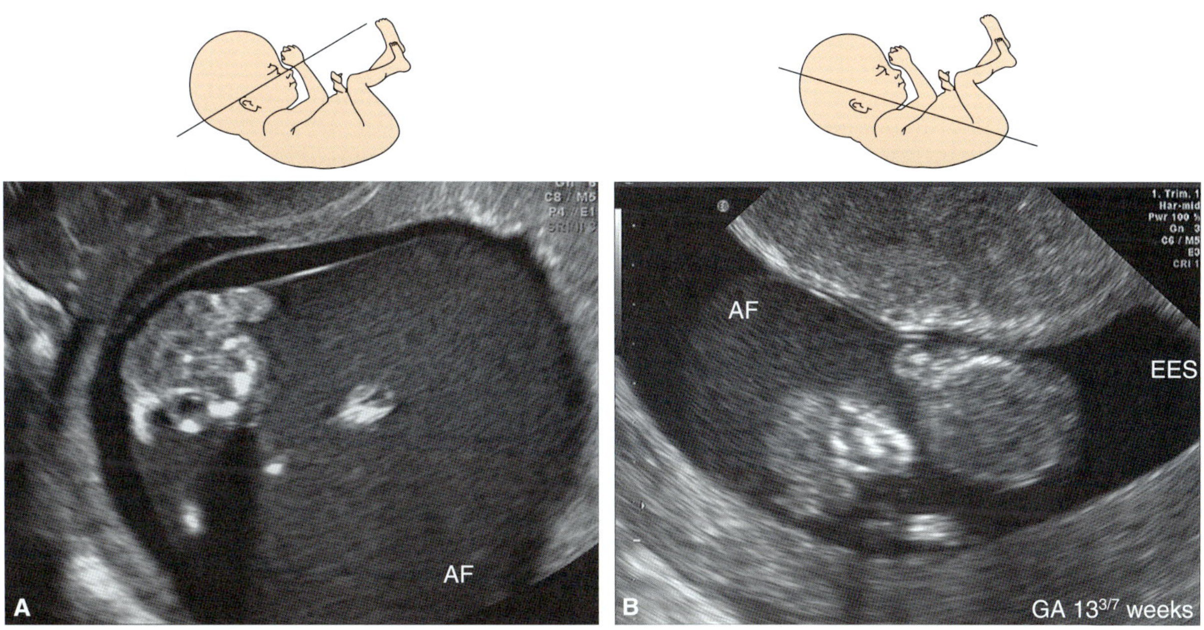


**Figure 5–6.** A fetus with exencephaly-anencephaly sequence at 13 weeks, 3 days. **(A), (B)** The amniotic fluid (AF) appears echogenic when compared with the extraembryonic space (EES), which is anechoic; due to the disintegrating brain tissue, eventually no brain tissue will be seen, and the typical anencephalic appearance will be evident.

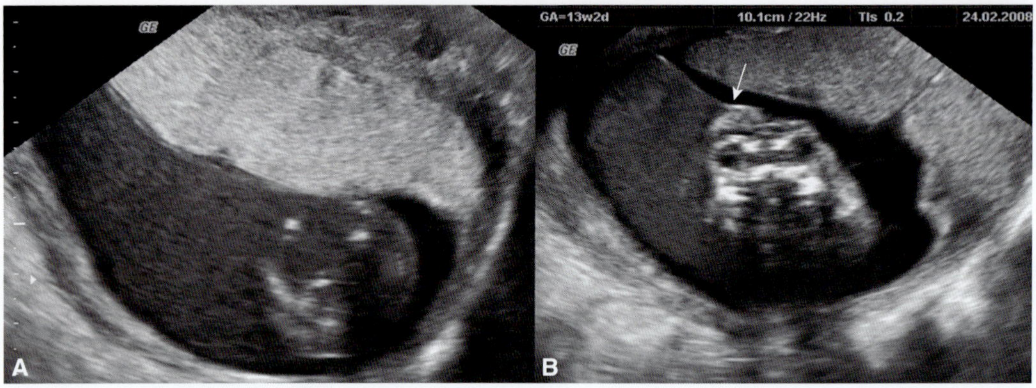


**Figure 5–7.** Transvaginal sonography at 13 weeks, 2 days in an anencephalic fetus. **(A)**"Milky" amniotic fluid. **(B)** Anencephaly, most probably due to amniotic band sequence. Note the continuity between the amnion and the brain remnants (*arrow*). (Courtesy of Gustavo Malinger.)

first trimester, specific structures, such as the ventricles and the choroid plexus, may be apparent (Figure 5–8). Usually, the first trimester exencephalic fetus has an apparently wide fetal head, with sonolucent spaces within the disintegrating brain.[29] The outer shape of the head is bilobed; we, as well as other authors, have referred to this appearance as a "Mickey Mouse"–shaped head[54] (see Figure 5–5). Exencephaly is rarely observed in human infants due to the disintegration of the exposed brain that occurs during intrauterine life. Most cases of exencephaly diagnosed in utero will have the typical anencephalic appearance at the time of delivery (Figure 5–9). Like anencephaly, exencephaly is a lethal malformation incompatible with postnatal life.

The anencephalic fetus is easy to detect using sonography due to the severity of the malformation. This is especially true during the second and third trimesters of pregnancy. During the first trimester, the typical anencephalic phenotypic picture may not be sonographically apparent. Instead, an exencephalic fetus with an abnormally shaped head and some brain tissue may be imaged by sonography.

Anencephaly is characterized by the symmetric partial or total absence of the cranial vault above the orbits. In addition, a variable degree of disintegrating brain tissue may be present. The parts of the brain that are missing are the prosencephalon, the mesencephalon, and the rostral part of the rhombencephalon.[18] In a sagittal view of a fetus with anencephaly, the profile of the chin, lips, nose, and orbits appears relatively normal, but superior to the area of the orbital ridges, the forehead and calvarium are obviously missing (Figure 5–10). A coronal view demonstrates the absence of the cranium above the prominent orbits with preservation of the base of the skull and facial features.[55] The prominent, bulging eyes give the anencephalic fetus its typical "frog's facies." Several other abnormalities involving the eye and orbit of anencephalic fetuses have been described in pathologic specimens, such as coloboma, corneal dermoids, and anophthalmia.[27] In addition, it has been reported that although the eyes of the anencephalic fetus may appear normal, often they have no connection to the brain centrally. Using sonography, we have noted the lenses of the anencephalic fetus to have an apparent strabismus, with both lenses located in the lower lateral aspect of the orbits. In most cases of anencephaly, a soft, spongy, red-colored vascular glial tissue simulating cerebral content is seen to protrude or to be exposed at the site of the defect. This tissue is commonly referred as the area cerebrovasculosa.

Anencephaly can be further divided in two types, depending on the severity of the skull defect:

1. Holoacrania (Greek *holos,* "entire"), in which most or all of the calvarium is missing to the level of the foramen magnum. This is the typical anencephaly that is easily recognized by sonography.[21,27,29] In addition, in holoacrania variable degrees of spinal rachischisis may be present.
2. Merocrania (Greek *meros,* "part"), in which there is a partial or incomplete median cranial defect with

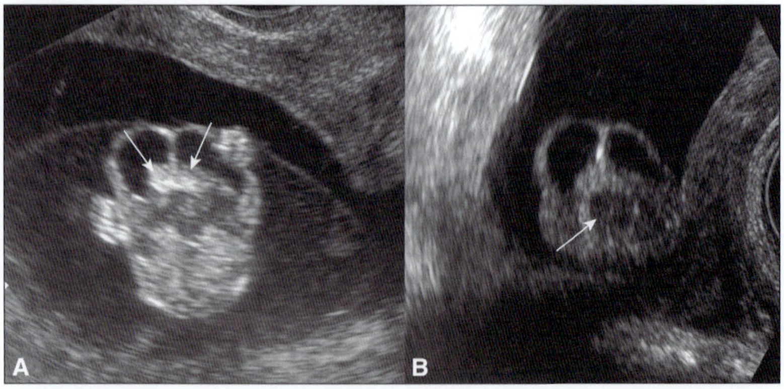


**Figure 5–8.** Merocrania in a fetus at 15 weeks, 6 days. Although the coronal plane **(A)** may produce the false impression of holoacrania, the medial plane **(B)** shows the presence of cranial bone. Note the relatively small anterior fontanelle with uncovered freely floating brain (*arrows*). (Courtesy of Gustavo Malinger.)

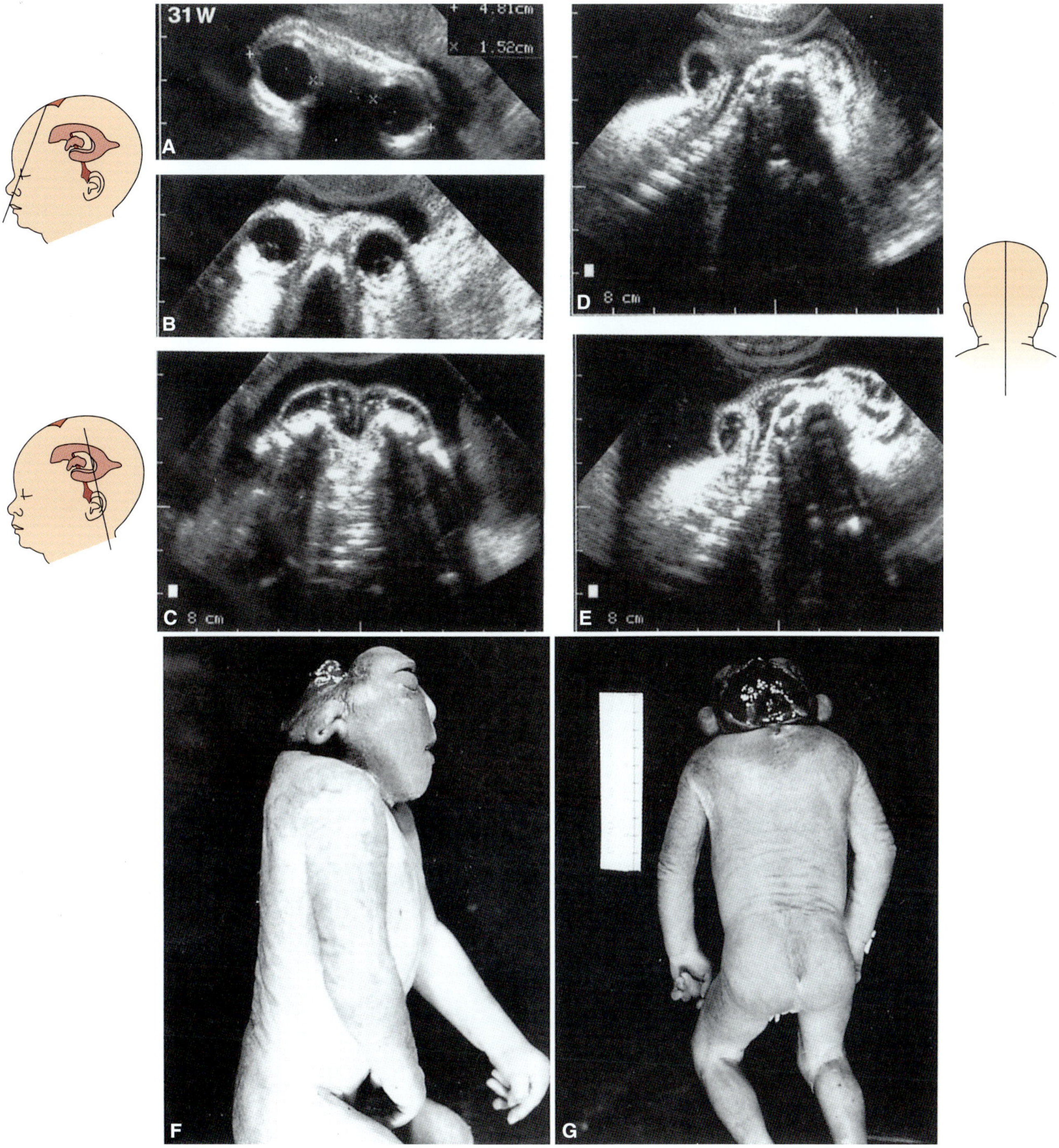


**Figure 5–9.** Anencephaly at 31 postmenstrual weeks. **(A)–(C)** Subsequent coronal sections from the front to the back showing the widely spaced orbits (hypertelorism), the lens in the dislocated position (strabismus), and the scant tissue at the base of the skull. **(D), (E)** Median views showing the upper end of the vertebral column covered by a small amount of tissue (cerebrovasculosa). **(F), (G)** Lateral and posterior views of the specimen after birth.

ectopia of the brain. The foramen magnum is not involved and no cervical lordosis is present. Merocrania may be confused with a cephalocele; however, it can be differentiated from it by the presence of cranial bones, sutures, and fontanelles and the absence of skin covering the ectopic brain[21,27,29] (Figure 5–8).

Three-dimensional (3D) US is not essential to make the diagnosis of exencephaly-anencephaly sequence because two-dimensional (2D) US will provide all of the information needed for the diagnosis. However, it plays a key role in the counseling of the couple whose fetus has this anomaly as it will help the patient understand the

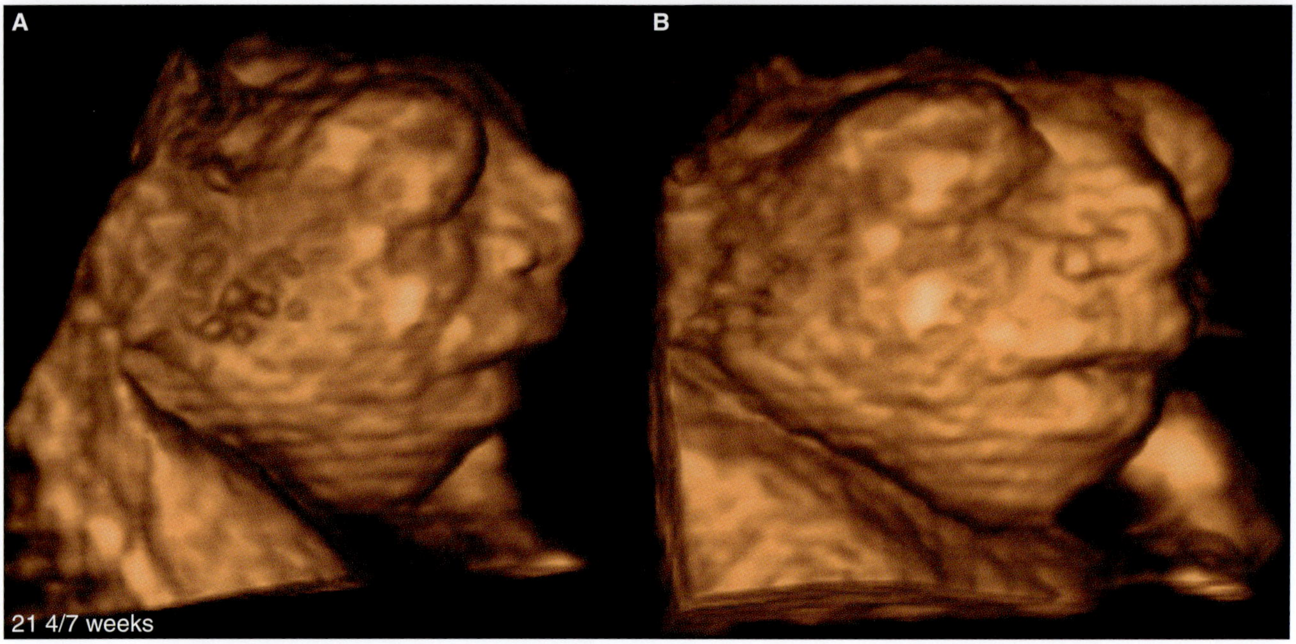


**Figure 5–10.** A 3D reconstruction of the fetal face (using the surface rendering display) of a fetus with anencephaly at 21 weeks, 4 days. **(A)** Profile that demonstrates the typical bulging eyes, as well as the lack of calvarium above the fetal orbits. **(B)** The nose, lips, and chin appear normal, but the calvarium is missing just above the prominent fetal eyes.

severity of the anomaly. In addition to the reconstruction of the face (Figures 5–10 and 5–11), tomographic sections of the brain can be obtained to clearly define the defect (Figures 5–12 and 5–13).

## Differential Diagnosis

Anencephaly or exencephaly may result as a consequence of amniotic bands (see Figure 5–7). This nonrecurring cause of anencephaly can be differentiated from the

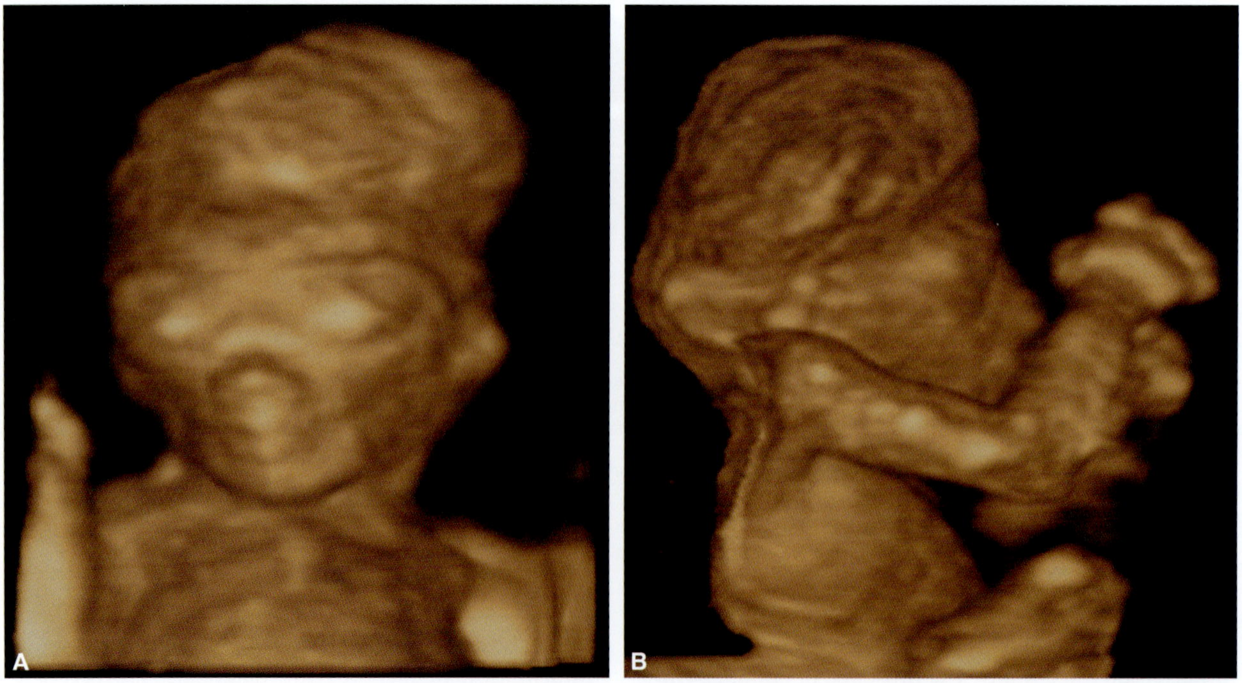


**Figure 5–11.** Using the surface-rendering modality of the 3D US machine, the face of a fetus with exencephaly-anencephaly sequence is displayed. **(A)** Frontal view of the face displaying a significant amount of abnormal-appearing brain tissue. **(B)** Lateral view.

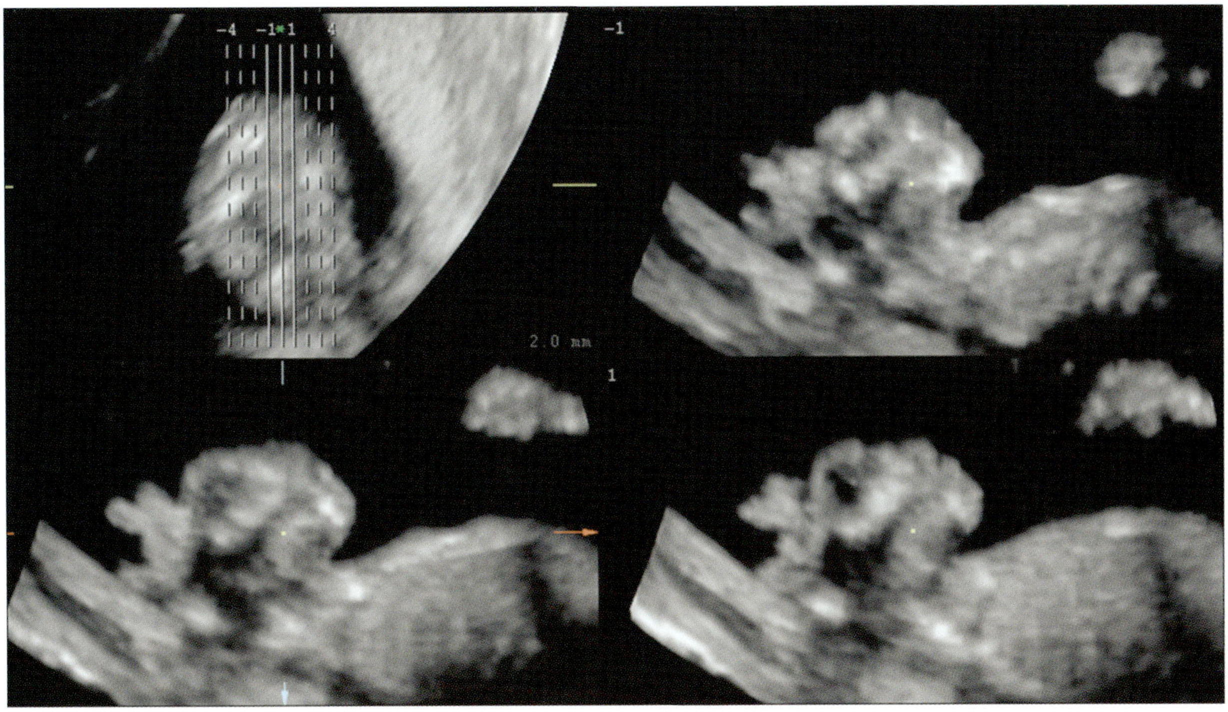

**Figure 5–12.** A typical-appearing fetus with exencephaly-anencephaly sequence is shown using the tomographic feature. Note that, compared with Figures 5–13 and 5–14, there is less visible brain tissue.

anencephaly occurring as a result of failure of the neural tube to close, in that the cranial lesion is asymmetric, and multiple amputations of the fingers or toes, as well as defects of the abdominal wall, may also be present. The key sonographic finding in making this diagnosis of amniotic band syndrome is the presence of a band between the fetal defect and the placenta.[53,56]

## Prognosis

Anencephaly is a lethal condition that more commonly affects female fetuses. It has been estimated that ~75% of fetuses with anencephaly are stillborn. Most infants born alive with anencephaly will die within the first 48 hours and the remaining within the first week of life,[57,58] although

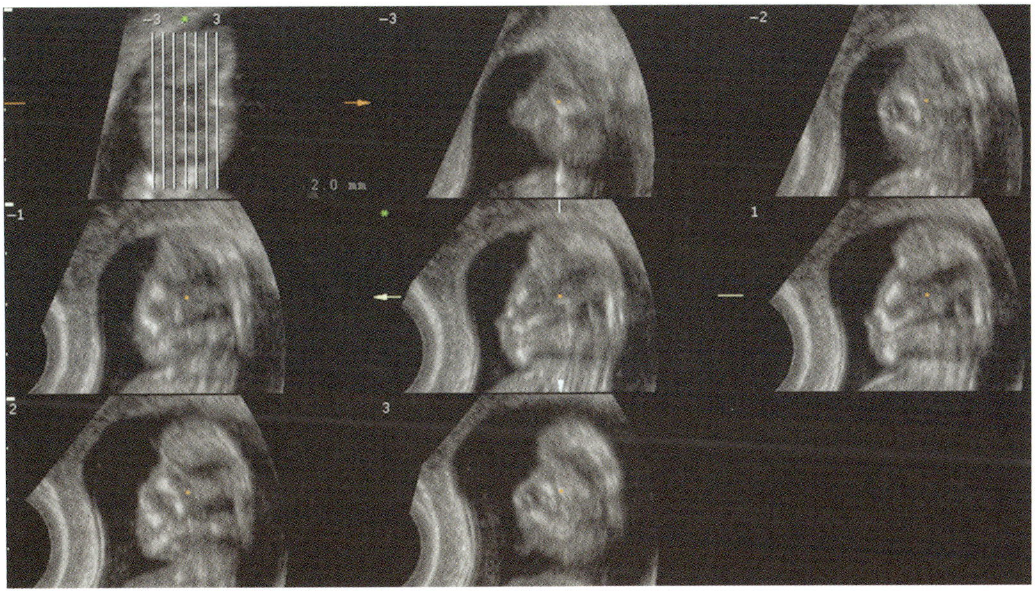

**Figure 5–13.** Using 3D US, the volume of a fetus with exencephaly-anencephaly sequence is displayed using the tomographic feature of the US machine. Serial sagittal sections are displayed that clearly show the absence of the bony skull, as well as the exposed and abnormal-appearing fetal brain.

rare prolonged cases of survival up to 14 months have been reported.[59]

### Obstetric Management

Termination should be offered at the time of diagnosis, given the fact that this is a lethal anomaly. For those fetuses diagnosed at the time of delivery, compassionate and comforting care should be given. Most fetuses with anencephaly die within the first week of life; however, survival has been reported.[60]

## INIENCEPHALY SEQUENCE

### Synonyms

None

### Definition

Iniencephaly is a complex and lethal malformation that has three main features: a defect in the occiput involving the foramen magnum, retroflexion of the entire spine that forces the fetus to look upward with its occiput directed toward the lumbar region, and open spinal defects of variable degree.[61–66]

### Incidence

Iniencephaly is a rare malformation. The reported incidence of iniencephaly ranges from 1 to 6 per 10,000 births. Like anencephaly, most of the affected fetuses are female (90%).[67]

### Pathogenesis

Iniencephaly, like anencephaly, results from a failure of fusion in the cervical and upper thoracic region of the upper spine. This lack of fusion secondarily results in a short neck and trunk, cervical and upper thoracic vertebral defects, defects of the thoracic cage, anterior spina bifida, diaphragmatic defects, and hypoplasia of the lung and/or heart.[68] The malformation results from developmental arrest of the embryo no later than 24 days after conception. This results in persistence of the embryonic cervical retroflexion that leads to failure of the neural groove to close in the area of the cervical spine or the upper thorax.[61,62,69] This defect most likely occurs only a few days later than anencephaly.

Iniencephaly has been divided into two types: iniencephalus clausus (or the closed type) and iniencephalus apertus (or the open type). In the latter, an occipital cephalocele protruding through the foramen magnum and occipital bone defect is present[67] (Figures 5–14, 5–15, and 5–16).

### Etiology

Iniencephaly, like all NTDs, has multifaceted causes, mostly a mix of genetic and environmental factors. Folic acid can decrease the recurrence rate.

### Associated Anomalies

Other malformations occur in up to 84% of fetuses with iniencephaly. Many of these associated malformations can only be diagnosed beyond the first trimester of the pregnancy. Among the associated anomalies, spina bifida is the most common, occurring in up to 50% of cases.[70] Other anomalies are anencephaly, hydrocephaly, microcephaly, ventricular atresia, holoprosencephaly, polymicrogyria, agenesis of the cerebellar vermis, occipital encephalocele, cleft lip and palate, absence of the mandible, diaphragmatic hernia, thoracic cage deformities, cardiac malformation, urinary tract anomalies, omphalocele, clubfoot, and p olyhydramnios.[62,63,66,69,71,72]

### Recurrence Risk

The recurrence risk of iniencephaly is 1.9%, which is similar to that quoted for most NTDs (see above).

### Sonographic Diagnosis

Using TVS, iniencephaly has been diagnosed as early as 12.5 weeks' gestation[73] (Figure 5–14). On the median plane, the head appears large and held in retroflexion, the neck is not visualized, and the spine is usually lordotic (Figure 5–15). In cases of iniencephalus apertus, a posterior cephalocele is present in the occipital area (Figure 5–16). On transverse views, the open spinal defect is present. On axial sections, the head circumference may be several standard deviations below the mean, consistent with microcephaly. In addition, a size/dates discrepancy in a well-dated pregnancy may be the first sign of an iniencephalic fetus.

### Differential Diagnosis

The main differential diagnosis is the Klippel-Feil syndrome (KFS). In the typical clinical scenario, there is a triad of findings consisting of a short neck, low posterior hairline, and limited neck movement, although <50% of patients demonstrate all three clinical features.[74] Findings detected by prenatal sonography are cervical vertebral anomalies, short neck, low-set ears, and facial asymmetry.[75] Other conditions that should be considered are Jarcho-Levin syndrome, Gorlin syndrome, anencephaly with raschischis, and cervical encephalocele.

### Prognosis

Iniencephaly, especially the open type, is essentially a lethal anomaly, with most of the fetuses with this condition being stillborn or dying shortly after birth. However, long-term survival has been reported of up to 2 years of age.[72]

### Obstetric Management

Termination should be offered at the time of diagnosis, given the fact that this is a lethal anomaly. For those fetuses diagnosed at the time of delivery, compassionate and comforting care should be given. Dystocia of labor may occur due to the abnormal head position.

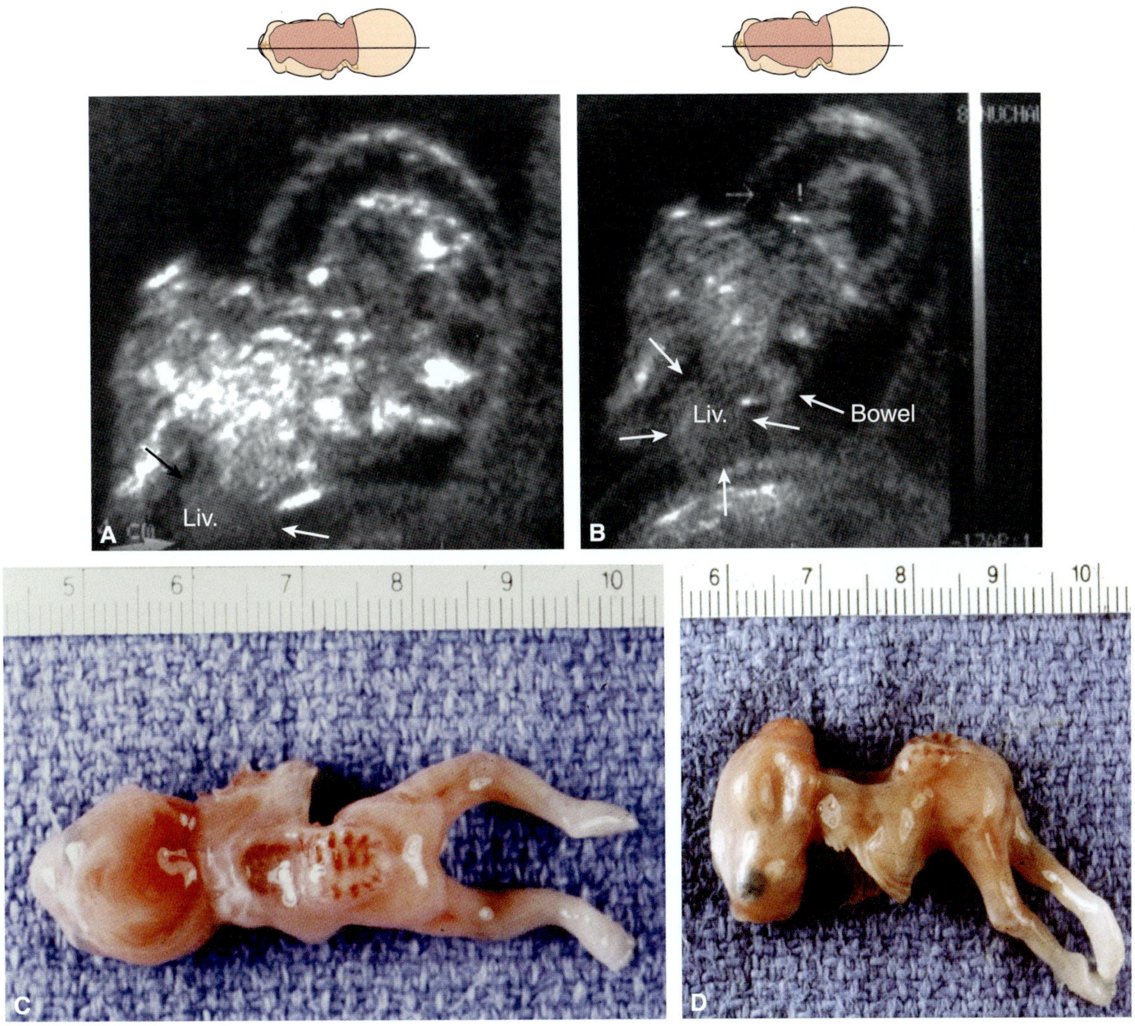


**Figure 5–14.** Iniencephaly at 12½ postmenstrual weeks. **(A)** Sonographic appearance in the median plane. Note the short body length due to the absence of the neck. Omphalocele was also present. L, liver. **(B)** The specimen from the side showing the shortened neck. **(C)** The dorsal view of the specimen showing the total spinal rachischisis. **(D)** Sagittal view of the specimen.

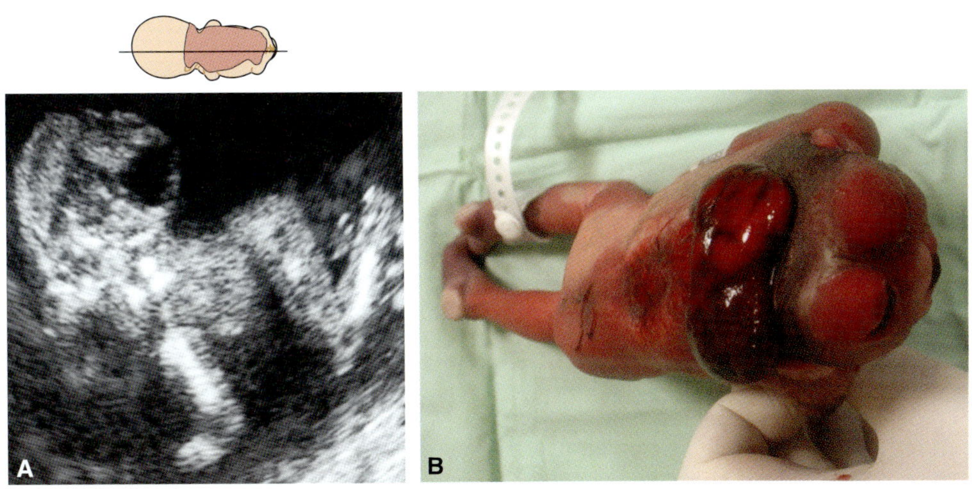


**Figure 5–15.** Iniencephaly at 19 postmenstual weeks. **(A)** The ultrasound image. Note the deviant brain structure and the extended head. **(B)** Pathologic specimen.

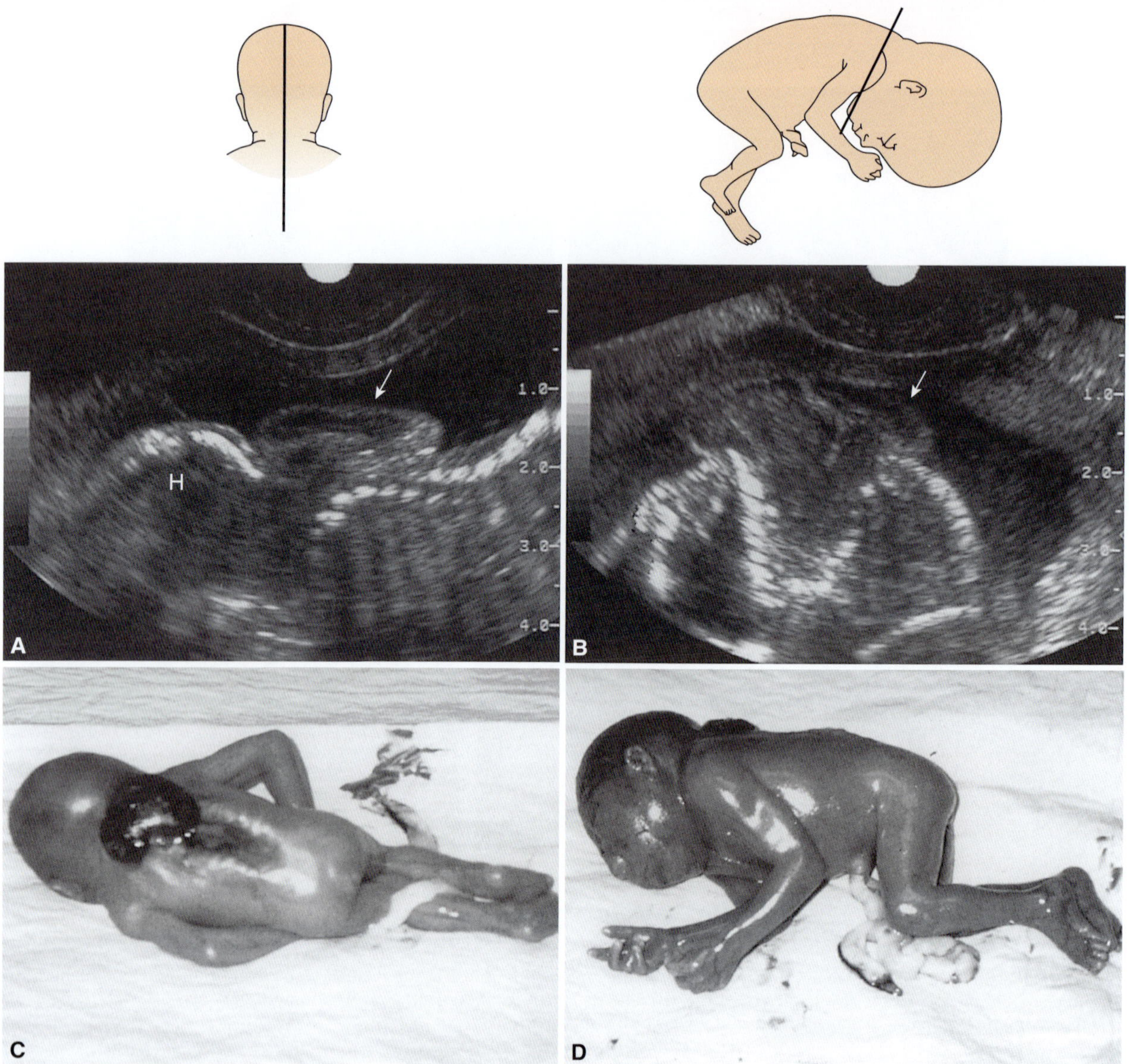


**Figure 5–16.** A fetus with iniencephaly at 22 postmenstrual weeks. **(A)** Longitudinal median section. On the left of the picture, the outline of the head (H); on the right, the distorted vertebral column with several kyphoscoliotic deformations. Note the bulging brain tissue (occipital meningomyelocele, *arrow*). **(B)** Transverse section with the open vertebral column (rachischisis) is seen with the bulging brain tissue (*arrow*). **(C), (D)** The aborted specimen demonstrating the absence of a neck (iniencephaly) and rachischisis with meningomyelocele.

# CEPHALOCELE

## Synonyms

Cranium bifidum, encephalocele

## Definition

Cephaloceles are cranial defects, along bony sutures, in which there is a herniation of the brain and/or meninges. Sporadic or nonsyndromic cephaloceles account for ~5% of all NTDs.[76] When the cephalocele sac contains brain tissue, it is termed an encephalocele; if only cerebrospinal fluid is present (CSF), it is termed a meningocele.

## Incidence

The reported incidence ranges from 1 per 3500 to 1 per 5000 live births.[77] It is estimated that meningoceles are approximately 10 times less common than encephalocele.[78] Cephalocele may involve the occipital, frontal, temporal, and parietal regions of the fetal head (Table 5–5). The occurrence of the different types of cephaloceles shows geographical variation. In Europe and North America, 66% to 89% of all cephaloceles are occipital, with the balance being equally distributed among frontal and parietal cephaloceles. In Thailand and countries of southern Asia, the frontal (sincipital) location is more common than the occipital.[14,32,55,78–82]

**Table 5–5. CLASSIFICATION OF CEPHALOCELE ACCORDING TO THE SITE OF THE BONE DEFECT**

| |
|---|
| Occipital |
| Anterior |
| Sincipital |
| Basal |
| Parietal |

Modified, with permission, from Simpson DA, David DJ, White J. Cephalocele: Treatment, outcome, and antenatal diagnosis. *Neurosurgery.* 1984;15:14–21.

## Pathogenesis

Occipital cephaloceles occur more commonly in female than in male fetuses, in contrast to parietal and sincipital cephaloceles, which are more prevalent in males (Figures 5–17, 5–18, 5–19, 5–20, 5–21, 5–22, and 5–23).[78] The development of most severe cephaloceles takes place no later than 26 days after conception, when the anterior neural tube closes.[11]

Anterior or sincipital cephaloceles are frontonasal herniations of the brain and/or meninges through a skull defect. Anterior cephaloceles always occur in the midline sagittal axis of the cranium. Cephaloceles occur at the sites of the fontanelles (frontal, sphenoidal) or at the cribriform plate of the ethmoid, the foramen cecum, the foramen magnum, or through a suture line.[54,81,83,84] They are divided into two main types: sincipital and basal. Sincipital cephaloceles are external lesions that occur near the root of the nose (glabella) and are subdivided into nasofrontal, nasoethmoidal, and nasorbital types (Figures 5–24, 5–25, 5–26, 5–27, and 5–28). Basal cephaloceles are internal lesions that occur within the nose, pharynx, or orbit. These are further subdivided into five types: sphenoorbital, sphenomaxillary, transethmoidal, sphenoethmoidal, and sphenopharyngeal.[83,85]

The pathogenesis of anterior cephaloceles is unclear. Anterior cephaloceles occur early in development at around 45 to 50 days of embryonic age. This is the time when the base of the occiput and the sphenoid body develop and assume their normal appearance.[86] Anterior cephaloceles, like occipital cephaloceles, may occur as a sporadic defect, associated with a chromosomal syndrome, or as part of a nonchromosomal developmental syndrome. Syndromes that include an anterior cephalocele are aberrant tissue band syndrome, frontonasal dysplasia, absent corpus callosum, clefting, craniostenosis, hypothalamic pituitary dysfunction, meningocele, and Roberts-SC phocomelia syndrome.[85,87,88]

Parietal cephaloceles are located in the midline between the lambda and the bregma. The size, shape,

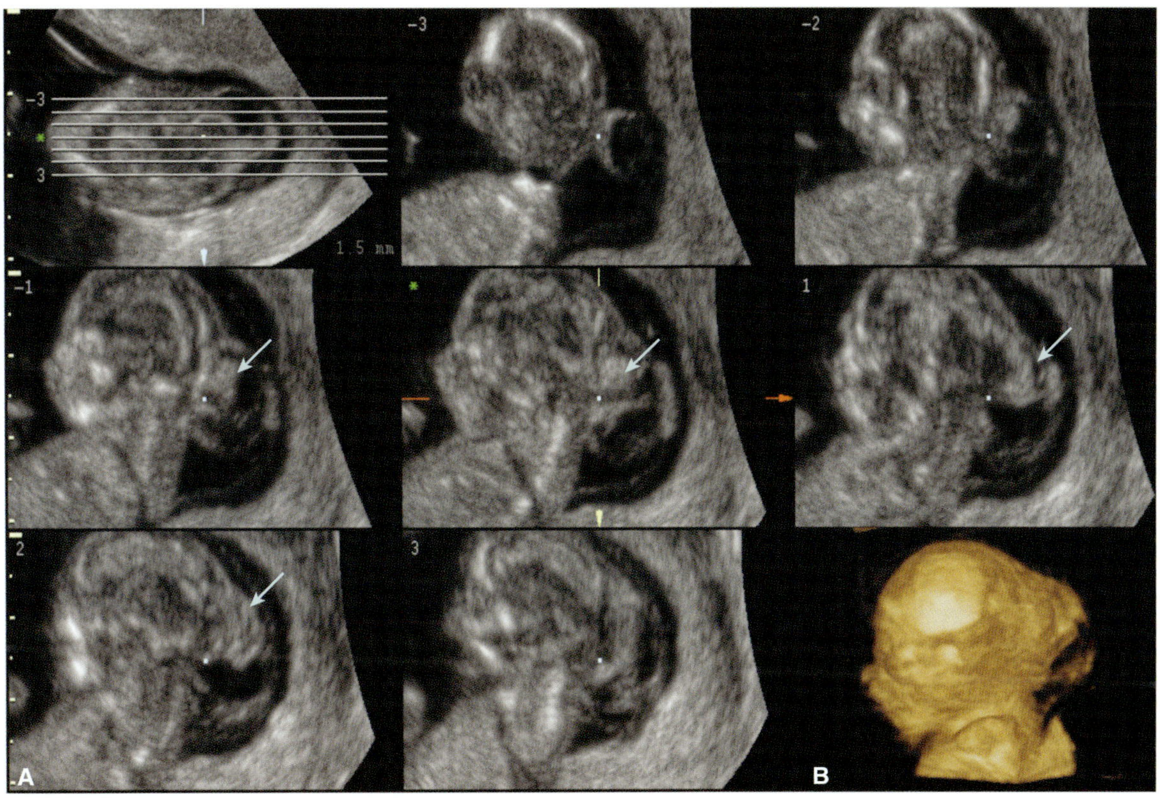


**Figure 5–17.** Posterior encephalocele at 12 weeks, 6 days. **(A)** Series of parallel sagittal sections as viewed using the tomographic imaging display showing the brain tissue extending into the amniotic sac (*arrow*). **(B)** Picture generated using surface rendering showing the head with the posterior encephalocele from a lateral view.

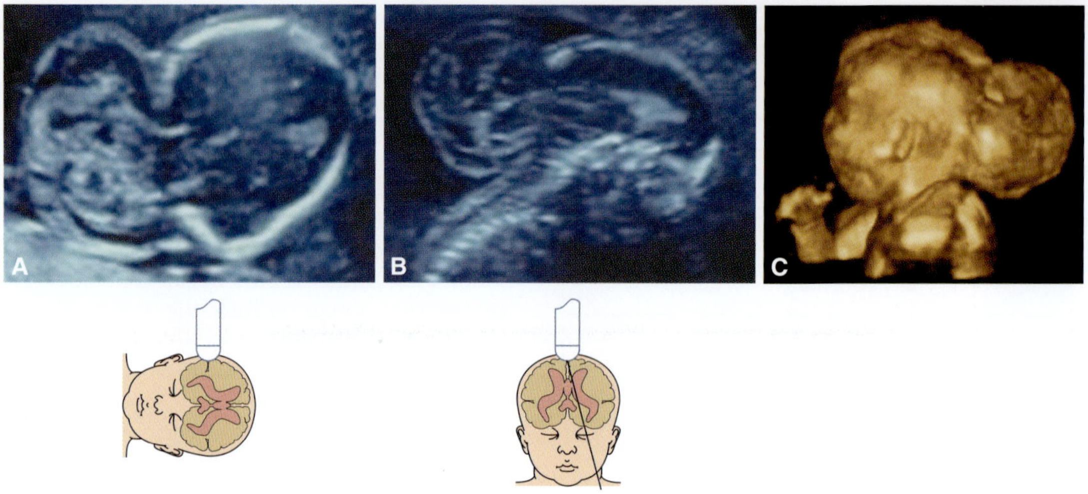


**Figure 5–18.** Using transabdominal sonography, a large posterior encephalocele is seen in this fetus at 19 postmenstrual weeks. **(A)** An axial section displays the large cephalocele sac. Brain tissue is seen extending into the sac. **(B)** Sagittal section displays the encephalocele. **(C)** A 3D reconstruction of the posterior encephalocele.

position, and content of the cephalocele sac may be variable.[78] The cephalocele sac may contain the parietal cortex.

Atretic meningoceles are extremely infrequent, affecting the parietal and positioned close to the lambda suture. Usually there is a round bone defect that contains meninges and neural rests.[89] Associated anomalies, including heterotopia, cerebellar dysgenesis, and venous anomalies, have been reported.[90,91]

## Etiology

Cephaloceles usually occur as an isolated lesion, but in a small percentage of cases, they may be part of a nonchromosomal or chromosomal syndrome. Chromosomal abnormalities associated with cephaloceles are trisomy 13; trisomy 18; mosaic trisomy 20; deletion (13q), (2)(q21→q24); monosomy X; duplication (6)(q21→qter), (7)(pter→p11), and (8)(q23→qter). We have encountered

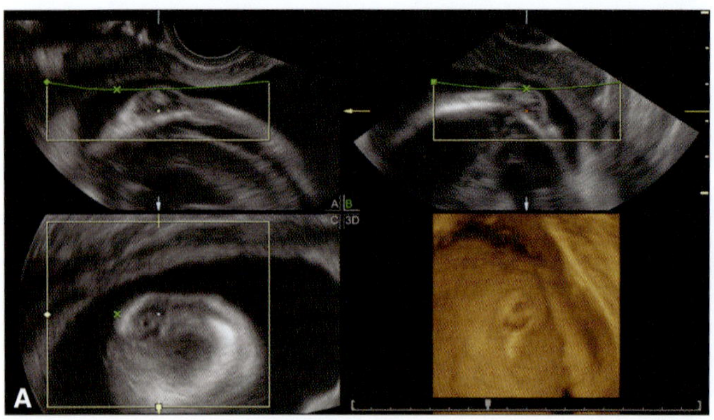


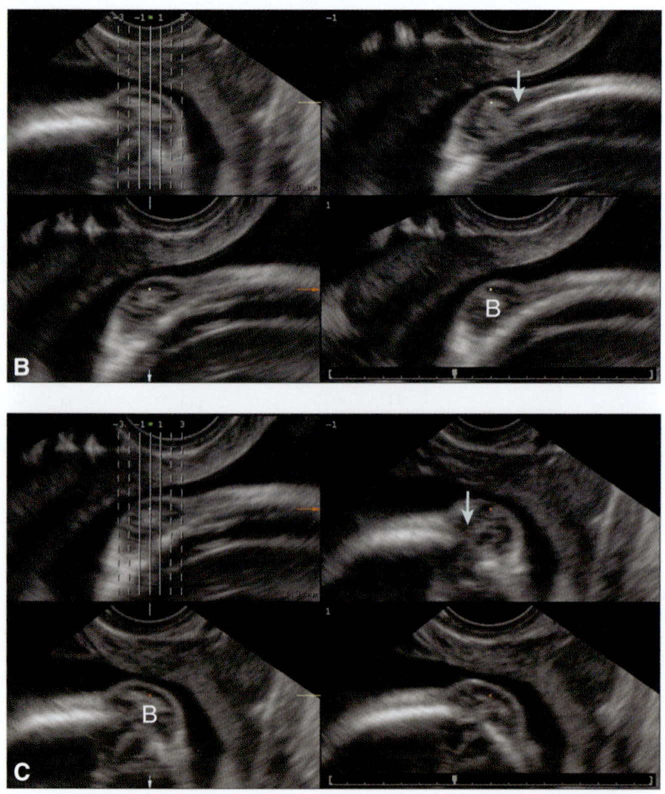


**Figure 5–19.** A small posterior encephalocele arising from the posterior aspect of the sagittal suture is seen using 3D transvaginal sonography in a patient at 21 weeks, 4 days, referred to our unit for evaluation of borderline ventriculomegaly. **(A)** The volume is displayed using the three orthogonal planes (Box A: sagittal; Box B: coronal; Box C: axial) the rendered imaged is seen in the lower right box. **(B), (C)** Volume displayed using tomographic imaging. In **B** the image is zoomed, and the small cranial defect (*arrow*) is seen in serial sagittal sections; in **C** in serial coronal sections. The herniated brain, B, is seen within the cephalocele sac.

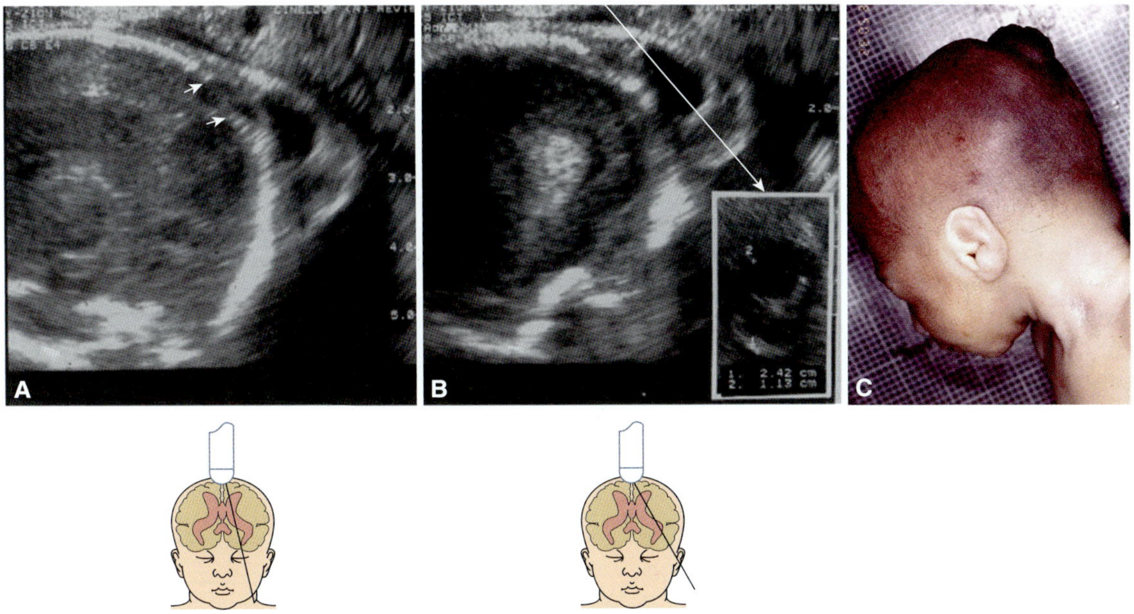


**Figure 5–20.** Parietal cephalocele at 22 postmenstrual weeks. **(A)** The small (7 mm) bony defect lies between the small white arrows. Note that this is evident in the oblique–1 sections. The brain tissue on all sections appeared normal. **(B)** A slightly more lateral section shows the posterior horn with a hyperechogenic choroid plexus and the skull defect with the sonolucent meningocele. The picture in the inlay was taken across the plain marked by the white line. The size of the lesion was 2.4 × 1.1 cm. **(C)** Posterior views of the lesion. The patient refused further testing and requested termination of the pregnancy.

two fetuses with large posterior encephalocele and a deletion of the short arm of chromosome 13 (13q) (see Figure 5–23). Besides the encephaloceles, these fetuses have skeletal malformations. The most remarkable malformation is the absence of the thumb.

Some of the nonchromosomal syndromes that feature a cephalocele are listed in Table 5–6. In these cases, the karyotype is normal, and the clues to the prenatal diagnosis are the sonographic findings. Therefore, it is imperative to perform a detailed targeted scan looking for other sonographic abnormalities. This is especially important if this is the first affected fetus.

## Associated Anomalies

In a recent study 65.6% of the fetuses/infants with cephaloceles had at least one major malformation, and 34.4% had an isolated cephalocele.[92] Joo et al[76] published their 26-year experience with nonsyndromic cephaloceles. In their series the extracranial malformations associated with cephaloceles were cardiovascular (VSD, coartaction of the aorta, single umbilical artery), urogenital tract (pyelectasis, ureteral agenesis), malformations of the extremities (talipes equinovarus), and malformations of the thorax and abdominal wall (gastroschisis, diaphragmatic hernia, costal malformations).

Of the syndromic causes of cephaloceles, Meckel-Gruber, Walker-Warburg and Knobloch syndromes are among the most common (Figures 5–29, 5–30, and 5–31). Meckel-Gruber syndrome is lethal. There are several types of Meckel-Gruber syndrome, of which type 1 is caused by mutation in a gene encoding a component of the flagellar apparatus basal body proteome (*MKS1;* 609883; gene map locus 17q23). Approximately 80% of the cases of Meckel-Gruber syndrome have an occipital cephalocele. The two other consistent findings in the typical triad of malformations are bilateral renal cystic dysplasia and postaxial polydactyly of both hands and feet (see Figure 5–30).[78,82] These latter malformations have been reported to be present in 95% and 75% of cases.[93] In order to make the diagnosis of Meckel-Gruber syndrome, at least two of the three major signs must be present. Using sonography, the diagnosis can be made by the early second trimester of pregnancy.[94] However, in patients with a prior history of Meckel-Gruber syndrome, the diagnosis could be made in the first trimester (see Figure 5–29). The cystic dysplastic kidney is the most consistent anomaly. The kidneys are up to 10 to 20 times larger than normal, are hyperechogenic, and contain multiple small cysts measuring between 2 and 5 mm.[82,95] As a result of the dysplastic kidneys, there is impaired renal function, and oligohydramnios is present. In addition, the fetal bladder is not imaged by US. The size of the cephalocele may be variable. In one of our cases of Meckel-Gruber syndrome, the skull defect measured 2 mm (see Figure 5–30). Other sonographic findings are microcephaly with a biparietal diameter (BPD) and head circumference lagging behind dates and hydrocephaly. Associated malformations that may present in Meckel-Gruber syndrome include renal agenesis, renal hypoplasia, ureteral duplication, cleft lip and palate, micrognathia, microphthalmia, ambiguous genitalia, congenital hepatic fibrosis, talipes equinovarus, short limb dwarfism, malformed tongue, intestinal malrotation, Dandy-Walker malformation, and congenital heart defects.[96,97] The heart defects include VSDr or ASD, aortic hypoplasia or coarctation, aortic valvular stenosis, and rotational anomalies.[82]

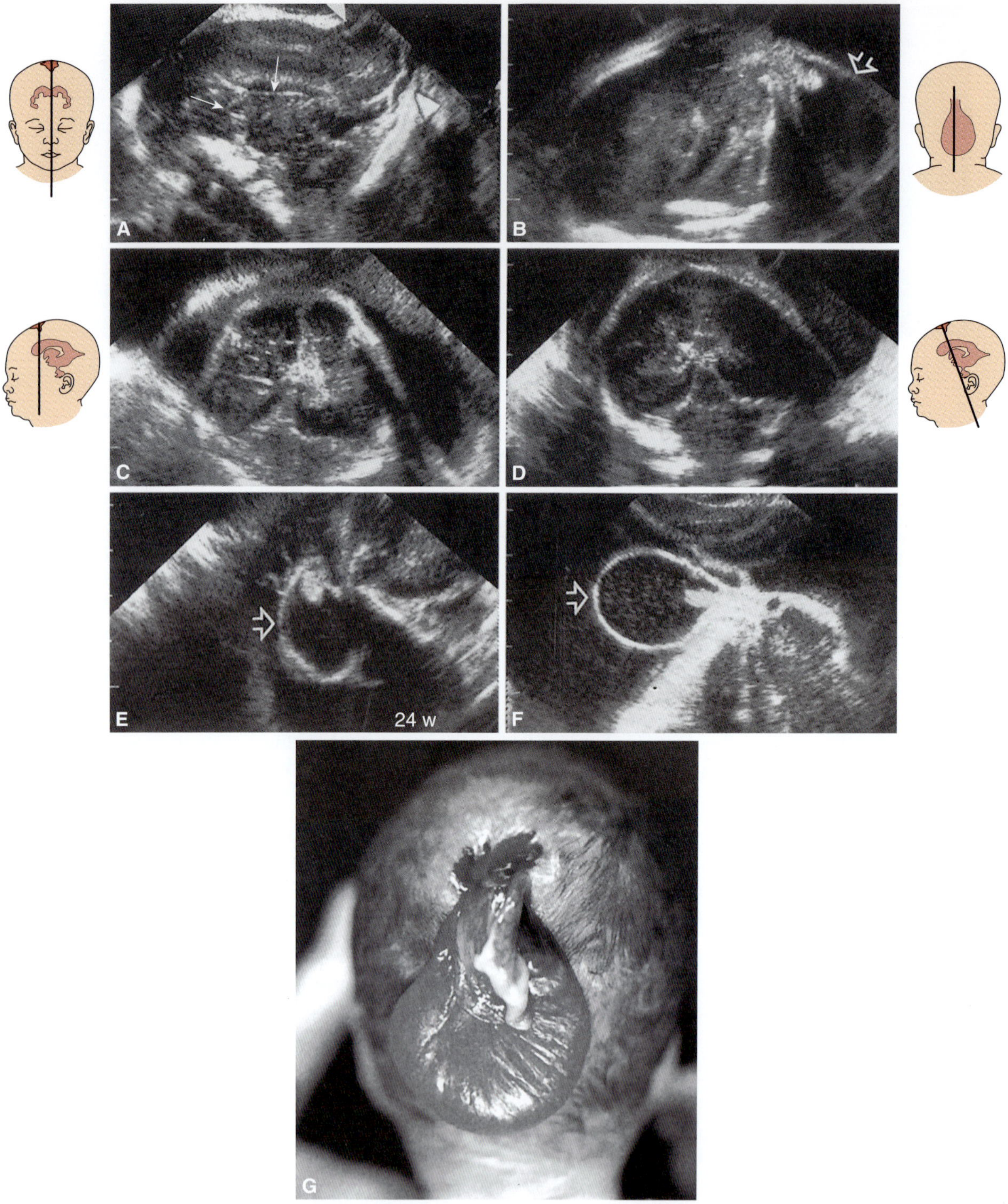


**Figure 5–21.** Occipital encephalocele. The patient presented at 24 postmenstrual weeks for dating US. The measurements revealed microcephaly and the occipital bulging structure. **(A)** Median section of the brain showing the bony lesion between the two white arrowheads. Note the typical shape of the corpus callosum (*small arrows*) and the small cavum septi pellucidi. **(B)** This view concentrates on the posterior herniated sac marked by an open arrow; a very small echogenic structure is bulging into the fluid. **(C)** Midcoronal–1 section: almost no anterior horns are seen on this section. **(D)** Midcoronal–3 section: very small lateral ventricles with echogenic choroid plexus is seen. **(E), (F)** Targeted views of the posterior cephalocele marked by open arrows inside a small (½ cm) echogenic tissue; this may correspond to meninges or a very minute amount of brain tissue. **(G)** The specimen showing the translucent thin membrane of the cephalocele bulging through the midline skull defect. In addition, this fetus had single umbilical artery, dilated renal pelves, cardiomegaly with pericardial infusion, and an interventricular septal defect with a wide pulmonary artery.

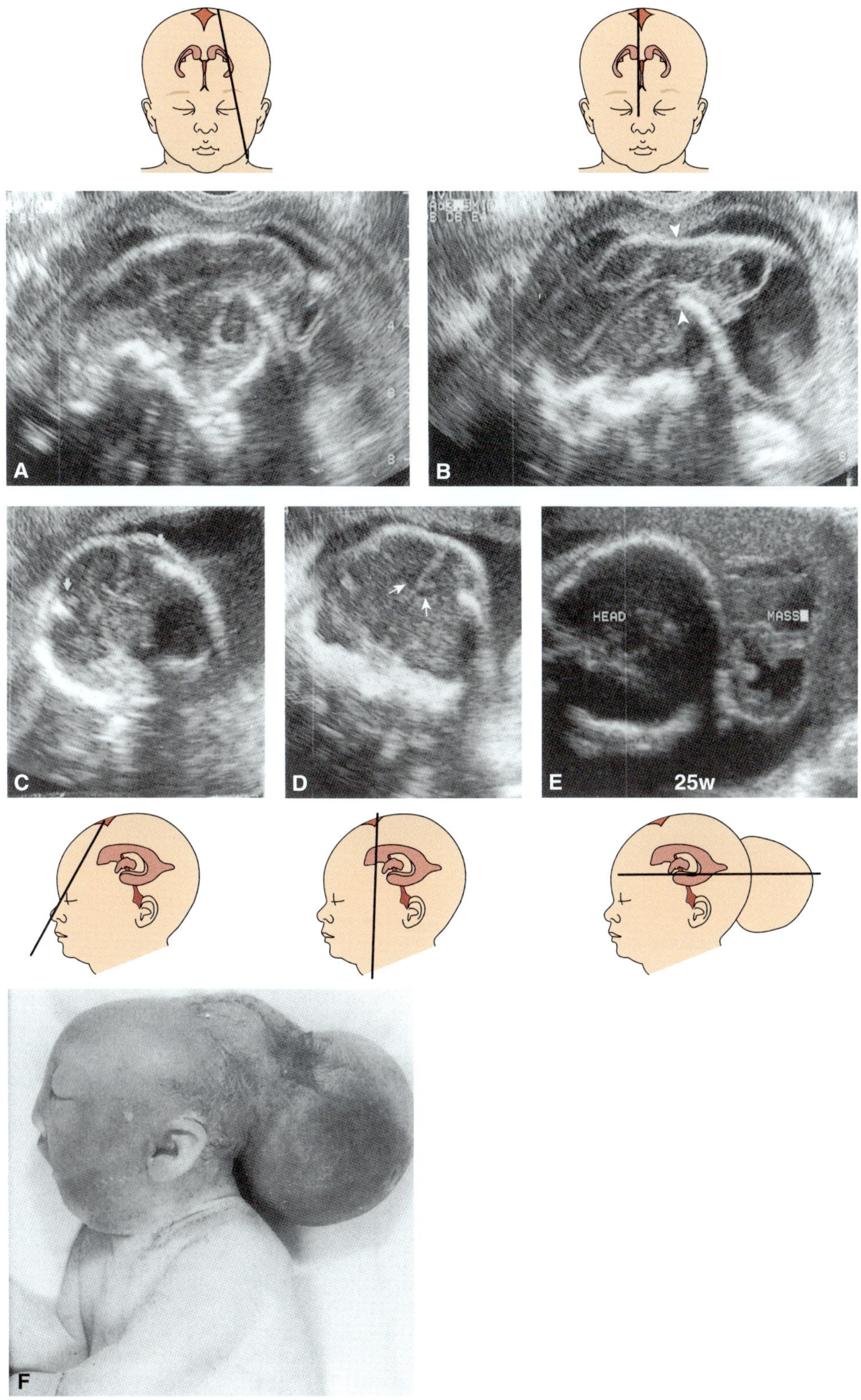


**Figure 5–22.** Sonographic pictures of an occipital encephalocele at 25 postmenstrual weeks. Delivery took place at 34½ postmenstrual weeks. **(A), (B)** Median views showing the skull defect between the two white arrows and the bulging brain and cerebrospinal fluid bulging into the sac. **(C), (D)** Frontal–1 and –2 views, showing what appears to be normal symmetrical brain tissue. Panel **(D)** shows the anterior horns (*small arrows*). **(E)** A horizontal section of the defect and the herniated mass. The head demonstrated severe microcephaly for the age. **(F)** The specimen demonstrating severe microcephaly and the large posterior encephalocele. The chromosomal studies demonstrated a 13q deletion.

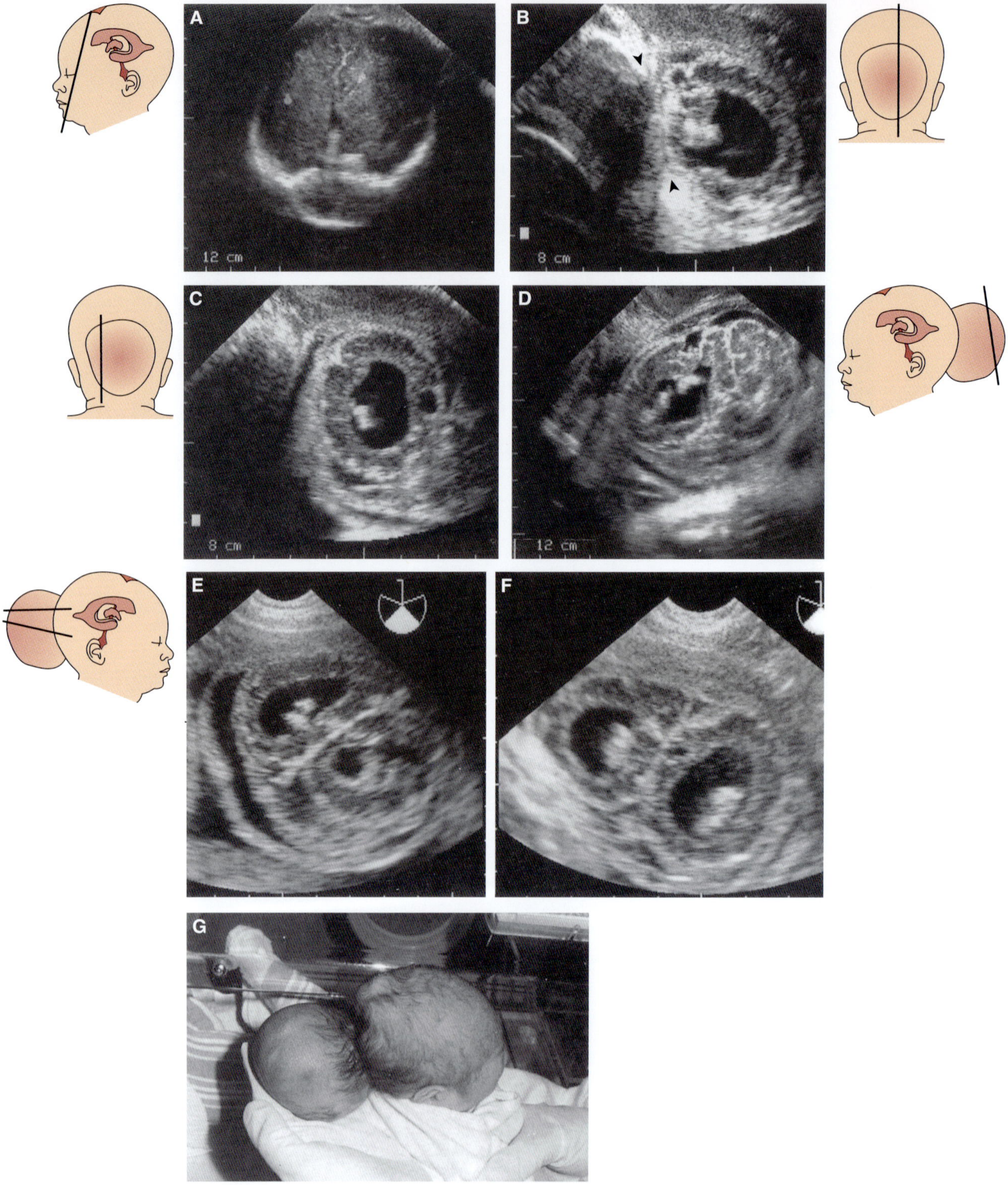


**Figure 5–23.** Occipital encephalocele in a fetus at 34 postmenstrual weeks. This patient presented for her first US exam at this gestational age. Microcephaly was also diagnosed (the biparietal diameter [BPD] and the head circumference were consistent with 26 postmenstrual weeks). **(A)** Frontal–2 section showing the longitudinal sulcus and apparently normal brain tissue. **(B)** Median section depicting the large bony defect in the occipital region marked by two black arrowheads. Brain tissue seems to protrude, pulling with it the posterior horn and the choroid plexus. **(C), (D)** Different sections of the encephalocele itself. **(E), (F)** Coronal sections by definition, showing the longitudinal sulcus and the dilated occipital horns and within it the choroid plexus. **(G)** A picture of the neonatal head showing the large occipital encephalocele. Clinical course: The neonate was found to have a chromosome 13q deletion and was admitted and discharged several times but reached the age of 1½ years. Another anomaly included absence of the thumbs. Cranioplasty was performed, which was complicated by wound infection and worsening hydrocephaly. A drain was placed; however, the infant was admitted several times to the hospital because of cerebrospinal fluid leak from the incision site. The infant had severe mental retardation and seizure disorder. The computed tomography (CT) studies showed that the encephalocele included the cerebellar hemispheres and a portion of the posterior horns (as diagnosed by the US pictures), in addition, partial agenesis of the corpus callosum with the splenium virtually absent was seen.

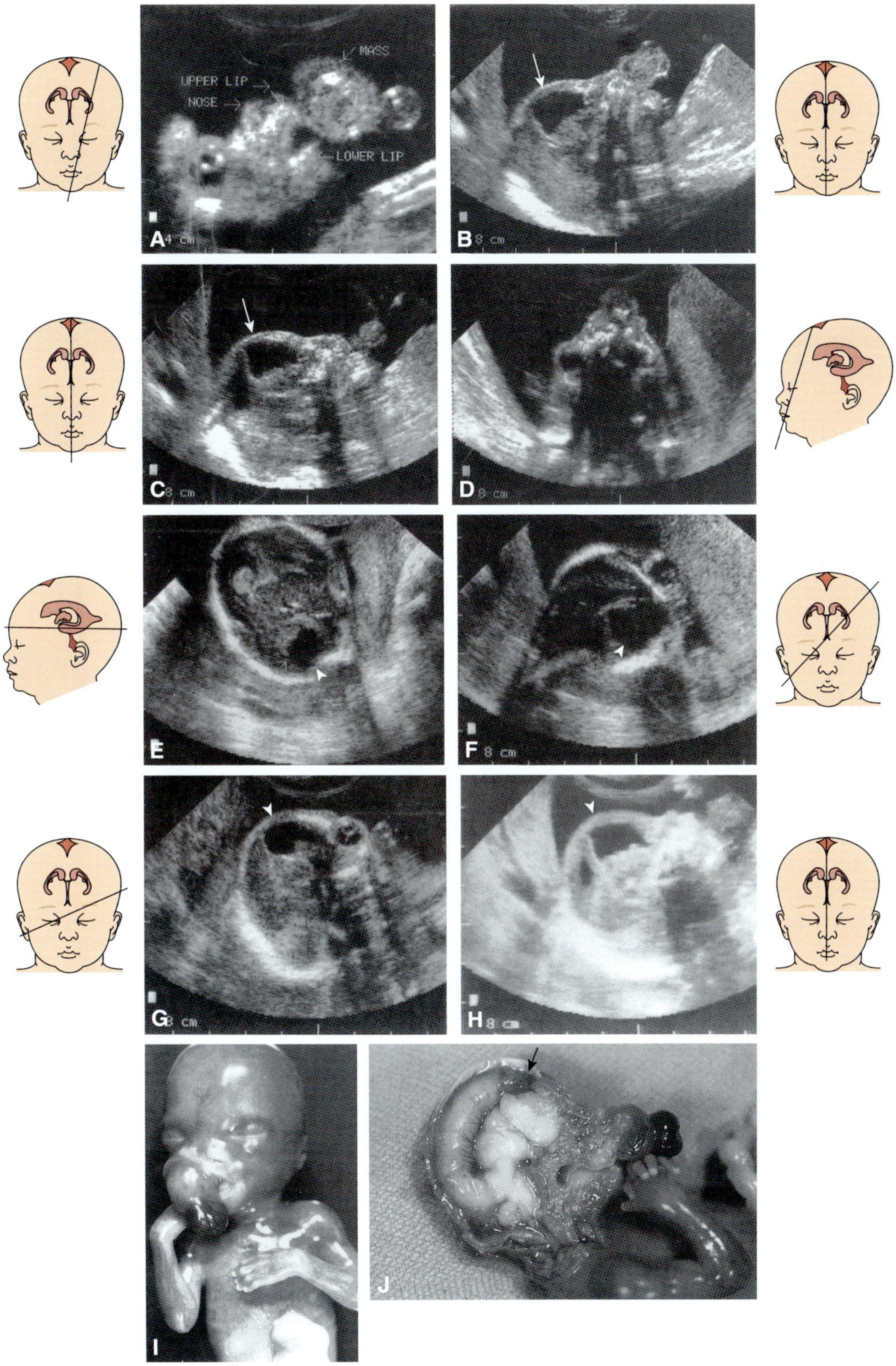


**Figure 5–24.** Anterior encephalocele at 13½ postmenstrual weeks. **(A)** Median section showing the eye, nose, upper and lower lips, and a lobulated mass protruding between the lips. **(B), (C)** Slightly and progressively lateral paramedian sections showing not only the lesion but also a sizable sonolucency in the skull probably left behind by the protruding mass, leaving that space vacant. **(D)** Horizontal section of the lesion showing the protruding mass between the two orbits. **(E)–(H)** Horizontal paramedian and median sections of the lesion. These pictures where aimed at determining the place of the sonolucency in the skull. This was finally located to be in the area of the anterior horn almost symmetrically between the two hemispheres (*arrowheads*). **(I)** The side view of the aborted specimen showing the bulging cephalocele emerging through the mouth. **(J)** A median transection of the head demonstrating the origin of the lesion protruding from the anterior horn. The sonolucent space in the area of the frontal horn detected by US is now clearly seen on this section (*black arrow*). (**A–G** from Monteagudo A, Timor-Tritsch IE, Cephalocele, Anterior. www.thefetus.net, (1992) with permission.)

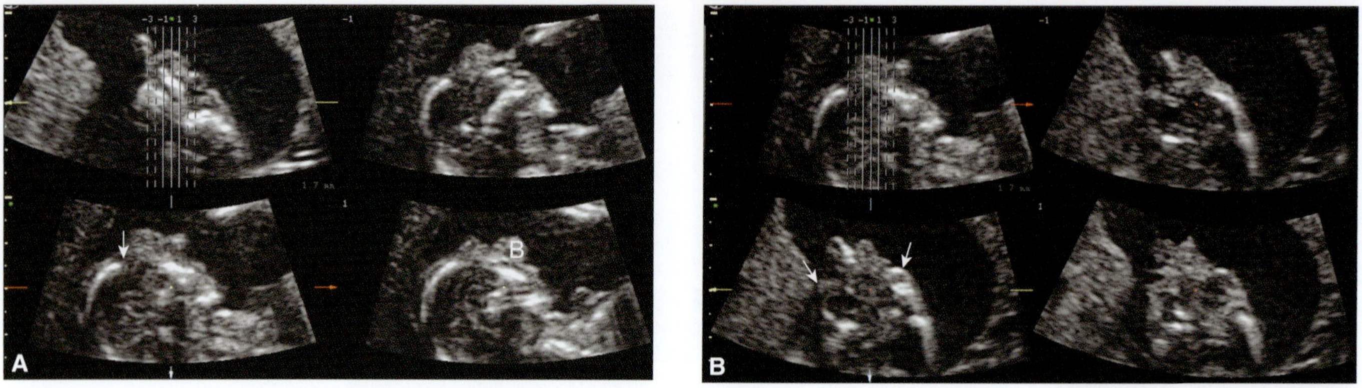

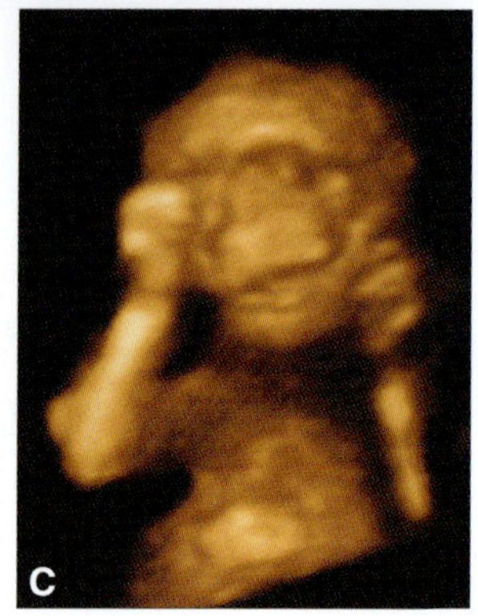

**Figure 5–25.** A transabdominal volume was obtained at 16 postmenstrual weeks of a fetus with an anterior encephalocele. This fetus was part of a twin pregnancy; the other fetus was normal. **(A), (B)** Volume displayed using the tomographic feature. In **(A),** median as well as parasagittal sections of the face are seen, showing an anterior facial mass (encephalocele). The large skull defect (*arrow*) as well as the brain extending into the mass is apparent. In **(B),** the orbits (*small arrows*) are seen to be widely separated by the encephalocele. **(C)** The surface rendering of the face reveals an abnormality with a large irregular mass (encephalocele) between the eyes.

Most fetuses with Meckel-Gruber syndrome are either stillborn or die within the first day of life due to the dysplastic kidneys that result in oligohydramnios and in turn result in hypoplastic lungs, although prolonged survival up to 28 months has been reported.[98] Kaplan et al[99] reported on a rare case of survival of a child with prenatally diagnosed Meckel syndrome variant. In that case, the child had an occipital cephalocele and a unilateral multicystic kidney, with the remaining kidney having normal renal function.

## Walker-Warburg Syndrome (Lissencephaly Type II, HARD (±E) Syndrome)

The descriptive acronym for this syndrome, HARD (±E), refers to the distinguishing features of this entity: hydrocephaly, agyria (lissencephaly), retinal dysplasia, Dandy-Walker malformation, and at times encephalocele. Cephalocele is not considered diagnostic for Walker-Warburg syndrome and is seen in ~26.7% of cases reported.[100] Walker-Warburg syndrome is caused by mutation in the genes encoding protein O-mannosyltransferase-1 (POMT1); and -2 (POMT2; gene map locus 14q24.3, 9q34.1, 9q31, 22q12.3-q13.1, 19q13.3). The prognosis of newborns with the syndrome is dismal[100,101](Figure 5–31).

## Knobloch Syndrome

Knobloch is a rare syndrome characterized by vitreoretinal degeneration and occipital encephalocele. This automosal syndrome is caused by mutation in the collagen XVIII, alpha-1 polypeptide (*COL18A1* gene; gene map locus 21q22.3). The encephalocele is mild and contains only a small amount of dysplastic glial or neuronal tissue. Usually there is normal cognitive development; however, eye pathology may be severe.[102]

## Sonographic Diagnosis

The sonographic appearance of an occipital cephalocele is that of a sac-like structure adjacent to the fetal head. The cephaloceles show a range in size not only of the skull defect but also of the cephalocele sac itself. The size of the cephalocele may range from a few millimeters to a mass exceeding the size of the normal cranial vault.[103] In infants the size distribution of cephaloceles are as follows: 16% are >20 cm, 14% are between 15 and 20 cm, 12% are between 10 and 15 cm, 30% are between 5 and 10 cm, and 28% are <5 cm.[78] The head circumference and BPD may be significantly smaller than expected for the fetal age. Microcephaly was reported to occur in 9% to 24% of cases,[78] and ventriculomegaly was reported in 47% of in utero cases.[104] Other malformations are agenesis of the corpus callosum, Dandy-Walker cyst, holoprosencephaly (lobar), and Arnold-Chiari type II malformation.[78] Closer inspection of the cranium reveals a defect through which the contents of the cephalocele sac communicate with the intracranial portion of the brain structures. The sac may contain brain tissue (encephalocele) (Figure 5–18), or it may be sonolucent, containing only CSF (meningocele).[55,105,106] Meningoceles account for ~10% to 20% of occipital lesions.[11] The brain tissues most often present in the encephalocele sac are the occipital

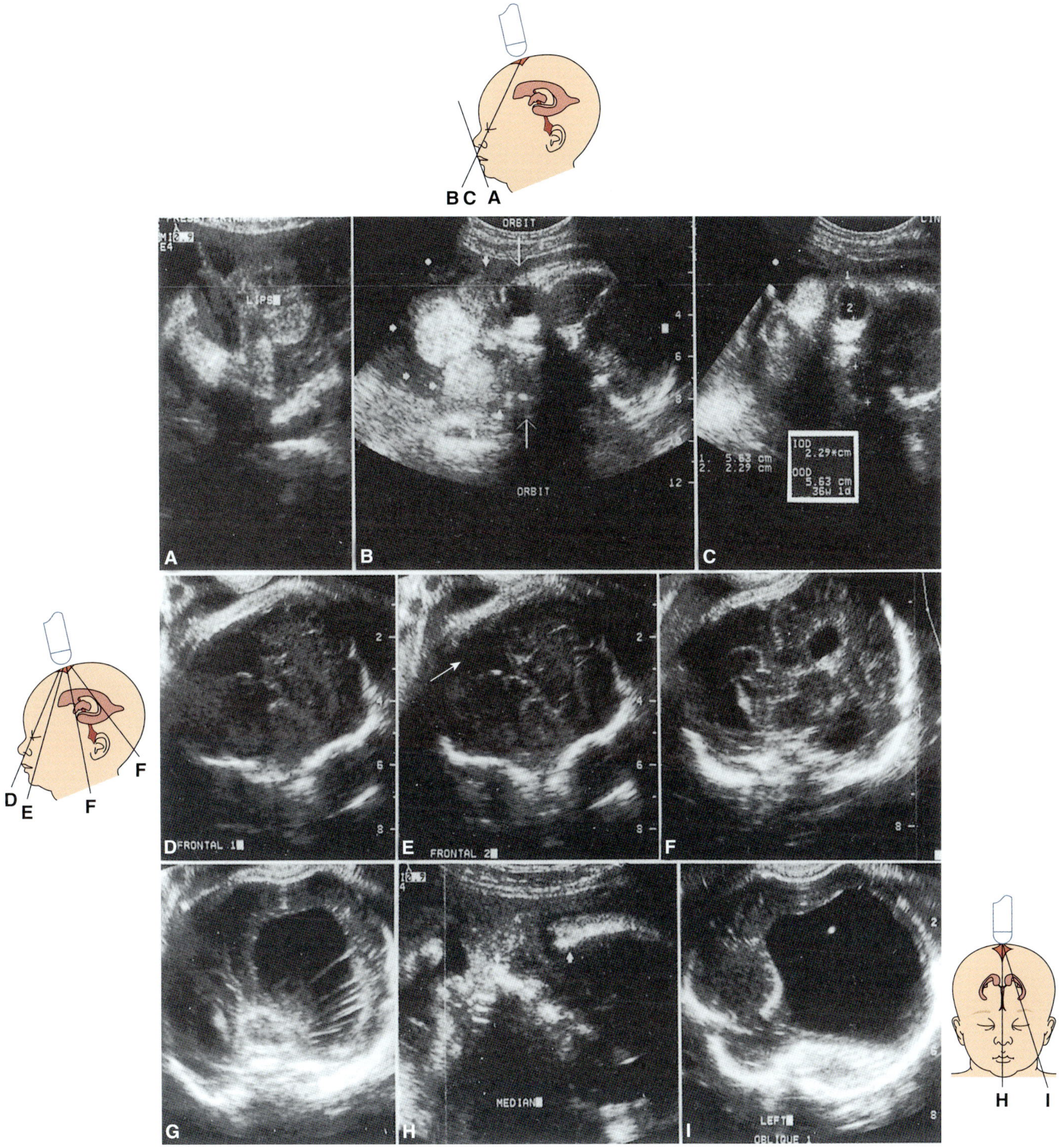


**Figure 5–26.** Anterior encephalocele at 35 weeks, 3 days. The patient was referred for a second-opinion US because of a suspected large subarachnoid cyst and microcephaly. **(A)–(C)** Hypertelorism is noted with a hyperchogenic mass protruding between the fetal orbits. IOD, interorbital distance; OOD, outer orbital distance. **(D)–(G)** Serial coronal sections from anterior to posterior of the fetal brain. **(D)** Frontal–1 section showing an irregularly shaped head and interhemispheric fissure. **(E)** Frontal–2 section here a sonolucent structure (*arrow*). **(F), (G)** The hemispheres are not symmetrical, and the ventricle is dilated and contains some adhesions. **(H)** Median section showing the cranial defect (*arrow*) through which the brain tissue has herniated. **(I)** Left oblique–1 sections showing the unilateral hydrocephaly.

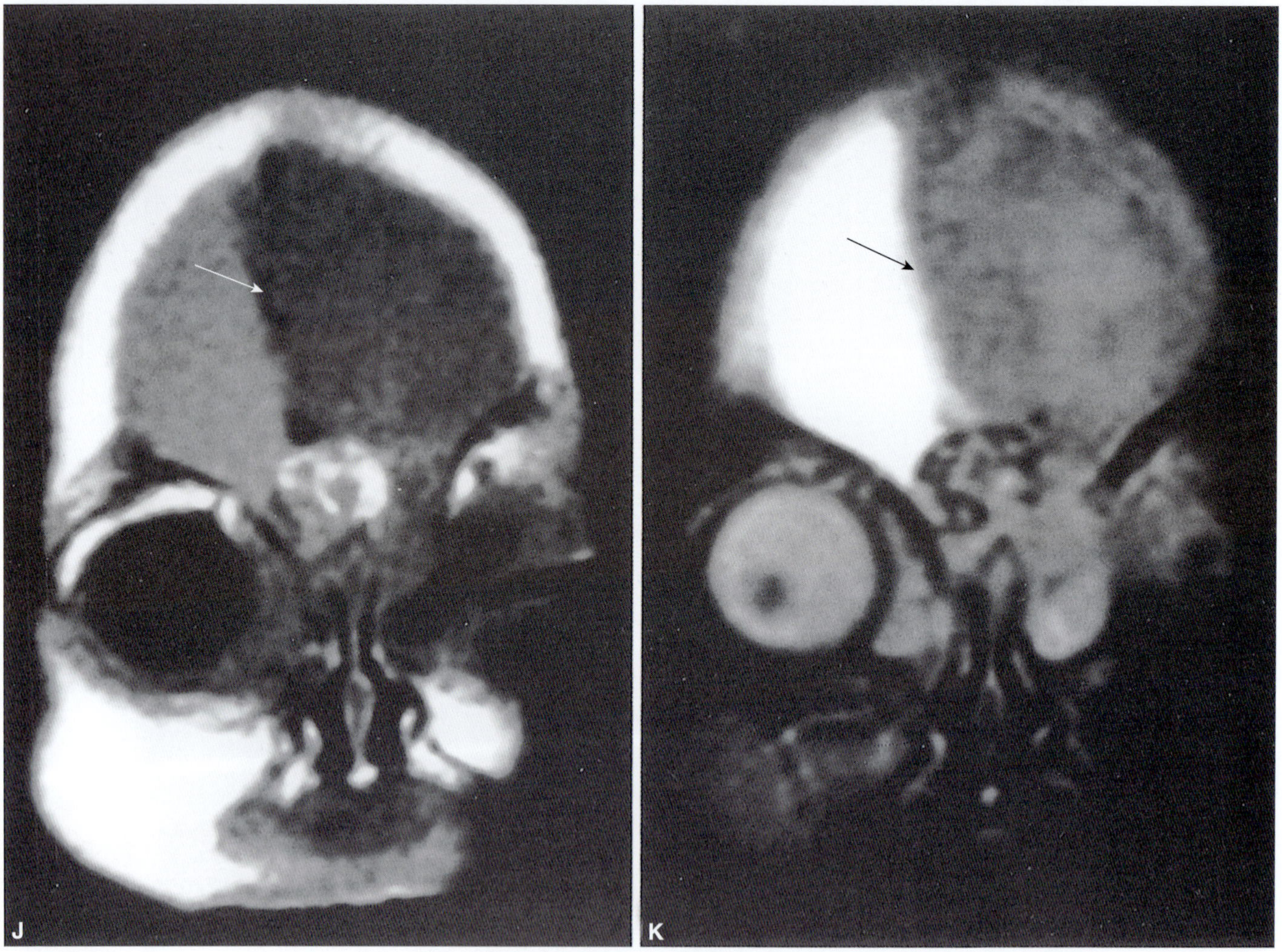


**Figure 5–26.** *(continued)* (J)–(M) Magnetic resonance imaging of the neonate. (J), (K) Coronal sections showing a large cystic area in addition to the encephalocele (*arrow*).

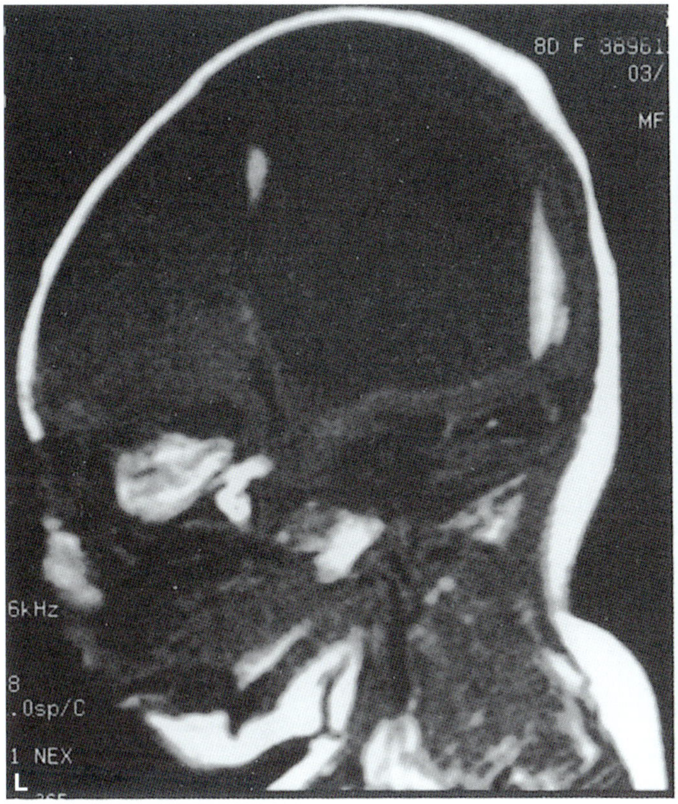


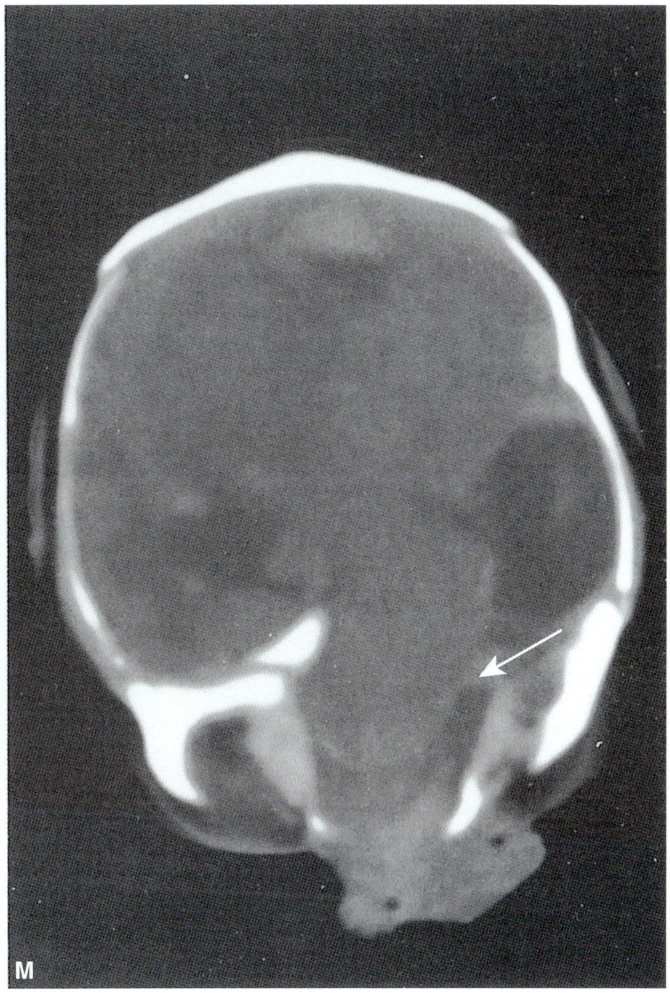


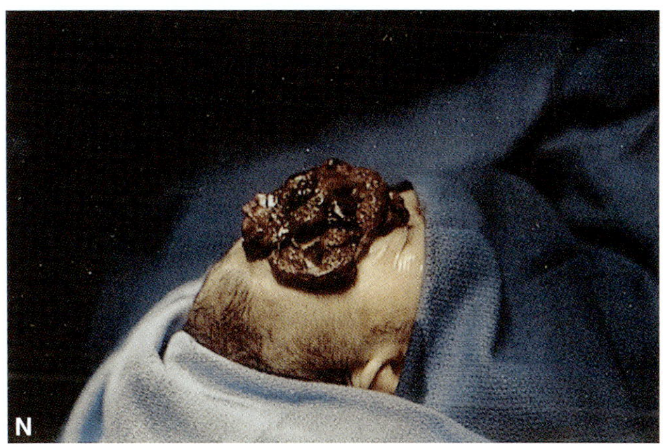


**Figure 5–26.** *(continued)* **(L)** Sagittal section showing unilateral hydrocephaly. **(M)** Axial section showing the nasoethmoidal skull defect (*arrow*) through which the brain is herniating. **(N)** Picture of the neonate at the time of surgical correction of the encephalocele. At birth, the neonate had multiple problems, including severe anemia, seizures, tonic posturing, and abnormal tongue movements. A ventriculoperitoneal shunt was subsequently placed. By the eighth month of life, the infant had had multiple hospital admissions and her problems included diabetes insipidus, epilepsy, and temperature instability.

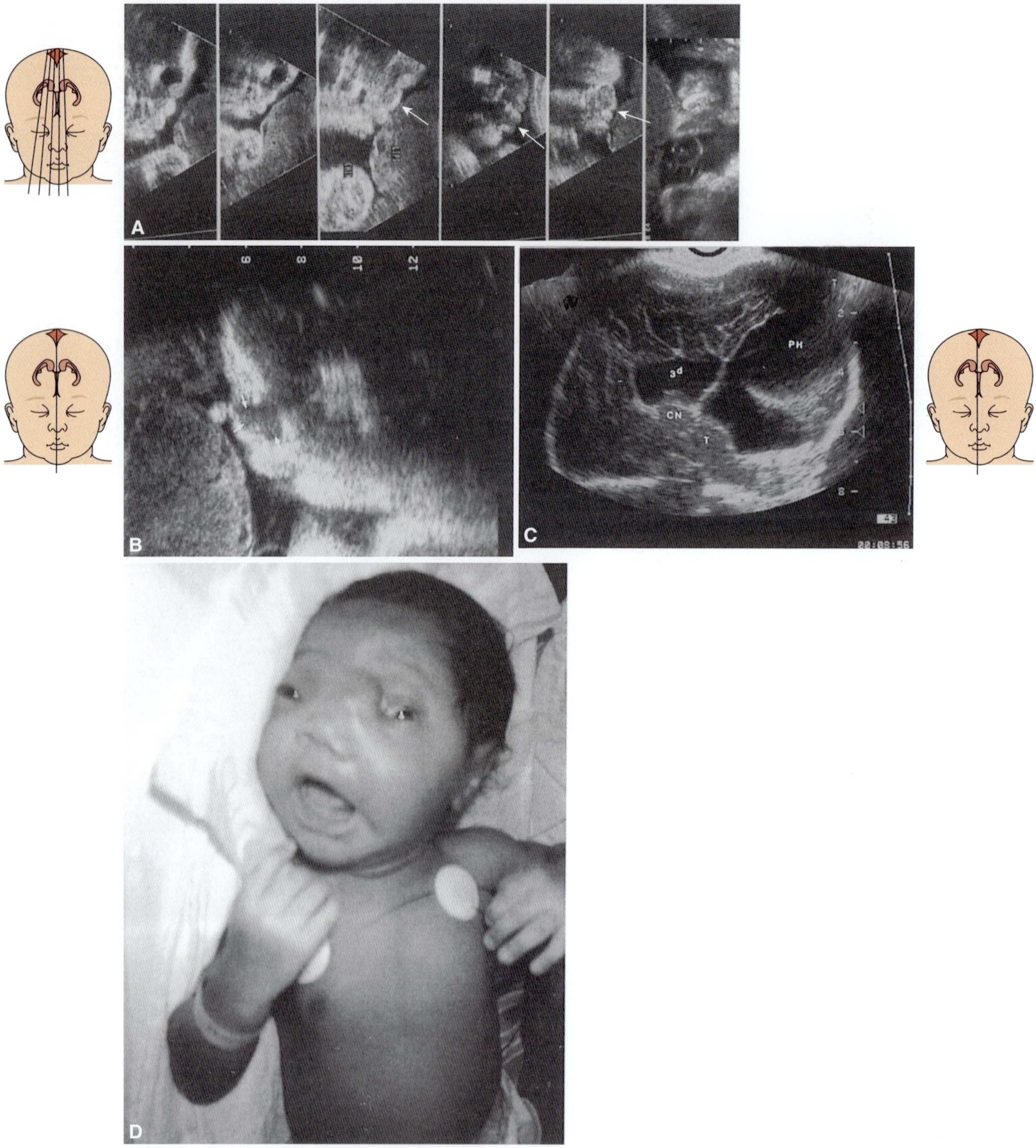


**Figure 5–27.** Anterior encephalocele in a fetus at 36 postmenstrual weeks. **(A)** Serial sections in the sagittal plane showing the profile and a mass bulging to distort the normal shape of the profile (*arrows*). **(B)** Median section of the face showing the sonolucent bulge marked by arrows just behind the prominence of the nose. **(C)** Median section of the brain showing the typical sunburst appearance of the gyri above the space representing the third ventricle. This is typical of the sonographic image of agenesis of the corpus callosum. The posterior horn (PH) is widely dilated. CN, caudate nucleus; T, thalamus. **(D)** The neonate clearly showing a distorted face and widely spaced eyes (hypertelorism), as well as a bulge in the midline or somewhat closer to the left eye. The slight distortion and slight displacement of the nose are evident.

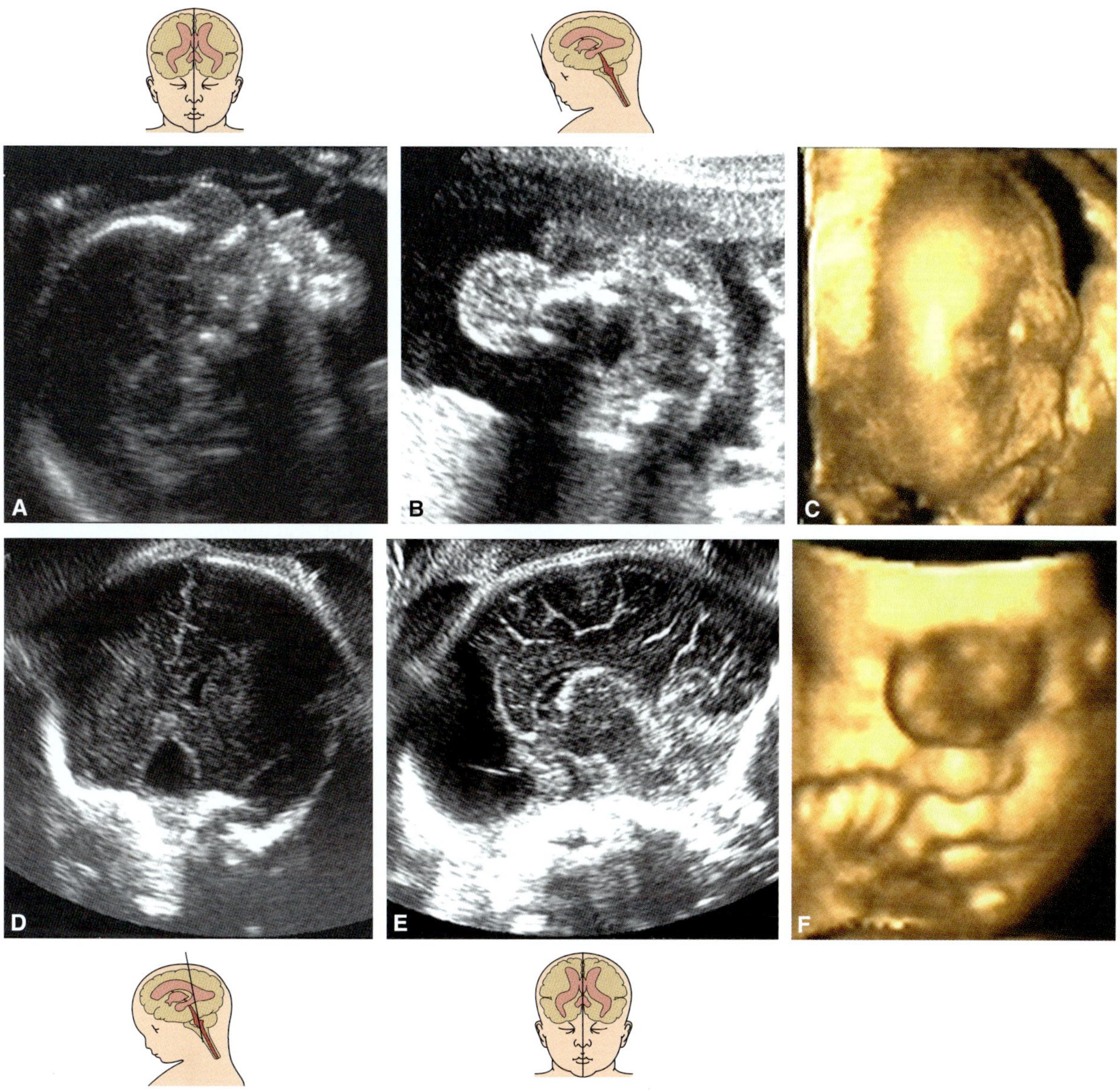


**Figure 5–28.** A fetus with an anterior encephalocele was scanned at 25 **(A)–(C)** and 32 **(D), (E)** postmenstrual weeks using 2D and 3D sonography. **(A)** The profile shows a mass superior to the nose and the nasal bone, as well as the skull defect. Although the brain is not clearly seen, it was normal. **(B)** Coronal section through the level of the anterior cephalocele. **(C)** The rendered face showing the mass. **(D), (E)** At 32 postmenstrual weeks in the anterior coronal and median section of the brain (E), a sonolucent space is seen; this is the result of the herniated brain into the cephalocele sac. **(F)** The rendered image of the fetus at 32 postmenstrual weeks.

lobes, which exhibit a normal gyral pattern (Figure 5–22 and 5–23). Approximately half of the cephaloceles situated "low" in the cervical region contain the occipital lobes of the hemispheres, but almost all contain the cerebellum.[11]

Hydrocephaly may be present in 20% to 65% of cases as a result of aqueductal stenosis or Chiari III malformation. The corpus callosum is usually present, but it may also be completely or partially missing. The septum pellucidum may be absent in up to 80% of cases.[78] Other associated malformations that may be apparent are cerebellar dysplasia, spinal dysraphism, diastematomyelia, Klippel-Feil deformity, Dandy-Walker malformation, cleft palate, microphthalmia, tracheoesophageal fistula, and cardiac malformations.[32,78,105,107]

Early diagnosis of occipital cephalocele is possible (Figure 5–17). Fleming et al[108] reported on the prenatal diagnosis of an occipital encephalocele using TVS at 12 postmenstrual weeks. It is important to note that some of the abnormalities associated with occipital cephaloceles (eg, agenesis of the corpus callosum) may only become sonographically apparent later on, during the late second or third trimester of pregnancy.

The sonographic appearance of an anterior cephalocele is that of an irregularly shaped mass protruding from the fetal face (Figures 5–24, 5–25, 5–26, 5–27, and 5–28). Associated anomalies include ocular hypertelorism, nasal widening, cleft lip and/or palate, median nasal fissure, spina bifida, agenesis of the corpus callosum,

**Table 5–6. SYNDROMES WITH ACEPHALOCELE**

| Syndrome | Other Features Detectable with Prenatal Ultrasound |
|---|---|
| Apert | Craniosynostosis, short skull base, syndactyly hands and feet, megalencephaly, encephalocele |
| Craniotelencephalic dysplasia | Craniosynostosis, frontal encephalocele at metopic region, microphthalmia, septo-optic dysplasia, agenesis of the corpus callosum, lissencephaly, arhinencephaly |
| Cranium bifidum occultum | Occipital encephalocele |
| Dyssegmental dysplasia | Clefting, encephalocele, micromelia, thick and bowed bones |
| Facio-auriculo-vertebral | Face hypoplasia, cardiac and vertebral anomalies, posterior cephalocele |
| Fried: Meckel like | Lobar holoprosencephaly, large occipital encephalocele, microcephaly, congenital heart disease. |
| Fronto-facio-nasal-dysplasia | Cranium bifidum occultum, anterior cephalocele, cleft lip and/or palate |
| Frontonasal dysplasia | Hypertelorism, frontonasal encephalocele, median cleft lip |
| Meckel-Gruber | Microcephaly, encephalocele, microphthalmia, cleft lip and palate, cystic dysplastic kidneys, polydactyly |
| Oculo-encephalo-hepato-renal | Micrognathia, postaxial polydactyly, cystic renal dysplasia, meningoencephalocele |
| Phocomelia-encephalocele-urogenital anomalies | Bilateral radial aplasia, absent right thumb, fused pelvic kidney, dextroposed heart, hypoplastic lung, thin corpus callosum, encephalocele |
| Roberts-SC phocomelia | Microbrachycephaly, growth restriction, cleft lip and palate, frontal encephalocele |
| von Voss-Cherstvoy: limb defects, thrombocytopenia | Occipital encephalocele, absent corpus callosum, hypoplastic thumbs, renal agenesis |
| Walker-Warburg | Type II lissencephaly, cerebellar malformations, vermis hypoplasia, micropthalmia, posterior encephalocele |
| Warfarin embryopathy | Micropthalmia, cardiac anomalies, occipital encephalocele |

Data from Hunter AG. Brain and spinal cord. In: Stevenson RE, Hall JG, Goodman RM, eds. *Human Malformations and Related Anomalies.* Vol 2. New York: Oxford University Press; 1993:109–137.

ventriculomegaly, and microcephaly.[81] The differential diagnosis of an anterior cephalocele includes teratoma, glioma, dermal sinus cyst, facial hemangioma, orbital duplication, and proboscis.

Three-dimensional ultrasound can render the fetal face and can therefore be useful in further evaluating cases in which an anterior cephalocele is present (see Figures 5–25C and 5–28). In addition, rendering can be applied to other types of cephalocele (see Figures 5–17C, 5–18, and 5–19A). The 3D orthogonal planes as well as the tomographic US imaging display can aid in the exact localization and extent of the cephalocele, as well as in the total evaluation of the intracranial anatomy (see Figures 5–19A, 5–19B, C, and 5–25).

There are no published reports of fetuses with atretic meningoceles. We have diagnosed two patients with this condition. In both cases the patients were referred for evaluation because of the presence of a parietal bone defect (Figure 5–32). The visualization of an abnormal falcine artery or an abnormally positioned straight sinus is indicative of an atretic meningocele and helps in the differential diagnosis.

## Risk of Recurrence

The recurrence risk for sporadic (nonsyndromic) occipital cephaloceles is 1% to 3%; however, if the cephalocele is the result of an autosomal recessive condition such as Meckel-Gruber or Walker-Warburg syndrome, the risk is 25%.

## Differential Diagnosis

Cephalocele must be distinguished from midline scalp masses, such as cysts, hemangiomas, nuchal tumors, cephalohematoma, cystic teratomas, scalp edema, cystic hygroma, branchiogenic cyst, and fetal hair (during the third trimester).[109–114] In all cases in which a cephalocele is suspected, a careful search for the cranial defect and possible associated anomalies must be undertaken.

## Prognosis

The prognosis for fetuses with a cephalocele depends on the location, size, and content of the lesion and on the concurrent intracranial as well as extracranial malformations (Table 5–7). The small defects can be easily corrected with

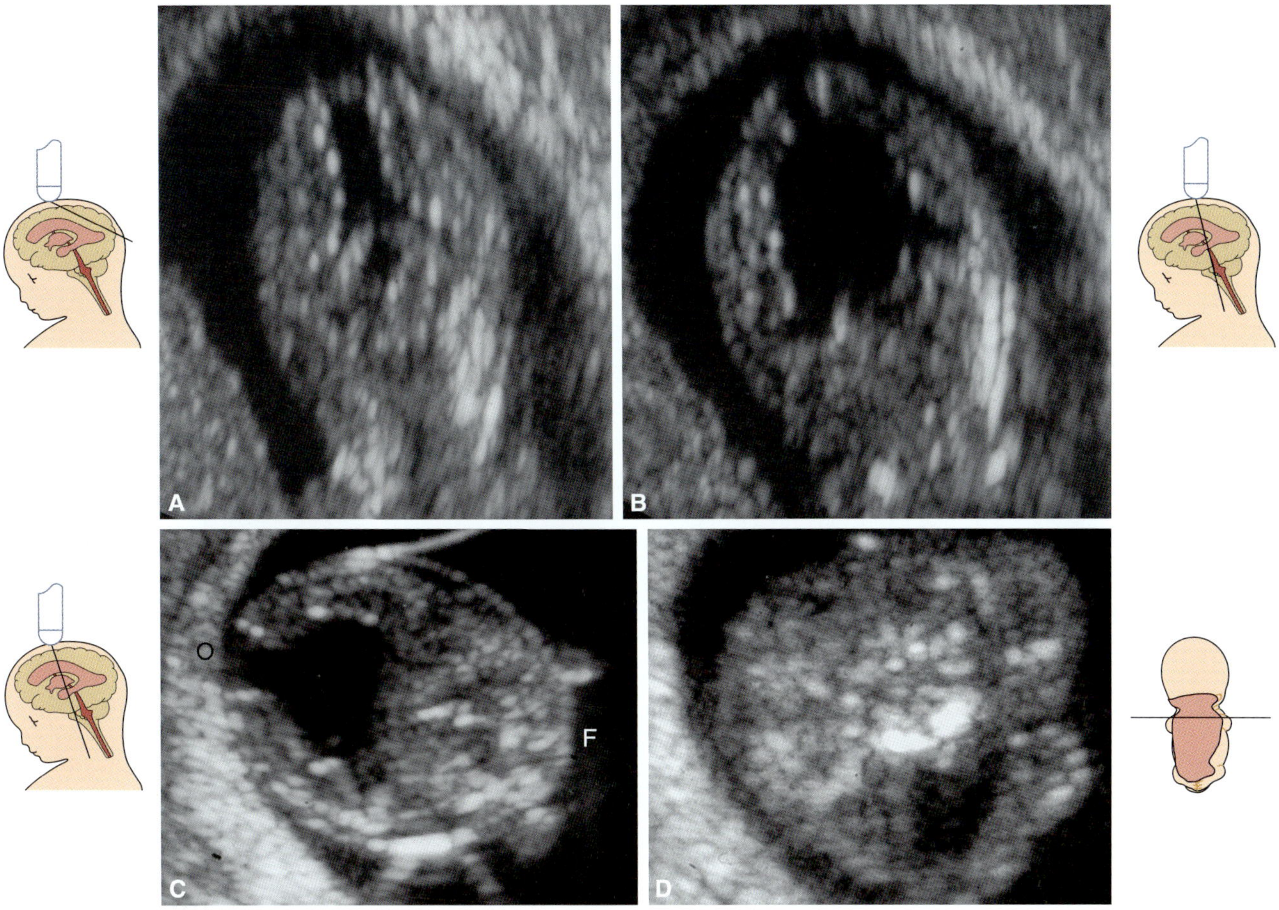


**Figure 5–29.** Meckel-Gruber syndrome (MGS) at 11 weeks, 3 days. This patient was at high risk for MGS because she had a previous child with this syndrome. At the time of this scan, a posterior skull defect was seen, as well as a large posterior fossa. There was no polydactyly (similarly, no polydactyly was present in the previous MGS infant). **(A), (B)** Posterior coronal sections showing a large sonolucent midline cystic area that is freely connected with the amniotic cavity. **(C)** Axial section showing the cranial defect and large cystic structure, which completely fill the area of the posterior fossa. O, occipital; F, frontal. **(D)** A view of the right arm and hand of the fetus showing five digits.

surgery, but larger lesions are usually not compatible with life or may result in a neurologically impaired infant.[115] The reported survival rate for infants with posterior cephalocele ranges from 40% to 75%.[107,116–118] Mortality is most commonly due to the severity of the other associated malformation or the inability to repair the defect. Meningocele has a lower mortality rate that ranges from 10% to 25%.[119] Disabilities occur in the surviving children. Brown et al[119] reported that 25% of the surviving infants with occipital cephalocele had severe long-term disability, and 38% had a mild handicap. These disabilities occurred in their series regardless of the defect size, as well as the presence or absence of brain tissue in the cephalocele.

Anterior cephaloceles appear to carry a relatively better prognosis than other types of cephaloceles. Brown and Sheridan-Pereira[119] found that 42% of children with anterior cephaloceles were normal, 17% had mild handicaps, and 25% had severe handicaps. The primary morbidity in children with anterior defects is facial disfigurement, anosmia, and visual problems.[118,120] Surgical procedures for anterior cephalocele offer only a very limited improvement of the facial deformity, and many of the children who have survived suffer cosmetic facial and eye deformities.[79,85,118,120,121]

The prognosis for the infant with a parietal cephalocele is the following: ~33% will die, 40% will have marked mental retardation, 13% will be able to get an education, and 15% will develop normally.[104]

### Obstetric Management

Delivery route needs to be individualized after consultation with the appropriate specialists, such as maternal-fetal medicine, neonatology, and pediatric neurosurgery.[25]

## SPINAL DYSRAPHISM AND CHIARI II MALFORMATION

### Synonyms

Spina bifida, Chiari II malformation, Arnold-Chiari malformation, open NTD

The term *Chiari II malformation* refers to a constellation of brain anomalies commonly associated with an open spinal defect; therefore, both entities will be described together.

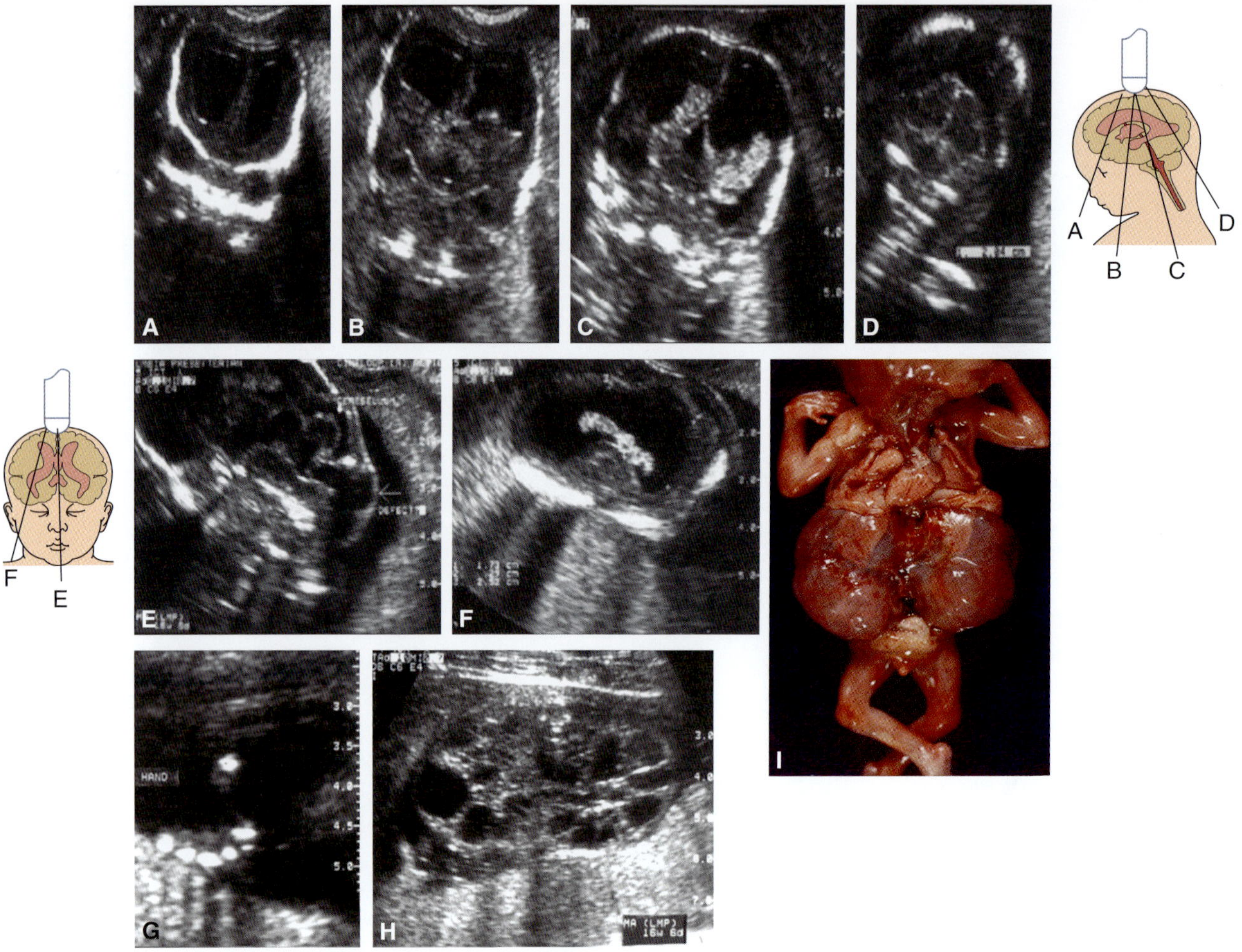


**Figure 5–30.** Meckel-Gruber syndrome at 16 weeks, 6 days. The systematic workup of the brain is shown in panels **(A)–(F)**. **(A)** Frontal–2 section showing the enlarged anterior horns. **(B)** Midcoronal–1 section: The severely dilated lateral ventricles are evident. **(C)** Midcoronal–2 section: The dangling hyperechogenic choroid plexus is seen (dangling choroid plexus sign); the dilated third ventricle is also seen. **(D)** Occipital–2 section showing the cerebellum. **(E)** Median section with an arrow pointing to a very small encephalocele. **(F)** Oblique–1 sections through the lateral ventricle; the anterior, posterior, and inferior horns are seen on the same section. The choroid plexus above the thalamus (T) is freely floating in the cerebrospinal fluid. **(G)** The additional feature of this syndrome is the postaxial polydactyly (*arrow*). **(H)** The enlarged multicystic kidneys. **(I)** The aborted specimen with the two large kidneys exposed.

## Definition

Spinal dysraphism refers to a defect in which the spine is open with protrusion of the spinal contents through the bony defect. Myelocele and myelomeningocele develop similarly, but the term *myelocele* refers to a midline plaque of neural tissue (neural placode) that is flush with the surface and is not covered by skin. In contrast, the myelomeningocele is a bulging defect in which the elevated neural plate and meninges are contiguous laterally with the subcutaneous tissue.[122] Approximately 10% to 15% of spinal dysraphic defects are closed, and normal skin covers the bony defect (Figure 5–33).

Chiari II malformation is a complex anomaly resulting from the presence of open spinal dysraphism in which there is herniation of the cerebellar vermis and brainstem through the foramen magnum.[123,124] The abnormal position of these structures causes effacement of the cisterna magna and abnormal placement of the tentorium; hydrocephaly and reduced amount of extra-axial CSF are usually present.

## Incidence

The birth prevalence of spina bifida in the United States is 1.90 per 10,000 live births.[125] This number reflects a downward trend from the 1970s, when the incidence was reported to be 0.5 to 0.6 per 1000 live births.[126] Approximately 80% of the lesions occur in the lumbar, thoracolumbar, or lumbosacral areas of the spine and the remaining 20% in the cervical and sacral areas.[127]

## Pathogenesis

The onset of myelomeningocele is probably around the fourth (postconceptual or postmenstrual) week of gestation at the time of closure of the posterior neural tube.

There are four main theories that have been proposed to explain the varied hindbrain anomalies seen in cases of Chiari II malformation.[128] Stevenson[128] summarized and eloquently discussed these four theories: The first theory is that of Chiari, which attributed the hindbrain herniation

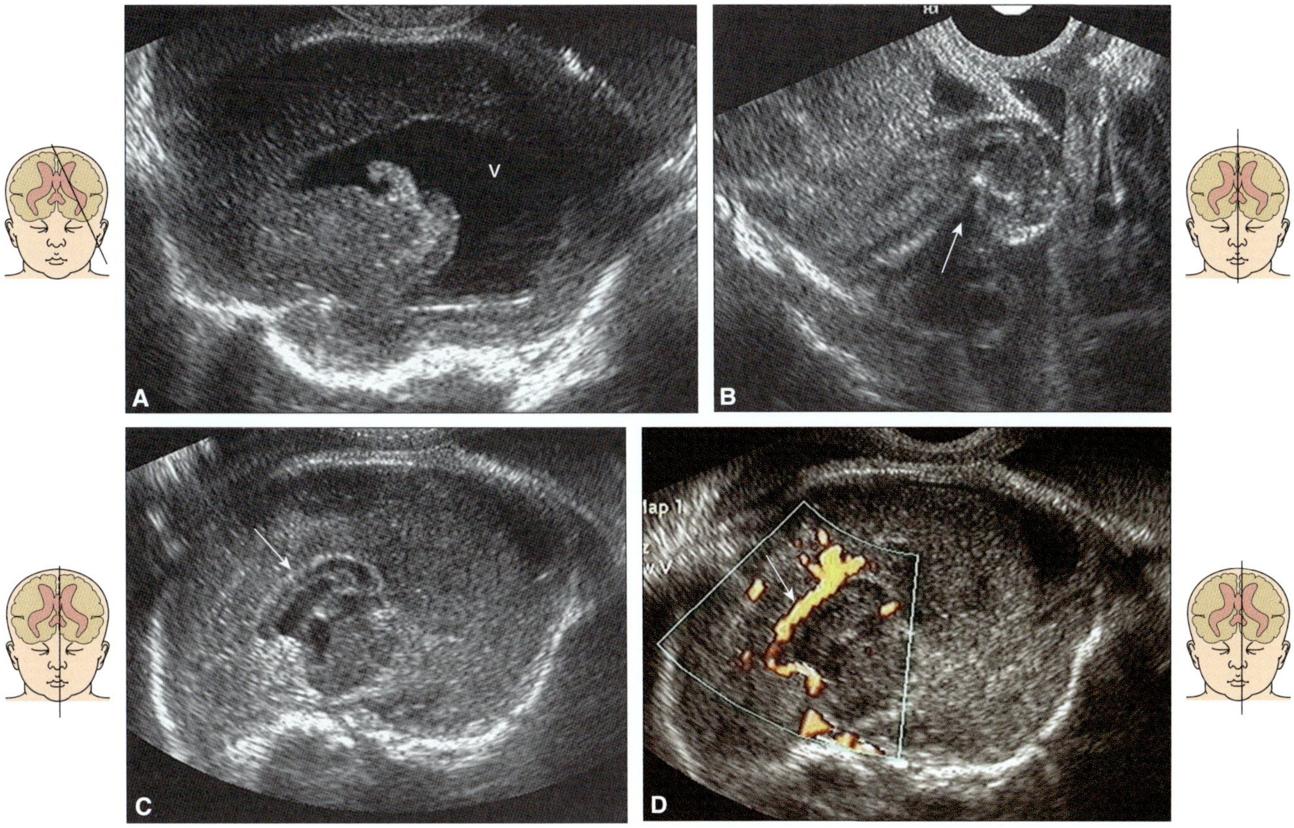


**Figure 5–31.** A 34-week fetus with Walker-Warburg syndrome. **(A)** An oblique section was obtained using transvaginal sonography, which demonstrates the dilated lateral ventricles, V. **(B)** The posterior encephalocele is seen protruding through the skull defect (*arrow*). **(C), (D)** Median section of the fetal brain showing the corpus callosum (*arrow*) and the pericallosal artery (*two arrows*). The brain surface is very smooth, and there is an absence of the cingulate gyrus that is consistent with lissencephaly.

to hydrocephaly;[129] however, prenatal sonography in many instances shows the abnormal posterior fossa and cerebellum ("banana" sign) before the hydrocephaly is seen. The second theory proposed by Cleland[130] is that of primary dysgenesis of the hindbrain; this theory does not explain the cranial and supratentorial anomalies that are commonly seen in patients with Chiari II malformation and spina bifida, but it explains the posterior fossa anomalies. The third theory suggests that the open and tethered spinal cord pulls the hindbrain posteriorly, resulting in the vermian and brainstem herniation seen in Chiari II malformation. The fourth theory is the unified theory of McLone and Knepper,[131] which includes aspects of all of the above theories. In the unified theory, the Chiari II malformation

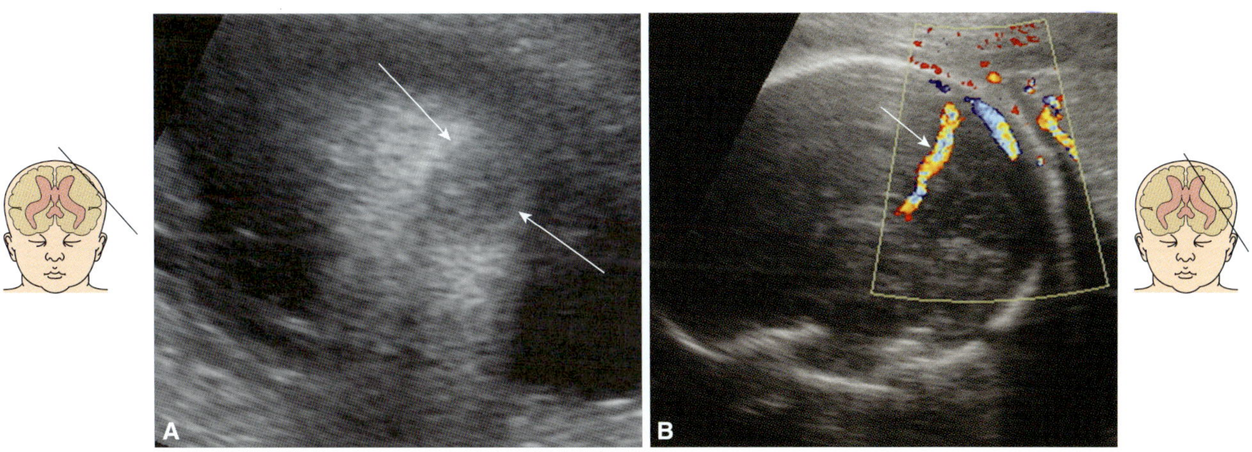


**Figure 5–32.** Transabominal songraphy at 29 weeks, 6 days. **(A)** Parietal bone round defect (*arrows*), **(B)** Color Doppler of the abnormally large vein (*arrow*) reaching the parietal bone at the level of the defect. (Courtesy of Gustavo Malinger.)

**Table 5–7. PROGNOSIS FOR FETUSES WITH CEPHALOCELE**

| Prognosis Better | Prognosis Worse |
|---|---|
| Cranial meningocele | Cranial meningoencephalocele |
| Small nubbing of dysplastic glial or neuronal tissue in hernia | Larger portions of clearly recognizable brain in hernia |
| Cephalocele diameter <5 cm | Cephalocele diameter >5 cm |
| No associated anomalies | Concurrent microcephaly or holoprosencephaly |
| Normal ventricles | In utero ventricular enlargement |

is a result of a series of interrelated time-dependent defects in the development of the ventricular system;[131] essentially, the inability to maintain distention of the ventricular system because of CSF leaks results in the lack of development of the posterior fossa, as well as abnormalities of neural and calvarial development.

## Etiology

The etiology for the Chiari II malformation is the open NTD itself. The etiology for the NTD has been described above.

## Associated Anomalies

Associated brain abnormalities seen with Chiari II malformation can be divided into those of the skull, which includes a small posterior fossa, low-lying tentorium cerebelli, and enlarged foramen magnum; those involving the cerebral hemispheres, such as polymicrogyria, cortical heterotopias, and dysgenesis of the corpus callosum; and those involving the posterior fossa, such as descent of the cerebellar vermis through the foramen magnum, displacement of the superior cerebellum through the tentorium, and aqueductal stenosis. Table 5–8 has a complete list of associated anomalies.[123] Approximately 80% to 90% of children with meningomyelocele and the Chiari II anomaly will develop hydrocephaly.[128] There are multiple reasons for the hydrocephaly in Chiari II, such as obstruction of the outlet of the fourth ventricle, blockage of the cerebellar aqueduct, and obstruction at the level of the abnormal tentorium.[131] Other non-CNS anomalies are congenital scoliosis or kyphosis, hip deformities, and clubfoot.[122,132]

## Sonographic Diagnosis

TVS can image the rudimentary neural tube by the seventh postmenstrual week of gestation (see Chapter 2). The vertebral column can be imaged by the 9th to 10th postmenstrual week; using a median plane, the posterior fetal contour, including the covering skin, can be imaged well enough to detect major neural tube abnormalities.[45,133,134] From the late first to the early second trimester, the fetal spine can be scanned in the three planes (sagittal, coronal, and transverse) using conventional 2D imaging; however, due to fetal position and/or maternal body habitus, not all planes may be accessible in all cases. However, 3D US presents obvious advantages (Figure 5–34). In the sagittal plane, the vertebral column appears as two echogenic, parallel lines, flaring toward the upper cervical spine and converging toward the sacrum (Figure 5–35).[135] In the coronal plane, it appears as two or three (depending on the depth of the scan) parallel bands of echoes corresponding to the body, one on each side of the posterior vertebrae arch (Figure 5–36). In the transverse plane, the intact vertebral arch is represented by a triangular configuration of three echoes, forming a closed circle around the neural canal (Figure 5–37).[115]

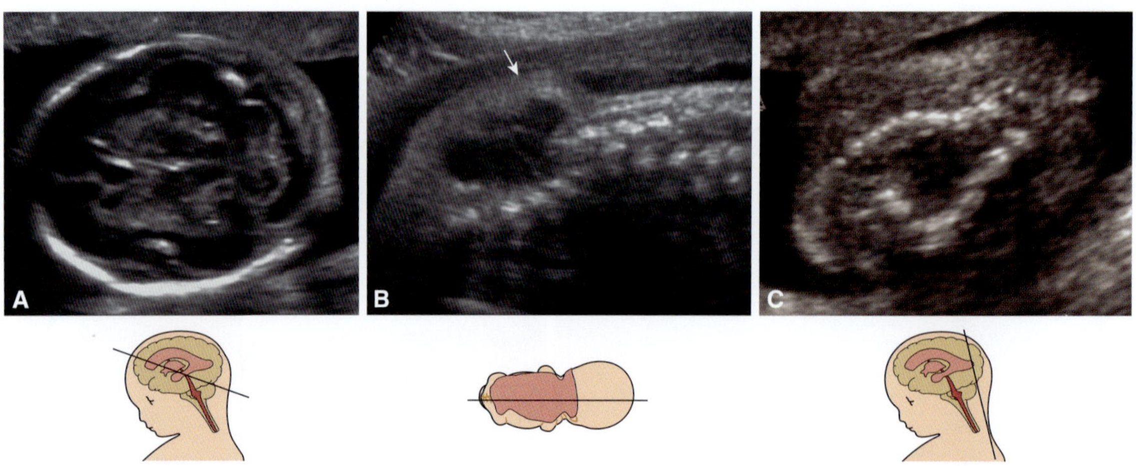


**Figure 5–33.** A patient with a normal maternal serum alpha-fetoprotein. The US revealed a closed neural tube defect. These pictures were taken at 31 weeks, 2 days. **(A)** The fetal head shape and the cerebellum and posterior fossa appear normal. **(B)** A sagittal view of the lumbosacral region of the fetal spine shows a large bulge (*arrow*). The fetal skin is contiguous, covering the myelomeningocele. **(C)** Coronal section shows the splayed vertebrae as the result of the spinal defect.

**Table 5–8. CHIARO-ASSOCIATED CENTRAL NERVOUS SYSTEM MALFORMATIONS**

| Malformation |
|---|
| **Disorders of the skull** |
| Lückenschädel of the skull |
| Small posterior fossa |
| Low-lying tentorium cerebelli with large incisura |
| Scalloping of the petrous bone |
| Shortening of the clivus |
| Enlargement of the foramen magnum |
| **Disorders of the cerebal hemisheres** |
| Polymicrogyria |
| Cortical heterotopias |
| Dysgnesis of the corpus callosum |
| Large massa intermedia |
| **Disorders of the posterior fossa** |
| Descent of the cerebellar vermis through the foramen magnum |
| Caudal displacement of pons and medulla |
| Rostral displacement of superior cerebellum through the tentorium |
| Kinking of the brainstem |
| Loss of pontine flexure |
| Aqueductal stenosis or forking |
| Beaking of the tectum |

Reproduced, with permission, from McLone DG, Dias MS. The Chiari II malformation: Cause and impact. *Childs Nerv Syst.* 2003;19:540–550.

Prenatal diagnosis of spina bifida is possible before the 12th postmenstrual week by noting irregularities of the bony spine or a bulging within the posterior contour of the fetal back in a sagittal view (Figure 5–38).[136] On transverse sections, the open spine has a U shape, and in the coronal section, the affected bony segment shows a divergent configuration replacing the normal parallel lines of the normal vertebral arches (Figures 5–39 to 5–48). The diagnostic sensitivities for the prenatal sonographic detection of open myelomeningocele are reported to be between 80% and 90% and even higher prior to the knowledge of the MSAFP results.[137–139] Determining the site and the extent of the spinal lesion is important because they correlate with the neurologic outcome of the fetus. The higher and the larger the lesion, the more severe the neurologic dysfunction the neonate will have. The vertebral level can be assessed in a sagittal view of the spine by (1) counting up from the last ossified vertebral segment (S4 in the second and S5 in the third trimester) (2) assuming that the last rib corresponds to T12, and the top of the iliac wing corresponds to L5 to S1.[140] Using this method, Kollias et al[140] reported that the pathology and the in utero US assessment of the spinal level agreed in 64% of cases, and in an additional 14% it correlated to within one vertebra of the lesion. Three-dimensional US can be used to count the ribs and determine the level of the spinal defect (Figures 5–42 and 5–43).

Spina bifida occulta refers to a spinal anomaly that is covered with skin and hence with no exposed neural tissue. If only the spinous process and neural arch of the vertebrae are affected, this is usually an asymptomatic condition, rarely diagnosed in utero, and not associated with elevated MSAFP. However, commonly *spina bifida occulta* is used as

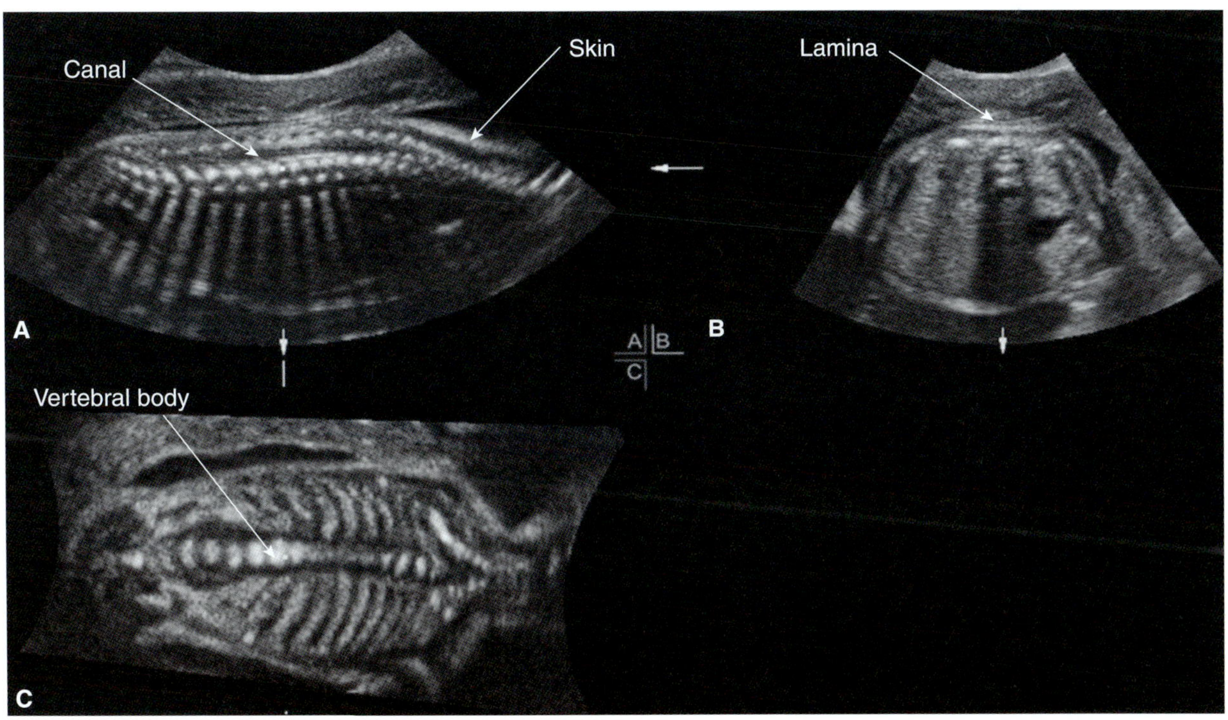


**Figure 5–34.** Using 3D sonography, the spine is displayed along three orthogonal scanning planes: sagittal (**A**), transverse (**B**), and coronal (**C**).

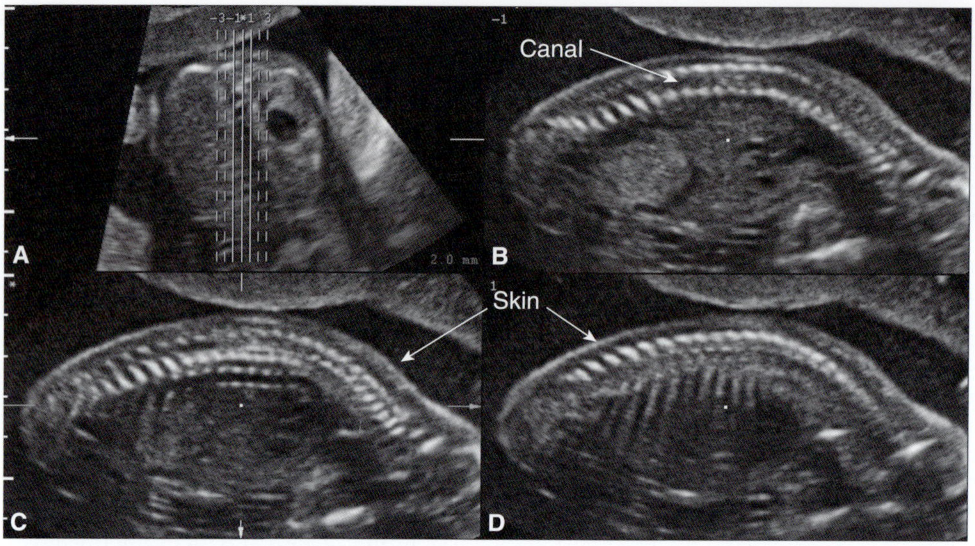


**Figure 5–35.** A volume of a normal fetal spine is displayed using 3D tomography. **(A)** Transverse section of the fetal abdomen at the level of the stomach; the parallel lines are placed 2 mm from each other. **(B)–(D)** Display of three sagittal sections of the fetal spine at 2 mm from each other. Note that the posterior contour of the spine (skin) is seen in its entirety. The bony components of the vertebrae are seen and are also parallel to each other.

a general term to include conditions such as tethered spinal cord, lipomyelomeningocele, lipomeningocele, thickened filum terminale, fatty filum terminale, diastematomyelia (split spinal cord), diplomyelia, and dermal sinus tract (with involvement of the spinal cord); these conditions can be associated with significant neurologic dysfunction.

After the 12th week, there are well-established intracranial sonographic findings that can enhance the detection of spina bifida, namely, the "lemon" sign, the "banana sign,"[141,142] and hydrocephaly (Figures 5–44, 5–45, 5–46, 5–47, and 5–48). The lemon sign refers to deformity of the frontal bone, and the banana sign refers to the

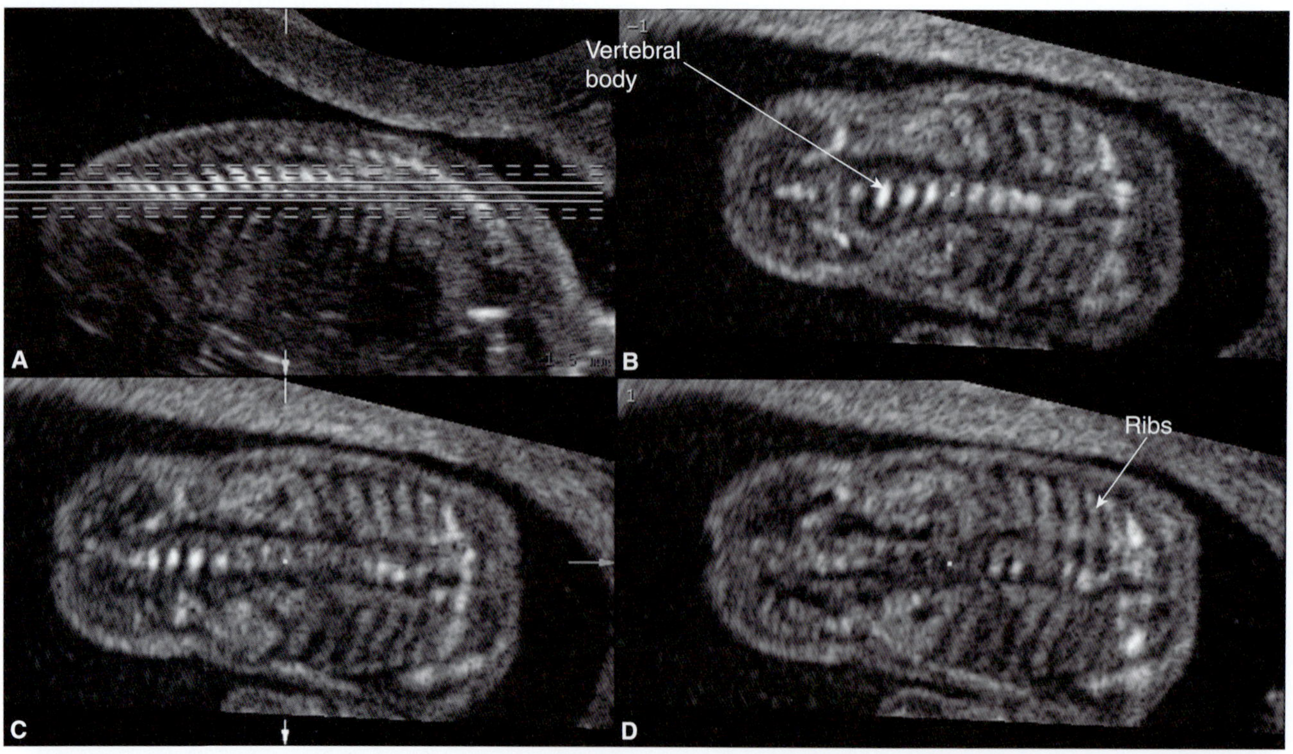


**Figure 5–36.** Volume of a normal fetal spine displayed using 3D tomography. **(A)** Sagittal section. The longitudinal lines are 1.5 mm from each other, the same distance between the sections in **(B)–(D)**. **(B)–(D)** Three coronal sections of the fetal spine at 1.5 mm from each other. **(B)** A coronal section demonstrating the vertebral bodies; due to the normal curvature of the spine, only a part of the vertebral bodies of the fetus are seen. **(C), (D)** Two more anterior coronal sections displaying the fetal ribs.

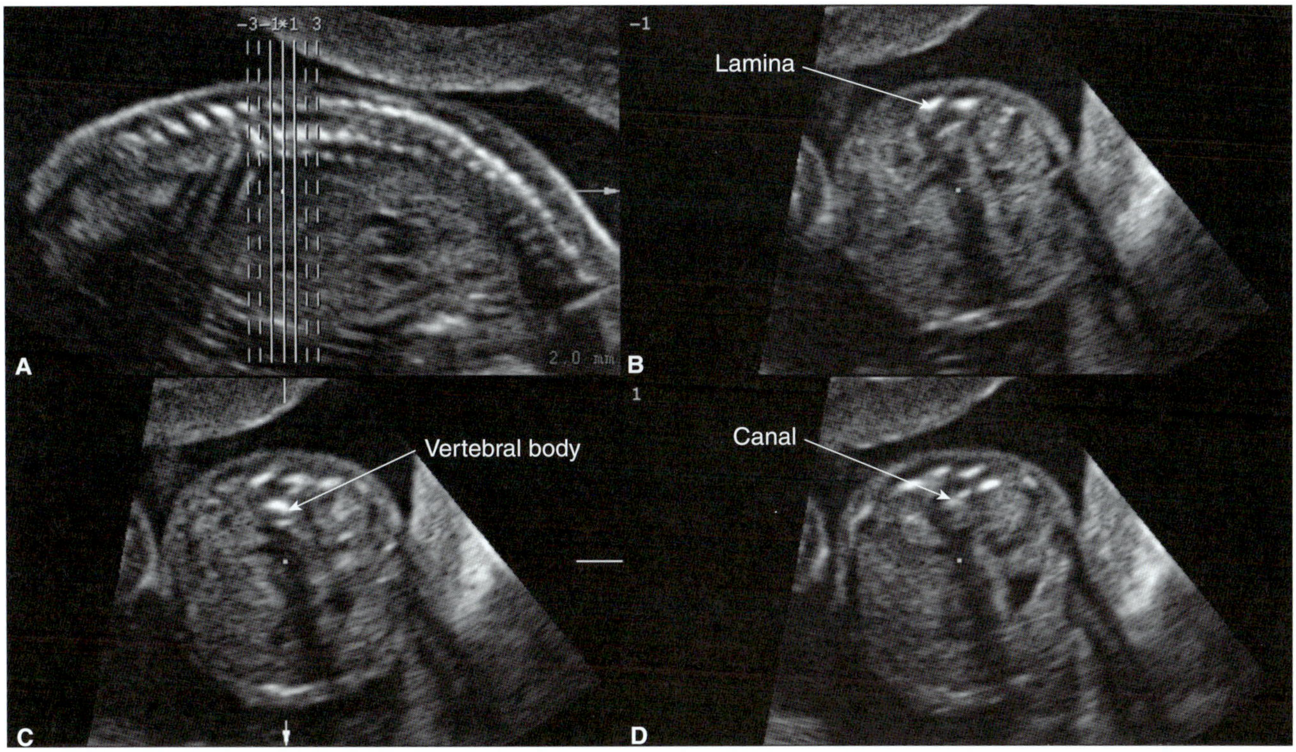


**Figure 5–37.** A volume of a normal fetal spine is displayed using 3D tomography. **(A)** Sagittal section: The lines are 2 mm from each other. **(B)–(D)** Three axial (transverse) sections of the fetal spine are 2 mm from each other. These transverse sections through the fetal spine demonstrate the triangular configuration of the lamina and vertebral bodies enclosing the spinal canal. Note the skin covering the vertebrae.

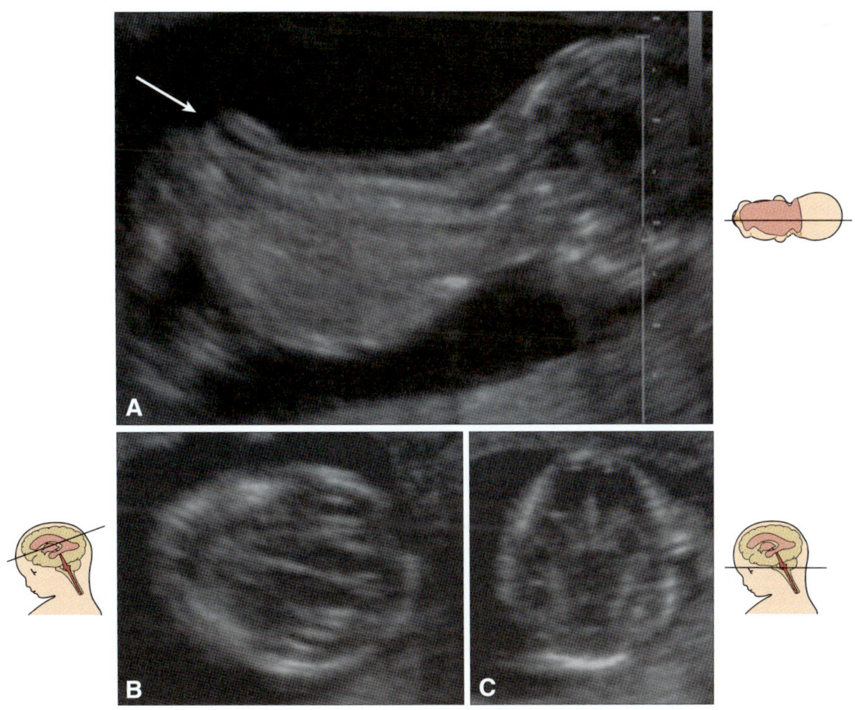


**Figure 5–38.** A fetus with a sacral spinal defect at 12 postmenstrual weeks. **(A)** Sagittal section demonstrating a defect over the sacral area of the spine (*arrow*). **(B), (C)** Because of the gestational age, the typical "lemon" sign is not seen; however, the cerebellum is not clearly seen.

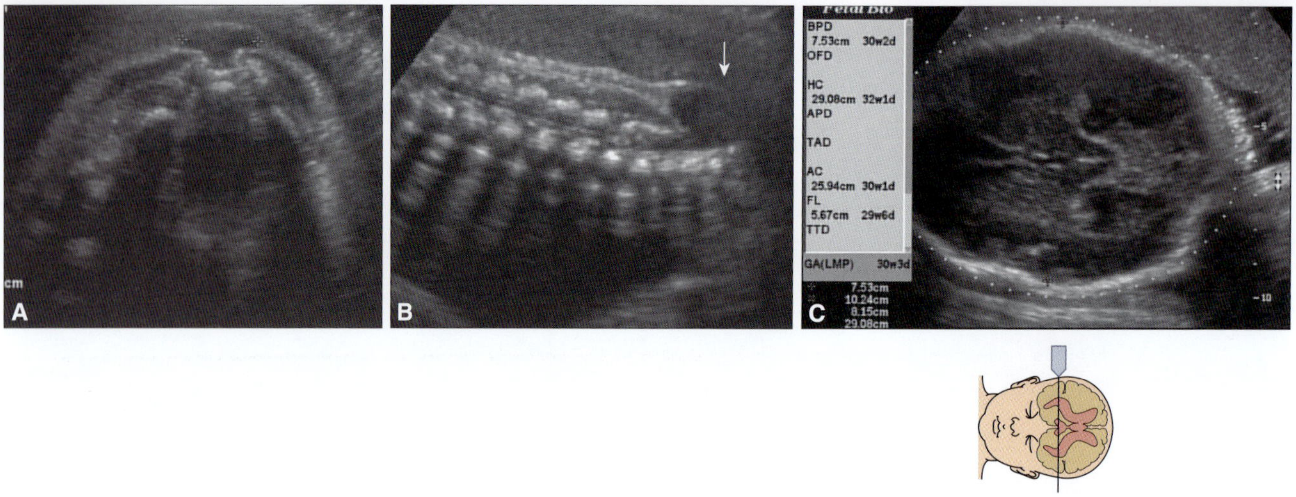


**Figure 5–39.** Transabdominal sonography shows a sacral defect of a fetus at 30 postmenstrual weeks. **(A)** Transverse sections through the spinal defect. Note that the defect is covered by a thin membrane; no skin is covering the defect. In addition, the vertebra has a U-shape. **(B)** Sagittal section showing the extent of the spinal lesion (*arrow*). **(C)** The cerebellum is not seen, as it has completely herniated.

abnormal shape of the flattened cerebellum, which obliterates the cisterna magna. Blumenfeld et al[143] reported on the diagnosis of NTDs between 12 and 17 weeks by using the banana and lemon signs. In one case followed serially from 10 weeks the cerebellum initially appeared normal, by 12 weeks there was a mild convexity of the cerebellum, and by 14 postmenstrual weeks, the typical banana and lemon signs were present. Although only a single report is currently available regarding the earliest appearance of these cranial findings, it seems that the "lemon" and "banana" signs may be imaged from 14 postmenstrual weeks. Therefore, from the early second trimester these indirect cranial findings may be used to enhance the detection of open NTDs. Because these findings may be subtle at 14 to 15 postmenstrual weeks, a follow-up scan later on in the second trimester may be indicated in cases at risk. The lemon sign is present in virtually all cases between 16 and 24 postmenstrual weeks, but after 24 postmenstrual weeks of gestation, the lemon sign is a less reliable marker and is present in only 13% to 50% of fetuses with spinal defects.[132,144–146] It is theorized that the loss of the lemon sign with advancing gestational age in fetuses with spina bifida is the result of maturation and "strengthening" of the fetal skull.[144,145] In contrast, cerebellar abnormalities with obliteration of the cisterna magna are present all through gestation in 95% to 100% of cases,[144,146–148] although after 24 postmenstrual weeks, cerebellar absence is more commonly seen than the banana sign.[132] These indirect cranial findings in conjunction with a spinal defect are referred to as the Chiari II malformation. This malformation is present in almost every case of thoracolumbar, lumbar, and lumbosacral myelomeningocele. In other words, the Chiari II malformation is exclusively found in cases of open spina bifida. The major features include (1) inferior displacement of the medulla and fourth ventricle into the upper cervical canal; (2) elongation and thinning of the upper medulla and lower pons and persistence of the embryonic flexures of these structures, (3) inferior displacement of the lower cerebellum through the foramen magnum (banana sign); and (4) a variety of bony defects of the foramen magnum, occiput, and upper cervical vertebrae.[11] The hydrocephaly probably results from either the hindbrain malformation that blocks the flow of CSF through the fourth ventricle or posterior fossa or from aqueductal stenosis that may be present in 40% to 75% of the cases.[11,12]

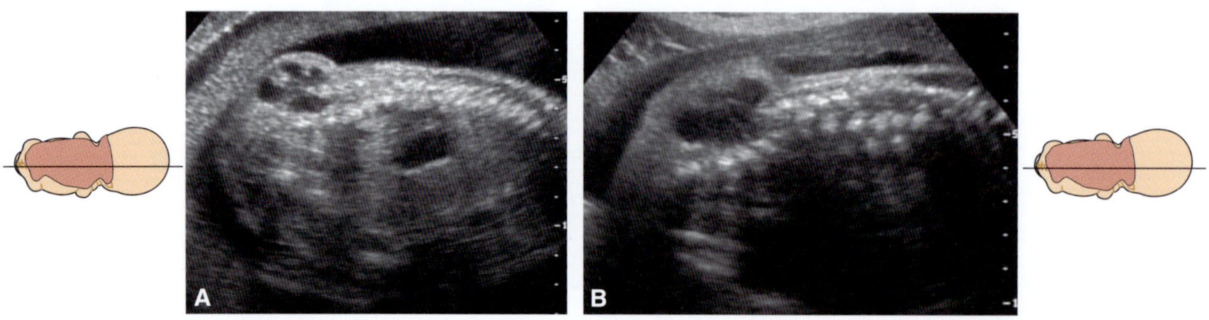


**Figure 5–40.** Two different cases of spina bifida covered by skin. **(A)**, **(B)** Sagittal sections showing the bulging defect covered by skin.

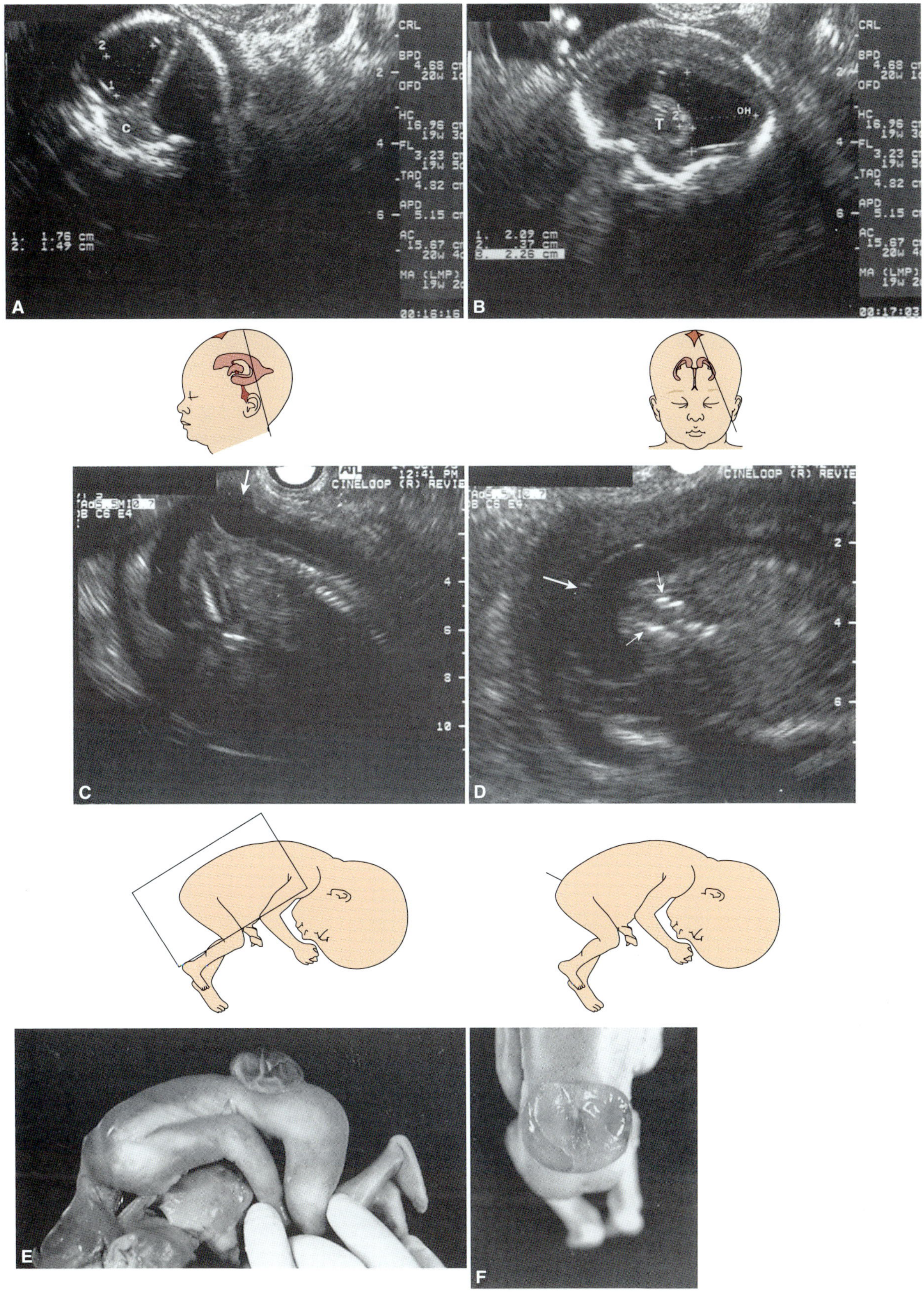


**Figure 5–41.** Arnold-Chiari type II malformation at 19 postmenstrual weeks. **(A)** An occipital–1 section of the brain demonstrating the dilation of the posterior horns and the extremely thin cerebellum, C. **(B)** An oblique–1 section showing the dilated ventricular system. Note the thin hyperechoic choroid plexus above the thalamus, T. Also note that the most dilated horn of the lateral ventricle is the posterior horn, OH. **(C)** The median section of the vertebral column showing the cystic appearance of the sacral meningocele (*white arrow*). **(D)** The transverse section of the lesion. The (*white long arrow*) points at the membranous coverage of the meningocele. Note the open vertebra (*small white arrow*). **(E), (F)** A view from the side of the aborted specimen.

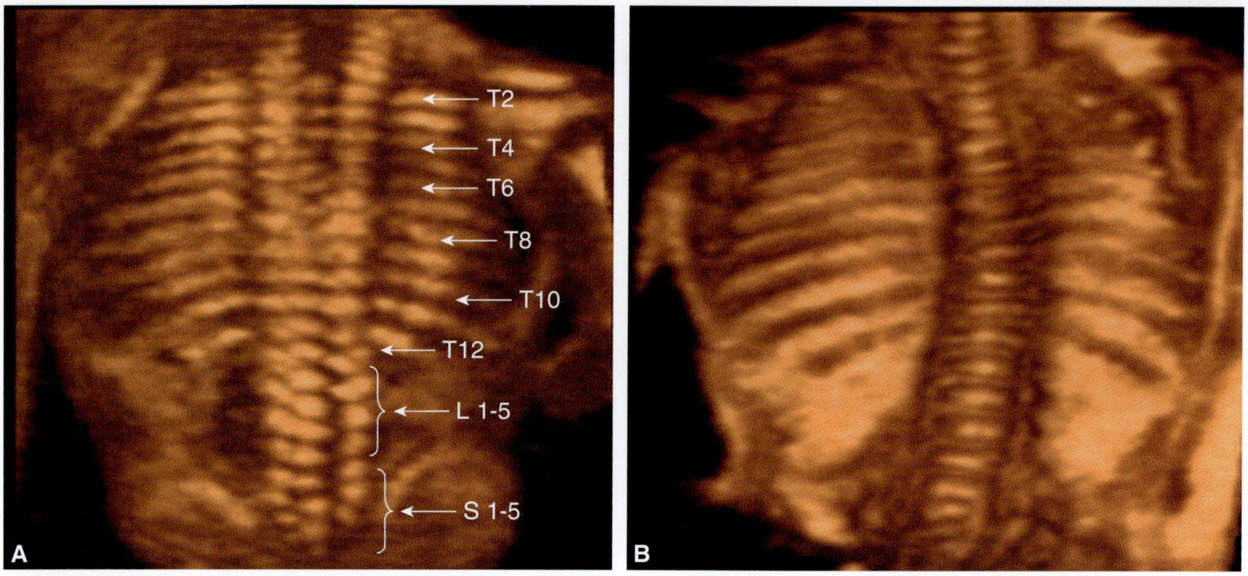


**Figure 5–42.** By using the 3D radiograph mode or bone display, the ribs and vertebrae are displayed. **(A)** Using this modality, the level of the spinal defect can be determined by counting the ribs and/or vertebral bodies. **(B)** The image looks at the spine from the inside, revealing the vertebrae and the interverteal spaces.

Recently, three other sonographically detectable supratentorial abnormalities that can be imaged with transabdominal sonography (TAS) when scanning in the axial plane during 2nd/3rd trimester have been described in fetuses with Chiari II malformation (Figure 5–49).[149–151] The first is the ventricular point, which refers to a pointed deformity of the posterior horn when scanning axially at the level of the lateral ventricles; this deformity has previously been described in the magnetic resonance literature (Figure 5–49A).[152,153] Callen et al[149] found the ventricular point in 70% of fetuses with myelomeningocele, although they believe that the real prevalence may be closer to that described by Levine et al[152] of 92%. Another important factor about the ventricular point is that it was seen in 75% of fetuses younger than 24 weeks of gestation. The second is tectal beaking, or abnormal elongation of the tectum

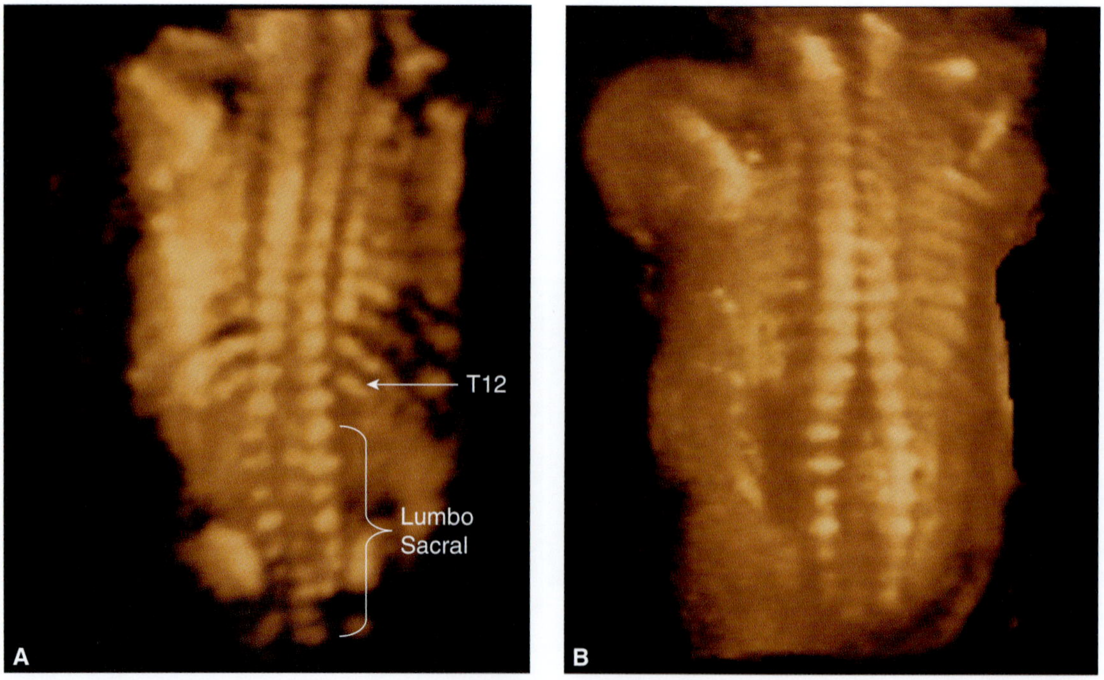


**Figure 5–43.** The 3D radiograph or bone display of a fetus at 18 weeks, 3 days, with a large lumbosacral spinal defect. **(A)** The level of the defect is localized by starting the count at the 12th vertebra. **(B)** The divergent vertebrae are seen at the level of the defect.

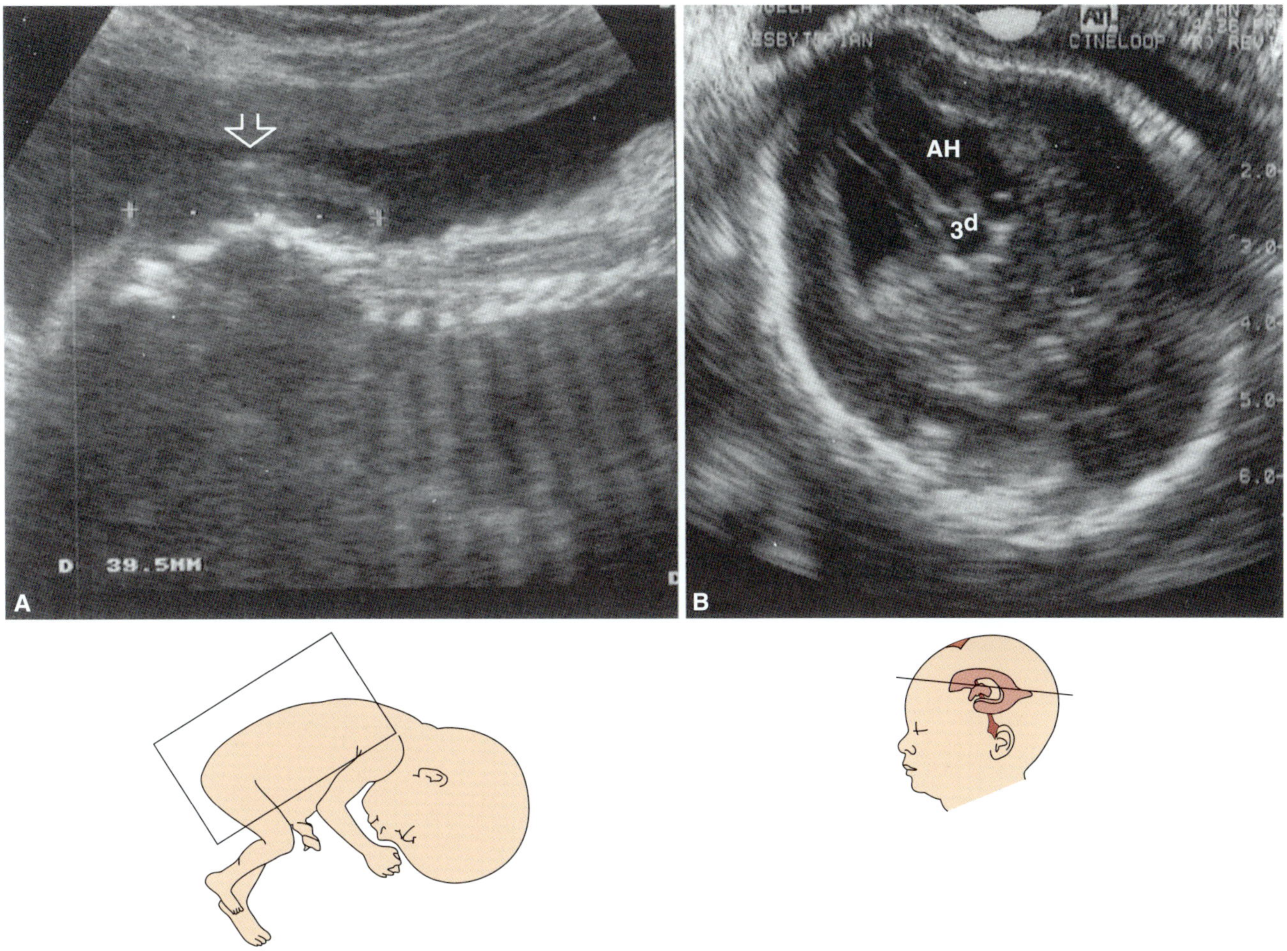


**Figure 5–44.** Arnold-Chiari type II malformation at 24 postmenstrual weeks. Diagnosis: sacral spina bifida. **(A)** Median section of the lower spine demonstrating the bulging membranes of the meningomyelocele measuring 3.9 × 3.1 × 3.7 cm (*arrow*). **(B)** The "lemon" sign of the deformed bone at the temporal region is shown, as well as dilation of the anterior horns (AH) and the third ventricle.

(Figure 5–49B); this finding has previously been described on magnetic resonance imaging (MRI) of neonates with Chiari II malformation.[154,155] The tectum is located in the dorsal region of the mesencephalon; it consists of the superior and inferior colliculi. The superior colliculi has visual receptors, and the inferior has auditory receptors. Callen et al[150] reported on tectal beaking when scanning in the axial plane; this is the same findings reported by others when using MRI. In their study, this finding was present in 66% of cases with Chiari II malformation; it was seen with equal frequency before or after 24 postmenstrual weeks, and even in fetuses with normal-size ventricles, tectal beaking could be seen. Tectal beaking correlates with the severity of the spinal defect as well as being the most likely cause of the oculomotor impairment in children with Chiari II defect.[150,155] The third abnormality is the interhemispheric cyst, although this can be seen in other conditions, such as interhemispheric arachnoid cyst, dorsal cysts associated with callosal dysgenesis, pineal cyst, and cavum vela interpositi, as well as in normal fetuses (Figure 5–49C).[151,156] Wong et al[151] found that 43% of fetuses with an open spinal defect had the interhemispheric cyst seen; they speculate in their article that this cyst is part of a dilated third ventricle that is unable to expand anteriorly due to the massa intermedia, so it expands posteriorly. Lack of visualization of the intracranial translucency between 11 and 13 postmenstrual weeks has recently been described by Chaoui[157,158] et al as a new sign of open spinal defect (Figure 5–50). The fourth ventricle is identifiable between 11 and 13 weeks as an intracranial translucency in the customary sagittal section used to measure the nuchal translucency. In their study, intracranial translucency could be seen in all normal fetuses; however, in the four cases in which a spinal defect was diagnosed during the second trimester, the intracranial translucency could not be seen.

Three-dimensional US has an important role in the assessment of fetuses with Arnold-Chiari II malformation; the volume that is obtained can be displayed in multiples types of display, such as multiplanar or orthogonal planes (Figure 5–34), tomographic US imaging (Figures 5–35, 5–36, 5–42, 5–43, 5–51, 5–52, and 5–53), radiograph mode (bone), and surface rendering (Figures 5–42 and 5–43), which may facilitate the diagnosis of Arnold-Chiari II malformation.

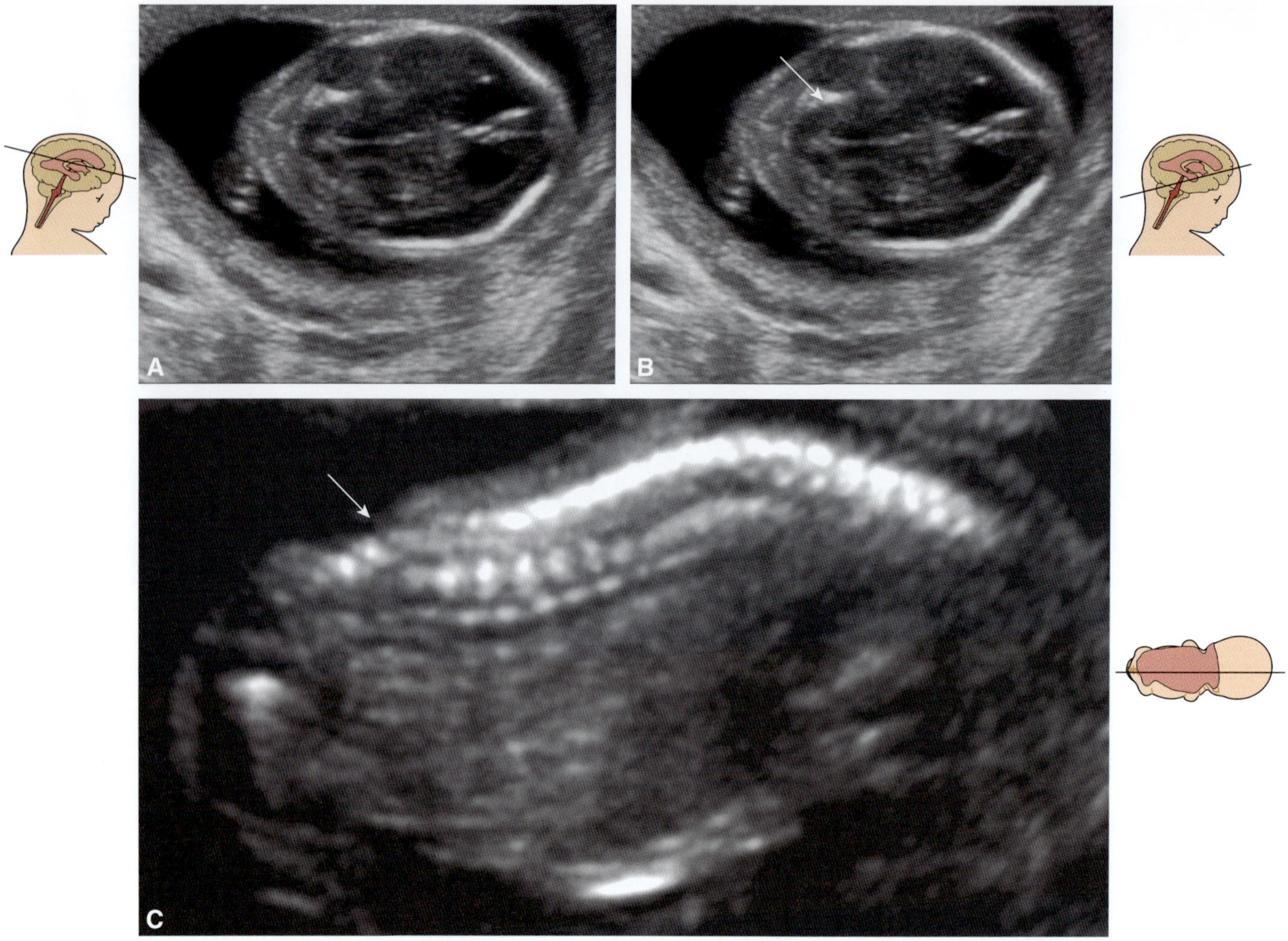

**Figure 5–45.** A transabdominal scan in a patient at 18 weeks, 3 days with elevated maternal serum alpha-fetoprotein showing the most common sonographic findings in cases of Chiari II malformation. **(A)** The fetal head clearly shows the "lemon" sign, which is a deformity of the frontal bones. **(B)** In the posterior fossa, the cerebellum *(arrow)* shows the "banana" sign, which is the result of an inferior displacement of the cerebellum and vermis obliterating the cisterna magna. **(C)** Sagittal view of the spine showing the large spinal defect *(arrow)*.

## Risk of Recurrence

The risk of spina bifida in the general population is ~0.3%.[159] However, once there is a family history, this risk increases. If one of the parents has spina bifida, the risk to the offspring is as high as 4.5%.[159] If a previous full sibling is affected, the recurrence risk is ~2% to 5%; if two previous siblings are affected, this risk increases to as high as 11%.[15] The recurrence risk among half-siblings is ~0.5% to 0.8%.[15] The risk for second-degree relatives (eg, grandparents and grandchildren, uncles and aunts, nephews and nieces) is 0.5%, and for third degree (eg, first cousins), it is similar to that of the general population.[15]

## Differential Diagnosis

The differential diagnosis of meningomyelocele includes sacrococcygeal teratoma or a mass affecting the spine that for Chiari II malformation includes aqueductal stenosis.

## Prognosis

Spinal dysraphism and Chiari II malformation are not lethal anomalies, although they are associated with a significant amount of morbidity and mortality. Approximately 14% of all children will die within the first 5 years of life in spite of aggressive treatment. Many of the deaths are related to shunt complications (malfunction and infection); among those with brainstem dysfunction secondary to the Chiari II malformation leading to respiratory and swallowing problems, the mortality rate rises to 35%.[160–162] In the past, renal failure as the result of recurrent urinary tract infection has been the most common cause of death among individuals who survive to adulthood.[162] Cognitive outcome is related to the hydrocephaly and shunt complications. About 70% of patients will have IQ >80; however, only about half of patients will be able to live independently as adults.[160,161] Independent mobility is related to the level of the defect. For those individuals with lesions above L2, there is

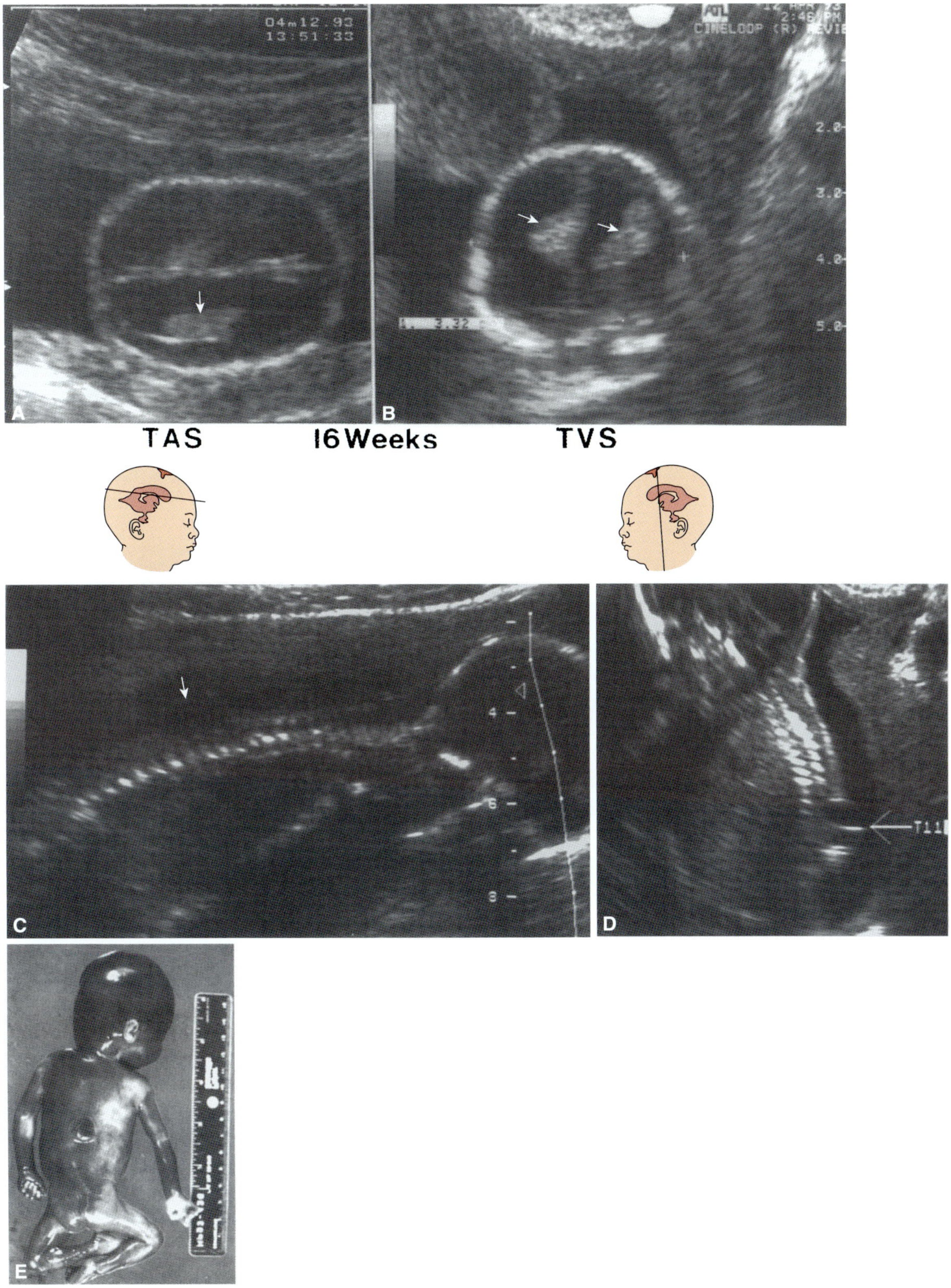


**Figure 5–46.** Arnold-Chiari type II malformation diagnosed at 16 postmenstrual weeks by transabdominal and transvaginal sonography. Diagnosis: thoracic spina bifida. **(A)** Horizontal transabdominal section of brain demonstrating the dilated lateral ventricles and the dangling choroid plexus (*arrow*). **(B)** Transvaginal scan using the mcoronal–1 section showing the dangling choroid plexus within the dilated ventricles (*arrow*). **(C)** The transabdominal scan with a 3.5 MHz probe demonstrates the faint outlines of the meningomyelocele (*arrow*). **(D)** The transvaginal picture was created by a 5MHz probe, which easily images the lesion at the 11th thoracic vertebra (*arrow*). **(E)** The aborted fetus with the lesion of the thoracic meningomyelocele and spina bifida.

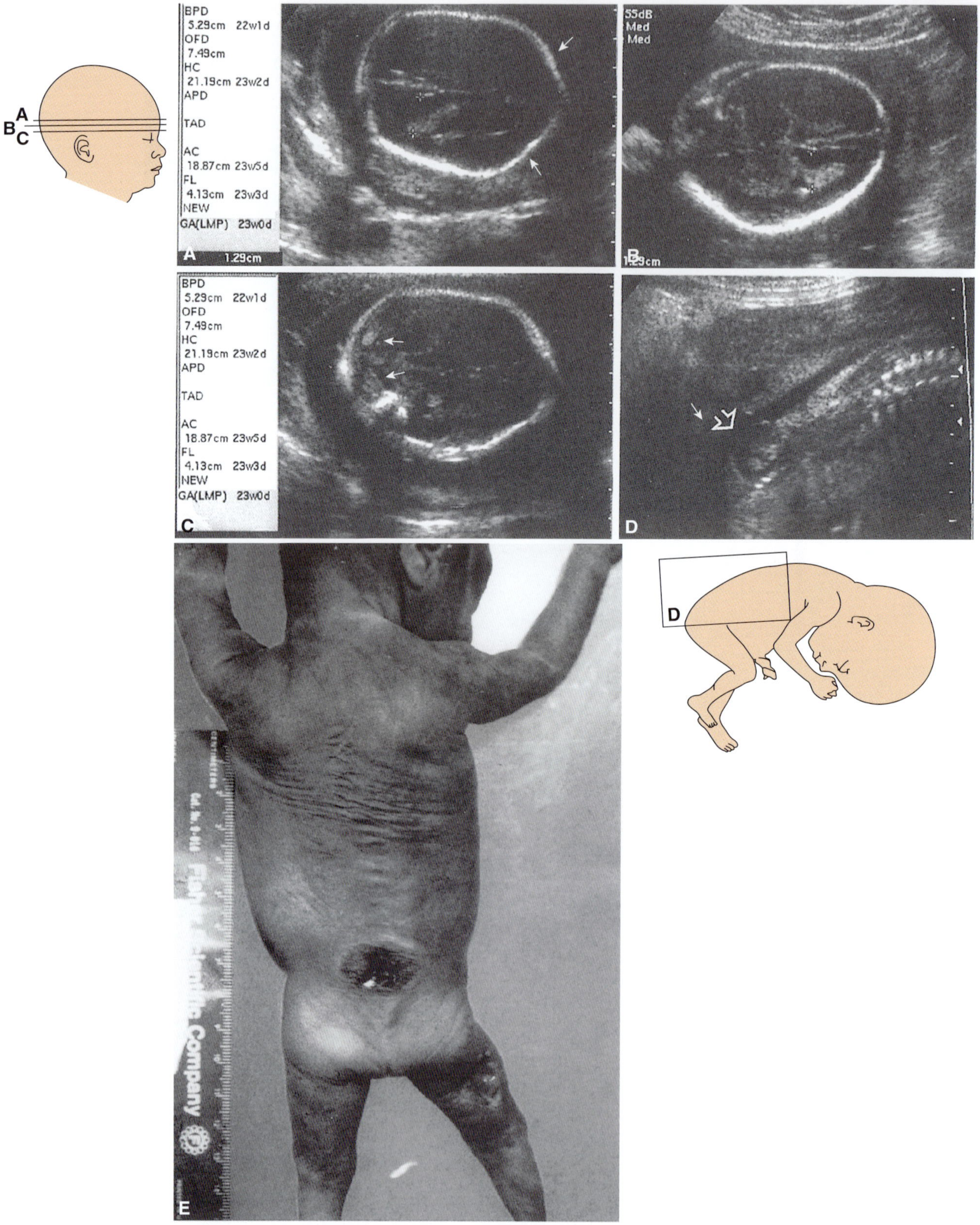


**Figure 5–47.** Workup of a patient with elevated maternal serum alpha fetoprotein. Biometry is consistent with 23 postmenstrual weeks. **(A)** The fetal head shows a very subtle "lemon" sign (*arrows*). In addition, the lateral ventricles are dilated measuring 1.3 cm. **(B)** Another view demonstrating the borderline dilation of the lateral ventricles. **(C)** The posteriorly tilted axial view used to image the posterior fossa. The cerebellum (*arrows*) has the typical "banana" shape seen in cases of open spinal defects. Also, note that the cistern magna is totally obliterated by the cerebellum. **(D)** A sagittal section of the fetal spine showing a sacral meningocele (*arrowhead*). **(E)** Pathology specimen demonstrating the defect that was imaged by US.

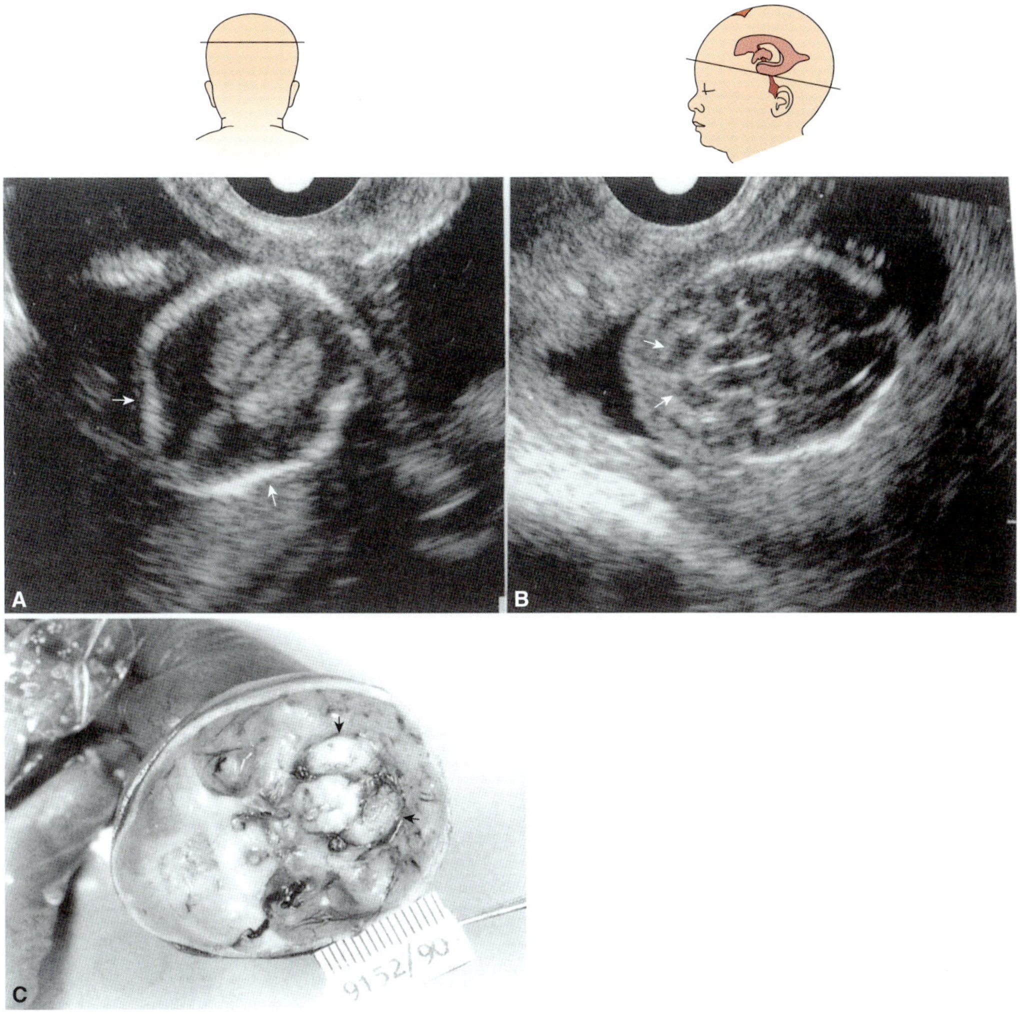

**Figure 5–48.** The "lemon" and banana" signs at 15 postmenstrual weeks. **(A)** Note the appearance of the frontal bones (*arrows*), including the typical lemon-shaped horizontal section of the skull. **(B)** The cerebellum (*arrows*) is impacted into the posterior fossa, which has obliterated the cisterna magna. **(C)** The base of the skull in a specimen of comparable age. Note the impacted hemispheres (*arrows*). The rest of the brain was removed. (Courtesy of M. Bronshtein, Al-Kol, Haifa, Israel.)

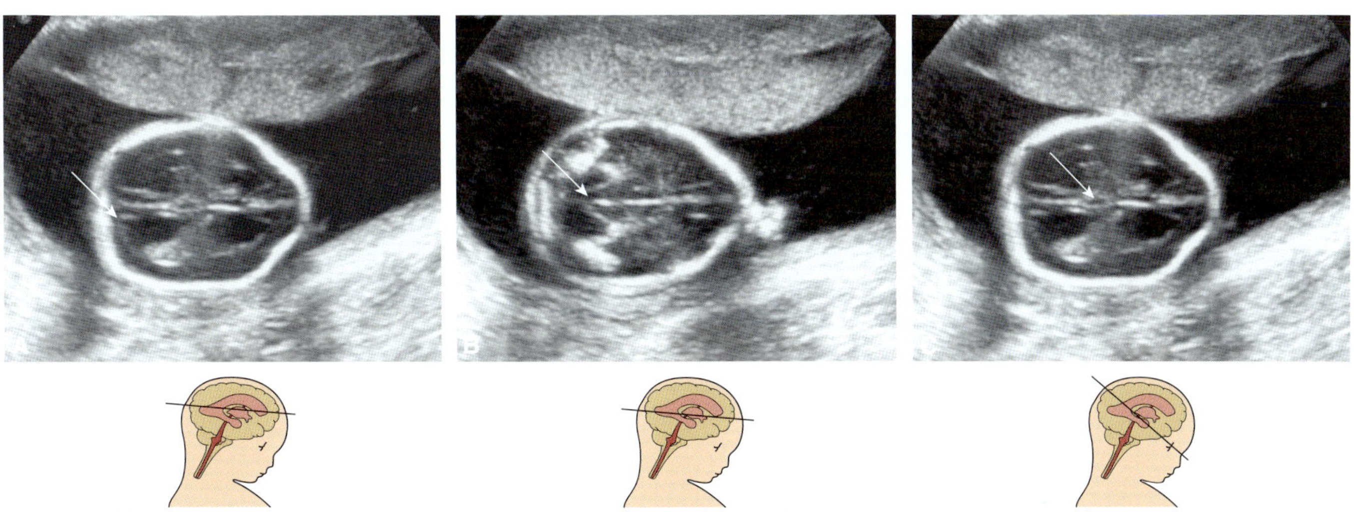

**Figure 5–49.** Additional sonographic findings seen by transabdominal sonography that help make the diagnosis of Chiari II malformation. **(A)** "Ventricular point" (*arrow*) a pointed deformity of the posterior horn. **(B)** "Tectal beaking" (*arrow*), the tectum is abnormally elongated as the result of the spinal defect. **(C)** Interhemispheric cyst (*arrow*).

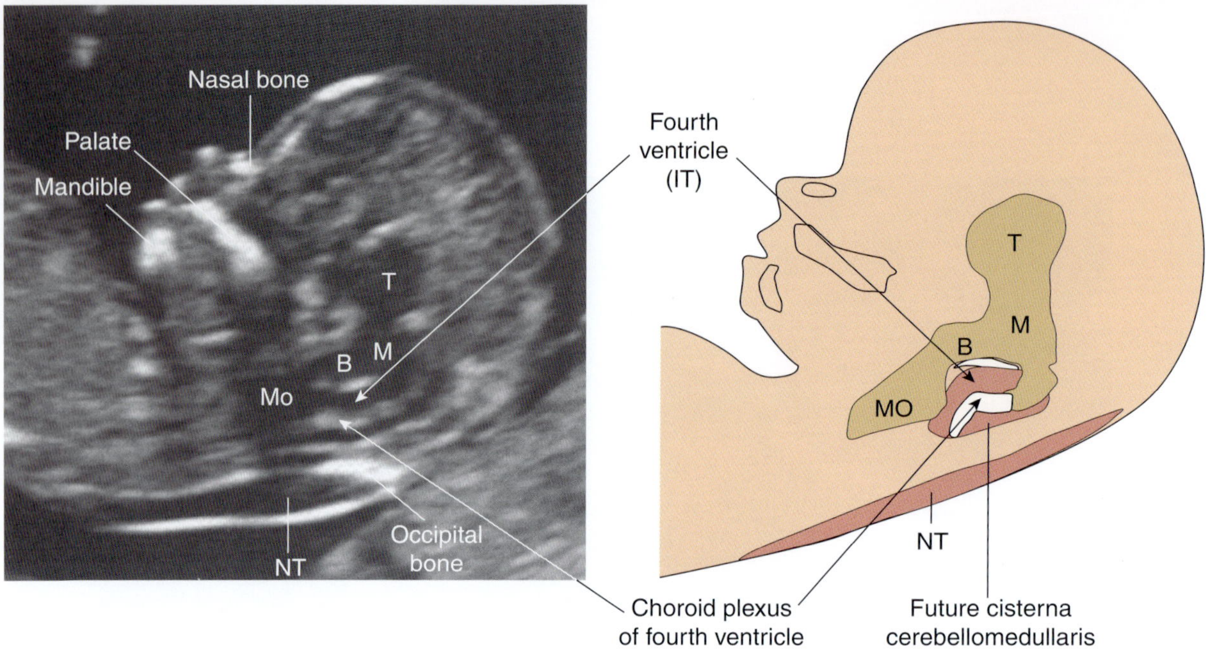


**Figure 5–50.** Ultrasound image in the mid-sagittal plane of the fetal face showing the nasal bone, palate, mandible, nuchal translucency (NT), thalamus (T), midbrain (M), brain steam (B) and medulla oblongata (MO). The fourth ventricle presents as an intracranial translucency (IT) between the brain stem and the choroid plexus. (Reproduced, with permission, from Chaoui R. UOG 2009;34:249–252.)

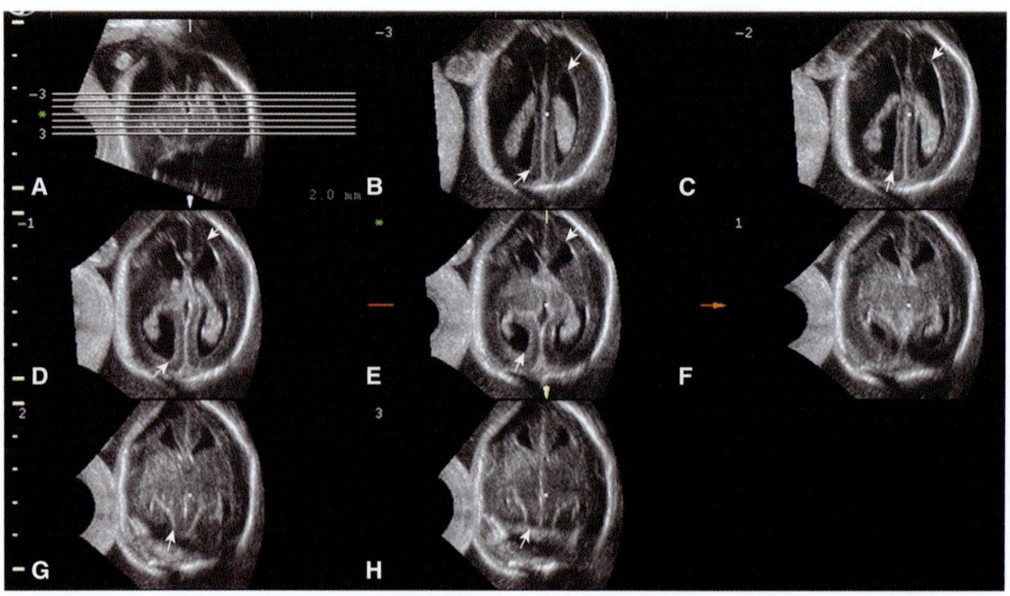


**Figure 5–51.** A volume of the head of a fetus with Chiari II malformation is displayed using the tomographic feature of 3D US. Using this format, most of the cranial sonographic findings that help in the diagnosis of a Chiari II malformation are seen. **(A)** Coronal section showing the localization of the axial sections displayed in **(B)–(H);** the sections are 2 mm apart. **(B)–(F)** Mild ventriculomegaly is present. The ventricular point sign (*small arrow*) is evident in the posterior horn of the lateral ventricle, as well as in the anterior horns (*arrow*). The head displays the "lemon" sign. The dot is over the interventricular cyst. **(G), (H)** Beaked tectum at the arrow. The cerebellum is not seen in this fetus, most likely because it has herniated through the foramen magnum.

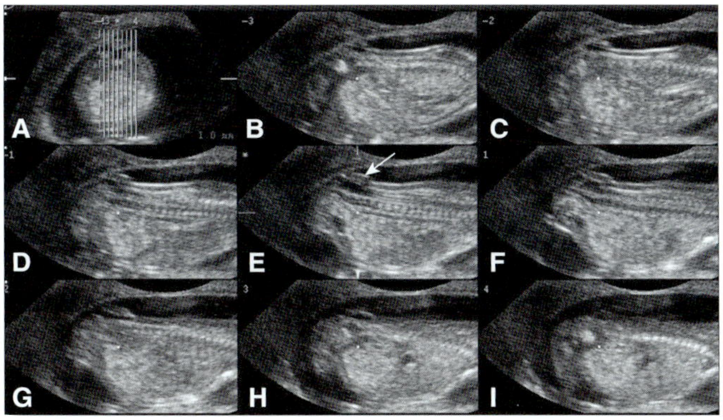


**Figure 5–52.** Volume of the spine of a fetus with Chiari II malformation displayed using the tomographic feature of 3D US. **(A)** Transverse section showing the 1 mm sections displayed in **(B)–(I)**. **(B)–(I)** The meningomeyelocele is seen involving the lower lumbar and all of the sacral area of the spine (*arrow*).

loss of the quadriceps and iliopsoas muscle; therefore, a wheelchair existence should be anticipated.[162] Social continence can be achieved in up to 80% of these children.[162]

## Obstetric Management

Management of a pregnancy with myelomeningocele should include genetic counseling and karyotyping. Over the past few years there has been some debate regarding the best method to deliver fetuses with spinal defects. Luthy et al[163] published a retrospective review of 160 cases of myelomeningocele. The results showed that those infants delivered by cesarean section before the onset of labor had better motor function when compared with infants who were delivered vaginally or if the cesarean section was performed after the onset of labor. In

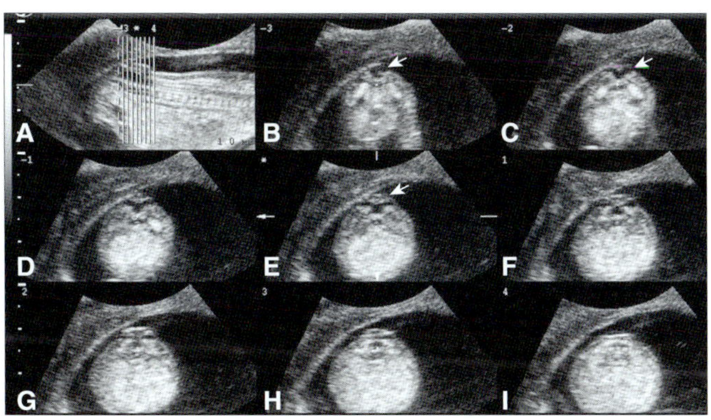


**Figure 5–53.** Volume of the spine of a fetus with Chiari II malformation is displayed using the tomographic feature of 3D US. The marker dot in all sections is over the vertebral body of the spine. **(A)** Sagittal section showing the 1 mm sections displayed in **(B)–(I)**. **(B)–(H)** The meningomeyelocele is seen with an obvious defect of the spine; the vertebrae display an abnormal U shape (*arrow*). **(I)** above the level of the meningomeyelocele, the transverse section appears normal.

our institution we electively section all infants at 37 to 38 postmenstrual weeks of gestation after confirmation of lung maturity. This is especially important for those infants with hydrocephaly because delaying the surgery may result in larger head size and worse cosmetic results.

Another option for patients is to undergo surgical treatment of the spinal defect in utero. This surgical treatment was reported to be associated with improving neurologic outcomes as well as reducing the morbidity associated with the Chiari II malformation.[161] In addition, fetuses treated with in utero surgery during the midtrimester may have lower rates of postnatal shunt placement compared with those operated after birth. Another potential benefit is the reversal of the hindbrain herniation.[160] An ongoing fact search, the Management of Myelomeningocele Study (MOMS), was designed to compare the two treatment approaches of babies with spina bifida: surgery before birth and surgery after birth.

## REFERENCES


1. Padmanabhan R. Etiology, pathogenesis and prevention of neural tube defects. *Congenit Anom (Kyoto)*. 2006;46:55–67.
2. O'Rahilly R, Müller F. Prenatal development of the brain. In: Timor-Tritsch IE, Monteagudo A, Cohen HL, eds. *Ultrasonography of the Prenatal and Neonatal Brain.* New York: McGraw-Hill; 2001, p.3.
3. O'Rahilly R, Müller F. The two sites of fusion of the neural folds and the two neuropores in the human embryo. *Teratology.* 2002;65: 162–170.
4. O'Rahilly R, Müller F. *The Embryonic Human Brain. An Atlas of Developmental Stages.* New York: Wiley-Liss; 1994.
5. Richards DS, Seeds JW, Katz VL, Lingley LH, Albright SG, Cefalo RC. Elevated maternal serum alpha-fetoprotein with normal ultrasound: Is amniocentesis always appropriate? A review of 26,069 screened patients. *Obstet Gynecol.* 1988;71:203–207.
6. Limb CJ, Holmes LB. Anencephaly: Changes in prenatal detection and birth status, 1972 through 1990. *Am J Obstet Gynecol.* 1994;170:1333–1338.
7. Reichler A, Hume RF Jr., Drugan A, et al. Risk of anomalies as a function of level of elevated maternal serum alpha-fetoprotein. *Am J Obstet Gynecol.* 1994;171:1052–1055.
8. Haddow JE. Prenatal screening for open neural tube defects, Down's syndrome, and other major fetal disorders. *Semin Perinatol.* 1990;14:488–503.
9. Bock JL. Current issues in maternal serum alpha-fetoprotein screening. *Am J Clin Pathol.* 1992;97:541–554.
10. Burton BK. Elevated maternal serum alpha-fetoprotein (MSAFP): Interpretation and follow-up. *Clin Obstet Gynecol.* 1988;31: 293–305.
11. Volpe J. Neuronal proliferation, migration, organization and myelination. In: *Neurology of the Newborn.* 3rd ed. Philadelphia: WB Saunders; 1995:3–42.
12. Carter CO, Evans KA, Till K. Spinal dysraphism: Genetic relation to neural tube malformations. *J Med Genet.* 1976;13:434–450.
13. Cunningham ME, Walls WJ. Ultrasound in the evaluation of anencephaly. *Radiology.* 1976;118:165–167.
14. Icenogle DA, Kaplan AM. A review of congenital neurologic malformations. *Clin Pediatr.* 1981;20:565–576.
15. Deak KL, Siegel DG, George TM, Gregory S, Ashley-Koch A, Speer MC. Further evidence for a maternal genetic effect and a sex-influenced effect contributing to risk for human neural tube defects. *Birth Defects Res A Clin Mol Teratol.* 2008;82:662–669.
16. Williams LJ, Rasmussen SA, Flores A, Kirby RS, Edmonds LD. Decline in the prevalence of spina bifida and anencephaly by race/ethnicity: 1995–2002. *Pediatrics.* 2005;116:580–586.
17. Prevalence of neural tube defects and folic acid knowledge and consumption—Puerto Rico, 1996–2006. *MMWR Morb Mortal Wkly Rep.* 2008;57:10–13.

18. O'Rahilly R, Müller F. The nervous system. In: *Human Embryology and Teratology.* 1st ed. New York: Wiley-Liss; 1992:253–291.
19. Marin-Padilla M. Cephalic axial skeletal-neural dysraphic disorders: Embryology and pathology. *Can J Neurolog Sci.* 1991;18:153–169.
20. Müller F, O'Rahilly R. Cerebral dysraphia (future anencephaly) in a human twin embryo at stage 13. *Teratology.* 1984;30:167–177.
21. Müller F, O'Rahilly R. Development of anencephaly and its variants. *Am J Anat.* 1991;190:193–218.
22. O'Rahilly R, Müller F. *Human Embryology and Teratology.* New York: Wiley-Liss; 1992.
23. Bronshtein M, Ornoy A. Acrania: anencephaly resulting from secondary degeneration of a closed neural tube: Two cases in the same family. *J Clin Ultrasound.* 1991;19:230–234.
24. Timor-Tritsch IE, Greenebaum E, Monteagudo A, Baxi L. Exencephaly-anencephaly sequence: Proof by ultrasound imaging and amniotic fluid cytology. *J Matern Fetal Med.* 1996;5:182–185.
25. Cheschier N. ACOG practice bulletin: Neural tube defects. (Replaces committee opinion no. 252, March 2001.) *Int J Gynaecol Obstet.* 2003;83:123–133.
26. Mitchell LE. Epidemiology of neural tube defects. *Am J Med Genet C Semin Med Genet.* 2005;135C:88–94.
27. Lemire RJ. Anencephaly. In: Myrianthopoulos N, ed. *Handbook of Clinical Neurology.* Vol 6. Amsterdam: Elsevier; 1987:71–95.
28. Joo JG, Beke A, Papp C, et al. Neural tube defects in the sample of genetic counselling. *Prenat Diagn.* 2007;27(10):912–921.
29. Salamanca A, Gonzalez-Gomez F, Padilla M. Prenatal ultrasound semiography of anencephaly: Sonographic-pathological correlations. *Ultrasound Obstet Gynecol.* 1992;2:95–100.
30. Johnson A, Losure TA, Weiner S. Early diagnosis of fetal anencephaly. *J Clin Ultrasound.* 1985;13:503–505.
31. Moore K. *Clinically Oriented Embryology.* Philadelphia: WB Saunders; 1988.
32. Pretorius DH, Russ PD, Rumack CM, Manco-Johnson ML. Diagnosis of brain neuropathology in utero. *Neuroradiology.* 1986;28:386–397.
33. Ceylaner S, Ceylaner G, Gunyeli I, et al. Postmortem evaluation of 220 prenatally diagnosed fetuses with neural tube defects: Detection of associated anomalies in a Turkish population. *Prenat Diagn.* 2006;26:147–153.
34. Neural tube defects. ACOG practice bulletin #44. American College of Obstetricians and Gynecologists. *Obstet Gynecol.* 2003;102:203–213.
35. Spina bifida and anencephaly before and after folic acid mandate—United States, 1995–1996 and 1999–2000. *MMWR Morb Mortal Wkly Rep.* 2004;53:362–365.
36. Czeizel AE, Dudas I. Prevention of the first occurrence of neural-tube defects by periconceptional vitamin supplementation. *N Engl J Med.* 1992;327:1832–1835.
37. Bower C, Stanley FJ. Dietary folate as a risk factor for neural-tube defects: Evidence from a case-control study in Western Australia. *Med J Aust.* 1989;150:613–619.
38. Werler MM, Shapiro S, Mitchell AA. Periconceptional folic acid exposure and risk of occurrent neural tube defects. *JAMA.* 1993;269:1257–1261.
39. Milunsky A, Jick H, Jick SS, et al. Multivitamin/folic acid supplementation in early pregnancy reduces the prevalence of neural tube defects. *JAMA.* 1989;262:2847–2852.
40. Prevention of neural tube defects: Results of the Medical Research Council Vitamin Study. MRC Vitamin Study Research Group. *Lancet.* 1991;338:131–137.
41. Use of supplements containing folic acid among women of childbearing age—United States, 2007. *MMWR Morb Mortal Wkly Rep.* 2008;57:5–8.
42. Trends in wheat-flour fortification with folic acid and iron—worldwide, 2004 and 2007. *MMWR Morb Mortal Wkly Rep.* 2008;57:8–10.
43. Bell KN, Oakley GP, Jr. Update on prevention of folic acid-preventable spina bifida and anencephaly. *Birth Defects Res A Clin Mol Teratol.* 2009;85:102–107.
44. Campbell S, Johnstone F, Holt E, May P. Anencephalus: Early ultrasonic diagnosis and active management. *Lancet.* 1972;2:1226.
45. Rottem S, Bronshtein M, Thaler, Brandes J. First trimester transvaginal sonographic diagnosis of fetal anomalies. *Lancet.* 1989;1: 444–445.
46. Inman V, Saunders JDC. The ossification of the human frontal bone. *J Anat.* 1937;71:383–394.
47. Kennedy KA, Flick KJ, Thurmond AS. First-trimester diagnosis of exencephaly. *Am J Obstet Gynecol.* 1990;162:461–463.
48. Bronshtein M, Weiner Z. Anencephaly in a fetus with osteogenesis imperfecta: Early diagnosis by transvaginal sonography. *Prenat Diagn.* 1992;12:831–834.
49. Cox GG, Rosenthal SJ, Holsapple JW. Exencephaly: Sonographic findings and radiologic-pathologic correlation. *Radiology.* 1985; 155:755–756.
50. Ganchrow D, Ornoy A. A pathological Anatomy and Histology: Possible evidence for secondary degeneration of central nervous system in the pathogenesis of anencephaly and brain dysraphia. A study in young human fetuses. *Virchows Arch.* 1979;384:285–294.
51. Padmanabhan R. Is exencephaly the forerunner of anencephaly? An experimental study on the effect of prolonged gestation on the exencephaly induced after neural tube closure in the rat. *Acta Anat (Basel).* 1991;141:182–192.
52. Vergani P, Ghidini A, Sirtori M, Roncaglia N. Antenatal diagnosis of fetal acrania. *J Ultrasound Med.* 1987;6:715–717.
53. Casellas M, Ferrer M, Rovira M, Pla F, Martinez MA, Cabero L. Prenatal diagnosis of exencephaly. *Prenat Diagn.* 1993;13:417–422.
54. Nishi T, Nakano R. First-trimester diagnosis of exencephaly by transvaginal ultrasonography. *J Ultrasound Med.* 1994;13: 149–151.
55. Hidalgo H, Bowie J, Rosenberg ER, Ram PC, Ford K, Lipsit E. Review. In utero sonographic diagnosis of fetal cerebral anomalies. *Am J Roentgenol.* 1982;139:143–148.
56. Mahony BS, Filly RA, Callen PW, Golbus MS. The amniotic band syndrome: Antenatal sonographic diagnosis and potential pitfalls. *Am J Obstet Gynecol.* 1985;152:63–68.
57. Pomerance JJ, Morrison A, Williams RL, Schifrin BS. Anencephalic infants: Life expectancy and organ donation. *J Perinatol.* 1989;9: 33–37.
58. Baird PA, Sadovnick AD. Survival in infants with anencephaly. *Clin Pediatr (Phila).* 1984;23:268–271.
59. McAbee G, Sherman J, Canas JA, Boxer H. Prolonged survival of two anencephalic infants. *Am J Perinatol.* 1993;10:175–177.
60. Nembhard WN, Waller DK, Sever LE, Canfield MA. Patterns of first-year survival among infants with selected congenital anomalies in Texas, 1995–1997. *Teratology.* 2001;64:267–275.
61. Aleksic S, Budzilovich G. Iniencephaly. In: Myrianthopoulos N, ed. *Malformations.* Vol 56. Amsterdam: Elsevier; 1987;6:129–136.
62. Foderaro AE, Abu-Yousef MM, Benda JA, Williamson RA, Smith WL. Antenatal ultrasound diagnosis of iniencephaly. *J Clin Ultrasound.* 1987;15:550–504.
63. Lemire R, Beckwith J, Shepard T. Iniencephaly and anencephaly with spinal retroflexion: A comparative study of eight human specimens. *Birth Defects.* 1987;23:225.
64. Nishimura H, Okamoto N. Iniencephaly. In: Vinken PJ, Bruyn GW, eds. *Handbook of Clinical Neurology.* Vol 30. Amsterdam: Elsevier-North-Holland; 1976;257–268.
65. Rodriguez MM, Reik RA, Carreno TD, Fojaco RM. Cluster of iniencephaly in Miami. *Pediatr Pathol.* 1991;11:211–221.
66. Shoham Z, Caspi B, Chemke J, Dgani R, Lancet M. Iniencephaly: Prenatal ultrasonographic diagnosis—a case report. *J Perinat Med.* 1988;16:139–143.
67. Aleksic S, Budzilovich G, Greco MA, Feigin I, Epstein F, Pearson J. Iniencephaly: A neuropathologic study. *Clin Neuropathol.* 1983;2:55–61.
68. Jones KL. *Smith's Recognizable Patterns of Human Malformation.* Philadelphia: Elsevier Saunders; 2006.
69. Romero R, Pilu G, Jeanty P, Ghidini A, Hobbins J. *Prenatal Diagnosis of Congenital Anomalies.* Norwalk: Appleton & Lange; 1988.
70. Joo JG, Beke A, Papp C, Szigeti Z, Csaba A, Papp Z. Major diagnostic and pathological features of iniencephaly based on twenty-four cases. *Fetal Diagn Ther.* 2008;24:1–6.
71. David TJ, Nixon A. Congenital malformations associated with anencephaly and iniencephaly. *J Med Genet.* 1976;13:263–265.
72. Aytar MH, Dogulu F, Cemil B, Ergun E, Kurt G, Baykaner K. Iniencephaly and long-term survival: A rare case report. *Childs Nerv Syst.* 2007;23:719–721.
73. Bromley B, Lieberman R, Benacerraf BR. Choroid plexus cysts: not associated with Down syndrome [see comments]. *Ultrasound Obstet Gynecol.* 1996;8:232–235.

74. Tracy MR, Dormans JP, Kusumi K. Klippel-Feil syndrome: Clinical features and current understanding of etiology. *Clin Orthop Relat Res.* 2004:183–190.
75. Benacerraf B. *Ultrasound of Fetal Syndromes.* Philadelphia: Churchill Livingstone–Elsevier; 2008.
76. Joo JG, Papp Z, Berkes E, Papp C, Rigo J. Non-syndromic encephalocele: A 26-year experience. *Dev Med Child Neurol.* 2008;50: 958–960.
77. Harley EH. Pediatric congenital nasal masses. *Ear Nose Throat J.* 1991;70:28–32.
78. Naidich TP, Altman NR, Braffman BH, McLone DG, Zimmerman RA. Cephaloceles and related malformations. *AJNR Am J Neuroradiol.* 1992;13:655–690.
79. Chervenak FA, Isaacson G, Mahoney MJ, Berkowitz RL, Tortora M, Hobbins JC. Diagnosis and management of fetal cephalocele. *Obstet Gynecol.* 1984;64:86–91.
80. McSherry J. Folic acid and the pill [letter]. *CMAJ.* 1998;159:218.
81. Monteagudo A. Cephalocele: Anterior. *Fetus.* 1992;2:1–4.
82. Nyberg DA, Hallesy D, Mahony BS, Hirsch JH, Luthy DA, Hickok D. Meckel-Gruber syndrome. Importance of prenatal diagnosis. *J Ultrasound Med.* 1990;9:691–696.
83. Whatmore WJ. Sincipital encephalomeningoceles. *Br J Surg.* 1973; 60:261–270.
84. Mood GF. Congenital anterior herniations of brain. *Ann Otorhinolaryngol.* 1938;47:391–401.
85. Cohen MM, Jr., Lemire RJ. Syndromes with cephaloceles. *Teratology.* 1982;25:161–172.
86. Rapport RL, Dunn RC, Alhady, F. Anterior encephalocele. *J Neurosurg.* 1981;54:213–219.
87. Diebler C, Dulac O. Cephaloceles: Clinical and neuroradiological appearance. Associated cerebral malformations. *Neuroradiology.* 1983;25:199–216.
88. Jones K. *Smith's Recognizable Patterns of Human Malformations.* Philadelphia: WB Saunders; 1988.
89. Patterson RJ, Egelhoff JC, Crone KR, Ball WS, Jr. Atretic parietal cephaloceles revisited: An enlarging clinical and imaging spectrum? *AJNR Am J Neuroradiol.* 1998;19:791–795.
90. Martinez-Lage JF, Poza M, Sola J, et al. The child with a cephalocele: etiology, neuroimaging, and outcome. *Childs Nerv Syst.* 1996;12: 540–550.
91. Brunelle F, Baraton J, Renier D, et al. Intracranial venous anomalies associated with atretic cephalocoeles. *Pediatr Radiol.* 2000;30: 743–747.
92. Wen S, Ethen M, Langlois PH, Mitchell LE. Prevalence of encephalocele in Texas, 1999–2002. *Am J Med Genet A.* 2007;143A: 2150–2155.
93. Moerman PH, Verbeken E, Fryns JP, Lauweryns JM. The Meckel syndrome:Pathological and cytogenetic observations in eight cases. *Hum Genet.*1982;62:240–245.
94. Pachi A, Giancotti A, Torcia F, Deprosperi V, Maggi E. Gruber syndrome: Ultrasonographic diagnosis at 13 weeks gestational age in a at-risk case. *Prenatal Diagnosis.* 1989;9:187–190.
95. Anderson VM. Meckel syndrome:Morphologic considerations. *Birth Defects.* 1982;18:145–160.
96. Herriot R, Hallam LA, Gray ES. Dandy-Walker malformation in the Meckel syndrome. *Am J Med Genet.* 1991;39:207–210.
97. Vernekar JA, Mishra GK, Pinto RGW, Bhandari M, Mishra M. Antenatal ultrasonic diagnosis of Meckel Gruber syndrome ( a case report with review of literature). *Australas Radiol.* 1991;35: 186–188.
98. Ramadani HM, Nasrat HA. Prenatal diagnosis of recurrent Meckelsyndrome. *Int JGynecol Obstet.* 1992;39:327–332.
99. Kaplan M, Ben-Neriah Z, Achiron R. Survival in an infant witha prenatally diagnosed Meckel syndrome variant. *Am J Perinat.* 1993;10:172–174.
100. Monteagudo A, Alayon A, Mayberry P. Walker-Warburg syndrome: Case report and review of the literature. *J Ultrasound Med.* 2001;20:419–426.
101. Low AS, Lee SL, Tan AS, Chan DK, Chan LL. Difficulties with prenatal diagnosis of the Walker-Warburg syndrome. *Acta Radiol.* 2005;46:645–651.
102. Wilson C, Aftimos S, Pereira A, McKay R. Report of two sibs with Knobloch syndrome (encephalocoele and viteroretinal degeneration) and other anomalies. *Am J Med Genet.* 1998;78:286–290.
103. McLaurin RL. Encephalocele and cranium bifidum. In: Myrianthopoulos NC ed. *Handbook of Clinical Neurology: Malformations.* Vol 6. Amsterdam: Elsevier; 1987;97–111.
104. Yokota A, Kajiwara H, Kohchi M, Fuwa I, Wada H. Parietal cephalocele: Clinical importance of its atretic form and associated malformations. *J Neurosurg.* 1988;69:545–551.
105. Fiske CE, Filly RA. Ultrasound evaluation of the normal and abnormal fetal neural axis. *Radiol Clin North Am.* 1982;20:285–296.
106. Nyberg D, Pretorius D. Cerebral malformations. In: Nyberg D, Mahoney B, Pretorius D, eds. *Diagnostic Ultrasound of Fetal Anomalies: Text and Atlas.* Chicago: Year Book; 1990:83–202.
107. Simpson DA, David DJ, White J. Cephaloceles: Treatment, outcome, and antenatal diagnosis. *Neurosurgery.* 1984;15:14–21.
108. Fleming AD, Vintzileos AM, Scorza WE. Prenatal diagnosis of occipital encephalocele with transvaginal sonography. *J Ultrasound Med.* 1991;10:285–286.
109. Chen CP, Hwu YM, Tsai FJ, Wang W. Occipital encephalocele associated with iniencephaly mimicking an unilateral nuchal tumor on prenatal ultrasound. *Genet Couns.* 2008;19:101–103.
110. van Tellingen V, Obihara CC, van Tilborg GF, van Dijken PJ. MRI diagnosis of occipital cephalohematoma mimicking an encephalocele. *Am J Perinatol.* 2008;25:153–155.
111. Baykaner MK, Ergun E, Cemil B, Bayik P, Emmez H. A mature cystic teratoma in pineal region mimicking parietal encephalocele in a newborn. *Childs Nerv Syst.* 2007;23:573–576.
112. Blanluet-Gerard M, Patkai J, Simon I, Levaillant JM, Haddad B. Prenatal skin edema mimicking a recurrence of meningo-encephalocele. *Prenat Diagn.* 2003;23:173–175.
113. Kuo MF, Wang HS, Chen MT. Sincipital encephalocele mismanaged as a facial hemangioma. *Pediatr Neurol.* 2002;26:408–410.
114. Noriega CA, Fleming AD, Bonebrake RG. A false-positive diagnosis of a prenatal encephalocele on transvaginal ultrasonography. *J Ultrasound Med.* 2001;20:925–927.
115. Sarnat HB, Mueller DL. Fetal neurology. In: Eden RD, Boehm FH, Haire M, eds. *Assessment and Care of the Fetus: Physiological, Clinical, and Medicolegal Principles.* Norwalk: Appleton & Lange; 1990;43–67.
116. Lorber J. The prognosis of occipital encephalocele. *Dev Med Child Neurol.* 1967;9(suppl b):75–86.
117. Lorber J, Schofield, J.K. The prognosis of occipital encephalocele. *Z Kinderchir.* 1979;28:347–351.
118. Mealey J, Dzenitis AJ, Hockey AA. The prognosis of encephaloceles. *J Neurosurg.* 1970;32:209–218.
119. Brown MS, Sheridan-Pereira M. Outlook for the child with a cephalocele. *Pediatrics.* 1992;90:914–919.
120. Suwanwela C, Hongsaprabhas C. Fronto-ethmoidal encephalomeningocele. *J Neurosurg.* 1966;25:172–182.
121. Lipschitz R, Beck JM, Froman C. An assessment of the treatment of encephalomeningoceles. *S Afr Med J.* 1969;43:609–610.
122. Osborn A. Normal anatomy and congenital anomalies of the spine an d spinal cord. In: *Diagnostic Neuroradiology.* St. Louis: Mosby-Year Book; 1994;799–807.
123. McLone DG, Dias MS. The Chiari II malformation: Cause and impact. *Childs Nerv Syst.* 2003;19:540–550.
124. Tubbs RS, Shoja MM, Ardalan MR, Shokouhi G, Loukas M. Hindbrain h3erniation: A review of embryological theories. *Ital J Anat Embryol.* 2008;113:37–46.
125. Racial/ethnic differences in the birth prevalence of spina bifida—United States, 1995–2005. *MMWR Morb Mortal Wkly Rep.* 2009;57:1409–1413.
126. Yen IH, Khoury MJ, Erickson JD, James LM, Waters GD, Berry RJ. The changing epidemiology of neural tube defects. United States, 1968–1989. *Am J Dis Child.* 1992;146:857–861.
127. Welch K, Winston K. Spina bifida. In: Myrianthopoulos N, ed. *Handbook of Clinical Neurology.* Vol 6. Amsterdam: Elsevier; 1987;6:477–508.
128. Stevenson KL. Chiari type II malformation: Past, present, and future. *Neurosurg Focus.* 2004;16:E5.
129. Chiari H. Ueber Veränderungen des Kleinhirns infolge von Hydrocephalie des Grosshirns. *Dtsch Med Wochenschr.* 1891; 17:1172–1175.
130. Cleland J. Contribution to the study of spina bifida, encephalocele, and anencephalus. *J Anat Physiol.* 1883;17:257–291.

131. McLone DG, Knepper PA. The cause of Chiari II malformation: A unified theory. *Pediatr Neurosci.* 1989;15:1–12.
132. Van den Hof MC, Nicolaides KH, Campbell J, Campbell S. Evaluation of the lemon and banana signs in one hundred thirty fetuses with open spina bifida. *Am J Obstet Gynecol.* 1990;162: 322–327.
133. Timor-Tritsch IE, Monteagudo A, Peisner DB. High-frequency transvaginal sonographic examination for the potential malformation assessment of the 9-week to 14-week fetus. *J Clin Ultrasound.* 1992;20:231–238.
134. Birnholz J. Smaller parts scanning of the fetus. *Radiol Clin North Am.* 1992;30:977–991.
135. Campbell S. Early prenatal diagnosis of neural tube defects by ultrasound. *Clin Obstet Gynecol.*1977;20:351–359.
136. Baxi L, Warren W, Collins MH, Timor-Tritsch IE. Early detection of caudal regression syndrome with transvaginal scanning. *Obstet Gynecol.* 1990;75:486–489.
137. Hogge WA, Thiagarajah S, Ferguson JED, Schnatterly PT, Harbert GM, Jr. The role of ultrasonography and amniocentesis in the evaluation of pregnancies at risk for neural tube defects [see comments]. *Am J Obstet Gynecol.* 1989;161:520–523; discussion 523–524.
138. Main DM, Mennuti MT. Neural tube defects: issues in prenatal diagnosis and counselling. *Obstet Gynecol.* 1986;67:1–16.
139. Thornton JG, Lilford RJ, Newcombe RG. Tables for estimation of individual risks of fetal neural tube and ventral wall defects, incorporating prior probability, maternal serum alpha-fetoprotein levels, and ultrasonographic examination results [see comments]. *Am J Obstet Gynecol.* 1991;164:154–160.
140. Kollias SS, Goldstein RB, Cogen PH, Filly RA. Prenatally detected myelomeningoceles: Sonographic accuracy in estimation of the spinal level. *Radiology.* 1992;185:109–112.
141. Campbell J, Gilbert WM, Nicolaides KH, Campbell S. Ultrasound screening for spina bifida: Cranial and cerebellar signs in a high-risk population. *Obstet Gynecol.* 1987;70:247–250.
142. Nicolaides KH, Campbell S, Gabbe SG, Guidetti R. Ultrasound screening for spina bifida: Cranial and cerebellar signs. *Lancet.* 1986; 2:72–74.
143. Blumenfeld Z, Siegler E, Bronshtein M. The early diagnosis of neural tube defects. *Prenat Diagn.* 1993;13:863–871.
144. Nyberg DA, Mack LA, Hirsch J, Mahony BS. Abnormalities of fetal cranial contour in sonographic detection of spina bifida: Evaluation of the "lemon" sign. *Radiology.* 1988;167:387–392.
145. Penso C, Redline RW, Benacerraf BR. A sonographic sign which predicts which fetuses with hydrocephalus have an associated neural tube defect. *J Ultrasound Med.* 1987;6:307–311.
146. Thiagarajah S, Henke J, Hogge WA, Abbitt PL, Breeden N, Ferguson JE. Early diagnosis of spina bifida: The value of cranial ultrasound markers. *Obstet Gynecol.* 1990;76:54–57.
147. Goldstein RB, Podrasky AE, Filly RA, Callen PW. Effacement of the fetal cisterna magna in association with myelomeningocele [see comments]. *Radiology.* 1989;172:409–413.
148. Pilu G, Romero R, Reece EA, Goldstein I, Hobbins JC, Bovicelli L. Subnormal cerebellum in fetuses with spina bifida. *Am J Obstet Gynecol.* 1988;158:1052–1056.
149. Callen AL, Filly RA. Supratentorial abnormalities in the Chiari II malformation:1. The ventricular "point."*J Ultrasound Med.* 2008;27: 33–38.
150. Callen AL, Stengel JW, Filly RA. Supratentorial abnormalities in the Chiari II malformation:2. Tectal morphologic changes. *J Ultrasound Med.* 2009;28:29–35.
151. Wong SK, Barkovich AJ, Callen AL, Filly RA. Supratentorial abnormalities in the Chiari II malformation:3. The interhemispheric cyst. *J Ultrasound Med.* 2009;28:999–1006.
152. Levine D, Trop I, Mehta TS, Barnes PD. MR imaging appearance of fetal cerebral ventricular morphology. *Radiology.* 2002;223:652–660.
153. Rickard S, Morris J, Paley M, Griffiths P, Whitby E. In utero magnetic resonance of non-isolated ventriculomegaly: Does ventricular size or morphology reflect pathology? *Clin Radiol.* 2006;61:844–853.
154. Wolpert SM, Anderson M, Scott RM, Kwan ES, Runge VM. Chiari II malformation: MR imaging evaluation. *AJR Am J Roentgenol.* 1987; 149:1033–1042.
155. Just M, Schwarz M, Ludwig B, Ermert J, Thelen M. Cerebral and spinal MR: Findings in patients with postrepair myelomeningocele. *Pediatr Radiol.* 1990;20:262–266.
156. Vergani P, Locatelli A, Piccoli MG, et al. Ultrasonographic differential diagnosis of fetal intracranial interhemispheric cysts. *Am J Obstet Gynecol.* 1999;180:423–428.
157. Chaoui R, Benoit B, Mitkowska-Wozniak H, Heling KS, Nicolaides KH. Assessment of intracranial translucency (IT) in the detection of spina bifida at the 11–13-week scan. *Ultrasound Obstet Gynecol.* 2009;34:249–252.
158. Chaoui R, Nicolaides KH. From nuchal translucency to intracranial translucency: Towards the early detection of spina bifida. *Ultrasound Obstet Gynecol.* 2010;35:133–138.
159. Bonaiti-Pellie C, Smith C. Risk tables for genetic counselling in some common congenital malformations. *J Med Genet.* 1974;11:374–347.
160. Chescheir NC. Maternal-fetal surgery: Where are we and how did we get here? *Obstet Gynecol.* 2009;113:717–731.
161. Adzick NS. Fetal myelomeningocele: Natural history, pathophysiology, and in-utero intervention. *Semin Fetal Neonatal Med.* 2010;15(1):9–14.
162. Thompson DN. Postnatal management and outcome for neural tube defects including spina bifida and encephalocoeles. *Prenat Diagn.* 2009;29:412–419.
163. Luthy DA, Wardinsky T, Shurtleff DB, et al. Cesarean section before the onset of labor and subsequent motor function in infants with meningomyelocele diagnosed antenatally. *NEJM.* 1991;324: 662–666.

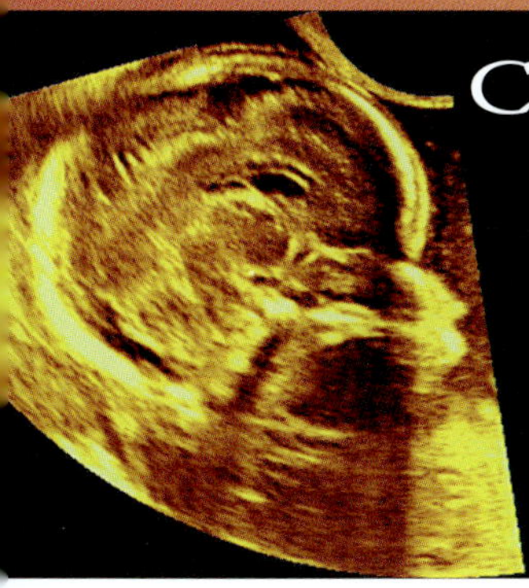

Chapter 6

# ANOMALIES OF VENTRAL INDUCTION

*Gianluigi Pilu • Selim Buyukkurt • Gustavo Malinger*

## KEY POINTS

1. Anomalies of ventral induction of the fetal brain include a group of conditions that share in common an anomalous process of cleavage of the brain and formation of midline structures, encompassing a wide spectrum of severity. They are frequently associated with other malformations and genetic conditions.
2. Holoprosencephaly is one of the most severe disorders of ventral induction; it features incomplete separation of the cerebral hemispheres and has a very severe prognosis in most cases.
3. Agenesis of the corpus callosum is either complete or limited to the posterior portion; the anatomy is variable, but enlargement of the lateral ventricles and the absence of the cavity of the septum pellucidum are frequently present. The prognosis is largely influenced by the the association with other anomalies; isolated agenesis of the corpus callosum may be associated with a normal intellectual development, although the experience is limited.
4. Agenesis of the septum pellucidum is frequently a part of other, often severe malformations, including holoprosenephaly, gross hydrocephaly, and schizencephaly. Isolated agenesis of the septum pellucidum may be a normal variant, although it may be the only antenatal finding of septo-optic dysplasia, a condtiion that is usually associated with visual impairment and endocrine disfunction.

The ontogenesis of the cerebral midline is frequently referred to as the process of ventral induction. It takes place between the fifth week after conception and midgestation.[1] Anomalies occurring during this period lead to the development of a wide range of malformations with a severity that is closely related with the time of occurrence. Beause ventral induction is closely related to facial development, many fetuses and children with prosencephalic disorders suffer from facial anomalies. A categorization of these anomalies is presented in Table 6–1. Disorders of prosencephalic formation, aprosencephaly and atelencephaly, will not be discussed in the following sections, as they are the extreme end of the spectrum of severity, and their occurrence is extremely rare. Aprosencephaly is the complete lack of development of the telencephalon and diencephalon, and in atelencephaly, the diencephalon is present but usually abnormal.[2] In all prenatal reports, a different brain malformation was diagnosed in utero, and the definitive diagnosis was reached only after pathologic examination.[3] Disorders of prosencephalic cleavage, holoprosencephaly and holotelencephaly, follow in the degree of severity. Disorders of prosencephalic midline development, agenesis of the corpus callosum, agenesis of septum pellucidum, and septo-optic dysplasia, usually have less severe presentations, but affected subjects may suffer from neurodevelopmental retardation and endocrinologic and visual disorders.

## DISORDERS OF PROSENCEPHALIC CLEAVAGE

### Holoprosencephaly

#### Definition

Holoprosencephaly is a genetically and phenotypically heterogeneous disorder involving the development of the forebrain and midface.

#### Synonyms

Arhinencephaly

#### Incidence

Holoprosencephaly is seen in 1.0 to 1.7 per 10,000 births and terminations.[4,5] The real incidence is probably higher than that, because the most severe forms of holoprosencephaly may result in early pregnancy loss,[6] and minor forms will not be recognized at birth, thus escaping epidemiologic surveys.

#### Pathogenesis

Holoprosencephaly is commonly regarded as the result of a failure of cleavage of the prosencephalon. The prosencephalon is the most rostrad of the three primitive cerebral vesicles and gives rise to the cerebral hemispheres and diencephalic structures (including the neurohypophysis, thalami, and third ventricle). This differentiation process

**Table 6–1. ANOMALIES OF VENTRAL INDUCTION**

| |
|---|
| Disorders of prosencephalic formation<br>Aprosencephaly<br>Atelencephaly |
| Disorders of prosencephalic cleavage<br>Holoprosencephaly<br>Holotelencephaly |
| Disorders of prosencephalic midline development<br>Agenesis of the corpus callosum, complete and partial<br>Agenesis of the septum pellucidum<br>Septo-optic dysplasia |

is thought to be induced by the precordal mesenchyma, which is probably also responsible for the differentiation of the median facial structures (forehead, nose, interorbital structures, premaxilla, and upper lip).

An interference with the activity of the prechordal mesenchyma would lead to defects in both the brain and midface. The cerebral anomalies are due to varying degrees of failure of cleavage of the derivatives of the prosencephalon, with incomplete division of the cerebral hemispheres and underlying structures. The facial anomalies encompass a broad range of defects that are due to aplasia or varying degrees of hypoplasia of the median structures (Table 6–2). Holoprosencephaly indeed fits the definition of a malformative sequence, featuring both cerebral and facial anomalies.

## Etiology

Holoprosencephaly is a genetically heterogeneous condition involving at least 12 known loci on 11 chromosomes. The known holoprosencephaly-associated genes include Sonic hedgehog (*SHH*) on 7q36 (MIM 600725), *ZIC2* on 13q32 (MIM 603073), *SIX3* on 2p21 (MIM 603714), and TG-interacting factor (*TGIF*) on 18p11.3 (MIM 602630). Hereditary holoprosencephaly has been reported with autosomal dominant inheritance with variable penetrance (MIM 142945), autosomal recessive (MIM 236100), and X-linked recessive (MIM 306990).[7,8] Holoprosencephaly is commonly associated with chromosomal abnormalities, mostly with trisomy 13 and triploidy.[9–11] Syndromes that include holoprosencephaly among their manifestations are DiGeorge, Meckel, Kallmann, campomelic dysplasia, Hall-Pallister, and Vasadi, among others. There are no environmental teratogens known to cause this malformation in humans, but in animals the condition can be induced by veratrum alkaloids and radiation. Ingestion of salicylates in pregnancy has also been reported in relation to holoprosencephaly.

**Table 6–2. FACIAL DEFECTS IN HOLOPROSENCEPHALY**

| | |
|---|---|
| Cyclopia | Single eye or single orbit<br>Arrhinia with prosboscis |
| Ethmocephaly | Extreme hypotelorism<br>Arrhinia with prosboscis |
| Cebocephaly | Orbital hypotelorism<br>Prosboscis-like nose, no cleft |
| Median cleft | Orbital hypotelorism<br>Flat nose |
| Agnathia-astomia | Hypoplasia or absence of the mandible<br>Small or absent mouth<br>Abnormal position of the ears |

## Pathology

Holoprosencephaly is a continuum of malformations (Figure 6–1). A widely accepted classification recognizes three major varieties: the alobar, semilobar, and lobar type.[9] Recently, a new variant, the middle interhemispheric variant, has been described,[12–14] and the term *holotencephaly* has been suggested to describe cases with less pronounced derangement, with hemispheres incompletely cleaved but normal diencephalon.[15] In the alobar variety, the most severe one, the interhemispheric fissure and the falx cerebri are totally absent, there is a single primitive ventricle, the thalami are fused on the midline, and there is absence of the third ventricle, neurohypophysis, and olfactory bulbs and tracts. The term *arhinencephaly* is indeed frequently used as a synonym of *holoprosencephaly.* In the semilobar variety, the two cerebral hemispheres are partially separated posteriorly, but there is still a single anterior ventricular cavity. In both the alobar and semilobar forms, the roof of the ventricular cavity, the tela choroidea, normally enfolded within the brain, may balloon out between the cerebral convexity and the skull to form a cyst of variable size, commonly referred to as the dorsal sac. With lobar holoprosencephaly, the anatomical derangement is much more subtle. In pathologic studies, this condition is usually described as a brain almost completely divided into two distinct hemispheres, with the only exception being a variable degree of fusion at the level of the cingulate gyrus and frontal horns of the lateral ventricles. The septum pellucidum is always absent. The olfactory bulbs and tracts and the corpus callosum may be absent, hypoplastic, or normal. An interesting aspect of lobar holoprosencephaly that has been described in studies employing magnetic resonance is the fusion of the fornices, which are seen as a solid fasicle running in the midline in the upper portion of the third ventricle.[16]

Pleomorphic facial anomalies are a part of the holoprosencephalic sequence[17] (Table 6–2). Facial anomalies are usually encountered with the alobar and semilobar types, rarely with lobar holoprosencephaly or holotelencephaly. It should be stressed that infants with any kind of holoprosencephaly may have a normal face.[9]

## Associated Anomalies

Holoprosencephaly reflects a very early derangement of embryogenesis and is very frequently associated with

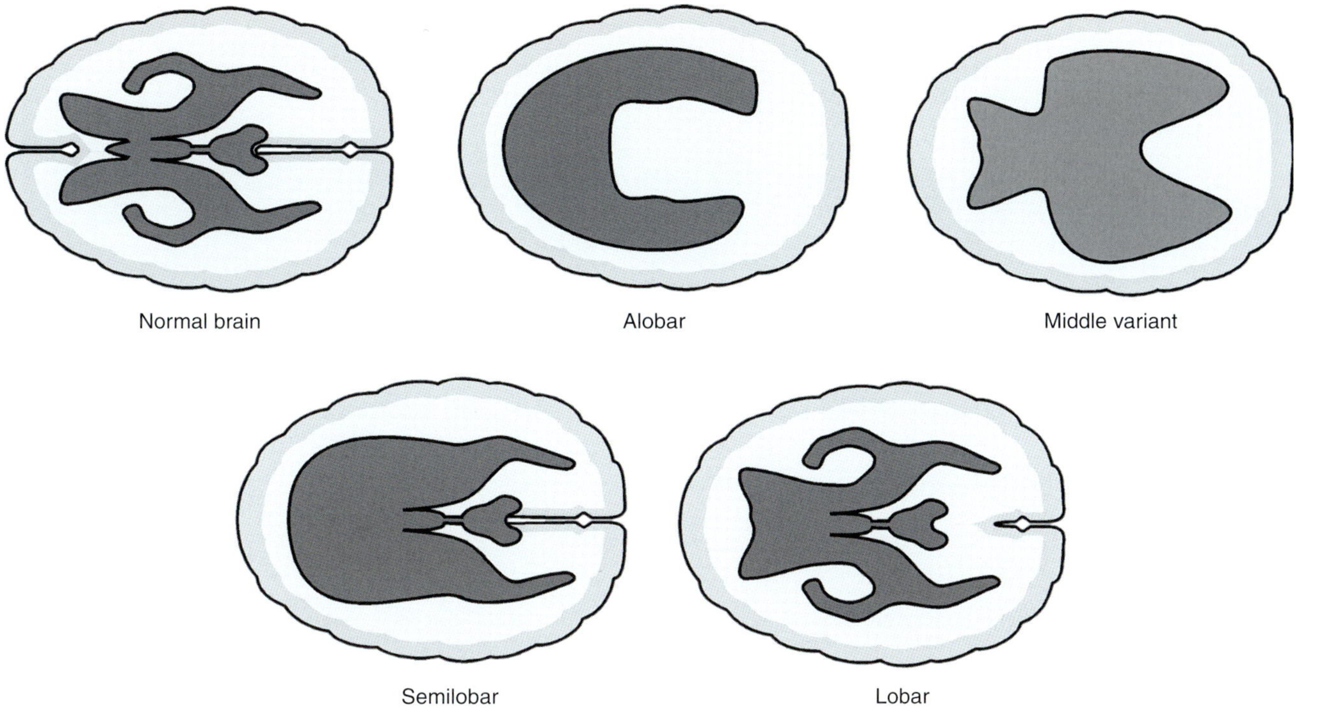


**Figure 6–1.** Schematic representation of a normal brain compared with different varieties of holoprosencephaly seen on an axial plane.

other malformations.[8] Apart from facial anomalies, which are considered a part of the malformative sequence, and other telencephalic anomalies, such as interhemispheric cysts and lipomas, holoprosencephaly has a striking association with two other conditions: chromosomal aberrations and Dandy-Walker malformation. The list of chromosomal aberrations found in patients with holoprosencephaly includes more than 35 conditions, but only 7 are frequently described: trisomy 13, del(13q), del(18p), trisomy 18, triploidy, dup(3p), and de1(7)(pter+q32).[8,10,11] It has been estimated that over 60% of infants with trisomy 13 have holoprosencephaly; conversely, holoprosencephaly is associated with trisomy 13 in ~20% of cases. All varieties of holoprosencephaly are often associated with microcephaly, less frequently with macrocephaly, which is invariably due to internal obstructive hydrocephaly.

## Recurrence Risk

Holoprosencephaly with normal chromosomes has an estimated recurrence risk in siblings of 6%, but this calculation is derived from both truly sporadic events and hereditary conditions with 25% to 50% risk.[8]

## Diagnosis

The most valuable clue to the diagnosis is the demonstration of the single primitive ventricle (Figure 6–2).[9,18,19] When present, the dorsal sac can be recognized (Figure 6–3). Depending on the degree of enfolding of the cortex over the ventricle, alobar holoprosencephaly may be further subdivided into a pancake, cup, and ball variety (Figure 6–4). Demonstration of facial anomalies such as cyclopia, hypotelorism, and median cleft lip strengthens the diagnosis of holoprosencephaly based on central nervous system (CNS) findings. Conversely, should any of the mentioned facial features be serendipitously encountered, a careful examination of the intracranial contents is recommended.

By using high-frequency transvaginal transducers, diverticulation of the forebrain can be demonstrated as early as the seventh week of amenorrhea. Indeed, by using this approach, a diagnosis of the alobar variety can be easily made at the onset of the second trimester,[20] and in some instances even during the first trimester[18,21] (Figure 6–5).

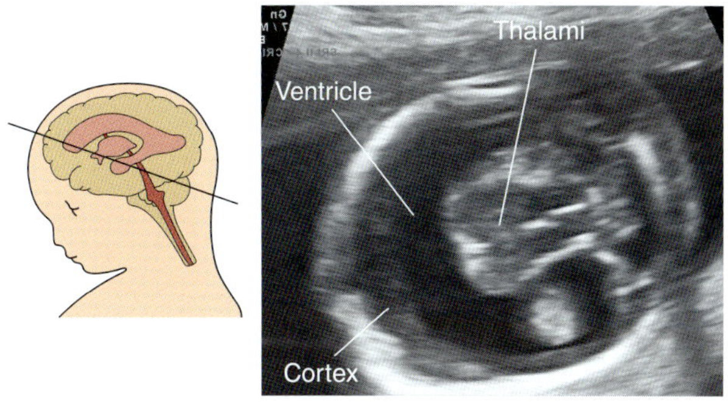


**Figure 6–2.** Most cases of alobar holoprosencephaly seen around midgestation will appear like this: In an axial scan at the level of the thalami, there is no midline echo, and a crescent-shaped ventricular cavity is seen between the anterior frontal cortex and the posterior bulb-shaped thalami. The posterior fossa may be normal. (Reproduced, with permission, from *Atlas of Obstetric Ultrasound*, 2009. The Global Library of Women's Medicine. www.glowm.com.)

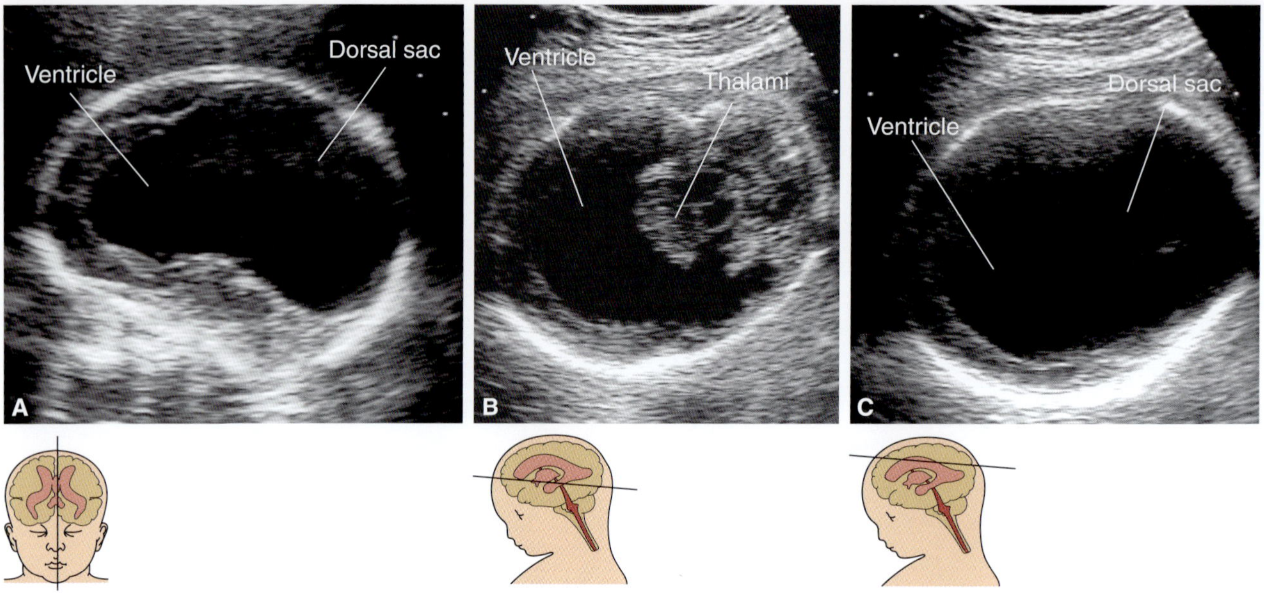


**Figure 6–3.** Multiplanar sonography of alobar holoprosencephaly in the midtrimester. (**A**) Median plane demonstrating the single ventricular cavity, which has a rim of cortex anteriorly and amply communicates posteriorly with a dorsal sac. (**B**) Axial scan at the level of the thalamus, demonstrating the crescent-shaped single ventricle and the absence of the midline in the anterior cortex. (**C**) In a slightly craniad axial plane than the previous one, the communication between the ventricular cavity and the dorsal sac is demonstrated. (Reproduced, with permission, from the *Visual Encyclopedia of Ultrasound in Obstetrics and Gynecology,* International Society of Ultrasound in Obstetrics and Gynecology, 2010, www.isuog.org.)

Timor-Tritsch et al[22] used three-dimensional (3D) inversion rendering in the first as well as the early second trimester as an aid to diagnose holoprosencephaly. It was possible to discern between alobar and semilobar holoprosencephaly (Figure 6–6).

The ultrasonic findings of semilobar holoprosencephaly are very similar to the ones described for the alobar type. The diagnosis of the semilobar variety is suggested by the presence of well-developed occipital horns. Although lobar holoprosencephaly is amenable to antenatal identification, a specific diagnosis is difficult. The typical case will present with absence of the septum pellucidum and slightly enlarged and dysmorphic lateral ventricles (Figure 6–7). The major problem resides in the differential diagnosis between lobar holoprosencephaly, agenesis of the septum pellucidum, and other hydrocephalic conditions associated

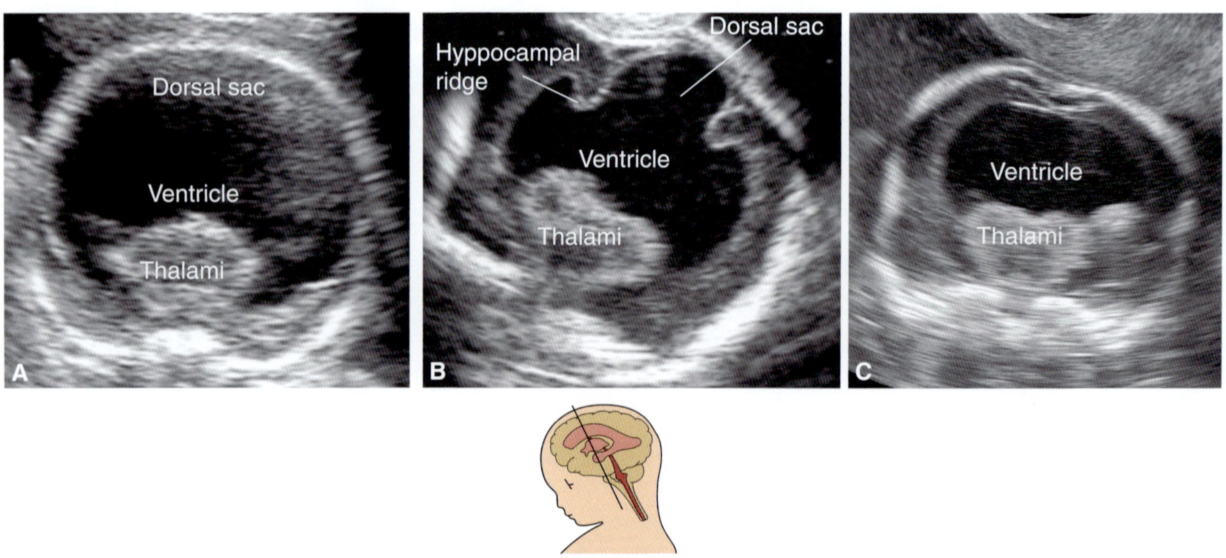


**Figure 6–4.** In alobal holoprosencephaly, a dorsal sac is frequently seen on top of the ventricular cavity; the degree of development of the cortex is variable. (**A**) In some cases, it forms a thin rim at the base of the ventricles (pancake). (**B**) In other cases, it is partially enfolded on top of the ventricular cavity. (**C**) In still other cases, the ventricle is completely covered, and there is no dorsal sac; frequently, these cases are pathologically diagnosed as belonging to the semilobar variety. (Reproduced, with permission, from the *Visual Encyclopedia of Ultrasound in Obstetrics and Gynecology,* International Society of Ultrasound in Obstetrics and Gynecology, 2010, www.isuog.org.)

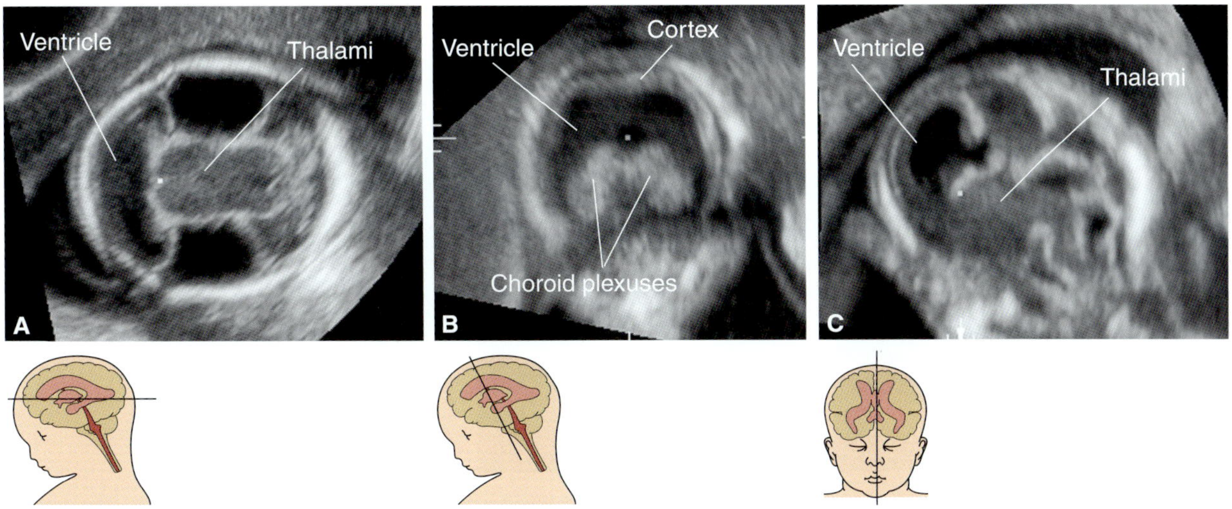


**Figure 6–5.** Alobar holoprosencephaly in a fetus at 13 postmenstrual weeks. The most striking findings, the absence of the midline echo and the presence of a single rudimentary ventricular cavity, are well demonstrated in a vaginal scan. (Reproduced, with permission, from Tutschek B, PiluG. Virtual reality ultrasound imaging of the normal and abnormal fetal central nervous system. *Ultrasound Obstet Gynecol.* 2009;34(3):259–267.)

with secondary disruption of the septum pellucidum. Failure to demonstrate a well-developed corpus callosum, poorly formed frontal horns, and incomplete separation of the inferior frontal lobes favor the diagnosis of lobar holoprosencephaly.[9,16,23,24] Recently, it has been suggested that color Doppler may be useful for a specific diagnosis. In lobar holoprosencephaly, the frontal horns are fused, and the anterior cerebral arteries run along the surface of the brain instead of coursing within the interhemispheric fissure. This sign has been defined as the serpent crawling under the skull.[23] The middle interhemispheric variant of holoprosencephaly is intermediate between the lobar and alobar variety. When compared with the alobar variety, the frontal lobes are more differentiated than usual with recognizable frontal horns. Posteriorly, however, there is one single large and undifferentiated ventricular cavity with a hypoplastic diencephalon (Figure 6–8).

A specific diagnosis of holotelencephaly is difficult. We have always found this condition with severe obstructive ventricular dilation, as well as well-formed but fused frontal horns because of the absence of the septum pellucidum. In all our cases, as well as in some cases of the lobar type, the fornices are fused and are seen in the midline as a thick fasicle running from the anterior to the posterior commissure.[16] In a midcoronal scan, the abnormal fornices result in a peculiar image: a small, round structure is seen in the midportion of the third ventricle (Figure 6–9). Fetal magnetic resonance imaging (MRI) may have a role in the elucidation of particularly difficult cases of lobar types or some of the nonclassical forms, such as the middle interhemispheric variant.[13,25]

## Differential Diagnosis

Alobar holoprosencephaly with a large ventricular cavity and/or dorsal sac has an appearance similar to that of hydranencephaly. Although in our experience demonstration of the remains of the frontal cortex and/or facial anomalies has always allowed a clear distinction between these two entities, it goes without saying that, from a practical perspective, a diagnostic error would be anyhow uneventful, given the very poor prognosis of both conditions. Lobar holoprosencephaly must be distinguished from simple hydrocephaly with secondary disruption of the septum pellucidum.[12] A midcoronal scan of the fetal head is the most important view to differentiate among these two conditions, because it allows identification of findings that are typical of lobar holoprosencephaly: the flat roof of the frontal horns and the possible presence of the fused fornices. Distinction between lobar holoprosencephaly and the absence of the septum pellucidum, isolated or associated with septo-optic dysplasia, is a much greater challenge, and the experience is limited. We have always found lobar holoprosencephaly associated with significant derangements of the anatomy of the hemispheres. The presence of well-formed and separated frontal horns and corpus callosum favors the diagnosis of absence of the septum pellucidum.[12]

## Implications for Sonographic Diagnosis

In many cases, expert vaginal sonography can diagnose alobar and possibly semilobar forms during the first trimester.[18,21] The lobar variety is probably difficult to identify prior to 16 to 18 weeks.

## Implications for Sonographic Screening

Alobar and semilobar holoprosencephalies are associated with profound distortion of intracranial architecture that should always be detected with a standard sonographic examination performed in the midtrimester. Findings associated with the lobar variety may be subtle. The cavum septi pellucidi, however, is always absent, with central fusion of the frontal horns. Identification of the absence of the septum pellucidum is not always easy.[26]

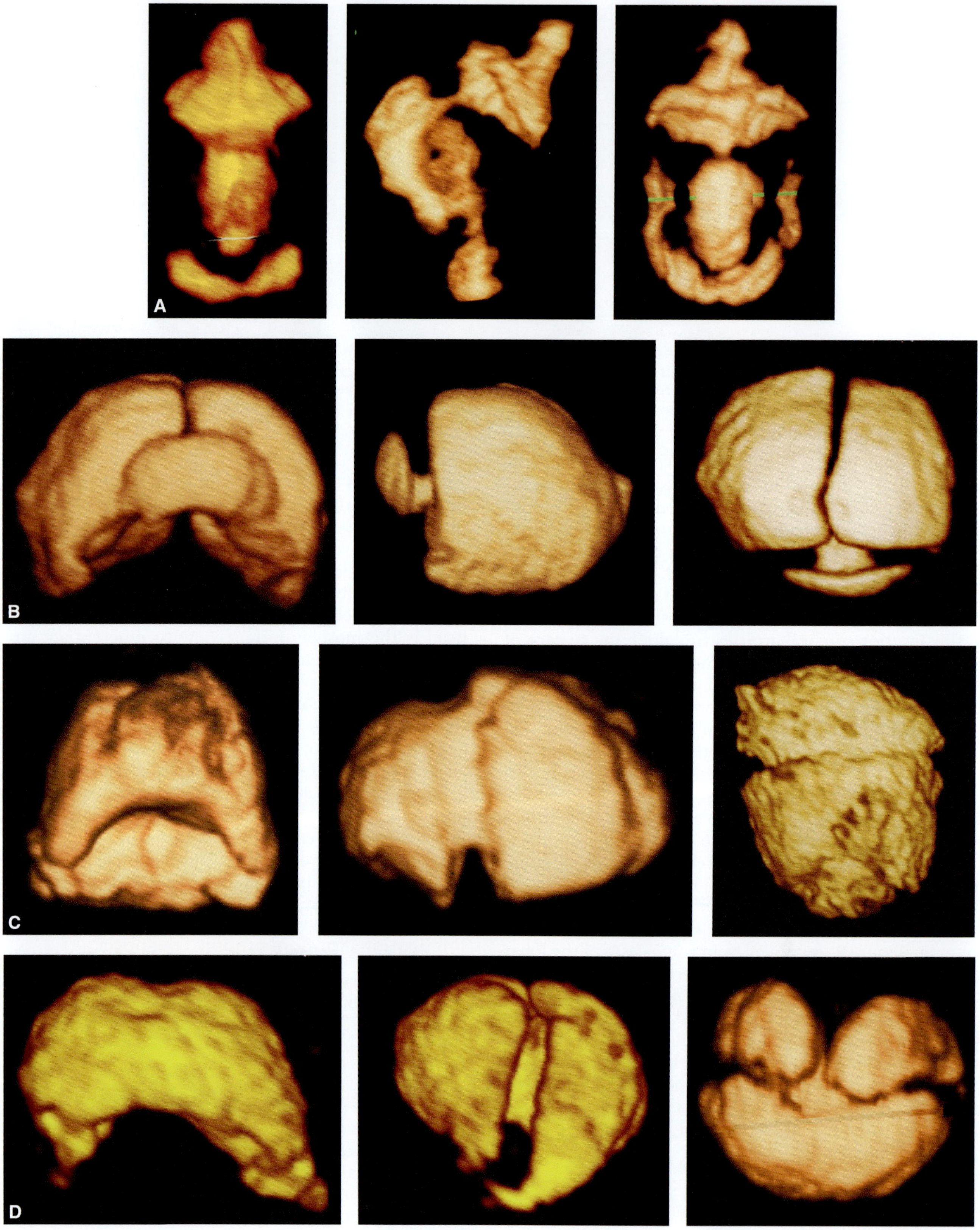


**Figure 6–6.** Pictorial table showing three-dimensional inversion rendering of the fluid in the ventricles of fetuses with holoprosencephaly in lateral, frontal, and superior views. (**A**) 9 weeks 2 days; (**B**) 10 weeks 2 days; (**C**) 13 weeks 5 days; (**D**) 14 weeks 5 days. (Reproduced, with permission, from Timor-Tritsch IE, Monteagudo A, Santos R. Three dimensional inversion rendering in the first and early second trimester fetal brain: Its use in holoprosencephaly. *Ultrasound Obstet Gynecol.* 2008;32:744–750.)

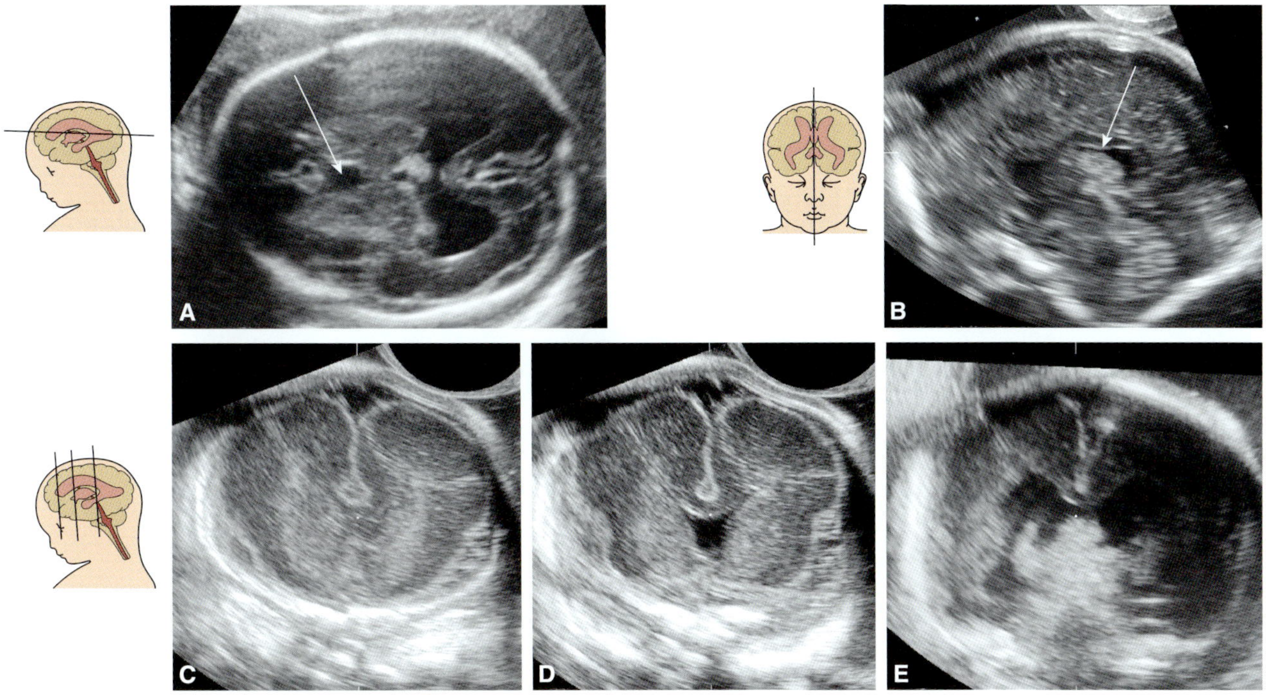


**Figure 6–7.** Lobar holoprosencephaly. (**A**) The cavum septi pellucidi is absent, and the lateral ventricles appear significantly dysmorphic and fused from the level of the frontal horns to the bodies. (**B**) In the sagittal plane, the corpus callosum is not clearly visible, and only an irregular ridge of tissue is seen bridging between the hemispheres posteriorly (*arrow*). (**C–E**) Coronal sections are most useful for the diagnosis in that they demonstrate inferior fusion of the frontal lobes, poorly developed fused frontal horns, and communication between the bodies of the lateral ventricles. (Reproduced, with permission, from the *Visual Encyclopedia of Ultrasound in Obstetrics and Gynecology,* International Society of Ultrasound in Obstetrics and Gynecology, 2010, www.isuog.org.)

## Prognosis

Alobar holoprosencephaly is lethal, although cases with long survival rates have been described. Semilobar holoprosencephaly is not necesserily lethal, but it is associated with extremely severe neurologic compromise. When these conditions are identified in utero, termination of pregnancy could be offered prior to viability. A conservative management is recommended in continuing pregnancies.

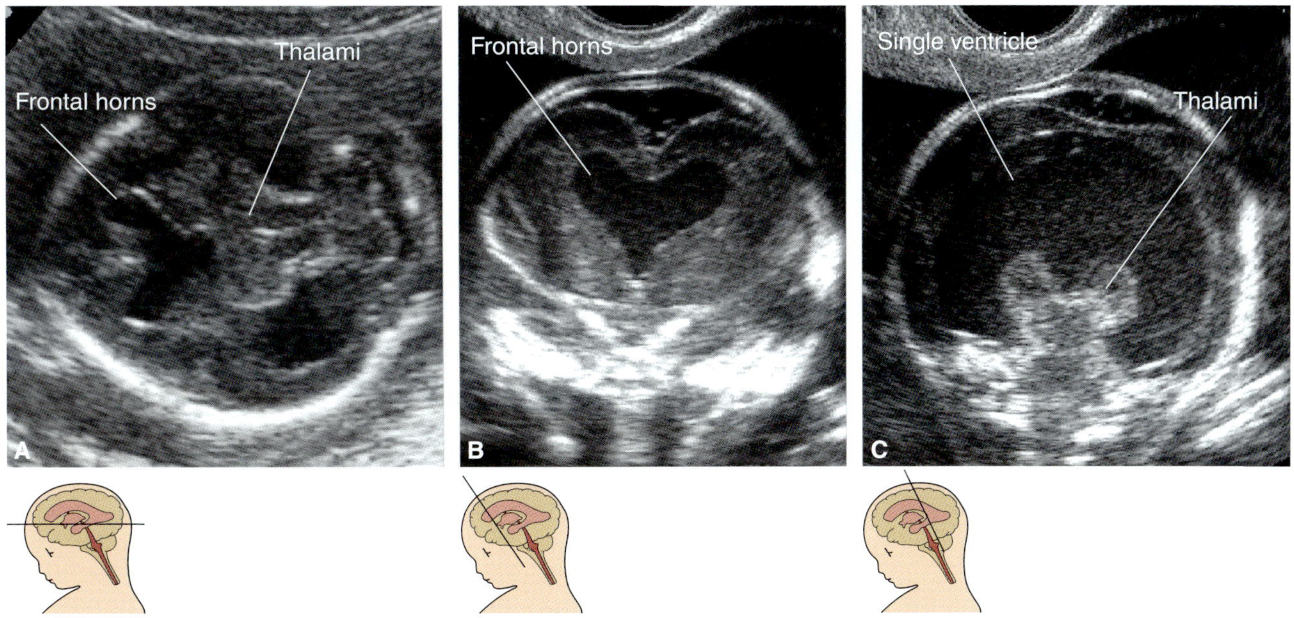


**Figure 6–8.** Middle interhemispheric variant of holoprosencephaly in the axial (**A**), anterior coronal (**B**), and midcoronal plane (**C**). The frontal horns are well developed, and there is a partial formation of the interhemispheric fissure. However, the midcoronal plane reveals a common ventricular cavity with hypoplastic undivided thalami.

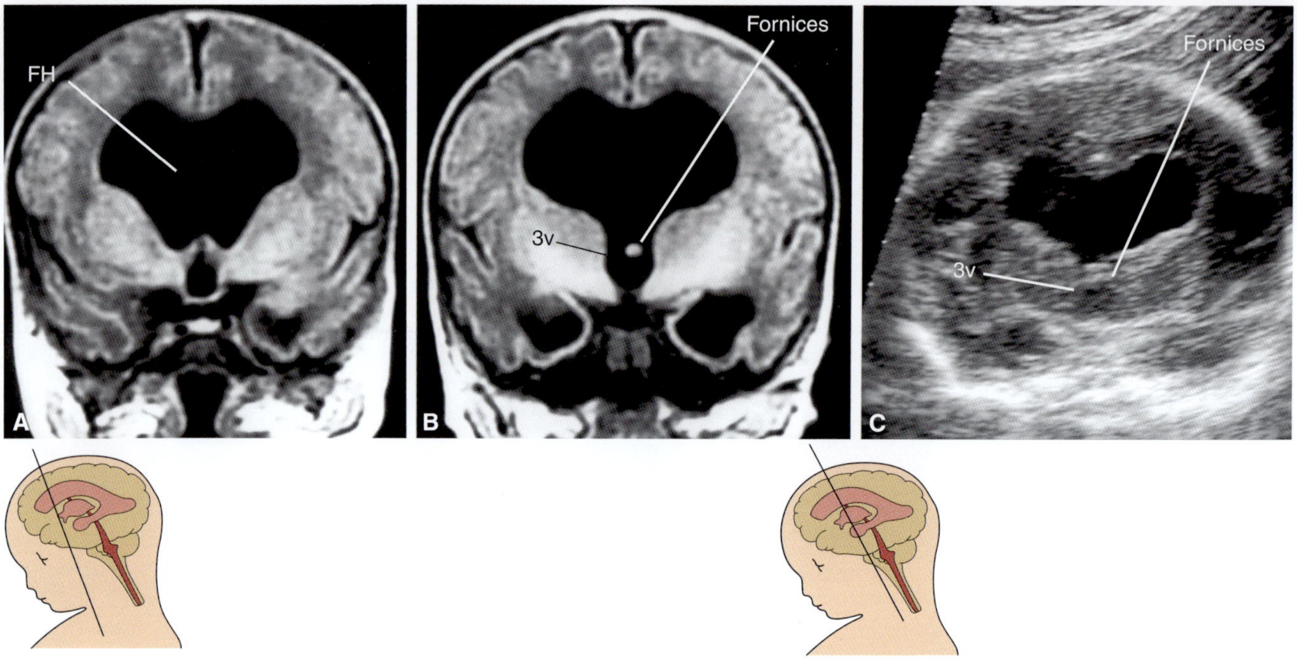


**Figure 6–9.** The appearance of a well-developed frontal cortex and ventricular system associated with obstructive dilation favors the diagnosis of holotelencephaly. The fornices (*arrow*) are fused and form a thick fascicle running in the floor of the ventricular cavity. (Reproduced, with permission, from Pilu G, Ambrosetto P, Sandri F, et al. Intraventricular fused fornices: A specific sign of fetal lobar holoprosencephaly. *Ultrasound Obstet Gynecol.* 1994;4[1]:65–67.)

The prognosis of lobar holoprosencephaly is uncertain. The available clinical data are limited. It has been reported that affected individuals may have a normal life span, but mental retardation and neurologic sequelae are common. Dysplasia of the aqueduct of Sylvius is presumably present in many cases, leading to obstructive hydrocephaly. The only available antenatal series includes five infants who were followed up after birth, and all had very abnormal developmental quotients. This series may be biased by the inclusion of fetuses with severe hydrocephaly and other associated anomalies.[24]

### Obstetric Management

Fetal karyotype is mandatory when holoprosencephaly is discovered by ultrasound (US). Termination of pregnancy can be offered to parents with previable fetuses. Because alobar and semilobar holoprosencephalies are associated with a dismal prognosis, in the presence of severe hydrocephaly, US-guided cephalocentesis could be considered to avoid the risk of dystocia.

## DISORDERS OF PROSENCEPHALIC MIDLINE DEVELOPMENT

### Agenesis of the corpus callosum

#### Definition

Agenesis of the corpus callosum is complete or partial absence of the corpus callosum. The corpus callosum is the largest commissure connecting the hemispheres and is composed of axonal tracts connecting between the right and left side of the brain. The corpus callosum starts its development relatively late in pregnancy, at around 10 weeks, and continues growing well after delivery.

#### Epidemiology

The incidence varies in different studies, depending on the population investigated and the method of ascertainment. Estimates of 0.3% to 0.7% in the general population[27] and 2% to 3% in the developmentally disabled are usually quoted.[28] In our own experience with low-risk patients assessed by US at 15 to 17 postmenstrual weeks and reassessed at 22 to 25 postmenstrual weeks, we found only one case of agenesis of the corpus callosum out of 2835 examinations (personal observation).

#### Etiology

The etiology is heterogeneous. Various teratogens have also been implicated as a possible cause of agenesis of the corpus callosum, including alcohol and maternal phenylketonuria. Genetic factors are probably predominant. Autosomal dominant, autosomal recessive, and sex-linked transmission have all been documented. Chromosomal anomalies, including autosomal trisomies and other rearrangements, are increasingly reported. Agenesis of the corpus callosum may also be associated with mendelian syndromes. Causative genes have not been found to date.[29] It is important to remember that congenital callosal pathologies may also develop after prenatal insults such as infections[30] or ischemic processes.[31]

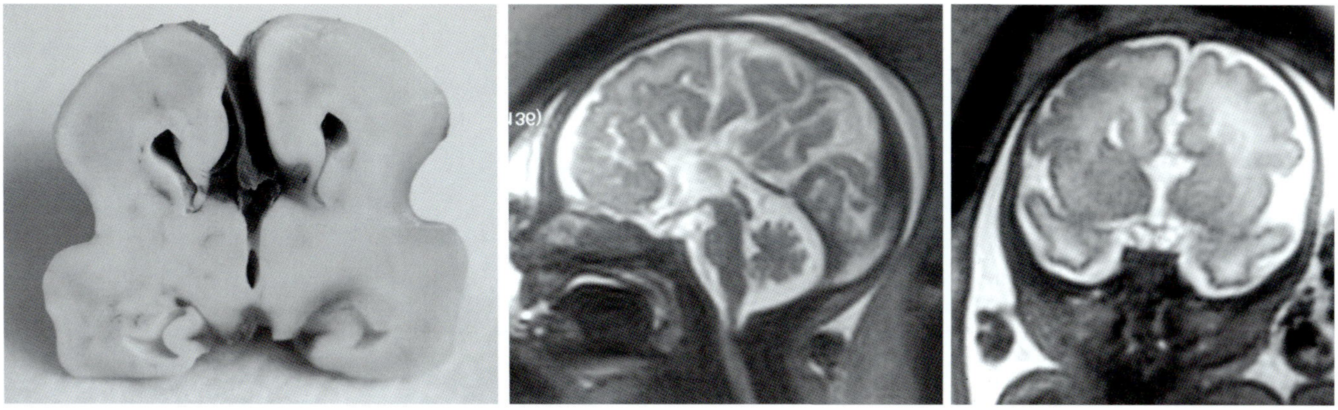

**Figure 6–10.** Complete agenesis of the corpus callosum. (**A**) Pathology in a midtrimester fetus. (**B,C**) Magnetic resonance imaging (MRI) at 32 postmenstrual weeks. Apart from the absence of the corpus callosum, a number of abnormal findings can be appreciated, including the enlarged interhemispheric fissure due to the separation of the hemispheres, the comma-shaped frontal horns, and the radiate array of sulci around the roof of the third ventricles. (Reproduced, with permission, from the *Visual Encyclopedia of Ultrasound in Obstetrics and Gynecology*, International Society of Ultrasound in Obstetrics and Gynecology, 2010, www.isuog.org.)

## Embryology/Pathology

The corpus callosum is a broad plate of dense myelinated fibers, located deep in the longitudinal fissure, that reciprocally interconnect regions of the cortex in all lobes with corresponding regions of the opposite hemispheres. It derives from the massa commissuralis, an embryologic structure formed by the fusion of the lateral margins of the groove that separates the primitive telencephalic vesicles. Formation of the corpus callosum is a late event in cerebral ontogenesis. Callosal fibers may be identified close to the lamina terminalis during the 10th gestational week, but the corpus callosum itself develops some weeks later. Histologic studies have shown the presence of callosal fibers crossing the midline at 13 weeks, but recent studies based on diffusion tensor MRI were able to demonstrate the presence of a clearly defined midline corpus callosum only at around 15 weeks; by this time only the anterior portions (rostrum, genu, and part of the body) are present.[32] In the same study, the corpus callosum was fully identified only 3 to 5 weeks later. The corpus callosum is in close anatomical and embryologic relationship with the underlyng septum pellucidum. Although there is no a priori evidence to suggest that the development of the septum pellucidum cannot proceed independently of the corpus callosum, most observers claim that there can be no septum pellucidum without a corpus callosum.

Agenesis of the corpus callosum may be either complete (Figure 6–10) or partial (Figure 6–11). When partial, the caudad portion (splenium and body) is most commonly missing to varying degrees (Figure 6–12), but some degree of anterior agenesis or dysmorphism may be present.

Complete agenesis of the corpus callosum is typically associated with significant distortion of the intracranial architecture. The lateral ventricles tend to be larger than normal, particularly at the level of the atria and occipital horns. It has been postulated that the absence of the posterior portion of the corpus callosum results in distortion of the array of white matter tracts in the occipital lobes, leading to caudad expansion of the ventricles.[33] Such ventricular enlargement tends to be stable and is not usually associated with intracranial hypertension. The frontal horns are usually normal in size but are more separated than usual from the midline. The third ventricle is often superiorly elongated, reaching the area normally occupied by the corpus callosum. At times, it may be found to communicate with a large interhemispheric cyst. On other

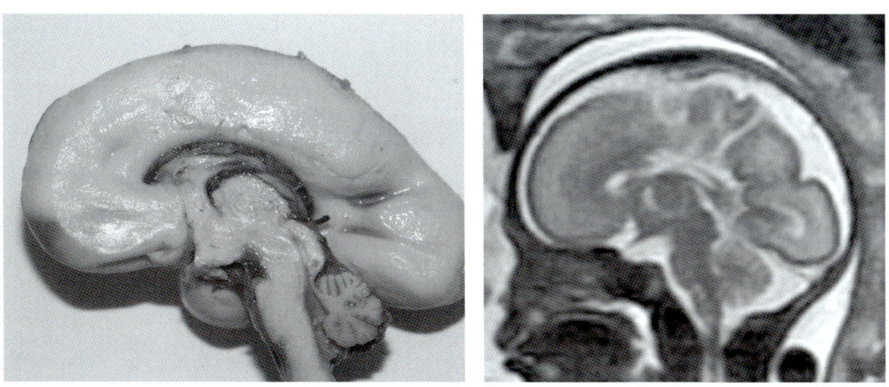

**Figure 6–11.** Partial agenesis of the corpus callosum. (**A**) Pathology in a midtrimester fetus. (**B**) MRI at 32 postmenstrual weeks. The corpus callosum does not arch over the entire area of the third ventricle but is interrupted about halfway. (Reproduced, with permission, from the *Visual Encyclopedia of Ultrasound in Obstetrics and Gynecology*, International Society of Ultrasound in Obstetrics and Gynecology, 2010, www.isuog.org.)

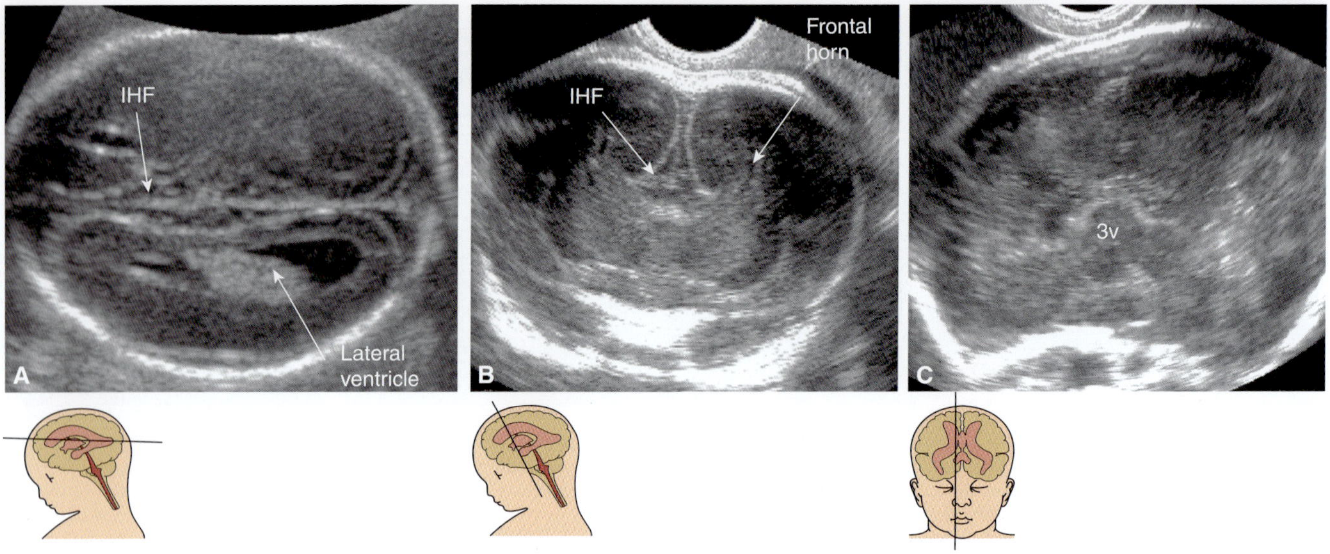


**Figure 6–12.** Sonography of fetal agenesis of the corpus callosum. (**A**) In the axial plane, the interhemispheric fissure (IHF) appears wider than usual without evidence of the cavum septi pellucidi. (**B**) In the coronal and sagittal plane, no corpus callosum and cavum septi pellucidi can be seen above the third ventricle (3v). (Reproduced, with permission, from the *Visual Encyclopedia of Ultrasound in Obstetrics and Gynecology,* International Society of Ultrasound in Obstetrics and Gynecology, 2010, www.isuog.org.)

occasions, a lipoma may be found at or above the position usually occupied by the corpus callosum. Absence of the corpus callosum also results in abnormal induction of medial cerebral convolutions determining during the third trimester a radiate arrangement of cerebral sulci around the roof of the third ventricle, extending through the zone normally occupied by the cingulate gyrus. The modification of the arterial vascular supply in infants with agenesis of the corpus callosum has been investigated in depth with both angiography and sonography and they are relevant for antenatal diagnosis. Under normal conditions, the callosal arteries, branches of the anterior cerebral arteries, run along the superior surface of the corpus callosum, describing a semicircular loop. When the corpus callosum is absent, such a loop is lost, and branches of the anterior cerebral artery are seen ascending linearly with a radiate arrangement.[34]

Hypoplasia of the corpus callosum refers to a corpus callosum that has a normal length but is thinner than normal.

## Diagnosis

Development of the corpus callosum is a late event, completed only by 18 weeks; therefore, an early diagnosis of its absence is difficult if not impossible. In one antenatal series, 10 of 15 affected fetuses were found to have an unremarkable intracranial sonogram at 16 to 22 postmenstrual weeks' gestation.[35] However, in expert hands complete agenesis of the corpus callosum can be realiably diagnosed as early as 18 to 20 postmenstrual weeks. Our earliest diagnosis was made in a pregnant patient at specific risk at 16 weeks. The demonstration of the normal corpus callosum is possible with US, starting from around 18 to 20 postmenstrual weeks of gestation, but requires some degree of technical skill, as this structure is not depicted using the standard axial planes, but coronal and particularly sagittal. In fetuses in the vertex presentation, the transvaginal approach is preferred;[36] in the breech presentation, we recommend a transfundal approach. Recently, the use of 3D multiplanar technique has been proposed.[37]

The anatomy of agenesis of the corpus callosum is variable. Definitive diagnosis depends on showing absence of the complex formed by the corpus callosum and cavum septum pellucidum. This should include multiplanar imaging to demonstrate the corpus callosum in both sagittal and coronal planes (Figure 6–13). Vaginal sonography is particularly helpful in vertex fetuses to obtain these views.

There are a number of other indirect clues to complete agenesis of the corpus callosum on standard transverve views. Failure to visualize the cavum septum pellucidum, which under normal conditions is seen without difficulty beyond 18 postmenstrual weeks, should raise the suspicion of agenesis of the corpus callosum. Other findings include

- Ventriculomegaly, typically mild. Prenatal studies suggest that agenesis of the corpus callosum is found in 3% of all fetuses with ventriculomegaly and in almost 10% of those with mild ventriculomegaly.[38–40]
- Disproportionate enlargement of the occipital horns (also referred to as colpocephaly) with a sharp anterior horn. This usually results in the typical teardrop configuration of the lateral ventricles[34] (Figure 6–13).
- Upward displacement of the third ventricle, which can be identified by demonstrating that this structure reaches superiorly the level of lateral ventricles[34] (Figure 6–14).

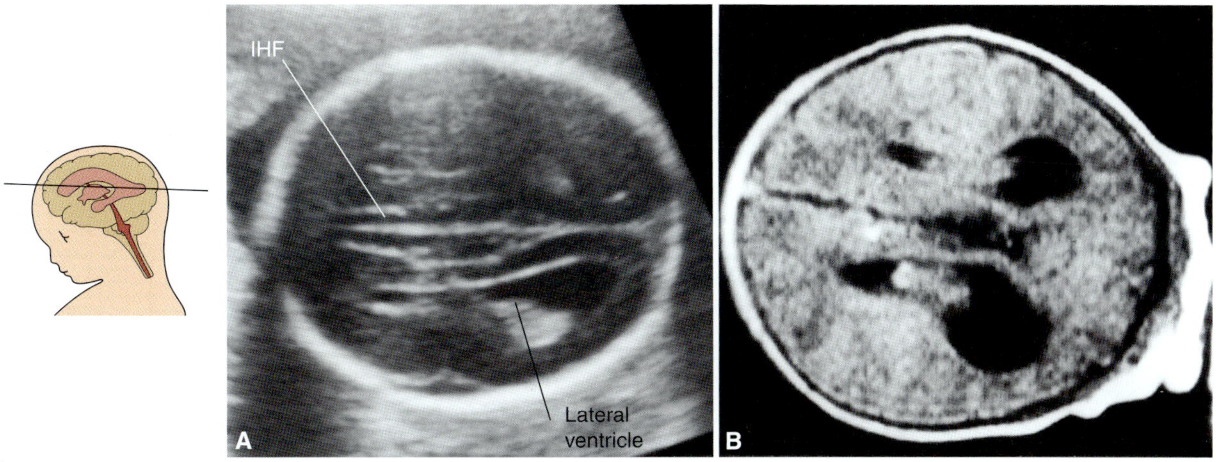


**Figure 6–13.** Ventriculomegaly with tear-shaped lateral ventricles is a very typical finding of agenesis of the corpus callosum. **(A)** fetal sonogram; **(B)** postnatal computed tomography (CT). The IHF is typically enlarged. (Reproduced, with permission, from Pilu G, Sandri F, Perolo A, et al. Sonography of fetal agenesis of the corpus callosum: A survey of 35 cases. *Ultrasound Obstet Gynecol.* 1993;3[5]:318–329.)

- Abnormal midline lesions occur frequently, including cysts (Figure 6–15)[41] and lipomas (Figure 6–16).[34,42] Lipomas appear as brightly echogenic lesions. A lipoma in the anterior midline is associated with agenesis of the corpus callosum in 50% of cases.[42] It is worth noting, however, that lipomas usually are not demonstrable in the second trimester and tend to appear only in late gestation.[34]
- Absence of the pericallosal arteries, branches of the anterior cerebral arteries that normally run along the superior surface of the corpus callosum in a semicircular loop. When the corpus callosum is absent, such a loop is lost, and branches of the anterior cerebral artery are seen ascending linearly with a radiate arrangement[34] (Figure 6–17).

Partial agenesis of the corpus callosum has been described antenatally.[34,43] The cerebral findings associated with it are usually more subtle than with the complete form. Ventriculomegaly and the teardrop sign are usually absent. The cavum septi pellucidi, although shorter, is present. In many cases, the diagnosis is only possible by demonstrating in a midsagittal plane that the corpus callosum is shorter than normal (Figure 6–18).

In addition to conventional US, 3D US may prove useful in evaluating fetuses with suspected agenesis of the corpus

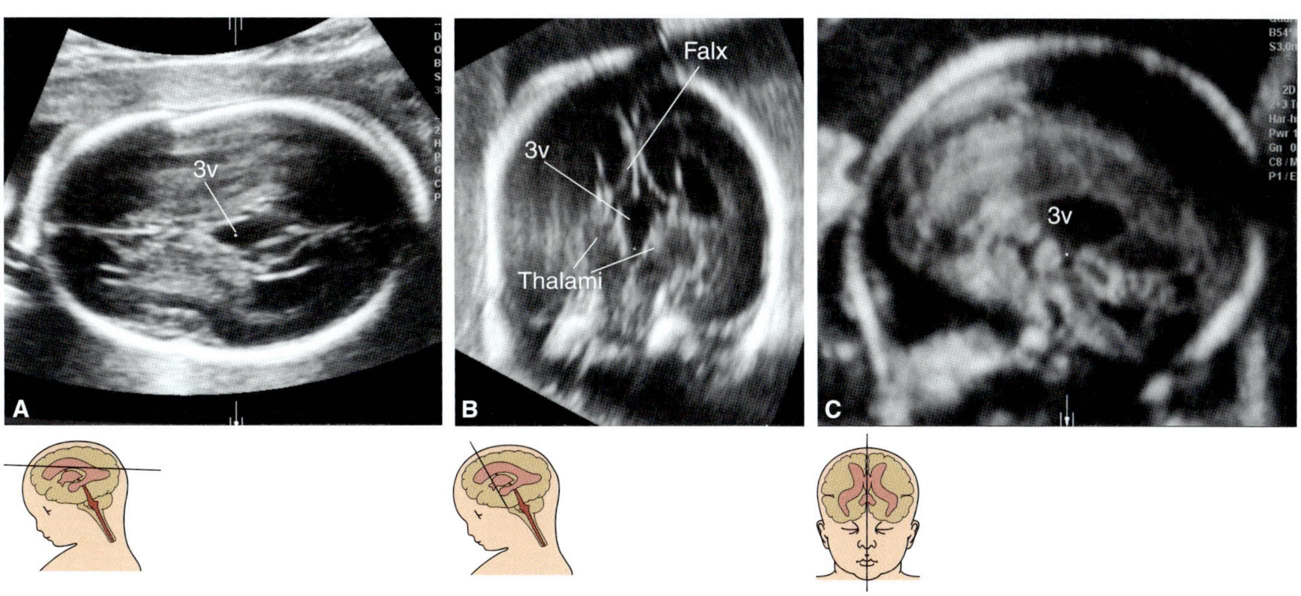


**Figure 6–14.** In this fetus with complete agenesis of the corpus callosum, the third ventricle is enlarged and superiorly displaced, coming into direct contact with the falx cerebri. (Reproduced, with permission, from the *Visual Encyclopedia of Ultrasound in Obstetrics and Gynecology,* International Society of Ultrasound in Obstetrics and Gynecology, 2010, www.isuog.org.)

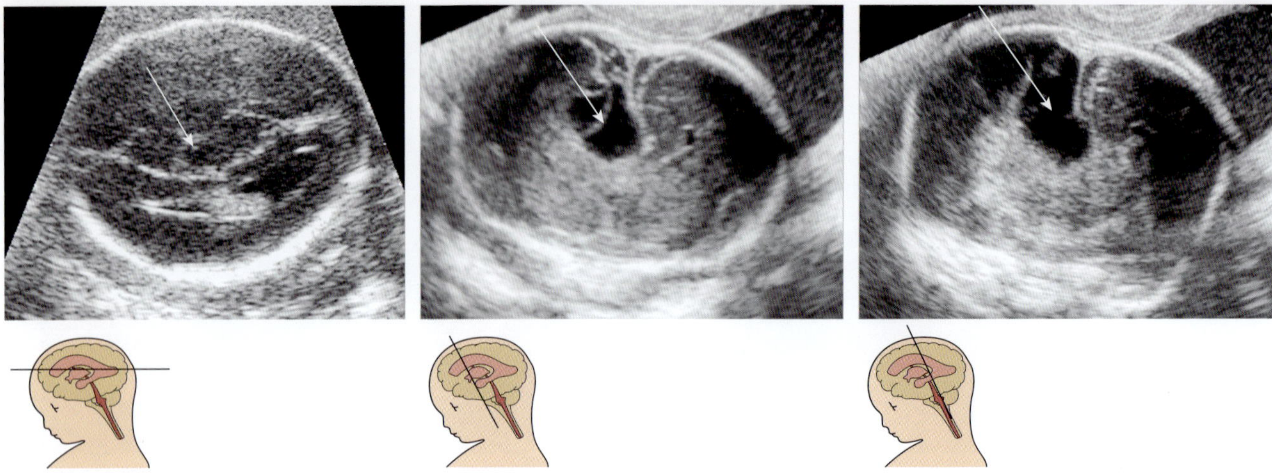

**Figure 6–15.** Agenesis of the corpus callosum with interhemispheric cysts. (Reproduced, with permission, from *the Visual Encyclopedia of Ultrasound in Obstetrics and Gynecology,* International Society of Ultrasound in Obstetrics and Gynecology, 2010, www.isuog.org.)

callosum by allowing the reconstruction of a sagittal plane even in cases where this is not easily accessible.[37,44] The role of MRI in the diagnosis and assessment of agenesis of the corpus callosum is controversial. Some authors have found it to be more informative than US.[45–47] In our experience, US provides a more detailed visualization of the corpus callosum than fetal MRI and enables better measurements of callosal length and thickness. We do agree, however, that MRI may be more informative regarding the presence of associated anomalies, and cortical malformations in particular.[45,46]

To our knowledge, hypoplasia of the corpus callosum has rarely been diagnosed in utero. In our own experience, we have recognized this condition in a handful of cases, but only in third trimester fetuses that had other CNS malformations.

## Differential Diagnosis

Agenesis of the corpus callosum must be distinguished from other causes of ventriculomegaly.[45] Agenesis of the corpus callosum with an interhemispheric cyst must be differentiated from other intracranial fluid-filled lesions, such as arachnoid cyst, porencephaly, or an aneurysm of the vein of Galen.

## Implications for Sonographic Diagnosis

In expert hands, complete agenesis of the corpus callosum can be demonstrated at midgestation. Our earliest diagnosis was made at 16 weeks. The lesion can be suspected in axial planes, but usually multiplanar imaging is required to diagnose the condition. Coronal views are

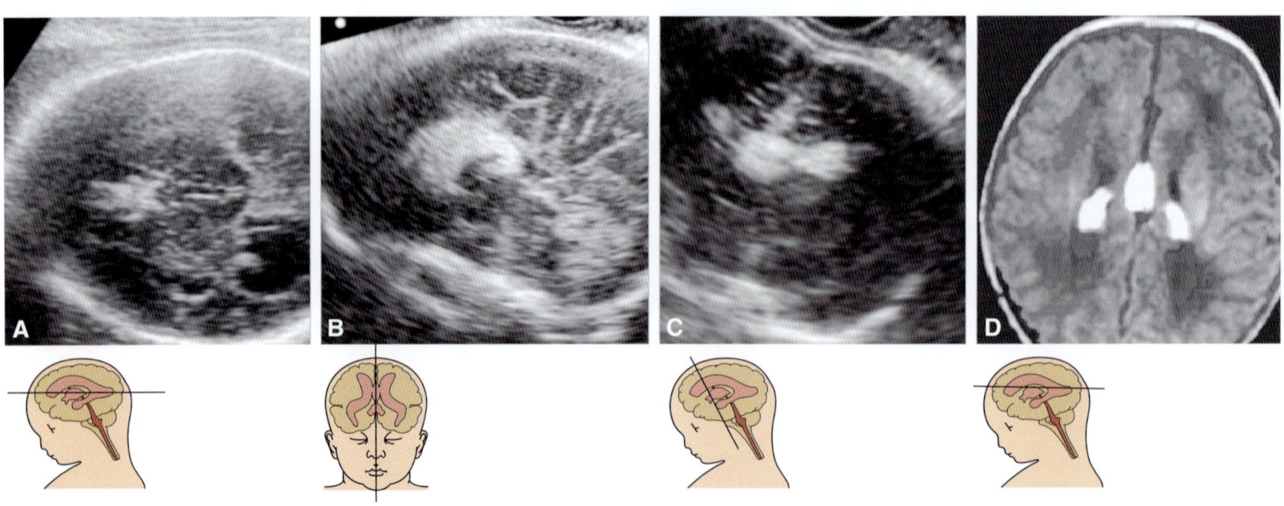


**Figure 6–16.** Agenesis of the corpus callosum with lipomas. In some cases, there is lateral extension of the midline lipomatous process to involve the choroid plexuses of the lateral ventricle. (**A–C**) Prenatal ultrasound. (**D**) Postnatal CT.

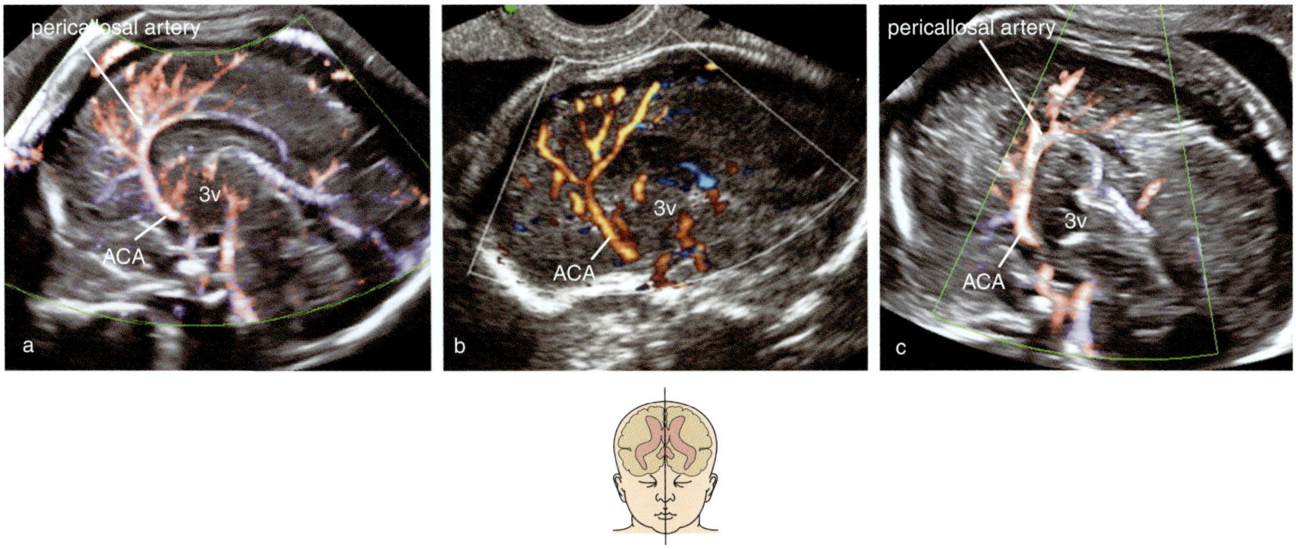


**Figure 6–17.** Color Doppler of the cerebral circulation in the midsagittal plane. (**A**) In normal fetuses, the anterior cerebral artery (ACA) forms the pericallosal artery that runs over the corpus callosum. (**B**) Complete agenesis of the corpus callosum. The ACA ascends vertically without forming the loop of the pericallosal artery. (**C**) Partial agenesis of the corpus callosum. The loop of the pericallosal artery is present but shortened. 3v, third ventricle. (Reproduced, with permission, from *Atlas of Obstetric Ultrasound,* 2009. The Global Library of Women's Medicine. www.glowm.com.)

helpful, but sagittal views are more important in that they allow recognition of at least some cases of partial agenesis. It is uncertain whether all cases of partial agenesis can be diagnosed in early gestation. It is important to stress that complete or partial absence of the corpus callosum is usually the consequence of a malformative process, but it may also derive from intrauterine-acquired insults. In these cases, diagnosis prior to the destructive event is impossible. Other anomalies of the corpus callosum, such as hypoplasia, usually are not identified antenatally.

## Implications for Sonographic Screening

Prenatal diagnosis of agenesis of the corpus callosum is difficult. In low-risk fetuses, which are usually examined only with axial sections,[48] the condition should be suspected in the presence of abnormal findings, including mostly ventriculomegaly and failure to visualize the cavum septi pellucidi. In one large series, the diagnosis could never be made in early gestation in low-risk patients.[35] In another series including both low- and high-risk cases, the findings in axial planes were found to be elusive.[34] We do expect, therefore, that the diagnostic

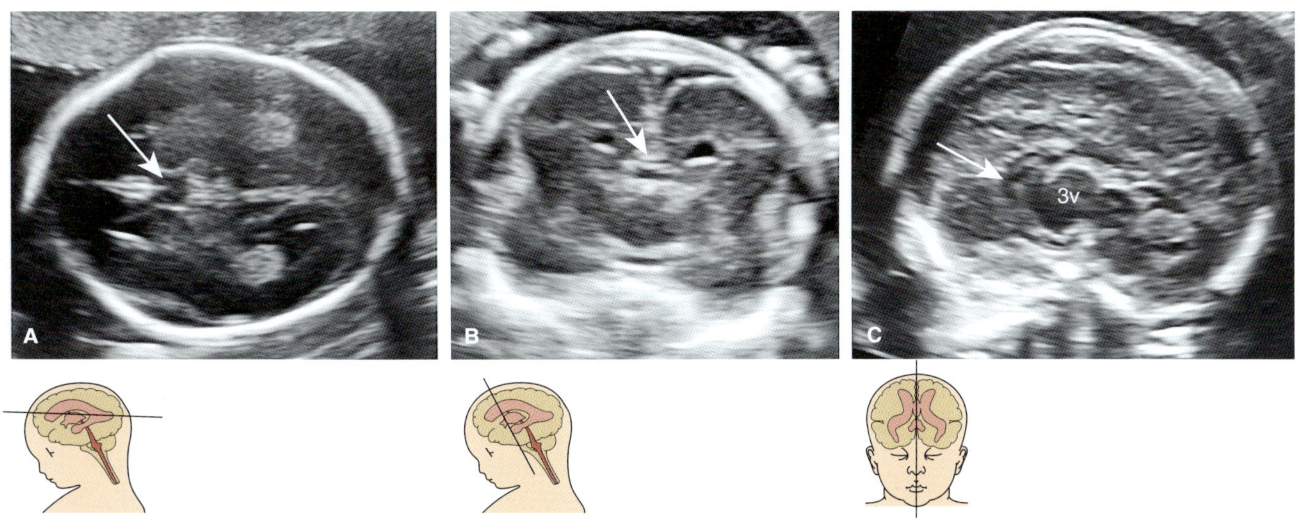


**Figure 6–18.** Partial agenesis of the corpus callosum. (**A**) In the axial plane, the cavum septi pellucidi (*arrow*) is present. (**B**) In the coronal plane, the corpus callosum (*arrow*) is seen bridging between the two hemispheres, although it appears thinner than usual. (**C**) Only in the sagittal plane is the anomaly clearly demonstrated. The cavum septi pellucidi/corpus callosum complex (*arrow*) is present but is much smaller than normal; it does form a complete arch over the third ventricle (3v), but only reaches about midway. (Reproduced, with permission, from Tutschek B, Pilu G: Virtual reality ultrasound imaging of the normal and abnormal fetal central nervous system. *Ultrasound Obstet Gynecol.* 2009;34(3):259–267.)

**Table 6–3. SYNDROMES FEATURING AGENESISOF THE CORPUS CALLOSUM**

| |
|---|
| **Frequently in** |
| Acrocallosal syndrome (AR) |
| Aicardi syndrome (X-linked dominant) |
| Andermann syndrome (AR) |
| Cerebro-oculo-facio-skeletal syndrome (AR) |
| Fryns syndrome (AR) |
| Marden-Walker syndrome (AR) |
| Meckel-Gruber syndrome (AR) |
| Microphtalmia—linear skin defects syndrome (X-linked dominant) |
| Miller-Dieker syndrome (lissencephaly syndrome) |
| Neu-Laxova syndrome (AR) |
| Septo-optic dysplasia sequence |
| Walker-Warburg syndrome (X-linked dominant) |
| Zellweger syndrome (AR) |
| **Occasionally in** |
| Apert syndrome (AR) |
| Baller-Gerold syndrome (AR) |
| Callosogenital dysplasia syndrome (AR) |
| Coffin-Siris syndrome (AR?) |
| Congenital microgastria—limb reduction complex (unknown) |
| Crouzon syndrome (AD) |
| Duplication 4p syndrome |
| Fetal alcohol syndrome |
| Fetal warfarin syndrome |
| FG syndrome (X-linked recessive) |
| Frontonasal dysplasia sequence (sporadic/AD) |
| Gorlin syndrome (AD) |
| Greig cephalopolysyndactyly syndrome (AD) |
| Hydrolethalus syndrome (AR, X-linked dominant) |
| Lens dysplasia (X-linked recessive) |
| Marshall-Smith syndrome (unknown) |
| Metabolic disorders |
| Oculoauricolovertebral spectrum (unknown) |
| Oculocerebrocutaneous syndrome (Delleman syndrome) (unknown) |
| Opitz syndrome (AD, X-linked recessive) |
| Orofaciodigital syndrome type 1 (X-linked dominant) |
| Peters plus syndrome (AR) |
| Radial aplasia-thrombocytopenia syndrome (AR) |
| Rubinstein-Taybi syndrome (sporadic) |
| Shapiro syndrome (X-linked recessive) |
| Simpson-Golabi-Behmel syndrome (X-linked recessive) |
| Trisomy 8 syndrome |
| Trisomy 13 syndrome |
| Trisomy 18 syndrome |
| X-linked hydrocephaly spectrum (X-linked recessive) |
| XO syndrome |
| XXXXY syndrome (hypoplastic) |
| Yunis-Varon syndrome |

AD, autosomal dominant; AR, autosomal recessive.

yield during routine second trimester US examinations will remain low. Should the demonstration of a median plane be routinely required by the governing bodies, the diagnosis of callosal anomalies would be significantly increased.

## Associated Anomalies

The high frequency of associated malformations suggests that agenesis of the corpus callosum is frequently part of a widespread developmental disturbance. In a large postnatal series, CNS anomalies, including microcephaly, abnormal convolutional patterns, heterotopia, intracranial lipomas, interhemispheric cysts, neural tube defects (NTDs), Dandy-Walker malformation, aplasia, and hypoplasia of the pyramidal tracts, were found in 85% of cases.[49] Among the CNS malformations that are amenable to prenatal identification, the ones that are most frequently encountered in conjunction with callosal anomalies are Dandy-Walker malformation, cortical malformations, and interhemispheric cysts.[41] Systemic anomalies, including a variety of musculoskeletal, cardiovascular, genitourinary, and gastrointestinal malformations, were found in 62% of cases.

Chromosomal anomalies are found in 20% of cases and mostly include trisomy 18, 8, and 13.[50] Agenesis of the corpus callosum is also a part of mendelian syndromes (Table 6–3). Callosal agenesis is found in two conditions with sex-linked dominant etiology and lethality in males: the orofaciodigital type I syndrome[51] and Aicardi syndrome.[52] Frontonasal dysplasia or median cleft face syndrome is also frequently associated with agenesis of the corpus callosum.[53–55] This condition is usually a sporadic disease, but a few familial cases consistent with an autosomal dominant transmission have been described.[56,57]

In antenatal series, anatomical anomalies were found in 50% of cases.[34] The anomaly most frequently encountered was Dandy-Walker malformation. Cardiovascular anomalies mainly included conotruncal malformations: tetralogy of Fallot and a double outlet right ventricle. A detailed list of syndromes associated with agenesis of the corpus callosum is given in Table 6–3.

## Prognosis/Clinical Manifestations

Associated anomalies are frequently found with agenesis of the corpus callosum, and they have a major impact on the final outcome. Knowledge of specific syndromes is important.[58] When a syndrome or associated malformations are diagnosed, the prognosis is severe, and termination of pregnancy should be considered. The worst outcomes are found in the presence of cortical malformation and Dandy-Walker malformation.[59]

Counseling couples with fetuses that have seemingly isolated nonfamilial agenesis of the corpus callosum is difficult. The corpus callosum is phylogenetically a recent structure, and its absence is not lethal. Isolated agenesis of the corpus callosum may be a completely asymptomatic event or revealed during the course of a neurologic examination by subtle deficits, such as inability to match stimuli using both hands or to discriminate differences in temperature, shape, and weight in objects placed in both hands.

Persons with agenesis of the corpus callosum may have neurologic problems, such as seizures, intellectual impairment, and psychoses. However, these conditions are believed to be caused by abnormalities in associated cerebral anomalies rather than in the corpus callosum per se. In postnatal series, children with isolated agenesis of the corpus callosum are more frequently free from neurologic compromise.

Pediatric series are based on investigation of symptomatic individuals and are therefore presumably biased. The experience with antenatal diagnosis thus far is limited, but it seems more favorable than expected from postnatal data. As an isolated finding, agenesis of the corpus callosum is associated with normal to borderline intellectual development in most cases.[34,60] However, long-term studies have reported a progressive decrease in intellectual capacity throughout the years, and most infants tend to have significant difficulties in school.[61] Abnormalities of the corpus callosum have also been linked to psychoses[62] and inborn errors of metabolism,[57] but the most frequent defect encountered in these patients is global or partial hypoplasia, which is unlikely to be identified in utero.

### Management

Agenesis of the corpus callosum is associated with an excess of both neural and extraneural malformations, as well as with chromosomal aberrations. Antenatal identification of callosal agenesis dictates the need for a careful survey of the entire fetal anatomy, including echocardiography, karyotype, TORCH (toxoplasmosis, other infections, rubella, cytomegalovirus, herpes simplex virus) tests, and in cases with apparently isolated agenesis, a fetal brain MRI. Isolated agenesis of the corpus callosum does not require any modification of standard obstetric management.

### Recurrence Risk

The risk of recurrence depends on the underlying etiology. In nonsyndromic cases, an empiric recurrence risk of 5% has been suggested.[63]

## AGENESIS OF THE SEPTUM PELLUCIDUM AND SEPTO-OPTIC DYSPLASIA

### Definition

Agenesis of the septum pellucidum is a cerebral anomaly that features the absence of the septum pellucidum; when this is associated with optic nerve hypoplasia and/or hypophyseal dysfunction, the condition is known as septo-optic dysplasia (or de Morsier syndrome). (See also chapter 2)

### Embryology and Pathology

The septum pellucidum is part of the midline structures at the level of the frontal horns of the lateral ventricles; it is made up of two leaves separated in the fetus by a fluid-containing cavity, the cavum septi pellucidi (CSP). Agenesis of the septum pellucidum is usually associated with other brain anomalies, including holoprosencephaly and cortical malformations,[12,64] the association with schizencephaly being particularly frequent.[65] Apparently isolated cases of agenesis of the septum pellucidum may be due to septo-optic dysplasia or represent an isolated anomaly. Septo-optic dysplasia, also known as de Morsier syndrome, is a rare condition characterized by optic nerve hypoplasia, pituitary hypoplasia, and agenesis of the septum pellucidum. The optic nerves and chiasm are affected by different degrees of hypoplasia, resulting in poor vision and nystagmus. A subset of these infants are blind, but they usually will develop a modest degree of vision function later in life. Signs of both anterior and posterior hypopituitarism are virtually always present. Deficiency of growth hormone and antidiuretic hormone may result in hypopituaric dwarfism and diabetes insipidus, respectively. Low levels of thyroid-stimulating hormone, luteinizing hormone, and follicle-stimulating hormone are usually present.

### Associated Anomalies

Ventriculomegaly, schizencephaly, agenesis of the corpus callosum, craniofacial anomalies, such as hypothelorism and clefting, are often present.

### Etiology

The etiology is unknown. Septo-optic dysplasia can be caused by a mutation in the homeobox gene *HESX1* or occur because of exposure to teratogens or viral infections.[66] Most cases are sporadic; standard counseling is that the risk of recurrence is low. Hereditary cases have been reported that were compatible with both autosomal recessive and autosomal dominant transmission; it is presently accepted that a genetic factor plays an important role, at least in some cases.[67]

### Recurrence Risk

Standard counseling is that the risk of recurrence is low, although a few cases suggesting mendelian transmission have been described.[67]

### Diagnosis

Septo-optic dysplasia should be suspected when the cavum septi pellucidi is absent in an otherwise normal brain.[12,25,67–69] Visualization of the cavum septi pellucidi is usually easy, but demonstration of the absence may be difficult at times and the ultrasound findings may be misleading.[25] The frontal horns are fused on the midline. The corpus callosum is usually present, although it is frequently described as thinned in postnatal studies. Ventriculomegaly may be present. Multiplanar imaging is essential to demonstrate this condition and particularly to differentiate it from other entities (Figures 6–19). Three-dimensional imaging usual orthogonal planes, tomographic imaging an inversion rendering of the CSP are additional and emerging tools to differentiate this condition from other entities (Figure 6–20).

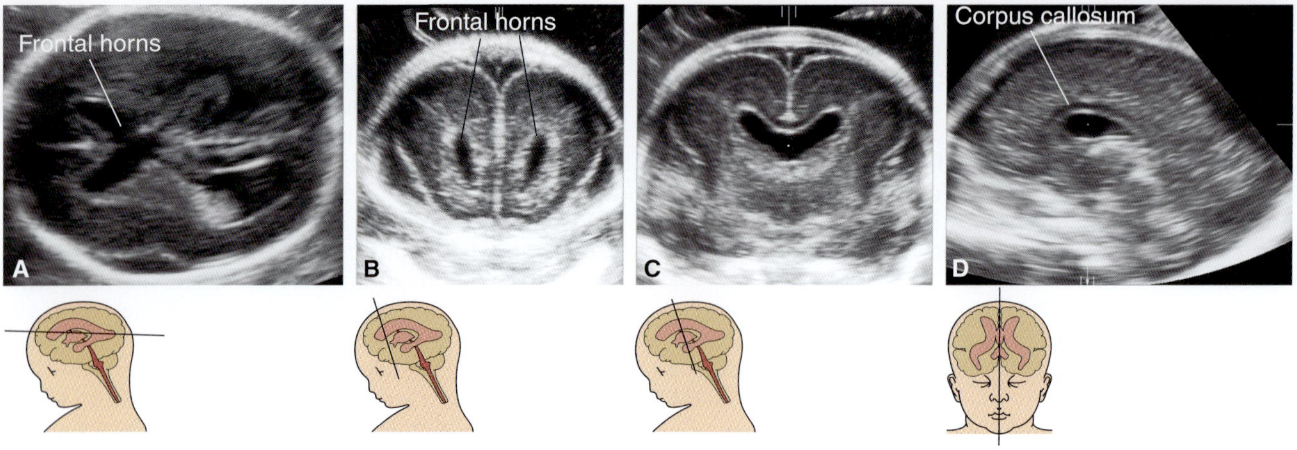


**Figure 6–19.** Agenesis of the septum pellucidum. In this case, a differential diagnosis than lobar holoprosencephaly is possible by demonstrating in the axial plane (**A**) as well as in an anterior coronal plane (**B**) that the frontal horns are separated anteriorly, with a well-developed IHF between the anterior hemispeheres. The demonstration of a normal corpus callosum also favors the diagnosis of agenesis of the septum pellucidum. (Reproduced, with permission, from Tutschek B, Pilu G. Virtual reality ultrasound imaging of the normal and abnormal fetal central nervous system. *Ultrasound Obstet Gynecol.* 2009 Sep;34(3):259–267.)

## Differential Diagnosis

The finding of an absent cavum septi pellucidi with central fusion and squaring of frontal horns is similar to the previously described lobar holoprosencephaly. The presence of well-formed albeit fused frontal horns that dicaricate anteriorly and the documentation of otherwise normal cerebral structures, including a regular corpus callosum, favor the diagnosis of absence of the septum pellucidum versus holoprosencephaly. After birth, a definitive diagnosis of septo-optic hypoplasia is made by the CT or MRI demonstration of optic tract hypoplasia, endocrine evaluation, and visual assessment. In the fetus, the differential diagnosis between SOD and isolated ASP may be attempted by evaluation of maternal urine and serum estriol levels and fetal blood assays for growth hormone, ACTH, and prolactin.[67] A specific diagnosis was made antenatally in one case demonstrating hypoplasia of the optic chiasms with MR in the third trimester of pregnancy[67] (Figure 6–21). The largest available antenatal experience has been made, however, with sonography. Three-dimensional ultrasound visualization and measurement of the optic chiasms and tracts (Figure 6–21) identified 4 of 5 cases of optic tract hypoplasia within a group of fetuses with ASP.[70–71]

## Implications for Sonographic Diagnosis

Although the recurrence risk is low, a familial history of septo-optic dysplasia is an indication for a targeted sonogram. It is important to stress that only those cases with absence of the septum pellucidum are currently amenable to antenatal sonographic recognition. We would recommend an examination at 18 weeks, when the anterior midline structures of the brain are usually clearly visualized.

## Implications for Sonographic Screening

The experience with the antenatal diagnosis of septo-optic dysplasia is limited. Absence of the cavum septi pellucidi with fusion of the frontal horns is theoretically recognizable by a standard sonographic examination performed after 18 weeks. However, we expect that this finding will be very subtle.

## Prognosis

Many fetuses with absence of the septum pellucidum have severe cerebral anomalies such as holoprosencephaly and schizencephaly that are rapidly identified and carry a poor prognosis. The main problem arises after the diagnosis of a seemingly isolated agenesis of the septum pellucidum that, in the majority of cases, cannot be differentiated from SOD. Isolated agenesis of the septum pellucidum has been identified in the fetus and had a good outcome.[68] The outcome of individuals affected by SOD is controversial. Visual impairment is usually present, but blindness is rare. Hypopituitarism is amenable to medical treatment. The developmental outcome is debated. Absence of the septum pellucidum and optic nerve hypoplasia are associated with an excess of cerebral palsy, mental retardation, and seizures. However, abnormal development is usually limited to those cases with coexistent cerebral hemispheric anomalies, such as schizencephaly. Of 7 infants with isolated septo-optic dysplasia, with no other brain abnormalities, only one was found to have moderate cognitive and language delays.[71] Antenatal series suggests that about 25% of fetuses with seemingly isolated ASP have septo-optic dysplasia, and the remaining are usually asymptomatic.[71,73] Although the available experience is limited, it would seem that within this group of fetuses, visualization of a normal optic chiasm with three-dimensional ultrasound does not rule out with septo-optic dysplasia, but significantly decreases the risk.[71]

## Obstetrical Management

Standard obstetric care.

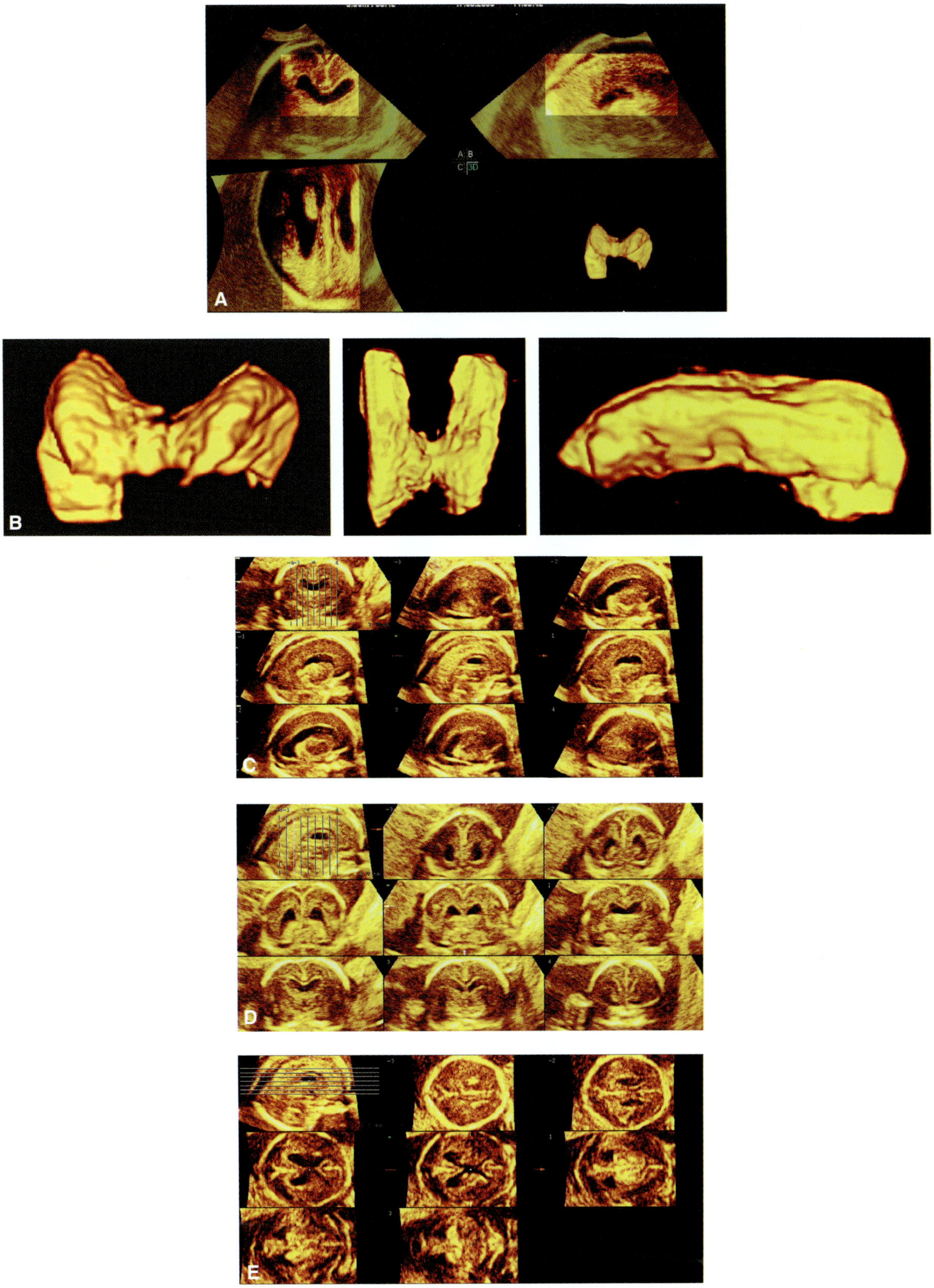

**Figure 6–20.** Sonography of fetal agenesis of the septum pellucidum: multiplanar imaging with three-dimensional rendering of the cavity of lateral ventricles (**A**); cast of the lateral ventricles obtained with three-dimensional ultrasound and inversion mode (**B**), tomographic images in the sagittal (**C**), coronal (**D**), and axial planes (**E**). (Courtesy Ilan Timor-Tritsch and Ana Monteagudo).

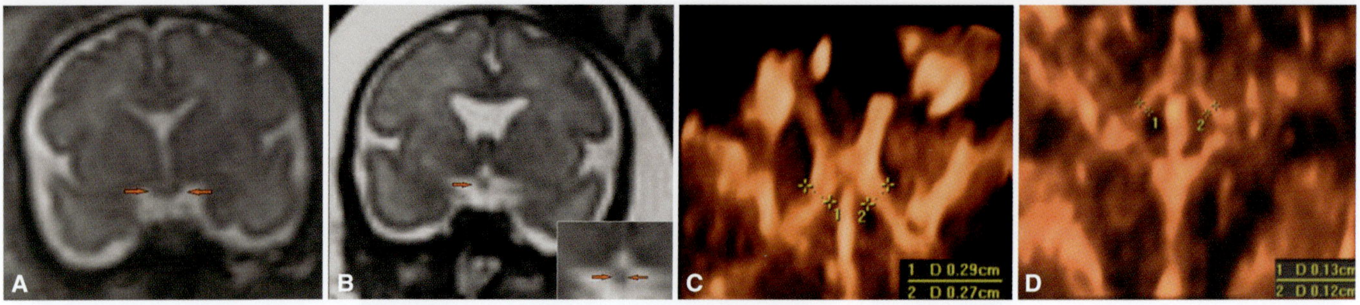


**Figure 6–21.** Demonstration of fetal optic chiasm. MR coronal sections demonstrating a normal chiasm (arrows) (**A**) compared with a hypoplastic one (arrows) in one fetus with septo-optic dysplasia. Three-dimensional sonograms demonstrating measurement of the posterior tracts in a normal optic chiasm (**C**) compared with an hypoplastic one (**D**). (**A, B** Reproduced from Lepinard C, Coutant R, Boussion F, Loisel D, Delorme B, Biquard F, et al. Prenatal diagnosis of absence of the septum pellucidum associated with septo-optic dysplasia. *Ultrasound Obstet Gynecol.* 2005 Jan;25(1):73–75.) (**C, D** Reproduced from Damaj L, Bruneau B, Ferry M, Moutard ML, Garel C, Odent S, Adamsbaum C, Avni F, Tréguier C, Lazaro L: Pediatric outcome of children with the prenatal diagnosis of isolated septal agenesis. *Prenat Diagn.* 2010;30(12-13):1143–1150.)

## REFERENCES


1. Volpe JJ. Human brain development. *Neurology of the Newborn,* 3rd ed. Philadelphia: W.B. Saunders Company; 1995. p. 1–43.
2. Harris CP, Townsend JJ, Norman MG, White VA, Viskochil DH, Pysher TJ, et al. Atelencephalic aprosencephaly. *J Child Neurol.* 1994;9(4):412–416.
3. Ippel PF, Breslau-Siderius EJ, Hack WW, van der Blij HF, Bouve S, Bijlsma JB. Atelencephalic microcephaly: a case report and review of the literature. *Eur J Pediatr.* 1998;157(6):493–497.
4. Forrester MB, Merz RD. Epidemiology of holoprosencephaly in Hawaii, 1986–97. *Paediatr Perinat Epidemiol.* 2000;14(1):61–63.
5. Ong S, Tonks A, Woodward ER, Wyldes MP, Kilby MD. An epidemiological study of holoprosencephaly from a regional congenital anomaly register: 1995–2004. *Prenat Diagn.* 2007;27(4):340–347.
6. Matsunaga E, Shiota K. Holoprosencephaly in human embryos: Epidemiologic studies of 150 cases. *Teratology.* 1977;16:261–272.
7. McKusick VA. Holoprosencephaly. *OMIM* [serial on the Internet]. 2009: Available from: http://www.ncbi.nlm.nih.gov/entrez/dispomim.cgi?id=236100.
8. Cohen MM, Jr. Perspectives on holoprosencephaly: Part I. Epidemiology, genetics, and syndromology. *Teratology.* 1989;40(2): 211–235.
9. Blaas HG, Eriksson AG, Salvesen KA, Isaksen CV, Christensen B, Mollerlokken G, et al. Brains and faces in holoprosencephaly: pre- and postnatal description of 30 cases. *Ultrasound Obstet Gynecol.* 2002;19(1):24–38.
10. Rizzo N, Pittalis MC, Pilu G, Orsini LF, Perolo A, Bovicelli L. Prenatal karyotyping in malformed fetuses. *Prenat Diagn.* 1990;10(1):17–23.
11. Rizzo N, Pittalis MC, Pilu G, Perolo A, Banzi C, Visentin A, et al. Distribution of abnormal karyotypes among malformed fetuses detected by ultrasound throughout gestation. *Prenat Diagn.* 1996;16(2):159–163.
12. Malinger G, Lev D, Kidron D, Heredia F, Hershkovitz R, Lerman-Sagie T. Differential diagnosis in fetuses with absent septum pellucidum. *Ultrasound Obstet Gynecol.* 2005;25(1):42–49.
13. Picone O, Hirt R, Suarez B, Coulomb A, Tachdjian G, Frydman R, et al. Prenatal diagnosis of a possible new middle interhemispheric variant of holoprosencephaly using sonographic and magnetic resonance imaging. *Ultrasound Obstet Gynecol.* 2006;28(2):229–231.
14. Lewis AJ, Simon EM, Barkovich AJ, Clegg NJ, Delgado MR, Levey E, et al. Middle interhemispheric variant of holoprosencephaly: a distinct cliniconeuroradiologic subtype. *Neurology.* 2002 24;59(12):1860–1865.
15. Stagnaro MG, Beluschi C, Della Cella G, Bellati R, Bacigalupo L, Maddaluno O, et al. [Holotelencephaly: description of a case]. *Pediatr Med Chir.* 1984;6(1):141–146.
16. Pilu G, Ambrosetto P, Sandri F, Tani G, Perolo A, Grisolia G, et al. Intraventricular fused fornices: a specific sign of fetal lobar holoprosencephaly. *Ultrasound Obstet Gynecol.* 1994;4(1):65–67.
17. DeMeyer W, Zeman W, Palmer CG. The face predicts the brain: Diagnostic significance of median facial anomalies for holoprosencephaly (archinencephaly). *Pediatrics.* 1964;34:256–263.
18. Blaas HG, Eik-Nes SH, Vainio T, Isaksen CV. Alobar holoprosencephaly at 9 weeks gestational age visualized by two- and three-dimensional ultrasound. *Ultrasound Obstet Gynecol.* 2000;15(1):62–65.
19. Pilu G, Romero R, Rizzo N, Jeanty P, Bovicelli L, Hobbins JC. Criteria for the prenatal diagnosis of holoprosencephaly. *Am J Perinatol.* 1987;4(1):41–49.
20. Bronshtein M, Wiener Z. Early transvaginal sonographic diagnosis of alobar holoprosencephaly. *Prenat Diagn.* 1991;11(7):459–462.
21. Blaas HG. Holoprosencephaly at 10 weeks 2 days (CRL 33 mm). *Ultrasound Obstet Gynecol.* 2000 Jan;15(1):86–87.
22. Timor-Tritsch IE, Monteagudo A, Santos R. Three-dimensional inversion rendering in the first-and early second-trimester fetal brain: its use in holoprosencephaly. *Ultrasound Obstet Gynecol.* 2008;32:744–750.
23. Bernard JP, Drummond CL, Zaarour P, Molho M, Ville Y. A new clue to the prenatal diagnosis of lobar holoprosencephaly: the abnormal pathway of the anterior cerebral artery crawling under the skull. *Ultrasound Obstet Gynecol.* 2002;19(6):605–607.
24. Pilu G, Sandri F, Perolo A, Giangaspero F, Cocchi G, Salvioli GP, et al. Prenatal diagnosis of lobar holoprosencephaly. *Ultrasound Obstet Gynecol.* 1992;2(2):88–94.
25. Garel C. MRI of the fetal brain. Normal development and cerebral pathologies. Berlin: Springer; 2004.
26. Pilu G, Tani G, Carletti A, Malaigia S, Ghi T, Rizzo N. Difficult early sonographic diagnosis of absence of the fetal septum pellucidum. *Ultrasound Obstet Gynecol.* 2005;25(1):70–72.
27. Grogono JL. Children with agenesis of the corpus callosum. *Dev Med Child Neurol.* 1968;10:613–616.
28. Jeret JS, Serur D, Wisniewski K, Fisch C. Frequency of agenesis of the corpus callosum in the developmentally disabled population as determined by computerized tomography. *Pediatr Neurosci.* 1985–1986;12(2):101–103.
29. Schell-Apacik CC, Wagner K, Bihler M, Ertl-Wagner B, Heinrich U, Klopocki E, et al. Agenesis and dysgenesis of the corpus callosum: clinical, genetic and neuroimaging findings in a series of 41 patients. *Am J Med Genet A.* 2008;146A(19):2501–2511.
30. Malinger G, Lev D, Zahalka N, Ben Aroia Z, Watemberg N, Kidron D, et al. Fetal cytomegalovirus infection of the brain: the spectrum of sonographic findings. *Am J Neuroradiol.* 2003;24(1):28–32.
31. Weinstein AS, Goldstein RB, Barkovich AJ. In utero disappearance of the corpus callosum secondary to extensive brain injury. *J Ultrasound Med.* 2003;22(8):837–840.
32. Ren T, Anderson A, Shen WB, Huang H, Plachez C, Zhang J, et al. Imaging, anatomical, and molecular analysis of callosal formation in the developing human fetal brain. *Anat Rec A Discov Mol Cell Evol Biol.* 2006;288:191–204.

33. Barkovich AJ, Norman D. Anomalies of the corpus callosum: correlation with further anomalies of the brain. *AJR Am J Roentgenol.* 1988;151(1):171–179.
34. Pilu G, Sandri F, Perolo A, Pittalis MC, Grisolia G, Cocchi G, et al. Sonography of fetal agenesis of the corpus callosum: a survey of 35 cases. *Ultrasound Obstet Gynecol.* 1993;3(5):318–329.
35. Bennett GL, Bromley B, Benacerraf BR. Agenesis of the corpus callosum: prenatal detection usually is not possible before 22 weeks of gestation. *Radiology.* 1996;199(2):447–450.
36. Malinger G, Zakut H. The corpus callosum: normal fetal development as shown by transvaginal sonography. *AJR Am J Roentgenol.* 1993;161(5):1041–1043.
37. Pilu G, Segata M, Ghi T, Carletti A, Perolo A, Santini D, et al. Diagnosis of midline anomalies of the fetal brain with the three-dimensional median view. *Ultrasound Obstet Gynecol.* 2006;27(5):522–529.
38. Filly RA, Cardoza JD, Goldstein RB, Barkovich AJ. Detection of fetal central nervous system anomalies: a practical level of effort for a routine sonogram. *Radiology.* 1989;172(2):403–408.
39. Patel MD, Filly AL, Hersh DR, Goldstein RB. Isolated mild fetal cerebral ventriculomegaly: clinical course and outcome. *Radiology.* 1994;192(3):759–764.
40. Goldstein RB, La Pidus AS, Filly RA, Cardoza J. Mild lateral cerebral ventricular dilatation in utero: clinical significance and prognosis. *Radiology.* 1990;176(1):237–242.
41. Barkovich AJ, Simon EM, Walsh CA. Callosal agenesis with cyst: a better understanding and new classification. *Neurology.* 2001;56(2):220–227.
42. Mulligan G, Meier P. Lipoma and agenesis of the corpus callosum with associated choroid plexus lipomas. In utero diagnosis. *J Ultrasound Med.* 1989;8(10):583–588.
43. Volpe P, Paladini D, Resta M, Stanziano A, Salvatore M, Quarantelli M, et al. Characteristics, associations and outcome of partial agenesis of the corpus callosum in the fetus. *Ultrasound Obstet Gynecol.* 2006;27(5):509–516.
44. Pilu G, Ghi T, Carletti A, Segata M, Perolo A, Rizzo N. Three-dimensional ultrasound examination of the fetal central nervous system. *Ultrasound Obstet Gynecol.* 2007;30(2):233–245.
45. Benacerraf BR, Shipp TD, Bromley B, Levine D. What does magnetic resonance imaging add to the prenatal sonographic diagnosis of ventriculomegaly? *J Ultrasound Med.* 2007;26(11):1513–1522.
46. Levine D, Barnes PD. Cortical maturation in normal and abnormal fetuses as assessed with prenatal MR imaging. *Radiology.* 1999;210(3):751–758.
47. Levine D, Barnes PD, Madsen JR, Li W, Edelman RR. Fetal central nervous system anomalies: MR imaging augments sonographic diagnosis. *Radiology.* 1997;204(3):635–642.
48. ISUOG guidelines. Sonographic examination of the fetal central nervous system: guidelines for performing the basic examination and the fetal neurosonogram. *Ultrasound Obstet Gynecol.* 2007;29(1):109–116.
49. Parrish ML, Roessmann U, Levinsohn MW. Agenesis of the corpus callosum: a study of the frequency of associated malformations. *Ann Neurol.* 1979;6(4):349–354.
50. Serur D, Jeret JS, Wisniewski K. Agenesis of the corpus callosum: clinical, neuroradiological and cytogenetic studies. *Neuropediatrics.* 1988;19(2):87–91.
51. Salinas CF, Pai GS, Vera CL, Milutinovic J, Hagerty R, Cooper JD, et al. Variability of expression of the orofaciodigital syndrome type I in black females: six cases. *Am J Med Genet.* 1991;38(4):574–582.
52. Donnenfeld AE, Packer RJ, Zackai EH, Chee CM, Sellinger B, Emanuel BS. Clinical, cytogenetic, and pedigree findings in 18 cases of Aicardi syndrome. *Am J Med Genet.* 1989;32(4):461–467.
53. Grover SB, Charan KA, Saxena NC. Frontonasal dysplasia with corpus callosum lipoma. *Indian Pediatr.* 1999;36(4):398–401.
54. Meguid NA. Frontonasal dysplasia, lipoma of the corpus callosum and tetralogy of Fallot. *Clin Genet.* 1993;44(2):95–97.
55. Toriello HV, Radecki LL, Sharda J, Looyenga D, Mann R. Frontonasal "dysplasia," cerebral anomalies, and polydactyly: report of a new syndrome and discussion from a developmental field perspective. *Am J Med Genet Suppl.* 1986;2:89–96.
56. Guion-Almeida ML, Richieri-Costa A. Frontonasal dysplasia, severe neuropsychological delay, and midline central nervous system anomalies: report of 10 Brazilian male patients. *Am J Med Genet A.* 2009;149A(5):1006–1011.
57. Bamforth F, Bamforth S, Poskitt K, Applegarth D, Hall J. Abnormalities of corpus callosum in patients with inherited metabolic diseases. *Lancet.* 1988;2(8608):451.
58. Paul LK, Brown WS, Adolphs R, Tyszka JM, Richards LJ, Mukherjee P, et al. Agenesis of the corpus callosum: genetic, developmental and functional aspects of connectivity. *Nat Rev Neurosci.* 2007;8(4):287–299.
59. Byrd SE, Radkowski MA, Flannery A, McLone DG. The clinical and radiological evaluation of absence of the corpus callosum. *Eur J Radiol.* 1990;10(1):65–73.
60. Gupta JK, Lilford RJ. Assessment and management of fetal agenesis of the corpus callosum. *Prenat Diagn.* 1995;15(4):301–312.
61. Moutard ML, Kieffer V, Feingold J, Kieffer F, Lewin F, Adamsbaum C, et al. Agenesis of corpus callosum: prenatal diagnosis and prognosis. *Childs Nerv Syst.* 2003;19(7–8):471–476.
62. Lewis SW, Reveley MA, David AS, Ron MA. Agenesis of the corpus callosum and schizophrenia: a case report. *Psychol Med.* 1988;18(2):341–347.
63. Young ID, Trounce JQ, Levene MI, Fitzsimmons JS, Moore JR. Agenesis of the corpus callosum and macrocephaly in siblings. *Clin Genet.* 1985;28(3):225–230.
64. Belhocine O, Andre C, Kalifa G, Adamsbaum C. Does asymptomatic septal agenesis exist? A review of 34 cases. *Pediatr Radiol.* 2005;35(4):410–418.
65. Raybaud C, Girard N, Levrier O, Peretti-Viton P, Manera L, Farnarier P. Schizencephaly: correlation between the lobar topography of the cleft(s) and absence of the septum pellucidum. *Childs Nerv Syst.* 2001;17(4–5):217–222.
66. Dattani ML, Martinez-Barbera J, Thomas PQ, Brickman JM, Gupta R, Wales JK, et al. Molecular genetics of septo-optic dysplasia. *Horm Res.* 2000;53 Suppl 1:26–33.
67. Wales JK, Quarrell OW. Evidence for possible Mendelian inheritance of septo-optic dysplasia. *Acta Paediatr.*1996;85(3):391–392.
68. Lepinard C, Coutant R, Boussion F, Loisel D, Delorme B, Biquard F, et al. Prenatal diagnosis of absence of the septum pellucidum associated with septo-optic dysplasia. *Ultrasound Obstet Gynecol.* 2005;25(1):73–75.
69. Celentano C, Prefumo F, Liberati M, Tartaro A, Gallo G, Lattanzio G, et al. Prenatal diagnosis of septal agenesis with normal pituitary function. *Prenat Diagn.* 2006;26(11):1075–1077.
70. Pilu G, Sandri F, Cerisoli M, Alvisi C, Salvioli GP, Bovicelli L. Sonographic findings in septo-optic dysplasia in the fetus and newborn infant. *Am J Perinatol.* 1990;7(4):337–339.
71. Bault JP, Salomon LJ, Guibaud L, Achiron R. Role of three-dimensional ultrasound measurement of the optic tract in fetuses with agenesis of the septum pellucidum. *Ultrasound Obstet Gynecol.* 2011;37(5):570–575.
72. Williams J, Brodsky MC, Griebel M, Glasier CM, Caldwell D, Thomas P. Septo-optic dysplasia: the clinical insignificance of an absent septum pellucidum. *Dev Med Child Neurol.* 1993;35(6):490–501.
73. Damaj L, Bruneau B, Ferry M, Moutard ML, Garel C, Odent S, Adamsbaum C, Avni F, Tréguier C, Lazaro L: Pediatric outcome of children with the prenatal diagnosis of isolated septal agenesis. *Prenat Diagn.* 2010;30(12-13):1143–1150.

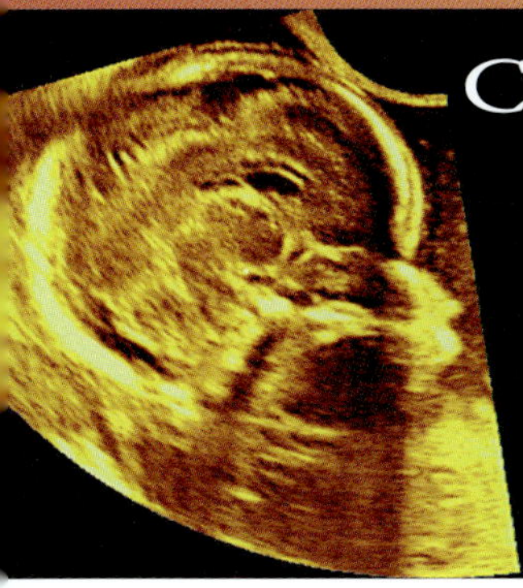

Chapter 7

# MALFORMATIONS OF CORTICAL DEVELOPMENT

*Gustavo Malinger • Ants Toi • Liat Ben-Sira • Tally Lerman-Sagie*

**KEY POINTS**

1. Proliferation, neuronal migration, and organization occur relatively late in pregnancy and do not end until after delivery.
2. Malformations of cortical development (MCD) may be diagnosed during fetal life; the chances for diagnosis are better in severe cases and in those with associated anomalies.
3. MCD assay may in same cases diagnosed by using ultrasound. Characteristic features are shown in Figure 7–1.
4. Even when MCD is suspected, a definitive diagnosis is usually difficult during pregnancy.
5. In patients at risk, search systematically for signs of MCD. Check for the size of the lateral ventricles and the regularity of their walls; also, the presence of abnormal underdeveloped or overdeveloped sulci.
6. When a suspicion is raised, consult with a genetician and a pediatric neurologist. In low-risk patients, these signs may be the only possibility for prenatal diagnosis.

The processes of primary neurulation and ventral induction that result in the formation of the neural tube and in the formation of the prosencephalon, respectively, are completed by the second month of gestation.[1] This is followed by three overlapping phases of cortical development, which are under the control of numerous genes: proliferation, migration, and organization. Stem cells at the surface of the ventricles proliferate and divide into glial cells and neuronal cells. The glial cells migrate to the cortex in a very regular radial pattern, leaving a radial scaffolding along which the neurons migrate (radial migration) to the surface. The later arriving neurons migrate in stages through the inner layers and ultimately lie outside them (inside out migration). Ultimately, six layers are formed. Once the neurons arrive at the cortex, they organize local connections. In addition to this radial migration, there is a tangential migration of neurons to form what are believed to be controlling tracts.[2] The genes that control neuronal development also function in other parts of the body, so it is not unusual to find cerebral malformations associated with diverse somatic manifestations, such as skeletal dysplasia as present in thanatophoric dysplasia. This normal orderly developmental process can be disturbed by genetic, teratogenic, and environmental conditions. Because the cerebrum develops simultaneously with other structures, an insult at a specific time can affect the normal development of all the structures that are vulnerable at that time, including the eyes, face, and hindbrain. Hence the importance of assessing all of these areas if abnormality is suspected in any one of them. Over the past decade, the knowledge regarding the genetics, morphology, and clinical aspects of these conditions has expanded significantly, and new developments in this field have occurred rapidly.

Different classifications of malformations of cortical development (MCD) have been proposed[3–5] (Table 7–1). Fundamentally, they are based on two factors: gene abnormality and timing of the first abnormal developmental event. Final phenotypic outcomes are often more dependent on the time that an insult occurs and interferes with normal development than its specific nature. Although Barkovich et al's[3] and Volpe's[5] classifications are particularly useful in clinical management, they are acknowledged to be in evolution and will change as new information becomes available. Sarnat's[4] classification is more centered on the genetic and embryologic mechanisms of the different diseases. The reader is referred to Chapter 2 for information on the normal sonographic appearance and development of the sulci and gyri.

## MALFORMATIONS DUE TO ABNORMAL NEURONAL PROLIFERATION

### Microcephaly

#### Synonym

Micrencephaly

#### Definition

*Microcephaly* means small head. More specifically, it is intended to mean small brain (micrencephaly). In children and adults, microcephaly is defined as low brain weight and a small occipitofrontal head circumference (HC) >2

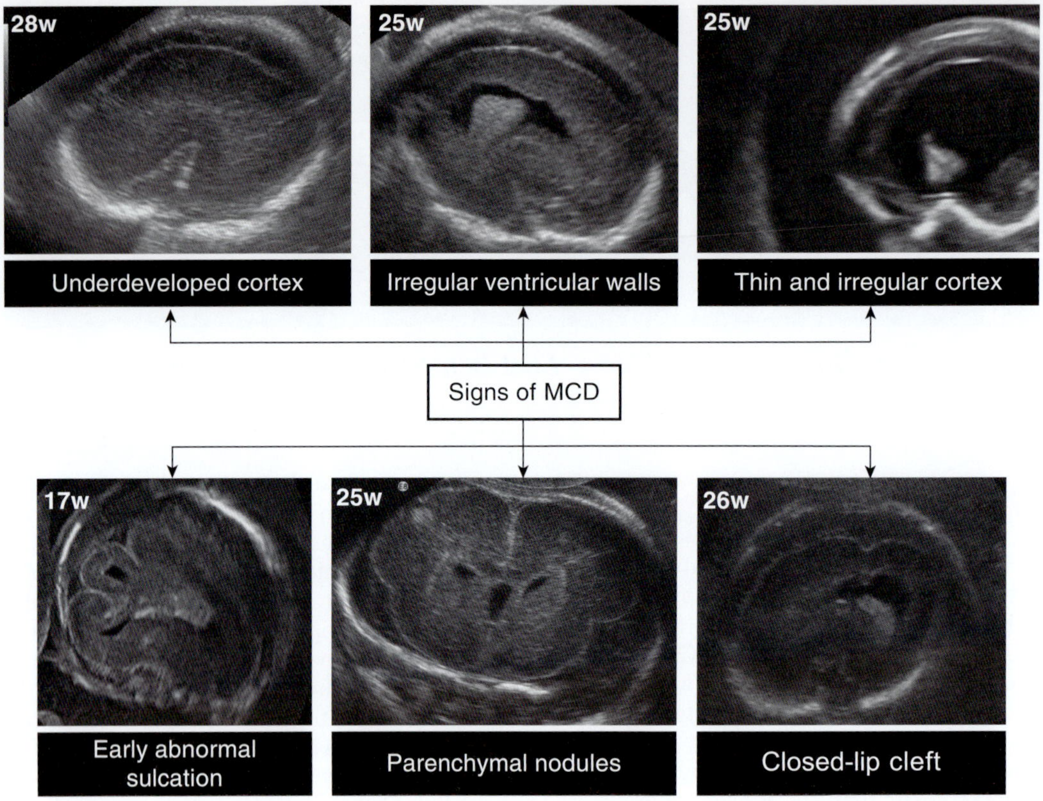


**Figure 7–1.** Ultrasound signs of malformations of cortical development.

**Table 7–1. MALFORMATIONS OF CORTICAL DEVELOPMENT**

| Malformations due to abnormal neuronal proliferation |
|---|
| Microcephaly<br>Macrocephaly<br>Hemimegalencephaly<br>Tuberous sclerosis complex |
| **Malformations due to abnormal neuronal migration or organization** |
| Lissencephaly/subcortical band heterotopia spectrum<br>Cobblestone complex syndromes<br>Heterotopia<br>Schizencephaly/polymicrogyria |

Data from Barkovich AJ, Kuzniecky RI, Jackson GD, Guerrini R, Dobyns WB. A developmental and genetic classification for malformations of cortical development. *Neurology.* 2005;65:1873–1887; Sarnat H, Flores-Sarnat L. Integrative classification of morphology and molecular genetics in central nervous system malformations. *Amer J Med Genet.* 2004;126A:386–392; Volpe JJ. Neuronal proliferation, migration, organization, and mielinization. In: *Neurology of the Newborn.* Philadelphia: Saunders; 2008:51–118.

standard deviations (SDs) below the mean or below the third percentile (see Chapter 3). The implications of a diagnosis of fetal microcephaly may be grave. Measurements should be carefully obtained, and normograms used should take into consideration fetal gender, ethnic background, parental size, and family history. Diagnosis using –2 SDs as the lower limit will automatically categorize 2% of the population inappropriately as microcephalic. Such a broad definition obviously includes normal individuals. It is clear that there is an inverse relationship between the HC and the probability of associated mental retardation. Prenatally, there is no consensus regarding the exact definition of an abnormally small HC; some authors propose the –2 SD cutoff,[3] whereas others propose the –3 SD cutoff.[6,7] Using the –3 SD definition, Chervenak et al[6] showed that prenatal HC measurement was sensitive for diagnosing microcephaly with no false-negatives; –4 SD was a specific test with no false-positive cases (see Chapter 3).

## Incidence/Prevalence

Seto et al[8] noted in a population-based study performed in Japan a significant increase in the incidence of microcephaly as reported on birth forms from 0.37 per 10,000 births to 0.86 per 10,000 when comparing two consecutive 10-year periods between 1981 and 2000. Similar results (0.67 per 10,000 births) were found in a large Chinese study that recorded all the cases of microcephaly in newborns and stillborns of more than 28 weeks' gestation diagnosed during the first 7 days of life.[9] In a Canadian study,[10] the incidence of microcephaly dropped from 0.3 per 10,000 live births to 0.1 per 10,000 when the diagnosis was made by HC measurements instead of relying only on the clinical impression. In 1999 in the United States, the nationwide rate of microcephaly was much higher and reached 5.9 per 10,000 live births;[11] epidemiologic data from a single U.S. state showed a rate of 7 per 10,000 children under the age of 1 year.[12] These differences are due to the fact that in the majority of cases, microcephaly is not present at birth but develops by the age of 1 year. In a study published in 1977, Sells[13] found that 1.9% of the children attending regular classes in Seattle had an HC measurement <2 D of the mean for age and sex, but their IQs were not significantly different than those of the control group.

## Pathogenesis

According to Rakic's[2,14] studies, cells in the ependymal layer of the lateral ventricle are the precursor of neuron and glial cells; during early proliferative stages, these progenitor cells start to divide symmetrically until the ventricular zone becomes highly cellular. A reduction in the total number of progenitor cells will cause a severe and lethal form of microcephaly known as radial microbrain. Decreased progenitor stem cell divisions result in microcephaly vera and reduced neuron numbers. In these cases, the weight of the brain is reduced, but macroscopically, it will appear almost normal.[5]

## Etiology

Microcephaly can result from many different processes, including chromosomal abnormalities, single gene defects, infections, and environmental effects, all of which can impair neuronal proliferation (Table 7–2). Microcephaly may be present as an isolated finding or it may be part of a more complex condition. Only some of these conditions may be apparent at prenatal examination. A search in the Online Mendelian Inheritance in Man (OMIM) database found 548 entries for microcephaly, but only some of these conditions are apparent in utero or in the neonatal period. When isolated, it is termed *primary microcephaly.* Autosomal recessive inheritance is described with gene mutations involving *MCPH, ASPM, CDK5RAP,* or *CENPJ* in some mild cases, and *ALM, ARFGEF2,* or *RAB3GAP* in more severe cases.[3]

The whole picture regarding the genetics of microcephaly is far from complete, and new genes have been described, some of them transmitted as an X-linked trait as *MRXS9* on chromosome Xq12-q21.31[15] or as an autosomal dominant trait with incomplete penetrance due to microdeletions on chromosome 1q21.1[16] or microduplications on chromosome 9q22.32.[17] It is likely that current microarray-based comparative genome hybridization (CGH) techniques will demonstrate additional gene abnormalities that are currently undetectable using conventional cytogenetic methods.

## Pathology

The information available in the literature regarding the pathology of microcephaly is scant. Reported cases consistently describe reduced brain weight with sulcal patterns ranging from normal to patterns described as "simplified gyral pattern" or microlissencephaly. The actual microscopic structure of the cortex in these cases is not clear. An example of the cerebral histology in a fetus at 26 postmenstrual weeks with microcephaly vera published by Evrard et al[18] showed a depleted germinal layer, white matter without migrating neurons, and abnormal superficial cortical layers. Garel described a fetus with microlissencephaly at 26 postmenstrual weeks showing normal myelination, cortical thickness, and neuronal differentiation with a very small number of cortical neurons and simplified gyration.[19]

**Table 7–2. SYNDROMES WITH POSSIBLE PRENATAL MICROCEPHALY**

| | Earliest Reported Diagnosis | Methods of Diagnosis | Associated Anomalies |
|---|---|---|---|
| Syndromes | | | |
| **Cerebrooculofacioskeletal syndrome (AR)[188]** | Second trimester | US, DNA repair analysis | Microphthalmia, CNS Skeletal |
| **Cockayne syndrome (AR)[189]** | First trimester | DNA analysis | IUGR, brain calcifications, cataracts, skeletal |
| **Cornelia de Lange syndrome (AD, S)[190]** | First trimester | US, mutation analysis | IUGR, GUT, CHD, facial, skeletal |
| **Meckel-Gruber syndrome (AR)[191]** | First trimester | US | Encephalocele, polycystic kidneys, polydactyly |
| **Mowat-Wilson syndrome (AD)[195]** | Birth | US, MRI | ACC, CHD, facial, megacolon, hypospadias. |
| **Neu-Laxova syndrome (AR)[193]** | Second trimester | US | IUGR, CNS, skeletal, facial |
| **Warburg micro syndrome (AR)[194]** | Birth | Clinical presentation | ACC, microphthalmia, cataracts |

*(continued)*

**Table 7–2. SYNDROMES WITH POSSIBLE PRENATAL MICROCEPHALY (CONTINUED)**

| | Earliest Reported Diagnosis | Methods of Diagnosis | Associated Anomalies |
|---|---|---|---|
| **Migration disorders with associated microcephaly** | | | |
| Galloway-Mowat syndrome (AR)[195] | Second trimester | US, MRI | IUGR, facial, MCD |
| Miller-Dieker lissencephaly syndrome (AD)[120,196] | Late second trimester | FISH, US, MRI | Lissencephaly, ventriculomegaly, MR |
| Norman-Roberts syndrome (AR)[197] | Second trimester | US, MRI | IUGR, facial, lissencephaly |
| **Metabolic diseases** | | | |
| 3-hydroxyisobutyric aciduria (AR)[198] | Second trimester<br>Third trimester | 3-OHB elevated in AF<br>US, MRI | MCD, brain calcifications, facial |
| Maternal phenylketonuria embryopathy[199] | Second trimester | US | IUGR, CHD, MR |
| Recessive hereditary methemoglobinemia type II (AR)[200] | Birth | Clinical presentation, low cytb5r activity | IUGR |
| Smith-Lemli-Opitz syndrome (AR)[201] | Second trimester | Low E3, elevated 7-dehydrocholesterol, mutation analysis, US | IUGR, CNS, facial, CHD, renal, micropenis, polydactyly |
| **Skeletal dysplasias** | | | |
| Microcephalic osteodysplastic primordial dwarfism type I (AR)[202,203] | Second trimester | US | IUGR, CNS, skeletal, CHD, facial, micropenis |
| Juberg-Hayward syndrome (AR)[204] | Second trimester | US | IUGR, CNS, facial, skeletal |
| Seckel syndrome (AR)[205] | Second trimester | US, MRI | IUGR, skeletal, facial |
| Chromosomal disorders | | | |
| Trisomy 21[71] | First trimester | US, karyotype | Increased NT, CHD |
| Trisomy 13[5] | First trimester | US, karyotype | CNS, facial, CHD |
| Trisomy 18[5] | First trimester | US, karyotype | CNS, facial, CHD, skeletal |
| 5p deletion (cri du chat)[206] | Second trimester | US, karyotype | IUGR, facial |
| Mosaic variegated mutation syndrome (AR)[207] | 22 weeks | US, karyotype | IUGR, ACC, CH, DWM, facial |
| Nijmegen breakage syndrome (AR)[208] | First trimester | DNA analysis | |
| Triploidy[209] | First trimester | Karyotype, US | |
| Wolf-Hirschhorn syndrome[210] | Second trimester | FISH, US, MRI | IUGR, PVPC, facial, CHD, MRI |

ACC, agenesis of corpus callosum; AD, autosomal dominant; AR, autosomal recessive; CH, cerebellar hypoplasia; CHD, congenital heart disease; CNS, central nervous system; DWM, Dandy-Walker malformation; FISH, fluorescent in-situ hybridization; GUT, genitourinary tract; IUGR, intrauterine growth retardation; MCD, malformations of cortical development; MR, mental retardation; MRI, magnetic resonance imaging; NT, nuchal translucency; OHB, hydroxybutiric acid; PVPC, periventricular pseudocyst; US, ultrasound.

## Associated Anomalies

The presence of associated anomalies and their identification using imaging or pathologic description is paramount in reaching a definitive diagnosis. The anomalies present in microcephalic individuals may be classified into three groups: associated anomalies directly related to the small brain (sloping forehead, apparent large ear size, and increased amount of extra-axial cerebrospinal fluid [CSF]) (Figures 7–2 and 7–3) or to abnormal cortical migration (microlissencephaly, periventricular heterotopia, and dysgenesis of the corpus callosum) (Figure 7–4), other brain anomalies (cerebellar or brainstem dysgenesis), and non–central nervous system (CNS) anomalies. Non-CNS abnormalities may involve any body system.

## Risk of Recurrence

Genetic counseling for families with known single-gene defects is straightforward. The genetic counseling recommendations for primary microcephaly are not yet clearly established. Based on the growing number of autosomal recessive microcephaly loci being reported, Dobyns recommends giving a 25% recurrence risk to parents of any child with microcephaly with simplified gyral pattern or primary microcephaly.[7] He believes that the lower risks suggested by older studies is probably due to inclusion of children with nonspecific mild microcephaly.

The recurrence risk may be as high as 50% when one of the parents is microcephalic with normal intelligence,[20,21] in these cases, the child will have normal or near-normal intelligence.

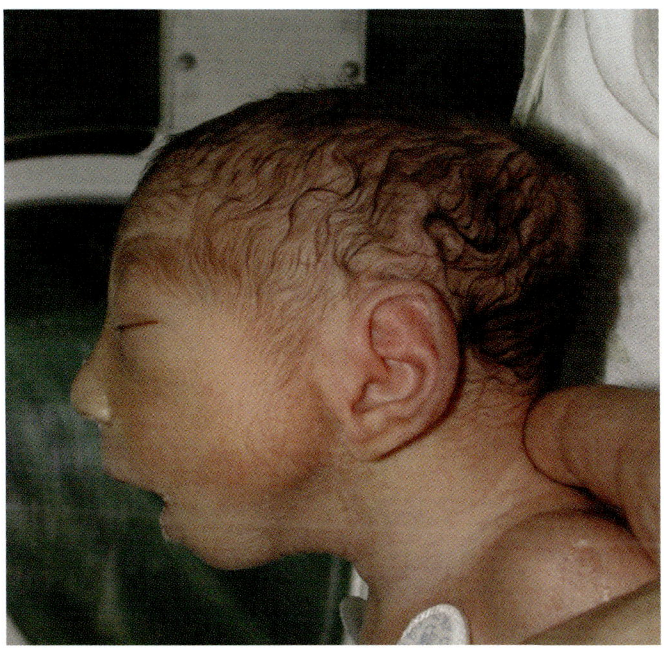

**Figure 7–2.** Newborn with severe microcephaly showing sloping forehead. The size of the ear is normal but when compared with the small head gives the impression as being big.

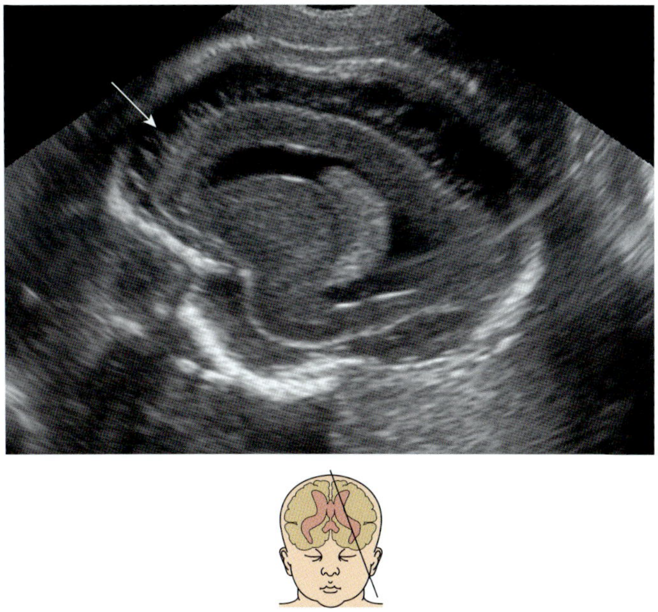

**Figure 7–3.** Increased amount of subarachnoid fluid due to the presence of a very small brain in a microcephalic fetus at 24 postmenstrual weeks. The abnormal subarachnoid space is particularly evident around the frontal lobe (*arrow*).

## Sonographic Diagnosis

The diagnosis of fetal microcephaly is mainly based on biometric measurements. An accurate diagnosis can be difficult, especially in borderline cases due to various factors, including gestational age uncertainties; lack of appropriate HC charts specific for gender, ethnic background, and fetal weight; influence of parental head circumference; and late development of microcephaly during the third trimester or postnatal period.[22–25]

Generally, suspicion should be aroused by any head size that is significantly smaller than expected for dates or in comparison to other body parts. Suspected cases should undergo detailed evaluation of the brain and all other body systems. Most significant cases will have additional findings beyond small head measurements, and these can help to confirm the diagnosis. Often intracranial brain structures are very difficult to see because the cranial sutures are very narrow (Figure 7–5). This limited visibility itself is a clue to failure of brain growth because skull growth depends on brain growth.

Chervenak et al[6] published in 1984 a paper on the diagnosis of fetal microcephaly. More than 25 years later, it continues to be the main reference for calculating abnormal HC size and counseling. According to their data, microcephaly was diagnosed when the HC is found to be $<-3$ SD. Using this cutoff, they had no false-negative diagnoses; an HC $<-4$ SD was a specific cutoff without false-positive patients. An HC/abdominal circumference ratio $<3$ SD and a femur length/head circumference ratio $>3$ SD were also helpful in the diagnosis[26] (see Chapter 3).

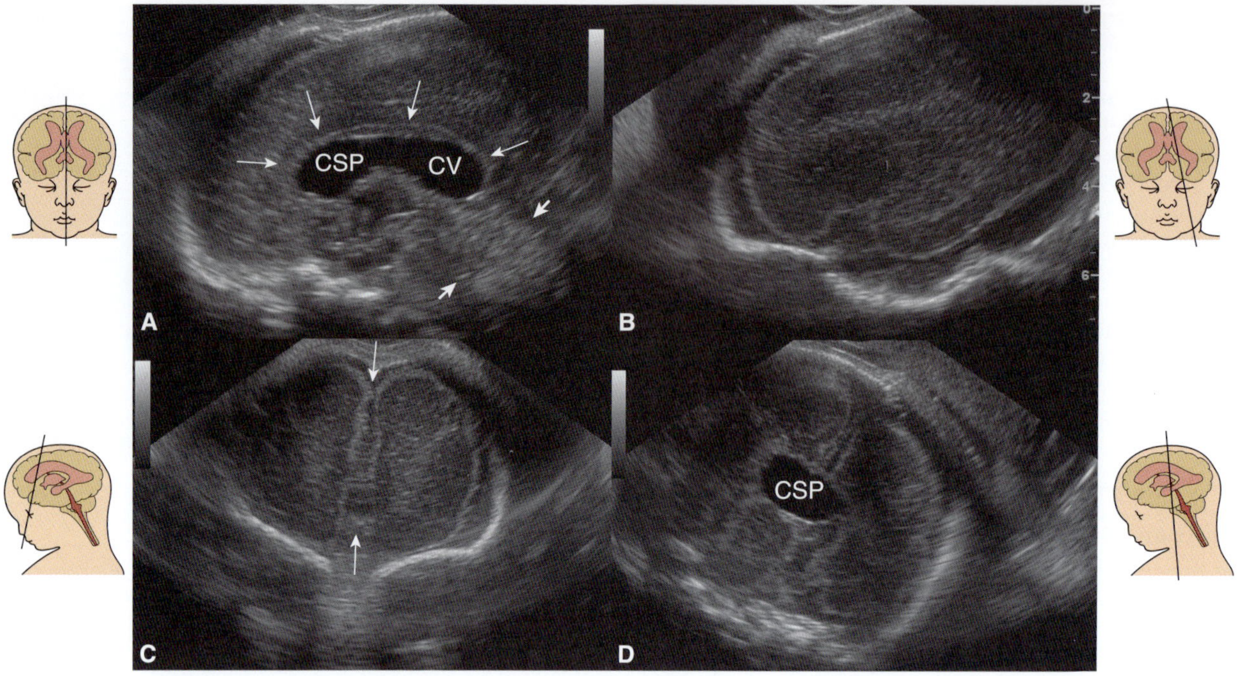


**Figure 7–4.** A fetus with microcephaly, lissencephaly, and dysgenesis of the corpus callosum at 33 weeks, 4 days. **(A)** Midsagittal plane shows a thin corpus callosum of irregular thickness (*arrows*) with a large cavum septi pellucidi (CSP) and cavum verga (CV); the vermis is not clearly defined (*arrowheads*). **(B)** Parasagittal plane at the level of the insula shows complete lack of sulcation. **(C)** Coronal plane at the level of the frontal lobes showing similar findings. Note the wide interhemispheric fissure with increased amount of cerebrospinal fluid (CSF) between the lobes (*arrows*). **(D)** In a more posterior coronal plane, the CSP is abnormally large.

Other measurements have been proposed in an effort to improve diagnostic accuracy,[27,28] but these have not been independently verified.[23]

Patients with extreme microcephaly have been diagnosed as early as 15 postmenstrual weeks of pregnancy, but this is the exception.[29] These patients usually have multiple malformations, and the diagnosis is straightforward (Figure 7–6). It is of paramount importance to remember that prenatal diagnosis consistently fails to diagnose most cases of primary microcephaly mainly because head growth is normal until late pregnancy. In a study of 9600 low-risk pregnancies evaluated using axial planes that included HC measurements, Reece and Goldstein[30] failed to diagnose all 5 cases with microcephaly. Bromely and Benacerraf[31] found that 6 out of 7 microcephalic children had a normal HC before 22 postmenstrual weeks of pregnancy, and microcephaly was detected between 27 and 33 postmenstrual weeks of pregnancy. Even in high-risk cases with recurrence risk of 25% to 50%, the likelihood of reaching a correct diagnosis during the last weeks of pregnancy may be impossible.[23,32]

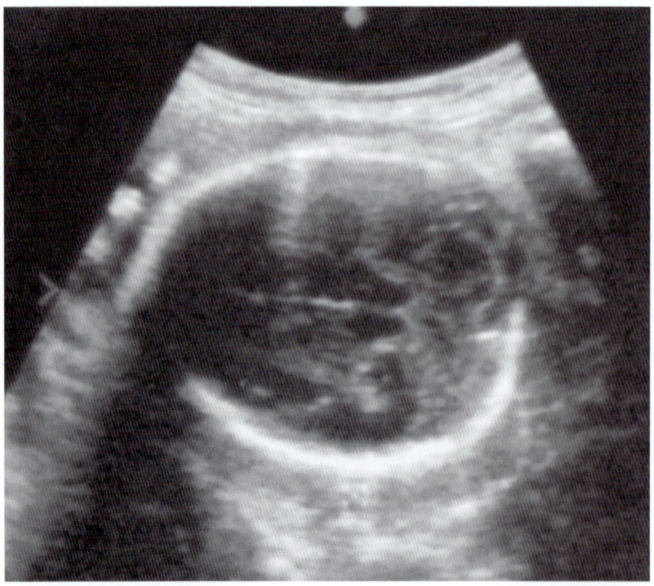

**Figure 7–5.** Difficult visualization of the brain in a fetus at 26 postmenstrual weeks with a small head circumference (HC <3 standard deviations [SD]). A similar picture in a fetus with normal HC should raise the suspicion of craniosynostosis.

Pilu and colleagues[33] reported on the prenatal diagnosis of microcephaly in two fetuses assisted by transvaginal sonography (TVS) and color Doppler. In these two cases, TVS revealed aberrant findings, including large subarachnoid spaces and a rudimentary shape of the lateral ventricles. In one of these fetuses, a sloping forehead was present; and in the other, power Doppler ultrasound (US) demonstrated a discrepancy in the size of the signals generated by the intracranial arteries branching from the internal carotid arteries and those branching from the vertebral arteries. This was interpreted as the consequence of a reduced blood supply to the undersized cerebral hemispheres.[33] The authors suggested that evaluation of intracranial anatomy by TVS and power Doppler examination of the cerebral vessels

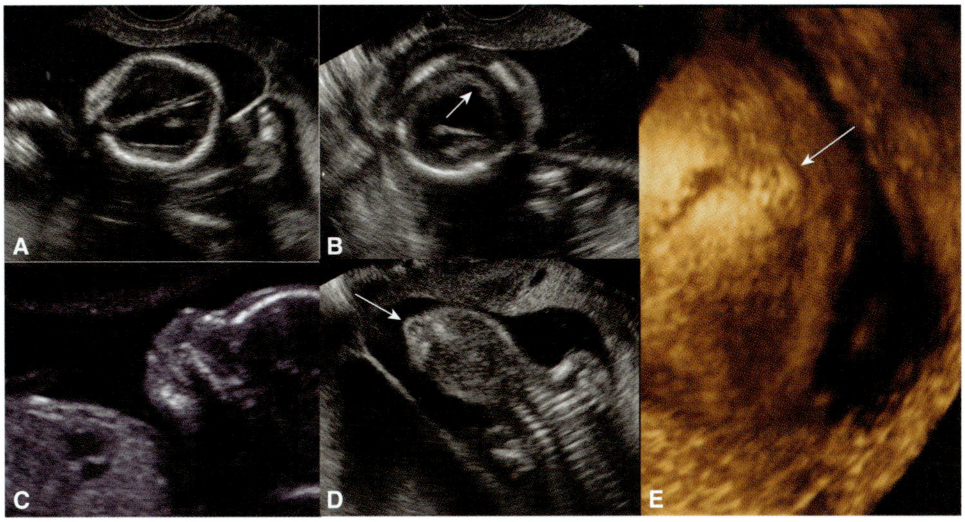


**Figure 7–6.** Discordant twin pregnancy at 18 postmenstrual weeks. Twin A, female with microcephaly, occipital encephalocele, ventriculomegaly, and facial dysmorphism; twin B, normal male (not shown). **(A)** Lemon-shaped calvarium with bilateral ventriculomegaly. Biparietal diameter (BPD) = 30 mm, well below the fifth percentile, HC = 117 mm, between −2 and −3 SD. **(B)** Ventriculomegaly with abnormal brain parenchyma and indentation of the ventricular wall (*arrow*). **(C)** Fetal profile shows an abnormal nose with mild micrognathia. **(D, E)** Occipital encephalocele (*arrow*).

may be of value in the diagnosis of fetal microcephaly. In fetuses with a small HC, the presence of an increased amount of CSF surrounding the brain, particularly when this fluid is prominent around the frontal horns and in the interhemispheric fissure, can be an indicator of congenital microcephaly (see Figure 7–3).

The accuracy of US in the diagnosis of fetal microcephaly has not been studied prospectively, but two retrospective analyses have been published. In the first study, den Hollander et al[34] reported on 30 fetuses referred at a mean gestational age of 27 postmenstrual weeks due to reduced head size or suspected intrauterine growth retardation (IUGR) or intra- or extracranial anomalies. Associated anomalies were present in 83.3% of the patients: holoprosencephaly (16.7%), chromosomal anomalies (23.3%), genetic syndromes (20%), and multiple anomalies (23.3%). Only five patients were considered as representing "isolated microcephaly," but a careful analysis of these cases showed that three of them had other anomalies, and only two represented patients with autosomal recessive primary microcephaly. The authors did not describe the number of fetuses with microcephaly diagnosed after delivery in their center.[34]

Dahlgren and Wilson[35] reviewed all cases of microcephaly diagnosed during a 10-year period at British Columbia Women's Hospital. They found 45 cases; in 21, the diagnosis was made prenatally and confirmed postnatally. In 15 patients, the second-trimester US was available, and 12 of these patients had a normal scan between 15 and 20 postmenstrual weeks of gestation. In nine patients (43%), the etiology of microcephaly remained unclear: possible viral infection based on placental signs of villitis or chorioamnionitis (four), multiple malformations (one), constitutional (one), and no specific etiology identified (one).

Our diagnostic approach to patients with suspected microcephaly is presented in Figure 7–7.

## Magnetic Resonance Imaging Diagnosis

Magnetic resonance imaging (MRI) can be very helpful and may add information regarding associated malformations and subtle differences in the gyration pattern that may be difficult to visualize by US. The characteristic receding forehead, increased amount of extra-axial fluid, and presence of a simplified gyral pattern have been reported using MRI[19,36] (Figure 7–8). It is important to remember that in all these patients, the MRI was performed following the measurement of an HC <−3 SD.

### Implications for Sonographic Screening, Including Earliest Recognition

Frustratingly, most children suffering from primary microcephaly will have normal HC when examined during the second trimester and even later on in pregnancy or at birth. The only chance to reach a diagnosis in at least some of the patients will be to perform follow-up examination of those fetuses with an HC in the low-normal range, but we doubt that such an approach is warranted. Another possibility should be rescreening at 32 to 34 postmenstrual weeks. Fetuses with syndromic microcephaly may be detected during routine second-trimester US based on the presence of associated anomalies.

### Implications for Targeted Ultrasound Examination

In families at risk of microcephaly following the diagnosis of the disease in a sibling or when one of the parents has microcephaly, it is important to obtain exact dating using first-trimester US measurements. An early

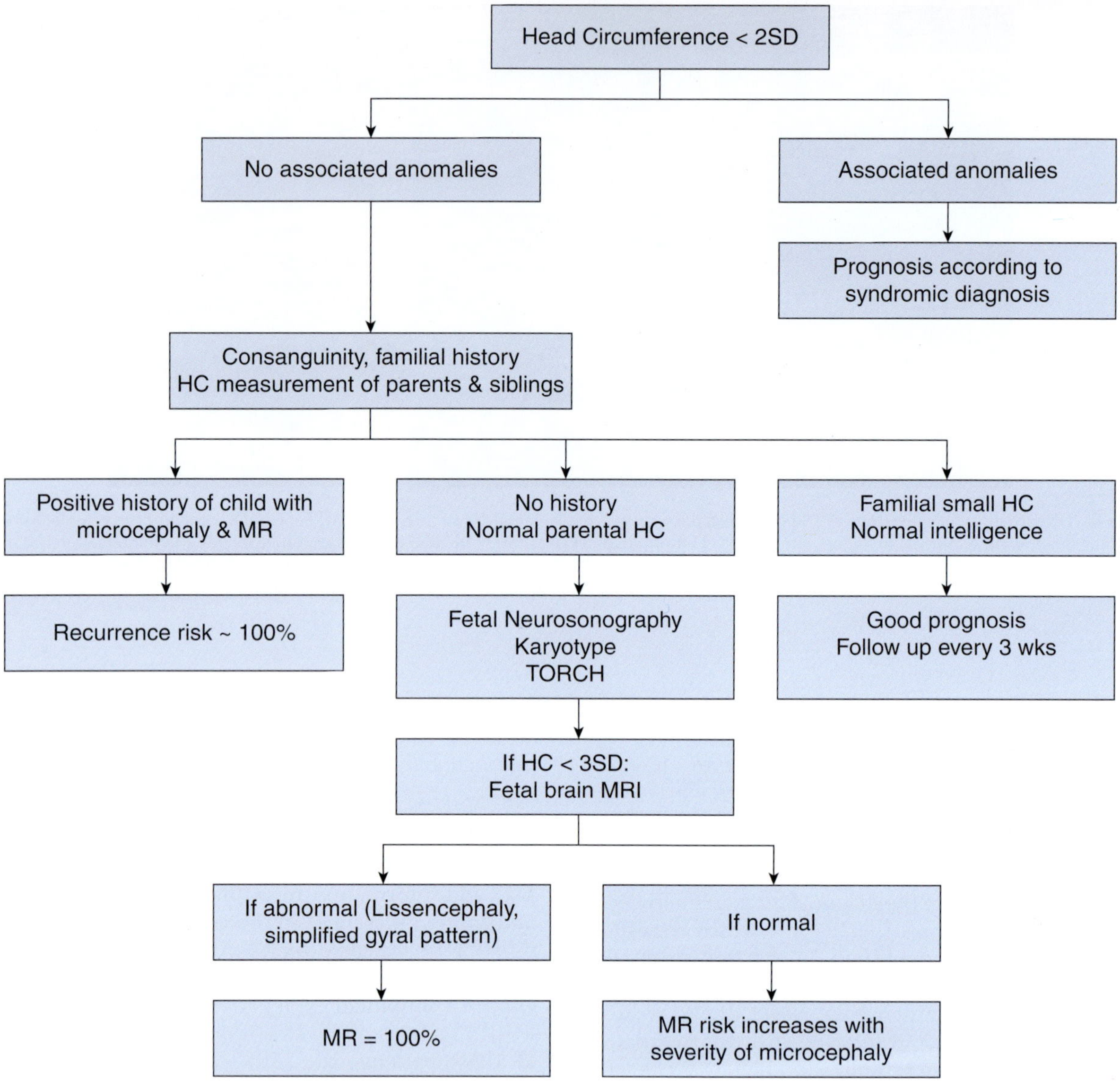


**Figure 7–7.** Proposed flowchart for the diagnosis of microcephaly.

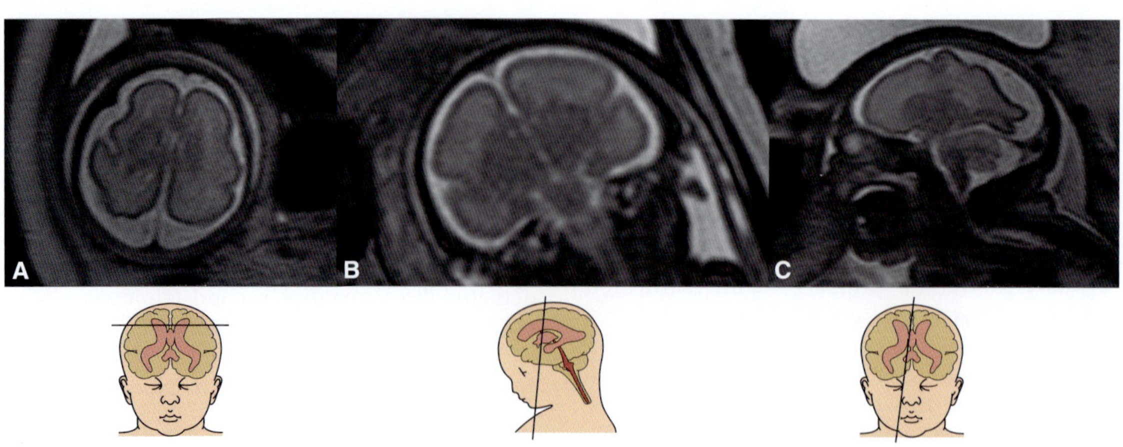


**Figure 7–8.** T2-weighted magnetic resonance imaging (MRI) at 31 postmenstrual weeks in a fetus with microcephaly and simplified cortical pattern. Axial **(A),** coronal **(B),** and sagittal **(C)** planes show sloping forehead and increased extra-axial fluid with abnormal, simplified sulcation pattern. (Courtesy of Dr. Atil Yuksel and Dr. Arda Lembet, Istanbul, Turkey.)

second-trimester anatomical US examination performed between 14 and 16 postmenstrual weeks of gestation may be used to rule out the presence of associated anomalies. Fetal measurements should be performed at 4-week intervals until term to evaluate the HC growth curve. A detailed neurosonogram or MRI is indicated at around 32 postmenstrual weeks if the HC is small.

The use of gender-specific charts[37] may be helpful in improving diagnostic accuracy.

### Prognosis

The fate of fetuses with an HC between −2 SD and −3 SD during pregnancy is still not clear. In a recent study,[38] we found that when excluding fetuses with associated malformations, there were no significant differences in neurodevelopmental performance at the ages of 2 to 4 years between children that had small HC (between −2 SD and −3 SD) in the prenatal period and controls. Studies have shown that children with an HC between −2 SD and −3 SD are more likely to have learning disabilities with near-normal intelligence.[38]

Arvey et al[39] found that in children with microcephaly, diagnosed during the first year of life, the risk of moderate to severe mental retardation increased from 33% to 62% when comparing children with a HC between −2 SD and −3 SD and those with an HC <−3 SD.

Outcomes in those syndromes and associated anomalies can depend on the associated abnormalities.

### Obstetric Management

Syndromic and autosomal recessive primary microcephalies are conditions associated with a high risk of moderate to severe mental retardation, and termination of pregnancy, when legally possible, should be offered. Milder cases will continue to be very difficult to manage.

Careful examination of the parents and family history is important because some normal families have members with small-appearing heads.

## Macrocephaly

### Synonyms

Macrocrania. Following exclusion of ventriculomegaly and enlarged subarachnoidal spaces, megalencephaly, megacephaly, megalocephaly may be used as synonyms.

### Definition

Macrocephaly is defined in children and adults as increased brain weight and an HC >2 SD above the mean or above the 98th percentile. The diagnosis excludes head enlargement that is secondary due to other causes, such as hydrocephaly, subdural hematoma, and tumors. As in microcephaly, the diagnosis of fetal macrocephaly may carry a grave prognosis, but the possibility of a false-positive diagnosis should be considered. Common pitfalls may be due to measurement errors and lack of normograms based on fetal gender, ethnic background, and parental HC. It should be remembered that using +2 SD as the upper limit automatically categorizes 2% of the population as macrocephalic. There is no consensus during fetal life regarding the exact definition of an abnormally large HC as there is no available literature on this issue.[32] The U.S. Centers for Disease Control and Prevention (CDC) growth charts for HC have recently defined the 97th percentile at birth as 39 cm for boys and 38 cm for girls (http://www.cdc.gov/growthcharts/). These charts are not concordant with the fetal charts.

### Incidence/Prevalence

Statistical data regarding the prevalence or incidence of macrocephaly at birth in the general population are scant. In a study performed in Sweden only in boys, it was found that the prevalence was 1 in 198.[40] In autopsy series, the rates of macrocephaly range from 1 in 1146 to 1 in 50,000.[41] Macrocephaly is more prevalent in selected populations, such as children with learning disorders,[42] developmental disabilities,[43] or autism.

### Pathogenesis

Macrocephaly is considered a defect of cell proliferation due to either a more rapid or prolonged time of cell replication or a reduced rate of cell apoptosis.[5] Although the total number of neurons is increased, the cells are morphologically normal.

In a mouse model, postnatal progressive megalencephaly has recently been linked to potassium channel dysfunction. The authors propose that a potassium ion channelopathy may be the cause of idiopathic megalencephaly and early-onset epilepsy in a group of infants or young children with or without cognitive impairments.[44]

### Etiology

Macrocephaly may be isolated or part of a syndrome. There is an isolated form known as familial benign macrocephaly which is due to enlargement of the subarachnoid space and may be transmitted as a dominant or recessive trait or be sporadic.

Macrocephaly associated with other malformations is usually due to specific syndromes, some of which may be diagnosed prenatally[45–69] (Table 7–3). Others, such as Weaver, Sturge-Weber, Alexander, and fragile X, may not manifest macrocephaly during fetal life.

### Pathology

There are no available data regarding histopathology of familial benign isolated macrocephaly.

### Associated Anomalies

The diagnosis of associated anomalies enables differentiation between syndromic and nonsyndromic cases, and a detailed search should be performed when macrocephaly develops in utero. Family history is important because about half the cases will be benign familial macrocephaly. The search for associated anomalies should be initially oriented toward differentiation between fetuses with

**Table 7–3. SYNDROMES WITH MACROCEPHALY IN WHICH PRENATAL DIAGNOSIS MAY BE POSSIBLE**

| | Earliest Reported Diagnosis | Method | References |
|---|---|---|---|
| **Syndromes** | | | |
| PTEN-related syndromes | Birth | Mutation analysis | Tekin et al[45] |
| Neurofibromatosis type 1 | 27 weeks | US, MRI | McEwing et al[46] |
| Linear epidermal nevus syndrome | 30 weeks | US | Neis et al [47] |
| Hemimegalencephaly | 25 weeks<br>32 weeks | US<br>MRI | Malinger et al[69]<br>Agid et al[48] |
| Frontal macrocephaly, polymicrogyria | 21 weeks | US, MRI | Parazzini et al[49] |
| Macrocephaly with thick corpus callosum | 23 weeks | US, MRI | Lerman-Sagie et al[68] |
| **Overgrowth syndromes** | | | |
| Macrocephaly, capillary malformation syndrome | 31 weeks | MRI, US | Gripp et al[50], Nyberg et al[51] |
| Sotos syndrome | 31 weeks | US | Thomas et al[52], Chen et al[53] |
| Simpson-Golabi-Behemel syndrome | Birth (34 weeks) | Clinical presentation | Yamashita et al[54], Hughes-Benzite et al[55] |
| Perlman syndrome | Birth | Clinical presentation | Schilke et al[56], Alessandri et al[57] |
| Megalencephaly, polymicrogyria, and hydrocephaly (MPPH) syndrome | 31 weeks | MRI, US | Gripp et al[50] |
| **Neuro cardio facio cutaneous syndromes** | | | |
| Costello syndrome | 27 weeks | US | Lin et al[58] |
| **Metabolic diseases** | | | |
| Glutaric aciduria, type 1 (GA-1) | 33 weeks | US, MRI | Mellerio et al[59] |
| D-2-hydroxyglutaric aciduria | 40 weeks | US, Mutation analysis | Zafeiriou et al[60]<br>Augoustides-Savvopoulou et al[67] |
| Canavan disease | Birth | Clinical presentation | Traeger et al[61] |
| Megalencephalic leukodystrophy with cysts (MLWC) | First trimester | Mutation analysis | Shukla et al[66] |
| **Skeletal dysplasias** | | | |
| Achondroplasia | 27 weeks | US | Huggins et al[62] |
| Thanatophoric dysplasia | 15 weeks<br>27 weeks | US<br>US | See Figure 7–9<br>Chen et al[63] |
| Campomelic acampomelic dysplasia | Birth (33 weeks) | Clinical presentation | Michel-Calemard et al[64] |
| Greig cephalosyndactyly syndrome | Birth | Clinical presentation | Sobetzko et al[65] |
| **Chromosomal disorders** | | | |
| 46XX del [3q]26.1-27.1 | 20 weeks | US | See Figure 7–10 |

MRI, magnetic resonance imaging; PTEN, Phosphatase and tensin homolog; US, ultrasound.

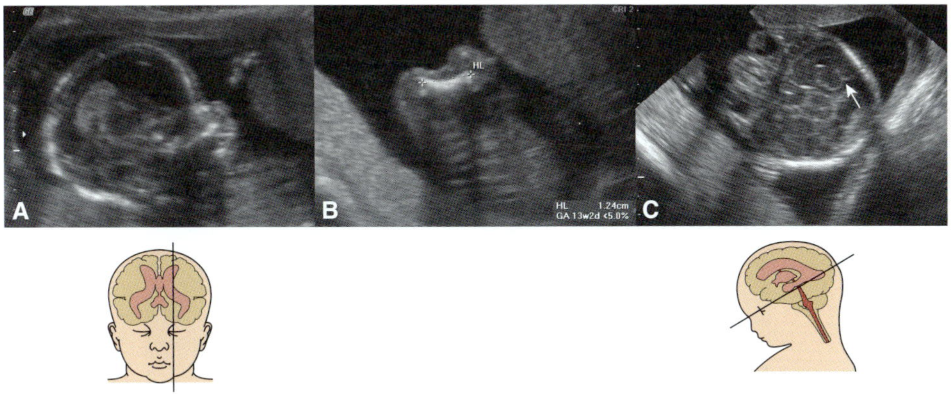

**Figure 7–9.** Thanatophoric dysplasia in a fetus at 15 postmenstrual weeks. **(A)** Frontal bossing with an HC above the 98th percentile. **(B)** Very small and bowed humerus. **(C)** Abnormal temporal sulcus (normally apparent by the early third trimester).

abnormal growth (overgrowth syndromes or skeletal dysplasias) and those who only have a large HC (Figure 7–9). As with microcephaly, macrocephalic individuals display craniofacial anomalies that may be directly related to the large brain (frontal bossing and increased amount of extra-axial fluid) (Figures 7–9 and 7–10) or associated with MCD (pachygyria, polymicrogyria, periventricular heterotopia, and dysgenesis of the corpus callosum) (Figures 7–9, 7–10, and 7–11), other brain anomalies (ventriculomegaly and cerebellar or brainstem dysgenesis) (Figure 7–10), or non-CNS anomalies (Figure 7–9).

When searching for non-CNS anomalies, particular attention should be given to the extremities (polydactyly and vascular malformations)[50] (Figure 7–11).

## Risk of Recurrence

Genetic counseling for families with known single-gene defects is straightforward. Familial isolated macrocephaly may have a recurrence risk of up to 50%, but this is usually a relatively benign condition. According to Arbour et al,[70] the inheritance pattern of nonsyndromic macrocephaly is considerably lower than expected for an autosomal dominant trait and should be considered multifactorial and not dominant. Similar findings were found in the Swedish study previously mentioned.[40]

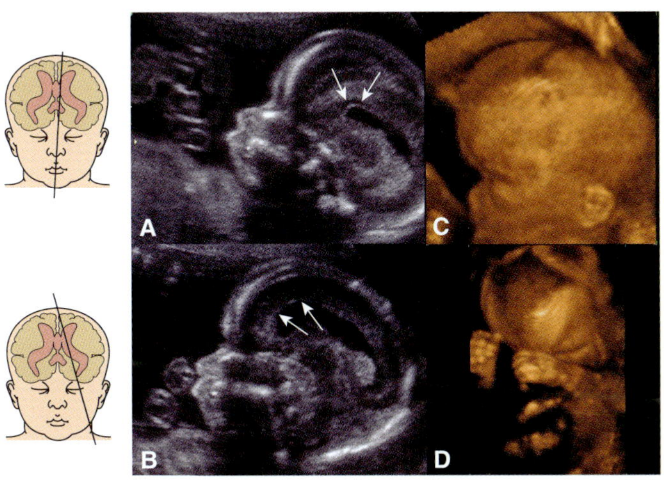

**Figure 7–10.** Macrocephaly (HC = +2 SD) in a fetus at 20 postmenstrual weeks with chromosome 3q deletion. **(A)** Median section of the brain shows dysgenesis of the corpus callosum (*arrows*). **(B)** Paramedian section shows ventriculomegaly; note the irregular ventricular wall (*arrow*). **(C, D)** Three-dimensional (3D) imaging of the fetal profile shows frontal bossing (C) and wide open anterior fontanelle (D).

## Sonographic Diagnosis

Due to its development in late pregnancy or after birth, macrocephaly is usually not diagnosed during pregnancy, and when suspected during the third trimester, biometric and anatomical evaluation are usually difficult. Accurate diagnosis can be limited due to gestational age uncertainties, lack of appropriate gender-specific fetal HC charts, ethnic background, weight, and influence of parental HC.

According to our experience, the vast majority of fetuses with apparently isolated macrocephaly with HC between 2.0 and 2.5 SD are males and most of them have a normal HC at birth.

Exceptionally, macrocephaly may be diagnosed during the second trimester. These patients are at increased risk of having one of the syndromic conditions (see Figures 7–9 and 7–10; Table 7–3). The prenatal diagnosis of familial isolated benign macrocephaly may be made when there is a family history and no associated malformations[71,72] (Figure 7–12).

Our diagnostic approach to patients with suspected macrocephaly is presented in Figure 7–13.

## MRI Diagnosis

MRI may add information regarding associated malformations and subtle differences in the gyration pattern that may be difficult to visualize by US. The characteristic frontal bossing, increased amount of extra-axial fluid, and presence of abnormal sulcation have been reported using MRI[19,36] (Figure 7–11).When evaluating patients with suspected macrocephaly, caution must be taken because increased extra-axial fluid may give a false impression of an abnormal oversulcation pattern (see Figure 7–12).

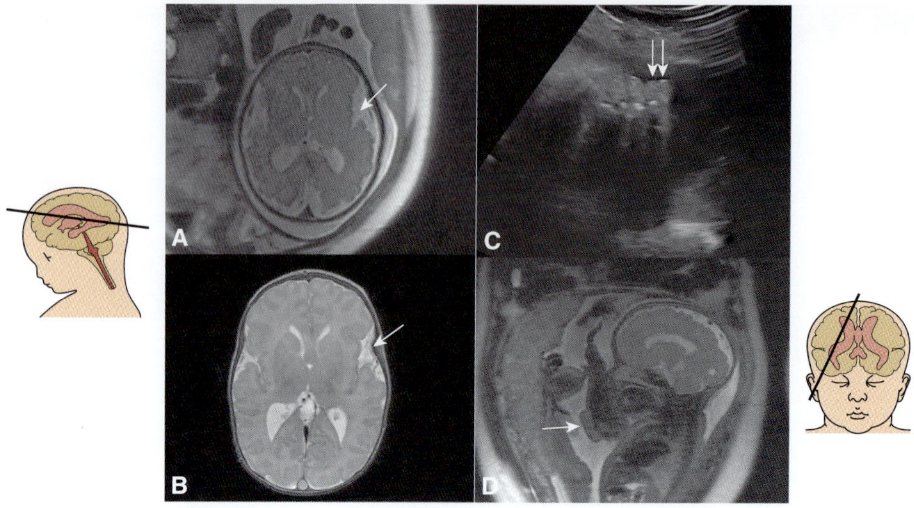

**Figure 7–11.** Macrocephaly/vascular malformations syndrome. Prenatal at 32 weeks of gestation **(A)** and postnatal at 2 months of age **(B)** axial T2-weighted MRI show an abnormally open operculum lined with an abnormal cortex (polymicrogyria) (*arrows*). **(C)** Ultrasound (US) at 33 postmenstrual weeks shows syndactyly of foot fingers 5 and 6 (*arrows*). **(D)** Fetal MRI shows a hemangioma of the elbow (*arrow*).

## Implications for Sonographic Screening, Including Earliest Recognition

Most of the children with isolated macrocephaly will have an age-appropriate HC when examined during the second trimester and even in later pregnancy or at birth. The only chance to reach a diagnosis in at least some of the patients will be to perform follow-up examination of fetuses with an HC in the high-normal range, but we doubt that such an approach is warranted.

Syndromic macrocephaly along with associated anomalies may present during routine second-trimester US.

## Implications for Targeted Examination

In families at risk of having syndromic macrocephaly, it is of paramount importance to establish accurate dating in the first trimester. An early second-trimester anatomical US examination performed between 14 and 16 postmenstrual weeks may be performed to rule out the presence of associated anomalies. Fetal measurements can be performed at 4-week intervals until term to evaluate the HC growth curve. A detailed neurosonogram or MRI may provide additional information if the HC is large.

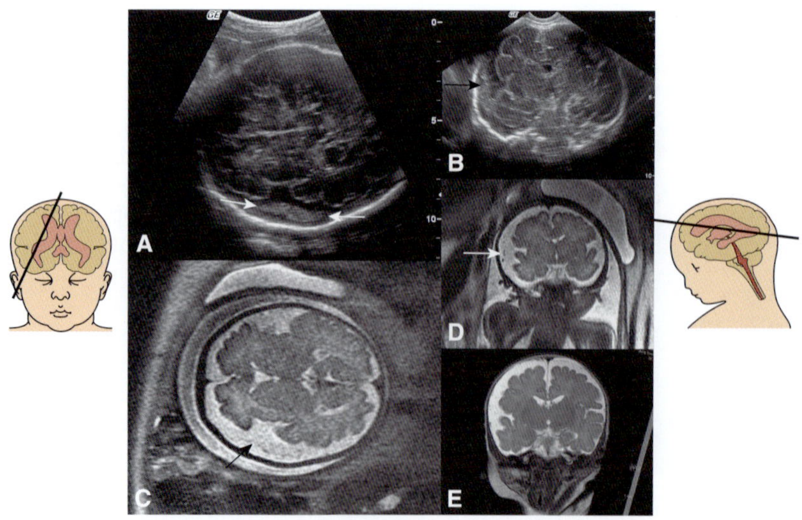

**Figure 7–12.** Prenatal US **(A, B)** and MRI **(C, D)** at 32 weeks' gestation and postnatal MRI **(E)** in a patient with apparently isolated macrocephaly showing subarachnoid enlarged spaces. A subdural hematoma was suspected by neurosonography due to the presence of floating echogenic material (*arrows* in **A** and **B**). MRI shows asymmetric amounts of CSF overlying the right hemisphere with residual dural thickening (*arrow*). The father is also macrocephalic; the child is developing normally at the age of 3 years. The subdural hematoma resolved shortly after birth.

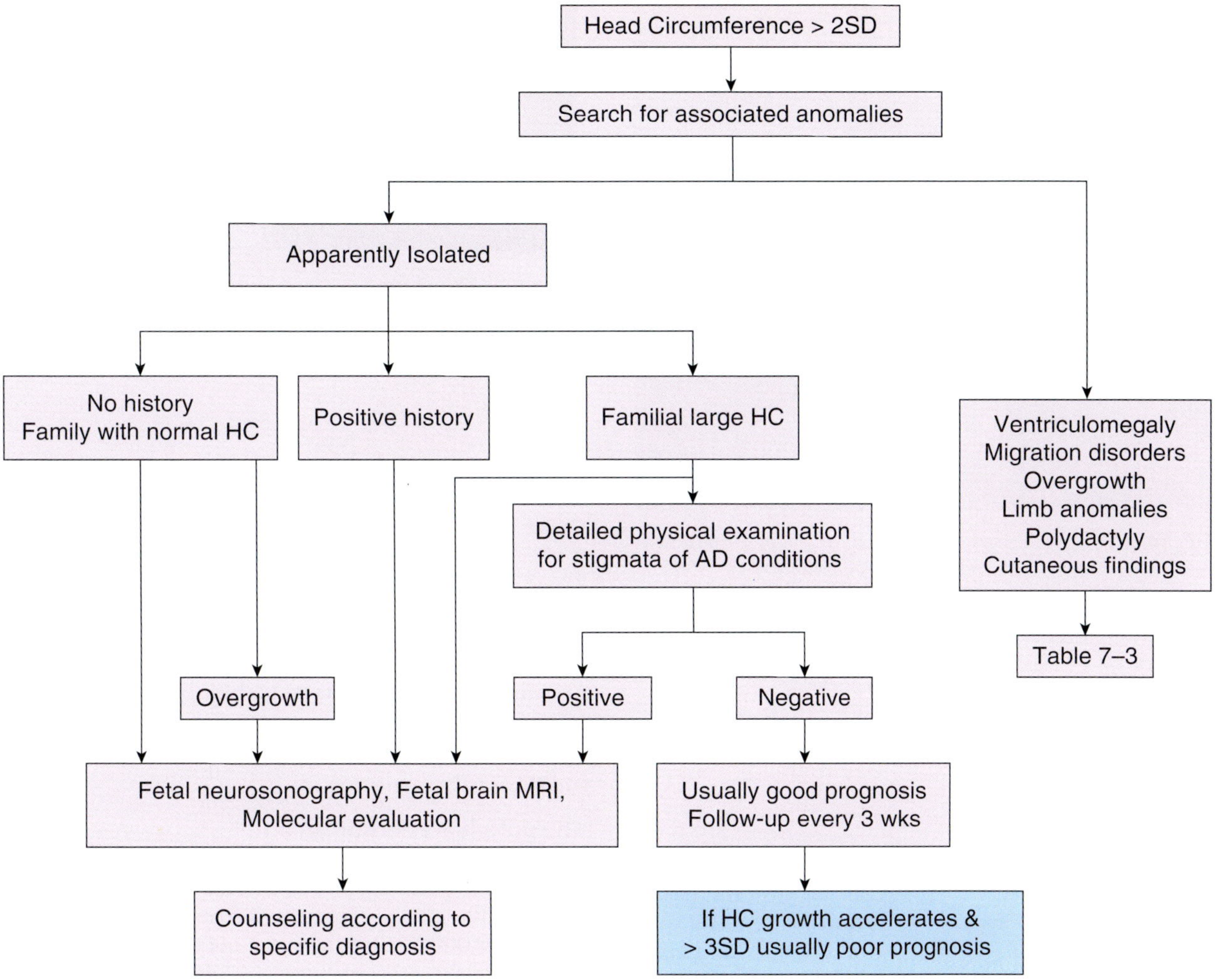


**Figure 7–13.** Proposed flowchart for the diagnosis of macrocephaly.

## Prognosis

The fate of fetuses with an HC between 2 and 3 SD during pregnancy is not clear. In a recent study we found that when excluding fetuses with associated malformations, there were no significant differences in the neurodevelopmental performance at the ages of 2 to 4 years between children with a large HC (between 2 and 3 SD) in the prenatal period and controls.[38]

A study in boys has shown that those with an HC above 2 SD have a significantly lower intelligence level (odds ratio, 1.32; 95% confidence interval [CI], 1.11–1.38), but not mental retardation (odds ratio, 1.31; 95% CI, 0.80–2.02).[40] Others found that the risk of mental retardation in children without apparent associated malformations was as high as 7% to 10%.[73,74]

## Obstetric Management

Syndromic macrocephalies are conditions associated with a high risk of moderate to severe mental retardation, and termination of pregnancy, when legally possible, should be offered. Isolated macrocephaly, particularly in patients with a family history and when the HC measurement is close to 2 SD, has a good prognosis.

# Hemimegalencephaly

Hemimegalencephaly describes abnormal hamartomatous enlargement of one hemisphere. It is regarded as an abnormality of neuronal proliferation and migration and may be due to abnormal function of left-right organizer genes. Most cases are sporadic with unknown etiology.

Isolated and syndromic forms are described. A group of syndromes known as neurocutaneous syndromes are frequently associated with hemimegalencephaly. Neurocutaneous syndromes include epidermal nevus syndrome, Proteus syndrome, Kippel-Tréaunay-Weber syndrome, neurofibromatosis type 1, and tuberous sclerosis complex, among others. The cerebral findings are similar in isolated and syndromic cases.[75,76] The clinical manifestations vary with the degree of brain abnormality and can include epilepsy, psychomotor retardation, and contralateral hemiparesis. Hemispherectomy may be needed for seizure control.[75]

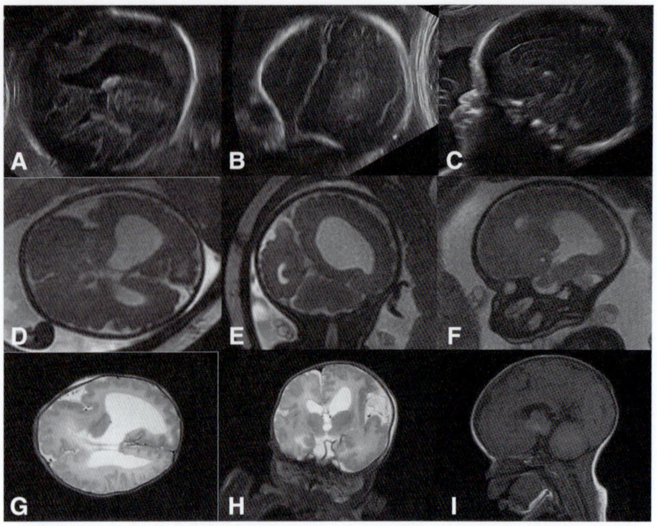


**Figure 7–14.** Hemimegalencephaly diagnosed by US at 28 postmenstrual weeks of gestation **(A–C)** with MRI confirmation at 29 weeks of gestation **(D–F)** and following delivery **(G–I)**. The clinical course was complicated by refractory epilepsy. Note the difference in the size of the cerebral hemispheres and lateral ventricles. The corpus callosum is thick (C, I), and the vermis not observed in the midline (E, I). Abnormal sulcation in the left hemisphere is suggested on fetal images and clearly depicted in both hemispheres on postnatal MRI (G, H). (Courtesy of Dr. Mauricio Herrera, Bogotá, Colombia.)

It has been detected as early as 18 weeks gestation.[77] At prenatal US the affected hemisphere shows increased volume, ventricular enlargement, abnormal texture, and occasional calcifications (Figure 7–14). The smaller hemisphere is compressed and distorted by the enlarged one, and characteristically abnormal findings are also present.[78] Note that normal fetuses can have a minimal 2 mm asymmetry at 20 to 22 postmenstrual weeks.[79]

Prenatal US findings can be confirmed by MRI (Figure 7–14). Differential diagnosis includes intracranial tumor or bleed and infections.

Prenatally diagnosed cases are offered pregnancy termination.

## Tuberous Sclerosis Complex

### Synonyms

Tuberous sclerosis, TSC, Bourneville disease, epiloia, phakomatosis TS

### Definition

Tuberous sclerosis complex (TSC) is a neurocutaneous syndrome characterized by abnormal proliferation of neurons and glia in the form of hamartomata or low-grade tumors with accompanying anomalies of migration and differentiation. The manifestations of TSC are not limited to the brain but usually involve other systems, particularly the skin, eyes, kidneys, lungs, heart, blood vessels, and bones. In the fetus, the presence

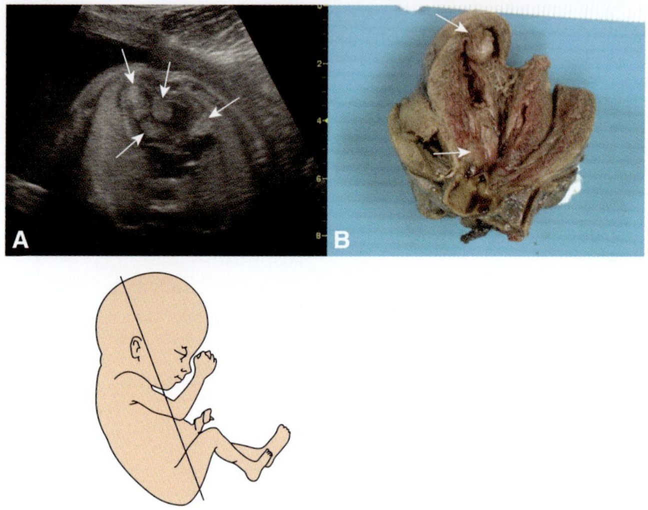


**Figure 7–15.** Multiple cardiac rhabdomyomata in a fetus with tuberous sclerosis. **(A)** Fetal US at 26 weeks' gestation shows the presence of at least four intracardiac tumors (*arrows*). **(B)** Coronal view of the heart at 30 weeks shows the cardiac rhabdomyomata (*arrows*).

of cardiac rhabdoyomata is highly suggestive of TSC (Figure 7–15).

### Incidence/Prevalence

The prevalence is estimated to be between 7 and 12 cases per 100,000 live births, with more than half of these cases undetected prenatally.[80] The total population prevalence figures have steadily increased from 1 in 150,000 in 1956, to 1 in 100,000 in 1968, to 1 in 70,000 in 1971, to 1 in 34,200 in 1984, to the present figure of 1 in 12,500 in 1998.

### Etiology and Pathogenesis

TSC is caused by mutations of the *TSC1* gene on chromosome 9[81] or of the *TSC2* gene on chromosome 16.[82] This autosomal dominant disease expresses the following two successive mutations: A germ line mutation produces a loss of heterozygocity in one of the alleles, followed by a somatic mutation of the other allele.[83] *TSC1* and *TSC2* encode for two proteins called hamartin and tuberin, respectively. Hamartin and tuberin are tumor suppressors acting as inhibitors in the mTOR cascade pathway. Hyperactivation of this pathway results in abnormal cell growth and proliferation.[84] Although most of the cases are due to sporadic mutations in *TSC2, TSC1* mutations are more common in familial cases.

### Pathology

TSC may affect the brain in different forms. The name of the disease originates from the presence of firm cortical masses with dimpling resembling potatoes with eyes. Similar nodules may be found in the periventricular zone. The tubers are composed of large, poorly differentiated cells of neuronal and glial origin. Similar cells may be found in the white matter. Abnormal cell differentiation may also produce benign giant cell astrocytomas. In the fetus, the only other organ frequently involved (in up to 50% of cases) is the heart by the development of rhabdomyomata.

### Risk of Recurrence

TSC is transmitted as an autosomal dominant trait with high penetrance but variable expression, which may cause mildly affected individuals to be undiagnosed. The vast majority of cases are sporadic (Table 7–4). Following the prenatal diagnosis or the birth of an affected patient, both parents should be evaluated for the presence of subclinical disease.

### Sonographic Diagnosis

The reported incidence of cardiac tumors in fetuses at fetal echocardiography is 0.14%; rhabdomyomata represents >90% of them.[85] The first prenatal diagnoses of TSC were reported by DeVore et al[86] and Crawford et al.[87] Crawford and colleagues based their diagnosis on the second-trimester detection of cardiac rhabdomyomata in a fetus at risk. The first examination at 18 postmenstrual weeks was considered normal, but by 22 postmenstrual weeks, the presence of cardiac tumors was evident.[87]

In 1986, Muller et al[88] reported the first US prenatal diagnosis of a fetus at 26 weeks with brain involvement. Since then a large number of case reports and small series of fetuses with TSC stigmata have been published.

Eight groups have studied the implications of the diagnosis of cardiac rhabdomyomata[89,96] (Table 7–4). In the majority of patients, the diagnosis was made relatively late in pregnancy, the mean time of diagnosis ranging between 26 and 30 postmenstrual weeks of pregnancy. Multiple rhabdomyomata were found more frequently than single ones (72% vs 28%); only 23% required postnatal medical or surgical treatment, and the vast majority decreased in size after delivery. The risk for a fetus with rhabdomyoma to suffer from TSC in the whole group was 75%, and a familial history was obtained in 17%. The risk for developmental disease was available from three studies showing that 20 out of 47 children (42.5%) were affected. Affected children were diagnosed either before or after delivery. Tworetzky et al[93] found neurodevelopmental deficits in 85% of children diagnosed before or after delivery.

Isolated reports on the US appearance of TSC-related brain lesions have been published. In most cases the findings were observed in patients at high risk for TSC (familial history or presence of rhabdomyomata).[88,97–99] Mirkin and colleagues[98] reported on the presence of a

**Table 7–4. PUBLISHED SERIES ON FETUSES WITH PRENATAL DIAGNOSIS OF CARDIAC RHABDOMYOMATA**

| Author (Year) | Number of Fetuses | Week of Diagnosis | Single, Multiple | Outcome | Need for Treatment | TSC in Family | Neurodevelopmental Delay |
|---|---|---|---|---|---|---|---|
| Pipitone et al[89] (2002) | 9 | 27–36 Mean 30.0 | 1 single, 8 multiple | 9 delivered (1 NND) | 5 | 7/80/9 | NS |
| D'Addario et al[90] (2002) | 6 | 23–37 Mean 30.0 | 3 single, 3 multiple | 6 delivered | 1 (died) | 3/60/6 | NS |
| Gamzu et al[91] (2002) | 18 | 21–33 Mean 27.1 | 12 single, 6 multiple | 12 delivered, 6 TOP | 0 | 7/123/18 | NS |
| Bader et al[92] (2003) | 20 | 19–37 Mean 28.4 | 2 single, 18 multiple | 18 delivered 2 TOP-IUFD | 7 | 15/194/20 | 6/18 |
| Tworetzky et al[93] (2003) | 42 | 15–38 Mean 28.5 | 9 single, 33 multiple | 34 delivered, 8 TOP-IUFD | 8 | 33/4210/42 | 85% (of prenatal + postnatal group) |
| Fesslova et al[94] (2004) | 13 | 21–36 Mean 26.0 | 5 single, 8 multiple | 9 delivered, 4 TOP | 0 | 9/112/13 | 5/9 2 neurosurgery |
| Chao et al[95] (2008) | 11 | 18–39 Mean 27.5 | 5 single, 6 multiple | 8 delivered (2 NND), 3 TOP-IUFD | 2 | 3/62/11 | NS |
| Saada et al[96] (2009) | 51 | 21–37 Mean 27.1 | 10 single, 41 multiple | 25 delivered, 26 TOP | 5 (1 died) | 39/518/51 | 9/20 With MRI + 67% With MRI – 33% |
| Total | 170 | 15–38 | 47 single, 123 multiple | 121 delivered (3 NND), 49 TOP-IUFD | 28/121 | 116/15529/170 | 20/47 |

IUFD, intrauterine fetal death; MRI, magnetic resonance imaging; NND, neonatal death; NS, not stated; TOP, termination of pregnancy; TSC, tuberous sclerosis complex.

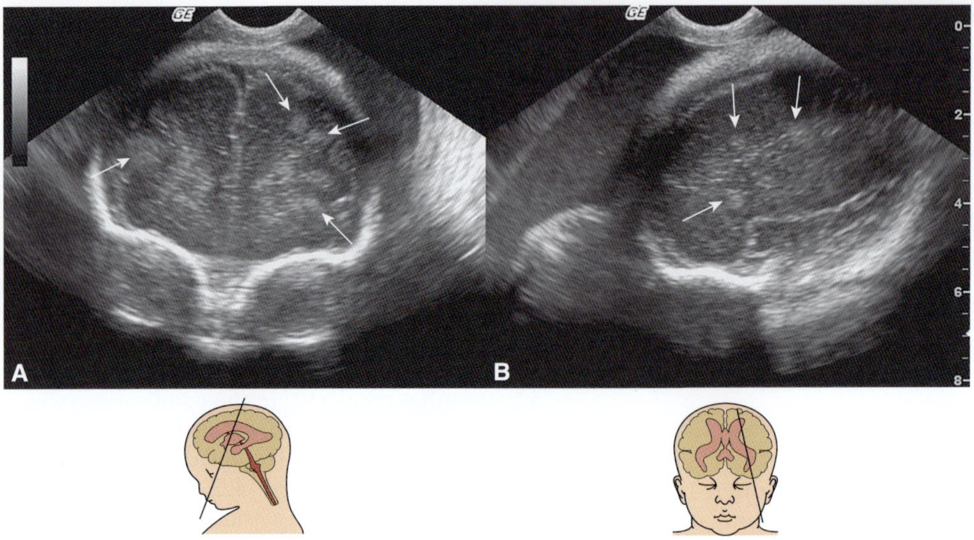


**Figure 7–16.** Brain transvaginal sonography (TVS) images in a fetus with tuberous sclerosis at 28 postmenstrual weeks (same patient as in Figure 7–14) show multiple parenchymal echogenic nodules (*arrows*). **(A)** Coronal section at the level of the frontal horns. **(B)** Paramedian section lateral to the lateral ventricle.

large subependymal tumor diagnosed at 27 postmenstrual weeks that was resected after birth and found to be a giant cell astrocytoma. The diagnosis of TSC was only made at 4 years of age.

In fetuses referred because of multiple cardiac rhabdomyomata (see Figure 7–15), the diagnosis of brain involvement is usually possible when multiple bilateral parenchymal and periventricular echogenic nodules are present[77] (Figure 7–16). Milder brain involvement may be very difficult or even impossible to visualize (Figure 7–17).

## MRI Diagnosis

Many authorities[100,101] consider fetal MRI more effective than US for the diagnosis of TSC brain lesions, but this issue has never been studied in an unbiased way.

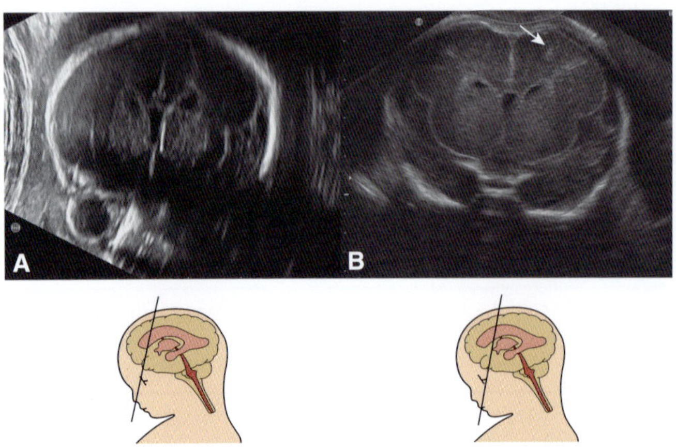


**Figure 7–17.** Tuberous sclerosis at 25 postmenstrual weeks in a fetus with multiple cardiac rhabdomyomata and no familiar history. **(A)** Apparently normal coronal transabdominal view. **(B)** Transvaginal coronal section showing the presence of at least one parenchymal nodule (*arrow*).

The largest published case series included 51 patients referred for fetal echocardiography because of the presence of cardiac rhabdomyomata during second- or third-trimester US examinations.[96] Although all the patients underwent a detailed US examination, the results of the examinations were not mentioned, and only data on fetal brain MRI were included. MRI was performed at a mean gestational age of 30 postmenstrual weeks (range 24–37 weeks), brain lesions were found in 25 (49%) patients, and 21 chose termination of pregnancy (TOP), with autopsy positive for TSC in all of them. MRI was considered normal in 26 (51%) patients, 5 underwent TOP, and TSC was diagnosed in 3. There were 25 deliveries, including four with positive MRI findings. Neurological complications were reported in 45% of the studied patients (9/20) and included seizures, mental retardation, nodding spasms, and language retardation; normal prenatal and even postnatal MRI did not rule out the development of neurological complications at latter stages[96] (Table 7–4).

### Implications for Sonographic Screening, Including Earliest Recognition

The presence of cardiac rhabdomyomata, particularly when multiple and large is highly indicative of the presence of TSC. In these patients a detailed neurosonographic examination and/or brain MRI are indicated. Although early second-trimester diagnosis may be posible,[93,102] it should be remembered that in more than two-thirds of cases the diagnosis is made after 24 postmenstrual weeks (Figures 7–15, 7–16, and 7–17).

### Implications for Targeted Examination

The role of fetal imaging in the diagnosis of TSC will become secondary following the introduction of molecular tests for deletion/duplication analysis of TSC1 and TSC2 genes.[103] Prenatal molecular diagnosis may be used when the disease is suspected early in pregnancy or when one of the parents is known to be affected.[103] When the suspicion of TSC is raised during the late second trimester or third trimester, a dedicated US or MRI examination, when positive, will continue to be the faster way to reach the diagnosis.

### Prognosis

TSC is a disease with multiorgan involvement but with a wide range of severity. The classic clinical triad of facial angiofibromas, mental retardation, and seizures is present in 30% of the patients. Mental retardation is present in 50% to 80% of patients. When diagnosed during fetal life or early infancy, neurodevelopmental disease may affect as much as 85% of patients.[93]

### Obstetric Management

The prenatal diagnosis of TSC poses a serious dilemma regarding continuation or termination of pregnancy, particularly when one of the parents is affected. Termination of pregnancy should be considered when legally possible and based on parents' desires. Postnatal neurosurgery may be needed to resect epileptogenic nodules or when giant cell astrocytoma produces hydrocephaly.

## MALFORMATIONS DUE TO ABNORMAL NEURONAL MIGRATION

### Lissencephaly Overview

*Lissencephaly* means "smooth brain." It describes a smooth pathologic appearance of the brain surface that lacks the normal gyri and sulci. There is spectrum of brain surface appearances ranging from completely smooth (agyria) to partially smooth with abnormally large gyri (agyria/pachygyria). Lissencephaly implies a major abnormality of neuron migration, secondary failure of normal gyration, and results in major neuromotor abnormality. There are two main processes or mechanisms by which migrational abnormality occurs: first, classical or type 1 lissencephaly and, second, type 2 or cobblestone cortex lissencephaly. In both there is major disruption of normal neuronal migration that starts in the first trimester, but the genetic and molecular disturbances are different. In type 1/classical, there is failure of neurons to migrate to the surface. In type 2, migration occurs but is not stopped at the surface by the pia limitans, allowing neurons to overmigrate into the subarachnoid space, where they cluster and partially cover brain surface vessels, resulting in a finely nodular surface that has been described as cobblestoned. The surface nodularity is so fine that to uninitiated observers, the brain surface appears smooth, but the partially covered surface vessels are more readily apparent.

There are two additional considerations. First, the genes and molecular mechanisms that control neuronal migration also have functions in the normal development of other tissues and organs. As a result, when they malfunction, it is common to see developmental abnormalities in other areas. For example, the genes associated with type 2 cobblestone cortex also function in normal muscle development. Fetuses with cobblestone cortex also have abnormal muscle structure clinically expressed as congenital muscular dystrophy and apparent with abnormal serum creatine kinase and abnormal muscle biopsy. Second, many structures, such as the eyes, cerebellum, and corpus callosum, are developing at the same time as neuronal migration is occurring. As a result, a teratologic insult (eg, infection) at a specific time can affect all of these structures at their stage of development. Therefore, it is not unusual to see MCD in association with abnormality involving the eyes, corpus callosum, and cerebellum. A corollary is that an abnormality detected in any of these structures should lead to evaluation of the other simultaneously developing areas.[3]

The performance of a detailed neurosonographic examination in search of migration disorders should be performed based on familial or clinical indications[104] (Table 7–5).

**Table 7–5. PATIENTS AT HIGH RISK OF ABNORMAL NEURONAL MIGRATION**

| | |
|---|---|
| Familiar history | Parents or siblings with MCD<br>Parents or siblings with non-diagnosed epilepsy<br>Maternal side siblings with MCD, epilepsy, early death of males |
| Abnormal US findings | Ventriculomegaly (including mild)<br>Suspected microcephaly or macrocephaly<br>Callosal anomalies<br>Agenesis of the septum pelucidum<br>Cerebellar anomalies<br>Ambiguous genitalia<br>Skeletal dysplasia |

MCD, malformations of cortical development; US, ultrasound.

### Lissencephaly/Subcortical Band Heterotopia Spectrum

#### Synonyms

Classical lissencephaly, lissencephaly type 1 (LIS1), X-linked lissencephaly, agyria/pachygyria, Miller-Dieker syndrome (MDS)

#### Definition

Type 1 or classical lissencephaly (smooth brain) is characterized by failure of migrating neurons to reach the cortical surface. As a result, there is total or partial failure to form cerebral convolutions or gyri and sulci. Subcortical band heterotopia (SBH) is a less severe phenotype of the same disease characterized by partial failure of the neurons to reach the cortex, resulting in a thin cortex with abnormal sulcation and a second layer/band of neurons underlying the outermost one.

## Incidence/Prevalence

In the period 1980 to 1988, the prevalence of lissencephaly type I in the Netherlands was 11.7 per 1 million births.[105] There are no available data from other countries on the incidence and prevalence of this disease.

## Pathogenesis

Neuronal migration occurs during and following the period of neuronal proliferation, starting at 6 to 7 postmenstrual weeks of gestation and is essentially finished by 30 weeks' gestation in the cerebral cortex. Neurons migrate from the ventricular and subventricular zone until they reach the pia surface in 6 successive waves; two different varieties of migration, tangential and radial, have been described.[2] Radial migration is responsible for the formation of most of the cortex; tangential migration is the way used by the interneurons to reach their place in the cortex.[2]

In patients with lissencephaly radial migration is disturbed between 11 and 13 postmenstrual weeks' gestation[106] due to abnormal function of genes that affect key molecular processes, in particular platelet-activating factor acetylhydrolase (PAFAH), doublecortin, and the glycoprotein reelin.[5] Different mutations affecting the same gene will result in different phenotypes.

## Etiology

Most of the known lissencephalies are transmitted as autosomal dominant or X-linked traits and only rarely as an autosomal recessive trait.

The lissencephaly/SBH spectrum includes four different genetic types: *LIS1* mutations, *DCX* mutations, *ARX* mutations, and reelin (*RELN*) mutations (Table 7–1).

*LIS1* mutations are the most frequent and result from deficiencies in PAFAH and affect the normal function of the cytoskeleton. Isolated lissencephaly and Miller-Dieker syndrome have a similar locus at 17p13.3. Mei et al[107] identified mutations in the *LIS1* gene in 20 (44%) of 45 patients with isolated lissencephaly. In 19 (76%) of 25 patients in whom FISH and direct sequencing had failed to detect mutations, multiplex ligation dependent probe amplification assay identified 18 small genomic deletions and 1 duplication.[107] Overall, small genomic deletions/duplications represented 49% of all *LIS1* alterations identified, and *LIS1* involvement was demonstrated in 39 (87%) of 45 patients. Cardoso et al[108] completed a physical and transcriptional map of the 17p13.3 region from LIS1 to the telomere. Using FISH, they mapped the deletion size in 19 children with isolated lissencephaly sequence (ILS), 11 children with MDS, and 4 children with 17p13.3 deletions not involving LIS1. They showed that the critical region that differentiates ILS from MDS at the molecular level can be reduced to 400 kB. Using somatic cell hybrids from selected patients, the authors identified eight genes that are consistently deleted in patients classified as having MDS.[108] In some reports, patients with large deletions and truncations of the *LIS1* mutations had diffuse or severe lissencephaly, whereas those with less severe *LIS1* mutations had posterior pachygyria only or posterior-predominant subcortical band heterotopia or even a normal brain MRI scan.[109] Others failed to find a similar correlation but instead found that the degree of severity correlates only with the degree of agyria and cortical thickening and with the standardized grading used currently in the interpretation of MRI.[110]

*DCX* mutations, located at Xq22.3, produce a deficiency in doublecortin, a protein essential in the formation of microtubules.[111] This X-linked lissencephaly results in males with lissencephaly of various grades of clinical severity, whereas affected females are clinically less affected, though they may have a double-cortex pattern or a normal MRI.

Aristaless-related homeobox protein (*ARX*) mutations are also located at Xq22 and result in lissencephaly with abnormal genitalia and anomalies of the corpus callosum (XLAG). In XLAG, the tangential neurons are affected. The severity of the malformation is determined by the size and the severity of the mutation. Conservative substitution in the homeo domain causes the Proud syndrome (X-linked mental retardation, callosal agenesis, and abnormal genitalia). Other mutations cause less severe phenotypes.[112]

*RELN* mutations cause lissencephaly with cerebellar hypoplasia. Reelin deficiency results in an abnormal stratification of the cortex with the first waves of neurons positioned in proximity to the pia surface. Abnormal migration in the cerebellum produces cerebellar hypoplasia. An autosomal recessive pattern of inheritance may be present in some of the affected families.[113]

## Pathology

In the classical form of lissencephaly, brain weight may be normal or low, and the brain has a "figure 9" shape with an open sylvian region because the frontal and temporal opercula fail to grow over the insula. However, variations in severity occur ranging from complete agyria to varying degrees of agyria and pachygyria. A morphological classification was developed to describe differences in severity of the gyral malformation. Lissencephaly grade 1 is complete agyria; grade 2 has widespread agyria with a few sulci restricted primarily to the frontal and temporal poles and basal frontal lobe; grade 3 has extensive areas of both agyria and pachygyria in which pachygyria is more common frontally and agyria posteriorly; and grade 4 has widespread pachygyria without areas of agyria[114] (Figure 7–18).

There are only a few reports of brain pathology in fetuses and newborns with lissencephaly/SBH spectrum, most with *LIS1* but also *XLIS.* A thick four-layer cortex is described composed of a superficial hypocellular "molecular" layer I, covering a cellular zone of heterotopic large pyramidal neurons in layer V and VI of normal cortex, often inverted; an underlying paucicellular layer; and a large rim of ectopic small neurons.[115] In another study that included 16 patients with lissencephaly type 1, the cortex was always thick, but the degree of involvement varied from patient to patient. The brains with *LIS1* mutations had the classic four-layer cortex, but patients with *DCX* and *ARX* mutations had different and distinct cytoarchitectural findings.[116]

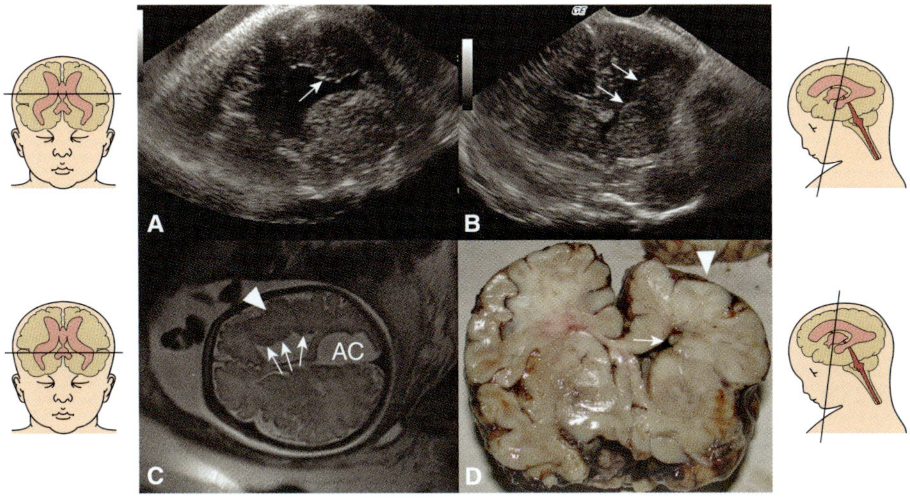


**Figure 7–18.** Focal unilateral parietal agyria with periventricular heterotopia in a fetus at 40 postmenstrual weeks referred for evaluation of a large interhemispheric arachnoid cyst. **(A)** Nonorthogonal view of the affected side shows irregular ventricular wall with abnormal brain tissue bulging into the ventricle (*arrow*). **(B)** Coronal view at the level of the third ventricle shows the irregular ventricular wall (*arrows*); note the lack of normal sulci on the affected side. **(C)** Axial MRI demonstrates the periventricular heterotopia (*arrow*), with the pachygyric overlying cortex (*arrowhead*) and the posterior interhemispheric arachnoid cyst (AC). **(D)** Macroscopic pathology confirms the presence of heterotopia (*arrow*) and pachygyria (*arrowhead*).

In brains with SBH, the outer cortex is normal with heterotopic, mainly pyramidal, neurons present in the deeper cortical layers and in the white matter.[117]

## Associated Anomalies

Children with lissencephaly have profound mental retardation. Isolated *LIS1* usually is not accompanied by any associated malformations.

In MDS the lissencephaly is always severe. Associated brain anomalies include dysgenesis of the corpus callosum and large cavum septi pellucidi. Some patients have an unusual midline calcification in the region of the corpus callosum or septum; the cerebellum is not affected.[114] Microcephaly is characteristically not present at birth but develops during the first year of life. Non-CNS changes include the face with prominent forehead, bitemporal hollowing, short nose with upturned nares, protuberant upper lip, thin vermilion border of the upper lip, and small jaw.[114] Some common findings amenable to prenatal diagnosis are cardiac malformations (20–25%), genital anomalies in males (70%), finger malformations (40–45%) (OMIM 247200) and Miller-Dieker lissencephaly syndrome (MDLS). Growth retardation and the presence of hydramnios have been retrospectively described in affected patients.

Patients with *RELN* mutations usually have severe cerebellar hypoplasia and may be differentiated from other types of lissencephaly by the prenatal development of microcephaly.

## Risk of Recurrence

In isolated *LIS1* and in 80% of the patients with MDS, the disease is caused by de novo mutations; thus, the recurrence risk is ~1%. Parental balanced chromosomal rearrangements and postzygotic mosaicism may be present in patients with MDS or *DCX-ARX*, respectively.

## Sonographic Diagnosis

The prenatal diagnosis of MDS may be possible, especially in patients known to be at risk of recurrence[118,119] or when a possible diagnosis is suspected during a US examination.[118,120,121] Diagnosis in low-risk patients depends on the recognition of abnormal sulcation patterns, but the differentiation between normal and abnormal sulcation may be difficult particularly during the second trimester[122–124] (Figure 7–19).

Saltzman et al[118] reported in 1991 the first two prenatal diagnoses of MDS. In one case, there was a prior child with lissencephaly, agenesis of the corpus callosum, right

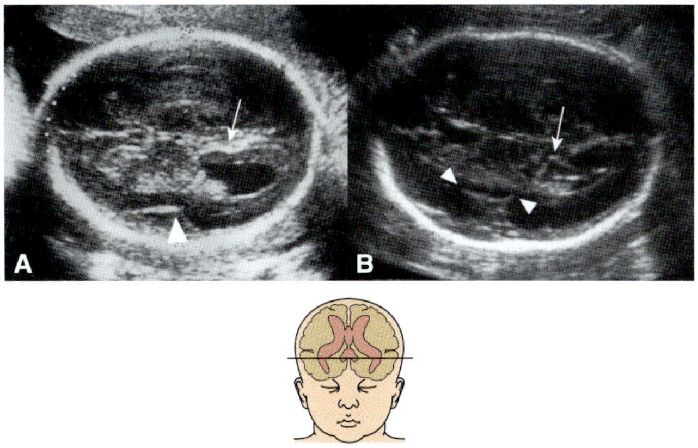


**Figure 7–19.** Abdominal transventricular axial planes in a fetus at 27 postmenstrual weeks with postnatal diagnosis of Miller-Dieker syndrome (MDS) **(A)** and in a normal fetus of the same gestational age **(B).** The arrows show the difference in shape between the parieto-occipital fissures and the well-developed temporal sulci forming the insula in **B,** and the shallow sylvian fissure resembling a fetus at 18 to 20 weeks' gestation in **A.** Note the borderline normal size of the lateral ventricle in the fetus with MDS.

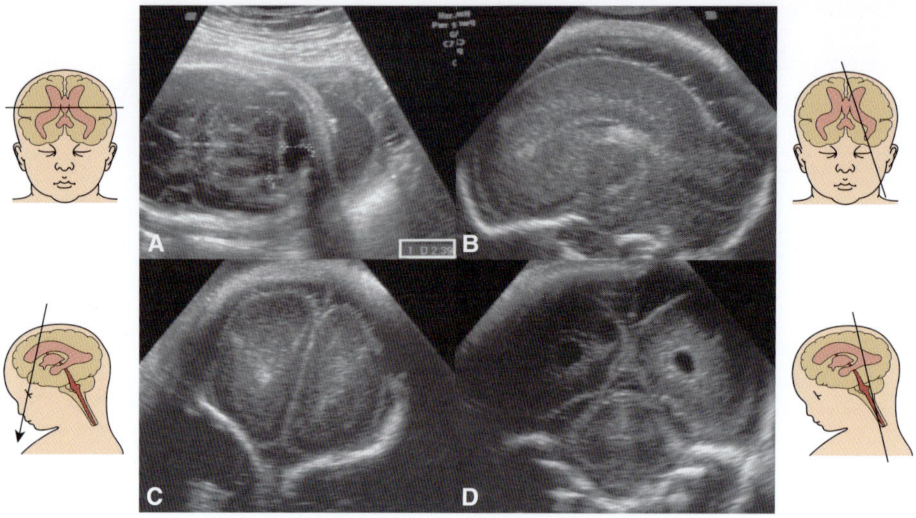


**Figure 7–20.** Lissencephaly with cerebellar hypoplasia at 28 postmenstrual weeks. **(A)** The transverse cerebellar diameter is well below the fifth percentile. Median **(B)** and coronal **(C, D)** planes showing the lack of sulcation. Note the abnormal shape and small size of the cerebellum **(D)**.

polycystic kidney, pulmonic stenosis, and a malrotated gut. The mother had a balanced translocation affecting chromosome 17p. The fetal karyotype was 46del(17)(13) mat. Hydramnios was present from 25 postmenstrual weeks, and a smooth cortical pattern was observed at 31 weeks' gestation. MDS was confirmed after delivery. The second patient diagnosed at 31 postmenstrual weeks had hydramnios, tetralogy of Fallot, and slightly small HC; the fetus was also slightly small for gestational age, and the sulci appeared smooth and underdeveloped. MDS was confirmed with fetal blood sampling.

The sonographic diagnosis of lissencephaly relies on the demonstration of an abnormal sulcation pattern. As shown in a retrospective study, fetuses with MDS had abnormal parieto-occipital and Sylvian fissures by the time of the second-trimester US examination.[120] The authors reported the ultrasonographic findings in a group of seven patients with postnatal cytogenetic diagnosis of lissencephaly associated with MDS; in six fetuses, mild ventriculomegaly was present at the time of the first US examination performed between 20 and 33 weeks' gestation, and a prenatal diagnosis of MCD was obtained in three fetuses with the additional use of MRI.[120]

During fetal life and even after termination of pregnancy, a specific diagnosis in these cases may be very difficult or even impossible without the use of molecular biology tests. In one of the first reports of MCD, Greco et al[125] reported a fetus with apparently isolated lissencephaly that was studied using prenatal US and prenatal and postnatal MRI, but when reviewing the images, the findings are more characteristic of hemimegalencephaly than of lissencephaly. In our experience, we were not able, even following autopsy, to reach a specific definitive diagnosis in the majority of our 23 patients with MCD.[77]

Sulcal development should be assessed in any fetus with mild ventricular enlargement as that may be the initial indicator of disruptions of cortical development. Failure to visualize normal sylvian and parieto-occipital fissures starting from 24 postmenstrual weeks should raise suspicion and prompt a detailed neurosonographic examination of the brain (Figure 7–19).

The detection of associated anomalies, particularly agenesis of corpus callosum (ACC), vermian hypoplasia, and abnormal male genitalia, helps in confirming suspicions (Figures 7–4 and 7–20).

## MRI Diagnosis

In adults and children, MRI is the method of choice for the detection of all MCD, specifically for the detection of lissencephaly. This is probably also true in the fetus, but interpretation should be by individuals experienced in fetal neurologic imaging with MRI and familiar with fetal brain development.

In reported cases, the patients were usually referred for brain MRI due to the visualization of ventriculomegaly or abnormal sulcation. MRI clearly depicts the smooth abnormal brain surface with abnormal operculization and thick cortex (Figure 7–21). Associated anomalies including dysgenesis of the corpus callosum, and abnormal cerebellum and brainstem are also clearly visualized.[19,120,126]

### Implications for Sonographic Screening, Including Earliest Recognition

As demonstrated by Toi et al,[124] the visualization of the parieto-occipital and sylvian fissures during the second-trimester US examination is feasible and potentially effective as a screening method to diagnose lissencephaly. The effectiveness of such an approach remains to be determined in the screening of a low-risk population.

### Implications for Targeted Examination

The diagnosis of lissencephaly should be possible when performing a targeted examination, but it may depend

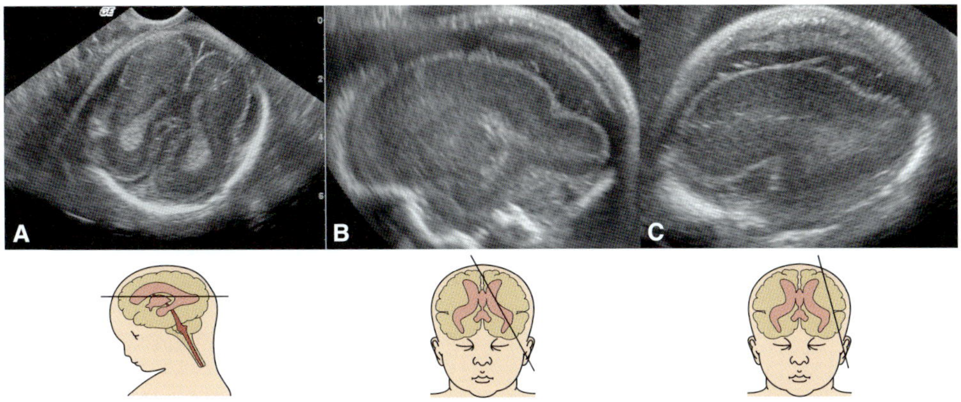


**Figure 7–21.** Autosomal recessive lissencephaly at 22 **(A, B)** and 25 **(C, D)** postmenstrual weeks of gestation. Two previous children were born with agyria and multiple malformations. At 22 weeks of gestation, the sylvian fissure is absent, and the shape of the brain is abnormal, but only at 25 weeks is the abnormal sulcation evident.

on the choice of the correct timing and on the severity of the disease and requires familiarity with normal brain and sulcal appearances at different gestational ages (see Chapter 2).

In suspicious cases it is helpful to compare the obtained images with these of a known normal fetus of a similar gestational age at the same plane[122–124] (Figure 7–19). Even in patients at risk due to a history of pachygyria/agyria in two previous pregnancies, we have found it extremely difficult to reach a decision before 24 to 25 weeks of pregnancy[77] (Figure 7–22).

Detailed neurosonographic evaluation and follow-up repeated examinations during the third trimester should be considered in patients with non-CNS anomalies and/or hydramnios in association with mild ventriculomegaly,[127] and there should be consideration for MRI examination in a center with fetal CNS MRI experience.

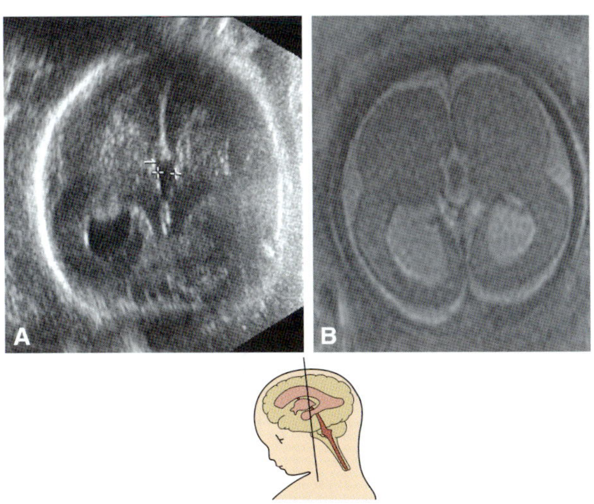


**Figure 7–22.** Lissencephaly at 33 postmenstrual weeks. Transabdominal US **(A)** and MRI **(B)** axial planes show the lack of sulcation colpocephaly with thick cortex and mild ventriculomegaly. Note the "figure eight" configuration in the MRI.

## Prognosis

Most patients exhibit moderate to severe developmental delay and neuromotor impairment. Isolated type I lissencephaly is characterized by profound mental retardation and seizures that are often intractable. Patients with MDS are the most severely affected and they usually die during the first years of life.

X-linked lissencephaly and XLAG in males have a similar prognosis. Females with SBH may present with epilepsy, developing during the second and third decades; some of them may be asymptomatic with normal MRI.

## Obstetric Management

In cases with a prenatal diagnosis, termination of pregnancy should be considered.

# Cobblestone Complex Syndromes

## Synonyms

Lissencephaly type II, α-dystroglycanopathies, Walker-Warburg syndrome (WWS), Chemke syndrome, hydrocephaly-agyria-retinal dysplasia +/– encephalocele (HARD-E) syndrome, congenital muscular dystrophy (CMD).

## Definition

The cobblestone complex syndromes (CCS) are characterized by abnormal migration of the neurons through the pia and into the meninges (overmigration) resulting in the "cobblestone" appearance of the cortex. The cellular layers of the cortex do not develop normally and heterotopic tissue is found between the white matter and the pia.

In this chapter, we will refer to the most common CCS, the Walker-Warburg syndrome (WWS), which is the most severe phenotypic manifestation of cobblestone cortex. Other syndromes associated with cobblestone lissencephaly are Fukuyama congenital muscular dystrophy and muscle-eye-brain disease.

## Incidence/Prevalence

WWS is a rare disease with a worldwide distribution; however, the overall incidence is unknown.[128] A survey in northeastern Italy reported an incidence rate of 1.2 per 100,000 live births.[129] One study has shown that 0.7% of the Ashkenazi Jews in Israel are carriers of a similar mutation at the Fukuyama congenital muscular dystrophy (FCMD) locus.[130]

## Pathogenesis

In these patients, normal neuronal migration is not stopped at the pial surface of the brain and overmigrates and invades the subarachnoid space, where surface brain vessels are enveloped. This results in a brain surface that is predominantly smooth with very subtle nodularity (called cobblestone cortex) and the characteristic finding of vessels that are partly buried in the brain surface.

At a molecular level, the data strongly support the hypothesis that defects in dystroglycan are central of structural and functional brain abnormalities seen in CMD.[130] A transmembrane glycoprotein, α-dystroglycan, interacts with several extracellular matrix components in the basal membrane, and disruption of its function is thought to underlie the severe defects in different tissues, including muscle, eye, and brain development in WWS patients.[131]

In mice, brain-selective deletion of dystroglycan is sufficient to cause CMD-like brain malformations, including disarray of cerebral cortical layering, fusion of cerebral hemispheres and cerebellar folia, and aberrant migration of granule cells. Additionally, high-affinity binding to laminin is lost, and there are discontinuities in the pial surface basal lamina (glia limitans) that probably underlie the neuronal migration errors.[132]

## Etiology

WWS is a genetically heterogeneous autosomal recessive disease characterized by congenital muscular dystrophy, cobblestone lissencephaly, and ocular malformations. Mutations in six genes involved in the glycosylation of α-dystroglycan (*POMT1, POMT2, POMGNT1, FCMD, FKRP,* and *LARGE*) have been identified in WWS patients, but these α-dystroglycanopathy genes are associated with extremely variable phenotypes ranging from mild CMD to WWS.

In a study of 43 WWS patients, Manzini et al[130] found that 40% of them had mutations of *POMT1, POMT2, FCMD,* and *FKRP.* In a population-based study that included all the Italian patients with CMD, homozygous and compound heterozygous mutations were detected in a total of 43 of 81 patients (53%) and included 7 novel variants. Mutations in *POMT1* were the most prevalent in this cohort (21%), followed by *POMT2* (11%), *POMGnT1* (10%), and *FKRP* (9%). One patient carried two heterozygous mutations in fukutin, and one harbored a new homozygous variant in *LARGE.*[133]

## Pathology

The macroscopic hallmark of the brain in WWS is the presence of lissencephaly with a very fine, "pebbly" surface with partly buried cerebral surface vessels in association with ventriculomegaly, thick meninges, and cerebellar anomalies.

The pathognomonic feature of cobblestone lissencephaly is represented by pial barrier disruption with neuronal and glial migration into the leptomeninges (Figure 7–23). This finding was observed as early as 18 to 20 weeks.[134] Cerebral and cerebellar cortical disorganization occur in parallel with pial barrier disruption.[135] At 34 weeks, the border between meningeal and neural structures becomes harder to discern; the leptomeninges are invaded by ectopic neuroglial cells and appear richly cellular; in addition, they become highly vascularized.[135]

Muscular and retinal involvements are also common in these patients (Figure 7–23).

## Associated Anomalies

According to Dobyns et al,[136] patients with WWS consistently present with cobblestone lissencephaly, pontocerebellar and retinal malformations, and CMD. CNS anomalies including ventricular dilation with or without hydrocephaly, macrocephaly, Dandy-Walker malformation, and cephaloceles are also relatively common. Non-CNS anomalies include anterior chamber malformations, microphthalmia, ocular colobomas, congenital cataracts, cleft lip and palate, and genital anomalies in males.[136] In a study on a cohort of patients with "dystroglycanopathies," Clement and colleagues[137] found that 8 out of 27 patients had no or minimal brain involvement on MRI studies, 4 patients had only cerebellar involvement, and 15 had different kinds of MCD. Only 2 had WSS, but 23 had abnormal cognitive development. This combination of findings with WWS has been described under the acronym HARD +/− E (hydrocephaly, agyria, retinal dysplasia +/− encephalocele).

## Risk of Recurrence

WWS is an autosomal recessive disease with a 25% risk of recurrence in families with an affected sibling.

## Sonographic Diagnosis

Prenatal diagnosis of WWS has been reported in families at risk.[138,139] Crowe et al[138] reported the first prenatal diagnosis in 1985, following the postnatal diagnosis in a sibling with hydrocephaly, bilateral microphthalmia, severe developmental retardation, and multiple brain anomalies. The affected fetus was diagnosed at 15 postmenstrual weeks because of the presence of a cephalocele.

Farrell et al[140] described the presence of hydrocephaly, encephalocele, abnormal vermis, and retinal detachment in a fetus from a nonconsanguinous pregnancy with recurrence in a second pregnancy. The same group reported another case diagnosed at 37 postmenstrual weeks with severe asymmetric hydrocephaly and signs of retinal detachment.[141]

Monteagudo et al[142] reported on the CNS findings in a patient referred at 34 postmenstrual weeks because of ventriculomegaly; the patient was studied using TVS, thus

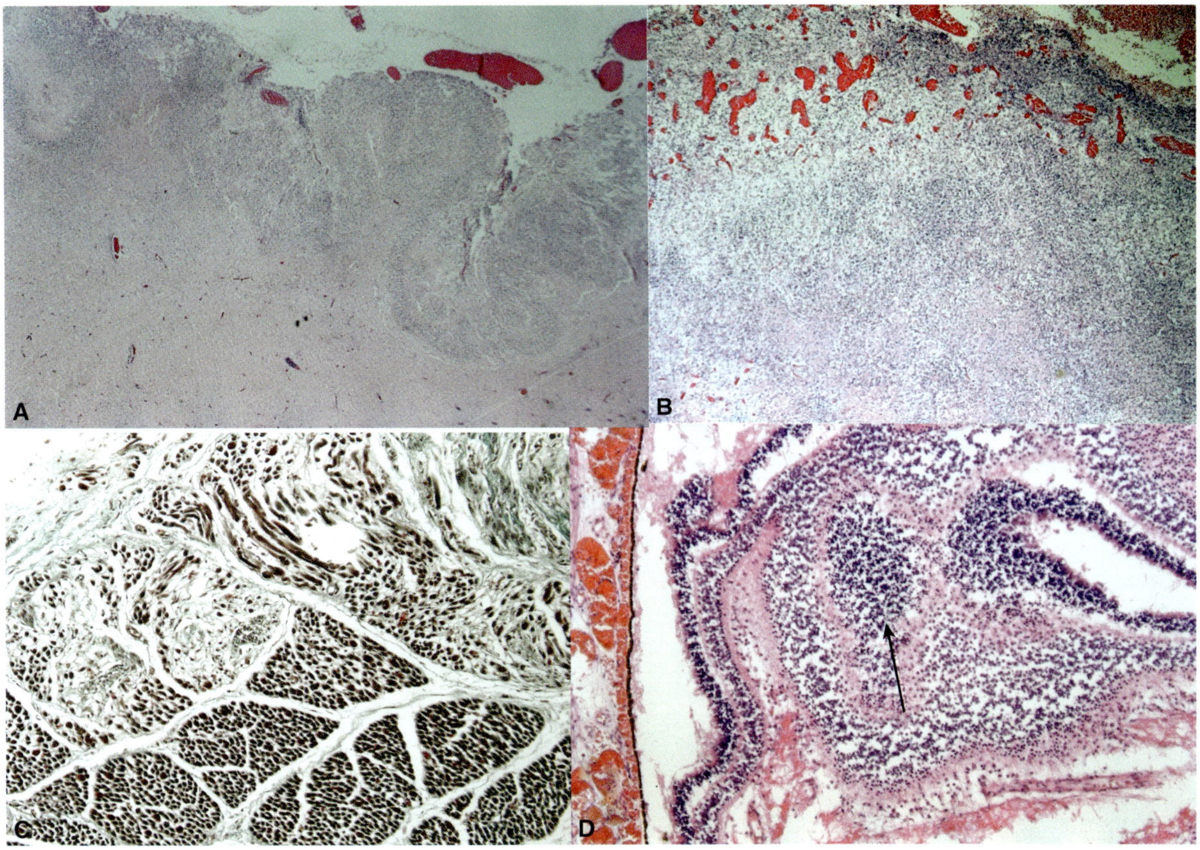


**Figure 7–23.** Microscopic findings in a fetus at 24 postmenstrual weeks with cobblestone complex syndrome. **(A)** Low magnification slide of the brain showing the unlayered cortex with neuronal invasion beneath the pia mater. **(B)** Neuronal invasion produces thickening of the meninges; the granular layer is absent. **(C)** Muscular involvement. Note the different sizes of the muscular fibers. **(D)** Retinal dysplasia (*arrow*). (Courtesy of Dr. Deborah Kidron, Kfar Saba, Israel.)

revealing for the first time the abnormal sulcation characteristic of WWS in conjunction with the presence of a cephalocele, vermian agenesis, micrognathia, and left eye cataract (Figure 7–24). The presence of abnormal sulcation may be demonstrated in patients with suspected WWS during the third trimester but in recurrent cases the early detection of ventriculomegaly or any other sign of CNS or eye anomaly should suffice to establish the diagnosis[143,144] (Figure 7–25). In low-risk patients, the same association should raise the suspicion of CCS (Figure 7–26).

In our published series of 23 patients with MCD, we suspected the presence of WWS in 1 patient without postnatal confirmation, and another patient with prenatal diagnosis of lissencephaly was found at necropsy to have WWS.[77]

## MRI Diagnosis

The prenatal diagnosis of WWS using MRI has been described several times[145,146] (Figure 7–27). Garel[19] believed the main asset of this MRI is its ability to analyze the posterior fossa and gyration that are not clearly visible in sonography. But a critical review of the cited papers is far from convincing regarding the prenatal demonstration of cobblestone lissencephaly. In one of the few articles that compare US and MRI in a fetus with WWS diagnosed at 20 weeks, the median images are quite similar, demonstrating the striking brainstem kinking, severe cerebellar and vermian dysgenesis associated with ocular changes, and small encephalocele. Brainstem kinking or Z malformation represents abnormal persistence of the normal mesencephalic folding that is present in normal fetuses in the first trimester. The folding normally straightens out by about 12 to 13 postmenstrual weeks. Kinking can be demonstrated by 3D US but can be difficult to show on 2D scans. Its persistence implies a severe disruption of brain development and failure of corticospinal tract development dating from the middle of the first trimester.[147] Strigini et al[148] reported a case with a homozygous mutation in the *POMT1* gene. US at 26 weeks showed ventriculomegaly with an abnormal cerebellum; MRI added information regarding the presence of a kinked brainstem and bifid pons. US at 31 weeks showed retinal nonattachment.

Even with the use of MRI a definitive diagnosis of WWS may be impossible, particularly during the second trimester, due to difficulties in the pathologic diagnosis of CMD and eye malformations at this early stage.[149] In highly suspicious cases, a search for putative WWS genes may help.[148]

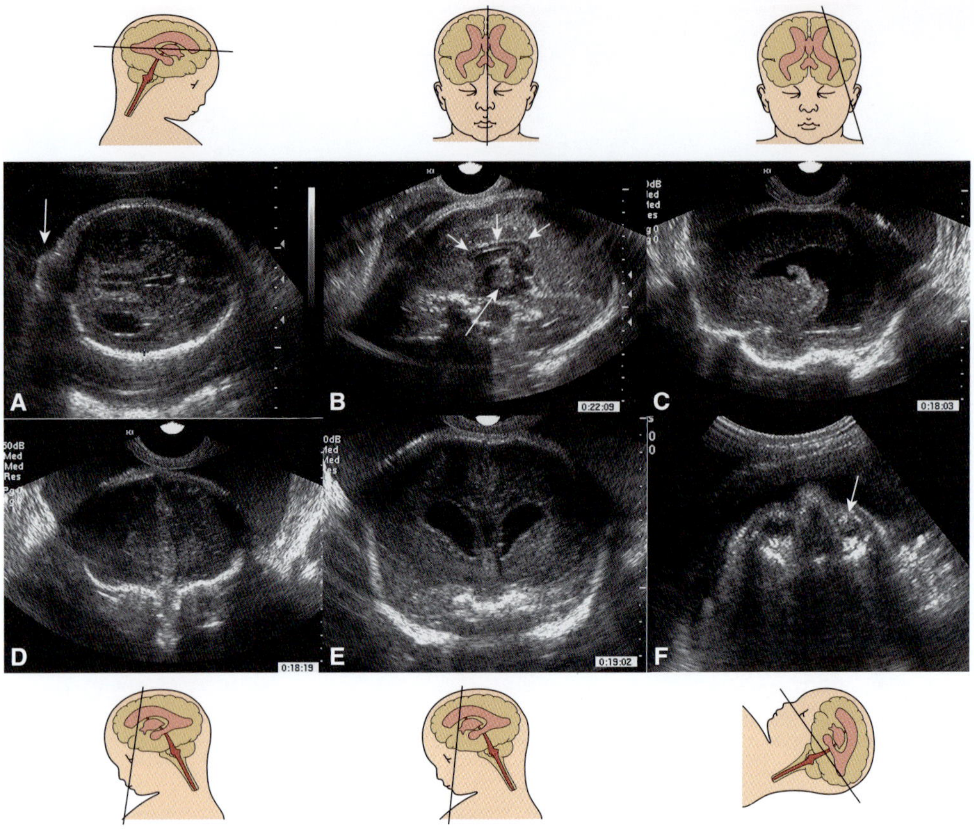

**Figure 7–24.** Walker-Warburg syndrome (WWS) in a fetus at 34 postmenstrual weeks referred because of ventriculomegaly. **(A)** Transabdominal axial plane shows the presence of a small occipital encephalocele (*arrow*). Note the apparently normal size of the distal lateral ventricle and the lack of sulcation on the same side. **(B)** Transvaginal median plane shows dysgenesis of the corpus callosum. The corpus callosum is shorter than usual, and the genu and splenium are poorly developed (*small arrows*). Note the clear visualization of the intrathalamic adhesion due to dilation of the third ventricle (*large arrow*). **(C)** Paramedian plane shows lateral ventricle dilation and lissencephalic cortex. **(D)** Frontal coronal plane shows almost a complete lack of sulcation. **(E)** Transcaudate coronal plane shows the dilated lateral ventricles and no sulci and gyri. **(F)** Left eye cataract (*arrow*). (With permission from Monteagudo A, 2001.[142])

### Implications for Screening, Including Time of Earliest Recognition

WWS is a rare disease, and in the majority of cases, the diagnosis will be possible only after delivery or in families at risk. During routine second- and third-trimester examinations, the first sign of the disease usually will be moderate to severe ventriculomegaly with or without associated anomalies. All patients with ventriculomegaly should be specifically scanned for the presence of cephalocele, cerebellar, and brainstem anomalies and dysmorphology signs, with particular attention to the eyes.

The presence of ventriculomegaly with abnormal brain and echogenic lenses may be present as early as 15 postmenstrual weeks (Figure 7–26). However, because of its rarity, WWS may remain undiagnosed in fetuses with ventriculomegaly until after delivery.[150]

### Implications for Targeted Examination

In families at risk, the presence of any brain or eye anomaly should be enough to reach a diagnosis. These findings may present as early as 12 to 14 postmenstrual weeks.[143,144] As previously mentioned, fetuses with ventriculomegaly must undergo a detailed multiplanar neurosonographic examination with particular emphasis in the depiction of the median plane for demonstration of the brainstem and the vermis (see Chapter 2). MRI may be helpful in patients in whom an optimal US evaluation is not possible[19,148] (Figure 7–27).

## Prognosis

Babies born with WWS have very poor tone (floppy baby) due to the associated abnormal muscle development. Muscle biopsy and molecular gene analysis can help with diagnosis. The condition is usually lethal within the first few months of life, with almost all children dying by the age of 3 years.[128]

## Obstetric Management

Following the prenatal diagnosis of WWS, termination of pregnancy should be considered.

# NEURONAL HETEROTOPIA

## Synonyms

Heterotopic gray matter, heterotopia

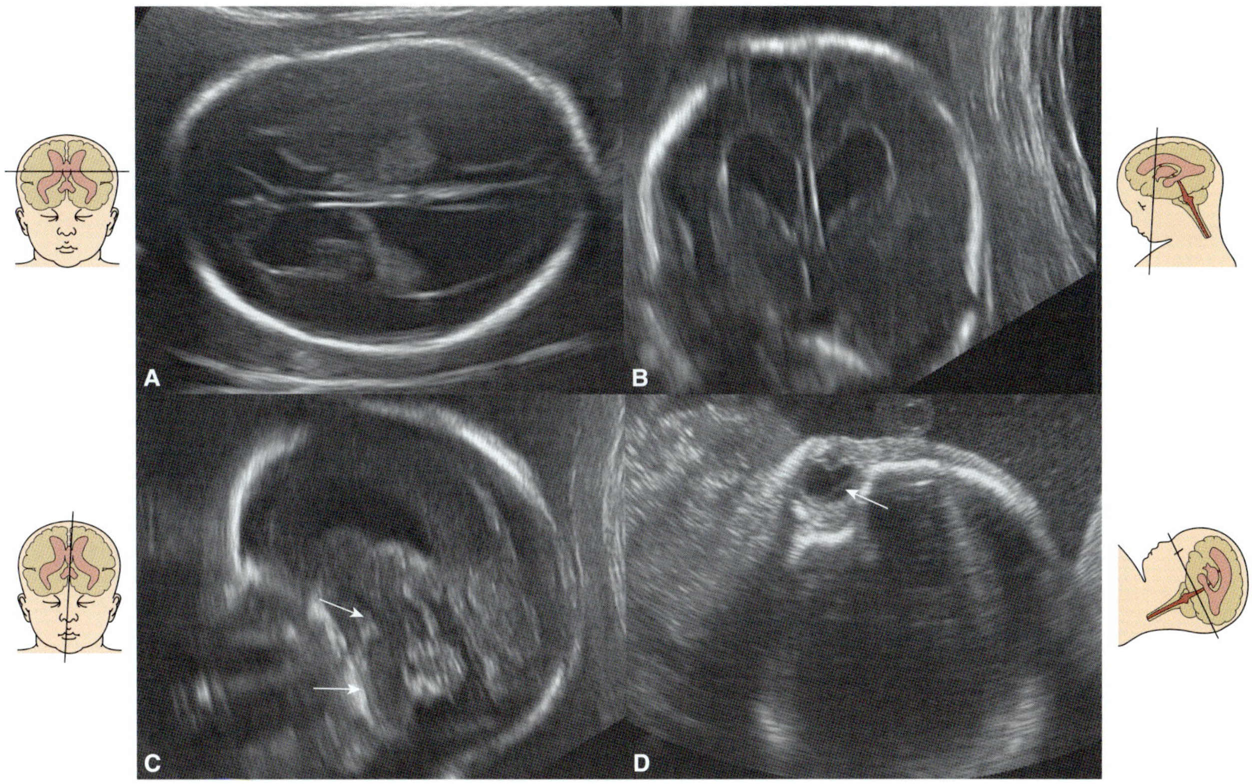


**Figure 7–25.** Neurosonographic transabdominal examination at 21 postmenstrual weeks consistent with recurrent WWS. In the previous pregnancy, a fetus with suspected WWS was diagnosed at 26 weeks of pregnancy. **(A)** Axial transventricular plane shows mild ventricular dilation (12.6 mm). **(B)** Coronal plane through the frontal horns shows dilation. **(C)** Median plane shows the abnormal shape of the kinked brainstem and lack of the anterior protuberance of the pons (*arrows*). **(D)** The presence of retinal detachment is confirmatory of the diagnosis (*arrow*).

## Definition

Neuronal heterotopia is characterized by the presence of clusters of neurons in any abnormal location in their pathway of migration from the periventricular germinal matrix to the cortex (Figure 7–28). In periventricular nodular heterotopia (PNH), neurons remain in the subependymal region of the ventricle, where they appear as a nodule at the surface of the ventricle. In nodular subcortical heterotopia, neuronal groups of neurons are located in the white matter. Subcortical band heterotopia results in the double cortex syndrome discussed under lissencephaly.

## Incidence/Prevalence

Clinically significant heterotopia is extremely rare; however, affected children may have epilepsy, variable intellectual

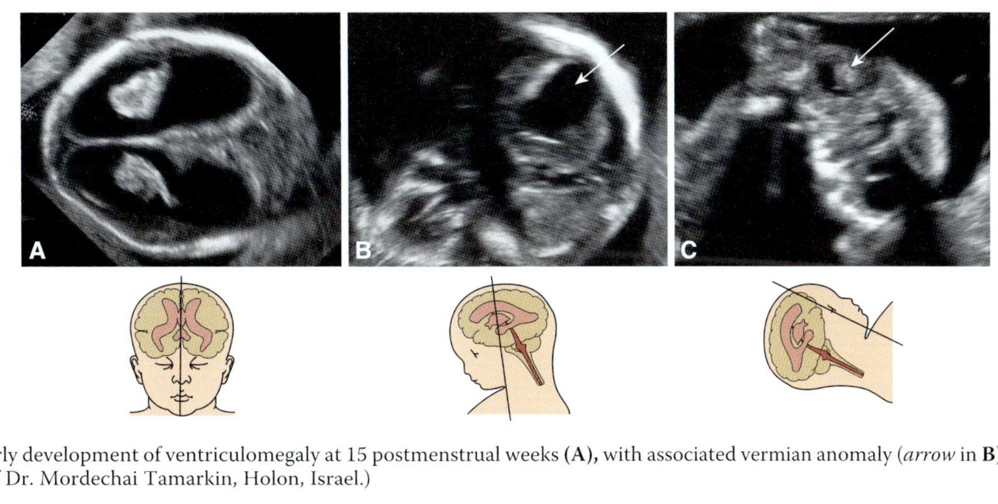


**Figure 7–26.** Early development of ventriculomegaly at 15 postmenstrual weeks **(A),** with associated vermian anomaly (*arrow* in **B**) and cataract (*arrow* in **C**). (Courtesy of Dr. Mordechai Tamarkin, Holon, Israel.)

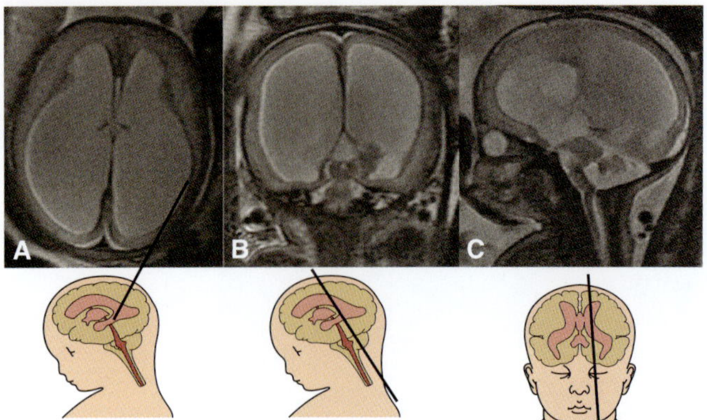


**Figure 7–27.** MRI at 34 postmenstrual weeks of a fetus with WWS. Axial **(A)** and coronal **(B)** sections show severe ventriculomegaly with thin lissencephalic cortex and dysplastic cerebellum. **(C)** Sagittal plane shows the characteristic Z shape of the brainstem and vermian dysgenesis. (Courtesy of Dr. Chen Hoffmann, Tel-Hashomer, Israel.)

deficits, other malformations, and genetic abnormalities or develop normally.[3] There are no data regarding its incidence or prevalence. Periventricular nodular heterotopia may be detected prenatally.

## Pathogenesis

PNH is mainly caused by defects of the Filamin A (*FLNA*) gene. The specific roles of Filamin A and its association with pathologic conditions are still to be fully understood.[151] Filamin homologues are implicated in the regulation of cell stability, protrusion, and motility across various biological systems.[152] *FLNA* likely influences neuroblast migration during cortical development in vertebrates, and heterotopia in humans likely results from disruption of this process.[153]

## Etiology

Periventricular heterotopia is a heterogeneous disease with 15 described phenotypes. Bilateral PNH is the most common subtype and was identified in a large series in 54% (98 of 182) of the patients.[154] Bilateral PNH is an X-linked dominant disorder far more frequent in females who present normal intelligence to borderline mental retardation, epilepsy of variable severity, and cardiovascular defects or coagulopathy. The disorder is generally associated with prenatal lethality in males, although a few cases of males with X-linked PNH due to germline and mosaic mutations have been reported.[154] X-linked PNH has been demonstrated to be associated with mutations in the Filamin A gene (*FLN1, FLNA,* or *ABP-280*). *FLN1* maps to Xq28 and codes for Filamin A, which binds to actin and a wide range of cytoplasmic signaling proteins. Additional phenotypes include PNH with Ehlers-Danlos syndrome (EDS), temporo-occipital PNH with hippocampal malformation and cerebellar hypoplasia, PNH with frontoperisylvian or temporo-occipital polymicrogyria, posterior PNH with hydrocephaly, PNH with microcephaly (autosomal recessive due to mutations of the *ARFGEF2* gene), PNH with frontonasal dysplasia, PNH with limb abnormalities, PNH with fragile X syndrome, PNH with ambiguous genitalia, micronodular PH, unilateral PNH, and laminar ribbonlike and linear PH.[154]

PNH has also been reported in a few patients with a chromosomal rearrangements in 5p15.1 and in 5p15.33[155] and as autosomal dominant disease affecting a father and his son.[156]

## Pathology

The data regarding the neuropathologic findings in patients with heterotopia are limited. In the largest published series (24 patients), Meroni et al[157] described two different groups of pathologies in nodular heterotopia. Patients in group 1 had clusters with large numbers of normal neurons in the white matter, suggesting the existence of a possible mechanism of neuroblast overproliferation. The overlying cortex was dysplastic but of normal thickness, suggesting that the neurons are overproduced during corticogenesis.[157] The nodules observed in group 2 patients were smaller than those observed in group 1, were always detected just below the gray matter, and were associated with cortical alterations that were particularly evident in the granular and supragranular layers. This suggests that the impaired neuronal migration occurred during the late phases of corticogenesis, in accordance with the inside-out mechanisms of cortical development.[157]

In a study of the prenatal diagnosis of MCD, Malinger et al[77] found that 12 out of 17 fetuses that underwent necropsy demonstrated heterotopia of different types and grades of severity, including 2 patients with cerebellar white matter heterotopia (Figure 7–28).

## Associated Anomalies

In female fetuses, PNH may be isolated and diagnosed incidentally or after the delivery of an affected child. Other described phenotypes may present with microcephaly, polymicrogyria, cerebellar hypoplasia, and ventriculomegaly.[151] Probably heterotopia is more frequent than previously recognized in fetuses with multiple congenital anomalies involving the CNS. In our series we found heterotopia to be associated with agenesis of the corpus callosum, lissencephaly, and cobblestone complex syndromes.[77]

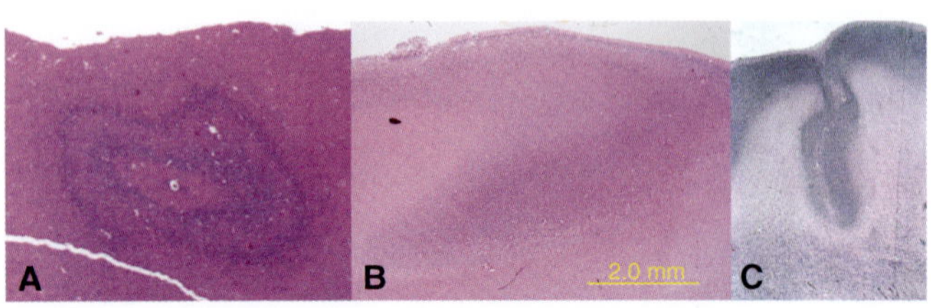


**Figure 7–28.** Microscopic findings in three different patients with heterotopia. **(A)** Cortical heterotopia. **(B)** White matter laminar heterotopia. **(C)** White matter nodular heterotopia.

Non-CNS anomalies include aortic valvulopathy, patent ductus arteriosus, aortic aneurism, frontonasal dysplasia, limb abnormalities, and ambiguous genitalia.[151] Mental retardation and epilepsy are common in these patients.

## Risk of Recurrence

Genetic counseling is straightforward in familial cases with a clear X-linked pattern of inheritance. The family should be informed regarding prenatal or early lethality in boys and a 50% recurrence risk in daughters. Although maternal transmission is much more likely, father-to-daughter transmission is possible, implying that either parent can transmit the mutation to a female proband. An affected man with PNH caused by an *FLN1* mutation would be expected to transmit the mutation to all his daughters, unless somatic mosaicism is present. If neither of the parents has epilepsy or cognitive impairment, the proband's mother should be studied first, in order to confirm the mutation or the brain abnormality. If the mother is negative, and the proband is a female, the father should also be studied, as germline and mosaic mutations have been reported.[154] In autosomal recessive cases, the risk of recurrence is 25%.

## Sonographic Diagnosis

The US prenatal diagnosis of PNH should be considered when the lateral ventricle wall is variably irregular with indentations of the periventricular heterotopic nodules (Figure 7–18). In cases where ventricle size is normal, it can be difficult to detect the nodularity. We have found a very small number of prenatal diagnosed cases, and all of them presented with associated anomalies. Mitchell et al[158] reported a female fetus referred for evaluation at 23 postmenstrual weeks for suspected Dandy-Walker malformation. Their US examination demonstrated the presence of a megacisterna magna and bilateral periventricular nodules consistent with heterotopia. The diagnosis was confirmed by pre- and postnatal MRI. Garel[19] described a patient with progressive ventriculomegaly initially detected at 22 weeks of gestation; at 30 weeks an irregular, "bumpy" ventricular wall raised the suspicion of PNH, which was confirmed by MRI. We reported on two patients with abnormal irregular lateral ventricle walls with associated malformations.[77] One patient was referred at 40 postmenstrual weeks because of a large interhemispheric arachnoid cyst, and a transvaginal examination showed the presence of focal abnormally wide gyri, atypical asymmetric lateral ventricles, and bulging of brain tissue into the lateral ventricle, confirmed by MRI (Figure 7–18). The second patient, referred at 22 postmenstrual weeks because of ACC, showed a unilateral irregular lateral ventricle wall with echogenic foci in the periventricular area. In both cases the diagnosis was confirmed at necropsy. Others have also reported finding PNH at neurosonography and confirmed by MRI during evaluation of fetuses with cerebral malformations, especially agenesis of the corpus callosum.[159] Heterotopia may not be recognized when the nodules are small or subcortical. The differential diagnosis includes tumors (especially tuberous sclerosis), hemorrhagic masses, and ventricular irregularity associated with infections such as cytomegalovirus. In some cases a definitive diagnosis will not be possible even after biopsy.[160] We studied two patients with asymmetric ventriculomegaly and hyperechogenic cortex who were postnatally diagnosed as suffering from nodular heterotopia; one of them developed epilepsy by the age of 8 months, but the definitive diagnosis was reached only at the age of 5 years[161] (Figure 7–29).

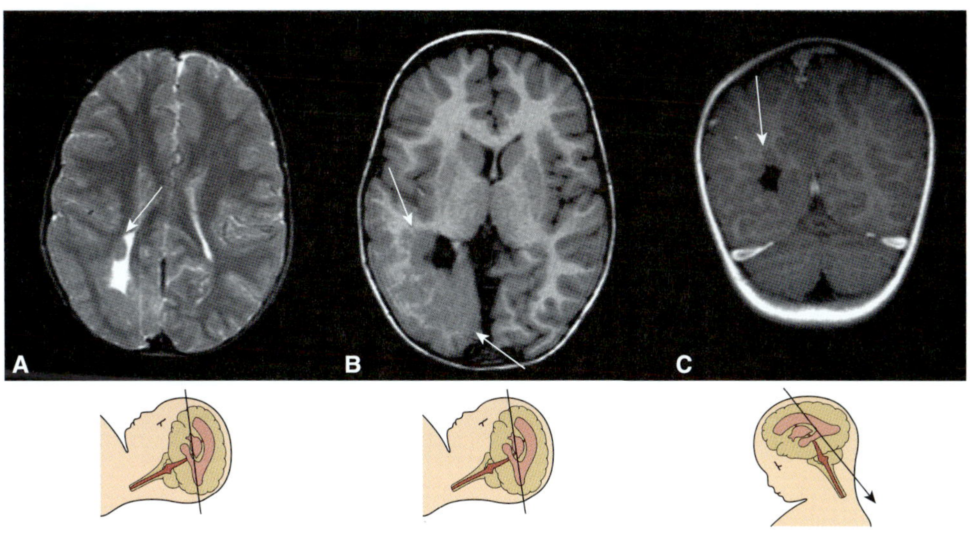


**Figure 7–29.** Periventricular nodular heterotopia initially evaluated due to fetal asymmetric ventriculomegaly and suspected white matter echogenicity. The girl developed complex partial seizures by the age of 2 years. The MRI was performed at the age of 5 years following the first episode of generalized seizures.T2 axial **(A)**, T1 axial **(B)**, and T1 coronal **(C)** images demonstrate periventricular heterotopia surrounding and protruding into the occipital horn and associated abnormal overlying cortex.

## MRI Diagnosis

Fetal MRI was used to confirm US diagnosis in three of the fetuses previously mentioned.[19,77,158] In other reported cases, an MRI diagnosis of PNH was obtained in patients referred for suspected CNS anomalies, including ventriculomegaly,[162] mega cisterna magna,[163] and thick corpus callosum.[164]

### Implications for Screening, Including Time of Earliest Recognition

According to isolated case reports, PNH may be diagnosed as early as 22 postmenstrual weeks, but most cases, especially if isolated, will remain undiagnosed during pregnancy.

### Implications for Targeted Examination

Visualization of the smoothness of the walls of the lateral ventricles and the periventricular zone is an integral part of the detailed neurosonographic examination. Axial planes alone may fail to depict subtle nodules, and we prefer to obtain coronal and parasagittal images of both ventricles (Figure 7–30).

Tuberous sclerosis (TS), periventricular hemorrhage (PVH), and irregularity associated with infections should be considered in the differential diagnosis. TS is usually associated with the visualization of intracardial rhabdomyomas, and the nodules are not only periventricular.[77] PVH occurs mainly around or at the caudate nuclei; the lesions evolve with time and are frequently associated with intraventricular bleeding and clots. In some cases, MRI with expert interpretation can be of help, along with evaluation of the remaining members of the family for subtle signs of TS.

## Prognosis

In families at risk, the identification of PNH is difficult to counsel due to the wide phenotypic and functional variations of the disease. Bilateral PNH in males is almost invariable lethal.

## Obstetric Management

Multispecialty counseling may be helpful, but limitations in the establishment of a prognosis make decisions difficult.

# Schizencephaly

## Synonyms

None

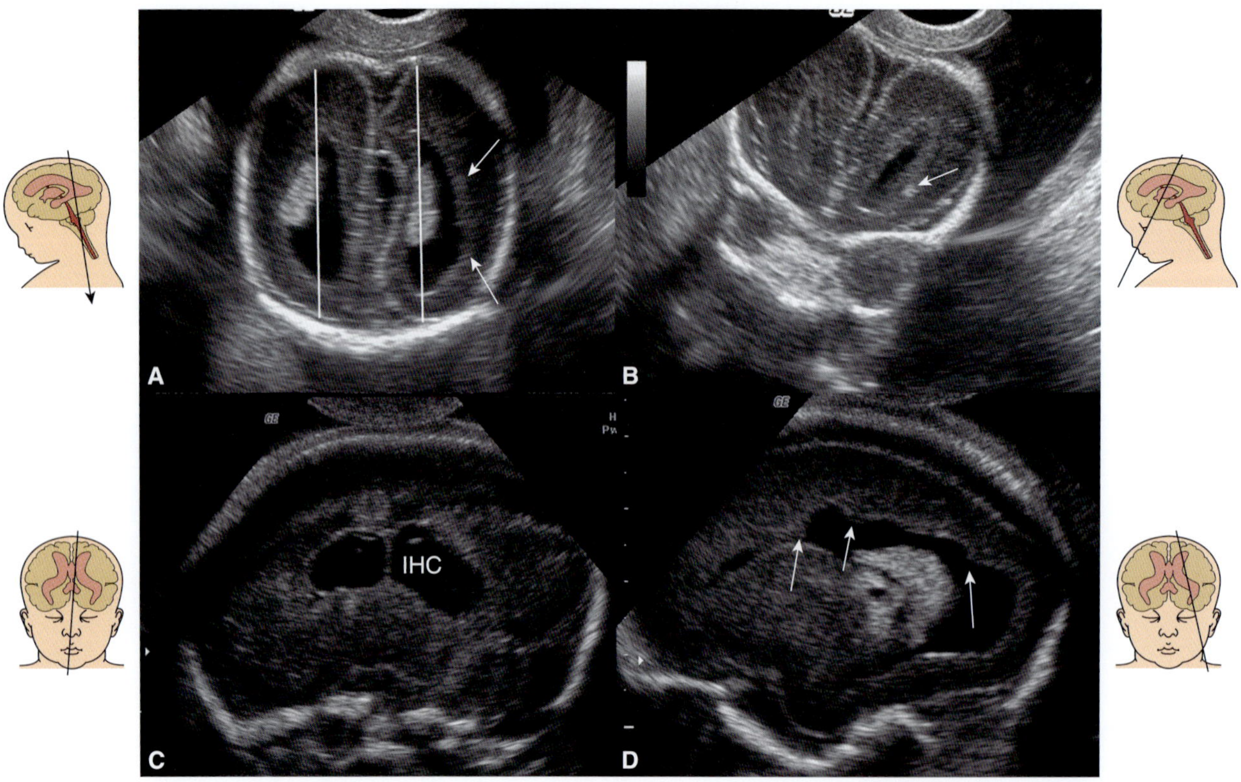


**Figure 7–30.** Histologically confirmed periventricular nodular heterotopia with agenesis of the corpus callosum in a female fetus at 22 postmenstrual weeks of gestation. Transvaginal technique. **(A)** Modified axial plane shows parallel colpocephalic lateral ventricles. Note the increase in echogenicity at the periventricular zone (*arrows*). **(B)** Frontal coronal plane shows a single hyperechogenic nodule. **(C)** Median plane fails to show the corpus callosum that has been replaced by large intrahemispheric cysts (IHC). **(D)** Paramedian plane at the level of the lateral ventricle shows the irregular ventricular wall with nodules protruding into the ventricle (*arrows*).

## Definition

Schizencephaly is a cerebral disorder characterized by the presence of a cleft of the cerebrum lined by abnormal gray matter and connecting the meningeal surface with the lateral ventricle (see Chapter 10). In closed-lip or type I schizencephaly, the walls of the defect are in contact, and a gray matter column is visible traversing the white matter between the cortex and ventricle, often with a dimple at the ventricle surface, but there is no communication between the ventricles and the subarachnoid space. Open-lip or type II schizencephaly refers to a wide open defect in which the gray matter–lined lips of the cleft are separated, allowing communication.[165]

## Incidence/Prevalence

In a population-based study of affected patients diagnosed before 1 year of age, Curry et al[166] reported a prevalence of 1.54 per 100,000. In about two-thirds of the patients the disease was isolated, and the remaining one-third had associated anomalies. In a pediatric population with MCD, only 5% had schizencephaly.[167]

## Pathogenesis

The developmental mechanism of schizencephaly is still not clear. The observed structural changes have been assumed to be a true malformation of cortical development by some authors;[168] however, similar lesions can result from arterial or venous circulatory disturbances, infections, or even maternal trauma. In any case, schizencephaly results from an early arrest of growth of parts of the hemispheric wall with quantitatively (if not qualitatively) normal growth or even overgrowth of the spared tissue occurring before or close after migration starts.[169] The possibility of a disruptive process in some of the patients is highlighted by the fact that in over half of the patients with a non-CNS abnormality, it was found to be secondary to vascular disruption.[166]

Barkovich et al[3] classified schizencephaly and polymicrogyria under the polymicrogyria/schizencephaly complex, as they are frequently observed together.[3]

It has been postulated that in some patients, schizencephaly may be the result of a mutation in the homeobox 2 gene (*EMX2*), which plays a role in the patterning of the developing neocortex.[170] But a recent study of 37 patients with schizencephaly failed to detect any pathogenic mutation.[171]

## Etiology

The etiology of schizencephaly is heterogeneous with well-documented cases of multiple occurrences within a family, but patients with schizencephaly have also been found following intrauterine viral infections, exposure to teratogens, or maternal trauma.[166] Schizencephaly has been found to be associated with some well-defined syndromes.[166] Common associations are absence of the septum pellucidum and septo-optic dysplasia.[168,172]

## Pathology

Transmantle gray matter connection from brain surface to ventricle surface characterizes this malformation (Figure 7–31). The abnormality may be unilateral or bilateral, and there may or may not be communication (closed or open lip) between the ventricles and subarachnoid space. When open, the walls of the defect are lined by gray matter. Schizencephaly is always accompanied by polymicrogyria (Figure 7–31). Pachygyria or heterotopia may be also found in some patients. Glial scarring is usually absent.

## Associated Anomalies

CNS anomalies are very common in these patients. Packard et al, in a series of 47 patients, found that 43 (91%) had associated cerebral developmental anomalies, most commonly absence of the septum pellucidum (45%) (Figures 7–31 and 7–32) and focal cortical dysplasia (40%).[173] Other anomalies commonly observed are dysgenesis of the corpus callosum, mega cisterna magna, hydrocephaly, gyral malformations, and optic nerve hypoplasia.[166,172] Non-CNS anomalies have been described, but in most cases they seem to occur sporadically. Arthrogryposis and ectrodactyly have been reported in more than isolated cases.[166]

## Risk of Recurrence

In the vast majority of cases this is a sporadic condition but some autosomal dominant and recessive cases have been reported.

## Sonographic Diagnosis

The prenatal US diagnosis of schizencephaly is possible but depends on the extent of cleft separation and on the presence of associated malformations (Figure 7–32). Closed-lip and open-lip variants with a very small gap may escape detection. In some patients the occipital median sulci in the visual cortex area may be erroneously suspected as a closed-lip defect.

The first prenatal diagnosis was performed in 1986 by Klingensmith and Cioffi-Ragan in a fetus at 31 postmenstrual weeks that presented with severe bilateral clefts.[174] Following this report, at least 17 fetuses with schizencephaly have been diagnosed at a mean gestational age of 29.3 postmenstrual weeks (range 21–28 weeks).[77,175–183] These fetuses were diagnosed during routine US examinations (4), following the visualization of enlarged lateral ventricles or unspecified suspicion of brain anomalies (9), following the diagnosis of septo-optic dysplasia (2), the inhalation of organic solvents (1), and due to lack of fetal movements (1). All the clefts were type II (open lip), 12 were bilateral and 5 unilateral.

Association with cerebral vascular occlusion and vasoconstrictive substances (cocaine) has been described.[184]

## MRI Diagnosis

The MRI diagnosis of fetal schizencephaly has been reported following US demonstration of diverse fetal

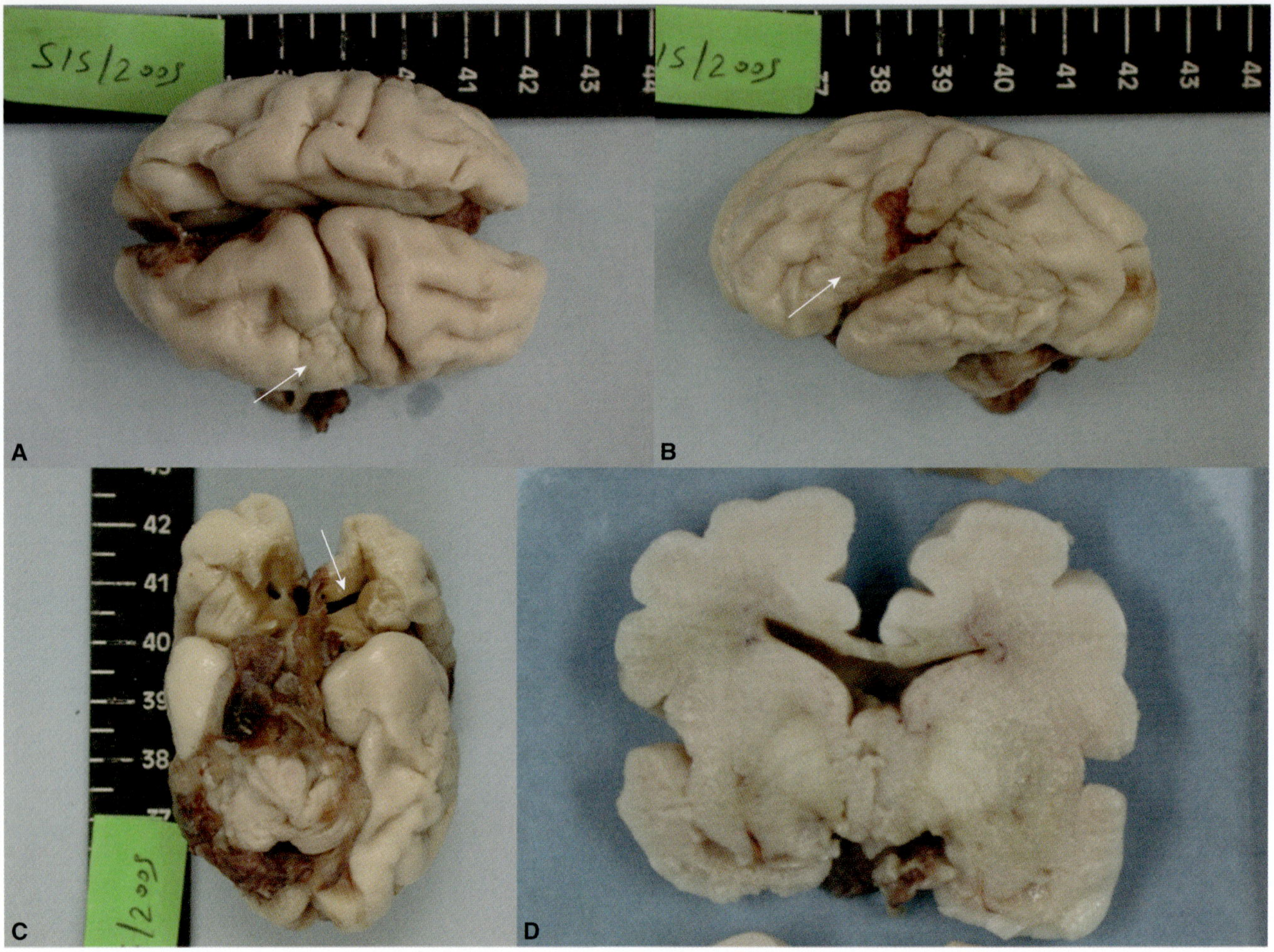


**Figure 7–31.** Macroscopic brain findings at 26 postmenstrual weeks in a fetus with schizencephaly. **(A, B)** Lateral and superior views of the brain demonstrate focal polymicrogyria (*arrows*). **(C)** Inferior view of the brain showing the communication between the frontal cortex and the lateral ventricles; the arrow points to the right lateral ventricle. **(D)** Associated agenesis of the septi pellucidi.

malformations.[77,178,179,182] MRI is indicated when the US depicts an abnormal sulcal pattern and rises the suspicion of schizencephaly or in patients with agenesis of the CSP to search for the presence of closed lip or small open lip defects that may remain undiagnosed after US examination[179] (Figure 7–33). Although large lesions are readily detected, the smaller closed ones can be missed by MRI.

### Implications for Sonographic Screening, Including Earliest Recognition

Schizencephaly has been diagnosed occasionally during routine sonographic examinations; careful examination of both hemispheres conducted at the three axial planes as recommended in the basic evaluation of the brain will depict at least some fetuses with large open-lip schizencephaly. The earliest diagnosis of a cortical cleft has been reported at 21 postmenstrual weeks in a fetus with osteogenesis imperfecta.[181] Successive "slicing" of a 3D US volume using the transgraphic display may be of help to localize and diagnose the pathology.

### Implications for Targeted Examination

The majority of the affected patients in postnatal series and in prenatal descriptions present with ventriculomegaly and/or agenesis of the CSP. Multiplanar neurosonographic examination may be helpful to investigate the brain parenchyma in search of abnormal continuity between the arachnoid space and the lateral ventricles (Figure 7–32). When the US examination is limited, or there is a suspicion of a closed-lip defect, MRI may help in the diagnosis but may also miss small closed lesions.

## Prognosis

Patients with schizencephaly commonly have delayed psychomotor development (57–80%), cerebral palsy (80–85%), and epilepsy (34–65%).[172,185,186] When the clefts are bilateral or unilateral but large, the prognosis is significantly worse. Patients with small unilateral schizencephaly may have a good developmental prognosis, particularly when the motor cortex is not involved.[187]

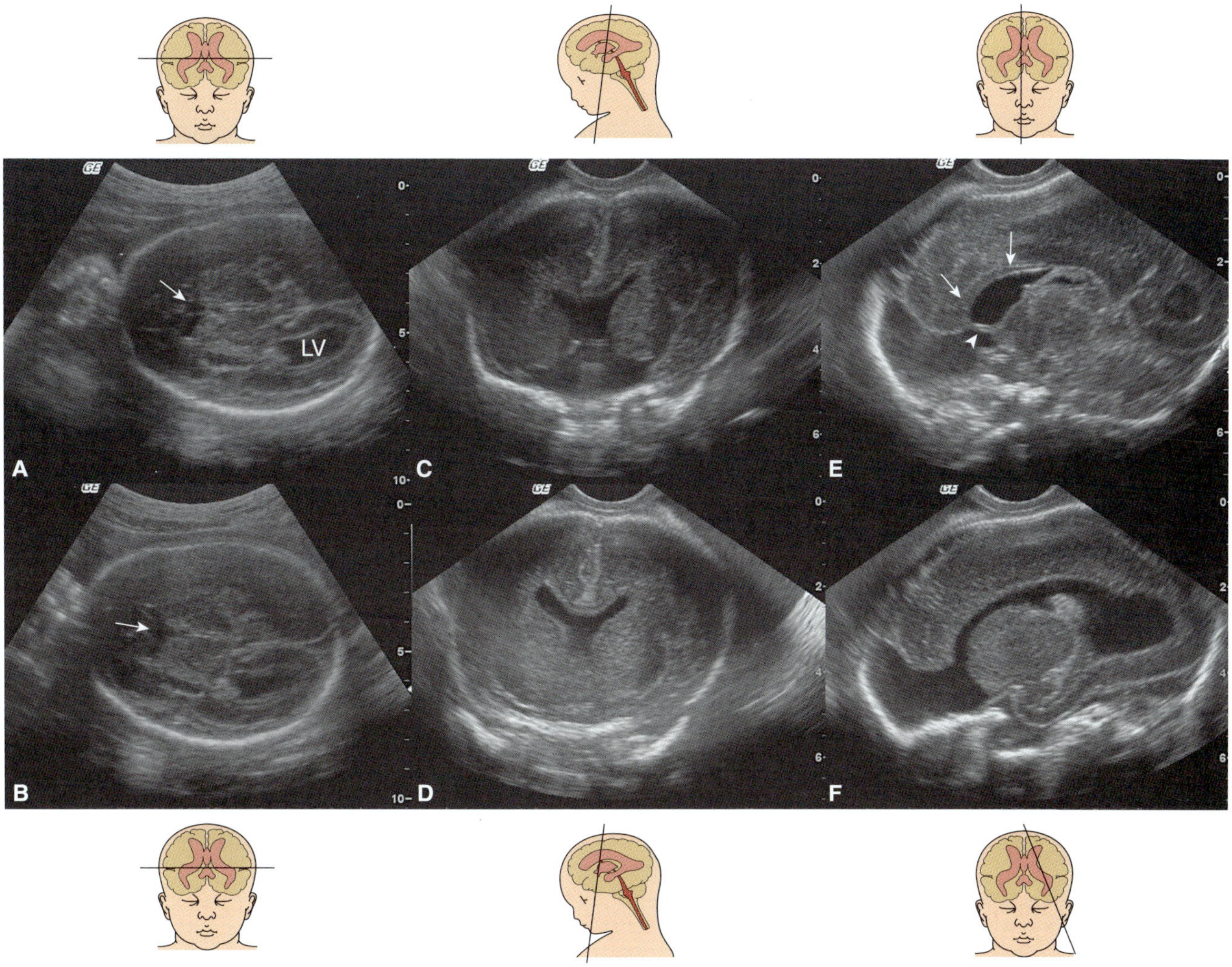


**Figure 7–32.** Transabdominal axial (**A, B**) and transvaginal coronal (**C, D**) and sagittal (**E, F**) US images in the same fetus as in Figure 7–30. Although the agenesis of the septi pellucidi may be suspected in **B** (*arrow*), these axial planes may be misinterpreted as normal. Note the apparent presence of the septi pellucidi in **A** (*arrow*) and the normal size of the lateral ventricle (LV). The diagnosis is evident in the coronal and axial planes. The corpus callosum is present and apparently normal (*arrows* in **E**).

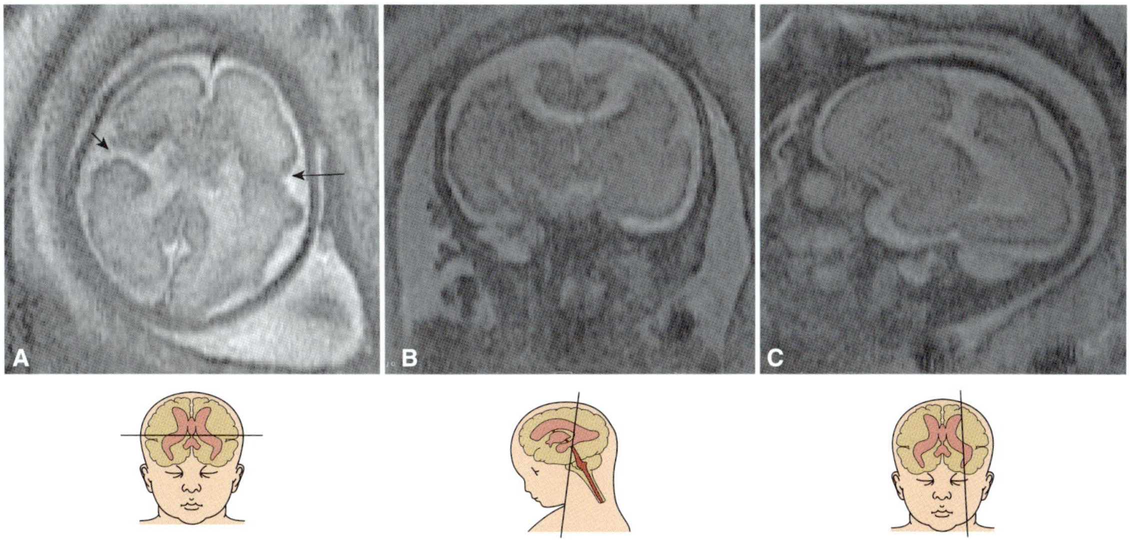


**Figure 7–33.** T2-weighted MRI at 28 postmenstrual weeks shows bilateral schizencephaly with multiple clefts lined by abnormal gray matter. **(A)** The axial section demonstrates the presence of an open lip (*arrowhead*) and a closed lip (*arrow*). Coronal **(B)** and sagittal **(C)** planes show open-lip defects lined with gray matter.

## Obstetric Management

Because all prenatally diagnosed cases tend to have bilateral or large unilateral clefts and a very poor prognosis, we believe that termination of pregnancy should be offered when legally possible, particularly when associated anomalies have been found. When unilateral closed-lip schizencephaly is diagnosed, it is difficult to give a straightforward recommendation, and the management should be individualized.

## REFERENCES


1. Volpe JJ. Neural tube formation and prosencephalic development. In: *Neurology of the Newborn.* Philadelphia: Saunders; 2008:3–50.
2. Rakic P. Specification of cerebral cortical areas. *Science.* 1988;241:170–176.
3. Barkovich AJ, Kuzniecky RI, Jackson GD, Guerrini R, Dobyns WB. A developmental and genetic classification for malformations of cortical development. *Neurology.* 2005;65:1873–1887.
4. Sarnat H, Flores-Sarnat L. Integrative classification of morphology and molecular genetics in central nervous system malformations. *Amer J Med Genet.* 2004;126A:386–392.
5. Volpe JJ. Neuronal proliferation, migration, organization, and mielinization. In: *Neurology of the Newborn.* Philadelphia: Saunders; 2008:51–118.
6. Chervenak FA, Jeanty P, Cantraine F, Chitkara U, Venus I, Berkowitz RL, Hobbins JC. The diagnosis of fetal microcephaly. *Am J Obstet Gynecol.* 1984;149:512–517.
7. Dobyns WB. Primary microcephaly: New approaches for an old disorder. *Am J Med Genet.* 2002;112:315–317.
8. Seto T, Nakagawa H, Morikawa Y, Nishijo M, Miura K and Kadoshima Y. Trend of congenital anomalies over 20 years ascertained by population-based monitoring in Ishikawa Prefecture, Japan. *Congenit Anom (Kyoto).* 2003;43:286–293.
9. Xiao KZ, Zhang ZY, Su YM, et al. Central nervous system congenital malformations, especially neural tube defects in 29 provinces, metropolitan cities and autonomous regions of China: Chinese Birth Defects Monitoring Program. *Int J Epidemiol.* 1990;19:978–982.
10. Trimble BK, Baird PA. Congenital anomalies of the central nervous system incidence in British Columbia, 1952–72. *Teratology* 1978;17:43–49.
11. Ventura SJ, Martin JA, Curtin SC, Menacker F, Hamilton BE. Births: Final data for 1999. *Natl Vital Stat Rep.* 2001;49:83.
12. Krauss MJ, Morrissey AE, Winn HN, Amon E, Leet TL. Microcephaly: An epidemiologic analysis. *Am J Obstet Gynecol.* 2003;188: 1484–1489.
13. Sells CJ. Microcephaly in a normal school population. *Pediatrics.* 1977;59:262–265.
14. Rakic P. Less is more: Progenitor death and cortical size. *Nat Neurosci.* 2005;8:981–982.
15. Shrimpton AE, Braddock BR, Hoo JJ. Narrowing the map of a gene (MRXS9) for X-linked mental retardation, microcephaly, and variably short stature at Xq12-q21.31. *Am J Med Genet.* 2000;92: 155–156.
16. Brunetti-Pierri N, Berg JS, Scaglia F, et al. Recurrent reciprocal 1q21.1 deletions and duplications associated with microcephaly or macrocephaly and developmental and behavioral abnormalities. *Nat Genet.* 2008;40:1466–1471.
17. Derwińska K, Smyk M, Cooper ML, Bader P, Cheung SW, Stankiewicz P. PTCH1 duplication in a family with microcephaly and mild developmental delay. *Eur J Hum Genet.* 2009;17:267–271.
18. Evrard P, de Saint-Georges P, Kadhim HJ, et al. Pathology of prenatal encephalopathies. In: French JH, Harel S, Casear P, eds. *Child Neurology and Developmental Disabilities.* Baltimore, MD: Paul H Brookes; 1989;153–176.
19. C. Garel. *MRI of the Fetal Brain: Normal Development and Cerebral Pathologies.* Berlin: Springer; 2004.
20. Persutte WH, Kurczynski TW, Chaudhuri K, Lenke RR, Woldenberg L, Brinker RA. Prenatal diagnosis of autosomal dominant microcephaly and postnatal evaluation with magnetic resonance imaging. *Prenat Diagn.* 1990;10:631–642.
21. R. Winter. Distinctive autosomal or X-linked dominant syndrome of microcephaly, mild developmental delay, short stature, and distinctive face. *Am J Med Genet.* 1993;47:917–920.
22. Leviton A, Holmes LB, Allred EN, Vargas J. Methodologic issues in epidemiologic studies of congenital microcephaly. *Early Hum Dev.* 2002;69:91–105.
23. Schwärzler P, Homfray T, Bernard JP, Bland JM, Ville Y. Late onset microcephaly: Failure of prenatal diagnosis. *Ultrasound Obstet Gynecol.* 2003;22:640–642.
24. Salomon LJ, Bernard JP, Duyme M, Buvat I, Ville Y. The impact of choice of reference charts and equations on the assessment of fetal biometry. *Ultrasound Obstet Gynecol.* 2005;25:559–565.
25. Berger I. Prenatal microcephaly: Can we be more accurate? *J Child Neurol.* 2009;24:97–100.
26. Chervenak FA, Rosenberg J, Brightman RC, Chitkara U, Jeanty P. A prospective study of the accuracy of ultrasound in predicting fetal microcephaly. *Obstet Gynecol.* 1987;69:908–910.
27. Goldstein I, Reece EA, Pilu G, O'Connor TZ, Lockwood CJ, Hobbins JC. Sonographic assessment of the fetal frontal lobe: A potential tool for prenatal diagnosis of microcephaly. *Am J Obstet Gynecol.* 1988;158:1057–1062.
28. Persutte WH, Coury A, Hobbins JC. Correlation of fetal frontal lobe and transcerebellar diameter measurements: The utility of a new prenatal sonographic technique. *Ultrasound Obstet Gynecol.* 1997;10:94–97.
29. Schinzel A, Litschgi M. Autosomal recessive severe congenital microcephaly: Antenatal ultrasonographic diagnosis and head growth from 15 to 24 weeks of gestation. *J Med Genet.* 1984;21: 355–358.
30. Reece EB, Goldstein I. Three-level view of fetal brain imaging in the prenatal diagnosis of congenital anomalies. *J Matern Fetal Med.* 1999;8:249–252.
31. Bromley B, Benacerraf BR. Difficulties in the prenatal diagnosis of microcephaly. *J Ultrasound Med.* 1995;14:303–306.
32. Malinger G, Lev D, Lerman-Sagie T. Assessment of fetal intracranial pathologies first demonstrated late in pregnancy: Cell proliferation disorders. *Reprod Biol Endocrinol.* 2003;1:110.
33. Pilu G, Falco P, Milano V, Perolo A, Bovicelli L. Prenatal diagnosis of microcephaly assisted by vaginal sonography and power Doppler. *Ultrasound Obstet Gynecol.* 1998;11:357–360.
34. den Hollander NS, Wessels MW, Los FJ, Ursem NT, Niermeijer MF, Wladimiroff JW. Congenital microcephaly detected by prenatal ultrasound: Genetic aspects and clinical significance. *Ultrasound Obstet Gynecol.* 2000;15:282–287.
35. Dahlgren L, Wilson RD. Prenatally diagnosed microcephaly: A review of etiologies. *Fetal Diagn Ther.* 2001;16:323–326.
36. Lembet A, Bodur H, Darnlacik A, et al. Microcephaly with simplified gyral pattern: The value of ultrasound and fetal MRI on management. *Ultrasound Obstet Gynecol.* 2007;30:595.
37. Schwärzler P, Bland JM, Holden D, Campbell S, Ville Y. Sex-specific antenatal reference growth charts for uncomplicated singleton pregnancies at 15–40 weeks of gestation. *Ultrasound Obstet Gynecol.* 2004;23:23–29.
38. Haslam RH. Microcephaly. In: Myrianthopoulos NC, ed. *Handbook of Clinical Neurology.* Amsterdam: Elsevier; 1987:267–284.
39. Arvey GB, Meneses L, Lodge A. The clinical significance of "measurement microcephaly." *Am J Dis Child.* 1972;123:214–217.
40. Petersson S, Pedersen NL, Schalling M, Lavebratt C. Primary megalencephaly at birth and low intelligence level. *Neurology.* 1999;53:1254–1259.
41. Hunter AG. Brain. In: Stevenson RE, Hall JG, Goodman RM, eds. *Human Malformations and Related Anomalies.* New York: Oxford University Press; 1993:2–19.
42. Smith RD, Ashley J, Hardesty RA, Tulley R, Hewitt J. Macrocephaly and minor congenital anomalies in children with learning problems. *J Dev Behav Pediatr.* 1984;5:231–236.
43. Nevo Y, Kramer U, Shinnar S, et al. Macrocephaly in children with developmental disabilities. *Pediatr Neurol.* 2002;27:363–368.
44. Almgren M, Schalling M, Lavebratt C. Idiopathic megalencephaly—possible cause and treatment opportunities: From patient to lab. *Eur J Paediatr Neurol.* 2008;12:438–445.

45. Tekin M, Hişmi BO, Fitoz S, et al. A germline PTEN mutation with manifestations of prenatal onset and verrucous epidermal nevus. *Am J Med Genet A.* 2006;140:1472–1475.
46. McEwing RL, Joelle R, Mohlo M, Bernard JP, Hillion Y, Ville Y. Prenatal diagnosis of neurofibromatosis type 1: Sonographic and MRI findings. *Prenat Diagn.* 2006;26:1110–1114.
47. Neis AE, Johansen KL, Harms RW, Watson WJ, Brost BC. Sonographic characteristics of linear nevus sebaceous sequence. *Ultrasound Obstet Gynecol.* 2006;27:323–324.
48. Agid R, Lieberman S, Nadjari M, Gomori JM. Prenatal MR diffusion-weighted imaging in a fetus with hemimegalencephaly. *Pediatr Radiol.* 2006;36:138–140.
49. Parazzini C, Righini A, Lalatta F, Bianchini E, Triulzi F. Frontal bilateral megalencephaly: Fetal and autopsy MR evaluation of an unclassified malformation. *Prenat Diagn.* 2005;25:489–491.
50. Gripp KW, Hopkins E, Vinkler H, et al. Significant overlap and possible identity of macrocephaly-capillary malformation and megalencephaly-polymicrogyria-polydactyly-hydrocephalus syndromes. *Amer J Med Genet A.* 2009;149A:868–876.
51. Nyberg RH, Uotila J, Kirkinen P, Rosendahl H. Macrocephaly-cutis marmorata telangiectatica congenita syndrome—prenatal signs in ultrasonography. *Prenat Diagn.* 2005;25:129–132.
52. Thomas A, Lemire EG. Sotos syndrome: Antenatal presentation. *Am J Med Genet A.* 2008;146A:1312–1313.
53. Chen CP, Lin SP, Chang TY, et al. Perinatal imaging findings of inherited Sotos syndrome. *Prenat Diagn.* 2002;22:887–892.
54. Yamashita H, Yasuhi I, Ishimaru T, Matsumoto T, Yamabe T. A case of nondiabetic macrosomia with Simpson-Golabi-Behmel syndrome: Antenatal sonographic findings. *Fetal Diagn Ther.* 1995;10:134–138.
55. Hughes-Benziete RM, Tolmie JL, McNay M, Patrick A. Simpson-Golabi-Behmel syndrome: Disproportionate fetal overgrowth and elevated maternal serum alpha-fetoprotein. *Prenat Diagn.* 1994;14:313–318.
56. Schilke K, Schaefer F, Waldherr R, et al. A case of Perlman syndrome: Fetal gigantism, renal dysplasia, and severe neurological deficits. *Am J Med Genet.* 2000;91:29–33.
57. Alessandri JL, Cuillier F, Ramful D, et al. Perlman syndrome: Report, prenatal findings and review. *Am J Med Genet A.* 2008;146A: 2532–2537.
58. Lin AE, O'Brien B, Demmer LA, et al. Prenatal features of Costello syndrome: Ultrasonographic findings and atrial tachycardia. *Prenat Diagn.* 2009;29:682–690.
59. Mellerio C, Marignier S, Roth P, et al. Prenatal cerebral ultrasound and MRI findings in glutaric aciduria type 1: A de novo case. *Ultrasound Obstet Gynecol.* 2008;31:712–714.
60. Zafeiriou DI, Ververi A, Salomons GS, et al. L-2-hydroxyglutaric aciduria presenting with severe autistic features. *Brain Dev.* 2008;30:305–307.
61. Traeger EC, Rapin I. The clinical course of Canavan disease. *Pediatr Neurol.* 1998;18:207–212.
62. Huggins MJ, Smith JR, Chun K, Ray PN, Shah JK, Whelan DT. Achondroplasia-hypochondroplasia complex in a newborn infant. *Am J Med Genet.* 1999;84:396–400.
63. Chen CP, Chern SR, Shih JC, et al. Prenatal diagnosis and genetic analysis of type I and type II thanatophoric dysplasia. *Prenat Diagn.* 2001;21:89–95.
64. Michel-Calemard L, Lesca G, Morel Y, Boggio D, Plauchu H, Attia-Sobol J. Campomelic acampomelic dysplasia presenting with increased nuchal translucency in the first trimester. *Prenat Diagn.* 2004;24:519–543.
65. Sobetzko D, Eich G, Kalff-Suske M, Grzeschik KH, Superti-Furga A. Boy with syndactylies, macrocephaly, and severe skeletal dysplasia: Not a new syndrome, but two dominant mutations (GLI3 E543X and COL2A1 G973R) in the same individual. *Am J Med Genet.* 2000;90:239–242.
66. Shukla P, Balakrishnan P, Agarwal N, et al. Prenatal diagnosis of megalencephalic leukodystrophy. *Prenat Diagn.* 2008;28:357–359.
67. Augoustides-Savvopoulou P, Salomons GS, Dotis J, et al. Mutation analysis a prerequisite for prenatal diagnosis of L-2-hydroxyglutaric aciduria? *Mol Genet Metab.* 2008;91:399–401.
68. Lerman-Sagie T, Ben-Sira L, Achiron R, et al. Thick fetal corpus callosum: An ominous sign? *Ultrasound Obstet Gynecol.* 2009;34:55–61.
69. Malinger G, Ben-Sira L, Lev D, Ben-Aroya Z, Kidron D, Lerman-Sagie T. Fetal brain imaging: A comparison between magnetic resonance imaging and dedicated neurosonography. *Ultrasound Obstet Gynecol.* 2004;23:333–340.
70. Arbour L, Watters GV, Hall JG, Fraser FC. Multifactorial inheritance of non-syndromic macrocephaly. *Clin Genet.* 1996;50:57–62.
71. Malinger G, Lerman-Sagie T, Achiron R, Lipitz S. The subarachnoid space: Normal fetal development as demonstrated by transvaginal ultrasound. *Prenat Diagn.* 2000;20:890–893.
72. DeRosa R, Lenke RR, Kurczynski TW, Persutte WH, Nemes JM. In utero diagnosis of benign fetal macrocephaly. *Am J Obstet Gynecol.* 1989;161:690–692.
73. Lorber J, Priestley BL. Children with large heads: A practical approach to diagnosis in 557 children, with special reference to 109 children with megalencephaly. *Dev Med Child Neurol.* 1982;23: 494–502.
74. Laubscher B, Deonna T, Uske A, van Melle G. Primitive megalencephaly in children: Natural history, medium term prognosis with special reference to external hydrocephalus. *Eur J Pediatr.* 1990;149:502–507.
75. Flores-Sarnat L. Hemimegalencephaly: 1. Genetic, clinical, and imaging aspects. *J Child Neurol.* 2002;17:373–384.
76. Tinkle BT, Schorry EK, Franz DN, Krone KR, Saal HM. Epidemiology of hemimegalencephaly: A case series and review. *Am J Med Genet.* 2005;139A:204–211.
77. Malinger G, Kidron D, Schreiber L, et al. Prenatal diagnosis of malformations of cortical development by dedicated neurosonography. *Ultrasound Obstet Gynecol.* 2007;29:178–191.
78. Woo CLF, Chuang SH, Becker L, et al. Radiologic-pathologic correlation in focal cortical dysplasia and hemimegalencephaly in 18 children. *Pediatr Neurol.* 2001;25:295–303.
79. Hering-Hanit R, Achiron R, Lipitz S, Achiron A. Asymmetry of fetal cerebral hemispheres: In utero ultrasound study. *Arch Dis Child Fetal Neonatal Ed.* 2001;85:F194–F196.
80. O'Callaghan FJK, Shiell AW, Osborne JP, Martyn CN. Prevalence of tuberous sclerosis estimated by capture-recapture analysis. *Lancet.* 1998;351:1490.
81. van Slegtenhorst M, de Hoogt R, Hermans C, et al. Identification of the tuberous sclerosis gene TSC1 on chromosome 9q34. *Science.* 1997;277:805–808.
82. European Chromosome 16 Tuberous Sclerosis Consortium. Identification and characterization of the tuberous sclerosis gene on chromosome 16. *Cell.* 1993;75:1305–1315.
83. Ess KC. The neurobiology of tuberous sclerosis complex. *Semin Pediatr Neurol.* 2006;13:37–42.
84. Napolioni V, Moavero R, Curatolo P. Recent advances in neurobiology of tuberous sclerosis complex. *Brain Dev.* 2009;31:104–113.
85. Holley DG, Martin GR, Brenner JI, et al. Diagnosis and management of fetal cardiac tumors: A multicenter experience and review of published reports. *J Am Coll Cardiol.* 1995;26:516–520.
86. DeVore GR, Hakim S, Kleinman CS, Hobbins JC. The in utero diagnosis of an interventricular septal cardiac rhabdomyoma by means of real-time-directed, M-mode echocardiography. *Am J Obstet Gynecol.* 1982;143:967–969.
87. Crawford DC, Garrett C, Tynan M, Neville BG, Allan LD. Cardiac rhabdomyomata as a marker for the antenatal detection of tuberous sclerosis. *J Med Genet.* 1983;20:303–304.
88. Muller L, de Jong G, Falck V, Hewlett R, Hunter J, Shires J. Antenatal ultrasonographic findings in tuberous sclerosis: Report of 2 cases. *S Afr Med J.* 1986;69:633–638.
89. Pipitone S, Mongiovì M, Grillo R, Gagliano S, Sperandeo V. Cardiac rhabdomyoma in intrauterine life: Clinical features and natural history. A case series and review of published reports. *Ital Heart J.* 2002;3:48–52.
90. D'Addario V, Pinto V, Di Naro E, Del Bianco A, Di Cagno L, Volpe P. Prenatal diagnosis and postnatal outcome of cardiac rhabdomyomas. *J Perinat Med.* 2002;30:170–175.
91. Gamzu R, Achiron R, Hegesh J, et al. Evaluating the risk of tuberous sclerosis in cases with prenatal diagnosis of cardiac rhabdomyoma. *Prenat Diagn.* 2002;22:1044–1047.
92. Bader RS, Chitayat D, Kelly E, et al. Fetal rhabdomyoma: Prenatal diagnosis, clinical outcome, and incidence of associated tuberous sclerosis complex. *J Pediatr.* 2003;143:620–624.

93. Tworetzky W, McElhinney DB, Margossian R, et al. Association between cardiac tumors and tuberous sclerosis in the fetus and neonate. *Am J Cardiol.* 2003;92:487–489.
94. Fesslova V, Villa L, Rizzuti T, Mastrangelo M, Mosca F. Natural history and long-term outcome of cardiac rhabdomyomas detected prenatally. *Prenat Diagn.* 2004;24:241–248.
95. Chao AS, Chao A, Wang TH, et al. Outcome of antenatally diagnosed cardiac rhabdomyoma: Case series and a meta-analysis. *Ultrasound Obstet Gynecol.* 2008;31:289–295.
96. Saada J, Hadj Rabia S, Fermont L, et al. Prenatal diagnosis of cardiac rhabdomyomas: Incidence of associated cerebral lesions of tuberous sclerosis complex. *Ultrasound Obstet Gynecol.* 2009;34:155–159.
97. Czechowski J, Langille EL, Varady E. Intracardiac tumour and brain lesions in tuberous sclerosis: A case report of antenatal diagnosis by ultrasonography. *Acta Radiol.* 2000;41:371–374.
98. Mirkin LD, Ey EH, Chaparro M. Congenital subependymal giant-cell astrocytoma: Case report with prenatal ultrasonogram. *Pediatr Radiol.* 1999;29:776–780.
99. Sgro M, Barozzino T, Toi A, Johnson J, Sermer M, Chitayat D. Prenatal detection of cerebral lesions in a fetus with tuberous sclerosis. *Ultrasound Obstet Gynecol.* 1999;14:356–359.
100. Mühler MR, Rake A, Schwabe M, et al. Value of fetal cerebral MRI in sonographically proven cardiac rhabdomyoma. *Pediatr Radiol.* 2007;37:467–474.
101. Sonigo P, Elmaleh A, Fermont L, Delezoide AL, Mirlesse V, Brunelle F. Prenatal MRI diagnosis of fetal cerebral tuberous sclerosis. *Pediatr Radiol.* 1996;26:1–4.
102. Brackley KJ, Farndon PA, Weaver JB, Dow DJ, Chapman S, Kilby MD. Prenatal diagnosis of tuberous sclerosis with intracerebral signs at 14 weeks' gestation. *Prenat Diagn.* 1999;19:575–579.
103. Milunsky A, Ito M, Maher TA, Flynn M, Milunsky JM. Prenatal molecular diagnosis of tuberous sclerosis complex. *Am J Obstet Gynecol.* 2009;200:e321–e326.
104. Malinger G, Lev D, Lerman-Sagie T. Abnormal sulcation as an early sign for migration disorders. *Ultrasound Obstet Gynecol.* 2004;24:704–705.
105. de Rijk-van Andel JF, Arts WF, Hofman A, Staal A, Niermeijer MF. Epidemiology of lissencephaly type I. *Neuroepidemiology.* 1991;10:200–204.
106. Sidman RL, Rakic P. Neuronal migration, with special reference to developing human brain: A review. *Brain Res.* 1973;62:1–35.
107. Mei D, Lewis R, Parrini E, et al. High frequency of genomic deletions and a duplication in the LIS1 gene in lissencephaly: Implications for molecular diagnosis. *J Med Genet.* 2008;45:255–361.
108. Cardoso C, Leventer RJ, Ward HL, et al. Refinement of a 400-kb critical region allows genotypic differentiation between isolated lissencephaly, Miller-Dieker syndrome, and other phenotypes secondary to deletions of 17p13.3. *Am J Hum Genet.* 2003;72:918–930.
109. Leventer RJ, Cardoso C, Ledbetter DH, Dobyns WB. LIS1 missense mutations cause milder lissencephaly phenotypes including a child with normal IQ. *Neurology.* 2001;57:416–422.
110. Uyanik G, Morris-Rosendahl DJ, Stiegler J, et al. Location and type of mutation in the LIS1 gene do not predict phenotypic severity. *Neurology.* 2007;69:442–447.
111. Caspi M, Atlas R, Kantor A, Sapir T, Reiner O. Interaction between LIS1 and doublecortin, two lissencephaly gene products. *Hum Molec Genet.* 2000;9:2205–2213.
112. Kato M, Das S, Petras K, et al. Mutations of ARX are associated with striking pleiotropy and consistent genotype–phenotype correlation. *Hum Mutat.* 2004;23:147–159.
113. Zaki M, Shehab M, El-Aleem AA, et al. Identification of a novel recessive RELN mutation using a homozygous balanced reciprocal translocation. *Am J Med Genet A.* 2007;143:939–944.
114. Dobyns WB, Reiner O, Carrozzo R, Ledbetter DH. Lissencephaly: A human brain malformation associated with deletion of the LIS1 gene located at chromosome 17p13. *JAMA.* 1993;270(23): 2838–2842.
115. Viot G, Sonigo P, Simon I, et al. Neocortical neuronal arrangement in LIS1 and DCX lissencephaly may be different. *Am J Med Genet A.* 2004;126A:123–128.
116. Forman MS, Squier W, Dobyns WB, Golden JA. Genotypically defined lissencephalies show distinct pathologies. *J Neuropathol Exp Neurol.* 2005;64:847–857.
117. Mai R, Tassi L, Cossu M, Francione S, et al. A neuropathological, stereo-EEG, and MRI study of subcortical band heterotopia. *Neurology.* 2003;60:1834–1838.
118. Saltzman DH, Krauss CM, Goldman JM, Benacerraf BR. Prenatal diagnosis of lissencephaly. *Prenat Diagn.* 1991;11:139–143.
119. Alvarado M, Bass HN, Caldwell S, Jamehdor M, Miller AA, Jacob P. Miller-Dieker syndrome: Detection of a cryptic chromosome translocation using in situ hybridization in a family with multiple affected offspring. *Am J Dis Child.* 1993;147:1291–1294.
120. Fong KW, Ghai S, Toi A, Blaser S, Winsor EJ, Chitayat D. Prenatal ultrasound findings of lissencephaly associated with Miller-Dieker syndrome and comparison with pre- and postnatal magnetic resonance imaging. *Ultrasound Obstet Gynecol.* 2004;24:716–723.
121. McGahan JP, Grix A, Gerscovich EO. Prenatal diagnosis of lissencephaly: Miller-Dieker syndrome. *J Clin Ultrasound.* 1994;22: 560–563.
122. Cohen-Sacher B, Lerman-Sagie T, Lev D, Malinger G. Developmental milestones of the fetal cerebral cortex: A longitudinal sonographic study. *Ultrasound Obstet Gynecol.* 2006;27:494–502.
123. Monteagudo A, Timor-Tritsch IE. Development of fetal gyri, sulci and fissures: A transvaginal sonographic study. *Ultrasound Obstet Gynecol.* 1997;9:222–228.
124. Toi A, Lister WS, Fong KW. How early are fetal cerebral sulci visible at prenatal ultrasound and what is the normal pattern of early fetal sulcal development? *Ultrasound Obstet Gynecol.* 2004;24:706–715.
125. Greco P, Resta M, Vimercati A, et al. Antenatal diagnosis of isolated lissencephaly by ultrasound and magnetic resonance imaging. *Ultrasound Obstet Gynecol.* 1998;12:276–279.
126. Fogliarini C, Chaumoitre K, Chapon F, et al. Assessment of cortical maturation with prenatal MRI: 2. Abnormalities of cortical maturation. *Eur Radiol.* 2005;15:1781–1789.
127. Chitayat D, Toi A, Babul R, et al. Omphalocele in Miller-Dieker syndrome: Expanding the phenotype. *Am J Med Genet.* 1997;69: 293–298.
128. Vajsar J, Schachter H. Walker-Warburg syndrome. *Orphanet J Rare Dis.* 2006;1:29.
129. Mostacciuolo ML, Miorin M, Martinello F, Angelini C, Perini P, Trevisan CP. Genetic epidemiology of congenital muscular dystrophy in a sample from the north-east Italy. *Hum Genet.* 1996;97: 277–279.
130. Manzini MC, Gleason D, Chang BS, et al. Ethnically diverse causes of Walker-Warburg syndrome (WWS): FCMD mutations are a more common cause of WWS outside of the Middle East. *Hum Mutat.* 2008;29:E231–E241.
131. Barresi R, Campbell KP. Dystroglycan: From biosynthesis to pathogenesis of human disease. *J Cell Sci.* 2006;119:199–207.
132. Moore SA, Saito F, Chen J, et al. Deletion of brain dystroglycan recapitulates aspects of congenital muscular dystrophy. *Nature.* 2002;418:422–425.
133. Mercuri E, Messina S, Bruno C, et al. Congenital muscular dystrophies with defective glycosylation of dystroglycan: A population study. *Neurology.* 2009;72:1802–1809.
134. Squier MV. Development of the cortical dysplasia of type II lissencephaly. *Neuropathol Appl Neurobiol.* 1993;19:209–213.
135. Gelot A, Billette de Villemeur T, Bordarier C, Ruchoux MM, Moraine C, Ponsot G. Developmental aspects of type II lissencephaly: Comparative study of dysplastic lesions in fetal and post-natal brains. *Acta Neuropath.* 1995;89:72–84.
136. Dobyns WB, Pagon RA, Armstrong D, et al. Diagnostic criteria for Walker-Warburg syndrome. *Am J Med Genet.* 1989;32:195–210.
137. Clement E, Mercuri E, Godfrey C, et al. Brain involvement in muscular dystrophies with defective dystroglycan glycosylation. *Ann Neurol.* 2008;64:573–582.
138. Crowe C, Jassani M, Dickerman L. The prenatal diagnosis of Warburg syndrome. *Am J Hum Genet.* 1985;37:A214.
139. Rodgers BL, Vanner LV, Pai GS, Sens MA. Walker-Warburg syndrome: Report of three affected sibs. *Am J Med Genet.* 1994;49:198–201.
140. Farrell SA, Toi A, Leadman ML, Davidson RG, Caco C. Prenatal diagnosis of retinal detachment in Walker-Warburg syndrome. *Am J Hum Genet.* 1987;28:619–624.
141. Chitayat D, Toi A, Babul R, et al. Prenatal diagnosis of retinal nonattachment in the Walker-Warburg syndrome. *Am J Hum Genet.* 1995;56:351–358.

142. Monteagudo A, Alayón A, Mayberry P. Walker-Warburg syndrome: Case report and review of the literature. *J Ultrasound Med.* 2001;20:419–426.
143. Gasser B, Lindner V, Dreyfus M, et al. Prenatal diagnosis of Walker-Warburg syndrome in three sibs. *Am J Med Genet.* 1998;76: 107–110.
144. Blin G, Rabbe A, Ansquer Y, Meghdiche S, Floch-Tudal C, Mandelbrot L. First-trimester ultrasound diagnosis in a recurrent case of Walker-Warburg syndrome. *Ultrasound Obstet Gynecol.* 2005;26:297–299.
145. Huppert BJ, Brandt KR, Ramin KD, King BF. Single-shot fast spin-echo MR imaging of the fetus: A pictorial essay. *Radiographics.* 1999;19:215–227.
146. Kojima K, Suzuki Y, Seki K, et al. Prenatal diagnosis of lissencephaly (type II) by ultrasound and fast magnetic resonance imaging. *Fetal Diagn Ther.* 2002;17:34–36.
147. Toi A, Chitayat D, Blaser S. Abnormalities of the foetal cerebral cortex. *Prenat Diagn.* 2009;29:355–371.
148. Strigini F, Valleriani A, Cecchi M, et al. Prenatal ultrasound and magnetic resonance imaging features in a fetus with Walker-Warburg syndrome. *Ultrasound Obstet Gynecol.* 2009;33:363–365.
149. Stroustrup Smith A, Levine D, Barnes PD, Robertson RL. Magnetic resonance imaging of the kinked fetal brain stem: a sign of severe dysgenesis. *J Ultrasound Med.* 2005;24:1697–1709.
150. Holzgreve H, Feil R, Louwen E, Miny P. Prenatal diagnosis and management of fetal hydrocephaly and iissencephaly. *Childs Nerv Syst.* 1993;9:408–412.
151. Parrini E, Ramazzotti A, Dobyns WB, et al. Periventricular heterotopia: Phenotypic heterogeneity and correlation with Filamin A mutations. *Brain.* 2006;129:1892–1906.
152. Ott I, Fischer EG, Miyagi Y, Mueller BM, Ruf W. A role for tissue factor in cell adhesion, migration mediated by interaction with actin-binding protein 280. *J Cell Biol.* 1998;140:1241–1253.
153. Sheen VL, Dixon PH, Fox JW, et al. Mutations in the X-linked filamin 1 gene cause periventricular nodular heterotopia in males as well as in females. *Hum Mol Genet.* 2001;10:1775–1783.
154. Guerrini R, Mei D, Sisodiya S, et al. Germline and mosaic mutations of FLN1 in men with periventricular heterotopia. *Neurology.* 2004;63:51–56.
155. Sheen VL, Wheless JW, Bodell A, et al. Periventricular heterotopia associated with chromosome 5p anomalies. *Neurology.* 2003;60:1033–1036.
156. McCann MV, Pongonis SJ, Golomb MR, Edwards-Brown M, Christensen CK, Sokol DK. Like father, like son: Periventricular nodular heterotopia and nonverbal learning disorder. *J Child Neurol.* 2008;23:950–953.
157. Meroni A, Galli C, Bramerio M, et al. Nodular heterotopia: A neuropathological study of 24 patients undergoing surgery for drug-resistant epilepsy. *Epilepsia.* 2009;50:116–124.
158. Mitchell LA, Simon EM, Filly RA, Barkovich AJ. Antenatal diagnosis of subependymal heterotopia. *AJNR Am J Neuroradiol.* 2000;21:296–300.
159. Glenn OA, Goldstein RB, Li KC, et al. Fetal magnetic resonance imaging in the evaluation of fetuses referred for sonographically suspected abnormalities of the corpus callosum. *J Ultrasound Med.* 2005;24:791–804.
160. Onyeije CI, Sherer DM, Jarosz CJ, Divon MY. Prenatal sonographic findings associated with sporadic subcortical nodular heterotopia. *Obstet Gynecol.* 1998;91:799–801.
161. Malinger G, Lerman-Sagie T, Watemberg N, Rotmensch S, Lev D, Glezerman M. A normal second-trimester ultrasound does not exclude intracranial structural pathology. *Ultrasound Obstet Gynecol.* 2002;20:51–56.
162. Sonigo PC, Rypens FF, Carteret M, Delezoide AL, Brunelle FO. MR imaging of fetal cerebral anomalies. *Pediatr Radiol.* 1998;28: 212–222.
163. Bargallo N, Puerto B, De Juan C, Martinez-Crespo JM, Lourdes Olondo M. Hereditary subependymal heterotopia associated with mega cisterna magna: Antenatal diagnosis with magnetic resonance imaging. *Ultrasound Obstet Gynecol.* 2002;20:86–89.
164. Rypens FF, Sonigo P, Aubry MC, Delezoide AL, Cessot F, Brunelle F. Prenatal MR diagnosis of a thick corpus callosum. *AJNR Am J Neuroradiol.* 1996;17:1918–1920.
165. Yakovlev PI, Wadsworth RC. Schizencephalies: A study of the congenital clefts in the cerebral mantle. 2. Clefts with hydrocepha!us and lips separated. *J Neunopathol Exp Neurol.* 1946;5:169–206.
166. Curry CJ, Lammer EJ, Nelson V, Shaw GM. Schizencephaly: Heterogeneous etiologies in a population of 4 million California births. *Am J Med Genet A.* 2005;137:181–189.
167. Leventer RJ, Phelan EM, Coleman LT, Kean MJ, Jackson GD, Harvey AS. Clinical and imaging features of cortical malformations in childhood. *Neurology.* 1999;53:715–722.
168. Raybaud C, Girard N, Lévrier O, Peretti-Viton P, Manera L, Farnarier P. Schizencephaly: Correlation between the lobar topography of the cleft(s) and absence of the septum pellucidum. *Childs Nerv Syst.* 2001;17:217–222.
169. Raybaud C. Destructive lesions of the brain. *Neuroradiology.* 1983;25:265–291.
170. Granata T, Farina L, Faiella A, Cardini R, D'Incerti L, Boncinelli E, Battaglia G. Familial schizencephaly associated with EMX2 mutation. *Neurology.* 1997;48:1403–1406.
171. Merello E, Swanson E, De Marco P, et al. No major role for the EMX2 gene in schizencephaly. *Am J Med Genet A.* 2008;146A: 1142–1150.
172. Denis D, Chateil JF, Brun M, et al. Schizencephaly: Clinical and imaging features in 30 infantile cases. *Brain Dev.* 2000;22:475–483.
173. Packard AM, Miller VS, Delgado MR. Schizencephaly: Correlations of clinical and radiologic features. *Neurology.* 1997;48:1427–1434.
174. Klingensmith WC III and Cioffi-Ragan DT. Schizencephaly: diagnosis and progression in utero. *Radiology* 1986;159:617–618.
175. Lituania M, Passamonti U, Cordone MS, Magnano GM, Toma P. Schizencephaly: Prenatal diagnosis by computed sonography and magnetic resonance imaging. *Prenat Diagn.* 1989;9:649–655.
176. Komarniski CA, Cyr DR, Mack LA, Weinberger E. Prenatal diagnosis of schizencephaly. *J Ultrasound Med.* 1990;9:305–307.
177. Ceccherini AF, Twining P, Variend S. Schizencephaly: Antenatal detection using ultrasound. *Clin Radiol.* 1999;54:620.
178. Denis D, Maugey-Laulom B, Carles D, Pedespan JM, Brun M, Chateil JF. Prenatal diagnosis of schizencephaly by fetal magnetic resonance imaging. *Fetal Diagn Ther.* 2001;16:354–359.
179. Oh KY, Kennedy AM, Frias AE, Jr., Byrne JL. Fetal schizencephaly: Pre- and postnatal imaging with a review of the clinical manifestations. *Radiographics.* 2005;25:647–657.
180. Huang WM, Monteagudo A, Bennett GL, Fowkes ME, Timor-Tritsch IE. Schizencephaly in a dysgenetic fetal brain: Prenatal sonographic, magnetic resonance imaging, and postmortem correlation. *J Ultrasound Med.* 2006;25:551–554.
181. Ozkur A, Kervancioglu R, Kervancioglu S, Dikensoy E, Bayram M. Second-trimester diagnosis of osteogenesis imperfecta associated with schizencephaly by sonography. *Saudi Med J.* 2007;28:1289–1290.
182. Witters I, Cannie M, Casaer P, Devriendt K, Fryns JP. Prenatal diagnosis of schizencephaly after inhalation of organic solvents. *Ultrasound Obstet Gynecol.* 2007;29:356–357.
183. Hung JH, Shen SH, Guo WY, et al. Prenatal diagnosis of schizencephaly with septo-optic dysplasia by ultrasound and magnetic resonance imaging. *J Obstet Gynaecol Res.* 2008;34:674–679.
184. Suchet IB. Schizencephaly: Antenatal and postnatal assessment with colour-flow Doppler imaging. *Can Assoc Radiol J.* 1994;45: 193–200.
185. Lopes CF, Cendes F, Piovesana AM, et al. Epileptic features of patients with unilateral and bilateral schizencephaly. *J Child Neurol.* 2006;21:757–760.
186. Mejía L, Gómez JC, Carrizosa J, Cornejo JW. Phenotypic characterization of 35 Colombian children with an imaging diagnosis of schizencephaly. *Rev Neurol.* 2008;47:71–76.
187. Barkovich AJ, Kjos BO. Schizencephaly: correlation of clinical findings with MR characteristics. *AJNR Am J Neuroradiol* 1992;13: 85–94.
188. Paladini D, D'Armiento M, Ardovino I, Martinelli P. Prenatal diagnosis of the cerebro-oculo-facio-skeletal (COFS) syndrome. *Ultrasound Obstet Gynecol.* 2000;16:91–93.
189. Conte C, D'Apice MR, Botta A, Sangiuolo F, Novelli G. Prenatal diagnosis of Cockayne syndrome type A based on the identification of two novel mutations in the ERCC8 gene. *Genet Test Mol Biomarkers.* 2009;13:127–131.

190. Barisic I, Tokic V, Loane M, et al; EUROCAT Working Group. Descriptive epidemiology of Cornelia de Lange syndrome in Europe. *Am J Med Genet A.* 2008;146A:51–59.
191. Ickowicz V, Eurin D, Maugey-Laulom B, et al. Meckel-Grüber syndrome: Sonography and pathology. *Ultrasound Obstet Gynecol.* 2006;27:296–300.
192. Adam MP, Schelley S, Gallagher R, et al. Clinical features and management issues in Mowat-Wilson syndrome. *Am J Med Genet A.* 2006;140:2730–2741.
193. Manning MA, Cunniff CM, Colby CE, El-Sayed YY, Hoyme HE. Neu-Laxova syndrome: Detailed prenatal diagnostic and post-mortem findings and literature review. *Am J Med Genet A.* 2004;125A: 240–249.
194. Graham JM, Jr., Hennekam R, Dobyns WB, Roeder E, Busch D. MICRO syndrome: An entity distinct from COFS syndrome. *Am J Med Genet A.* 2004;128A:235–245.
195. Horton AL, Smith JK, Strauss RA. Recurrence of Galloway Mowat syndrome and associated prenatal imaging findings. *Prenat Diagn.* 2009;29:280–282.
196. Lenzini E, D'Ottavio G, Città A, Benussi DG, Petix V, Pecile V. Prenatal diagnosis of Miller-Dieker syndrome by ultrasound and molecular cytogenetic analysis. *Clin Genet.* 2007;72:487–489.
197. Natacci F, Bedeschi MF, Righini A, et al. Norman-Roberts syndrome: acterization of the phenotype in early fetal life. *Prenat Diagn.* 2007;27:568–572.
198. Chitayat D, Meagher-Villemure K, Mamer OA, et al. Brain dysgenesis and congenital intracerebral calcification associated with 3-hydroxyisobutyric aciduria. *J Pediatr* 1992;121:86–89.
199. Levy HL, Lobbregt D, Platt LD, Benacerraf BR. Fetal ultrasonography in maternal PKU. *Prenat Diagn.* 1996;16:599–604.
200. Ewenczyk C, Leroux A, Roubergue A, et al. Recessive hereditary methaemoglobinaemia, type II: Delineation of the clinical spectrum. *Brain.* 2008;131:760–761.
201. Goldenberg A, Wolf C, Chevy F, et al. Antenatal manifestations of Smith-Lemli-Opitz (RSH) syndrome: A retrospective survey of 30 cases. *Am J Med Genet A.* 2004;124A:423–426.
202. Nadjari M, Fasouliotis SJ, Ariel I, Raas-Rothschild A, Bar-Ziv J, Elchalal U. Ultrasonographic prenatal diagnosis of microcephalic osteodysplastic primordial dwarfism types I/III. *Prenat Diagn.* 2000;20:666–669.
203. Yüksel D, Senbil N, Yilmaz D, Yarali N, Gürer YK. A rare cause of mental motor retardation: Recessive congenital methemoglobinemia type II. *Turk J Pediatr.* 2009;51:187–189.
204. Couvreur-Lionnais S, Rousseau T, Laurent N, et al. Prenatal diagnosis of Juberg-Hayward syndrome. *Prenat Diagn.* 2005;25:172–175.
205. Napolitano R, Maruotti GM, Quarantelli M, Martinelli P, Paladini D. Prenatal diagnosis of Seckel Syndrome on 3-dimensional sonography and magnetic resonance imaging. *J Ultrasound Med.* 2009;28: 369–374.
206. Chen CP, Lee CC, Chang TY, Town DD, Wang W. Prenatal diagnosis of mosaic distal 5p deletion and review of the literature. *Prenat Diagn.* 2004;24:50–57.
207. Chen CP, Lee CC, Chen WL, Wang W, Tzen CY. Prenatal diagnosis of premature centromere division-related mosaic variegated aneuploidy. *Prenat Diagn.* 2004;24:1.
208. Muschke P, Gola H, Varon R, et al. Retrospective diagnosis and subsequent prenatal diagnosis of Nijmegen breakage syndrome. *Prenat Diagn.* 2004;24:111–113.
209. Philipp T, Grillenberger K, Separovic ER, Philipp K, Kalousek DK. Effects of triploidy on early human development. *Prenat Diagn.* 2004;24:276–281.
210. Boog G, Le Vaillant C, Collet M, et al. Prenatal sonographic patterns in six cases of Wolf-Hirschhorn (4p-) syndrome. *Fetal Diagn Ther.* 2004;19:421–430.

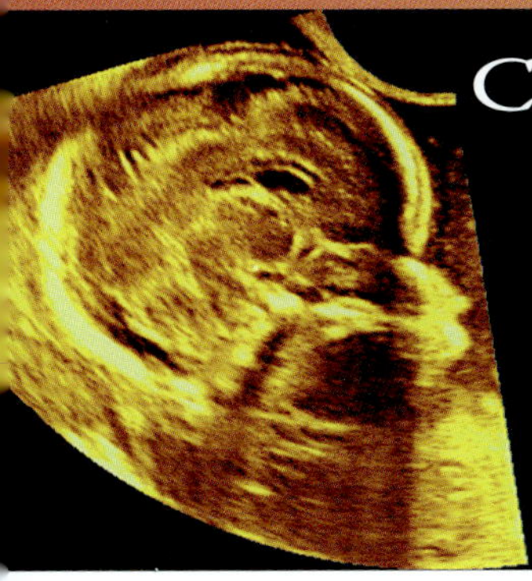

Chapter 8

# ANOMALIES OF THE CEREBELLUM

*Gianluigi Pilu • Gustavo Malinger • Selim Buyukkurt*

**KEY POINTS**

1. A wide variety of congenital anomalies can affect the cerebellum. The antenatal findings overlap among different pathologies and normal variants. Consequently, a specific diagnosis is often not possible.
2. One of the most common abnormal findings that is encountered is the impression of a communication between the fourth ventricle and the posterior cisterna magna. When this is seen after 20 postmenstrual weeks' gestation, it identifies a group of conditions that are commonly referred to as the Dandy-Walker complex.
3. Within the Dandy-Walker complex, cases with a normal appearance of the vermis and cisterna magna most frequently have a normal outcome. Fetuses with an enlarged cisterna magna and/or an abnormal vermis frequently exhibit abnormal development, but a precise prognosis is difficult to predict.
4. A large cisterna magna (> 10 mm) when isolated, usually has a good outcome.
5. Other cerebellar anomalies can be encountered, but the diagnosis is often difficult or impossible and the prognosis difficult to predict.

Abnormal sonographic findings of the posterior fossa are among the most common reasons for referral in tertiary care centers for fetal neuroimaging. They represent a major diagnostic challenge, and inaccurate interpretation with significant implications for counseling and management has been reported.[1,2] The problem is two fold: On the one hand, sonography is not an ideal tool for the visualization of the posterior fossa structures, particularly in the second trimester of gestation; on the other hand, many different entities, ranging from normal variants to severe anomalies, may have a similar sonographic appearance.[1–5] Categorization of these entities is still controversial, and there is no uniform approach.[2,6,7] In this chapter, we report our own vision of the problem and our own approach, which is summarized in Table 8–1.[4]

We stress that many difficulties are encountered in assessing antenatally this area of the brain and that frequently an accurate diagnosis cannot be made in utero.

## DANDY-WALKER COMPLEX

### Includes

Dandy-Walker malformation, vermian agenesis, vermian hypoplasia, Blake's pouch cyst

### Excludes

Megacisterna magna, Joubert and related cerebellar syndromes (vermian agenesis/hypoplasia with "molar tooth" sign)

### Definition and Classification

The term *Dandy-Walker syndrome,* subsequently modified to *Dandy-Walker malformation,* was originally introduced to indicate the association of (1) ventriculomegaly of variable degree, (2) a large cisterna magna with elevation of the tentorium, and (3) a defect in the cerebellar vermis through which the cyst communicates with the fourth ventricle.[8] The term *Dandy-Walker complex* (or *continuum*) was later introduced to indicate a spectrum of anomalies that also include other conditions with anatomical similarities to the classic description of Dandy-Walker malformation.[3,6] At present, the categorization of posterior fossa anomalies remains controversial, and there is no general consensus. We will include in this section three entities that share in common one sonographic finding: the impression that in an axial plane of the head the fourth ventricle is open posteriorly and communicates with the cisterna magna. In the following we will refer to this finding as the "open fourth ventricle." The anomalies that demonstrate this sign are heterogeneous and include the Blake's pouch cyst, vermian agenesis/hypoplasia, and Dandy-Walker malformation.[4] The rationale for grouping them together is that they are often difficult to differentiate, and they overlap clinically.

**Table 8–1. DIFFERENTIAL DIAGNOSIS OF CEREBELLAR DISORDERS**

| Diagnosis | TCD | Vermis Biometry | Superior/ Inferior Ratio | Fastigium | Fourth Ventricle | Pons | Prognosis |
|---|---|---|---|---|---|---|---|
| Delayed "closure" | N | N | N | N | Open | N | Good |
| Vermian hypoplasia | N | Small | N | N | Open/ closed | N | Variable |
| Vermian agenesis | N/S | Small | Abnormal | Abnormal | Abnormal | N | Malformations |
| Dandy-Walker malformation | N | –/Small | Abnormal | Abnormal | Abnormal | N | Poor |
| Joubert and related syndromes | N/S | –/Small | Abnormal | Abnormal | Abnormal | ? | Poor |
| Pontocerebellar hypoplasia | S | S | N | No | Normal | Abnormal | Poor |
| Rhombencephalosynapsis | S | – | – | Abnormal | Abnormal | N | Poor |

TCD, transverse cerebellar diameter; N, normal; S, small.
Modified from Malinger et al, 2009 with permission.[4]

## Incidence

Dandy-Walker malformation has an estimated prevalence of about 1 in 30,000 births and is found in 4% to 12% of all cases of infantile hydrocephaly.[9] The incidence of the other varieties of the Dandy-Walker complex is unknown.

## Pathogenesis

Different theories have been proposed. The element in common to the Dandy-Walker complex is an expansion of the fourth ventricle that displaces superiorly the cerebellar vermis. Prior to midgestation, the fourth ventricle is large, and the cerebellum does not cover it entirely. Only after 20 weeks does the cerebellum completely enfold the fourth ventricle. Many cases of the mildest anomaly in this group, the Blake's pouch cyst, resolve spontaneously throughout gestation and therefore probably represent a delay in normal anatomical development. In other cases, the expansion of the fourth ventricle is concomitant with aberrant development of the cerebellum, and of the vermis in particular, and these cases are more likely to be associated with neurologic compromise. The Dandy-Walker malformation was originally described in individuals with obstructive hydrocephaly and was postulated to arise from a primary atresia of the foramina of Luschka and Magendie.[8–10] A similar explanation was proposed for the Blake's pouch cyst.[11] It is now clear that most patients with the Dandy-Walker complex do not develop hydrocephaly, suggesting that the pathogenesis is more complex and is not merely the consequence of obstruction and overdistention of the fourth ventricle.[3,4,6,12,13] Several hypotheses have been formulated, but there is no clear evidence supporting any of them.

## Pathology

Blake described a normal embryological remain, a finger-like outpouch of the fourth ventricle, that is commonly found below the cerebellar vermis. This structure is now referred to as the Blake's pouch and can be sonographically demonstrated in most fetuses, particularly during the early second trimester.[14] Enlargement of the Blake's pouch (or of the entire fourth ventricle in the most severe forms) is responsible for the superior displacement of the vermis that is encountered in the Dandy-Walker complex. The enlarged Blake's pouch/fourth ventricle balloons into the cisterna magna and in the most severe cases obliterates it and distends the posterior fossa. With most techniques of diagnostic imaging, whether prenatal or postnatal, the thin walls of the Blake's pouch/fourth ventricle are difficult to visualize, and the impression is that of a communication between the fourth ventricle and the cisterna magna (Figure 8–1).

In this chapter, the term *Blake's pouch cyst* is reserved for cases in which the cisterna magna is not enlarged, and the cerebellar vermis is intact. Typically in these cases, the superior displacement is mild (Figure 8–2).[4,6,12,13]

*Vermian agenesis/hypoplasia* is characterized by a small vermis (Figure 8–3); the term *hypoplasia* should be reserved for cases in which the vermis is small but has a normal appearance (all the lobules are present); the term *partial agenesis* should indicate those cases in which a part, typically the most inferior portion, is absent. In these patients, the cisterna magna has a normal size. This condition was originally defined as Dandy-Walker variant, a term no longer in use.[7,15,16]

Dandy-Walker malformation is characterized by the enlargement of the cisterna magna, with elevation of the tentorium and torcular herophili. The cerebellar vermis

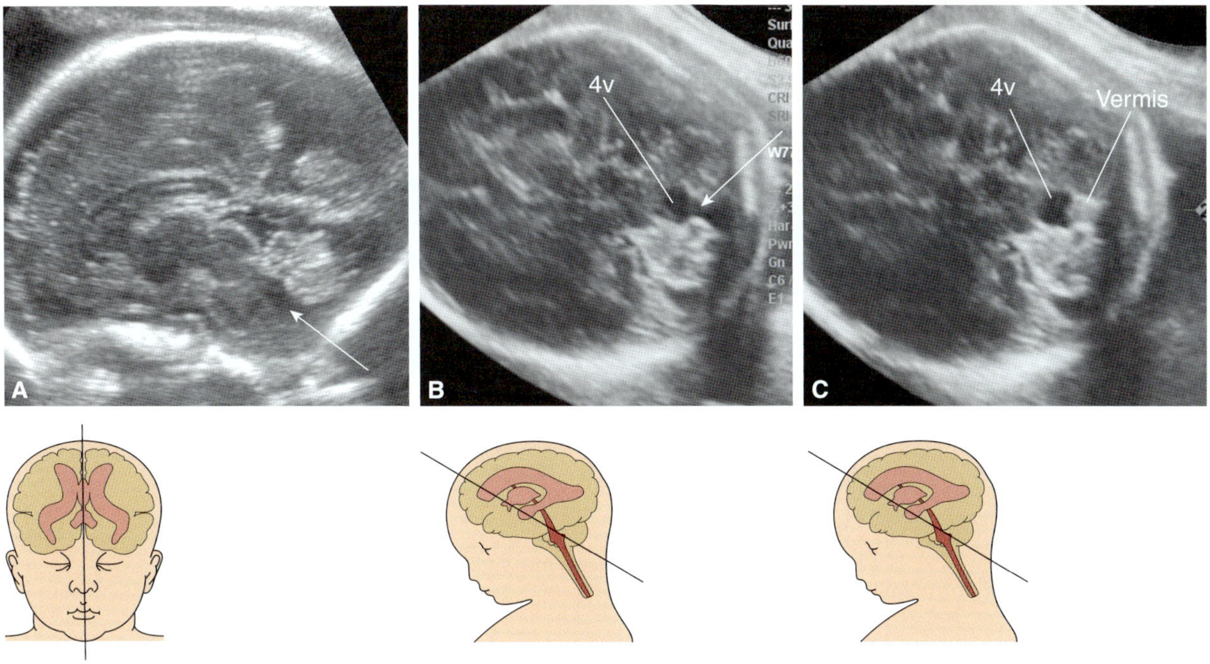


**Figure 8–1.** The open fourth ventricle sign. **(A)** A sagittal view demonstrates the slight superior rotation of the cerebellar vermis that results in the presence of a fluid between the brainstem and the inferior surface of the vermis (*arrow*). **(B)** A low axial section in the same case as A. The presence of fluid between the cerebellar hemispheres suggests communication between the fourth ventricle (4v) and the posterior cisterna magna (*arrow*). **(C)** In a slightly higher section, the vermis is seen closing the fourth ventricle posteriorly.

may be intact or incompletely formed but is usually significantly displaced upward (Figure 8–4). Hydrocephaly was classically considered an essential diagnostic element of this condition, but more recent evidence suggests that it is not present at birth in most patients, although it may develop in later life.[8,9]

## Etiology

Genetic factors have a major role in the etiology of the Dandy-Walker complex. Dandy-Walker malformation and vermian hypoplasia/agenesis may occur as a part of mendelian disorders and chromosomal aberrations.[17] In rare

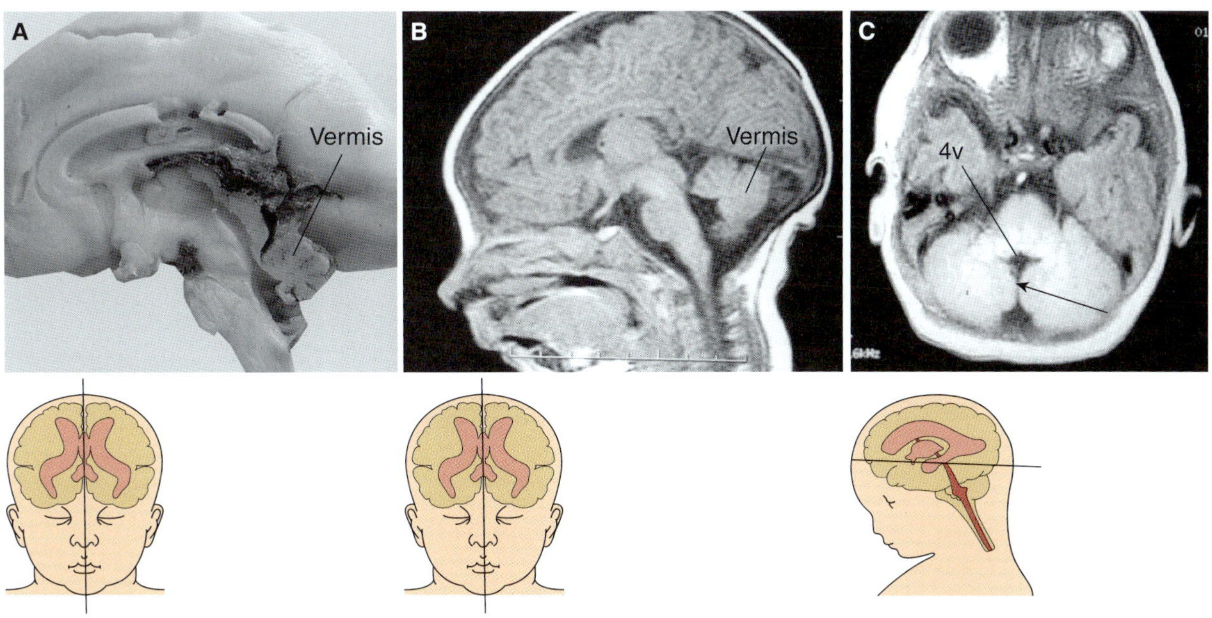


**Figure 8–2.** Blake's pouch cyst. **(A)** Pathologic specimen of a fetus at 20 weeks. An intact cerebellar vermis is slightly displaced superiorly; the thin walls of the Blake's pouch have been disrupted in the preparation of the specimen. **(B, C)** Magnetic resonance imaging (MRI) of a neonate; slight superior displacement of the vermis with the open fourth ventricle (4v) sign in the axial plane (*arrow*). (Reproduced, with permission, from the *Visual Encyclopedia of Ultrasound in Obstetrics and Gynecology*, International Society of Ultrasound in Obstetrics and Gynecology, 2010, www.isuog.org.)

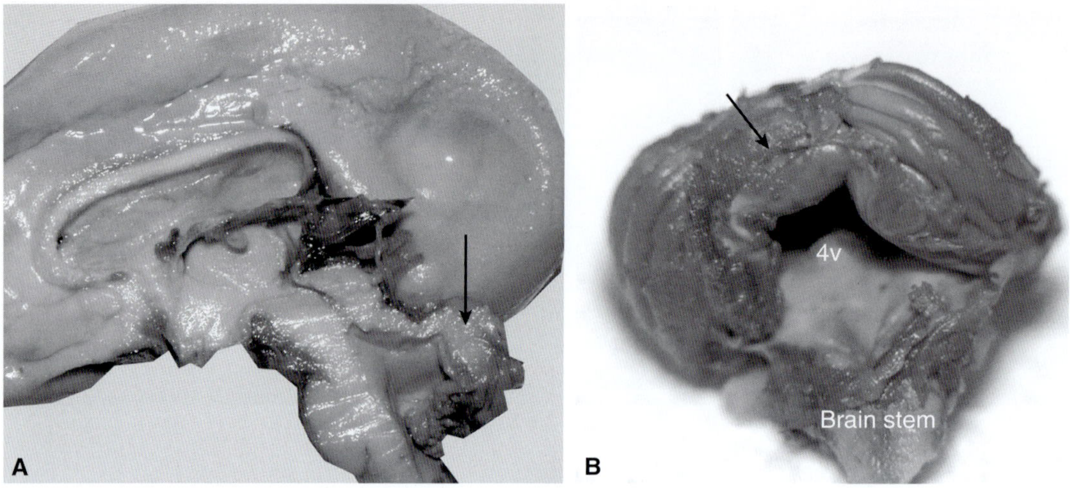


**Figure 8–3.** Vermian hypoplasia. **(A, B)** Pathologic specimens of two affected fetuses at midgestation. In both cases, the vermis (*arrow*) is superiorly displaced and appears small and rudimentary with no evidence of lobulation. There is a prominent aditus to the fourth ventricle (4v). As in the previous figures, the thin walls of the Blake's pouch have been disrupted in the preparation of the specimen. (Reproduced, with permission, from the *Visual Encyclopedia of Ultrasound in Obstetrics and Gynecology,* International Society of Ultrasound in Obstetrics and Gynecology, 2010, www.isuog.org.)

cases, the disease is inherited as an autosomal recessive or dominant trait. Environmental factors, including viral infections, alcohol abuse, and diabetes, have also been suggested as playing a role in the genesis of Dandy-Walker malformation, but the evidence is uncertain.[17]

## Recurrence Risk

In the absence of a recognizable syndrome, a recurrence risk of 1% to 5% is suggested for Dandy-Walker malformation and vermian hypoplasia/agenesis.[17] Autosomal transmission, both dominant and recessive, has been documented. There is no available information on Blake's pouch cyst.

## Associated Anomalies

The Dandy-Walker complex (particularly Dandy Walker malformation and vermian hypoplasia/agenesis) is frequently associated with chromosomal aberrations, syndromes and other cerebral malformations (mostly ventriculomegaly, agenesis of the corpus callosum, holoprosencephaly, and cephaloceles), polycystic kidneys, cardiovascular defects, and facial clefting.[15,18,19] Postnatal studies of infants with the classic type of Dandy-Walker malformation indicate a frequency of associated malformation ranging from 50% to 70%.[8–10] A detailed list of conditions found in association with Dandy-Walker malformation is given in Table 8–2.

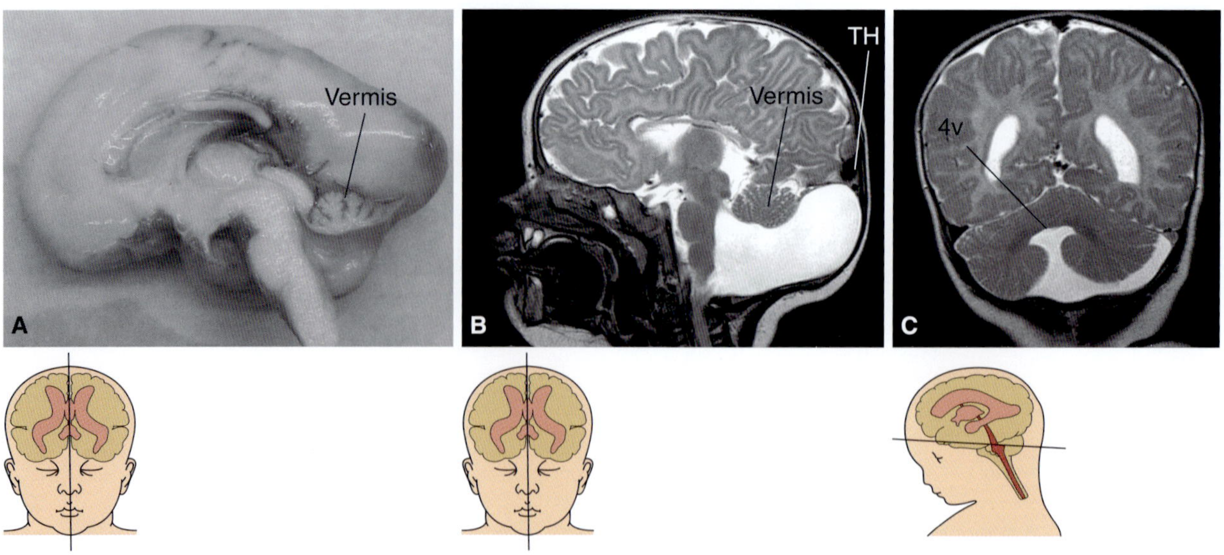


**Figure 8–4.** Dandy-Walker malformation. **(A)** Pathologic specimen from a midtrimester fetus. **(B, C)** MRI of an affected infant. There is a major displacement of the vermis that forms a right angle to the brain stem and the cisterna magna is enlarged; the tentorium cerebellii and the torcular herophili (TH) are displaced cranially as well. The fourth ventricle (4v) appears open. (Reproduced, with permission, from the *Visual Encyclopedia of Ultrasound in Obstetrics and Gynecology,* International Society of Ultrasound in Obstetrics and Gynecology, 2010, www.isuog.org.)

**Table 8–2. ABNORMALITIES ASSOCIATED WITH DANDY-WALKER MALFORMATION**

| Mendelian | Environmental |
|---|---|
| Warburg (AR) | Rubella |
| Aase-Smith (AD) | Coumadin |
| Ruvalcaba syndrome (AD/X-linked) | Alcohol |
| Coffin-Siris (AR) | Cytomegalovirus |
| Orofaciodigital syndrome type II (AR) | Diabetes |
| Meckel-Gruber syndrome (AR) | Isotretinoin |
| Aicardi syndrome (X-linked dominant) | **Multifactorial** |
| Ellis-Van Creveld (AR) | Congenital heart disease |
| Fraser cryptophthalmus (AR) | Neural tube defects |
| **Chromosomal** | Cleft lip/palate |
| 45, X | **Sporadic** |
| 6p– | Holoprosencephaly |
| 9q+ | Cornelia de Lange syndrome |
| Dup 5p | Goldenhar syndrome |
| Dup 8p | Kidney abnormalities |
| Dup 8q | Facial hemangiomas |
| Trisomy 9 | Klippel-Feil syndrome |
| Triploidy | Polysyndactyly |
| Dup 17q | |

AD, autosomal dominant; AR, autosomal recessive.

Modified from Murray et al, 1985.[17]

## Diagnosis

The landmark of the Dandy-Walker complex is the open fourth ventricle. This is demonstrated by sweeping the transducer in the posterior fossa along the axial plane and visualizing a fluid-filled tract connecting the cavity of the fourth ventricle to the cisterna magna (see Figure 8–1).[5,6,13,19] In early gestation, this is a normal finding, as the developing cerebellar vermis has not yet completely enfolded the fourth ventricle.[20,21] It is therefore imprudent to make a diagnosis of the Dandy-Walker complex at this gestational age, with the possible exception of those (rare) cases in which there is an obvious cystic enlargement of the cisterna magna or other abnormal findings.[22] After 20 weeks, the vermis has normally "closed" the fourth ventricle; therefore, the demonstration of an opening is indicative of the Dandy-Walker complex.[15,21]

The varieties of the Dandy-Walker complex have much different prognostic implications An alarmingly high rate of erroneous diagnoses was reported in one series in which only axial transabdominal sonography had been used;[1] this prompted a number of studies that have now established a systematic approach to the diagnosis involving multiplanar examinations possibly aided by magnetic resonance imaging (MRI).[3,4,6,13,14] It is now well accepted that a specific diagnosis requires assessment of the vermis (absent, hypoplastic, or intact) and the torcular herophili (normal position or elevated).[3,6,7] The evaluation of these findings is difficult and involves an element of subjectivity. There is potential for misinterpretation, particularly in early gestation, but an expert examiner using either sonography or MRI (or both) is able to make a precise diagnosis in the majority of cases.[3,4]

To assess the presence of the vermis, the best approach is to sweep the transducer in the posterior fossa along the axial plane. The vermis appears as an oval echogenic structure interposed between the fourth ventricle and the cisterna magna (see Figure 8–1). When this is not seen, and the area of the fourth ventricle is seen to communicate with the cisterna magna at any level, vermian agenesis can be inferred.

To assess the integrity of the vermis and the position of the torcular herophili, a median view is required. This can be obtained directly by multiplanar imaging, preferably through the posterior fontanelle, as this allows better visualization of the posterior fossa and brainstem. Three-dimensional ultrasound (3D US) can also be utilized.[12,23] Indeed, one of the major shortcomings in the median view is the difficulty to obtain with absolute precision the exact plane of section and to confuse the cerebellar hemispheres with the vermis. The advantage of 3D US is the ability to control the sections using as reference the orthogonal planes. The use of volume contrast imaging may also facilitate visualization of subtle anatomical details.[12,23] Once the vermis has been identified in the median plane, both a qualitative and a quantitative evaluation should be performed. It has been suggested that if the posterior apex (fastigium) of the fourth ventricle and the two main fissures of the vermis can be identified, the vermis is presumably intact.[3,6,12,23–25] The secondary fissure is at times difficult to define in early gestation, and a semiquantitative approach can be used alternatively (normally, twice as much vermis is found below rather than above the primary fissure).[6] Measurements of the fetal cerebellar vermis have been reported.[26,27] Most cases of defective vermis involve agenesis of the caudal portion; therefore, the vertical diameter is probably the most relevant one. A small vermis with an abnormal configuration (absence of fastigium and/or fissure) indicates partial agenesis. Conversely, a small vermis with a normal configuration indicates hypoplasia.[27] In practice, the distinction between these two entities in the fetus is difficult.

A word of caution is needed regarding the possibility of obtaining a truly, apparently normal median plane by

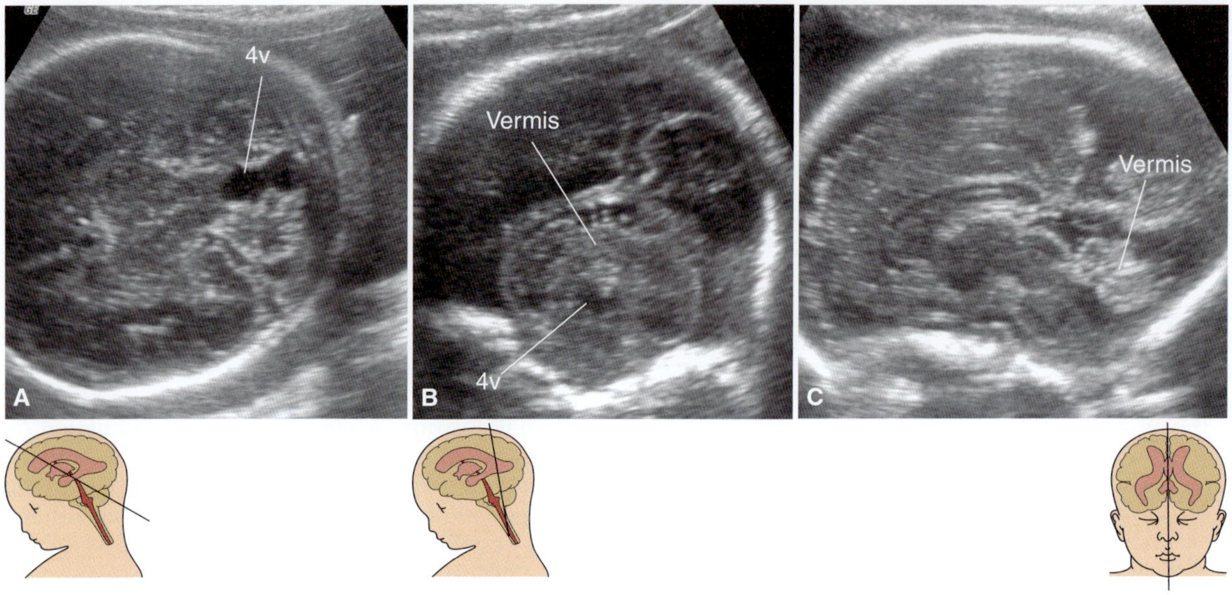


**Figure 8–5.** Sonography of Blake's pouch cyst. **(A)** An axial scan demonstrates an open fourth ventricle (4v). **(B)** A coronal scan reveals that the vermis is present. **(C)** A sagittal scan demonstrates a seemingly intact and slightly rotated vermis. The cisterna magna is not enlarged. Downslanting of the tentorium suggests a normal insertion of the torcular herophili. (Reproduced, with permission, from the *Visual Encyclopedia of Ultrasound in Obstetrics and Gynecology*, International Society of Ultrasound in Obstetrics and Gynecology, 2010, www.isuog.org.)

two-dimensional (2D) or 3D US in a fetus with complete vermian agenesis as the cerebellar hemispheres may be displaced into the midline and be in contact with each other. In these patients, the coronal plane may be used to demonstrate that the vermis is absent and that the folia are abnormally oriented.[27,28]

Normally, the tentorium has a posterior inclination of roughly 45°, and the torcular herophili is implanted in the inner skull at the same level of neck muscles. In our experience, MRI is usually more effective than sonography in identifying the torcular herophili. The nuchal region is usually poorly visualized with US in the median plane because of acoustic shadowing, and one has to rely on the direction of the tentorium. A posterior inclination suggests a normal position, a horizontal direction, or a superior displacement. Upward dislocation of the tentorium indicates indirectly an enlargement of the cisterna magna that is usually found to exceed a depth of 10 mm.[29,30] MRI has been advocated by many for the assessment of any cerebellar malformation identified with sonography.[31]

The Blake's pouch cyst, which is by far the most frequent variety encountered prenatally, features an upward rotation of the cerebellar vermis (usually a slight one, <45°). The cerebellar vermis, cisterna magna, and torcular herophili are in a normal position (Figures 8–5 and 8–6).[3,6,12,14] Vermian hypoplasia/partial agenesis is identified by an upward displacement of a small vermis, whereas the cisterna magna and torcular herophili are normal (Figure 8–7).[4,31] The landmark of the Dandy-Walker malformation is the large cisterna magna and the consequent superior displacement of the torcular herophili. The vermis is always significantly rotated superiorly (≥45°) and may be either normal or defective (Figures 8–8 and 8–9).[4,6,7,16,24,25]

It has been suggested that the shape of the opening of the fourth ventricle in the axial plane is relevant for the differential diagnosis of the different varieties of the Dandy-Walker complex.[18] Also in our experience, an

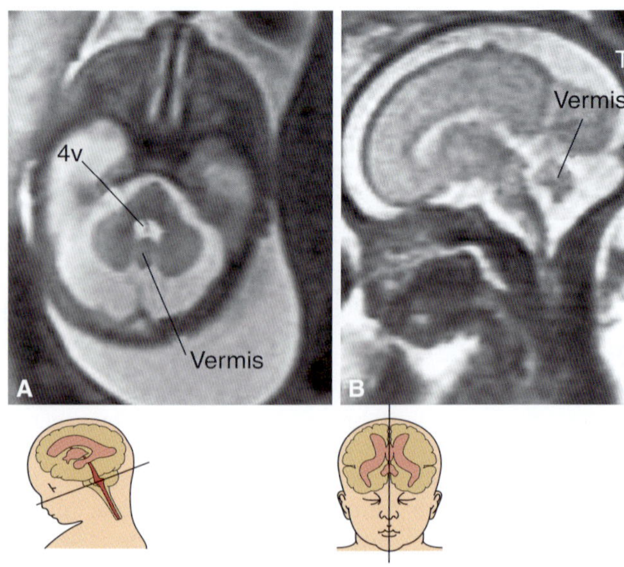


**Figure 8–6.** MRI of Blake's pouch cyst. When compared with the sonograms in the previous figures that were obtained from the same fetus, the most important contribution of MRI is the clear demonstration of the torcular herophili (TH) that is normally inserted. (Reproduced, with permission, from *Atlas of Obstetric Ultrasound*, 2009. The Global Library of Women's Medicine. www.glowm.com.)

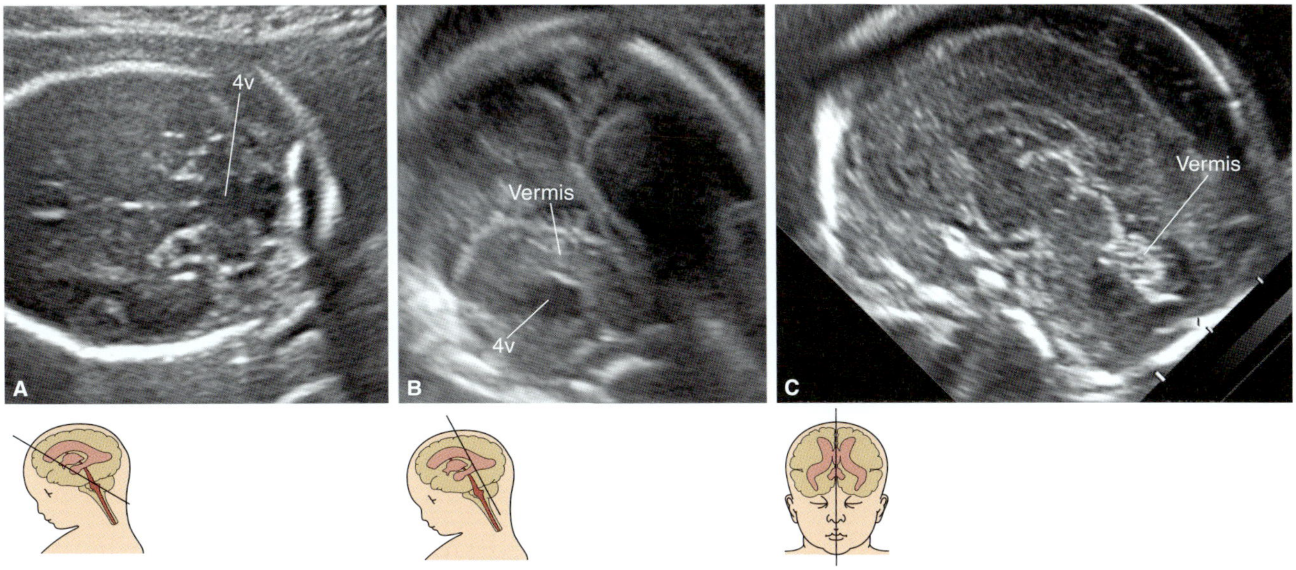


**Figure 8–7.** Sonography of vermian hypoplasia. The fourth ventricle (4v) is open; the vermis is present but is about half the normal size and does not demonstrate any of the typical anatomical landmarks, the fastigium point and the main fissures. The cisterna magna is not enlarged. Downslanting of the tentorium suggests a normal insertion of the torcular herophili (TH). (Reproduced, with permission, from *Atlas of Obstetric Ultrasound,* 2009. The Global Library of Women's Medicine. www.glowm.com.)

hourglass opening ("buttock" sign) is typical of the Blake's pouch. A triangular or square-shaped opening is indicative of either vermian hypoplasia or Dandy-Walker malformation (see Figures 8–5, 8–7, and 8–8).

Other cerebral anomalies, including ventriculomegaly and agenesis of the corpus callosum, can be found, particularly with vermian hypoplasia/partial agenesis and Dandy-Walker malformation. Most frequently, a Blake's pouch cyst is an isolated finding.[12,13,32]

## Differential Diagnosis

The Dandy-Walker complex should be differentiated from other cystic anomalies of the posterior fossa. In cases of megacisterna magna, the cisterna magna is large, but the cerebellum is intact, and the fourth ventricle is triangular and closed.[3,4,6,12] Cerebellar hypoplasia results in an ex vacuo large cisterna magna,[33] but the main feature of the condition is a global reduction in the size of an otherwise

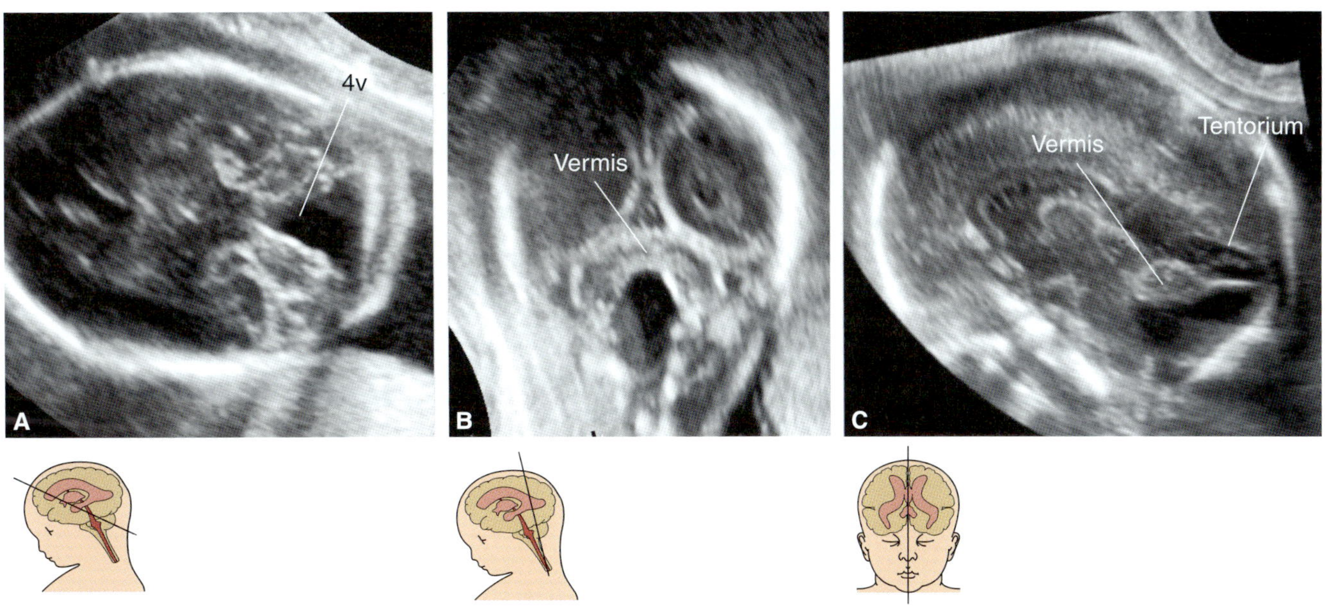


**Figure 8–8.** Sonography of Dandy-Walker malformation showing an open fourth ventricle (4v), enlarged cisterna magna, superior rotation of the small dysmorphicvermis, and cranial displacement of the tentorium. (Reproduced, with permission, from the *Visual Encyclopedia of Ultrasound in Obstetrics and Gynecology,* International Society of Ultrasound in Obstetrics and Gynecology, 2010, www.isuog.org.)

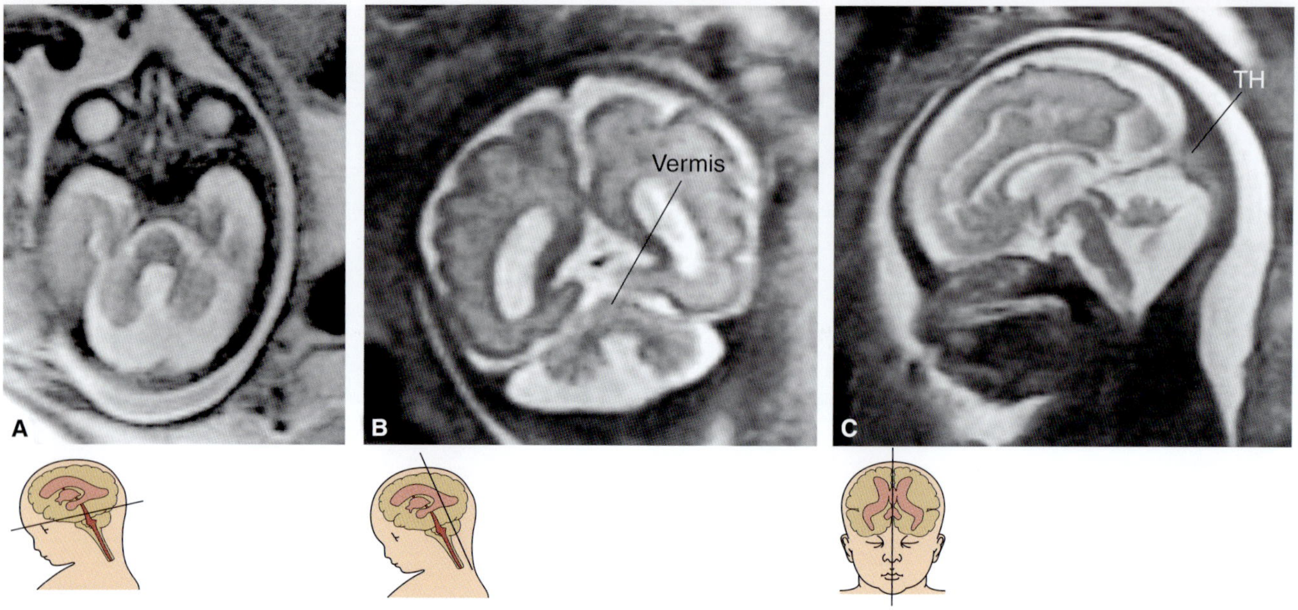


**Figure 8–9.** MRI of fetal Dandy-Walker malformation. The information is similar to that provided with ultrasound in Figure 8–8. There is a better demonstration of the high-riding tentorium and torcular herophili (TH). (Reproduced, with permission, from the *Visual Encyclopedia of Ultrasound in Obstetrics and Gynecology,* International Society of Ultrasound in Obstetrics and Gynecology, 2010, www.isuog.org.)

normally shaped cerebellum[4] (Figure 8–10). Arachnoid cysts growing in the posterior fossa have a mass effect and cause asymmetrical distortion of the cerebellum or pressure on the vermis, resulting in flattening of its dorsal border and in severe cases compression of the aqueduct and ventriculomegaly[34] (Figure 8–11). The greatest difficulty encountered is posterior fossa hemorrhage, which results at times in destruction of the cerebellar vermis and enlargement of the cisterna magna, mimicking very closely a Dandy-Walker malformation or vermian hypoplasia (Figure 8–12).[35]

## Implications for Targeted Examination

The Dandy-Walker complex has genetic implications, and sonography is usually offered to couples at risk. Although the most severe forms of this condition can be recognized as early as 14 weeks,[22] caution is necessary because of

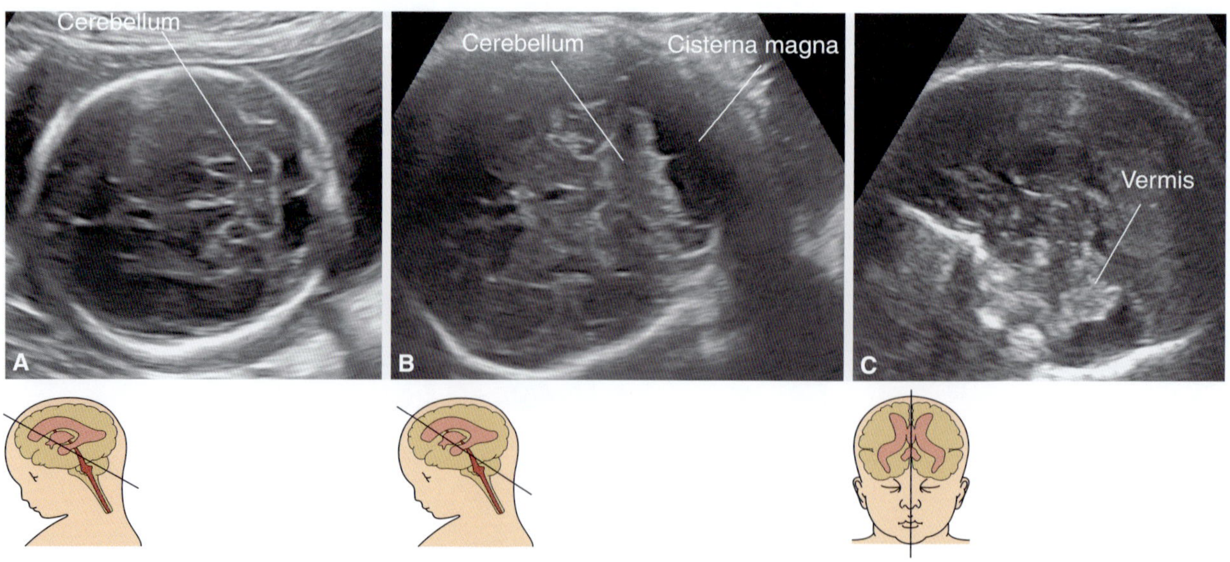


**Figure 8–10.** Sonography of cerebellar hypoplasia. **(A)** Second trimester fetus with multiple anomalies. The cerebellum has a normal shape, but the transverse diameter is about –3 standard deviations (SDs) from the mean. **(B, C)** Third trimester fetus with severe cerebellar hypoplasia. The transverse cerebellar diameter is below –4 SDs from the mean, and the cisterna magna is enlarged ex vacuo. (Reproduced, with permission, from the *Visual Encyclopedia of Ultrasound in Obstetrics and Gynecology,* International Society of Ultrasound in Obstetrics and Gynecology, 2010, www.isuog.org.)

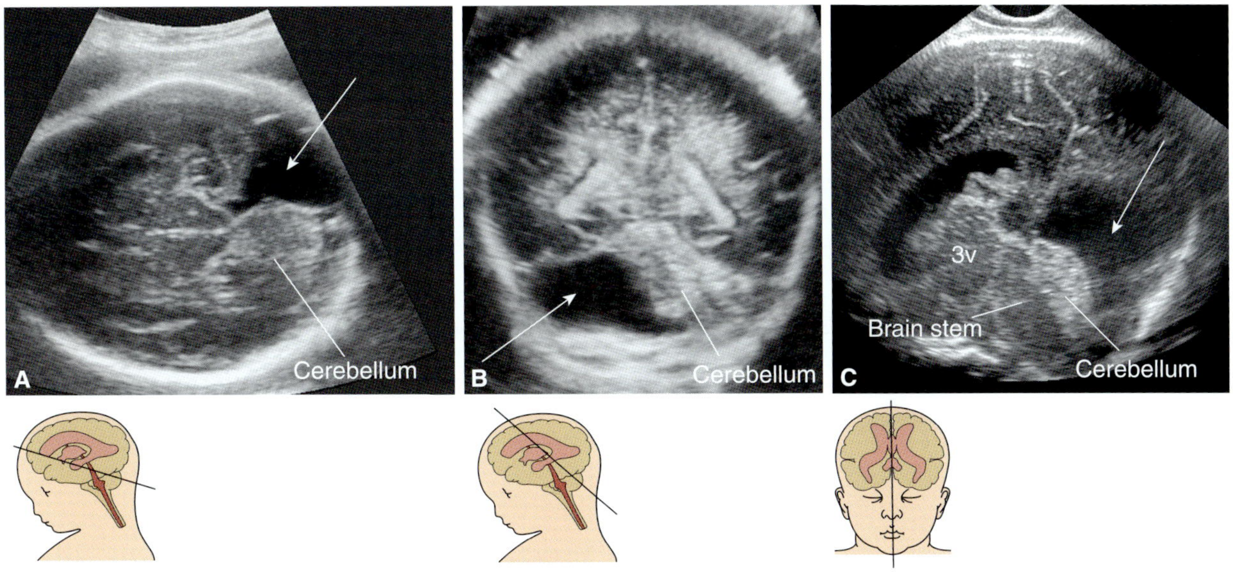


**Figure 8–11.** Sonography of a posterior fossa arachnoid cyst. **(A, B)** The cerebellum is displaced laterally by a fluid collection (*arrow*). **(C)** A cyst is interposed between the tentorium and the surface of the cerebellum (*arrow*) (3v, third ventricle). (Reproduced, with permission, from the *Visual Encyclopedia of Ultrasound in Obstetrics and Gynecology*, International Society of Ultrasound in Obstetrics and Gynecology, 2010, www.isuog.org.)

the ambiguous images caused by the incomplete development of the cerebellum at this gestational age.[20,21] We recommend limiting the diagnosis of Dandy-Walker complex to those cases in which either a very large cisterna magna or other abnormal findings are encountered. In the midtrimester, it is stressed that the transcerebellar view only demonstrates the superior part of the vermis and therefore is not sufficient to rule out the Dandy-Walker complex. A lower scan is required to demonstrate the "closure" of the inferior vermis.[4,12,23,36] In cases at risk, a median view should be obtained as well.[4,23,36] Couples should be informed that false-negative and false-positive cases have been reported and that an antenatal diagnosis is not possible in all cases, particularly with minor anatomical alterations.

## Implications for Sonographic Screening

In the midtrimester, a cisterna magna measuring > 10 mm[30,37] and/or an "open" fourth ventricle[5,19,38] alert to the possibility of Dandy-Walker complex. The transcerebellar view, which is recommended as part of the standard sonographic examination of the fetal brain,[29] will not detect all cases of Dandy-Walker complex.

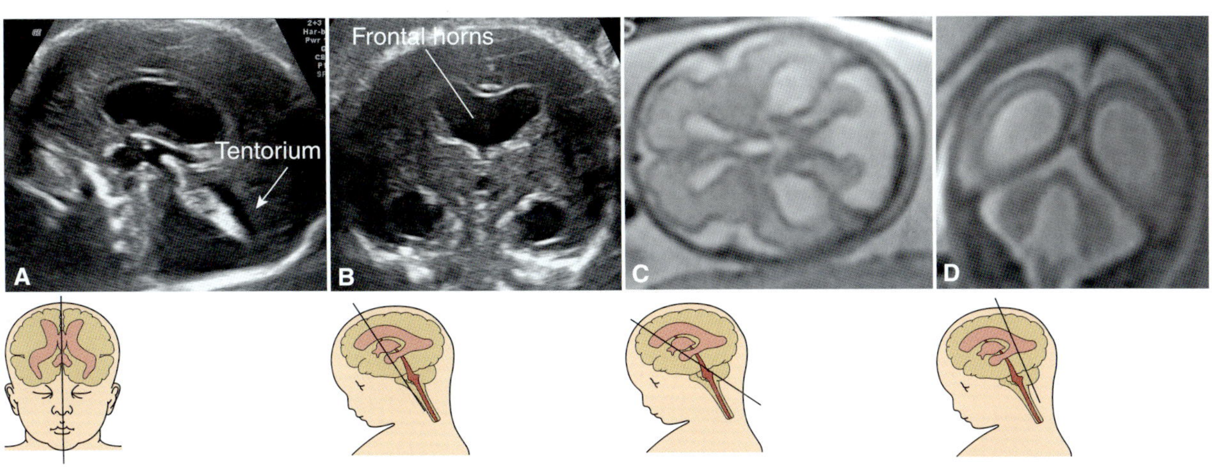


**Figure 8–12.** In this third trimester fetus, the association of severe ventriculomegaly, open fourth ventricle, small rotated vermis, and communication of the frontal horns had prompted the diagnosis of Dandy-Walker malformation associated with obstructive hydrocephaly and possibly a telencephalic malformation. After birth autopsy demonstrated the sequelae of a posterior fossa hemorrhage with secondary hydrocephaly and disruption of the septum pellucidum. In retrospect, the normal insertion of the tentorium was in contrast with the diagnosis of Dandy-Walker malformation. (Reproduced, with permission, from the *Visual Encyclopedia of Ultrasound in Obstetrics and Gynecology*, International Society of Ultrasound in Obstetrics and Gynecology, 2010, www.isuog.org.)

## Prognosis

Neurosurgical series that report the combination of Dandy-Walker malformation and hydrocephaly describe abnormal neurologic development in 40% to 70% of survivors.[8–10]

Dandy-Walker malformation is also part of many genetic syndromes, with a wide spectrum of outcomes. The clinical significance of Dandy-Walker malformation without ventriculomegaly is debated.[39] It would seem, however, that the neurologic outcome is mainly related to the appearance of the cerebellar vermis.[20,30,39] When this is of normal size and morphology, a normal development has been reported in 85% of cases. Conversely, when the vermis is abnormally lobulated, and/or there are associated cerebral anomalies, the prognosis is poor.[24,25]

Vermian hypoplasia/agenesis is also frequently part of multiple anomalies and genetic syndromes. When isolated, it may be asymptomatic, but precise risk figures are not available.[31,39]

Despite small series in the pediatric literature in which Blake's pouch cyst has been found in association with obstructive hydrocephaly,[11,40] cases diagnosed prenatally have in general a good outcome and tend to undergo intrauterine remission.[5,12–14,39] In our experience, associated anomalies, including chromosomal aberrations, are not infrequent. Indeed, in our own, albeit limited experience, the main difference between the three varieties of Dandy-Walker complex depends mostly on the rate of associated anomalies. Isolated cases usually have a good outcome.

## Obstetric Management

The diagnostic workup must include a detailed search for associated anomalies, including karyotyping. In counseling couples, it is stressed that any of these anomalies can have a good outcome when isolated and that Blake's pouch cyst is most frequently a normal variant. Serial scans are suggested because of the potential for cerebral maldevelopment, including ventriculomegaly. With the exception of those cases associated with hydrocephaly and macrocrania that may require cesarean delivery,[19] no modification of the standard obstetric management is indicated.

# MEGACISTERNA MAGNA

## Excludes

Dandy-Walker complex, cerebellarhypoplasia

## Definition

A large cisterna magna, in the absence of cerebellar anomalies

## Incidence

Unknown. If the obstetric definition of cisterna magna is used (a depth ≥10 mm in fetuses at 20–40 weeks' gestation),[29,30,37] a prevalence of ~2% is expected.

## Etiology, Pathogenesis, and Pathology

This condition is most frequently recognized by diagnostic imaging (Figure 8–13), and pathologic data are scant. It has been suggested that the enlargement of the cisterna magna may be secondary to a distention of the Blake's pouch that does not displace the cerebellar vermis.[14]

## Associated Anomalies

Megacisterna magna is usually an isolated finding. When the diagnosis is made in fetal life, an association with trisomy 18 has been reported.[37] This, however, may represent the consequence of cerebellar hypoplasia, which is seen frequently in these cases, rather than a primary enlargement.[33]

## Diagnosis

Megacisterna magna was originally described in postnatal patients using purely subjective criteria. In the obstetric literature, the term has been used to indicate cases with a cisterna magna depth in excess of 2 standard deviations (SDs) above the mean, or 10 mm (Figures 8–14 and 8–15).[30,37] The definition is now well established.[29] However, there is most likely a discrepancy between the classic postnatal radiologic definition of the condition (that identifies a rare finding) and the obstetric one (that implies a prevalence of ~2.5%). Indeed, most fetuses with a prenatal diagnosis of megacisterna magna are found to be normal after birth. The value of the obstetric definition

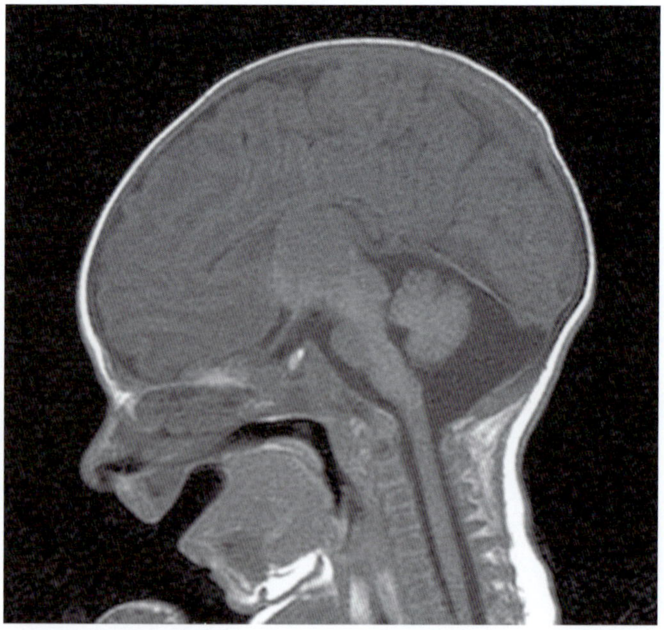

**Figure 8–13.** In the late second trimester, the depth of the cisterna magna of this infant was found to be in excess of 4 SDs above the mean. It progressively diminished in size, and at birth it was found to be only at the upper limit of normal by the neuroradiologist who performed this scan. The infant had a normal neurologic and intellectual postnatal follow-up. (Reproduced, with permission, from the *Visual Encyclopedia of Ultrasound in Obstetrics and Gynecology*, International Society of Ultrasound in Obstetrics and Gynecology, 2010, www.isuog.org.)

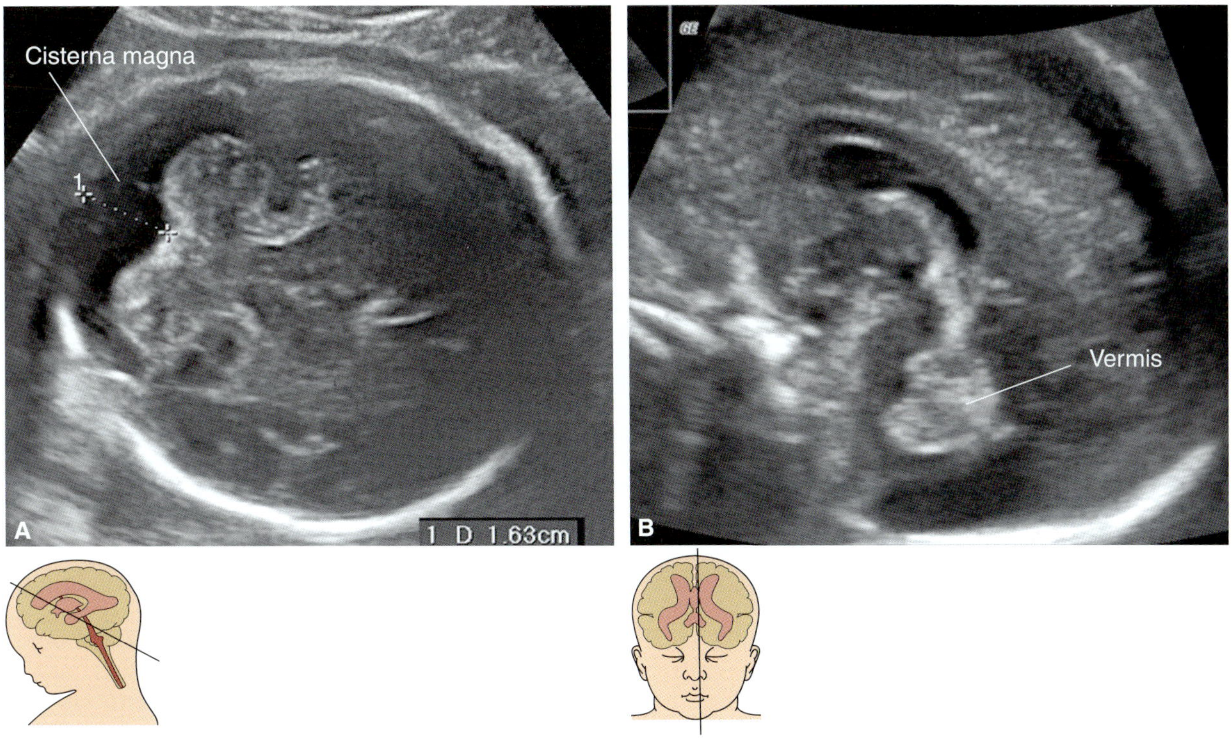


**Figure 8–14.** Sonography of megacisterna magna at 30 weeks' gestation (same case as in Figure 8–12). (Reproduced, with permission, from the *Visual Encyclopedia of Ultrasound in Obstetrics and Gynecology,* International Society of Ultrasound in Obstetrics and Gynecology, 2010, www.isuog.org.)

appears to be the identification of a generic risk factor for associated anomalies.

## Differential Diagnosis

This condition should be differentiated from the Dandy-Walker complex (which is characterized by an open fourth ventricle) (see Figure 8–1), cerebellar hypoplasia (small cerebellum) (Figure 8–10), and posterior fossa arachnoid cysts (mass effect with asymmetric distortion of the cerebellum) (Figure 8–11).

## Prognosis

In the absence of associated anomalies, the prognosis is good.[39] The largest antenatal series thus far available

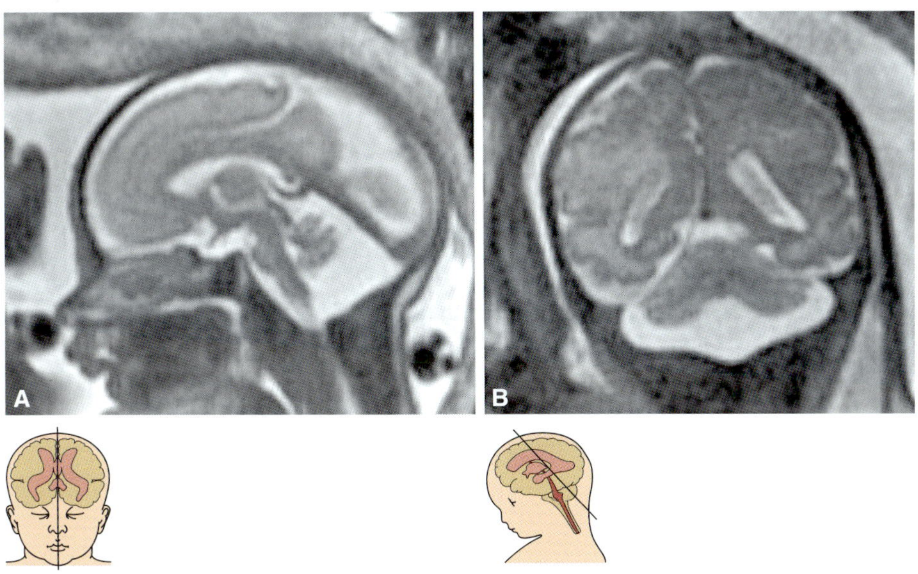


**Figure 8–15.** MRI of a neonatal megacisterna magna. (Reproduced, with permission, from the *Visual Encyclopedia of Ultrasound in Obstetrics and Gynecology,* International Society of Ultrasound in Obstetrics and Gynecology, 2010, www.isuog.org.)

does suggest that these infants may be at a slightly increased risk of mild developmental delay.[41] However, severe neurologic complications are rarely encountered. Indeed, megacisterna magna is frequently an incidental finding in radiologic examinations performed after birth.

### Obstetric Management

Other than the need for a detailed US scan, no modification of standard obstetric management is indicated. It remains uncertain whether fetal karyotyping is indicated. It would seem that the risk is only increased for trisomy 18, which is unlikely to result in a completely normal sonogram (Figure 8–16).

## CEREBELLAR HYPOPLASIA/ATROPHY

### Excludes

Dandy-Walker malformation, megacisterna magna, unilateral cerebellar hemisphere hypoplasia

### Definition

A small cerebellum

### Incidence

Rare

### Etiology and Pathogenesis

Variable. Cerebellar hypoplasia or atrophy may be the consequence of many different processes, including acquired lesions.[42] In our experience, it is usually found either in the context of multiple anomalies or as a consequence of pontocerebellar hypoplasia. This is a group of neurodegenerative disorders featured by the concomitance of cerebellar and brainstem hypoplasia with autosomal recessive transmission. Different types exist, and they usually develop either postnatally or in late gestation[43,44] (Table 8–3).

### Pathology

*Hypoplasia* refers to a morphologically normal but small cerebellum; *atrophy* refers to inadequate growth of the cerebellum with a progressive increase in the size of the fissures in comparison to the size of the foliae.[4] Differentiation of these two rare entities prenatally is probably impossible.

### Diagnosis

Hypoplasia of the cerebellum, with a secondary increase in the size of the cisterna magna, may be obvious, particularly in late gestation (Figures 8–10 and 8–17). Associated cerebral anomalies, including microcephaly and cortical malformations, may be present. The association with a thin brainstem that does not display the typical protrusion of the pons is indicative of pontocerebellar hypoplasia.[4] Normative data of the fetal pons have been published.[26] In our own experience, however, the diagnosis is more easily made using MRI (Figure 8–18).

Polyhydramnios, fetal paralysis, and seizures may be present. Particularly in early gestation, the diagnosis is extremely difficult or impossible. In at least one of our cases, the cerebellum had a normal appearance and dimensions at 20 weeks, and the condition could only be demonstrated in late gestation. Even in familial cases with

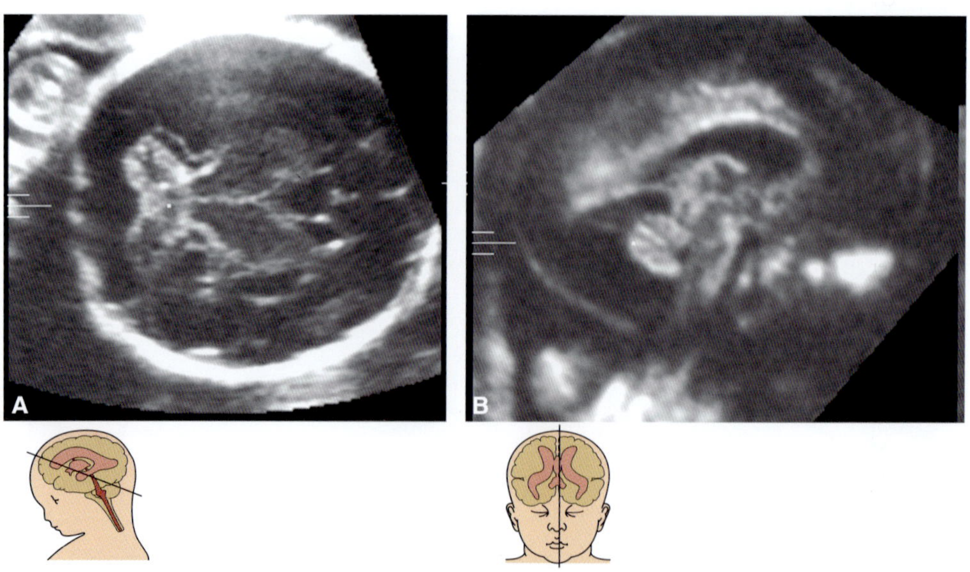


**Figure 8–16.** Megacisterna magna in a fetus with trisomy 18. The head appears round, the cavum septi pellucidi is enlarged, the vermis has an unusual appearance, and multiple extracranial anomalies were present. (Reproduced, with permission, from *Atlas of Obstetric Ultrasound,* 2009. The Global Library of Women's Medicine, www.glowm.com.)

**Table 8–3. PONTOCEREBELLAR HYPOPLASIAS: DIFFERENTIAL DIAGNOSIS OF THE THREE MOST COMMON TYPES**

| | Type 1 | Type 2 | Type 4 |
|---|---|---|---|
| **Presentation at birth** | | | |
| Polyhydramnios | +/– | Rare | +/– |
| Jitteriness, clonus | – | + | ++ |
| Muscle stiffness | – | – | ++ |
| Respiratory insufficiency | +/– | Rare | + |
| **Follow-up findings** | | | |
| Microcephaly | + | + | + |
| Gross delay of all milestones | + | + | + |
| Spinal anterior horn involvement | + | – | – |
| Chorea or spasticity | – | + | – |
| **Main findings at autopsy** | | | |
| Pontocerebellar hypoplasia | + | + | + |
| Regressive neuronal changes | + | + | + |
| Demyelination | – | – | – |
| Spinal anterior horn cells affected | + | – | – |
| Genes affected | Unknown | tRNA endonuclease subunit TSEN54; less frequently TSEN2, TSEN3 | TSEN54 |

Modified from Barth P. Pontocerebellar hypoplasia. In: Gilman S, editor-in-chief. MedLink Neurology. San Diego: MedLink Corporation. Available at http://www.medlink.com. Republished by permission.

an increased risk of recurrence, the diagnosis may be very difficult or even impossible during pregnancy.

Cerebellar hypoplasia is a rare condition, and it is unclear which is the optimal quantitative threshold to make this diagnosis. Most growth curves of the cerebellum report the 90% prediction interval,[45,46] and certainly the 5th centile is not a reasonable cutoff to use, as it would include a disproportionate number of normal fetuses. The most difficult clinical problem is certainly represented by second trimester fetuses with borderline measurement. The available experience is limited to a handful of cases diagnosed in utero, and providing risk estimates is impossible. It is likely, however, that most cases will not be positively identified in early gestation.

## Implications for Sonographic Screening

Most cases of cerebellar hypoplasia tend to develop throughout gestation, and we anticipate that it will be impossible to recognize them in utero, particularly in early gestation. The identification of a small or borderline cerebellum in a fetus represents a diagnostic dilemma. The available experience does not allow for establishing an optimal quantitative cutoff. A reasonable approach is to use −2 SD from the mean (2.5th centile). A careful search for associated anomalies, including the visualization of the brainstem, is indicated in these cases.

## Implication for Sonographic Diagnosis

Cerebellar hypoplasia should be suspected when a small cerebellum is seen, usually with an ex vacuo enlargement of the cisterna magna.[33] In borderline cases, polyhydramnios, other cerebral anomalies, and abnormal fetal movements, including contractures and seizure activity, increase the index of suspicion. It is important to stress that cerebellar hypoplasia is frequently evolutive, and sonographic diagnosis may fail particularly in early gestation. Follow-up examinations in patients with a familial history or with apparently small cerebellums during second trimester routine examinations seem indicated. Genetic testing is available for some of the conditions associated with cerebellar hypoplasia, and it should be considered in pregnancies at risk.[44]

## Prognosis

In general, prognosis is poor. Most fetuses we have diagnosed in utero died in the early postnatal period.[39,43,44] One exception was the case of a fetus with cerebellar hypoplasia from a mother who had cerebellar hypoplasia herself and moderate mental retardation. The infant survived and is doing well.

## Obstetric Management

When the diagnosis is made within the temporal limits of voluntary pregnancy termination, this can be offered to the couples. We recommend storing fetal DNA for subsequent analysis, as cerebellar hypoplasia is frequently part of genetic conditions with a high recurrence rate.

# RHOMBENCEPHALOSYNAPSIS

## Excludes

Dandy-Walker complex, vermian agenesis

## Definition

Fusion of the cerebellar hemispheres with vermian agenesis

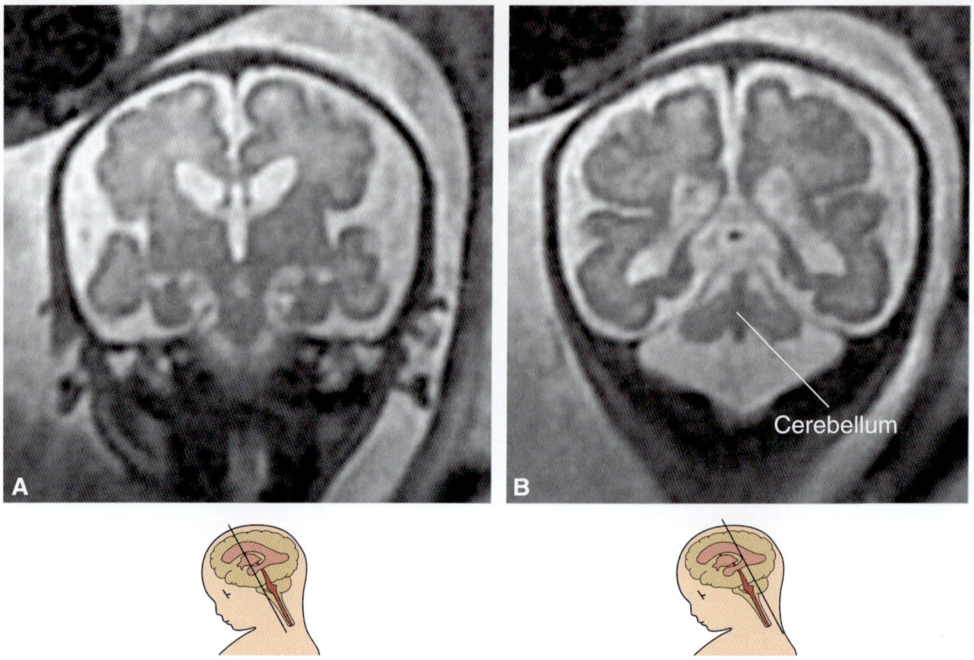


**Figure 8–17.** **(A, B)** Magnetic resonance of cerebellar hypoplasia, same case of the Figure 8–10 **(B, C)**. The cisterna magna is enlarged *ex vacuo*, as well as the entire subarachnoid space. (Reproduced, with permission, from the *Visual Encyclopedia of Ultrasound in Obstetrics and Gynecology,* International Society of Ultrasound in Obstetrics and Gynecology, 2010, www.isuog.org.)

## Etiopathogenesis

The formation and development of the midline portion of the cerebellum is thought to be controlled by the "isthmic organizer," a band of neuroepithelium that is located between the mesencephalon and the metencephalon. A defect in the isthmic organizer is considered to be the primary cause of rhombencephalosynapsis, and *FGF8* and *Lmx1a* have been suggested as candidate genes. The condition, however, seems to occur sporadically, and the recurrence risk is probably very small.[47–50]

## Pathology

Rhombencephalosynapsis is featured by variable degrees of agenesis of the vermis, dorsal fusion of the cerebellar

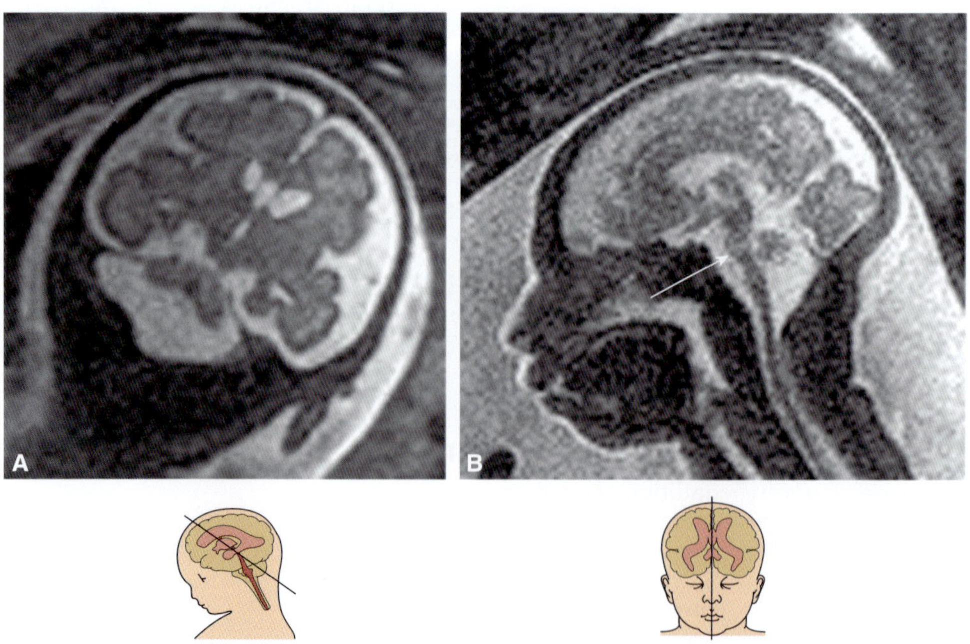


**Figure 8–18.** In this fetus with cerebellar hypoplasia, MRI demonstrated a very thin brainstem with no bulging of the pons (*arrow*). The forehead is sloping, suggesting microcephaly. This is an example of pontocerebellar hypoplasia. (Courtesy Rabih Chaoui, Berlin, Germany.)

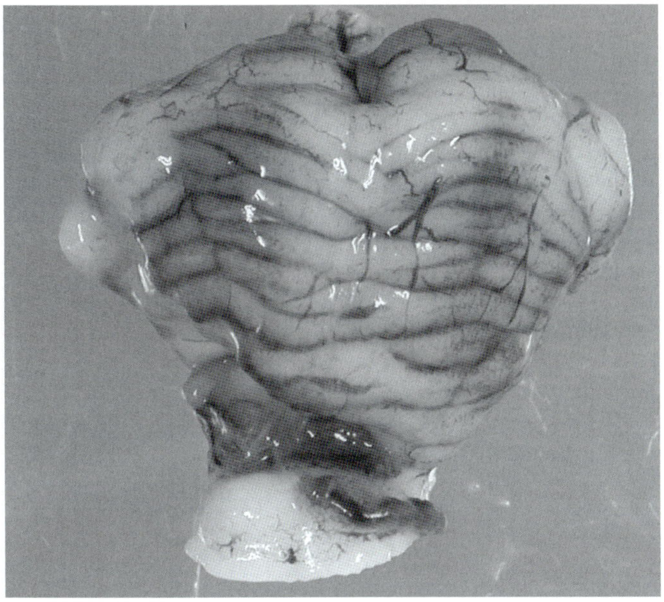

**Figure 8–19.** Rhombencephalosynapsis. Autoptic specimen demonstrates the absence of the vermis and the dorsal fusion of the cerebellar hemispheres. (Reproduced, with permission, from the *Visual Encyclopedia of Ultrasound in Obstetrics and Gynecology,* International Society of Ultrasound in Obstetrics and Gynecology, 2010, www.isuog.org.)

hemispheres and of the dentate nuclei, and superior cerebellar peduncles (Figure 8–19).[47,49]

## Associated Anomalies

Other central nervous system (CNS) anomalies are frequently found, and these cases are predominant in prenatal series.[49] Association with extraneural anomalies is also well established, including Gomez-Lopez-Hernandez syndrome, or cerebello-trigeminal-dermal dysplasia (OMIM 601853) and VACTERL-H association (spinal and forearm abnormalities).[49]

## Diagnosis

Postnatally, the diagnosis with MRI is prompted by the presence of a single-lobed cerebellum with a small keyhole shaped fourth ventricle. The most important views are the axial and coronal, which demonstrate a single cerebellar mass without the typical cleavage lines that are normally seen between the vermis and hemispheres.[3,42] The cerebellum is usually smaller than normal. The sagittal views are not diagnostic for the diagnosis, but they are helpful in that they demonstrate the absence of the normal anatomical landmarks of the vermis: the fastigium points and vermian fissures. Only a few cases have been recognized antenatally; these probably represent the most severe end of the spectrum of this condition and usually are seen in association with other cerebral and extracerebral anomalies.[4,48,49] The main sonographic finding is a small triangular cerebellum (Figure 8–20). However, there are no absolute sonographic criteria to differentiate the vermis from the surrounding hemispheres, and the diagnosis of rhombencephalosynapsis in the fetus is usually difficult and at times may be impossible.[4] Demonstration of an abnormal folial pattern crossing from one hemisphere to the other in a coronal view is an important clue to the diagnosis, but this is usually possible only in late gestation.[4]

## Differential Diagnosis

The differential diagnosis includes cerebellar hypoplasia (identification of rhombencephalosynapsis within a small cerebellum may be impossible) and vermian agenesis with molar tooth abnormality (again, a very difficult differential

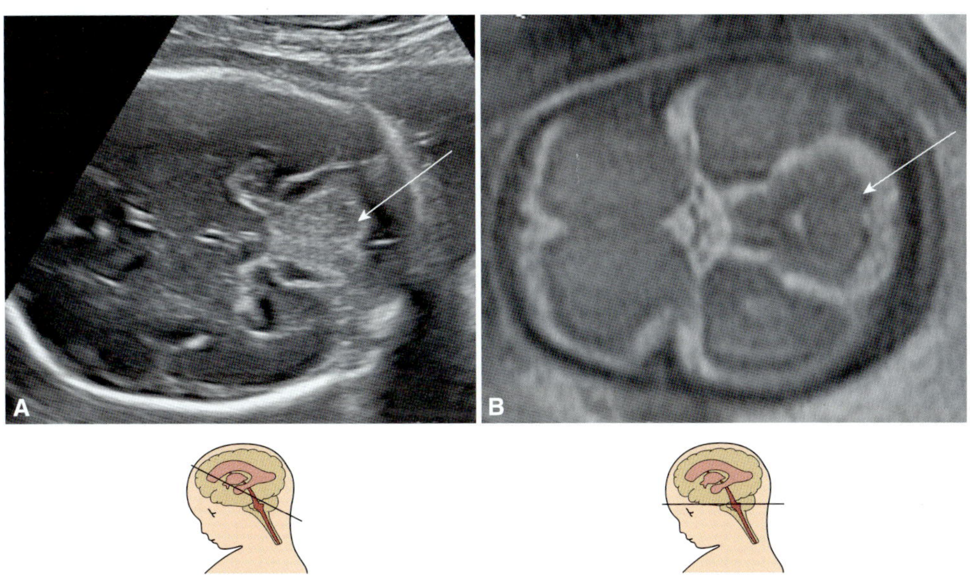


**Figure 8–20.** Prenatal findings of rhombencephalosynapsis. **(A)** Sonography. **(B)** MRI. The cerebellum is small, with an abnormal triangular shape, and the cleavage lines between the hemispheres and vermis are not demonstrated. (Reproduced, with permission, from the *Visual Encyclopedia of Ultrasound in Obstetrics and Gynecology,* International Society of Ultrasound in Obstetrics and Gynecology, 2010, www.isuog.org.)

diagnosis; however,vermian agenesis is usually associated with an open fourth ventricle).

### Prognosis

When associated anomalies are identified, such as severe ventriculomegaly, the prognosis is poor. Infants with isolated rhombencephalosynapsis usually have impairment of cognitive functions. The extent of the deficit, however, is variable and in some cases may be mild. Out of five isolated cases, two were indeed found to have normal IQs.[50] Truncal and/or limb ataxia, muscular hypotonia, abnormal eye movements, and head stereotypies are the most common neurologic disturbances. Attention problems are the most common behavioral disturbances.[50,53]

### Implications for Sonographic Screening

It is likely that in the absence of other intracranial anomalies or cerebellar hypoplasia, rhombencephalosynapsis can not be identified in a nontargeted examination of the fetal brain.

### Implications for Sonographic Diagnosis

The diagnosis of rhombecephalosynapsis is a difficult one even for expert sonologists. The most important views for the diagnosis are the axial and coronal ones, demonstrating an abnormal triangular configuration of the cerebellum. The condition should be suspected whenever the cerebellar dimensions are small.

### Obstetric Management

Exclusion of associated anomalies is the most important part of management. Some of the cerebral anomalies that have been found in association with rhombencephalosynapsis are difficult or impossible to demonstrate antenatally, particularly in early gestation. In continuing pregnancies, no modification of standard obstetric management is required.

## JOUBERT SYNDROME AND RELATED CEREBELLAR DISORDERS

### Includes

Vermian agenesis with Joubert syndrome; vermian agenesis with "molar tooth" anomaly; coloboma, oligophrenia/developmental delay, ataxia, cerebellar vermis hypoplasia, and hepatic fibrosis (COACH); cerebello-oculo-renal syndrome (CORS); oral-facial-digital syndrome type VI (OFD-VI); Senior-Løken syndrome.[51,52]

### Excludes

Vermian hypoplasia

### Definition

Hypoplasia of the cerebellar vermis associated with the characteristic neuroradiologic "molar tooth" sign; these neuroradiologic features are associated with extraneural anomalies and constitute different syndromes.

### Etiopathogenesis and Associated Anomalies

Joubert and related cerebellar disorders are transmitted as an autosomal recessive trait. The genetics is complex, with at least eight genes involved.[51–53] The different genotypes are responsible for the different clinical manifestations that have been categorized in a number of syndromes: Joubert syndrome,[52] COACH, CORS, OFD-VI, and Senior-Løken syndrome. The gene products that are affected in these conditions are known to take part in the development of the primary cilium and/or basal body and centrosome apparatus. Essentially, Joubert and related disorders are now considered part of the general group of ciliopathies.[52,53]

### Pathology

There is a variable degree of deficit of the cerebellar vermis, from hypoplasia to complete agenesis; consequently, the two hemispheres come in close contact in the midline.[54] The frequency of breathing disorders suggests the coexistence of lesions of the brainstem. Dysmorphic features are usually present, including a large head, prominent forehead, and typical facies (high, rounded eyebrows, epicanthal folds, and upturned nose).[51]

### Diagnosis

Postnatally, the predominant finding in neuroimaging of the head is the typical appearance of the mesencephalon in the axial plane (commonly referred to as the molar tooth sign) that is the consequence of a deep posterior interpeduncular fossa with thick and elongated superior cerebellar peduncles, associated with hypoplasia or agenesis of the cerebellar vermis (Figure 8–21).[28,54,55] Prenatal diagnosis with sonography is difficult.[4,28] In our own experience in a handful of cases, we have never been able to demonstrate with certainty the molar tooth sign, probably because of the limited contrast resolution of US, which does not allow a clear view of the cisterns surrounding the mesencephalon. In pregnancies at risk, an open fourth ventricle in the axial plane has been described as the most important finding.[28] The authors of the original report have not found sagittal planes to be of value. Indeed, the absence of the vermis results in apposition of the two cerebellar hemispheres in the midline that mimics the presence of a normal vermis. In low-risk pregnancies, this condition can be easily missed. An open fourth ventricle may be identified at least in some cases, but in our experience it is extremely difficult to assess the underdevelopment of the vermis (Figure 8–22). Furthermore, in the absence of a proband, the clinical manifestation of these disorders cannot be clearly predicted. Molecular genetics can be helpful in some cases.[56]

### Differential Diagnosis

The main intrauterine finding may be an open fourth ventricle; therefore, the entity that is most similar to Joubert

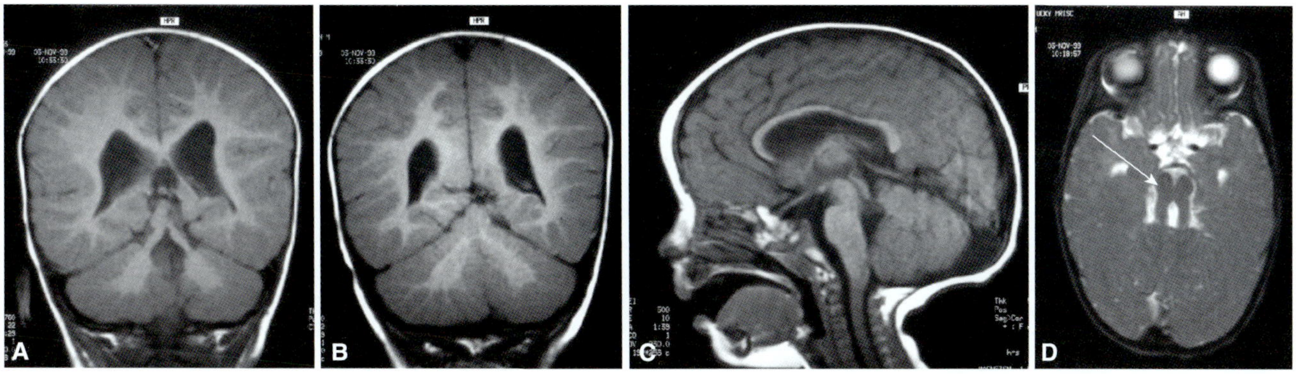


**Figure 8–21.** Joubert syndrome. **(A, B)** Postnatal MRI in the coronal planes demonstrates the absence of the vermis. **(C)** In the midsagittal plane, the anatomical landmarks of the vermis (fastigium point of the fourth ventricle, fissures) could not be demonstrated. **(D)** In the axial plane, the pathognomonic "molar tooth" sign is demonstrated (*arrow*). (Reproduced, with permission, from the *Visual Encyclopedia of Ultrasound in Obstetrics and Gynecology,* International Society of Ultrasound in Obstetrics and Gynecology, 2010, www.isuog.org.)

syndrome and related disorders is the Dandy-Walker complex. Careful examination in the axial and sagittal planes usually allows identification of a superiorly displaced vermis in the latter condition. MRI may be helpful because of its unique ability to document the molar tooth sign, which is pathognomonic of Joubert syndrome.[55]

## Implications for Targeted Examinations

In pregnancies at increased risk because of a previous affected child, neurosonography should be performed to assess the presence and integrity of the vermis. An open fourth ventricle after 20 weeks' gestation and failure to visualize the main landmarks of the cerebellar vermis are strongly suggestive of a recurrence. On the basis of the available evidence, MRI should be performed in that it allows a better demonstration of the abnormalities of the mesencephalon (molar tooth sign). In the absence of a familial history, the diagnosis of Joubert and related syndromes is a major challenge even for an expert using either US or MRI.

## Implications for Sonographic Screening

Joubert and related syndromes are associated with very subtle prenatal findings, and we expect that in low-risk

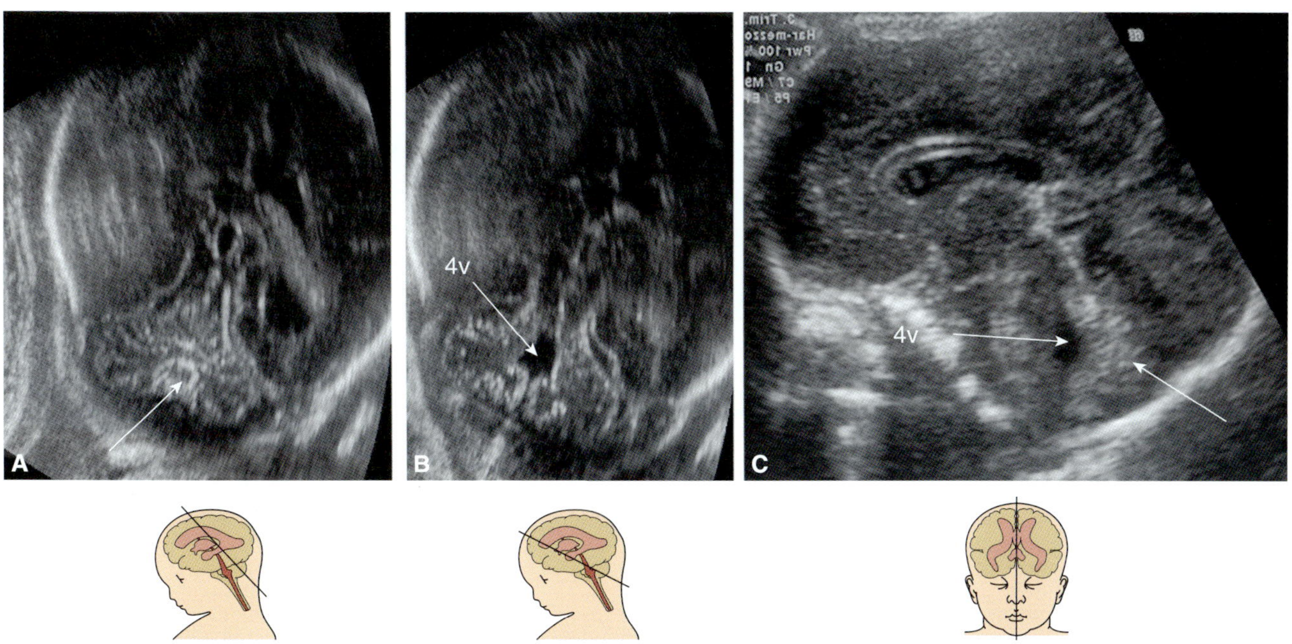


**Figure 8–22.** Sonography of Joubert syndrome. In this third trimester fetus, we were unable to clearly identify the cerebellar vermis between the two cerebellar hemispheres (*arrow*) **(A)**, and the fourth ventricle appeared open **(B)**. **(C)** In the midsagittal plane, the anatomical landmarks of the vermis (fastigium point of the fourth ventricle, fissures) could not be demonstrated (*arrows*). The diagnosis of Joubert syndrome was considered and was confirmed after birth. (Reproduced, with permission, from the *Visual Encyclopedia of Ultrasound in Obstetrics and Gynecology,* International Society of Ultrasound in Obstetrics and Gynecology, 2010, www.isuog.org.)

pregnancies, most cases will escape detection. In some cases, an open fourth ventricle can be identified. After 20 weeks' gestation, this finding requires an expert evaluation by either neurosonography or MRI.

### Prognosis

Most infants have severe intellectual impairment, and early death is common. Neurologic dysfunction typically includes ataxia, abnormal breathing patterns (hyperpnea intermixed with central apnea in the neonatal period), and abnormal behavior (temperament, hyperactivity, aggressiveness, and dependency).[51,54]

### Obstetric Management

When a confident diagnosis is made, termination of pregnancy may be offered to the couples. Otherwise, no modification of standard obstetric management is indicated.

## UNILATERAL CEREBELLAR LESIONS

### Definition

Echogenicity of one cerebellar hemisphere usually evolving into unilateral hypoplasia

### Excludes

Global cerebellar hypoplasia

### Etiopathogenesis

Echogenicity of one cerebellar hemisphere has been found as a consequence of hemorrhage, although in some cases the lesion may have an ischemic cause; in time the affected hemisphere becomes atrophic.[27,57] Two of the cases thus far described have occurred in severely anemic fetuses that were salvaged with intrauterine transfusions.[57] An association with cytomegalovirus (CMV) infection has been reported.[58] We have also documented this finding in otherwise normal fetuses, typically in the second trimester of gestation.

### Diagnosis

One of the cerebellar hemispheres is initially brightly echogenic and in the following weeks becomes hypoplastic and/or develops into a cystic lesion (Figure 8–23).

### Differential Diagnosis

Global cerebellar hypoplasia characterized by an overall reduction in cerebellar size.

### Associated Anomalies

Intracranial hemorrhage at other sites, CMV infection.

### Prognosis

The experience thus far is limited, and it is impossible to draw on specific figures. The handful of cases we have

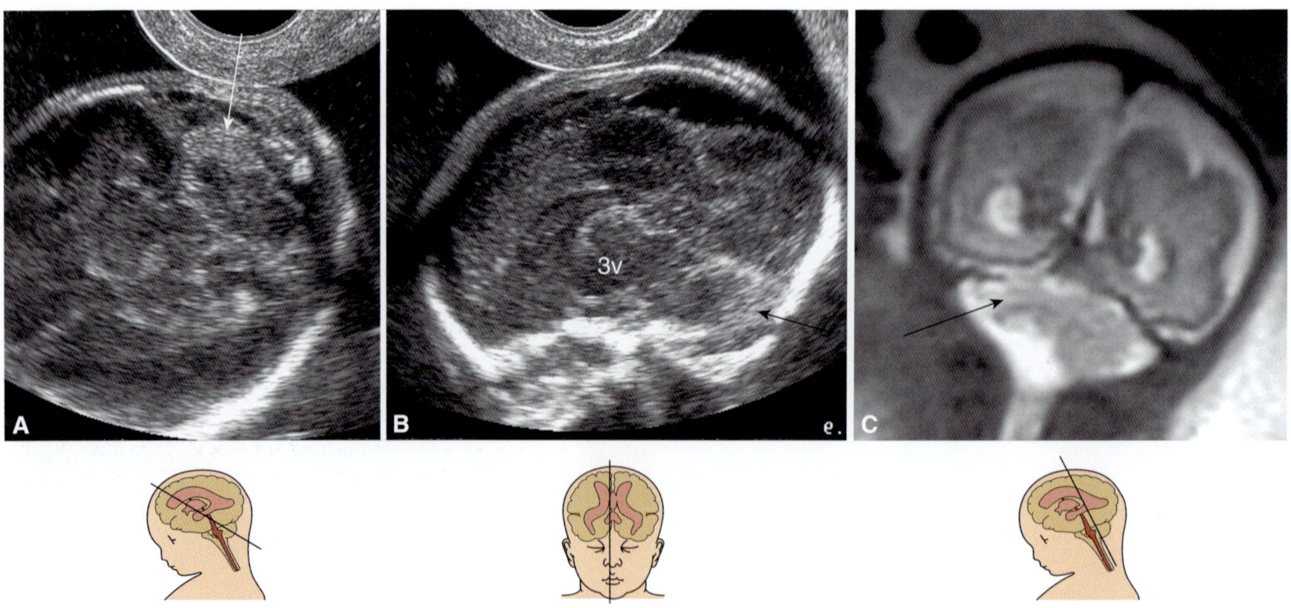


**Figure 8–23.** Acquired intrauterine lesion of one cerebellar hemisphere. This fetus developed severe anemia and hydrops as a consequence of anti-D alloimmunization. It was resuscitated with intrauterine transfusions but developed an intense echogenicity of one cerebellar hemisphere that eventually became atrophic. The vermis and contralateral hemisphere appeared intact. The neurologic and intellectual development was normal at long-term postnatal follow-up. (Reproduced, with permission, from Ghi T, Brondelli L, Simonazzi G, Valeri B, Santini D, Sandri F, Ancora G, Pilu G. Sonographic demonstration of brain injury in fetuses with severe red blood cell alloimmunization undergoing intrauterine transfusions. *Ultrasound Obstet Gynecol.* 2004;23(5):428–431.)[57]

seen in which the lesion was isolated demonstrated normal neurologic follow-up. Involvement of the vermis is usually associated with a worse prognosis.[59]

## Obstetric Management

CMV infection usually results in multiple abnormal cerebral findings. Alloimmune thrombocytopenia typically causes hemorrhages in the cerebral hemispheres. However, it would seem prudent to exclude both conditions. In continuing pregnancies, there is no indication to modify standard obstetric care.

## REFERENCES


1. Carroll SG, Porter H, Abdel-Fattah S, Kyle PM, Soothill PW. Correlation of prenatal ultrasound diagnosis and pathologic findings in fetal brain abnormalities. *Ultrasound Obstet Gynecol.* 2000;16(2):149–153.
2. Limperopoulos C, Robertson RL, Jr., Khwaja OS, Robson CD, Estroff JA, Barnewolt C, Levine D, Morash D, Nemes L, Zaccagnini L, du Plessis AJ. How accurately does current fetal imaging identify posterior fossa anomalies? *Am J Roentgenol.* 2008;190(6):1637–1643.
3. Guibaud L, des Portes V. Plea for an anatomical approach to abnormalities of the posterior fossa in prenatal diagnosis. *Ultrasound Obstet Gynecol.* 2006;27(5):477–481.
4. Malinger G, Lev D, Lerman-Sagie T. The fetal cerebellum. Pitfalls in diagnosis and management. *Prenat Diagn.* 2009;29(4):372–380.
5. Pilu G, Visentin A, Valeri B. The Dandy-Walker complex and fetal sonography. *Ultrasound Obstet Gynecol.* 2000;16(2):115–117.
6. Adamsbaum C, Moutard ML, Andre C, Merzoug V, Ferey S, Quere MP, Lewin F, Fallet-Bianco C. MRI of the fetal posterior fossa. *Pediatr Radiol.* 2005;35(2):124–140.
7. Barkovich AJ, Millen KJ, Dobyns WB. A developmental and genetic classification for midbrain-hindbrain malformations. *Brain.* 2009;132(Pt 12):3199–3230.
8. Hirsch JF, Pierre-Kahn A, Renier D, Sainte-Rose C, Hoppe-Hirsch E. The Dandy-Walker malformation. A review of 40 cases. *J Neurosurg.* 1984;61(3):515–522.
9. Osenbach RK, Menezes AH. Diagnosis and management of the Dandy-Walker malformation: 30 years of experience. *Pediatr Neurosurg.* 1992;18(4):179–189.
10. Sawaya R, McLaurin RL. Dandy-Walker syndrome. Clinical analysis of 23 cases. *J Neurosurg.* 1981;55(1):89–98.
11. Calabro F, Arcuri T, Jinkins JR. Blake's pouch cyst: an entity within the Dandy-Walker continuum. *Neuroradiology.* 2000;42(4):290–295.
12. Pilu G, Segata M, Ghi T, Carletti A, Perolo A, Santini D, Bonasoni P, Tani G, Rizzo N. Diagnosis of midline anomalies of the fetal brain with the three-dimensional median view. *Ultrasound Obstet Gynecol.* 2006;27(5):522–529.
13. Zalel Y, Gilboa Y, Gabis L, Ben-Sira L, Hoffman C, Wiener Y, Achiron R. Rotation of the vermis as a cause of enlarged cisterna magna on prenatal imaging. *Ultrasound Obstet Gynecol.* 2006;27(5):490–493.
14. Robinson AJ, Goldstein R. The cisterna magna septa: vestigial remnants of Blake's pouch and a potential new marker for normal development of the rhombencephalon. *J Ultrasound Med.* 2007;26(1):83–95.
15. Ecker JL, Shipp TD, Bromley B, Benacerraf B. The sonographic diagnosis of Dandy-Walker and Dandy-Walker variant: associated findings and outcomes. *Prenat Diagn.* 2000;20(4):328–332.
16. Has R, Ermis H, Yuksel A, Ibrahimoglu L, Yildirim A, Sezer HD, Basaran S. Dandy-Walker malformation: a review of 78 cases diagnosed by prenatal sonography. *Fetal Diagn Ther.* 2004;19(4):342–347.
17. Murray JC, Johnson JA, Bird TD. Dandy-Walker malformation: etiologic heterogeneity and empiric recurrence risks. *Clin Genet.* 1985;28(4):272–283.
18. Phillips JJ, Mahony BS, Siebert JR, Lalani T, Fligner CL, Kapur RP. Dandy-Walker malformation complex: correlation between ultrasonographic diagnosis and postmortem neuropathology. *Obstet Gynecol.* 2006;107(3):685–693.
19. Pilu G, Romero R, De Palma L, Rizzo N, Jeanty P, Copel JA, Bovicelli L, Hobbins JC. Antenatal diagnosis and obstetric management of Dandy-Walker syndrome. *J Reprod Med.* 1986;31(11):1017–1022.
20. Babcook CJ, Chong BW, Salamat MS, Ellis WG, Goldstein RB. Sonographic anatomy of the developing cerebellum: normal embryology can resemble pathology. *Am J Roentgenol.* 1996;166(2):427–433.
21. Bromley B, Nadel AS, Pauker S, Estroff JA, Benacerraf BR. Closure of the cerebellar vermis: evaluation with second trimester US. *Radiology.* 1994;193(3):761–763.
22. Achiron R, Achiron A. Transvaginal ultrasonic assessment of the early fetal brain. *Ultrasound Obstet Gynecol.* 1991;1(5):336–344.
23. Pilu G, Ghi T, Carletti A, Segata M, Perolo A, Rizzo N. Three-dimensional ultrasound examination of the fetal central nervous system. *Ultrasound Obstet Gynecol.* 2007;30(2):233–245.
24. Boddaert N, Klein O, Ferguson N, Sonigo P, Parisot D, Hertz-Pannier L, Baraton J, Emond S, Simon I, Chigot V, Schmit P, Pierre-Kahn A, Brunelle F. Intellectual prognosis of the Dandy-Walker malformation in children: the importance of vermian lobulation. *Neuroradiology.* 2003;45(5):320–324.
25. Klein O, Pierre-Kahn A, Boddaert N, Parisot D, Brunelle F. Dandy-Walker malformation: prenatal diagnosis and prognosis. *Childs Nerv Syst.* 2003;19(7-8):484–489.
26. Achiron R, Kivilevitch Z, Lipitz S, Gamzu R, Almog B, Zalel Y. Development of the human fetal pons: in utero ultrasonographic study. *Ultrasound Obstet Gynecol.* 2004;24(5):506–510.
27. Malinger G, Ginath S, Lerman-Sagie T, Watemberg N, Lev D, Glezerman M. The fetal cerebellar vermis: normal development as shown by transvaginal ultrasound. *Prenat Diagn.* 2001;21(8):687–692.
28. Doherty D, Glass IA, Siebert JR, Strouse PJ, Parisi MA, Shaw DW, Chance PF, Barr M, Jr., Nyberg D. Prenatal diagnosis in pregnancies at risk for Joubert syndrome by ultrasound and MRI. *Prenat Diagn.* 2005;25(6):442–447.
29. ISUOG. Sonographic examination of the fetal central nervous system: guidelines for performing the 'basic examination' and the 'fetal neurosonogram'. *Ultrasound Obstet Gynecol.* 2007;29(1):109–116.
30. Mahony BS, Callen PW, Filly RA, Hoddick WK. The fetal cisterna magna. *Radiology.* 1984;153(3):773–776.
31. Limperopoulos C, Robertson RL, Estroff JA, Barnewolt C, Levine D, Bassan H, du Plessis AJ. Diagnosis of inferior vermian hypoplasia by fetal magnetic resonance imaging: potential pitfalls and neurodevelopmental outcome. *Am J Obstet Gynecol.* 2006;194(4):1070–1076.
32. Paladini D, Volpe P. Posterior fossa and vermian morphometry in the characterization of fetal cerebellar abnormalities: a prospective three-dimensional ultrasound study. *Ultrasound Obstet Gynecol.* 2006;27(5):482–489.
33. Ghidini A, Fromberg RA, Tiernan J, Wieneke JA, Manz HJ, Sherer DM. Dilated subarachnoid cisterna ambiens: a potential sonographic sign predicting cerebellar hypoplasia. *J Ultrasound Med.* 1996;15(5):413–415.
34. Pilu G, Falco P, Perolo A, Sandri F, Cocchi G, Ancora G, Bovicelli L. Differential diagnosis and outcome of fetal intracranial hypoechoic lesions: report of 21 cases. *Ultrasound Obstet Gynecol.* 1997;9(4):229–236.
35. Yuksel A, Batukan C. Fetal cerebellar hemorrhage in a severely growth-restricted fetus: natural history and differential diagnosis from Dandy-Walker malformation. *Ultrasound Obstet Gynecol.* 2003;22(2):178–181.
36. Pilu G, Romero R, De Palma L, Jeanty P, Burdine C, Hobbins JC. Ultrasound investigation of the posterior fossa in the fetus. *Am J Perinatol.* 1987;4(2):155–159.
37. Nyberg DA, Mahony BS, Hegge FN, Hickok D, Luthy DA, Kapur R. Enlarged cisterna magna and the Dandy-Walker malformation: factors associated with chromosome abnormalities. *Obstet Gynecol.* 1991;77(3):436–442.
38. Pilu G, Goldstein I, Reece EA, Perolo A, Foschini MP, Hobbins JC, Bovicelli L. Sonography of fetal Dandy-Walker malformation: a reappraisal. *Ultrasound Obstet Gynecol.* 1992;2(3):151–157.

39. Bolduc ME, Limperopoulos C. Neurodevelopmental outcomes in children with cerebellar malformations: a systematic review. *Dev Med Child Neurol.* 2009;51(4):256–267.
40. Cornips EM, Overvliet GM, Weber JW, Postma AA, Hoeberigs CM, Baldewijns MM, Vles JS. The clinical spectrum of Blake's pouch cyst: report of six illustrative cases. *Childs Nerv Syst.*
41. Dror R, Malinger G, Ben-Sira L, Lev D, Pick CG, Lerman-Sagie T. Developmental outcome of children with enlargement of the cisterna magna identified in utero. *J Child Neurol.* 2009;24(12):1486–1492.
42. Poretti A, Wolf NI, Boltshauser E. Differential diagnosis of cerebellar atrophy in childhood. *Eur J Paediatr Neurol.* 2008;12(3):155–167.
43. Barth PG. Pontocerebellar hypoplasias. An overview of a group of inherited neurodegenerative disorders with fetal onset. *Brain Dev.* 1993;15(6):411–422.
44. Barth PG. Pontocerebellar hypoplasia--how many types? *Eur J Paediatr Neurol.* 2000;4(4):161–162.
45. Goldstein I, Reece EA, Pilu G, Bovicelli L, Hobbins JC. Cerebellar measurements with ultrasonography in the evaluation of fetal growth and development. *Am J Obstet Gynecol.* 1987;156(5):1065–1069.
46. Snijders RJ, Nicolaides KH. Fetal biometry at 14-40 weeks' gestation. *Ultrasound Obstet Gynecol.* 1994;4(1):34–48.
47. Chemli J, Abroug M, Tlili K, Harbi A. Rhombencephalosynapsis diagnosed in childhood: clinical and MRI findings. *Eur J Paediatr Neurol.* 2007;11(1):35–38.
48. McAuliffe F, Chitayat D, Halliday W, Keating S, Shah V, Fink M, Nevo O, Ryan G, Shannon P, Blaser S. Rhombencephalosynapsis: prenatal imaging and autopsy findings. *Ultrasound Obstet Gynecol.* 2008;31(5):542–548.
49. Pasquier L, Marcorelles P, Loget P, Pelluard F, Carles D, Perez MJ, Bendavid C, de La Rochebrochard C, Ferry M, David V, Odent S, Laquerriere A. Rhombencephalosynapsis and related anomalies: a neuropathological study of 40 fetal cases. *Acta Neuropathol.* 2009;117(2):185–200.
50. Poretti A, Alber FD, Burki S, Toelle SP, Boltshauser E. Cognitive outcome in children with rhombencephalosynapsis. *Eur J Paediatr Neurol.* 2009;13(1):28–33.
51. Parisi M, Glass I. Joubert syndrome. In: Pagon RA, Bird TD, Dolan CR, Stephens K, eds. GeneReviews [Internet]. 2010/03/20 ed. Seattle (WA): University of Washington; 2003.
52. Parisi MA. Clinical and molecular features of Joubert syndrome and related disorders. *Am J Med Genet C Semin Med Genet.* 2009;151C(4):326–340.
53. Doherty D, Parisi MA, Finn LS, Gunay-Aygun M, Al-Mateen M, Bates D, Clericuzio C, Demir H, Dorschner M, van Essen AJ, Gahl WA, Gentile M, Gorden NT, Hikida A, Knutzen D, Ozyurek H, Phelps I, Rosenthal P, Verloes A, Weigand H, Chance PF, Dobyns WB, Glass IA. Mutations in 3 genes (MKS3, CC2D2A and RPGRIP1L) cause COACH syndrome (Joubert syndrome with congenital hepatic fibrosis). *J Med Genet.*;47(1):8–21.
54. Zaki MS, Abdel-Aleem A, Abdel-Salam G, Marsh SE, Silhavy JL, Barkovich AJ, Ross ME, Saleem SN, Dobyns WB, Gleeson JG. The molar tooth sign: a new Joubert syndrome and related cerebellar disorders classification system tested in Egyptian families. *Neurology.* 2008;70(7):556–565.
55. Saleem SN, Zaki MS. Role of MR Imaging in prenatal diagnosis of pregnancies at risk for Joubert syndrome and related cerebellar disorders. *Am J Neuroradiol.*;31(3):424–429.
56. Edvardson S, Shaag A, Zenvirt S, Erlich Y, Hannon GJ, Shanske AL, Gomori JM, Ekstein J, Elpeleg O. Joubert syndrome 2 (JBTS2) in Ashkenazi Jews is associated with a TMEM216 mutation. *Am J Hum Genet.*;86(1):93–97.
57. Ghi T, Brondelli L, Simonazzi G, Valeri B, Santini D, Sandri F, Ancora G, Pilu G. Sonographic demonstration of brain injury in fetuses with severe red blood cell alloimmunization undergoing intrauterine transfusions. *Ultrasound Obstet Gynecol.* 2004;23(5):428–431.
58. Malinger G, Lev D, Zahalka N, Ben Aroia Z, Watemberg N, Kidron D, Sira LB, Lerman-Sagie T. Fetal cytomegalovirus infection of the brain: the spectrum of sonographic findings. *Am J Neuroradiol.* 2003;24(1):28–32.
59. Poretti A, Limperopoulos C, Roulet-Perez E, Wolf NI, Rauscher C, Prayer D, Muller A, Weissert M, Kotzaeridou U, DUP AJ, Huisman TA, Boltshauser E. Outcome of severe unilateral cerebellar hypoplasia. *Dev Med Child Neurol.* 2010;52:(8):718–724.

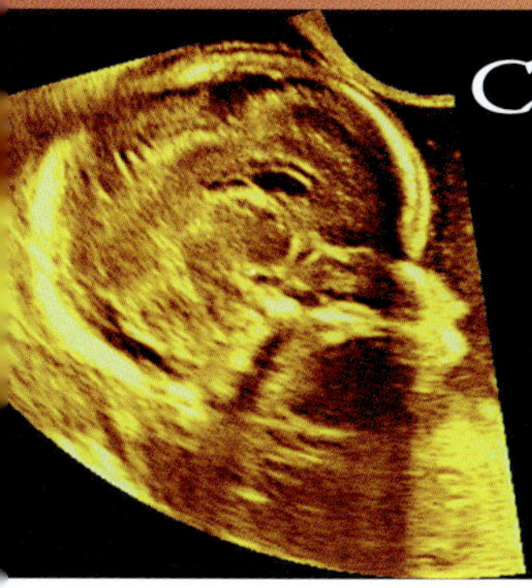

# Chapter 9

# INTRAUTERINE INFECTIONS AFFECTING THE BRAIN

***Gustavo Malinger • Tally Lerman-Sagie***

**KEY POINTS**

1. Depending on geographic factors, cytomegalovirus (CMV) and toxoplasmosis are the more frequent intrauterine infections (IUIs).
2. The pattern of brain involvement in CMV-IUI may range from minimal (small periventricular cysts, intrathalamic vasculopathy) to severe damage (brain atrophy, malformations of cortical development, and hemorrhages).
3. The prognosis is usually poor in the presence of intracranial findings.
4. Infected fetuses without brain findings are generally asymptomatic at birth but may develop sensorineural deafness.

The fetus may become infected with a variety of organisms through transplacental passage or as a result of an ascending infection. In some patients, the infection may involve the central nervous system (CNS), causing lesions in different areas and grades of severity (Table 9–1).

Cytomegalovirus (CMV) and *Toxoplasma gondii* are the most common pathogens affecting the brain. Other organisms that may infect the developing fetal brain are rubella virus,[1] varicella zoster virus,[2] herpes simplex virus,[3,4] parvovirus B19,[5,6] lymphocytic choriomeningitis virus,[7] West Nile virus,[8] *Treponema pallidum,*[9] *Trypanosoma cruzi,*[10] and the nematode filarial.[11] This chapter reviews each of these sources of infection.

## CYTOMEGALOVIRUS

### Definition

Cytomegalovirus (CMV) is a large DNA virus with a wide infectious clinical spectrum ranging from subclinical to severe multisystem involvement. CMV is transmitted by person-to-person contact. Following maternal infection, it may be transmitted through the placenta to the fetus.

### Synonyms

Herpesvirus 5, cytomegalic inclusion disease

### Incidence/Prevalence

Following the almost complete disappearance of congenital rubella after the introduction of widespread immunization programs, CMV infection has become the most common infection affecting the developing fetus.

The prevalence of CMV-seropositive pregnant women or at reproductive age ranges from >99% in Turkey[12] to between 43.6% and 57.2% in France[13] and England,[14] respectively.

A meta-analysis study of 27 culture-based universal study groups found a birth prevalence of congenital CMV of 0.64% (95% CI: 0.60–0.69%).[15] The same study found that from 954 infants identified with congenital CMV infection, only 103 (11%) were considered symptomatic.[15] A primary infection during pregnancy carries a significantly higher risk of fetal transmission than a recurrent infection (32.3% vs 1.4%).[15]

### Pathogenesis

Maternal viremia, placental infection, and hematogenous dissemination to the fetus are the most likely sequence of events leading to congenital CMV infection.[16] During the viremic phase, the virus circulates and disseminates, carried by leukocytes. The exact way in which CMV infects the placenta is not clearly understood, but once it reaches the fetal compartment, hematogenous dissemination ensues.[16] A direct effect on placental development causing placental insufficiency has been described as a possible factor in the pathogenesis of fetal disease.[17] CMV may also act as a teratogen, producing chromosomal injury or altering modulation of developmental gene expression.[18]

### Etiology

CMV infection is caused by a large double-stranded DNA herpesvirus. Geneotypically different CMV strains have been reported.[19] Preconceptional immunity against CMV provides only partial protection against intrauterine

**Table 9–1. ULTRASOUND CENTRAL NERVOUS SYSTEM FINDINGS FOLLOWING INTRAUTERINE INFECTIONS**

| Pathogen | CNS involvement | Reported in | Ventriculomegaly | Abnormal PVWM | Calcifications | Microcephaly | Others |
|---|---|---|---|---|---|---|---|
| CMV | Common | Fetus, infant | Common | Common | Frequent | Frequent | MCD, CC, cerebellum, hemorrhage |
| Toxoplasma | Common | Fetus, infant | Common | Rare | Common | Rare | Hydranencephaly |
| Rubella | Common | Infant | Rare | Common | Common | Common | – |
| Varicella zoster | Extremely rare | Fetus, infant | Rare | – | Rare | Rare | Encephalitis, cerebellum, MCD |
| Herpes simplex | Extremely rare | Fetus, infant | Common | Common | Rare | Rare | Encephalitis |
| Parvovirus B19 | Extremely rare | Fetus, infant | Rare | – | – | – | Hemorrhage, stroke, MCD |
| LCMV | Common | Fetus, infant | Common | Rare | Common | – | – |
| West Nile virus | Extremely rare | Fetus, infant | – | Rare | – | – | Meningitis, encephalitis |
| Syphilis | Extremely rare | Fetus, infant | Rare | Rare | – | Rare | MCD |
| Trypanosoma | Extremely rare | Fetus, infant | – | – | – | – | Meningoencephalitis |

CC, corpus callosum; CMV, cytomegalovirus; LCMV, Lymphocytic choriomeningitis virus; MCD, malformations of cortical development; PVWM, periventricular white matter, including cysts.

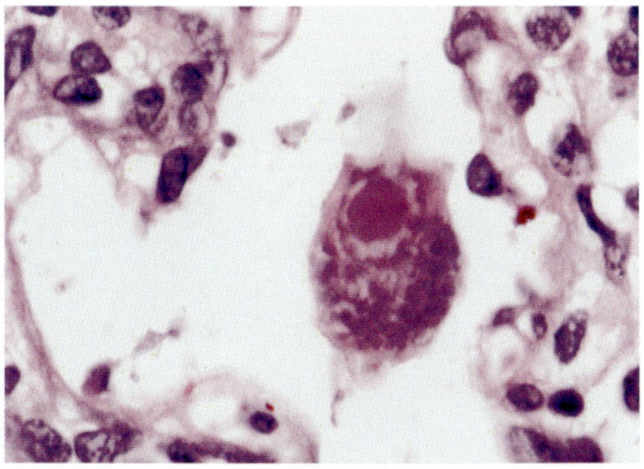

**Figure 9–1.** Cytomegalovirus (CMV) inclusion body in the white matter at 24 postmenstrual weeks. (Courtesy of Dr. Deborah Kidron, Kfar Saba, Israel.)

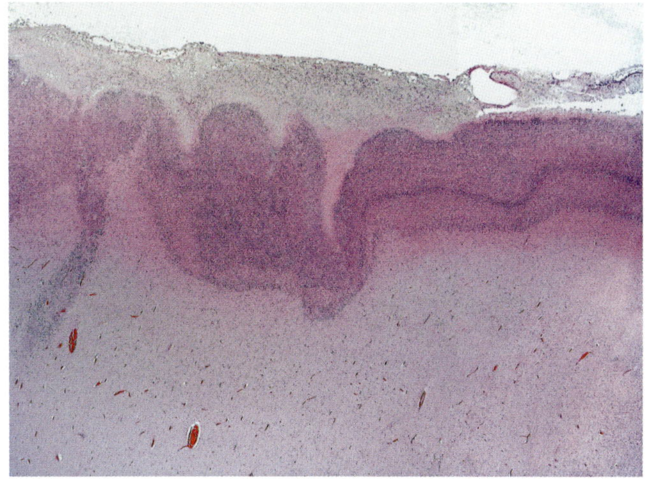

**Figure 9–2.** Polymicrogyria in a fetus at 31 postmenstrual weeks with CMV infection. Low field magnification. Note the transition from an almost normal six-layer cortex to the zone with polymicrogyria. Similar foci of polymicrogyria were found in other locations. (Courtesy of Dr. Letizia Schreiber, Holon, Israel.)

transmission of the virus, as reinfection with a different strain of CMV may lead to intrauterine transmission and symptomatic congenital infection.[20]

## Pathology

Intrauterine CMV infection frequently affects the fetal brain; the motif of this predilection is not clear, and the cellular targets not well defined. The presence of intracellular inclusion bodies in the brain (Figure 9–1) is considered diagnostic of CMV infection, but there are almost no histologic data regarding the type of cells affected.[21] From human and animal cell line cultures, it seems that neural stem cells in the fetal brain are the predominant cell type affected during development by CMV. Cheeran et al[21] proposed possible mechanisms of CMV developmental disruption, including direct damage followed by reduction in the number of neural stem cells or intermediate progenitors; alterations in stem cell migration and fate of cell differentiation; infection of astroglia, causing disruption of their normal supportive functions; and alterations in the microenvironment of the developing brain due to cytokines and soluble factors generated by resident glial cells.

These combined factors may produce not only malformative pathologies of different severity, including microcephaly and malformations of cortical development[22] (Figure 9–2), but also direct injury to the brain, resulting in ventriculomegaly, calcifications, brain atrophy, cyst formation, or hemorrhage.[22,23]

## Associated Anomalies

Fetal CMV infection may affect other systems and organs. Reported gastrointestinal findings include hyperechogenic intestines,[24–26] bowel dilation,[27] hepatomegaly and/or splenomegaly,[24,26,28,29] and liver calcifications.[25] In our experience, a frequent early sign of infection is hyperechogenic intestines. It is rarely observed as an isolated finding, and it is usually transient.

Rarely, fetal CMV infection may involve the heart and cause cardiomegaly,[29] endocardial fibroelastosis with hypoplastic left heart,[29] and cardiomyopathy.[24] Growth restriction, hydrops, and oligohydramnios are frequently present;[24–26,29] however, hydrops and oligohydramnios may be transient and resolve following the acute stages of the fetal disease. Placental thickness is significantly increased in infected fetuses.[29,30]

When a diagnosis is reached during pregnancy, multiple organ involvement may be present in as much as 42% of the patients.[29]

## Risk of Recurrence

Although uncommon recurrent maternal CMV infection may produce fetal disease, this may be due to reactivation of the disease or more probably to infection by a different strain.[20] It is usually recognized that in these fetuses the infection may be mild or even subclinical, but according to our personal experience and also to isolated cases reports, this assumption may not necessarily be true.[31–34] During a 3-year period, Zalel et al[34] found six fetuses with sonographic findings characteristic of CMV infection whose mothers were known to be CMV seropositive before or at the beginning of the index pregnancy; five out of six fetuses had severe brain involvement.

Well-documented cases of the consecutive occurrence of fetal CMV infection in the same woman are extremely rare. Stagno et al[35] described in 1973 two pregnant women who delivered affected siblings. The interval between the pregnancies was 17 and 14 months, respectively, and in both cases, the younger children were asymptomatic.

It is important to remember that, in these cases, the differential diagnosis includes the possibility of fetal disease due to a different infective agent and the autosomal recessive Aicardi-Goutières (pseudo-TORCH

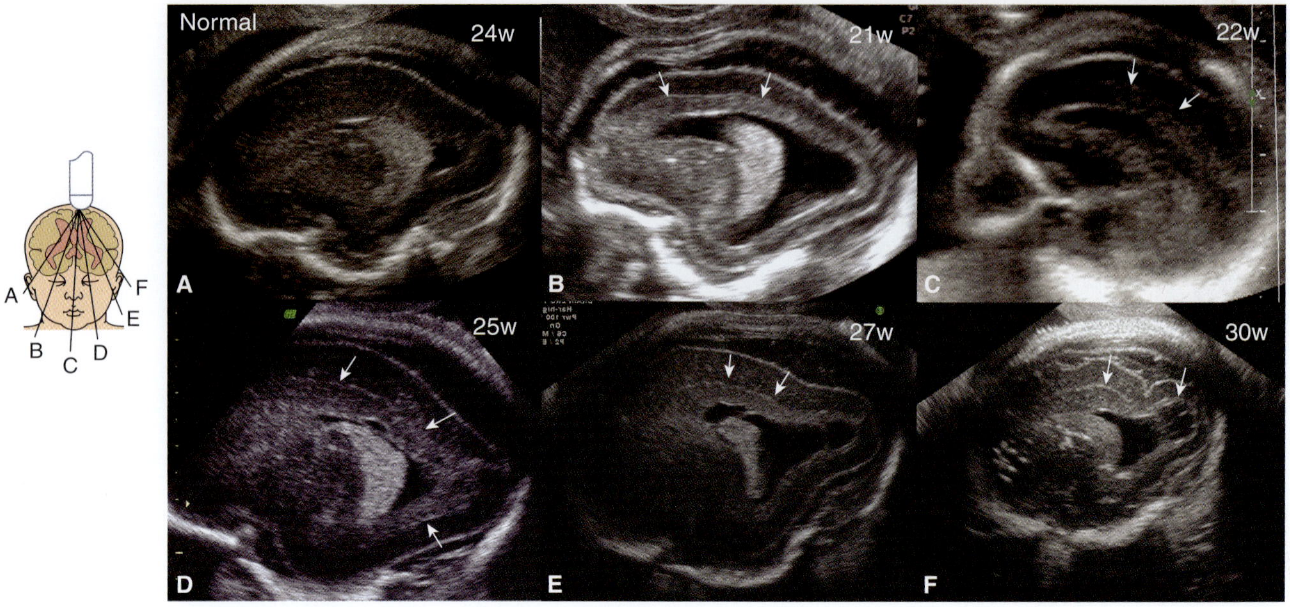


**Figure 9–3.** Transvaginal parasagittal planes. **(A)** Normal fetus at 24 postmenstrual weeks. The echogenicity of the brain parenchyma is similar throughout the whole surface. **(B–F)** Five fetuses with proven CMV at different gestational ages showing a clearly demarcated hyperechogenic periventricular zone (*arrows*). Not all of the affected fetuses have ventriculomegaly. Note the presence of punctuate calcifications **(B, F)**, periventricular cysts **(D, E)**, and intraventricular adhesions **(E, F)**.

[toxoplasmosis, other infections, rubella, cytomegalovirus, and herpes simplex virus) syndrome.[36]

## Sonographic Diagnosis

Fetal CNS signs of congenital CMV infection were first described in the 1980s[37] and are similar to those reported in newborns.[38] Although ventriculomegaly of different grades of severity, calcifications, and microcephaly are the more frequent presenting signs, abnormal periventricular echogenicity with or without cysts is consistently present in severely affected fetuses.

CMV may produce a very wide spectrum of brain pathologies according to the period of brain development in which the infection starts and probably also to the virulence of the virus or the immunological status of the mother and fetus. The general understanding is that early infection produces a more severe and generalized pattern of disease, whereas late infection produces a milder disease.[39]

Increased periventricular echogenicity is best depicted by transvaginal sonography (Figures 9–3 and 9–4). Characteristically, it involves the whole periventricular zone of both hemispheres, and it is well demarcated from the remaining brain parenchyma. Cysts and calcifications may be found within the zones of increased echogenicity. Cyst formation may be the result of parenchymal necrosis or liquefaction of small zones of hemorrhage; we have observed that in some cases the cyst walls, when adjacent, undergo lysis, and a larger porencephalic cyst is formed[40] (Figure 9–5). The presence of abnormal periventricular findings may be depicted in some, but not all, patients during a routine transabdominal examination using axial planes (Figure 9–6).

Intracranial calcifications involving the brain parenchyma, thalami, basal ganglia, and cerebellum can be demonstrated in at least some cases, starting from the second trimester. The calcifications may be punctuate or coarse; regional, isolated, diffuse, or in clusters (see Figures 9–3 and 9–4). Coarse echogenicities adjacent to the lateral ventricles may represent an end stage of periventriculitis. The differential diagnosis of intracranial calcifications includes other infectious agents, intracranial teratomas, tuberous sclerosis, Sturge-Weber syndrome, Aicardi-Goutières syndrome, and sagittal or transverse sinus thrombosis.[36,41–46]

Microcephaly is consistently observed but may not be obvious during the second trimester or even the early third trimester; in many cases, microcephaly is accompanied by brain atrophy (Figure 9–7). Migration and organization disorders ranging from focal sulcal anomalies to generalized lesions[40,47] (see Figures 9–4 and 9–7) are usually found in fetuses with severe involvement.

Congenital CMV may affect the white matter; this pattern of disease has been described in children and adults[48] but may also be depicted during fetal life, usually late in the third trimester (Figure 9–8). Callosal dysgenesis may be the result of this type of insult.[22,40]

Estroff and colleagues[49] reported the presence of branching linear echogenic areas in the thalami of a fetus with CMV. This entity is frequent in the neonatal period and was initially considered a characteristic sign of infection.[50,51] The current approach is that it represents a nonspecific sign, as it has also been described in children with asphyxia, chromosomal anomalies, metabolic diseases, maternal heroin abuse, and in the recipient in twin-to-twin transfusion syndome.[38] Single or ramified linear echo densities, produced by hyalinization or mineralization of

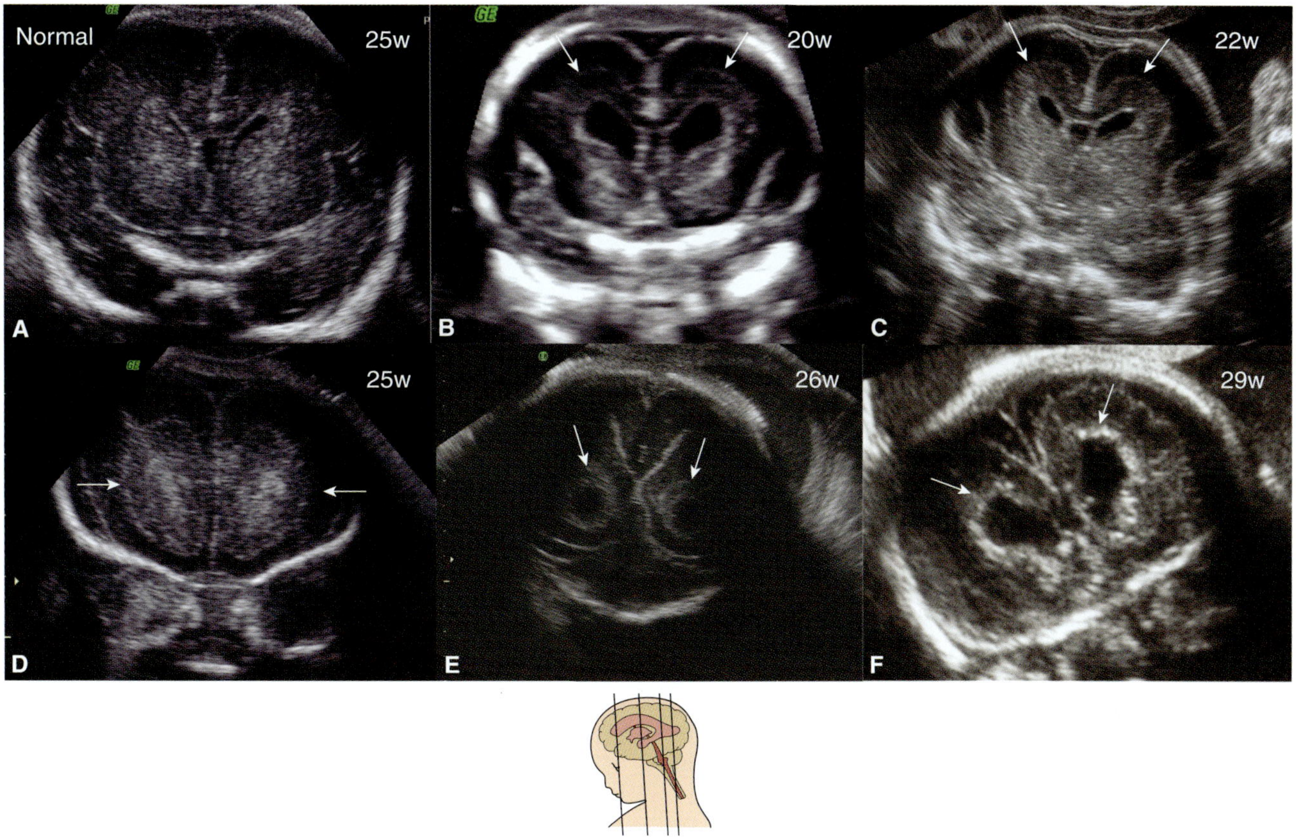


**Figure 9–4.** Transvaginal coronal planes. **(A)** Normal transthalamic section at 25 postmenstrual weeks. The thalami are slightly more echogenic than the brain. **(B–F)** Increased periventricular echogenicity with clear demarcation from the remainder of the brain (*arrows*) in five fetuses with CMV at different gestational weeks. Transfrontal plane **(D)**, transcaudate plane **(B, F)**, transthalamic plane **(C)**, and transoccipital plane **(E)**. Coarse calcifications and abnormal sulcation with early development of numerous shallow sulci are present in the fetus at 29 weeks of gestation **(F)**.

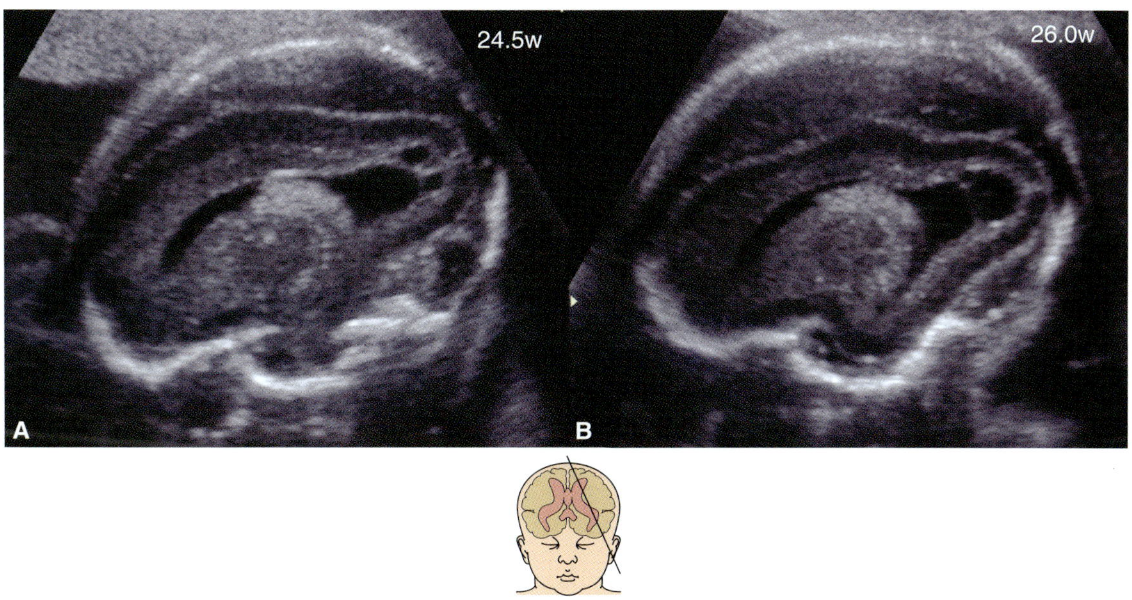


**Figure 9–5.** Transvaginal parasagittal planes. Periventricular occipital cysts **(A)** at 24.5 postmenstrual weeks converting into a larger porencephalic occipital cyst or intraventricular adhesion **(B)** 2 weeks later. (From Malinger G, Lerman-Sagie T. Fetal cytomegalovirus infection: The brain as a window in the establishment of prognosis. In: Ramenghi A, Evrard P, Mercuri E, eds. *Mariani Foundation Paediatric Neurology. Perinatal brain damage: From Pathogenesis to Neuroprotection.* Vol 19. Montrouge: Editions John Libbey Eurotext; 2008;49–54, with permission.)

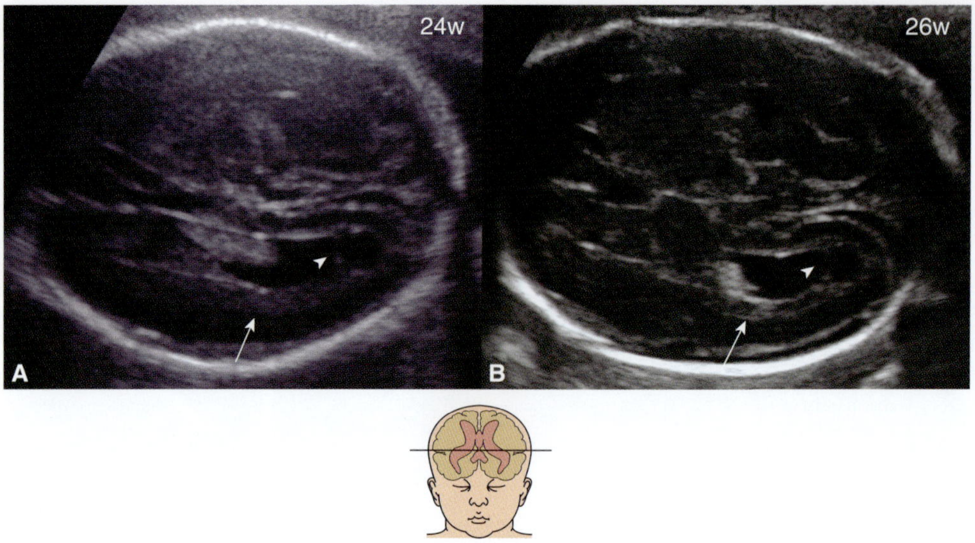


**Figure 9–6.** Transabdominal axial planes at the level of the lateral ventricles. **(A–B)** Images of fetuses with known CMV infection and periventricular hyperechogenicity show that it is clearly differentiated from the surrounding brain (*arrows*). Both fetuses **(A)** at 24 weeks, **(B)** at 26 weeks, presented with porencephalic occipital cysts (*arrowheads*) but without ventriculomegaly.

the perforating striatal arteries, are better visualized in the parasagittal plane (Figure 9–9). Striatal arteries originate from the middle cerebral arteries and irrigate the germinal matrix and when normal are not depicted.

Although extremely uncommon, isolated cases of cerebral[52,53] and cerebellar[54] hemorrhages have been reported. The cerebellum may also be involved demonstrating calcifications, cysts,[22,40] or a reduction in size.

## Magnetic Resonance Imaging Diagnosis

Two recent retrospective studies have compared fetal ultrasound (US) and magnetic resonance imaging (MRI) findings in patients with CMV. Picone and colleagues[55] studied 38 fetuses in which CMV polymerase chain reaction (PCR) was positive in the amniotic fluid.[55] MRI failed to show any sign of brain infection in 11 fetuses with normal US examinations. In 13 fetuses in which US only depicted extracerebral findings, MRI detected brain lesions in 46%. MRI confirmed the presence of cerebral signs found by US in the remaining 14 fetuses and in some of them added new information that was not depicted by US.[55] Benoist and colleagues[23] studied by targeted US and MRI 49 fetuses with proven CMV infection and compared the results to the postnatal US or post mortem examinations; the best positive predictive value (88.9%) was obtained when both US and MRI showed abnormal findings, and the best negative predictive value (93.5%) was obtained when the US was normal.

We have seen five CMV PCR-positive fetuses in whom there was a discrepancy between the US and MRI findings. The US was normal, whereas the MRI raised the suspicion of white matter abnormalities. Three children were delivered and were developing normally at ages 2 to 4 years; two pregnancies were terminated, and the autopsies were

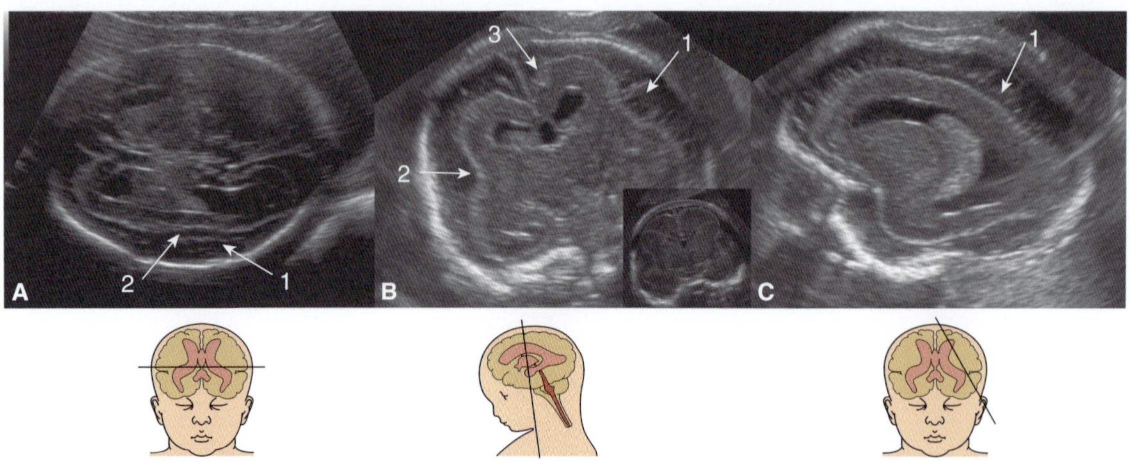


**Figure 9–7.** Orthogonal views of a fetus with CMV at 24 weeks, 2 days; the head circumference (HC) was 20 cm (<–2 SDs [standard deviations]). Axial **(A)**, coronal **(B)**, and sagittal **(C)** views. Note the enlarged subarachnoidal space (1), the underdeveloped sylvian fissure (2), and the presence of an abnormal sulcus in the frontal lobe (3). The small coronal figure provides an image for comparison of a normal fetus at 22 weeks of pregnancy.

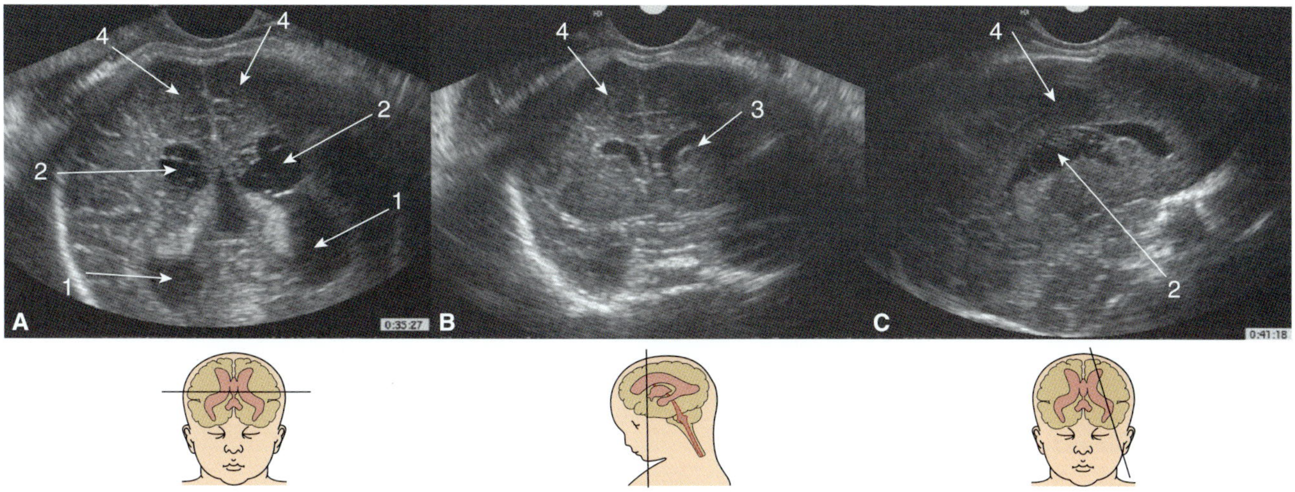


**Figure 9–8.** CMV in a fetus at 35 postmenstrual weeks; **(A)** axial, **(B)** coronal, **(C)** sagittal. The mother was CMV seropositive during the first trimester and was referred because of ventriculomegaly (1) at a routine ultrasound (US) examination. Bilateral large intraventricular cysts (2) and small periventricular pseudocysts (3) are depicted. The sulci and gyri are not observed due to white matter involvement (4).

negative for brain CMV; but in one patient microglial nodules consistent with an inflammatory reaction were found. Garel[56] reported that in all patients with a normal US the MRI was also normal.

Neurosonography and MRI perform equally in the demonstration of morphological anomalies (Figures 9–10 and 9–11).

### Implications for Sonographic Screening, Including Earliest Recognition

Due to the low prevalence of symptomatic congenital CMV infection, the low sensitivity and specificity of the available tests, and the lack of proven intrauterine treatments, universal screening for CMV infection is not an integral part of prenatal care. In these patients, second- or third-trimester US examinations are the only opportunity to raise the suspicion of fetal disease. The presence of any of the extracerebral findings described previously should prompt the performance of serological tests and a detailed brain examination for CMV signs. Before 20 weeks, the only described sign of fetal infection is intestinal hyperechogenicity; later on the presence of hepatosplenomegaly, ascites, or cardiomegaly should be considered suspicious. During routine second-trimester examinations, the presence of ventriculomegaly or

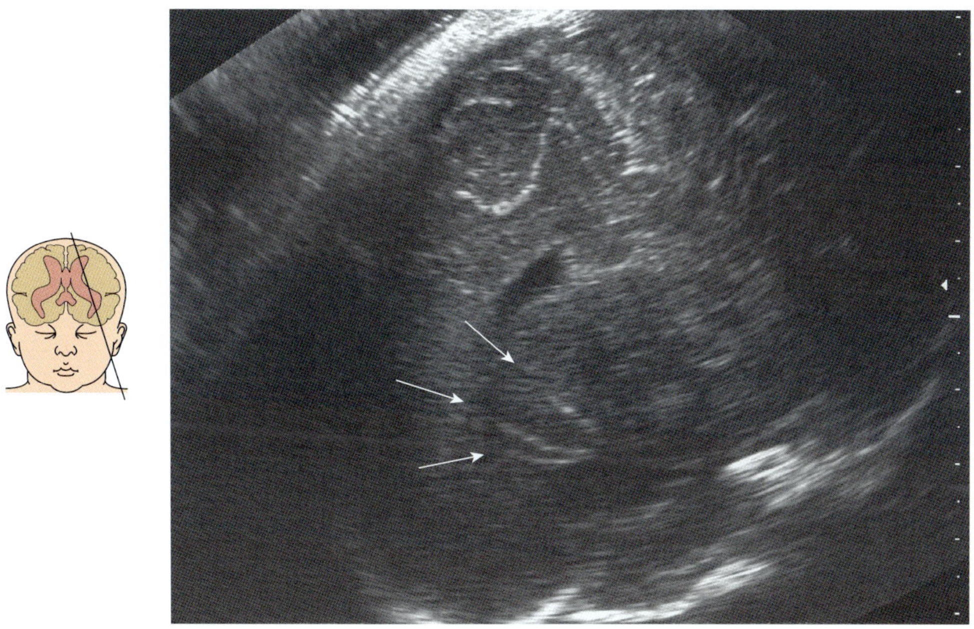

**Figure 9–9.** Linear striatal vasculopathy (*arrows*) at 35 postmenstrual weeks in an otherwise apparently normal fetus with positive polymerase chain reaction (PCR) CMV amniotic fluid.

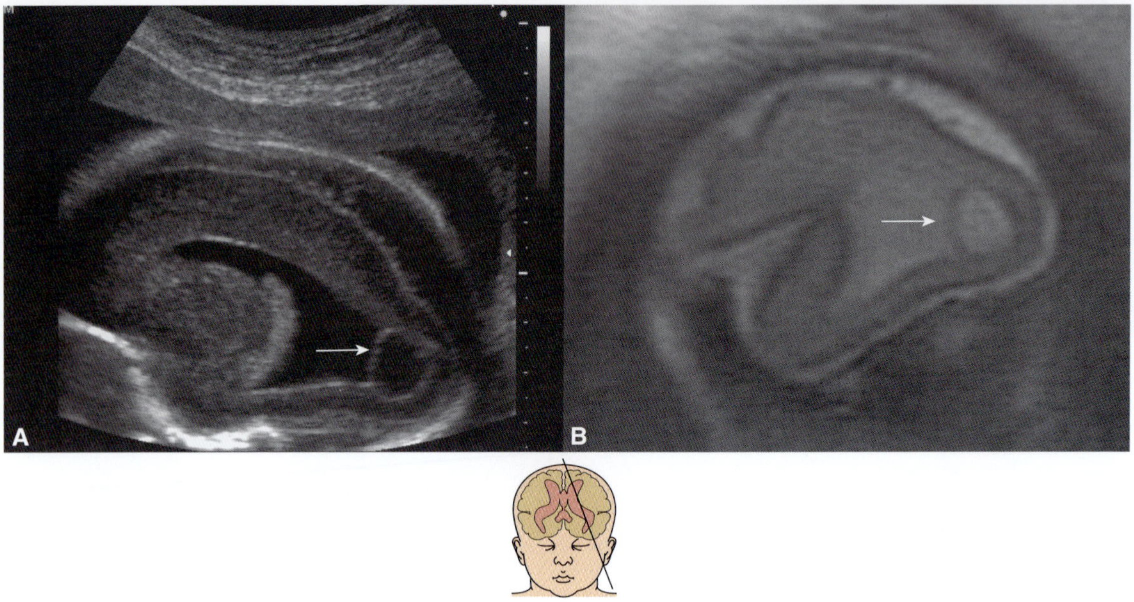


**Figure 9–10.** Sagittal transvaginal US **(A)** and MRI **(B)** at 24 postmenstrual weeks in a fetus with CMV. Note the similarity between the images showing the presence of a large occipital porencephalic cyst (*arrows*) and mild ventriculomegaly.

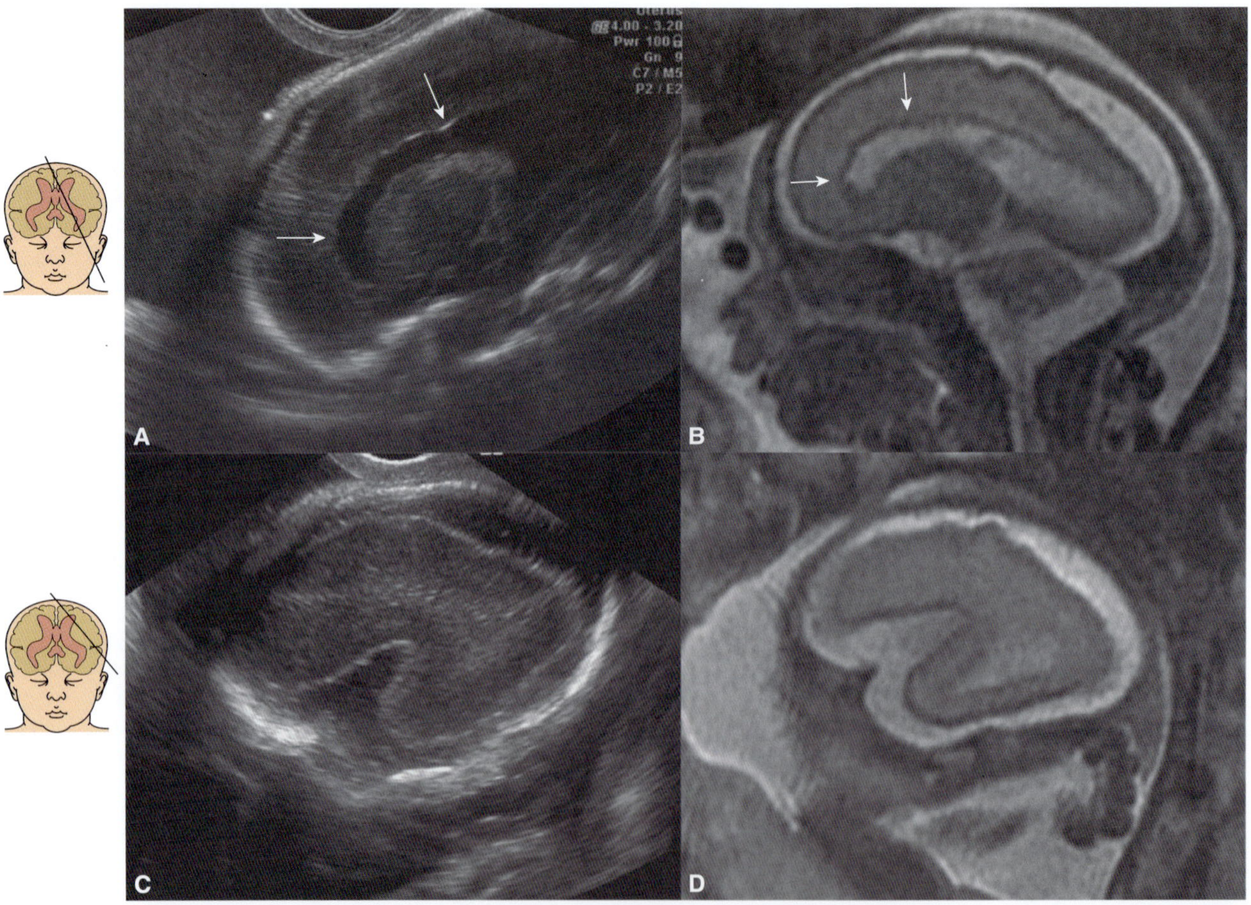


**Figure 9–11.** Sagittal transvaginal US and magnetic resonance imaging (MRI) at 29 postmenstrual weeks in a fetus with CMV. The MRI examination was performed 3 days after the US. Parasagittal US **(A)** and MRI **(B)** show mild ventriculomegaly with irregular, dentate ventricular walls (*arrows*) due to ventriculitis and ependymal damage. More lateral US **(C)** and MRI **(D)** views show a wide sylvian fissure and almost complete lack of sulcation.

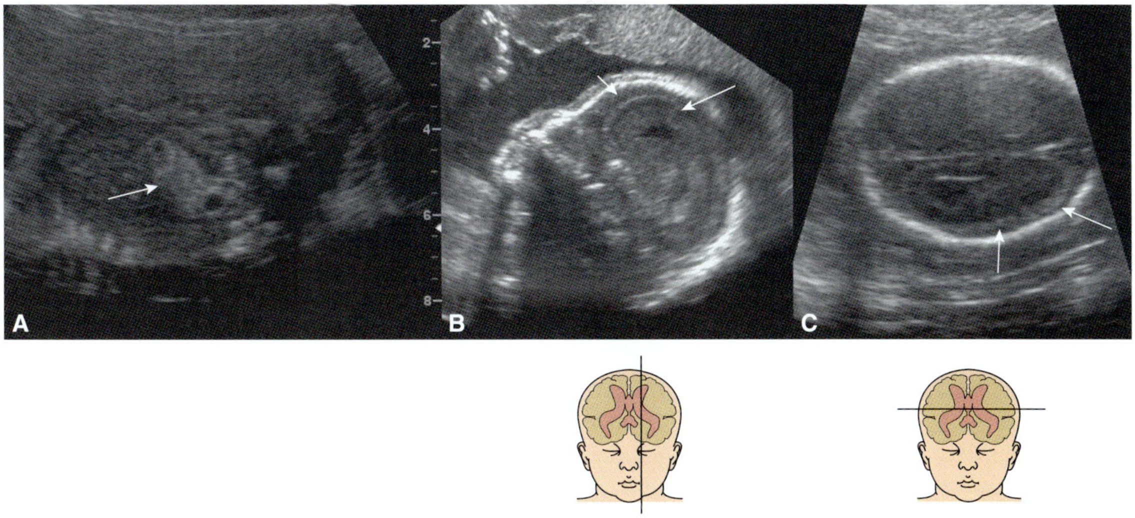


**Figure 9–12.** Early detection of CMV infection in a fetus at 20 postmenstrual weeks. **(A)** Transabdominal image showing hyperechogenic intestines (*arrow*). **(B)** Sagittal plane. Note the well demarcated periventricular echogenicity (*arrow*) with increased amount of subarachnoid fluid due to reduced cerebral size (*arrowhead*). **(C)** Axial plane at the level of the lateral ventricle. Hyperechogenic cerebral surface is consistent with early abnormal sulcation and probable polymicrogyria (*arrows*).

intracranial calcifications is a clear indication for further investigation. In these patients, a careful analysis of the periventricular zone is of paramount importance, as in the vast majority of patients with CMV, this region will be involved.[22,40]

The earliest reports of US recognition of CMV-related findings are at 19–20 weeks.[27,53] In our series, the earliest diagnosis was suspected at 20 weeks in a fetus with echogenic bowel, increased periventricular echogenicity, and abnormal sulcation (Figure 9–12).

### Implications for Targeted Ultrasound Examination

Targeted US examinations are of paramount importance in the management of fetuses with proven intrauterine infection and of those in whom maternal seroconversion has occurred during pregnancy, but the fetal status is unknown. Although not conclusively proven, most authorities believe that the presence of microcephaly or intracranial findings is associated with a poor prognosis, and in these cases termination of pregnancy or experimental antiviral treatments may be considered.[20,57]

Affected fetuses with normal targeted US examinations should be followed with repeated targeted examinations at 3- to 4-week intervals.

### Prognosis

Prognosis is based on the extent of involvement, particularly of the brain. If the examination remains normal, the prognosis appears to be excellent.[40] It is important to remember that a normal US examination will never be able to rule out sensorineural hearing loss (SNHL).

Although not always feasible, accurate knowledge of the gestational week in which the fetus was infected is an important parameter in counseling.[58] Maternal seroconversion during the third trimester implies fetal infection, as CMV is highly transmissible but is almost invariably asymptomatic.[59]

Recently, Foulon and colleagues[60] described the follow-up of 28 delivered children who had proven intrauterine fetal infection; 4 out of 5 children with first-trimester infection had SNHL, but all 12 children with third-trimester infection were unaffected.

Because most of the infected newborns are asymptomatic and thus not diagnosed, it is difficult to predict the risks of an abnormal neurodevelopmental outcome and/or SNHL in the whole affected population. Based on longitudinal studies, 85% to 100% of patients with asymptomatic disease will develop normally,[48,61–63] and only 1 out of 100 children will develop SNHL per year of follow-up.[64] The prognosis of affected fetuses with abnormal neurosonography during pregnancy can be predicted by extrapolating from existing data regarding the bad prognosis in newborns with symptomatic CMV and brain computed tomography or US signs of infection.[57,65] The prognosis remains unclear in patients with positive detection of CMV in the amniotic fluid who present with either isolated minor brain findings, such as periventricular pseudocysts or striatal vasculopathy, or isolated systemic findings.

Extrapolation of results of postnatal studies to fetal imaging is possible and enables counseling.[23,40,55,56] Counseling based on fetal blood platelet count,[66] viral load in the amniotic fluid,[67] viral strain subtypes,[68,69] and even fetal gender has been proposed.[70]

## Obstetric Management

Prevention of CMV infection by universal or selective vaccination of women before conception, as done in the case of congenital rubella, should be considered the optimal way of management, but the development of an effective vaccine has proven to be extremely complicated. Pass and colleagues[71] published the results of a phase 2, placebo-controlled, randomized, double-blind trial on the use of a vaccine consisting of recombinant CMV envelope glycoprotein B; they found that the vaccine has the potential to decrease the incidence of maternal and congenital CMV. CMV infection was observed in 18 women who received the CMV vaccine, and 1 newborn had asymptomatic congenital CMV compared with 31 women and 3 newborns (1 of them with severe symptomatic infection) in the placebo group.[71] Until the performance of large phase 3 trials, hygienic measures implemented in women of childbearing age will be the leading intervention for preventing CMV infection.[72,73] Patient information on this and other issues regarding CMV are available at http://www.cdc.gov/cmv.

In cases of known CMV seroconversion, amniocentesis may be performed starting from 22 weeks of pregnancy but not before 6 to 8 weeks have elapsed from the moment of the first positive CMV test. Because the presence of CMV in the amniotic fluid does not mean that the fetus will necessarily be affected, an alternative option would be to perform serial US examinations during pregnancy.[40]

Fetal MRI may be used when US visualization is suboptimal, when the operator is unsure regarding the presence or absence of findings, and probably as a backup for US late in pregnancy to rule out white matter disease or early myelinization abnormalities.

Preliminary results on antiviral treatment with valaciclovir[74] and with intravenous hyperimmune globulin[75] have been published, but the results are still controversial. Until effective antiviral treatments are developed, termination of pregnancy may be considered in fetuses with microcephaly and/or signs of brain infection.

## TOXOPLASMOSIS

### Definition

Congenital toxoplasmosis is the result of a transplacental infection with the protozoa *Toxoplasma Gondii.* In humans the most common source of infection is exposure to the domesticated cat or the ingestion or handling of contaminated meat.

### Incidence/Prevalence

The reported incidence of congenital toxoplasmosis ranges from 0.07 to 5.0 per 1000 live births.[76–81] It appears to be more prevalent in some countries (France,[76] Argentina,[79] Holland,[80] and Brazil[81]) than in others (Sweden,[77] Denmark,[78] and Ireland[80]). In the United States, data are available from the New England Regional Newborn Screening Program.[82] All infants in the program were tested for evidence of congenital toxoplasmosis; from 1986 to 1992, of 635,000 infants who underwent serologic testing, 52 were infected, representing an infection rate of ~1 per 10,000 live births. Only two (4%) of these infants were recognized as having congenital toxoplasmosis before the screening results were known; however, follow-up examinations of 19 (40%) of the 48 infants evaluated revealed signs of disease (eg, abnormal cerebrospinal fluid [CSF] examinations, hydrocephaly, and retinal lesions).

### Pathogenesis

The cat and other animals play an essential role in the life cycle of the parasite. The sexual cycle of the parasite takes place in the gastrointestinal tract of the cat. Oocysts are produced, which are then excreted in the feces.[83] Women may become exposed while cleaning the litter box of an infected cat or by handling soil or meat that has been contaminated. The oocysts are then ingested, with subsequent circulation of the parasites in the blood (tachyzoites). The tachyzoites penetrate into tissues such as muscle and brain and can be transmitted across the placenta. Fetal infection occurs when the mother has a primary infection with circulating tachyzoites.[84] The placenta becomes infected, and following a lag period there is a subsequent hematogenous spread to the fetus.

### Etiology

Women infected with toxoplasmosis before conception do not transmit the infection to their fetuses. If the infection occurs after conception, it can be transmitted across the placenta to the fetus. Fetal involvement results from acute infection in the mother.

The risk of fetal infection depends on the timing of primary maternal infection; the overall risk of transmission is ~40%.[85] If maternal infection occurs during the first and second trimesters, only ~10% to 25% and 30% to 54%, respectively, of the fetuses will become infected.[86] However, if infection occurs during the third trimester, the risk of fetal infection increases to 65%.[86–88] In contrast, the severity of the disease decreases with increasing gestational age at the time of infection, the most severe cases occurring following early infection. This risk of severe involvement decreases from 80% during the first[t] trimester to 0% during the third trimester. The diagnosis of primary disease in the mother is made based on documentation of seroconversion, a marked increase in antibody titer, or the presence of toxoplasmosis-specific immunoglobulin M (IgM).[89]

The clinical features of congenital toxoplasmosis include increased risk of premature delivery, seizures, meningoencephalitis, microcephaly, hydrocephaly, intracranial calcifications, chorioretinitis, hepatosplenomegaly, anemia, petechiae, hyperbilirubinemia, and pneumonitis.

### Pathology

The intracranial calcifications of fetal toxoplasmosis are multifocal and present in many areas of the brain, such as the basal ganglia, periventricular zone, white matter, and cerebral cortex, unlike CMV infection, which has a predilection for the periventricular zone.[90,91] The toxoplasmosis lesions in the brain start as vasculitis, subsequently followed by necrosis and cellular infiltration in the cortex, meninges, white matter, basal ganglia, brainstem, and spinal cortex. The necrosis is followed by calcification.[92]

### Risk of Recurrence

Rarely, a latent infection in an immunocompromised mother[93] or the ingestion of raw meat infected with

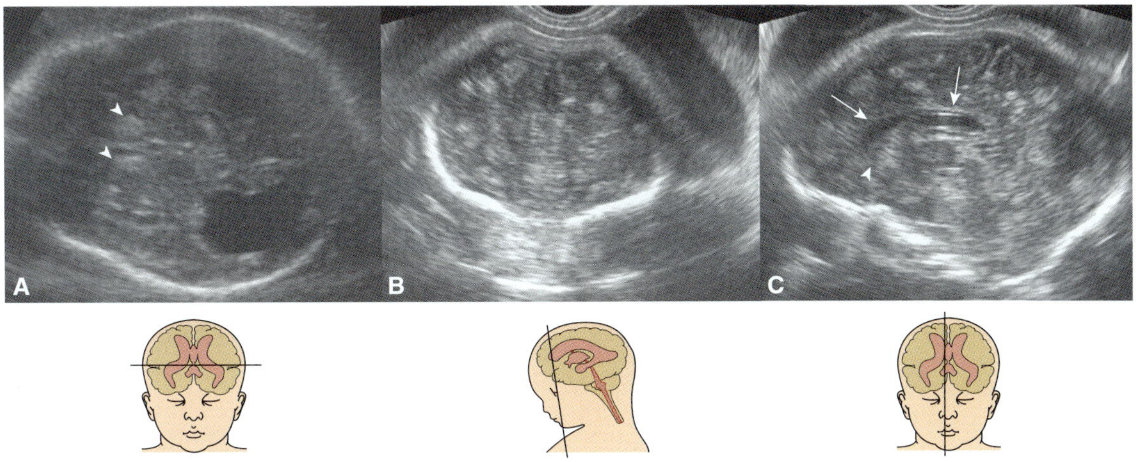


**Figure 9–13.** Toxoplasmosis with severe brain involvement diagnosed at 34 postmenstrual weeks. Axial **(A)**, coronal **(B)**, and sagittal **(C)** planes. Multiple noncalcified echogenic nodules are depicted in all the brain regions, including the caudate nuclei (*arrowheads* in A and C). Note the presence of ventriculomegaly (A) and dysgenesis of the corpus callosum (*arrow* in C). (Courtesy of Dr. Mauricio Herrera, Bogotá, Colombia.)

an extremely virulent strain in a seropositive woman[94] may result in fetal infection.

## Sonographic Diagnosis

The intracranial sonographic findings of fetal toxoplasmosis include intracranial calcifications, hydrocephaly, microcephaly, brain atrophy, and hydranencephaly. Hohlfeld and coworkers[95] reported on 89 cases of fetal toxoplasmosis, in 34 of which the pregnancy was electively terminated. In this subgroup, the most common brain sonographic finding was cerebral ventricular dilation, which was present in 74%, followed by intracranial calcifications in 18%. The ventricular dilation was bilateral and symmetrical, evolved very rapidly, and did not result in an increase in biparietal diameter (BPD).

Abboud and coworkers[96] analyzed the data from 2168 seroconversions during pregnancy, including 168 with proven fetal infection. They found that only 2.2% of the fetuses presented US signs of infection. Forty-four percent of the fetuses had multiple findings, including calcifications and ventriculomegaly; microcephaly was not diagnosed in any patient.

Although large studies describing the diagnosis of congenital toxoplasmosis have been published, the number of articles in which US brain images of affected fetuses are presented is surprisingly low. Couto and Ferreira[97] described a patient diagnosed during the second trimester with ventriculomegaly and large multiple periventricular echogenic nodules. Cuillier and Avignon[98] were able to compare the CNS findings in a 30-week fetus as demonstrated by transvaginal sonography (TVS), neurosonography, and MRI. TVS depicted ventriculomegaly, increased periventricular echogenicity with multiple intraparenchymal echogenic nodules, and brain abscess formation; MRI confirmed the findings and showed also partial left cerebellar hypoplasia. Garel[56] showed a good correlation between US and MRI in a fetus diagnosed at 31 weeks. The presence of multiple noncalcified echogenic nodules was also apparent in a fetus studied in Bogotá, Colombia (Figure 9–13).

## Associated Anomalies

Other sonographic findings reported in fetuses with congenital toxoplasmosis are a thickened placenta with hyperechoic areas, liver echogenicities, hepatomegaly, ascites, and pericardial or pleural effusions.[95,97,99,100] Although very common, most ocular lesions will not be detected during pregnancy; fetal cataract[101] and microphtalmia may be present.

## MRI Diagnosis

Barkovich and Girard[102] considered the use of fetal MRI extremely important as a diagnostic tool in patients with suspected fetal infection. They declared that MRI "gives the best assessment of the extent of brain damage" and should be used "when clinical suspicion is high in the setting of a normal ultrasound or to better define abnormalities detected by ultrasound"; it should be "routinely used in toxoplasmosis seroconversion to definitively rule out brain lesions, even when the ultrasound scan is considered normal."[102] These conclusions are not validated by previous investigations, and even the presented data cited do not enable reaching such categorical conclusions and are contradictory to published data showing that repeated normal US examinations were able to predict normal development in 35 out of 36 children with CT.[103] In treated patients, the presence of calcifications or moderate ventriculomegaly is not always associated with poor neurodevelopmental outcome.[101]

Examples of fetal MRI findings in patients with congenital toxoplasmosis showed in one case the presence of an abnormal periventricular signal with unilateral vebntriculomegaly[104] and in another, signs of intraventricular hemorrhage, left sylvian infarct with temporal atrophy, and hyperintense parenchyma.[56]

In our opinion, the main role of MRI resides in its ability to detect acute events in the form of white matter signal abnormalities.[102,104]

#### Implications for Sonographic Screening, Including Earliest Recognition

In countries without a screening policy of all pregnant women, US remains the only opportunity for detection of congenital toxoplasmosis. There are no published studies on this issue, but the US diagnosis of ventriculomegaly, increased periventricular echogenicities, multiple echogenic nodules, brain or liver calcifications, ascites, hepatosplenomegaly, or cataracts should prompt the performance of toxoplasma serology.

#### Implications for Targeted Examination

A detailed neurosonographic examination should be performed when the suspicion of congenital toxoplasmosis is raised by serologic studies; follow-up examinations at 3- to 4-week intervals are indicated even in patients with negative amniocentesis.[105]

### Prognosis

Most authors suggest that the presence of brain anomalies at birth carries an adverse outcome.[106,107] Roizen and colleagues[108] found that 8 out of 10 children with congenital hydrocephaly developed severe disabilities. In contrast to these results, Berrebi and collaborators[101] found that all 27 infants with proven congenital toxoplasmosis, including 10 with one or more clinical signs, 5 with isolated or multiple intracranial calcifications, 7 with peripheral chorioretinitis, and 2 with moderate ventricular dilations, were free from symptoms and had normal neurologic development at 15 to 71 months of age. It should be remembered that asymptomatic infants at birth carry an increased risk for developing ocular lesions, neurodevelopmental problems, and/or epilepsy during the first years of life.

### Clinical Management

Confirmation of fetal infection after maternal primary infection relies on the use of a PCR test performed on amniotic fluid.[109,110] Amniocentesis should not be performed until at least 4 weeks after the acute disease in the mother because testing too soon may result in a false-negative result.[109] Diagnostic tests are not warranted if maternal infection occurred within the first 2 weeks of pregnancy, due to only a slight risk of fetal infection.

Fetal therapy in cases of primary maternal infection includes treatment of the mother with spiramycin (1 g three times daily) until the diagnosis is confirmed by a PCR test of the amniotic fluid. Most authors recommend starting treatment quickly, before fetal infection occurs. This may be possible as there is a lag period between the onset of maternal and fetal infection. Following the confirmation of fetal infection, spiramycin may be continued until delivery, or it may be replaced by a combination of pyrimethamine, sulfadiazine, and folinic acid. A large meta-analysis of treated children with congenital toxoplasmosis has questioned the effectiveness of prenatal treatment. The study did not find an association between early treatment and a reduced risk of symptomatic congenital toxoplasmosis.[111] In addition, prenatal treatment did not reduce the risk of retinochoroiditis in children.[112]

Following confirmation of fetal infection with associated CNS involvement, termination of pregnancy should be considered.

## INFREQUENT INFECTIONS AND EMERGING INFECTIOUS DISEASES AFFECTING THE BRAIN

### Rubella

Congenital rubella syndrome is now a rarity because of the widespread use of immunization. The reported incidence is <1 per 1 million live births. The congenital syndrome is characterized by cataracts, glaucoma, chorioretinitis, microphthalmus, cardiac malformations, microcephaly, and deafness. Primary maternal disease can be asymptomatic. Maternal viremia results in infection of the placenta, with subsequent infection of the fetus. Infection can occur at any time during pregnancy, but first-trimester infection results in more severely affected infants. Congenital rubella lesions are found in 50% of fetuses affected in the first month of gestation, in 22% of those in the second month, and in 7% of those between the third and fifth months.[90,113]

CNS involvement in affected infants includes microcephaly, calcifications, subependymal caudate and striatothalamic cysts, and echogenic foci in the basal ganglia,[114,115] but to the best of our knowledge, there is a lack of such documentation in fetal studies.

The prognosis depends on the clinical features. Symptomatic children at birth usually have neurodevelopmental abnormalities. A group of 100 infants with congenital rubella syndrome showed microcephaly in 81%, severe neuromotor deficits in 47%, hearing loss in 72%, and ocular manifestations in 78%; only 9% appeared to be free of deficits at 18 months of age.[116]

### Varicella Zoster Virus

Varicella, or chickenpox, is usually a mild childhood disease characterized by fever, lymphadenitis, and skin rash. Reactivation of the disease may produce herpes zoster. Varicella is a highly contagious disease, and only a small proportion of the population reaches adulthood unaffected. It is difficult to determine the incidence of varicella in pregnant women, as it depends on its prevalence in the studied general population during the time of the study. Balducci et al[117] found in a prospective study performed between 1986 and 1990 that the estimated incidence was 7 in 10,000 pregnancies.

Transplacental transmission of the virus may result in fetal or neonatal disease. According to large series published during the last 25 years, the risk of congenital varicella syndrome ranges from 0%[117] to 9%.[118] In the largest prospective study published until now, Enders et al[119] followed 1739 pregnancies with varicella and herpes zoster and found that the fetuses were at a higher risk between

13 and 20 weeks of gestation, with 7 out of 351 (2%) affected fetuses. Similar results were found in another two large series.[120,121]

The congenital varicella syndrome includes skin scar lesions, limb deformities, CNS findings, hepatosplenomegaly, and gastrointestinal, eye, and urinary tract anomalies. Hydrops fetalis, growth restriction, hydramnios, and increased risk of prematurity may also be present. Neurologic deficits and herpes zoster may develop during infancy. Varicella infection after 20 weeks' gestation does not jeopardize the fetus.

CNS involvement has been reported in isolated cases,[122,123] but upon review of the four largest series on maternal varicella/zoster infection during pregnancy, it is evident that CNS involvement is very rare. From a total of 1925 cases of varicella and 395 cases of herpes zoster infection during pregnancy, only 1 patient was diagnosed as suffering from encephalitis and microcephaly.[117–121]

As in other intrauterine infections, it is important to realize that the US signs of brain involvement may develop late in pregnancy. Meyberg-Solomayer and colleagues[2] described a well-documented case following maternal infection at 16 weeks. At 21.3 weeks, the lateral ventricle width was 9 mm, and hepatic and myocardial calcifications and limb involvement were observed; at 33 weeks, brain calcifications were apparent. MRI performed at the age of 8 days showed ventricular dilation, calcifications, and porencephalic cysts. In another patient with chickenpox at 21.3 weeks' gestation, the fetus was apparently unaffected until 36 weeks' gestation, when isolated liver calcifications were depicted; after birth the infant presented with skin lesions all over the body and scalp and bilateral chorioretinitis. At 12 months, the infant had delayed psychomotor acquisitions, cortical atrophy, and blindness.[124] The development of cerebellar involvement, pachygyria, and abnormal operculization has been demonstrated using MRI in a fetus at 32 weeks of pregnancy.[125]

## Herpes Simplex Virus

Herpes simplex virus types 1 and 2 (HSV-1 and HSV-2) are among the most common human viral infections. Neonatal infection occurs due to direct contact with the virus during labor or ascending infection following premature rupture of membranes. It may cause a wide range of symptoms and involve diverse organs, including the newborn brain.

Intrauterine infection remote from birth and due to transplacental transmission is extremely rare. In a systematic review of the literature published between 1960 and 2004, Avgil and Ornoy[126] found 11 case reports describing affected newborns. CNS involvement was present in four: brain necrosis and ventriculomegaly were present in two, meningoencephalitis, cystic lesions in the brain parenchyma, and abnormal cerebellum in one each. At least three other newborns with cystic encephalomalacia and associated findings have been reported.[4,127]

Recently, Duin et al[3] reported a pregnant woman with primary HSV-2 infection during the first trimester and a normal US examination at 20 weeks' gestation. At 31 weeks, the fetus developed bilateral ventriculomegaly involving the frontal horns, frontal thinning of the cerebral cortex, and a wavering midline. At 35 weeks, the fetus was found to have intrauterine growth retardation below the fifth percentile and stable cerebral ventriculomegaly, but with a slight disruption of the cortical mantle. Fetal brain MRI at the same time showed severe parenchymal destruction, particularly in the temporal and parietal lobes, with frontal cortical thinning to 2 mm. No cerebral mantle could be seen. The occipital cortex was globally thinned with microgyria. Because of the rarity of fetal involvement, invasive diagnostic tests should be reserved for cases with clinical or laboratory evidence of maternal HSV infection.

Occasionally, generalized fetal herpes virus infection may be diagnosed in an otherwise normal and asymptomatic pregnancy by the presence of neurosonographic imaging signs similar to intrauterine CMV infection (Figure 9–14).

## Parvovirus B19

Although not considered a teratogenic virus, parvovirus B19 infection during pregnancy may produce different types of fetal brain insults. Isumi and colleagues[6] demonstrated marked neuropathologic changes in the fetal brain at the midembryonal period expressed by the presence of multinucleated giant cells of macrophage/microglia lineage and many small calcifications around vessels, predominantly in the cerebral white matter. Parvovirus B19 genome DNA was detected in the nucleus of the multinucleated giant cells and solitary endothelial cells by PCR amplification and in situ PCR methods. Insults may also be related to the development of severe fetal anemia with high-output cardiac failure and thrombocytopenia followed by intraventricular hemorrhage. It should be mentioned that the only available study on this issue failed to find a relationship between thrombocytopenia in parvovirus B19–infected fetuses and brain hemorrhage.[128]

Case reports of fetal cerebellar hemorrhage[129] and mild malformation of cortical development[130] are difficult to attribute to the virus teratogenicity or to the performance of blood transfusion in severely anemic fetuses. A case report on fetal stroke in congenital parvovirus B19 infection may be associated with the fact that the patient had activated protein C resistance.[131]

Nagel and collaborators[132] reported the long-term outcome of infected children after fetal transfusion for hydrops. The initial group consisted of 24 infants. There were 16 survivors, and only 11 (68%) were normal; 5 children (32%) demonstrated delayed psychomotor development with a suboptimal neurologic examination (mild delay $n = 3$, severe delay $n = 2$).

## Lymphocytic Choriomeningitis Virus

Lymphocytic choriomeningitis virus (LCMV) is an arenavirus transmitted by rodents through contact with their secretions. The infection may remain asymptomatic or cause fever, myalgia, headache, nausea, and vomiting. Some patients develop aseptic meningitis or meningoencephalitis.[133] Vertical transmission from an acutely infected

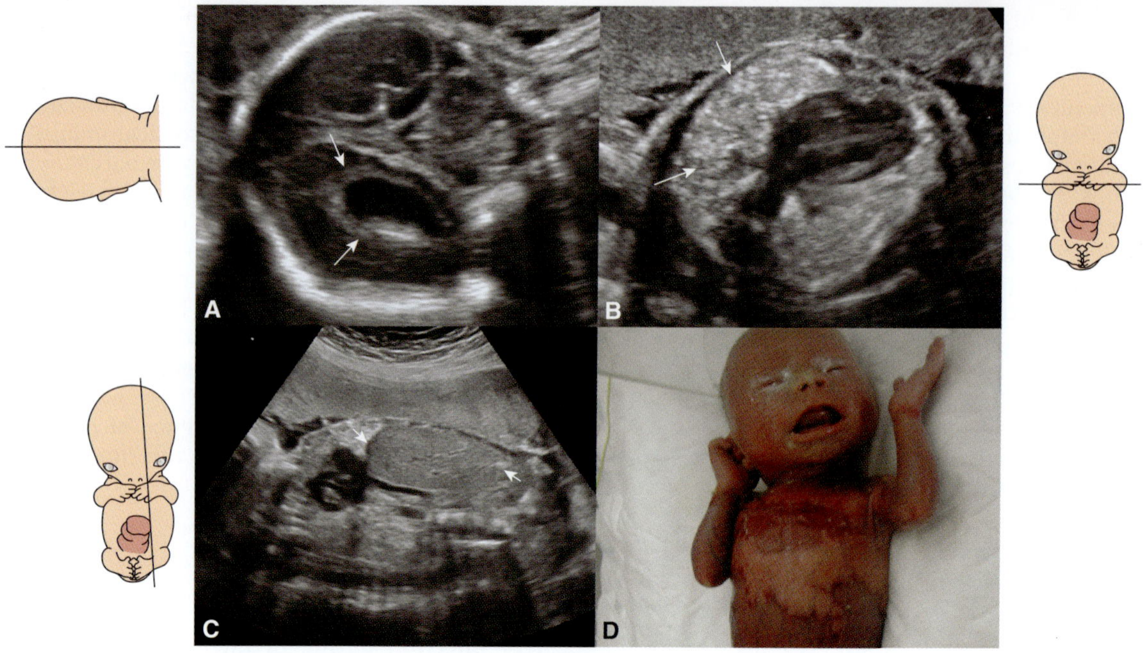


**Figure 9–14.** Herpes simplex infection at 29 postmenstrual weeks in a fetus referred for investigation due to the presence of oligohydramnios. During the examination, the amount of amniotic fluid was normal but highly particulate, probably due to severe herpetic dermatitis. **(A)** Coronal view at the level of the occipital lobes showing hyperechogenic periventricular white matter (*white arrows*). **(B)** Abnormal echogenicity of the lungs (*white arrows*). **(C)** Hepatomegaly (*arrowheads*). **(D)** Severe disseminated herpetic dermatitis in the newborn. (Courtesy of Dr. Mauricio Herrera, Bogotá, Colombia.)

mother to the fetus has been reported and is known to increase the risk of abortion and fetal insult. Chorioretinitis and ventriculomegaly are the predominant characteristics among children diagnosed with congenital LCMV infection; other described neuroimaging abnormalities are microcephaly, periventricular calcifications, pachygyria, cerebellar hypoplasia, and porencephalic and periventricular cysts.[7] According to Bonthius and colleagues,[7] the combination of micrencephaly and periventricular calcifications was the most common neuroimaging abnormality, and all children with this combination had profound mental retardation, epilepsy, and cerebral palsy.

Chorioretinitis was described in 48 of 54 infants and hydrocephaly or periventricular calcifications in 23 of 25 infants in whom neuroimaging studies were obtained.[134,135] Mortality among infants diagnosed with congenital LCMV is ~30%, and two-thirds of the survivors have long-term neurologic abnormalities.[136] However, it is possible that previously reported cases are biased toward the more severe end of the spectrum. A recent report of 2 children with evidence of chorioretinitis and presumed congenital LCMV infection without neurologic manifestations supports this possibility.[137]

The prenatal diagnosis of LCMV infection may be considered in fetuses with signs of intrauterine infection after exclusion of other, more common pathogens or when there is evidence of contact with rodents during pregnancy.[138]

## West Nile Virus

West Nile virus (WNV) is a mosquito-borne flavivirus and a human neuropathogen; WNV epidemics have occurred worldwide since 1999.[139] The disease affects predominantly adults, but affected children have been reported.[140]

Fetal infection with neurologic involvement was described for the first time in 2002 following maternal WNV disease at 27 weeks of pregnancy.[141] The WNV seropositive–infant was delivered at 38 weeks' gestation and was asymptomatic, but an ophthalmologic examination revealed bilateral chorioretinitis. MRI of the brain indicated severe cerebral abnormalities, including severe bilateral white matter loss in the temporal and occipital lobes and cystic change in one temporal lobe consistent with focal cerebral destruction.[141,142]

A follow-up study of all the WNV diagnosed cases (77 patients) in the United States during 2002–2003 found that at least three newborns were symptomatic (one with neurologic involvement), and another infant developed meningitis at the age of 10 days.[143] Seven infants had major malformations, but only three of these had defects that could have been caused by maternal WNV infection based on the timing of the infection.

A study of 566 pregnant women delivered in a single Colorado hospital found that 4% of them were seropositive, but WNV infection during pregnancy did not seem to affect adversely infant health at birth.[144]

## Syphilis

Syphilis, caused by *Treponema pallidum,* has been affecting women and their offspring for hundreds of years. The introduction of antibiotic treatment has made the disease less common but still present around the world.

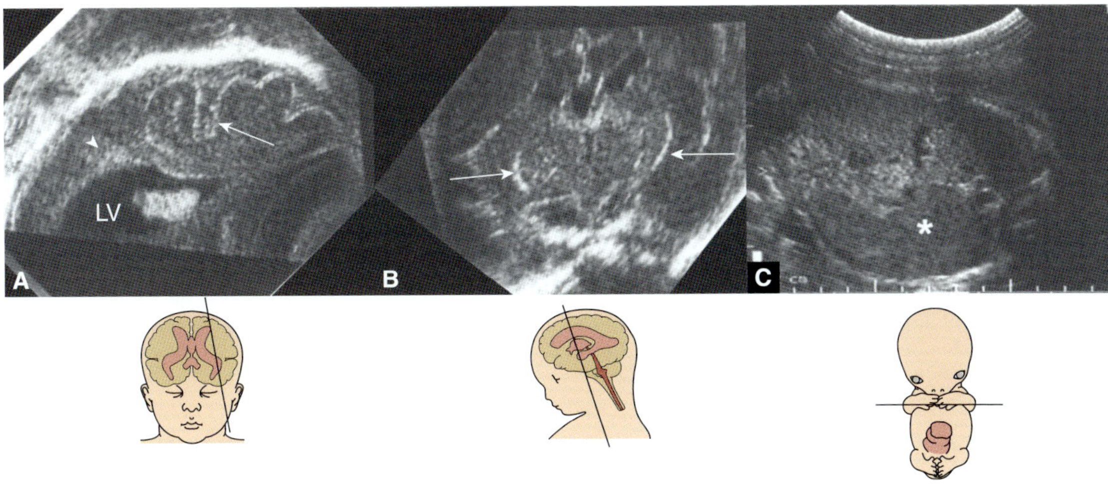


**Figure 9–15.** Ultrasonographic appearance of the fetal brain and spleen in a patient with congenital syphilis at 34 postmenstrual weeks. **(A)** Parasagittal transvaginal sonography (TVS) section at the level of the lateral ventricle (*) shows pachygyria (*arrow* ) and abnormal periventricular echogenicity (*arrowhead* ). **(B)** Coronal TVS section at the level of the thalami shows striatal vasculopathy (*arrows* ). **(C)** Splenomgaly (*).

Congenital syphilis is characterized by dermatologic anomalies; hepatosplenomegaly; lymphadenopathy; hematological, renal, CNS, ocular, and skeletal manifestations; and growth restriction. Fetal CNS involvement has rarely been reported in series or case reports. Hollier and colleagues[145] described 24 patients with untreated syphilis with a vertical transmission rate of 66%; 13 fetuses had hepatomegaly, and 3 had hepatosplenomegaly with ascites. CNS involvement was not reported in any of the patients. Mavrov and Goubenko[9] described 23 fetuses with US signs of infection from a group of 155 woman with syphilis. Ventriculomegaly was diagnosed in two and US changes in brain vessels in nine.

We have observed the presence of ventriculomegaly, pachygyria, and abnormal periventricular white matter in a fetus at 34 weeks following untreated first-trimester maternal infection; hepatosplenomegaly was present, and the newborn died on the first day of life[146] (Figure 9–15).

## Trypanosoma Cruzi (Chagas Disease)

*Trypanosoma cruzi* is an endemic South and Central American protozoa causing Chagas disease. The majority of persons infected remain in a subclinical stage, and only 30% to 40% develop the classical clinical picture affecting the heart and gastrointestinal tract. Migration and traveling have exported the disease to the United Sates and Europe. In a recent study from Barcelona performed on 1350 pregnant Latin American women and their offspring, the rate of seroprevalence was 3.4%, and 7.3% of the newborns were infected.[147] Vertical transmission from mother to fetus is believed to occur mainly in the acute phase of the disease, and only a few cases of fetal infection have been reported.[148] Okumura and colleagues[10] reported a patient diagnosed at 31 weeks because of the presence of ascites, hydrocele, and thickened placenta. Pathologic examination following fetal demise demonstrated the presence of meningoencephalitis.

## REFERENCES


1. Parisot S, Droulle P, Feldmann M, Pinaud P, Marchal C. Unusual encephaloclastic lesions with paraventricular calcification in congenital rubella. *Pediatr Radiol.* 1991;21(3):229–230.
2. Meyberg-Solomayer GC, Fehm T, Muller-Hansen I, et al. Prenatal ultrasound diagnosis, follow-up, and outcome of congenital varicella syndrome. *Fetal Diagn Ther.* 2006;21(3):296–301.
3. Duin LK, Willekes C, Baldewijns MM, Robben SG, Offermans J, Vles J. Major brain lesions by intrauterine herpes simplex virus infection: MRI contribution. *Prenat Diagn.* 2007;27(1):81–84.
4. Vasileiadis GT, Roukema HW, Romano W, Walton JC, Gagnon R. Intrauterine herpes simplex infection. *Am J Perinatol.* 2003;20(2):55–58.
5. Pistorius LR, Smal J, de Haan TR, et al. Disturbance of cerebral neuronal migration following congenital parvovirus B19 infection. *Fetal Diagn Ther.* 2008;24(4):491–494.
6. Isumi H, Nunoue T, Nishida A, Takashima S. Fetal brain infection with human parvovirus B19. *Pediatr Neurol.* 1999;21(3):661–663.
7. Bonthius DJ, Wright R, Tseng B, et al. Congenital lymphocytic choriomeningitis virus infection: spectrum of disease. *Ann Neurol.* 2007;62(4):347–355.
8. Centers for Disease Control and Prevention (CDC). Intrauterine West Nile virus infection—New York, 2002. *MMWR Morb Mortal Wkly Rep.* 2002;51(50):1135–1136.
9. Mavrov GI, Goubenko TV. Clinical and epidemiological features of syphilis in pregnant women: The course and outcome of pregnancy. *Gynecol Obstet Invest.* 2001;52(2):114–118.
10. Okumura M, Aparecida dos Santos V, Camargo ME, Schultz R, Zugaib M. Prenatal diagnosis of congenital Chagas' disease (American trypanosomiasis). *Prenat Diagn.* 2004;24(3):179–181.
11. Fonticiella M, López-Negrete L, Prieto A, et al. Congenital intracranial filariasis: A case report. *Pediatr Radiol.* 1995;25(3): 171–172.
12. Hizel S, Parker S, Onde U. Seroprevalence of cytomegalovirus infection among children and females in Ankara, Turkey, 1995. *Pediatr Int.* 1999;41(5):506–509.
13. Grangeot-Keros L, Simon B, Audibert F, Vial M. Should we routinely screen for cytomegalovirus antibody during pregnancy? *Intervirology.* 1998;41(4–5):158–162.
14. Griffiths PD, Campbell-Benzie A, Heath RB. A prospective study of primary cytomegalovirus infection in pregnant women. *Br J Obstet Gynaecol.* 1980;87(4):308–314.
15. Kenneson A, Cannon MJ. Review and meta-analysis of the epidemiology of congenital cytomegalovirus (CMV) infection. *Rev Med Virol.* 2007;17(4):253–276.
16. Revello MG, Gerna G. Pathogenesis and prenatal diagnosis of human cytomegalovirus infection. *J Clin Virol.* 2004;29(2):71–83.

17. Adler S P, Nigro G, Pereira L. Recent advances in the prevention and treatment of congenital cytomegalovirus infections. *Semin Perinatol.* 2007;31:10–18.
18. Fortunato EA, Dell'Aquila ML, Spector HD. Specific chromosome 1 breaks induced by human cytomegalovirus. *Proc. Natl. Acad. Sci. USA.* 2000;97:853–858.
19. Pang X, Humar A, Preiksaitis JK. Concurrent genotyping and quantitation of cytomegalovirus gB genotypes in solid-organ-transplant recipients by use of a real-time PCR assay. *J Clin Microbiol.* 2008;46(12):4004–4010.
20. Boppana SB, Rivera LB, Fowler KB, Mach M, Britt WJ. Intrauterine transmission of cytomegalovirus to infants of women with preconceptional immunity. *N Engl J Med.* 2001;344(18):1366–1377.
21. Cheeran MC, Lokensgard JR, Schleiss MR. Neuropathogenesis of congenital cytomegalovirus infection: Disease mechanisms and prospects for intervention. *Clin Microbiol Rev.* 2009;22(1): 99–126.
22. Malinger G, Lev D, Zahalka N, et al. Fetal cytomegalovirus infection of the brain: The spectrum of sonographic findings. *AJNR Am J Neuroradiol.* Jan 2003;24(1):28–32.
23. Benoist G, Salomon LJ, Mohlo M, Suarez B, Jacquemard F, Ville Y. Cytomegalovirus-related fetal brain lesions: Comparison between targeted ultrasound examination and magnetic resonance imaging. *Ultrasound Obstet Gynecol.* 2008;32(7):900–905.
24. Enders G, Bäder U, Lindemann L, Schalasta G, Daiminger A. Prenatal diagnosis of congenital cytomegalovirus infection in 189 pregnancies with known outcome. *Prenat Diagn.* 2001;21(5):362–377.
25. Lipitz S, Achiron R, Zalel Y, Mendelson E, Tepperberg M, Gamzu R. Outcome of pregnancies with vertical transmission of primary cytomegalovirus infection. *Obstet Gynecol.* 2002;100(3): 428–433.
26. Picone O, Costa JM, Leruez-Ville M, Ernault P, Olivi M, Ville Y. Cytomegalovirus (CMV) glycoprotein B genotype and CMV DNA load in the amniotic fluid of infected fetuses. *Prenat Diagn.* 2004;24(12):1001–1006.
27. Cuillier F. Cytomegalovirus infection. www.*TheFetus.net.* 2004. Accessed October 17, 2011.
28. Chaoui R, Zodan-Marin T, Wisser J. Marked splenomegaly in fetal cytomegalovirus infection: detection supported by three-dimensional power Doppler ultrasound. Ultrasound Obstet Gynecol. 2002;20(3):299–302.
29. Drose JA, Dennis MA, Thickman D. Infection in utero: US findings in 19 cases. *Radiology.* 1991;178(369–374).
30. La Torre R, Nigro G, Mazzocco M, Best AM, Adler SP. Placental enlargement in women with primary maternal cytomegalovirus infection is associated with fetal and neonatal disease. *Clin Infect Dis.* 2006;43(8):994–1000.
31. Gaytant MA, Rours GI, Steegers EA, Galama JM, Semmekrot BA. Congenital cytomegalovirus infection after recurrent infection: case reports and review of the literature. *Eur J Pediatr.* 2003;162(4):248–253.
32. Henrich W, Meckies J, Dudenhausen JW, et al. Recurrent cytomegalovirus infection during pregnancy: Ultrasonographic diagnosis and fetal outcome. *Ultrasound Obstet Gynecol.* 2002;19(6):608–611.
33. Rousseau T, Douvier S, Reynaud I, et al. Severe fetal cytomegalic inclusion disease after documented maternal reactivation of cytomegalovirus infection during pregnancy. *Prenat Diagn.* 200;20(4):333–336.
34. Zalel Y, Gilboa Y, Berkenshtat M, et al. Secondary cytomegalovirus infection can cause severe fetal sequelae despite maternal preconceptional immunity. *Ultrasound Obstet Gynecol.* 2008;31(4):417–420.
35. Stagno S, Reynolds DW, Lakeman A, Charamella LJ, Alford CA. Congenital cytomegalovirus infection: consecutive occurrence due to viruses with similar antigenic compositions. *Pediatrics.* 1973;52(6):788–794.
36. Leshinsky-Silver E, Malinger G, Ben-Sera L, et al. A large homozygous deletion in the SAMHD1 gene casues atypical Aicardi-Goutiéres syndrome associated with mtDNA deletions. *Eur J Hum Genet.* 2010;19(3):287–292.
37. Graham D, Guidi SM, Sander RC. Sonographic features of in utero periventricular calcification due to cytomegalovirus infection. *J Ultrasound Med.* 1982;1:171–172.
38. Govaert P, de Vries LS. *An Atlas of Neonatal Brain Sonography.* London: MacKeith Press; 1997.
39. Meyer U, Yee BK, Feldon J. The neurodevelopmental impact of prenatal infections at different times of pregnancy: The earlier the worse? *Neuroscientist.* 2007;13(3):241–256.
40. Malinger G, Lerman-Sagie T. Fetal cytomegalovirus infection: The brain as a window in the establishment of prognosis. In: Ramenghi A, Evrard P, Mercuri E, eds. *Mariani Foundation Paediatric Neurology. Perinatal brain damage: From Pathogenesis to Neuroprotection.* Vol 19. Montrouge: Editions John Libbey Eurotext; 2008;49–54.
41. Ghidini A, Sirtori M, Vergani P, Mariani S, Tucci E, Scola GC. Fetal intracranial calcifications. *Am J Obstet Gynecol.* 1989;160(1):86–87.
42. Degani S. Sonographic findings in fetal viral infections: A systematic review. *Obstet Gynecol Surv.* 2006;61(5):329–336.
43. Sherer DM, Onyeije CI. Prenatal ultrasonographic diagnosis of fetal intracranial tumors: a review. *Am J Perinatol.* 1998;15(5):319–328.
44. Kei OC, Duncan WJ, Human DG. Pulmonary arterial and intracranial calcification in the recipient of a twin-twin transfusion. *Cardiol Young.* 2002;12(5):488–490.
45. Malinger G, Kidron D, Schreiber L, et al. Prenatal diagnosis of malformations of cortical development by dedicated neurosonography. *Ultrasound Obstet Gynecol.* 2007;29(2):178–191.
46. Grant EG, Williams AL, Schellinger D, Slovis TL. Intracranial calcification in the infant and neonate: Evaluation by sonography and CT. *Radiology.* 1985;157(1):63–68.
47. Dhombres F, Nahama-Allouche C, Gelot A, et al. Prenatal ultrasonographic diagnosis of polymicrogyria. *Ultrasound Obstet Gynecol.* 2008;32(7):951–954.
48. van der Knaap MS, Vermeulen G, Barkhof F, Hart AA, Loeber JG, Weel JF. Pattern of white matter abnormalities at MR imaging: use of polymerase chain reaction testing of Guthrie cards to link pattern with congenital cytomegalovirus infection. *Radiology.* 2004;230(2):529–536.
49. Estroff JA, Parad RB, Teele RL, Benacerraf BR. Echogenic vessels in the fetal thalami and basal ganglia associated with cytomegalovirus infection. *J Ultrasound Med.* 1992;11(12):686–688.
50. Ben-Ami T, Yousefzadeh D, Backus M, Reichman B, Kessler A, Hammerman-Rozenberg C. Lenticulostriate vasculopathy in infants with infections of the central nervous system sonographic and Doppler findings. *Pediatr Radiol.* 1990;20(8):575–579.
51. Teele RL, Hernanz-Schulman M, Sotrel A. Echogenic vasculature in the basal ganglia of neonates: A sonographic sign of vasculopathy. *Radiology.* 1988;169(2):423–427.
52. Tongsong T, Sukpan K, Wanapirak C, Phadungkiatwattna P. Fetal cytomegalovirus infection associated with cerebral hemorrhage, hydrops fetalis, and echogenic bowel: case report. *Fetal Diagn Ther.* 2008;23(3):169–172.
53. Nigro G, La Torre R, Sali E, et al. Intraventricular haemorrhage in a fetus with cerebral cytomegalovirus infection. *Prenat Diagn.* 2002;22(7):558–561.
54. Ortiz JU, Ostermayer E, Fischer T, Kuschel B, Rudelius M, Schneider KT. Severe fetal cytomegalovirus infection associated with cerebellar hemorrhage. *Ultrasound Obstet Gynecol.* 2004;23(4):402–406
55. Picone O, Simon I, Benachi A, Brunelle F, Sonigo P. Comparison between ultrasound and magnetic resonance imaging in assessment of fetal cytomegalovirus infection. *Prenat Diagn.* 2008;28(8):753–758.
56. Garel C. *MRI of the Fetal Brain: Normal Development and Cerebral Pathologies.* Berlin: Springer; 2004;237–241.
57. Ancora G, Lanari M, Lazzarotto T, et al. Cranial ultrasound scanning and prediction of outcome in newborns with congenital cytomegalovirus infection. *J Pediatr.* 2007;150(2):157–161.
58. Pass RF, Fowler KB, Boppana SB, Britt WJ, Stagno S. Congenital cytomegalovirus infection following first trimester maternal infection: Symptoms at birth and outcome. *J Clin Virol.* 2006;35(2): 216–220.
59. Gindes L, Teperberg-Oikawa M, Sherman D, Pardo J, Rahav G. Congenital cytomegalovirus infection following primary maternal infection in the third trimester. *BJOG.* 2008;115(7):805–807.
60. Foulon I, Naessens A, Foulon W, Casteels A, Gordts F. Hearing loss in children with congenital cytomegalovirus infection in relation to the maternal trimester in which the maternal primary infection occurred. *Pediatrics.* 2008;122(6):e1123–e1127.
61. Zhang XW, Li F, Yu XW, Shi XW, Shi J, Zhang JP. Physical and intellectual development in children with asymptomatic congenital cytomegalovirus infection: A longitudinal cohort study in Qinba mountain area, China. *J Clin Virol.* 2007;40(3):180–185.

62. Ivarsson SA, Lernmark B, Svanberg L. Ten-year clinical, developmental, and intellectual follow-up of children with congenital cytomegalovirus infection without neurologic symptoms at one year of age. *Pediatrics.* 1997;99(6):800–803.
63. Conboy TJ, Pass RF, Stagno S, et al. Intellectual development in school-aged children with asymptomatic congenital cytomegalovirus infection. *Pediatrics.* 1986;77(6):801–806.
64. Rosenthal LS, Fowler KB, Boppana SB, et al. Cytomegalovirus shedding and delayed sensorineural hearing loss: results from longitudinal follow-up of children with congenital infection. *Pediatr Infect Dis J.* 2009;28(6):515–520.
65. Noyola DE, Demmler GJ, Nelson CT, et al. Early predictors of neurodevelopmental outcome in symptomatic congenital cytomegalovirus infection. *J Pediatr.* 2001;138(3):325–331.
66. Benoist G, Salomon LJ, Jacquemard F, Daffos F, Ville Y. The prognostic value of ultrasound abnormalities and biological parameters in blood of fetuses infected with cytomegalovirus. *BJOG.* 2008;115(7):823–829.
67. Goegebuer T, Van Meensel B, Beuselinck K, et al. Clinical predictive value of real-time PCR quantification of human cytomegalovirus DNA in amniotic fluid samples. *J Clin Microbiol.* 2009;47(3):660–665.
68. Rasmussen L, Geissler A, Winters M. Inter- and intragenic variations complicate the molecular epidemiology of human cytomegalovirus. *J Infect Dis.* 2003;187(5):809–819.
69. Pignatelli S, Dal Monte P. Epidemiology of human cytomegalovirus strains through comparison of methodological approaches to explore gN variants. *New Microbiol.* 2009;32(1):1–10.
70. Picone O, Costa JM, Dejean A, Ville Y. Is fetal gender a risk factor for severe congenital cytomegalovirus infection? *Prenat Diagn.* 2005;25(1):34–38.
71. Pass RF, Zhang C, Evans A, et al. Vaccine prevention of maternal cytomegalovirus infection. *N Engl J Med.* 2009;360(12):1250–1252.
72. Cannon MJ, Davis KF. Washing our hands of the congenital cytomegalovirus disease epidemic. *BMC Public Health.* 2005;5:70.
73. Harvey J, Dennis CL. Hygiene interventions for prevention of cytomegalovirus infection among childbearing women: systematic review. *J Adv Nurs.* 2008;63(5):440–450.
74. Jacquemard F, Yamamoto M, Costa JM, et al. Maternal administration of valaciclovir in symptomatic intrauterine cytomegalovirus infection. *BJOG.* 2007;114(9):1113–1121.
75. Nigro G, Torre RL, Pentimalli H, et al. Regression of fetal cerebral abnormalities by primary cytomegalovirus infection following hyperimmunoglobulin therapy. *Prenat Diagn.* 2008;28(6):512–517.
76. Ancelle T, Goulet V, Tirard-Fleury V, Baril L. La toxoplasmose chez la femme enceinte en France en 1995. *Bulletin Epidemiologique Hebdomadiare.* 1996;51:227–229.
77. Evengard B, Petersson K, Engman ML, et al. Low incidence of *Toxoplasma* infection during pregnancy and in newborns in Sweden. *Epidemiol Infect.* 2001;127:121–127.
78. Schmidt DR, Hogh B, Andersen O, Fuchs J, Fledelius H, Petersen E. The national neonatal screening programme for congenital toxoplasmosis in Denmark: Results from the initial four years, 1999–2002. *Arch Dis Child.* 2006;91:661–665.
79. Durlach R, Kaufer F, Carral L, et al. Argentine consensus of congenital toxoplasmosis. *Medicina (B Aires).* 2008;68(1):75–87.
80. Kortbeek LM, Hofhuis A, Nijhuis CD, Havelaar AH. Congenital toxoplasmosis and DALYs in the Netherlands. *Mem Inst Oswaldo Cruz.* 2009;104(2):370–373.
81. Varella IS, Canti IC, Santos BR, et al. Prevalence of acute toxoplasmosis infection among 41,112 pregnant women and the mother-to-child transmission rate in a public hospital in South Brazil. *Mem Inst Oswaldo Cruz.* 2009;104(2):383–388.
82. Guerina NG, Hsu H-W, Meissner H, et al. Neonatal serologic screening and early treatment for congenital *Toxoplasma gondii* infection. *N Engl J Med* 1994;330:1858–1863.
83. Sullivan WJ Jr, Smith AT, Joyce BR. Understanding mechanisms and the role of differentiation in pathogenesis of Toxoplasma gondii: a review. *Mem Inst Oswaldo Cruz.* 2009;104(2):155–161.
84. Dubey JP. The history of Toxoplasma gondii—the first 100 years. *J Eukaryot Microbiol.* 2008;55(6):467–475.
85. Peckham CS, Logan S. Screening for toxoplasmosis during pregnancy. *Arch Dis Child.* 1993;69(Special Issue 1):3–5.
86. Lynfield R, Guerina NG. Toxoplasmosis. *Pediatr Rev.* 1997;18(3):75–83.
87. Desmonts G, Couvreur J. Toxoplasmosis in pregnancy and its transmission to the fetus. *Bull N Y Acad Med.* 1974;50(2):146–159.
88. Desmonts G, Couvreur J. Congenital toxoplasmosis. A prospective study of 378 pregnancies. *N Engl J Med.* 1974;290(20):1110–1116.
89. Foulon W, Pinon JM, Stray-Pedersen B, et al. Prenatal diagnosis of congenital toxoplasmosis: a multicenter evaluation of different diagnostic parameters. *Am J Obstet Gynecol.* 1999;181(4):843–847.
90. Becker LE. Infections of the developing brain. *AJNR Am J Neuroradiol.* 1992;13(2):537–549.
91. Fitz CR. Inflammatory diseases of the brain in childhood. *AJNR Am J Neuroradiol.* 1992;13(2):551–557.
92. Gordon N. Toxoplasmosis: A preventable cause of brain damage. *Dev Med Child Neurol.* 1993;35(7):567–573.
93. Bachmeyer C, Mouchnino G, Thulliez P, Blum L. Congenital toxoplasmosis from an HIV-infected woman as a result of reactivation. *J Infect.* 2006;52(2):e55–57.
94. Elbez-Rubinstein A, Ajzenberg D, Dardé ML, et al. Congenital toxoplasmosis and reinfection during pregnancy: Case report, strain characterization, experimental model of reinfection, and review. *J Infect Dis.* 2009;199(2):280–285.
95. Hohlfeld P, MacAleese J, Capella-Pavlovski M, et al. Fetal toxoplasmosis: ultrasonographic signs. *Ultrasound Obstet Gynecol.* 1991;1(4):241–244.
96. Abboud P, Harika G, Saniez D, et al. Ultrasonic signs of fetal toxoplasmosis: Review of the literature. *J Gynecol Obstet Biol Reprod.* 1995;24(7):733–738.
97. Couto JC, Ferreira QT. Fetal toxoplasmosis infection. *www.TheFetus.net.* 2006.
98. Cuillier F, Avignon MS. Case of the week #168. *www.TheFetus.net.* 2006.
99. Blaakaer J. Ultrasonic diagnosis of ascites and toxoplasmosis. *Acta Obstet Gynecol Scand.* 1986;65:653–654.
100. Friedman S, Ford-Jones LE, Toi A, Ryan G, Blaser S, Chitayat D. Congenital toxoplasmosis: prenatal diagnosis, treatment and postnatal outcome. *Prenat Diagn.* 1999;19(4):330–333.
101. Berrebi A, Kobuch WE, Bessieres MH, et al. Termination of pregnancy for maternal toxoplasmosis. *Lancet.* 1994;344(8914):36–39.
102. Barkovich AJ, Girard N. Fetal brain infections. *Childs Nerv Syst.* 2003;19(7–8):501–507.
103. Berrebi A, Bardou M, Bessieres MH, et al. Outcome for children infected with congenital toxoplasmosis in the first trimester and with normal ultrasound findings: A study of 36 cases. *Eur J Obstet Gynecol Rep Biol.* 2007;135(1):53–57.
104. Brunel H, Girard N, Confort-Gouny S, et al. Fetal brain injury. *J Neuroradiol.* 2004;31(2):123–137.
105. Gay-Andrieu F, Marty P, Pialat J, Sournies G, Drier de Laforte T, Peyron F. Fetal toxoplasmosis and negative amniocentesis: Necessity of an ultrasound follow-up. *Prenat Diagn.* 2003;23(7):1098–1099.
106. McAuley J, Boyer KM, Patel D, et al. Early and longitudinal evaluations of treated infants and children and untreated historical patients with congenital toxoplasmosis: the Chicago Collaborative Treatment Trial. *Clin Infect Dis.* 1994;18(1):38–72.
107. McLeod R, Boyer K, Karrison T, et al. Outcome of treatment for congenital toxoplasmosis, 1981–2004: The National Collaborative Chicago-based Congenital Toxoplasmosis Study. *Clin Infect Diseases.* 2006;42(10):1383–1394.
108. Roizen N, Swisher CN, Stein MA, et al. Neurologic and developmental outcome in treated congenital toxoplasmosis. *Pediatrics.* 1995;95(1):11–20.
109. Hohlfeld P, Daffos F, Costa JM, Thulliez P, Forestier F, Vidaud M. Prenatal diagnosis of congenital toxoplasmosis with a polymerase-chain-reaction test on amniotic fluid. *N Engl J Med.* 1994;331(11):695–699.
110. Antsaklis A, Daskalakis G, Papantoniou N, Mentis A, Michalas S. Prenatal diagnosis of congenital toxoplasmosis. *Prenat Diagn.* 2002;22(12):1107–1011.
111. SYROCOT (Systematic Review on Congenital Toxoplasmosis) study group, Thiébaut R, Leproust S, Chêne G, Gilbert R. Effectiveness of prenatal treatment for congenital toxoplasmosis: a meta-analysis of individual patients' data. *Lancet.* 2007;369(9556):115–122.
112. Freeman K, Tan HK, Prusa A, et al. Predictors of retinochoroiditis in children with congenital toxoplasmosis: European, prospective cohort study. *Pediatrics.* 2008;121(5):e1215–1222.

113. Fucillo DA, Sever JL. Viral teratology. *Bacterial Rev.* 1973;37:19–31.
114. Yamashita Y, Matsuishi T, Murakami Y, et al. Neuroimaging findings (ultrasonography, CT, MRI) in 3 infants with congenital rubella syndrome. *Pediatr Radiol.* 1991;21(8):547–549.
115. Numazaki K, Fujikawa T. Intracranial calcification with congenital rubella syndrome in a mother with serologic immunity. *J Child Neurol.* 2003;18(4):296–297.
116. Desmond MM, Montgomery JR, Melnick JL, Cochran GG, Verniaud W. Congenital rubella encephalitis: Effects on growth and early development. *Am J Dis Child.* 1969;118(1):30–31.
117. Balducci J, Rodis JF, Rosengren S, Vintzileos AM, Spivey G, Vosseller C. Pregnancy outcome following first-trimester varicella infection. *Obstet Gynecol.* 1992;79(1):5–6.
118. Paryani SG, Arvin AM. Intrauterine infection with varicella-zoster virus after maternal varicella. *N Engl J Med.* 1986;314(24):1542–1546.
119. Enders G, Miller E, Cradock-Watson J, Bolley I, Ridehalgh M. Consequences of varicella and herpes zoster in pregnancy: Prospective study of 1739 cases. *Lancet.* 1994;343(8912):1458–1451.
120. Pastuszak AL, Levy M, Schick B, et al. Outcome after maternal varicella infection in the first 20 weeks of pregnancy. *N Engl J Med.* 1994;330(13):901–905.
121. Harger JH, Ernest JM, Thurnau GR, et al. Frequency of congenital varicella syndrome in a prospective cohort of 347 pregnant women. *Obstet Gynecol.* 2002;100(2):260–265.
122. Harding B, Baumer JA. Congenital varicella-zoster: A serologically proven case with necrotizing encephalitis and malformation. *Acta Neuropathol.* 1988;76(3):311–315.
123. Al-Katawee YA, Al-Hasoun YA, Taha MN, Al-Moslem K. Congenital varicella-zoster virus infection: A rare case of severe brain and ocular malformations without limb or cutaneous involvement in a newborn after maternal subclinical infection. *Saudi Med J.* 2005;26(5):869–871.
124. Boumahni B, Kauffmann E, Laffitte A, Randrianaivo H, Fourmaintraux A. Congenital varicella: limits of prenatal diagnosis. *Arch Pediatr.* 2005;12(9):1361–1363.
125. Verstraelen H, Vanzieleghem B, Defoort P, Vanhaesebrouck P, Temmerman M. Prenatal ultrasound and magnetic resonance imaging in fetal varicella syndrome: correlation with pathology findings. *Prenat Diagn.* 2003;23(9):705–709.
126. Avgil M, Ornoy A. Herpes simplex virus and Epstein-Barr virus infections in pregnancy: consequences of neonatal or intrauterine infection. *Reprod Toxicol.* 2006;21(4):436–445.
127. Gray PH, Tudehope DI, Masel J. Cystic encephalomalacia and intrauterine herpes simplex virus infection. *Pediatr Radiol.* 1992;22(7):520–532.
128. de Haan TR, van den Akker ES, Porcelijn L, Oepkes D, Kroes AC, Walther FJ. Thrombocytopenia in hydropic fetuses with parvovirus B19 infection: Incidence, treatment and correlation with fetal B19 viral load. *BJOG.* 2008;115(1):76–81.
129. Glenn OA, Bianco K, Barkovich AJ, Callen PW, Parer JT. Fetal cerebellar hemorrhage in parvovirus-associated non-immune hydrops fetalis. *J Matern Fetal Neonatal Med.* 2007;20(10):769–772.
130. Pistorius LR, Smal J, de Haan TR, et al. Disturbance of cerebral neuronal migration following congenital parvovirus B19 infection. *Fetal Diagn Ther.* 2008;24(4):491–494.
131. De Haan TR, Van Wezel-Meijler G, Beersma MF, Von Lindern JS, Van Duinen SG, Walther FJ. Fetal stroke and congenital parvovirus B19 infection complicated by activated protein C resistance. *Acta Paediatr.* 2006;95(7):863–867.
132. Nagel HT, de Haan TR, Vandenbussche FP, Oepkes D, Walther FJ. Long-term outcome after fetal transfusion for hydrops associated with parvovirus B19 infection. *Obstet Gynecol.* 2007;109(1):42–47.
133. Jamieson DJ, Kourtis AP, Bell M, Rasmussen SA. Lymphocytic choriomeningitis virus: an emerging obstetric pathogen? *Am J Obstet Gynecol.* 2006;194(6):1532–1536.
134. Greenhow TL, Weintrub PS. Your diagnosis, please. Neonate with hydrocephalus. *Pediatr Infect Dis J.* 2002;22(12):1099, 1111–1112.
135. Barton LL, Mets MB, Beauchamp CL. Lymphocytic choriomeningitis virus: Emerging fetal teratogen. *Am J Obstet Gynecol.* 2002;187:1715–1716.
136. Wright R, Johnson D, Neumann M, et al. Congenital lymphocytic choriomeningitis virus syndrome: A disease that mimics congenital toxoplasmosis or cytomegalovirus infection. *Pediatrics.* 1997;100(1):e9.
137. Brezin AP, Thulliez P, Cisneros B, Mets MB, Saron MF. Lymphocytic choriomeningitis virus chorioretinitis mimicking ocular toxoplasmosis in two otherwise normal children. *Am J Ophthalmol.* 2000;130:245–247.
138. Meritet JF, Krivine A, Lewin F, et al. A case of congenital lymphocytic choriomeningitis virus (LCMV) infection revealed by hydrops fetalis. *Prenat Diagn.* 2009;29(6):626–627.
139. Davis LE, DeBiasi R, Goade DE, et al. West Nile virus neuroinvasive disease. *Ann Neurol.* 2006;60(3):286–300.
140. Lindsey NP, Hayes EB, Staples JE, Fischer M. West Nile virus disease in children, United States, 1999–2007. *Pediatrics.* 2009;123(6):e1084–1089.
141. Centers for Disease Control and Prevention (CDC). Intrauterine West Nile virus infection—New York, 2002. *MMWR Morb Mortal Wkly Rep.* 2002;51(50):1135–1136.
142. Alpert SG, Fergerson J, Noël LP. Intrauterine West Nile virus: Ocular and systemic findings. *Am J Ophthalmol.*136(4):733–735.
143. O'Leary DR, Kuhn S, Kniss KL, et al. Birth outcomes following West Nile virus infection of pregnant women in the United States: 2003–2004. *Pediatrics.* 2006;117(3):e537–545.
144. Paisley JE, Hinckley AF, O'Leary DR, et al. West Nile virus infection among pregnant women in a northern Colorado community, 2003 to 2004. *Pediatrics.* 2006;117(3):814–820.
145. Hollier LM, Harstad TW, Sanchez PJ, Twickler DM, Wendel GD Jr. Fetal syphilis: clinical and laboratory characteristics. *Obstet Gynecol.* 2001;97(6):947–953.
146. Malinger G, Pilu G. Sonography of the central nervous system. In: Rodech CH, Whittle MJ, eds. *Fetal Medicine: Basic Science and Clinical Practice.* 2nd ed. London: Elsevier; 2009:379–411. (Chap 30).
147. Muñoz J, Coll O, Juncosa T, et al. Prevalence and vertical transmission of Trypanosoma cruzi infection among pregnant Latin American women attending 2 maternity clinics in Barcelona, Spain. *Clin Infect Dis.* 2009(48):12.
148. Riera C, Guarro A, Kassab HE, et al. Congenital transmission of *Trypanosoma cruzi* in Europe (Spain): a case report. *Am J Trop Med Hyg.* 2006;75(6):1078–1081.

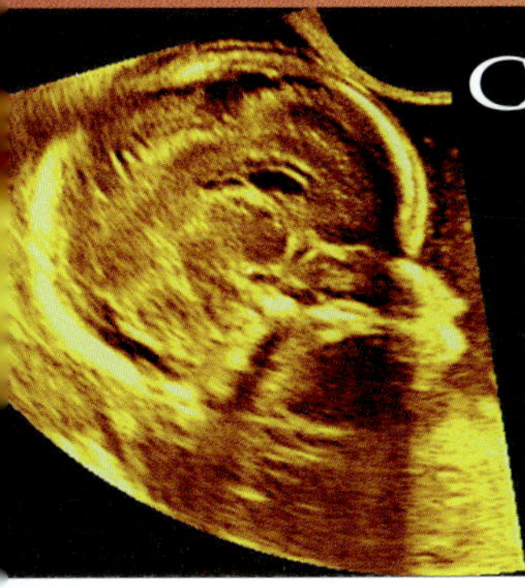

Chapter 10

# INTRAUTERINE INSULTS: FETAL STROKE AND DESTRUCTIVE PROCESSES

*Ana Monteagudo • Gianluigi Pilu • Gustavo Malinger*
*Selim Buyukkurt • Ashwin Jadhav*

**KEY POINTS**

1. Many congenital anomalies of the brain do not derive from abnormal embryogenesis but are the consequence of destructive processes that may occur any time in gestation, particularly in the third trimester.
2. Most of these destructive processes are the consequence of vascular accidents, hemorrhage, or occlusion. The etiology is often unknown, but they may derive from a variety of obstetric complications, such as placental insufficiency, coagulation disorders, drug consumption, and transplacental infections.
3. Disruptive lesions of the fetal brain are clinically important because they may have severe consequences, but they frequently escape early detection.
4. Intracranial hemorrhage is probably the most common and therefore the best known of all intrauterine disruptions of the fetal brain. The hemorrhage occurs usually into the lateral ventricles, and the sonographic pictures change with time. An echogenic collection is first seen, and in the following days it develops into a complex mass frequently complicated by severe ventriculomegaly.
5. Prenatal stroke is considered the most important determinant of cystic destruction of the cortex that, depending on the time of occurrence and the severity, may result in a spectrum of conditions, including porencephaly (single or multiple cysts replacing brain parenchyma), schizencephaly (a gray matter–lined cleft in the cerebral mantle connecting the cavity of lateral ventricles to the subarachnoid space), and hydranencephaly (complete destruction of the cerebral hemispheres).
6. Cerebellar lesions are discussed separately even though they also deal with intracranial hemorrhage. However, they deserve more focused attention.

Intrauterine insults may lead to brain ischemia (stroke), which is a major contributor to the sonographic brain findings that we will discuss in this chapter. Prenatal stroke can be the result of an arterial ischemic event, a venous thrombosis, or hemorrhage. The end-stage lesion is a cavity in the brain tissue of variable size and location.[1] The location of the cavity is predictable and stable depending on the vessel that was affected.[2] For example, stroke affecting the middle cerebral artery (MCA) will result in porencephaly and that affecting both internal carotid arteries (ICAs) in hydranencephaly. There are several factors determining the propensity of the immature brain to undergo dissolution and eventually cavitation: (1) the high water content of the unmyelinated brain, (2) the relative paucity of myelinated fibers, and (3) deficient glial response. The first two factors result in dissolution of the brain, and the latter is responsible for the cavitation.

## PORENCEPHALY

### Definition

*Porencephaly* is a collective term for a variety of cystic lesions of the brain. Some of these cavities communicate with the ventricular system, the subarachnoid space, or both. These defects have many similarities in etiopathogenesis with schizencephaly and hydranencephaly.[1] It is the outcome of an insult such as ischemic stroke, infection, hemorrhage, or trauma occurring between the second trimester of pregnancy and the early postnatal period. This insult results in focal or multifocal areas of brain necroses, which subsequently undergo dissolution and cavity formation.[1–3]

### Synonyms

Perencephaly, porencephalia; schizencephaly, porencephalic cyst.

### Incidence

Perinatal arterial ischemic stroke (PAIS) is estimated to occur in 1 in 2500 to 1 in 5000 term neonates. The perinatal period spans from the 28th postmenstrual week of gestation to a week after delivery; it is during this period that stroke is more likely to occur when compared with any other time during childhood. Porencephaly is the end result of a PAIS, and the neonatal outcome is significant neurologic morbidities, such as hemiplegic cerebral palsy (CP).[4,5]

## Pathogenesis

Porencephaly can be the end-stage result of an ischemic stroke following either an arterial or venous infarction or an intraparenchymal hemorrhage. Areas affected by the infarct undergo tissue necrosis and eventually resorption, leaving behind a cavity in the brain or porencephalic cyst. In "simple" porencephaly, the end result of a venous medullary infarction, typically there is a single cavity along the frontal, parietal, or temporal horns that communicates with the ipsilateral ventricle. Often this ventricle is dilated.[1] In preterm neonates, the parenchymal lesions associated with germinal matrix and intraventricular hemorrhages are the result of venous infarct (see below). Eventually these infarcts undergo cystic degeneration; small lesions are seen as periventricular leukomalacia, and large lesions that connect with the ventricles as porencephalic cysts. In most of these cases, the cortical mantle is spared, and the cysts take the shape of the area of the infarct.[1]

In the arterial type or clastic porencephaly, there is occlusion of an artery often on the left side of the brain; typically, a cavity is seen along the path of the MCA, which is the vessel most commonly involved. However, any arteries, such as the anterior cerebral, posterior cerebral, or anterior choroidal artery, can be affected.[1] As eluded above, arterial ischemic stroke occurs in the left hemisphere in ~55% of cases; bilaterally, in ~6%.[6] Benders et al[6] theorize that this may be the result of the hemodynamic differences from the patent ductus arteriosus or right-to-left intracardiac shunt involving the more direct route of the left common carotid artery.

Thrombophilias, specifically factor V Leiden and antiphospholipid antibodies, may play an important role in the pathogenesis of perinatal stroke; however, at present their role is not completely understood.[7]

## Etiology

The etiology of ischemic perinatal stroke that eventually may result in porencephaly has not been clearly elucidated. However, there are multiple potential risk factors both maternal and fetal/neonatal that have been associated with this condition (Table 10–1). In addition, thrombotic events on the fetal side of the placenta may potentially result in a thrombotic event due to the patency of the foramen ovale and to the right-to-left direction of the blood flow in the fetal system.[5] It has been proposed that in symptomatic cases of ischemic perinatal stroke, a workup similar to that performed on neonates should be done (Table 10–2).[5]

Porencephaly has also been described as the result of several other types of intrauterine exposures or insults. A more recent report[8] documents maternal carbon monoxide poisoning at 22 postmenstrual weeks resulting in the prenatal diagnosis of porencephaly. Another case report[9] described a patient who was treated with warfarin for a prosthetic heart valve and at 22 postmenstrual weeks suddenly had a surge on the prothrombin International Normalized Ratio (INR) to double its previous values. At 26 postmenstrual weeks, an ultrasound (US) demonstrated a large intracranial echogenic lesion suggestive of a subdural hematoma, and at birth the magnetic resonance imaging (MRI) revealed porencephalic cyst and mild ipsilateral ventriculomegaly. A case report[10] documents a prenatally detected case of porencephaly at 28 weeks following inadvertent penetration of the fetal skull during an amniocentesis unguided by continuous US at 16 weeks. Initially, the head US was normal, but at 28 weeks a left-sided ventriculomegaly and an anechoic mass in the area of the lateral ventricle were noted and confirmed at birth by computed tomography (CT) and MRI studies. Other reported events that have resulted in porencephaly are chorionic villus sampling, cocaine, vitamin A, and valproate use.[8] Porencephaly and other cystic brain lesions are seen frequently in monozygotic twins.[1] Familial cases of porencephaly have also been described.[11–14]

**Table 10–1. POTENTIAL RISK FACTORS ASSOCIATED WITH ISCHEMIC PERINATAL STROKE (IPS)**

| |
|---|
| Maternal factors/conditions |
| Thrombotic disorders (see Table 10–2) |
| Infertility and infertility treatment |
| Preeclampsia |
| Prolonged rupture of membrane (>24 h) |
| Chorioamnionitis |
| Maternal autoimmune conditions and autoantibodies (platelet alloantigen-1) |
| Antiphospholipid syndrome |
| Fetal/neonatal disorders |
| Mutations in procollagen IVa1 |
| Inherited thrombophilia |
| Twin-to-twin transfusion syndrome |
| Fetal/neonatal polycythemia |
| Congenital heart disease |
| Neonatal hypoglycemia (in preterm infants) |
| Persistent fetal circulation and extracorporeal membrane oxygenation therapy |
| Intrauterine growth restriction |
| Fetal/neonatal infections and meningitis |
| Nonspecific factors |
| Ethnicity and race (higher incidence in black infants compared with non-Hispanic white infants) |
| Infant gender (higher incidence in boys) |

Reproduced, with permission, from Raju TN, Nelson KB, Ferriero D, Lynch JK; NICHD-NINDS Perinatal Stroke Workshop Participants. Ischemic perinatal stroke: Summary of a workshop sponsored by the National Institute of Child Health and Human Development and the National Institute of Neurological Disorders and Stroke. *Pediatrics.* 2007;120:609–616.

**Table 10–2. SCREENING FOR RISK FACTORS: ACQUIRED OR INHERITED THROMBOTIC DISORDER IN PEDIATRIC PATIENTS WITH ISCHEMIC STROKE**

| Plasma/Protein Based | DNA Based |
|---|---|
| Activated protein C resistance | Factor V G1691A |
| Protein C activity/antigen | Prothrombin G20210A |
| Free and total protein S antigen | |
| Antithrombin activity/antigen | |
| Lipoprotein (a) | |
| Fasting homocysteine | |
| Lupus anticoagulant/ antiphospholipid antibodies | |
| Fibrinogen (Clauss) | |
| Plasminogen | |
| Factor VIIIC | |

Some experts make these recommendations for screening in pediatric stroke cases[38]; however, no such recommendations exist for IPS cases, and their cost versus benefits are not known.

Reproduced, with permission, from Raju TN, Nelson KB, Ferriero D, Lynch JK; NICHD-NINDS Perinatal Stroke Workshop Participants. Ischemic perinatal stroke: Summary of a workshop sponsored by the National Institute of Child Health and Human Development and the National Institute of Neurological Disorders and Stroke. *Pediatrics.* 2007;120:609–616.[5]

## Associated Anomalies

With the exception of ventriculomegaly, there are no typical associated anomalies in cases of porencephaly, but in the arterial type or classic porencephaly, areas of polymicrogyria may border the cysts.[1]

## Risk of Recurrence

At present there are no data regarding the risk of recurrence of a perinatal stroke, but recurrent stroke is rare among infants who have suffered a perinatal stroke.[15] The risk of recurrence of stroke in children who have suffered a perinatal stroke ranges from 3% to 30%.[15,16]

Among fetuses/neonates who have suffered a perinatal arterial stroke and their mothers, there is a high rate of thrombophilias when compared with the general population. Simchen et al[7] found that 64% of infants with perinatal arterial stroke had at least one thrombophilic marker, and among the mothers, 68% were carriers of a thrombophilia. In their study, factor V Leiden mutation, protein C deficiency, and the presence of antiphospholipid antibodies were significant factors for perinatal stroke. The authors recommended that any child that has suffered a perinatal arterial stroke have both parents tested for thrombophilias.

A mutation in collagen IV A1 (*COL4A1*) gene has been reported in a few families with an autosomal dominant form of porencephaly in which the porencephalic cyst is the result of a perinatal hemorrhage.[17] In cases of familial autosomal dominant porencephaly (OMIM 175780), the inheritance is similar to any dominant disease in which each baby has a 50% chance of receiving the affected mutation.

## Sonographic Diagnosis

The sonographic appearance of porencephaly is that of a cystic lesion that communicates with the lateral ventricle (Figure 10–1). The term *porencephaly* is derived from the Latin word *porus,* meaning communication between the ventricular and extracerebral space. The ipsilateral ventricle is dilated. The porencephalic cyst never causes a mass effect and is typically located along the distribution of the middle cerebral artery or other arteries (see above). This helps differentiate it from arachnoid and interhemispheric cysts.[18]

### Implications for Sonographic Screening

Porencephaly may be missed by antenatal sonography, particularly in early gestation, because of two reasons. First, it is usually a unilateral lesion; this makes it difficult to demonstrate when it occurs in the hemisphere proximal to the transducer, being usually obscured by sound reverberation and artifacts.[19] Second, it usually occurs only in late gestation.[1]

## Differential Diagnosis

The differential diagnosis of porencephaly includes all cystic brain lesions (see Chapter 9), but the most important differential diagnosis is the arachnoid cysts and unilateral schizencephaly. Arachnoid cysts are collections of cerebrospinal fluid (CSF). They are usually benign, congenital, space-occupying lesions; unlike porencephaly they do not communicate with the ventricles. The cyst wall is lined with collagen and cells of the arachnoid matter. In the arachnoid cyst, the CSF is located within the layers of the arachnoid membrane, which may or may not communicate with the subarachnoid space. In unilateral schizencephaly, the cyst communicates with the subarachnoid space, and the cavity is lined by gray matter; this is easily seen during a fetal MRI. Cystic neoplasms are rare, and these usually have mass effects with both solid and cyst components.

## Prognosis

Porencephaly is associated with significant morbidity and mortality. Ischemic perinatal stroke resulting in porencephaly is the leading cause of cerebral palsy (CP), and congenital hemiplegia is the most common type of CP.[5,20] Hemiparesis and motor deficits are seen in >80% of the presumed perinatal ischemic stroke.[5,20] In addition, 50% to 75% of survivors of perinatal ischemic stroke will have neurologic deficits or epilepsy. Moreover, ~20% to 60% of survivors will have deficits in language, vision, cognition, and behavior.[5] Unfortunately, there are no clearcut figures. Most prenatally diagnosed cases tend to have a poor outcome.[21–23]

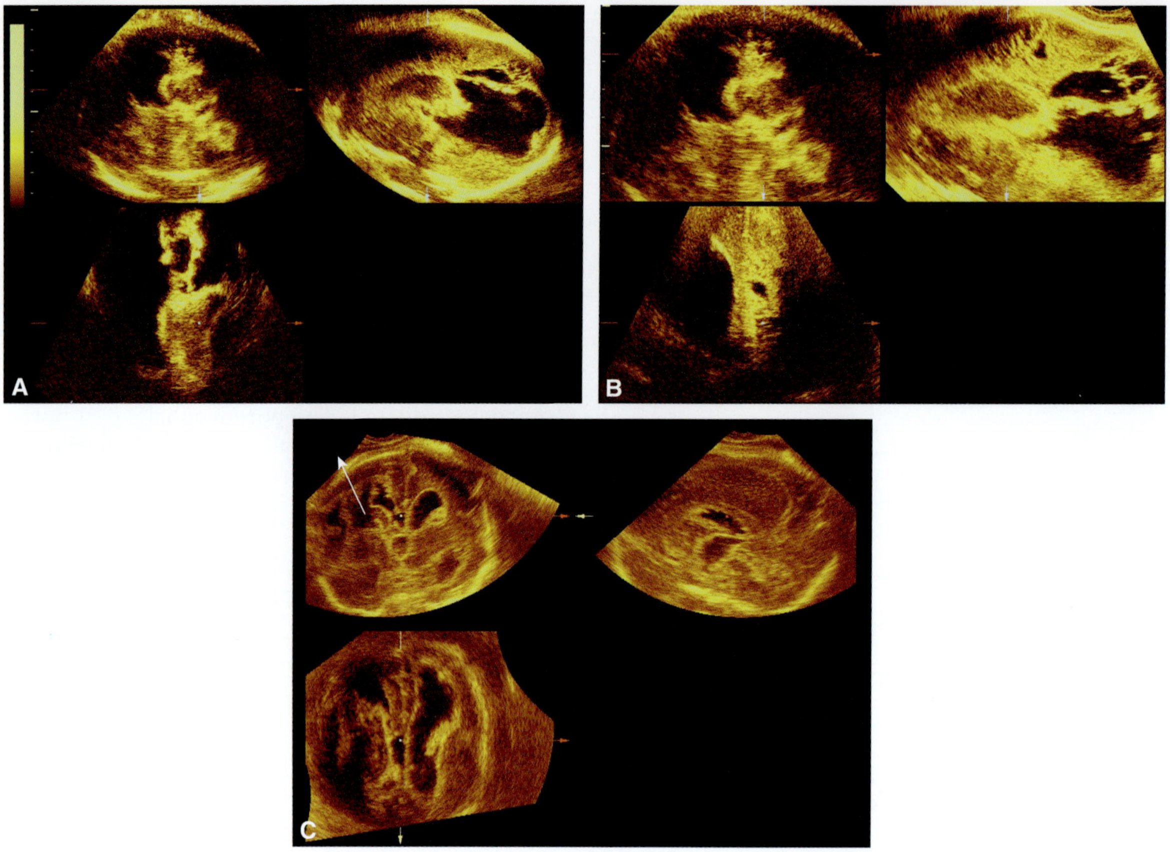

**Figure 10–1.** Porencephalic insult to the fetal brain imaged using three-dimensional (3D) transvaginal ultrasound (US). Observe the irregular anechoic spaces representing infarcted areas, as well as the dilated ventricles. Coronal **(A)**, sagittal **(B)**, and axial **(C)** sections.

Advances in neuroimaging have facilitated outcome prediction in cases of perinatal stroke, as described by Kirton and deVeber.[20] Outcome prediction provides important information for the family and allows patients to be entered into appropriate clinical trials. For example, lesion size and location are somewhat correlated with clinical outcomes. Poor motor outcomes can be predicted by infarction lesions of the MCA, periventricular venous lesions, or basal ganglia involvement, whereas isolated subcortical lesions carry a low risk of language, cognitive deficits, or epilepsy.

### Obstetric Management

In cases where porencephaly is diagnosed early (earlier than 24 weeks' gestation), termination of pregnancy should be offered to the patient; however, in the vast majority of cases, porencephaly will be diagnosed only during the third trimester; in these cases, management of the pregnancy with porencephaly should include a thrombophilia workup ideally of both parents, fetal MRI to further evaluate the fetal brain, and consultations with a geneticist, neonatologist, pediatric neurologist, and neurosurgeon. Given the fact that porencephaly is a relatively rare condition, there are no standard recommendations at this time regarding the best route of delivery. It is our opinion that, given the significant morbidities associated with porencephaly, cesarean section should be performed for routine obstetric indications.

## SCHIZENCEPHALY

### Definition

Schizencephaly is defined as a transcerebral, full-thickness, gray matter–lined clefts or defects extending from the lateral ventricles to the pial surface of the brain. The clefts of schizencephaly can be unilateral or bilateral and open or closed. In closed-lip schizencephaly (or type I), the lips of the cleft touch or are fused with each other (Figure 10–2); in contrast, in open-lip schizencephaly (or type II), the walls of the clefts are widely separated, and the space is filled with CSF, which is contiguous from the lateral ventricles to the subarachnoid space (Figure 10–2). Type II is frequently seen with hydrocephaly. Although schizencephaly can occur anywhere in the cerebral hemispheres, it is more commonly seen in the perisylvian area.[24]

### Synonyms

True porencephaly; early fetal porencephaly.

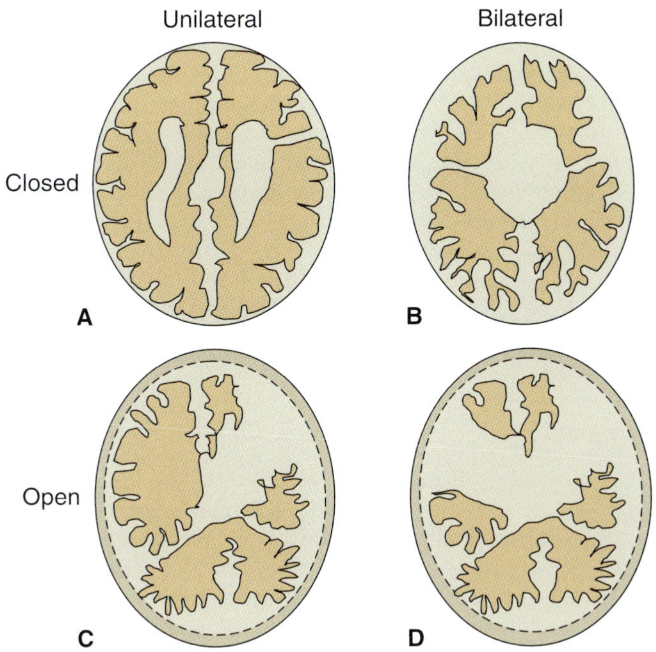


**Figure 10–2.** Graphic representations of the four types of schizencephaly. **(A)** Unilateral closed lip. **(B)** Bilateral closed lip. **(C)** Unilateral open lip. **(D)** Bilateral open lip.

## Incidence

Schizencephaly is a rare brain abnormality that was first described by Yakovlev and Wadsworth in 1946.[25] A recent publication of the birth prevalence of schizencephaly in south-eastern Hungary found it to be present in 0.54 per 10,000 live births;[26] this is in contrast with a study from the California Birth Defects Monitoring Program that found a prevalence of 1.54 per 100,000 (0.15 per 10,000).[27] A major difference between the studies was that the California study included patients up to 1 year of age, whereas in the Hungarian study, the average age at confirmation was 28.7 months; as a result, the California study may have underreported mild cases.[26] In the majority of patients, schizencephaly is sporadic, but familial schizencephaly has been reported.[24]

## Pathogenesis

There are two main theories regarding the pathogenesis of schizencephaly. The first is that of a failure of induction of neuronal migration; the second is that of vascular disruption and hypoxia-ischemia at critical points during the neuronal development (acquired). These processes usually occur before the 24th week of the pregnancy.[26,28]

## Etiology

The etiology of schizencephaly is heterogeneous and is not clear at present. Etiologies reported in the literature include viral teratogenicity as the result of in utero exposure to cytomegalovirus (CMV), warfarin exposure, alcohol abuse, cocaine use, trauma during the first and second trimesters, syndromic associations, association with the *EMX2* gene, maternal and/or infant thrombophilia, and alloimmune thrombocytopenia (hemorrhage).[27]

## Associated Anomalies

Curry et al[27] reported on 63 cases of schizencephaly from the California Birth Defects Monitoring Program; 43 cases had schizencephaly and central nervous system (CNS) anomalies only. The more common CNS anomalies present were hypoplastic or absent corpus callosum, absence of the septum pellucidum, hydrocephaly, gyral malformations (including heterotopias and polymicrogyria), and optic nerve hypoplasia. Rarely seen CNS anomalies included fusion of the thalami, accompanying porencephaly, arachnoid cyst, and cerebellar malformations. There were 20 cases that in addition to the associated CNS anomalies had non-CNS anomalies, such as amniotic band disruptive sequence, arthrogryposis, death of a monozygotic twin, septo-optic dysplasia, gastroschisis, cleft lip and/or palate, Aicardi syndrome, meningocele, 8p+, VATER association (vertebral defects, imperforate anus, tracheoesophageal fistula, radial and renal dysplasia), craniosynostosis, microphthalmia, cataracts, and hydronephrosis. In a more recent study by Szabo et al,[26] ~50% of the cases of schizencephaly had associated agenesis of the septum pellucidum; however, none of the patients had optic nerve hypoplasia or endocrinological abnormalities, which are typically seen in septo-optic dysplasia. In ~20% there was polymicrogyria contralateral to the cleft and agenesis or dysgenesis of the corpus callosum; there was also one case each of crossed cerebellar diaschisis and intracerebral calcification in the absence of any intrauterine infections.

## Risk of Recurrence

The risk of recurrence is uncertain at this time, as most cases are sporadic; familial cases of schizencephaly have been described. Some patients with schizencephaly have been found to have mutations in the *EMX2* gene (OMIM 269160).

## Diagnosis

The sonographic diagnosis is that of bilateral or unilateral wedge like defects or clefts in the cerebral cortex extending from the lateral ventricles to the subarachnoid space (Figure 10–3). The cavum septi pellucidi and the corpus callosum may be absent; there may be optic nerve hypoplasia. The thalami typically are not fused. The ventricles may be dilated. The circle of Willis is normal.[29]

Fetal MRI is helpful in identifying the gray matter. In open-lip schizencephaly, the gray matter is seen lining the walls of the clefts. In addition, it can help in identifying areas of polymicrogyria and heterotopias, which are common in cases of schizencephaly.[30] Oh et al[30] described the following postnatal MRI findings in schizencephaly: (1) a defect that extends from the pial surface to the ventricle; (2) the walls of the defect are lined with gray matter; (3) the ventricle may be tented, thus pointing to the defect; (4) absent cavum septi pellucidi in as many as 75% of cases of schizencephaly; (5) the corpus callosum is focally thinned or may be absent; (6) polymicrogyria and heterotopias are common; and (7) a roofing membrane covering the defect is infrequent (Figures 10–4, 10–5, and 10–6). Three-dimensional (3D) US helps to better define the defect, and pictures are comparable to MRI (Figures 10–7, 10–8, and 10–9).

### Implications for Sonographic Screening

Schizencephaly occurs very early in gestation. It is therefore likely that the cerebral clefts associated with the type II variety can be recognized by the midtrimester. Absence of the corpus callosum and ventriculomegaly are also frequently present, and this would facilitate the diagnosis. An exception could be represented by cases with unilateral clefts involving the cerebral hemisphere proximal to the transducer that is commonly not seen during standard examinations.[19] Most cases thus far have been recognized only in late gestation.

## Differential Diagnosis

The main differential diagnoses include holoprosencephaly, hydrocephaly, hydranencephaly, porencephaly, and arachnoid cysts (see Chapter 9). In holoprosencephaly, there is absence of the midline structures, fused thalami, and facial abnormalities (alobar and semilobar type); however, in schizencephaly, although the cavum septi pellucidi and corpus callosum may be absent, there are large cortical abnormalities, and typically the thalami are not fused. In hydrocephaly, the dilated lateral ventricles do not communicate with the subarachnoid space. In cases of hydranencephaly, the cerebral hemispheres may be completely or almost completely absent, and CSF fills the space. In porencephaly, although it may have a similar appearance, the porencephalic cavities are not lined by gray matter; this can be diagnosed by using MRI. Arachnoid cysts are not symmetrical and do not communicate with the lateral ventricles.

## Prognosis

The clinical symptoms correlate with the degree and severity of the cleft coupled with the severity of the cortical abnormalities.[24] Clinically, schizencephaly is typically characterized by a triad of abnormalities of neuronal migration, namely, motor disorder, such as hemi- or tetraparesis; intellectual impairment; and seizures.[31] Epilepsy is usually seen in children with unilateral closed schizencephaly, and microcephaly, spastic quadriplegia, and mental retardation in children with bilateral open clefts.[1] In a recent study by Szabo et al,[26]

A

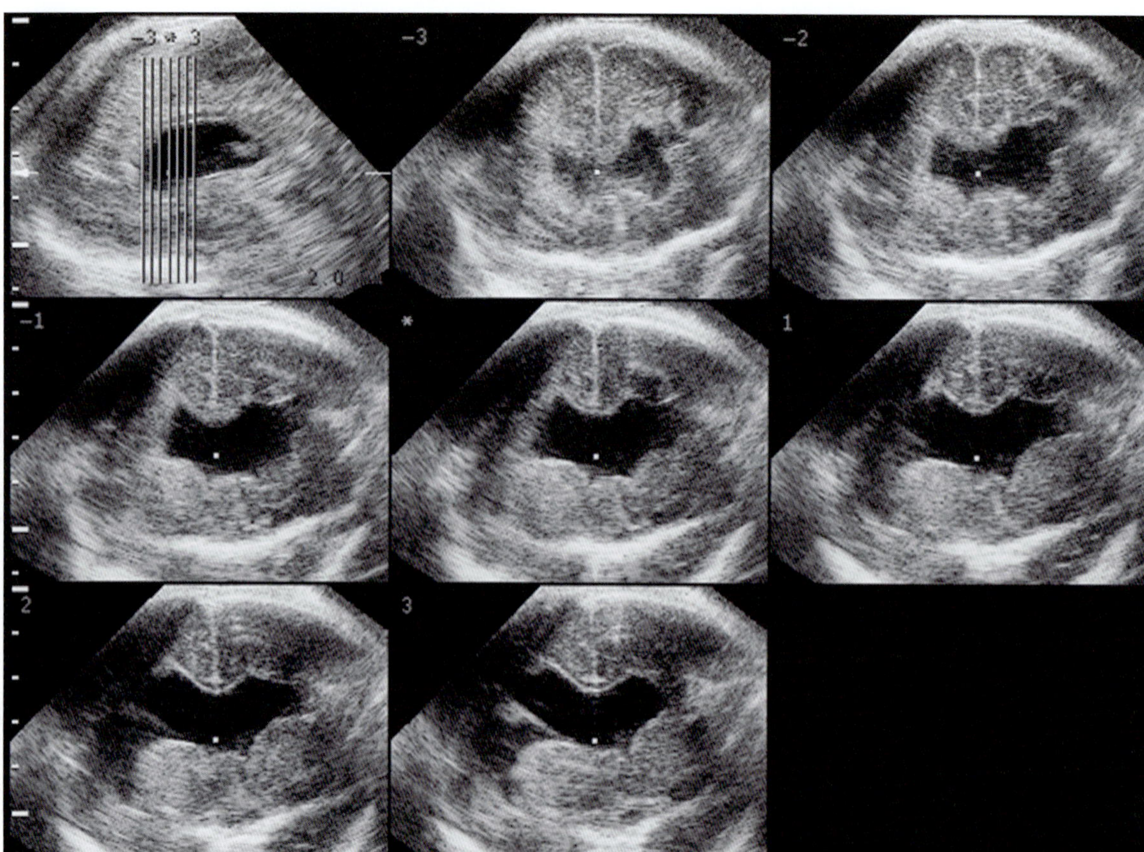

**Figure 10–3.** Tomographic images of bilateral open-lip schizencephaly detected at 21 postmenstrual weeks. **(A)** Coronal section.

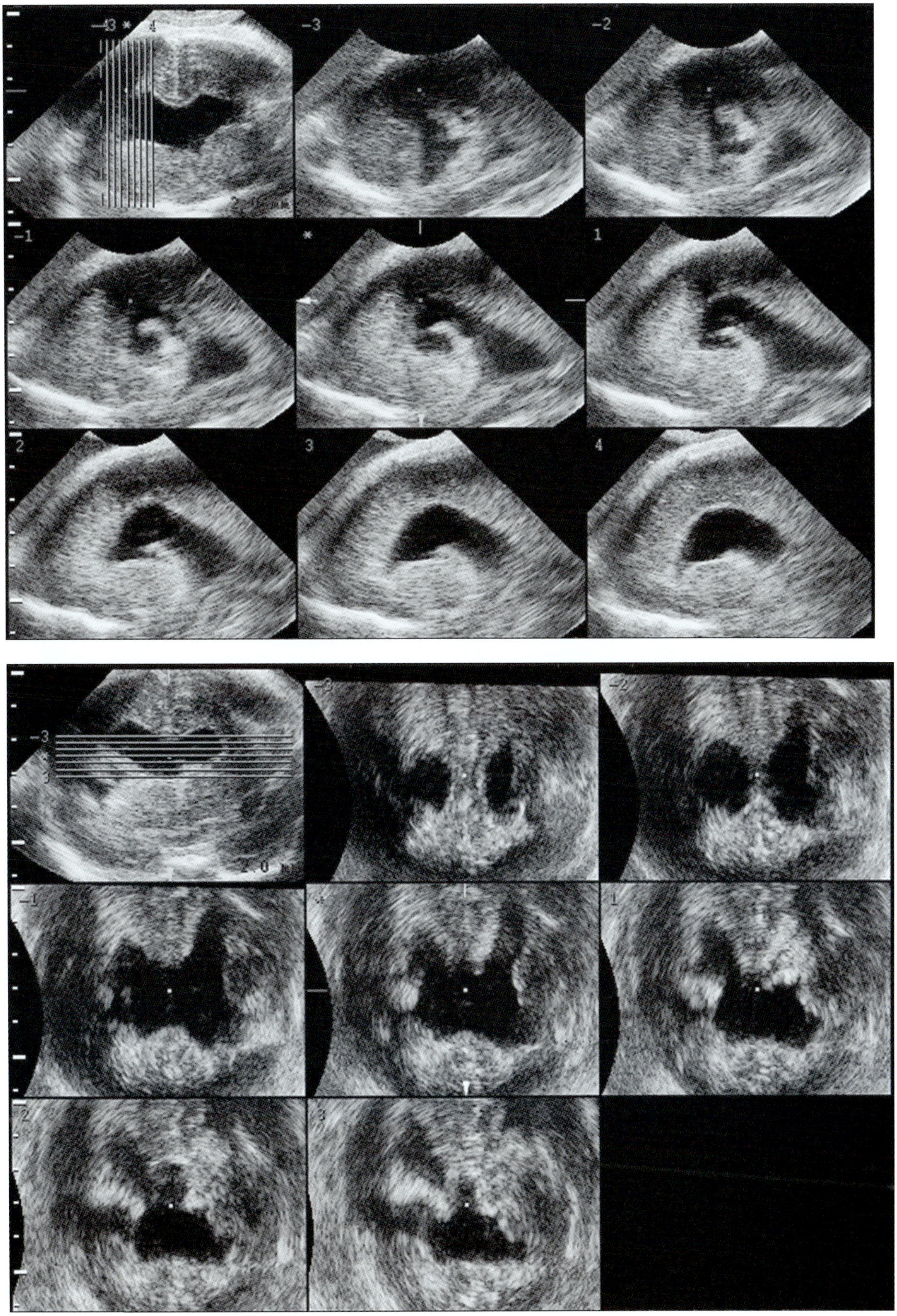

B

C

**Figure 10–3.** *(continued)* **(B)** Sagittal section. **(C)** Axial (horizontal section).

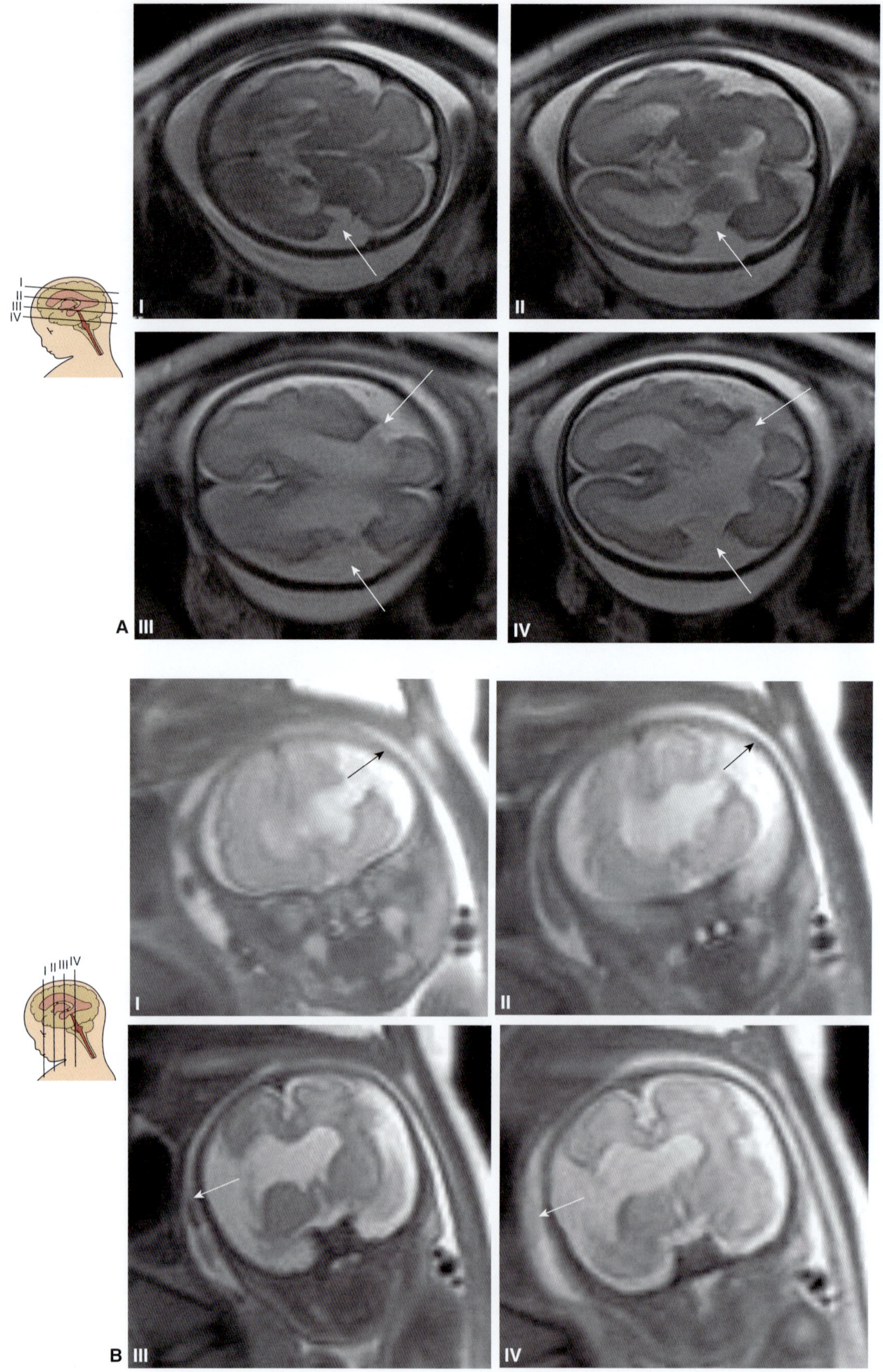


**Figure 10–4.** Serial magnetic resonance imaging (MRI) of bilateral open-lip schizencephaly. The arrows point to the clefts. **(A)** Axial plane. **(B)** Coronal plane.

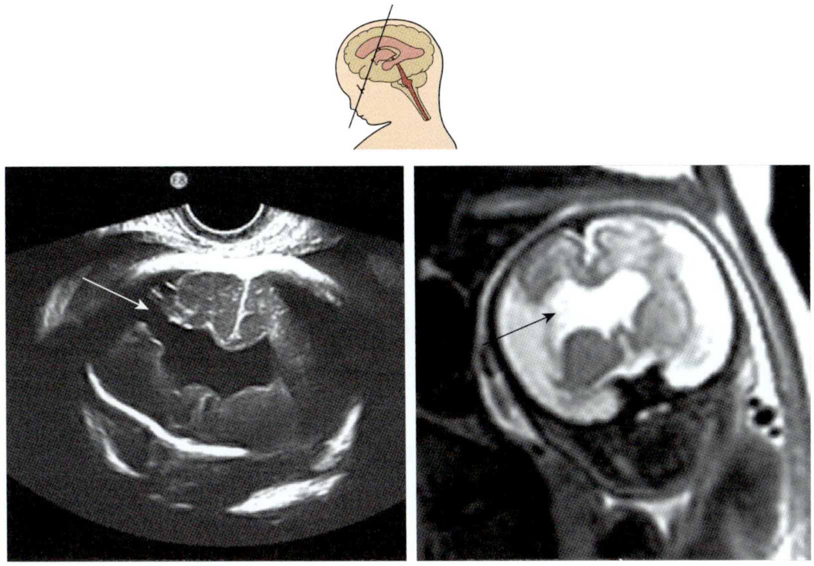

**Figure 10–5.** Comparison of US (*left*) and MRI (*right*) of a right-sided, open-lip schizencephaly. The arrows point to the cleft.

of 10 children with schizencephaly, 7 exhibited unilateral schizencephaly, and 3 had bilateral. Of the seven children with unilateral schizencephaly, six had contralateral spastic hemiplegia, and one had spastic tetraplegia; five of the seven had delayed development and intellectual disability, and two of the seven had seizures. Of the three children with bilateral schizencephaly, two had spastic tetraplegia, and the other had generalized hypotonia; all three had delayed developmental and intellectual disability, and one had seizures.

## Obstetric Management

Schizencephaly is a rare heterogeneous disease; if diagnosed early (earlier than 24 postmenstrual weeks), termination of pregnancy should be offered to the patient;

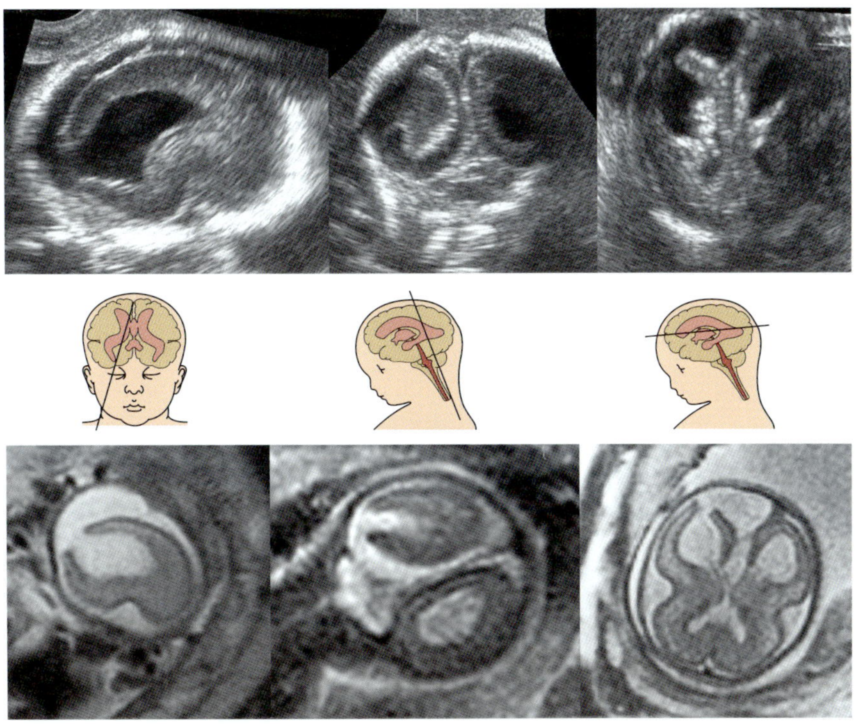

**Figure 10–6.** Comparative US (*upper row*) and MRI (*lower row*) of a unilateral, right-sided, open-lip schizencephaly. Sagittal, coronal, and axial planes, respectively (same case as in Figures 10–7 and 10–8).

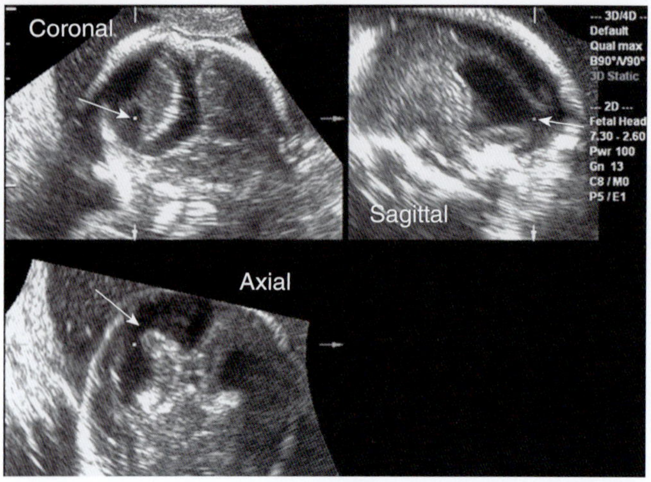


**Figure 10–7.** 3D US images of a unilateral, right-sided, open-lip schizencephaly. The arrows point to the cleft (same case as in Figures 10–6 and 10–8).

however, in the vast majority of cases, schizencephaly, like porencephaly, will be diagnosed only during the third trimester of pregnancy. In these cases, management should include fetal MRI to further evaluate the fetal brain, a thrombophilia workup (for both parents),[32] and consultations with a geneticist, neonatologist, pediatric neurologist, and neurosurgeon. Given the fact that schizencephaly is a rare condition, there are no standard recommendations at this time regarding the best route of delivery.

## HYDRANENCEPHALY

### Definition

Hydranencephaly is a rare brain malformation, the result of an encephaloclastic (destructive) process in which both cerebral hemispheres may be completely or almost completely absent, and CSF fills the space; essentially, the cerebral hemispheres have been reduced to a CSF-filled sac. The falx may be incomplete or absent, and the head size may be normal. The cerebellum and brainstem are normal but subject to intracranial pressure and are therefore deformed.

### Synonyms

Hydrocephalic anencephaly, hydroencephalodysplasia, cystencephaly hydromercencephaly, encephaloclastic proliferative vasculopathy (EPV), hydranencephaly, Fowler syndrome

### Incidence

Hydranencephaly occurs rarely, with a reported prevalence of 1 to 2 per 10,000 births. Most cases are sporadic; however, familial types of hydranencephaly have been described, such as (1) proliferative vasculopathy and hydranencephaly-hydrocephaly syndrome (MIM 225790), also known as Fowler syndrome, which is a recessive condition (gene map locus14q24.3); another feature of the syndrome is fetal akinesia deformation sequence, which can be seen from the late first to early second trimester;[33] (2) micro hydranencephaly (MIM 605013), in which there is microcephaly and hydranencephaly (gene map locus16p13.3-p12.1); and (3) hydranencephaly with renal aplasia-dysplasia (MIM 236500).

### Pathogenesis

Hydranencephaly is the result of an ischemic stroke of both internal carotid arteries (ICAs) occurring as early as the 11th postmenstrual week.[1,34] The areas affected by the infarct undergo tissue necrosis and eventually resorption, leaving behind a cavity in the brain. In hydranencephaly, the previously normal cerebral hemispheres are replaced by a thin-walled, fluid-filled cyst. The aqueduct is usually atretic, and increased fluid pressure causes the cyst (and the head) to enlarge as the result of hydrocephaly. There is variable preservation of the inferior frontal, temporal, and occipital lobes and of the basal ganglia and diencephalon.

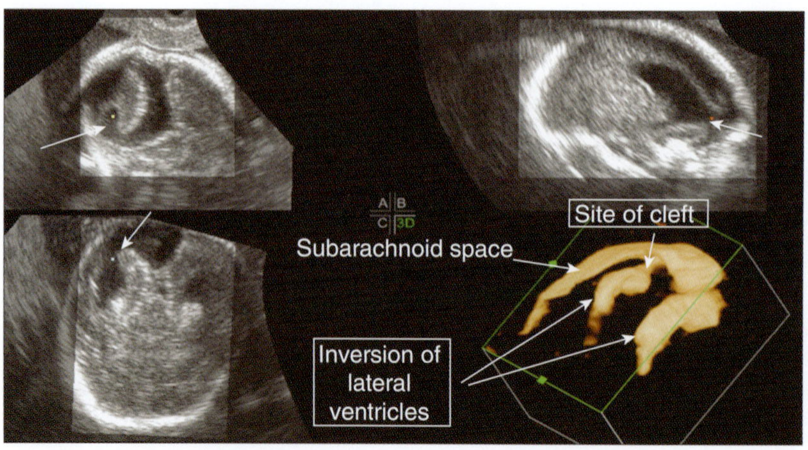


**Figure 10–8.** 3D inversion rendering of the fluid in a fetal brain demonstrating the fluid connected between the lateral ventricles and the subarachnoid space through the cleft (same case as in Figures 10–6 and 10–7).

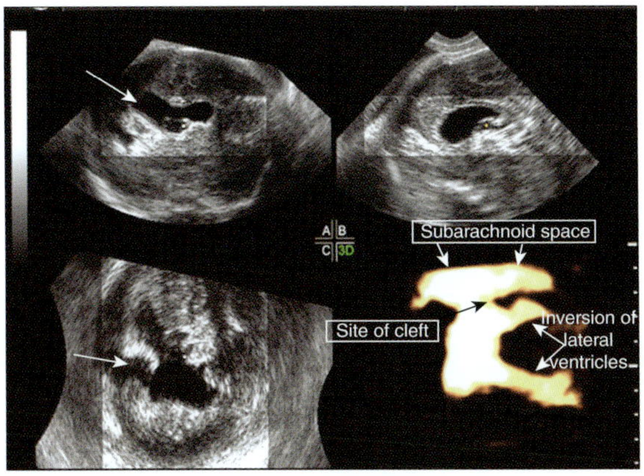


**Figure 10–9.** 3D US of unilateral, open-lip schizencephaly. Coronal **(A)**, sagittal **(B)**, and axial **(C)** orthogonal planes. The 3D rendering box represents the inversion of the fluid within the lateral ventricles with the connection (through the cleft) to the subarachnoid space.

The brainstem and cerebellum are usually preserved. If a unilateral internal carotid stroke occurs, the result is hemihydranencephaly; usually the left side is affected. In contrast, with children with hydranencephaly, those with hemihydranencephaly have a relatively good outcome.[1]

## Etiology

Hydranencephaly can be the result of a developmental or an encephaloclastic process secondary to an insult, such as vascular occlusion of a vessel of the anterior circulation (eg, the vein of Galen or ICAs), resulting in ischemia; intracranial hemorrhage, as in cases of coagulation disorder or thrombocytopenia; intrauterine infection (eg, herpes, CMV, or toxoplasmosis); and maternal-fetal hypotension, such as in the death of a monochorionic co-twin, maternal trauma, or abruption.[1,35,36]

## Associated Anomalies

Hydranencephaly can be associated with other brain anomalies, such as hydrocephaly, polymicrogyria, and microcephaly. When non-CNS abnormalities, such as fetal akinesia deformation sequence, are seen, the diagnosis of Fowler syndrome should be entertained. Renal abnormalities, such as hypoplastic kidneys, can also be observed with hydranencephaly as part of extremely rare syndromes.

## Risk of Recurrence

The risk of recurrence is uncertain, as most cases are sporadic. However, when hydranencephaly is part of a syndrome, such as Fowler (proliferative vasculopathy and hydranencephaly-hydrocephaly), it has a recessive inheritance.

## Sonographic Diagnosis

The sonographic findings of hydranencephaly include a normocephalic or macrocephalic fetus with a large fluid-filled intracranial cavity (Figures 10–10 and 10–11). Several reports on the in utero evolution of hydranencephaly resulting from an intracranial hemorrhage are present in the literature.[37,38] The usual presentation is the finding of a bright, homogeneous, hyperechoic mass most consistent with an intracranial hemorrhage. As the cases are followed prospectively with serial sonography, the echo-dense mass becomes more sonolucent with the development of the hydranencephaly. As a rule, no cerebral cortex is present, but there is partial preservation of portions of the occipital lobe. The falx cerebri is usually intact. The midbrain and basal ganglia are variably preserved. The brainstem and cerebellum are usually intact.[38] Polyhydramnios is usually present.

In cases of hydranencephaly as the result of Fowler syndrome in the first trimester, the brain appears to be totally replaced by a fluid-filled cavity, and the fetal limbs

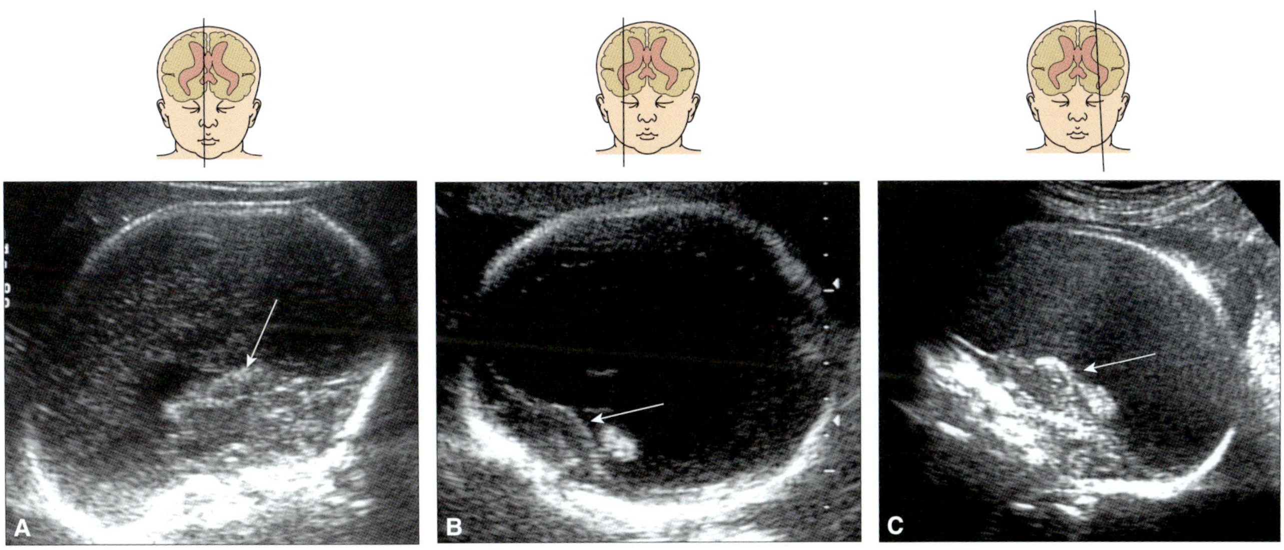


**Figure 10–10.** Hydranencephaly in a fetus at 22 weeks' gestation. **(A)** Median section along the falx. **(B, C)** Parasagittal sections showing structures of the midbrain (*arrows*).

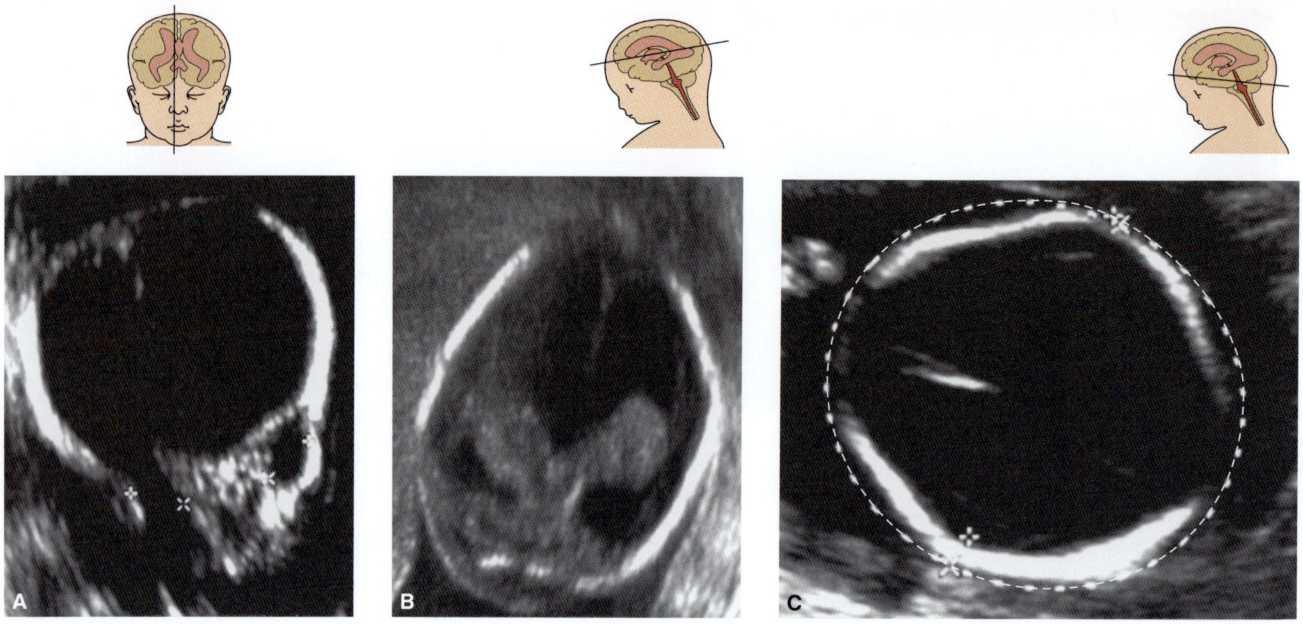


**Figure 10–11.** Hydranencephaly at 17 weeks, 3 days of gestation. **(A)** Anterior coronal view showing the fluid-filled head and falx. **(B)** Axial view at the level of the thalami. **(C)** Axial view at the level of the biparietal diameter. Note that there is no brain parenchyma, but the falx cerebri is still present.

will demonstrate abnormal positioning (arthrogryposis). Also apparent are thick nuchal translucency mild polyhydramnios, and lack of fetal movements (akinesia).[33]

## Differential Diagnosis

The differential diagnosis of hydranencephaly is massive hydrocephaly and alobar holoprosencephaly. Holoprosencephaly can be differentiated from hydranencephaly by the fact that the thalami are never fused in hydranencephaly. In hydrocephaly all parts of the ventricular system will become dilated, but in hydranencephaly, the third ventricle is present and visible but is not enlarged.[36] Belfar et al[39] reported on a case of evolving hydranencephaly in which the differential diagnosis included a fetal teratoma. In their case, the sonographic appearance was that of abnormal conglomeration of disorganized tissue replacing both cerebral hemispheres.

### Implications for Sonographic Screening

Hydranencephaly is easily identified by standard sonography at midgestation, when present. It has been noted, however, that this condition is the consequence of a disruptive event that may occur even in relatively late gestation. Several case reports exist that document a normal sonographic appearance of the brain at midgestation in fetuses that later developed hydranencephaly.

## Prognosis

Hydranencephaly is usually lethal, and fetuses with this condition are at an increased risk of being stillborn or dying within the first year of life. A baby born with hydranencephaly may appear normal initially because the brainstem is intact with normal head size, and they have spontaneous reflexes, such as sucking, swallowing, crying, and moving the arms and legs; on physical exam, the empty cranial cavity transilluminates. However, after a few weeks of life, the baby becomes irritable and has increased muscle tone; subsequently, seizures and hydrocephaly may appear. In addition, the baby will have failure to thrive, deafness, blindness, spastic quadriparesis, difficulty in feeding, and severe neurologic impairment. Most children will die in their first year of life, although survival past the age of 10 years can occur; there are several reports in the literature of individuals surviving into their 20s with hydranencephaly.[35,40]

## Obstetric Management

At the time of diagnosis, a complete anatomical survey, including a fetal echocardiogram, should be performed to look for associated anomalies, as these may point to the etiology of the hydranencephaly. The patient should receive counseling with maternal-fetal medicine, neonatology, neurology, and genetics. Fetal infection with CMV and toxoplasmosis should be excluded. Amniocentesis for karyotype and/or microarray testing should be offered as well. Termination of the pregnancy should be discussed, given the poor prognosis for fetuses/babies with hydranencephaly. In cases in which the patient elects to have a termination of pregnancy, fetal autopsy is recommended; however, if a destructive procedure is contemplated, a fetal MRI may be helpful in identifying associated anomalies. For those fetuses diagnosed at the time of delivery, after extensive counseling, compassionate care should be given.

## DURAL SINOVENOUS THROMBOSIS

### Definition

Cerebral sinovenous thrombosis (CSVT) involves a thrombus (blood clot) that forms within one of the venous sinuses that drain blood from the brain. The brain is drained by multiple large sinuses, such as the superior and inferior sagittal sinus, the superior and inferior petrosal sinus, the transverse sinus, the sigmoid sinus, the straight sinus, the cavernous sinus, and the confluence of sinuses (torcular herophili). The thrombosis can result in a stroke (venous infarct), or it may cause intracranial hemorrhage.

### Synonyms

Perinatal stroke, fetal stroke, thromboembolic, dural sinus thrombosis, infantile dural arteriovenous fistula (AVF).

### Incidence

CSVT is a rare condition in fetuses, and the incidence is largely unknown. It is often diagnosed late during the second trimester. Nevertheless, because of the increased use of prenatal sonography, this condition is now diagnosed in uterus with greater frequency. In neonates based on the Canadian Childhood Stroke Registry, the reported incidence is 41 per 100,000 live births per year.[41] Males are affected slightly more often than females, and the superior sagittal sinus and lateral sinuses are the most commonly affected structures.[42]

### Pathogenesis

Sinus thrombosis in neonates, infants, and adults has been associated with trauma and dural sinus malformation. It also has been associated with hypercoagulable states and thrombophilias (eg, antithrombin, protein C and S, and factor V Leiden mutation).[43] In fetuses, the pathogenesis is largely unknown, but it may be due to similar etiologies as in the neonate, such as dural sinus malformation.[1,44] Dural sinus malformations are congenital dural arteriovenous shunts, which are characterized by the presence of a giant dural sinus pouch that communicates with other sinuses and drains cerebral veins; they are often associated with slow blood flow velocities in arteriovenous shunts.[45,46] Spontaneous thrombosis of these sinuses can occur. These malformations are classified into two types: midline involving the torcular herophili and adjacent posterior and lateral sinuses involving even the jugular bulb with otherwise normal sinus.[45,46] Grange et al[47] reported progressive formation of a thrombus in a dilated torcular. The authors concluded that a primary venous malformation led to aberrant flow and progressive clot formation. Our group recently reported a case of torcular ectasia with a large thrombus. On pathologic examination, the clot displayed organized layering consistent with progressive growth of the thrombus, potentially due to turbulent flow patterns in the abnormally dilated vessels. These findings are consistent with the above hypothesis.[48]

### Etiology

The etiology of a dural sinus malformation is not fully understood; however, it is believed to arise as the result of a normal ballooning of the transverse sinus that takes place between the fourth and sixth month of intrauterine life; postnatally, the transverse sinus slowly undergoes remodeling until it reaches its final stage.[49] It is believed that posterior dural sinus malformation in the neonatal period is the result of the persistence of the ballooning sinus.[49] According to Barbosa et al,[49] dural sinus malformation is a disease involving a deviant development of the sinuses; eventually, this progresses to sinus wall overgrowth, abnormal development of venous spaces leading to the formation of giant lakes followed by secondary thrombosis of the spaces. If the venous drainage is rerouted, subsequent remodeling of the "channels" will take place. Often dural sinus malformation is associated with multiple slow arteriovenous shunts.

### Associated Anomalies

Besides dural sinus malformations, no other associated anomalies have been reported so far in these cases.

### Risk of Recurrence

The risk of recurrence is uncertain but likely is very low.

### Sonographic Diagnosis

Dural sinus thrombosis appears as a supratentorial space-occupying mass in the occipital region of the brain (Figures 10–10, 10–11, and 10–12). The mass may appear hyperechoic, located in the midline above the cerebellum. However, the appearance of the mass on US may be heterogeneous because the thrombus may be at different stages of evolution. Recently, a case of dural sinus thrombosis at the torcular diagnosed in our unit had the following normal intracranial findings: normal biometry, including biparietal diameter, head circumference, transverse cerebellar diameter, and lateral ventricle, as well as normal falx, corpus callosum, cavum septi pellucidi, posterior fossa, cerebellum, vermis, and cisterna magna. The abnormal findings were a supratentorial space-occupying mass in the occipital region of the brain, with a brightly echogenic nodule within the mass (Figure 10–13); no flow was seen when using color Doppler (Figure 10–14). The fetal MRI using T1-weighted images showed a hypersignal on the occipital region of the head and a central hyposignal on T2-weighted images (Figures 10–15 and 10–16). Over the following 2 weeks the size of the thrombus increased in size, and the fetus developed mild ventriculomegaly (Figure 10–17). In a recently reported case of torcular ectasia by our group, the US image using two-dimensional (2D) and 3D sonography revealed a large thrombus in the occipital region of the head; on color Doppler, no flow was seen (Figure 10–18A–D). On pathologic examination, the clot displayed organized layering consistent with progressive growth of the thrombus (Figure 10–18E–H). As described before, a thrombus may reside in one of the

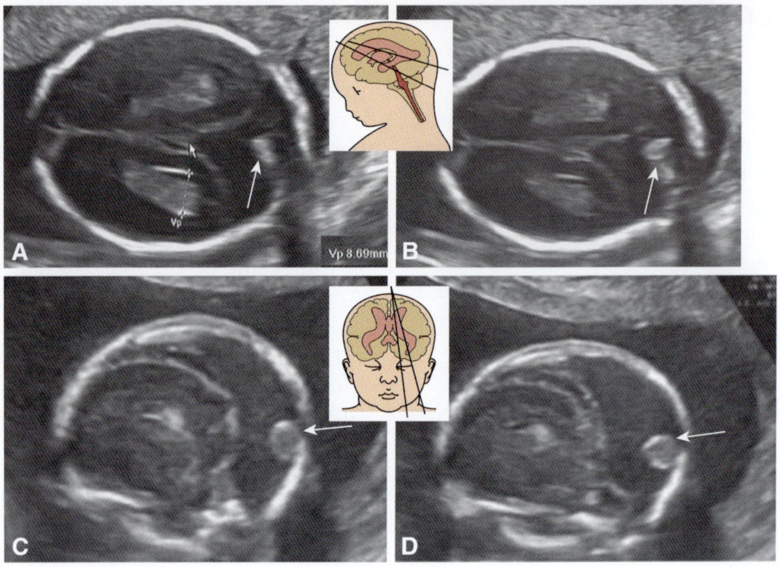


**Figure 10–12.** Thrombosis of the torcular herophili (confluence of the sinuses). **(A, B)** Higher and lower axial plane respectively. **(C, D)** Paramedian and slightly more lateral sagittal plane, respectively. (The arrow points to the hyperechoic spherical dot within the dilated sinus.)

transverse sinuses. Figure 10–19 depicts such an occurrence. Obliteration of one of the transverse sinuses carries a better prognosis than that of the confluence of the sinuses.

## Differential Diagnosis

The main differential diagnosis is based on space-occupying lesions in the posterior fossa, such as intracranial tumor, vein of Galen aneurysm, Dandy-Walker malformation, arachnoid cyst, and subdural hematoma. Intracranial tumors of the posterior fossa typically are teratomas that have a heterogeneous appearance. A vein of Galen aneurysm can be easily diagnosed by multiple facts. It is located in front of the posterior fossa and not within, and when color Doppler is applied, there is typically high and turbulent flow; additionally, these fetuses may present with hydrops. Arachnoid cysts are cystic anechoic structures, unlike a thrombus, which is heterogeneous in appearance. Dandy-Walker malformation involves the cerebellar vermis and in a median section of the posterior fossa is usually elevated and rotated. In cases of dural sinus thrombosis, the cerebellum, vermis, and posterior fossa may be displaced forward but are anatomically normal.

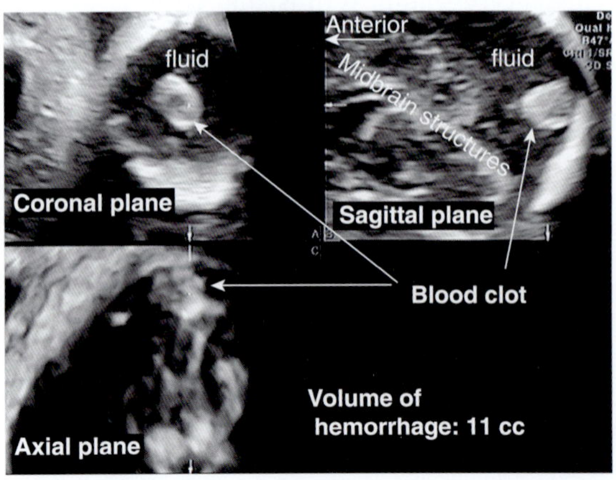


**Figure 10–13.** 3D picture of a thrombosis of the torcular herophili. The blood clot (*arrows*) and the approximate volume of the hemorrhage are shown. **(A)** Coronal plane. **(B)** Sagittal plane. **(C)** Axial plane.

## Prognosis

Prognosis of the fetus with a dural sinus thrombosis is unpredictable. However, midline thrombus at the torcular herophili has a worse postnatal prognosis than the lateral type, as the lateral type benefits from collateral drainage, usually has a benign course, and may remain asymptomatic for a long time.[46,49] A good prognostic sign is regression or decreasing size of the hematoma. Poor prognostic signs include enlargement of the thrombus, congestive heart failure, and development of hydrocephaly. Based on several case reports and series, ~50% of prenatally diagnosed cases will have a good outcome.[44,45,47,48,50–54] In the neonate, a good prognostic sign is the dural sinus malformation away from the torcular. Poor prognostic signs are midline dural sinus malformation involving the torcular, large size of the pouch, and spontaneous thrombosis that compromises the venous drainage with subsequent venous infarction and intraparenchymal hemorrhage; other complications, such as cardiac failure, macrocrania, venous thrombosis, and cerebral atrophy, are associated with poor outcomes.[46] The prognosis for dural sinus thrombosis identified postnatally is poor. Two large series of 19 and 30 cases showed 26% to 37% of the children died, 3% to 26% had poor neurologic outcome, 30% to 37% had mild neurologic deficit, and only 7% to 10% had no neurologic deficit (normal).[49,55]

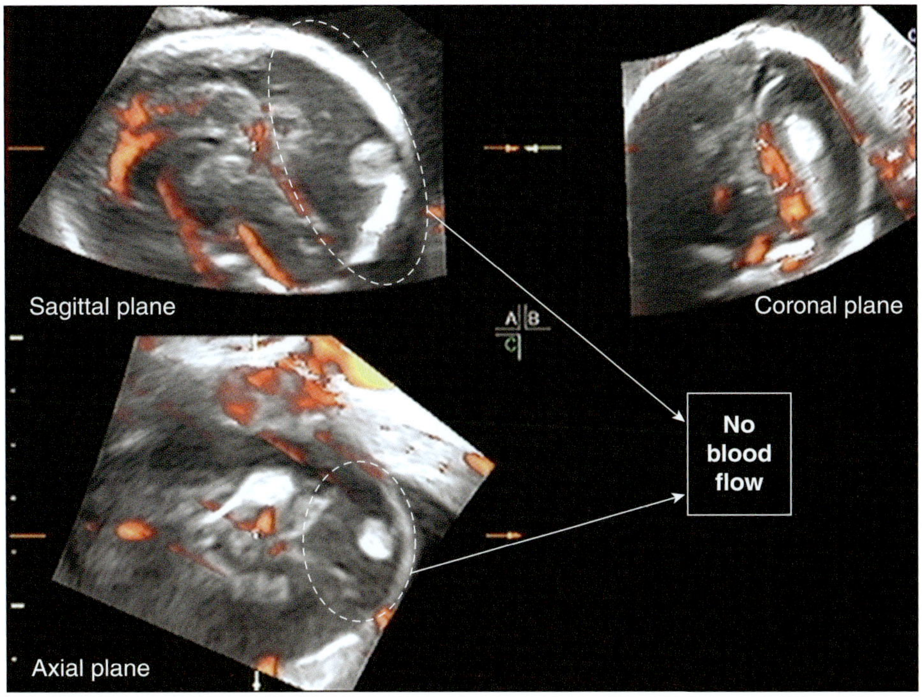


**Figure 10–14.** 3D power Doppler image of a sinus thrombosis demonstrating the dilated sinus devoid of Doppler signals.

## Obstetric Management

Because these are rare events, there are no large studies describing optimal obstetric management. However, if the sinovenous thrombosis is diagnosed early in the pregnancy, it is possible to follow these fetuses over the course of several weeks if the size of the thrombus increases and hydrocephaly develops; because these findings are associated with poor outcomes, a termination of pregnancy should be offered. In cases in which the patient decides to continue the pregnancy, fetal MRI to further evaluate the fetal brain and multidisciplinary consultations with a maternal-fetal medicine specialist, geneticist, neonatologist, pediatric neurologist, and neurosurgeon are suggested. An association has been reported with thrombophilias but not documented;[1] nevertheless, if a thrombophilia workup is done, it should be performed on both parents. A fetal

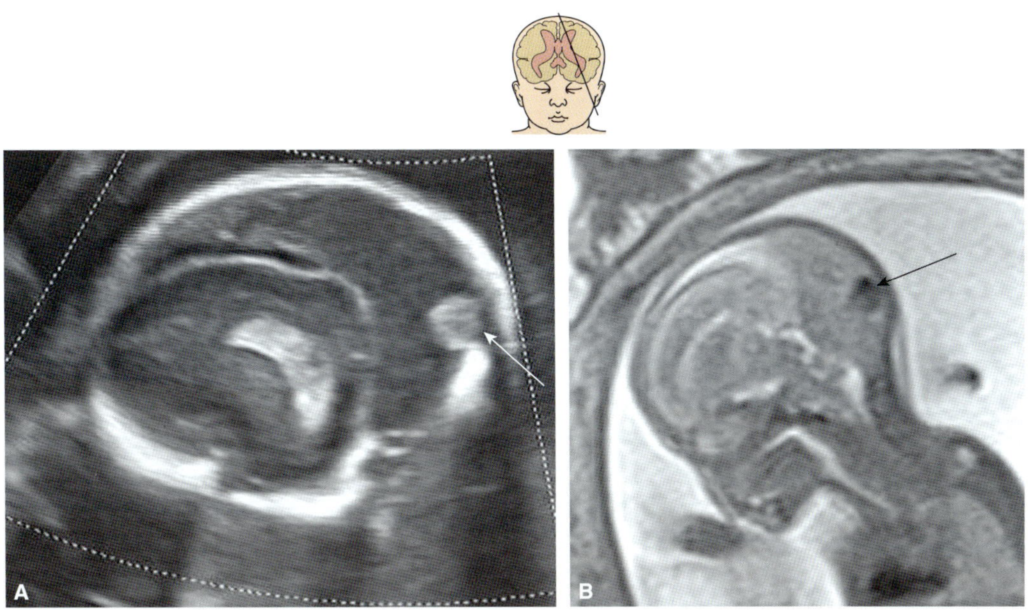

**Figure 10–15.** Juxtaposition of the same sagittal planes of the sinus thrombosis seen on Figure 10–14. (The arrows point to the thrombus). **(A)** Ultrasound. **(B)** MRI.

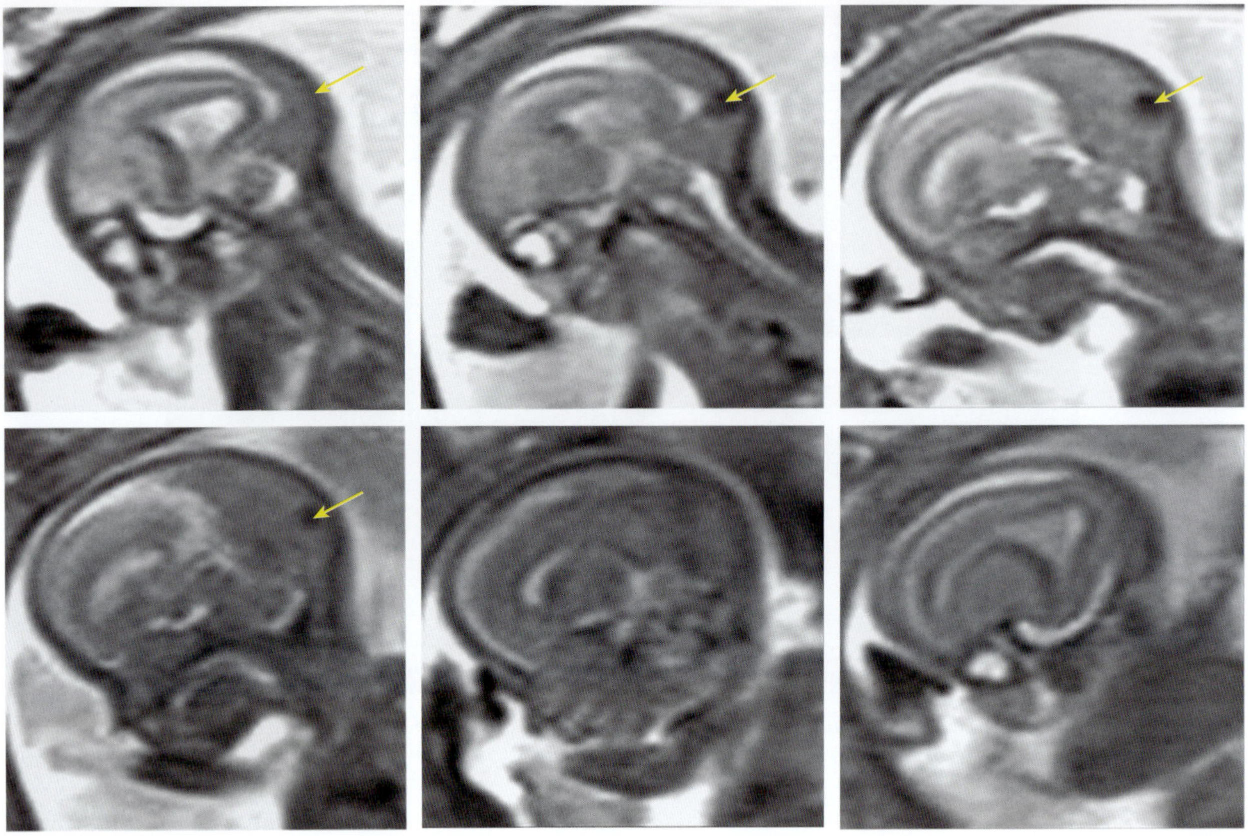

**Figure 10–16.** Serial sagittal MRI of the torcular thrombosis seen in Figures 10–12 to 10–15. (The arrow points to the thrombus.)

echocardiogram and serial US during the pregnancy to assess the size of the thrombus and lateral ventricles, and to rule out ascites, as well as MRI before delivery, can help in the management of the pregnancy. Because dural sinus thrombosis is a rare condition, there are no standard recommendations at this time regarding the best route of delivery. It is our opinion that cesarean section should be performed for obstetric indications.

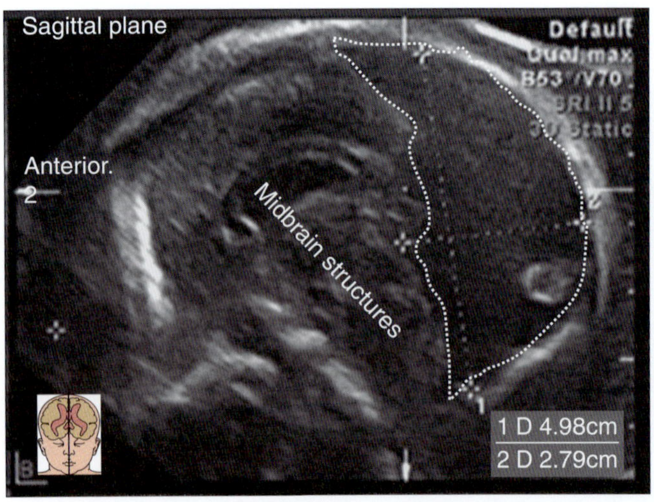


**Figure 10–17.** Follow-up sagittal image of the progressive nature of the torcular thrombosis depicted in Figures 10–12 to 10–14. The increasing volume of the lesion was obvious 1 week after the initial detection. This prompted the couple to ask for a termination of the pregnancy.

## IN UTERO INTRACRANIAL HEMORRHAGE

Subependymal germinal matrix hemorrhage–intraventricular hemorrhage (GMH-IVH) is the most commonly diagnosed type of intracranial hemorrhage in preterm neonates; however, in utero intracranial hemorrhage is a rare event, and in many cases the etiology is not identified.[43] Posthemorrhagic hydrocephaly is commonly associated with intracranial hemorrhage.[56] The hydrocephaly results from blockage of the CSF by the blood (posthemorrhagic hydrocephaly) and/or obliterative arachnoiditis.

## GERMINAL MATRIX HEMORRHAGE–INTRAVENTRICULAR HEMORRHAGE

### Definition

GMH-IVH is an intracranial hemorrhage confined to periventricular cerebral tissue. The term refers to hemorrhage within the fetal cranium. Intracranial hemorrhage is a common occurrence in the premature infant. In the fetus, the condition is rare, and the pathophysiology probably different. Only a few cases of fetal intracranial hemorrhage have been reported.[9,57–70]

## Synonyms

None

## Incidence

The exact incidence of fetal GMH-IVH is unknown. Vergani et al[68] suggested that fetal intracranial hemorrhage occurs in ~1 in 10,000 pregnancies. In contrast, in neonates, the frequency of GMH-IVH increases with decreasing gestational age; for example, in very low birth weight (VLBW) infants, GMH-IVH occurs in 15% to 25% of babies compared with 1% of term neonates.[71–74]

## Pathogenesis

In fetuses, the pathogenesis of intracranial hemorrhage has not been as clearly elucidated as in neonates; however, it is speculated that the pathogenesis is comparable to that of neonates. In neonates, the place of origin of intracranial hemorrhage is the germinal matrix. This area is a highly vascularized zone, with fragile blood vessels with little supporting stroma, especially between 24 and 32 postmenstrual weeks. In cases of "stress," such as sudden changes in cerebral blood pressure or perinatal asphyxia, which is associated with blood pressure fluctuations, damage and rupture of these vessels may take place, resulting in hemorrhage.[68,75] Intracranial hemorrhage is believed to cause obstruction of terminal veins, resulting in hemorrhagic venous infarction.[76] Hemorrhagic infarcts are seen in ~15% of neonates with intracranial hemorrhage; these infarcts are typically asymmetric and usually unilateral. Periventricular venous hemorrhagic infarcts can coexist with periventricular leukomalacia, which tend to be ischemic, symmetrical, and usually nonhemorrhagic.[77] The posthemorrhagic ventricular dilation is most likely the end result of obstruction by blood clots at the level of the interventricular foramina (Monro).[61]

## Etiology

Intracranial hemorrhages as the result of a venous hemorrhagic infarct or GMH-IVH share similar etiologies. Etiologies for in utero intracranial hemorrhage that have

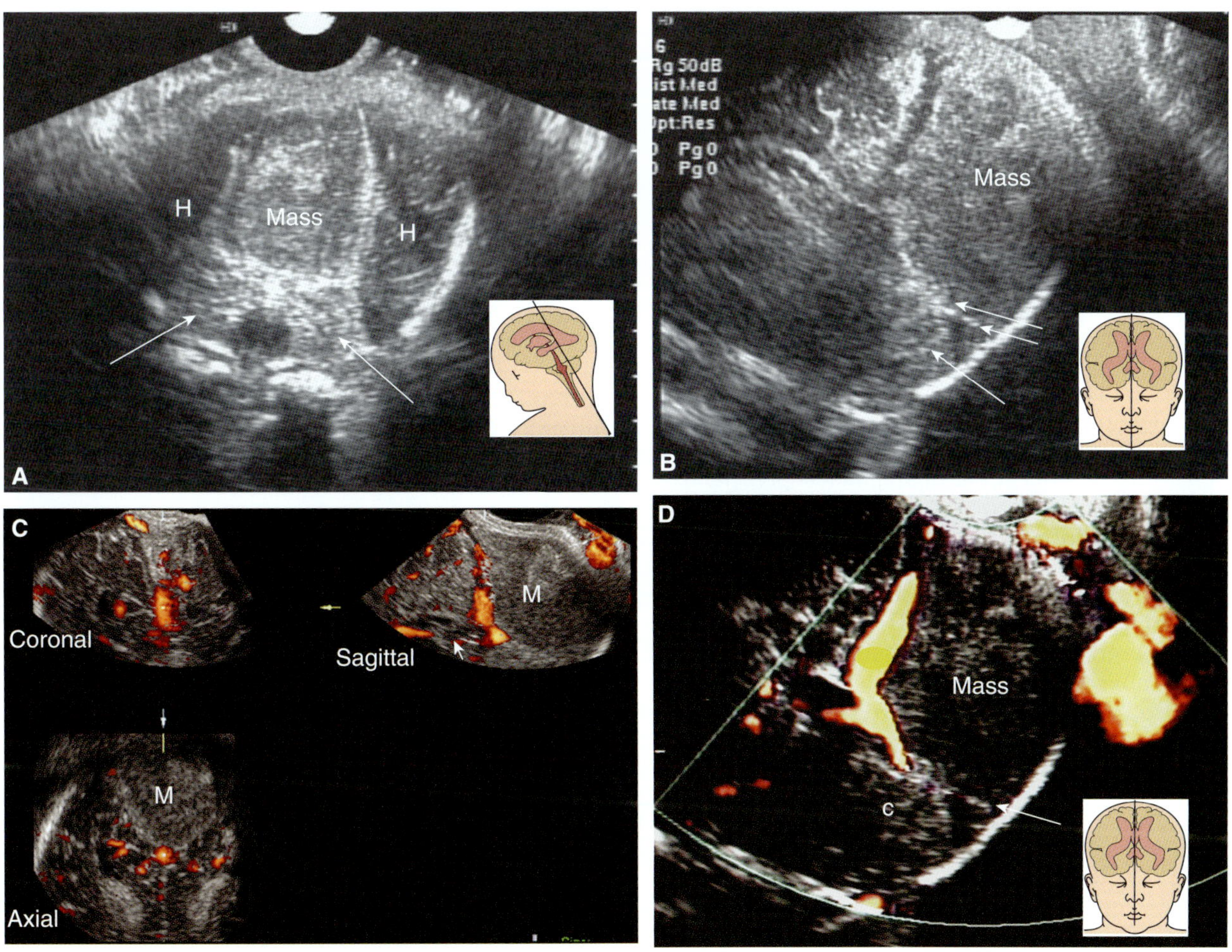


**Figure 10–18.** Another case of thrombosis of the torcular herophili at 38 postmenstrual weeks. The neonate died hours after delivery. **(A)** Posterior coronal plane. The mass displays the hemispheres (H). The arrows point to the cerebellum. **(B)** Sagittal section demonstrating the pressure of the mass on the posterior fossa and the cerebellum (*arrows*). **(C, D)** 3D power Doppler image showing displacement of the vessels by the mass (M).

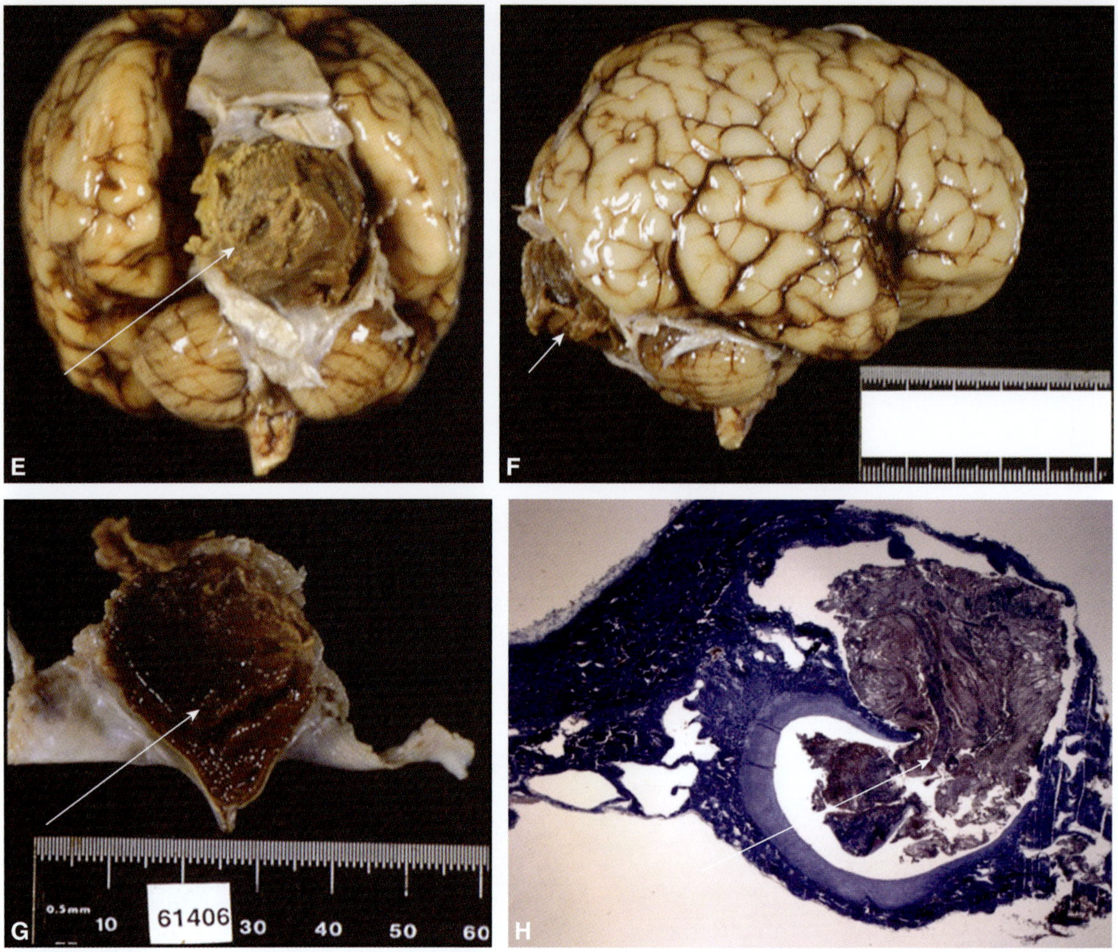


**Figure 10–18.** (*continued*) **(E)** The specimen posterior view of the thrombus (*arrow*) in the open sinus. **(F)** Lateral view of the brain with the thrombus (*arrow*). **(G)** The thrombus after its exposure by opening the sinus (*arrow*). **(H)** Histologic slide showing the thrombus (*arrow*) within the dilated sinus. (Reproduced, with permission, from Schwartz N, et al. JUM 2008;27:989).

been described in the literature include maternal trauma, hypoxia, infection (eg, CMV and toxoplasmosis), congenital vascular defects, ingestion of anticoagulant drugs (warfarin), maternal complications of pregnancy (preeclampsia, abruptio placenta, and seizure), maternal vitamin K deficiency, fetal blood dyscrasia, twin–twin or maternal-fetal transfusion, thrombocytopenia, fetal thrombophilia (factor V Leiden, protein C gene mutation, and 5,10-methylenetetrahydrofolate reductase [MTHFR] mutation), thrombosis of the umbilical cord, umbilical cord entanglement, and alloimmune thrombocytopenia.[57,65,78–85] Nonimmune hydrops also has been reported with in utero intracranial hemorrhage as a result of fetal anemia due to significant intracranial blood loss.[86] In ~50% of cases, however, the cause of the intracranial hemorrhage is not identified.[61]

## Risk of Recurrence

The risk of recurrence depends on the etiology, but because most cases occur sporadically, the risk of recurrence is very low.[61] However, if the intracranial hemorrhage occurred as the result of fetal/neonatal alloimmune thrombocytopenia, there is a 70% to 80% chance that the next child will also be affected by an intracranial hemorrhage.[87] If the pregnancy involved alloimmune thrombocytopenia but not intracranial hemorrhage, the risk of an intracranial hemorrhage in the next pregnancy is <10%.[87]

## Sonographic Diagnosis

The sonographic appearance of blood is brightly echogenic; therefore, whether the blood is located within the ventricle or the brain parenchyma, hemorrhage can be diagnosed in utero (Figures 10–20 and 10–21). The sonographic features of a fetal intracranial hemorrhage change over time in a predictable manner. The initial sonographic appearance of "fresh" blood clots is that of homogeneous hyperechoic areas that are distinct from the choroid plexus; the ventricles may show a "castlike" pattern that is brightly echogenic without posterior shadowing (Figures 10–21, 10–22, and 10–23). At this time, a mildly dilated lateral ventricle or hydrocephaly may be evident (Figures 10–24, 10–25, and 10–26). Over a period of a few days to 2 weeks the inner portions of the hematoma become hypoechoic (during the process of liquefaction), while the outer border remains echogenic and becomes sharply demarcated from the surrounding parenchyma (see Figure 10–25). Subsequently, the clot undergoes retraction and progressively becomes smaller; ventriculomegaly may resolve in some cases. As the clot retracts, as in cases of intraparenchymal hemorrhage, the developing porencephalic cyst becomes evident.[61,88,89] Color Doppler may help differentiate blood clots from other masses, as they do not have flow (see Figures 10–18 and 10–25C).

Fetal MRI is useful in assessing fetal intracranial bleeding. The most common reasons for obtaining a fetal MRI are ventriculomegaly, suspected posterior fossa anomaly, and agenesis of the corpus callosum.[90] Fetal MRI typically demonstrates blood or intracranial hemorrhage as areas of decreased signal on gradient echo-planar imaging, decreased signal on single-shot fast spin-echo (SSFSE) T2-weighted images, and increased signal intensity on T1-weighted images[91] (Figures 10–27 and 10–28). The advantages of MRI over US include higher contrast resolution, which is not affected by shadowing from the fetal skull or low amniotic fluid; however, fetal motion, small size of the structures being imaged, and significant distance between the coil and the structure being imaged are important limiting factors.[91]

## Differential Diagnosis

The main differential diagnosis is an intracranial tumor. Usually the tumor is heterogeneous and may grow rapidly in size; when using color Doppler, it will be vascular.

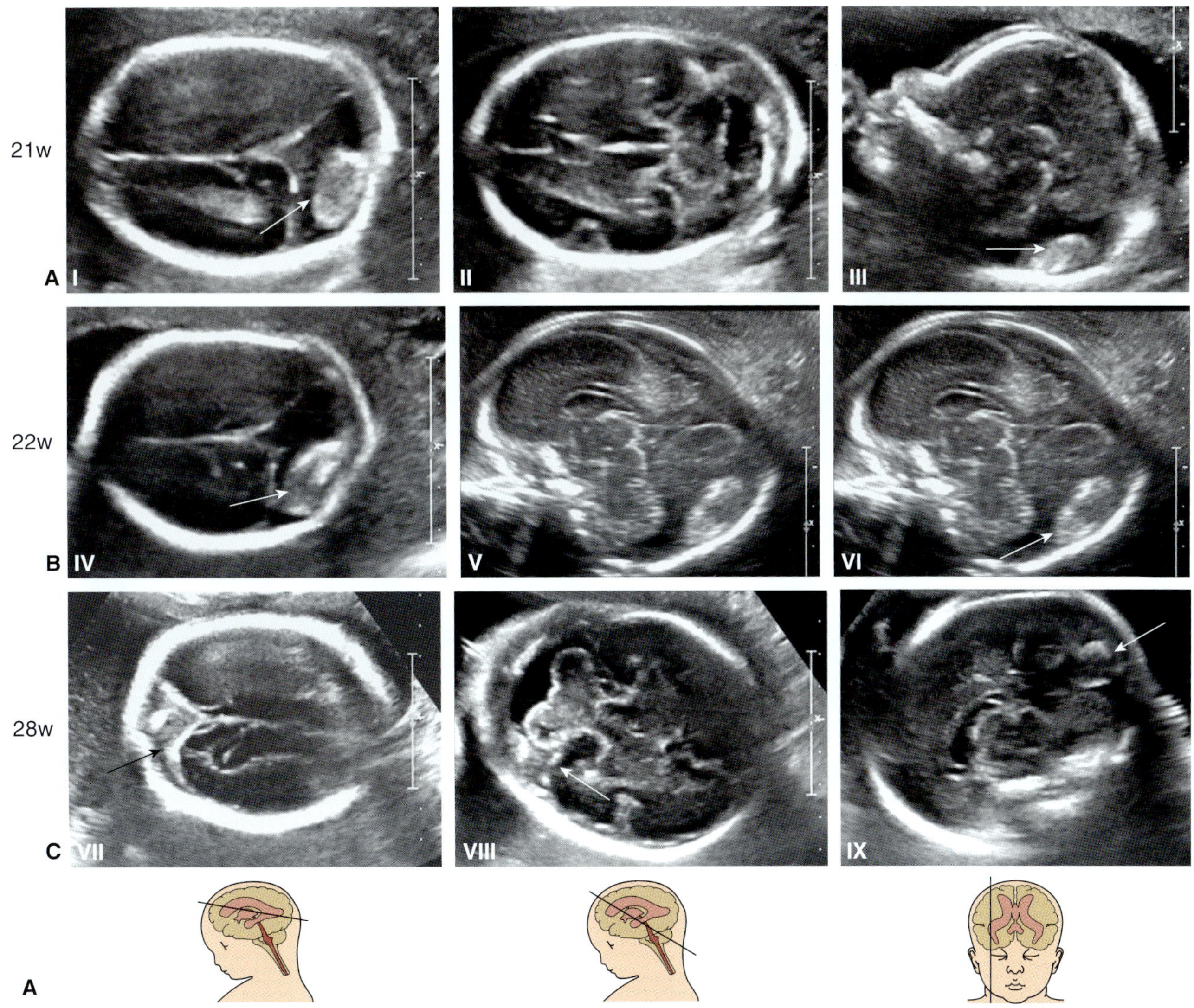


**Figure 10–19** **(A)** Thrombosis of the lateral sinus in a patient detected at 21 postmenstrual weeks during an otherwise uneventful pregnancy. The posterior hyperechogenic, oval mass is just above the cerebellum and appears to be supratentorial, with absence of signals on color Doppler imaging. There was no ventriculomegaly, and the brain appeared otherwise normal.The mass was surrounded by a sonolucent area. Clinically, there were no signs of fetal anemia. Chromosomal abnormalities, infections, and thrombophilic disorders were ruled out. (Courtesy of Maria Del Rio, Barcelona, MD, Spain.) Axial **(A)** **(I, II)** and parasagittal **(III)** sections at 21 postmenstrual weeks demonstrating the hyperechoic clot (*arrows*). **(B)** **(IV–VI)** Images obtained through the same planes at 22 weeks showing almost no changes. **(C)** **(VII–IX)** Follow-up images at 28 postmenstrual weeks using the previous planes for comparison. One can hardly see the lesion (*arrows*), and it looks as if the clot is decreasing in size. The rest of the anatomy appears to be normal.

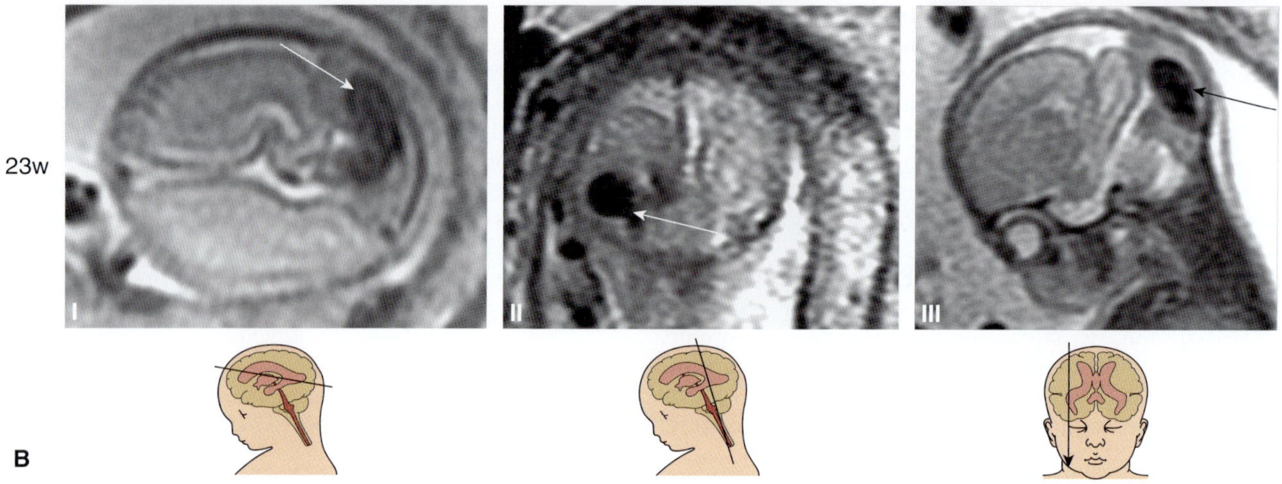


**Figure 10–19** *(continued)* **(B)** MRI images of the patient with thrombosis of the lateral sinus at 23 postmenstrual weeks. **(I)** Axial plane through the thrombus (*arrow*). **(II)** Posterior coronal plane. **(III)** Parasagittal plane across the thrombus (*arrow*). (Courtesy of Caterina Montull, Barcelona, MD, Spain.)

A choroid plexus papilloma is a rare tumor of the choroid plexus that may mimic a blood clot; however, the mass is well defined within the lateral ventricle and has blood flow when using color Doppler. Additionally, the associated hydrocephaly may be progressive.

## Prognosis

In the neonate, the neurodevelopmental outcome is related to the severity of the hemorrhage and the presence of intraparenchymal hemorrhagic infarcts. Papile et al[92] classified

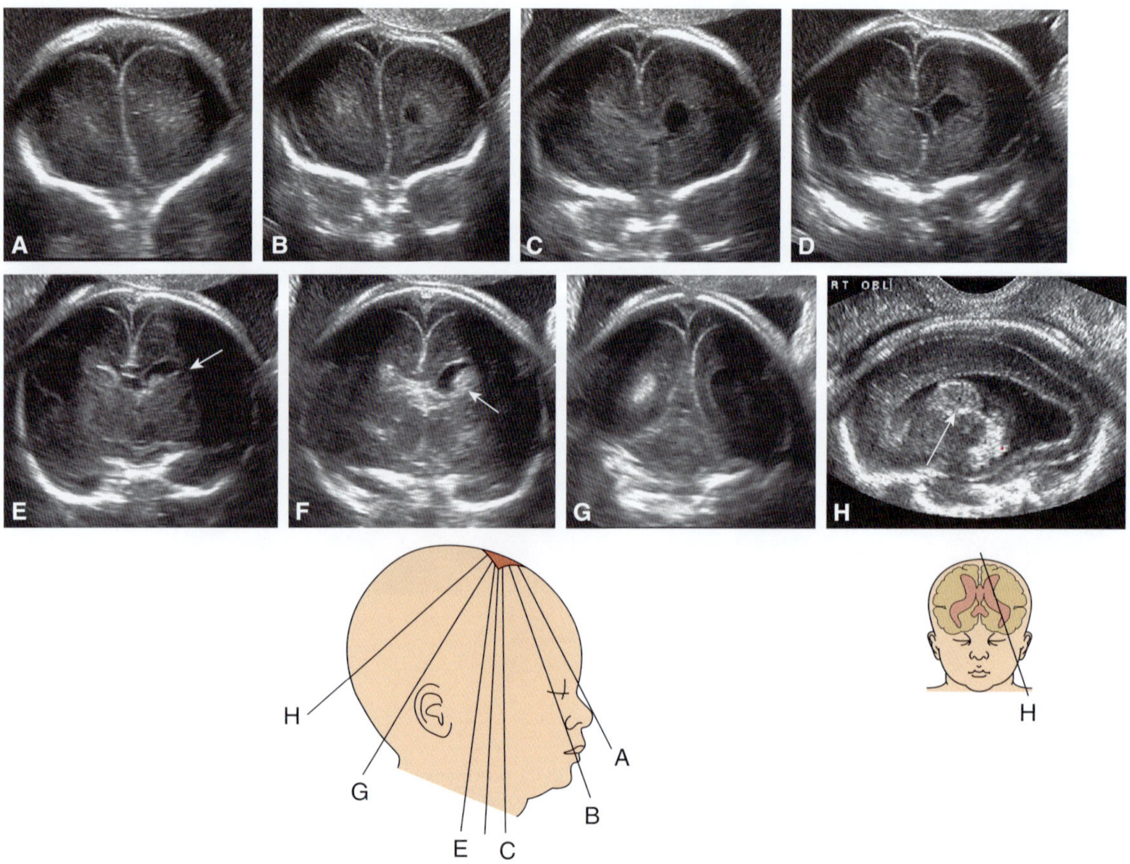


**Figure 10–20.** Serial coronal **(A –G)** and parasagittal or oblique **(H)** sections of a grade I intraventricular hemorrhage. (The short arrows point to the mild dilation of the left lateral ventricle. The long arrow points to the hemorrhage.)

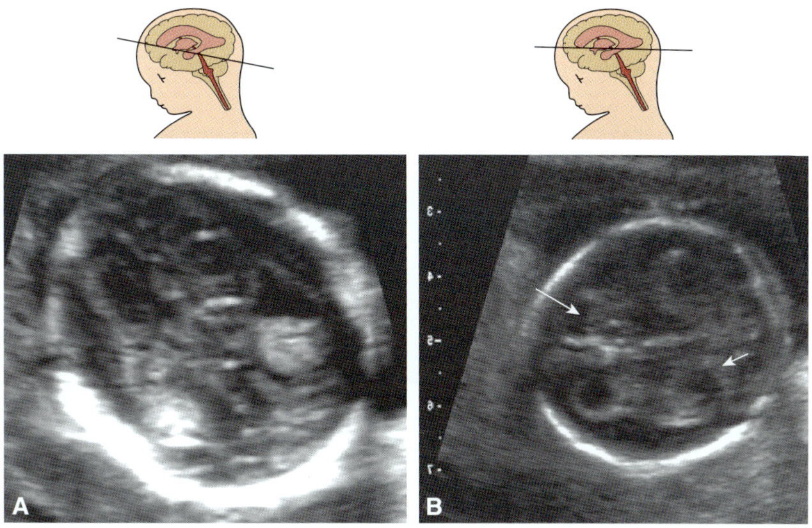


**Figure 10–21.** Intracranial hemorrhage at 16 postmenstrual weeks. **(A), (B)** The initial sonographic appearance of the "fresh" blood clots is that of homogeneous hyperechoic areas (*large arrow*), which are distinct from the choroid plexus (*small arrow*). The lateral ventricles show a castlike pattern that is brightly echogenic, most likely as the result of blood.

the intracranial hemorrhage of the neonate using four grades. Grade I is a GMH or a hemorrhage that is confined to the subependymal area of the brain. Grade II is an IVH, but there is no associated hydrocephaly. Grade III is an IVH with ventricular dilation. Grade IV is an IVH with parenchymal hemorrhage and hydrocephaly. The intraparenchymal lesions are the result of periventricular hemorrhagic infarction.[76] This scoring system has proven to be a useful tool in prognosticating outcomes in neonates; however, in fetuses, it has not been fully validated. The outcome of infants with grade I or II IVH is similar to other premature babies without a hemorrhage. However, neonates with grade III or IV have significantly long-term adverse neurodevelopmental outcomes. For neonates with grade III, the percentage of those with adverse outcomes approaches 35%; for those neonates with grade IV, it can be as high as 90%.[93]

The number of cases of documented fetal intracranial hemorrhage is limited, although with the increased use of prenatal sonography and MRI, this number is growing. Consequently, outcome data of fetal hemorrhage are slowly emerging. Achiron et al[57] reported on five cases of intracranial hemorrhage diagnosed in utero. Of the five affected fetuses, one was stillborn, and two died after birth. Two were reported to be developing normally at 12 and 18 months of life. Vergani et al[68] reported on the outcome of six fetuses with intracranial hemorrhage, three of whom had parenchymal involvement. Two had normal development at 30 months, one had mild left hemiparesis,

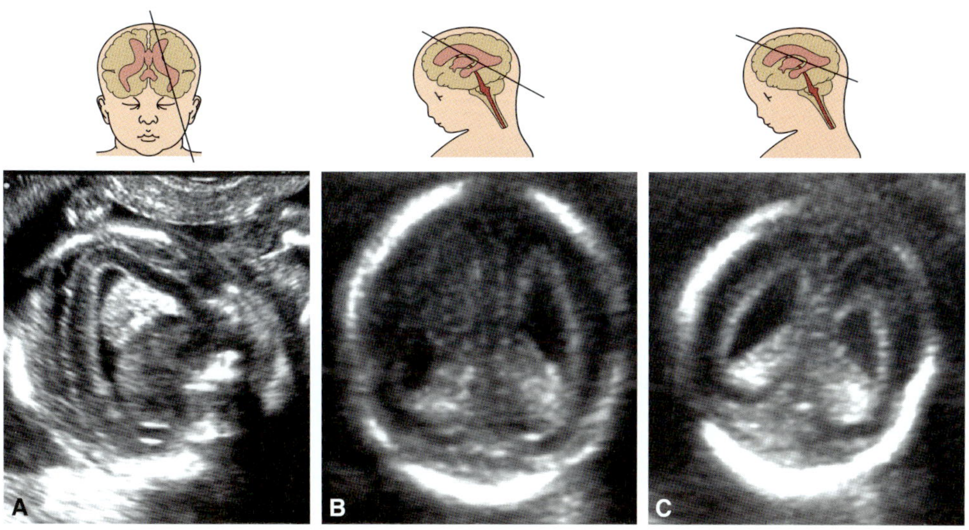


**Figure 10–22.** Intraventricular hemorrhage grade II at 17 postmenstrual weeks (same patient as in Figures 10–20, 10–21, and 10–23). **(A)** Parasagittal section. **(B, C)** Coronal sections. The features of the pathology are the heterogeneous choroid plexus, low-level echoic fluid in the ventricles, and a hyperechoic "coating" of the ventricular walls, in addition to various levels of ventriculomegaly.

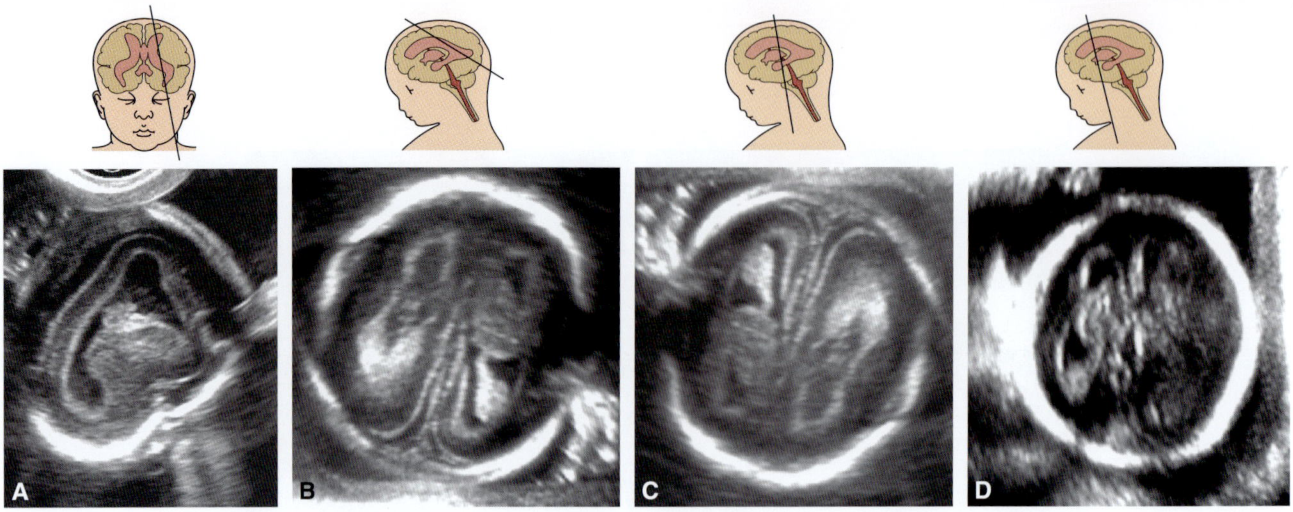

**Figure 10–23.** Intraventricular hemorrhage grade II at 23 postmenstrual weeks (same patient as in Figures 10–20 to 10–22). **(A)** Parasagittal section. **(B–D)** Axial section. The features of the pathology are the heterogeneous choroid plexus, low-level echoic fluid in the ventricles, and a hyperechoic "coating" of the ventricular walls, in addition to various levels of ventriculomegaly.

and two had adverse neurodevelopmental outcomes. There was one intrauterine fetal death. In this study, those fetuses with parenchymal involvement had the worst prognosis. Morioka et al[74] reported on five cases of fetal GMH-IVH. Two had a good outcome, one had a borderline outcome, and two had significant adverse neurologic outcomes (psychomotor and mental delays). The two fetuses with the worst neurologic outcomes had severe parenchymal damage (encephalomalacia and periventricular leukomalacia). Ghi et al[61] reported on their own experience, as well as a review of the literature. They found that intracranial hemorrhage diagnosed in utero is associated with a poor outcome. Approximately 40% of the fetuses dying in utero or within the first weeks of life and among the survivors, less than half were neurologically and developmentally normal. In their study, neonates with grade III or IV hemorrhages exhibited higher mortality (44%) and worse neurodevelopmental outcomes, with only 41% considered normal. However, in their study, data on Grades I and II were limited, with mortality reported as 7.1%; the study did not provide adequate prognostic data on this group of fetuses.[61] Nevertheless, the authors noted that resolution of the hemorrhage is associated with good outcomes, and progression of the hematoma is associated with worse outcomes. In neonates and fetuses, the end result of intraparenchymal hemorrhage/infarct is porencephaly. The size of the original hemorrhage correlates with the size of the porencephalic cyst. It must be pointed out that thus far the capability of US instrumentation has only allowed the detection of very severe intracranial hemorrhage. It is likely that technological improvements and the widespread use of high-resolution vaginal probes will allow detection of less severe lesions, which have a better outcome.

### Obstetric Management

A detailed anatomical survey to evaluate for associated anomalies is indicated. Blood work to rule out infectious etiology, maternal platelet count, maternal antiplatelet antibodies (alloimmunity), blood type and screen (isoimmunity), and a thrombophilia workup should be considered. Genetic counseling and amniocentesis for karyotype analysis could aid in further diagnosis. In addition, a good history should be taken that includes drug usage and recent trauma. Consultations with neonatology, pediatric neurology, pediatric neurosurgery, and maternal-fetal medicine should be included. MRI may be helpful in further evaluating the extent of the hemorrhage and to search for parenchymal involvement. Given the poor prognosis associated with large fetal intracranial hemorrhage, termination of pregnancy should be offered to the patient. At present, there are no established guidelines regarding the delivery route for fetuses with an intracranial hemorrhage. However, in cases in which the lesions are severe and are associated with a poor neonatal outcome, conservative management may be offered. There are no available data regarding the use of cesarean section in cases with less severe hemorrhage.[61]

## CEREBELLAR HEMORRHAGE

### Definition

Intracranial hemorrhage involving the cerebellum and posterior fossa

### Synonyms

None

### Incidence

The incidence of cerebellar hemorrhage in the fetus is unknown; however, prenatal diagnosis has been reported.[80,94–96] Limperopoulos and colleagues[97] reported overall incidence of up to 3% in preterm infants, with

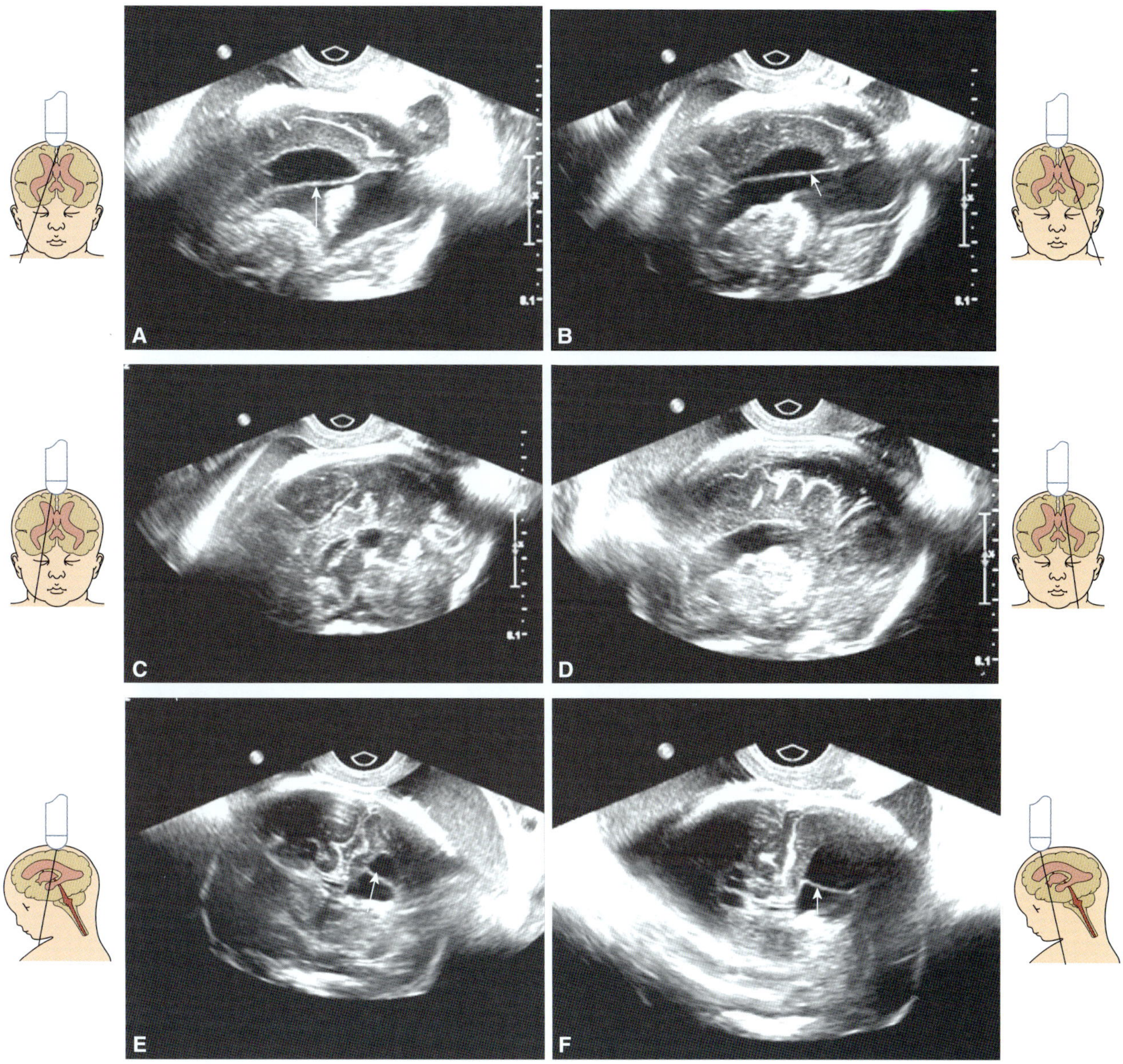

**Figure 10–24.** Intraventricular hemorrhage grade II US images. Note the adhesions in the lateral ventricle (*arrows*). **(A–D)** Sagittal sections. **(E), (F)** Coronal sections.

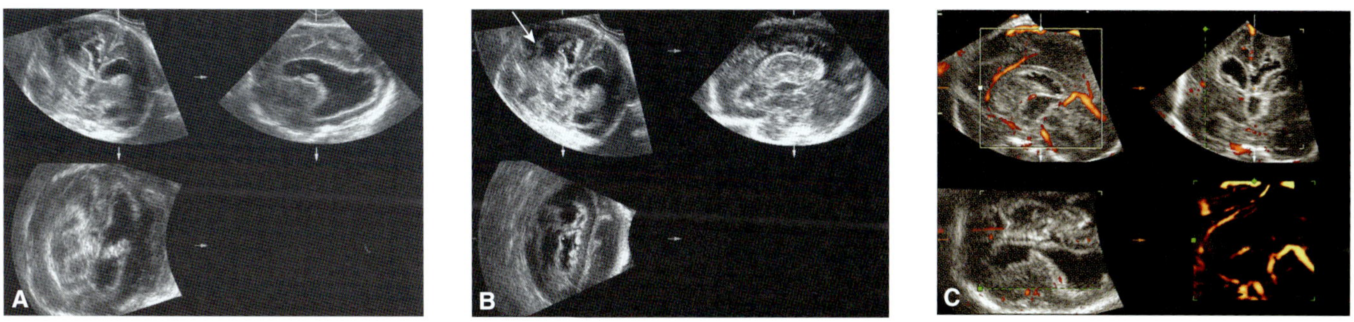

**Figure 10–25** 3D orthogonal images of grade IV intraventricular hemorrhage showing parenchymal involvement at 29 postmenstrual weeks. In **(A),** the head is tilted to the right to allow visualization of the entire ventricle in the oblique section (*upper right*). The axial section is the reconstructed plane. Note the dilation of the lateral ventricles, as well as the brightly echogenic periventricular area. **(B)** In the coronal section (*upper left*) (*lower left*), involvement of the parenchyma is demonstrated (*arrow*). **(C)** Power Doppler imaging of the brain. Doppler allows easy evaluation of the pericallosal artery in this fetus with a grade IV intracranial hemorrhage. Note that the areas of intracranial bleeding have no flow.

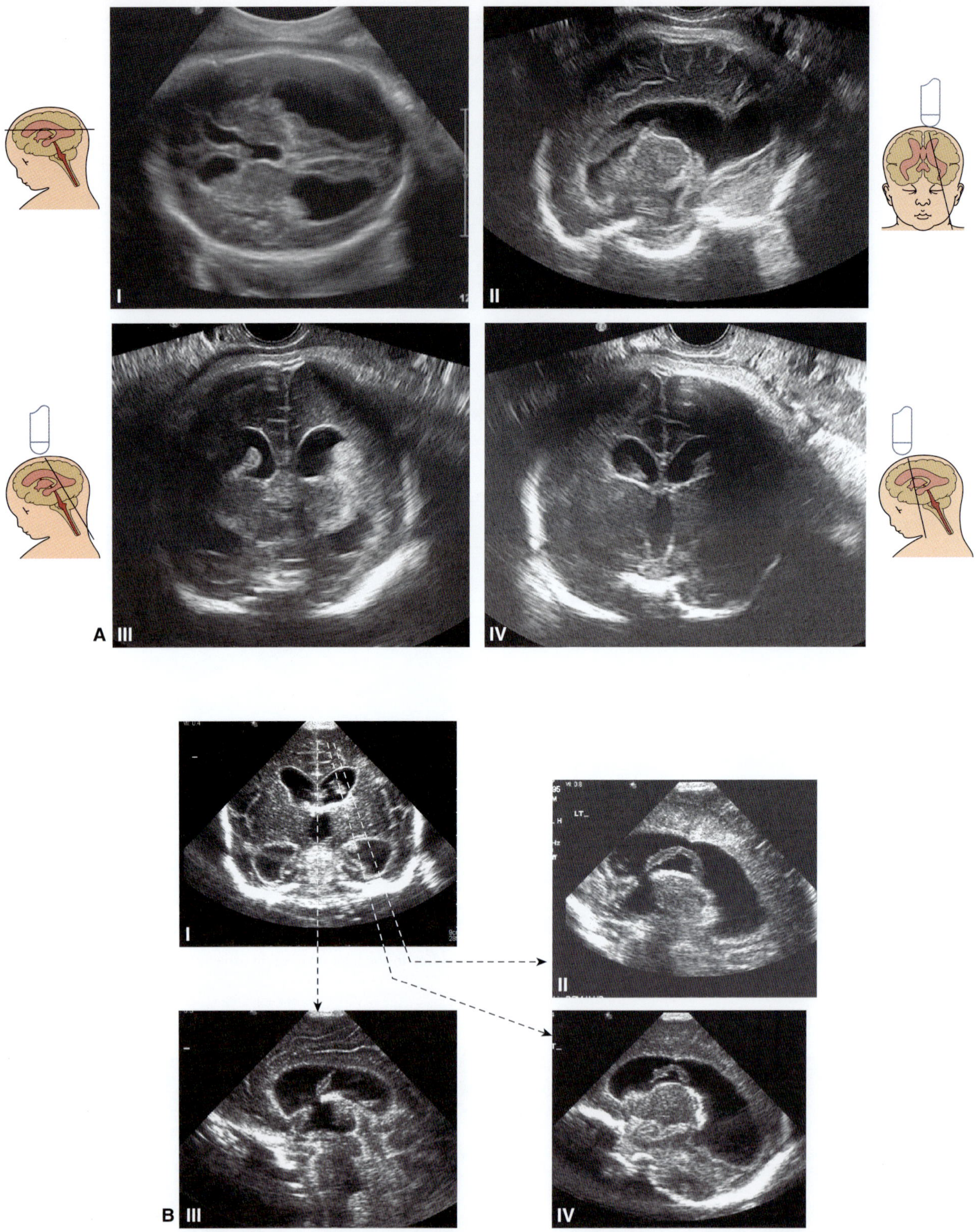


**Figure 10–26** **(A)** Intracranial hemorrhage diagnosed at 35 postmenstrual weeks, 5 days. Note the ventriculomegaly, the heterogeneous fluid in the lateral ventricles, and the hyperechoic coating of the ventricular walls and choroids. Diagnosis: intraventricular hemorrhage grade III. Axial **(I)**, parasagittal **(II)**, coronal **(III, IV)** planes. **(B)** US of the neonate **(I)** coronal section demonstrating the planes at which **(II, III)** and **(IV)** were obtained. The lateral ventricles are dilated, consistent with the posthemorrhagic hydrocephaly.

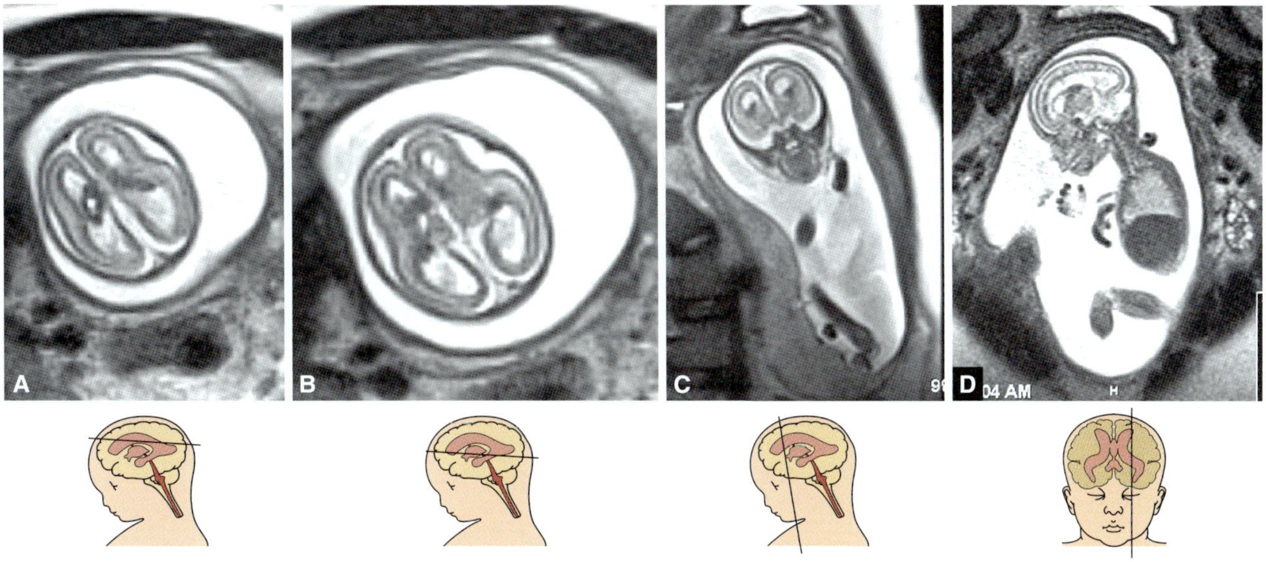


**Figure 10–27.** T2-weighted fetal MRI at 19 postmenstrual weeks depicting grade II intraventricular hemorrhage. **(A, B)** Axial sections. **(C)** Coronal section. **(D)** Sagittal section.

60% of all cerebellar hemorrhages occurring in infants weighing <750 g. Cerebellar hemorrhages are reported in up to 21% of cases at autopsy.[98]

## Pathogenesis

The exact pathogenesis of cerebellar hemorrhage is unknown.

## Etiology

Cerebellar hemorrhages are likely multifactorial in origin, including circulatory events of prematurity, presence of local pathology (eg, hemangiomas), trauma related to delivery, or other intracranial pathology (eg, IVH).

## Associated Anomalies

Associated anomalies in the reported cases include ventriculomegaly and frank hydrocephaly.

## Risk of Recurrence

Unknown

## Sonographic Diagnosis

The sonographic appearance is that of a highly echogenic area in the cerebellum. Cerebellar/vermis hypoplasia could be an associated finding and is appreciated in the typical axial view of the cerebellum and the midsagittal view of

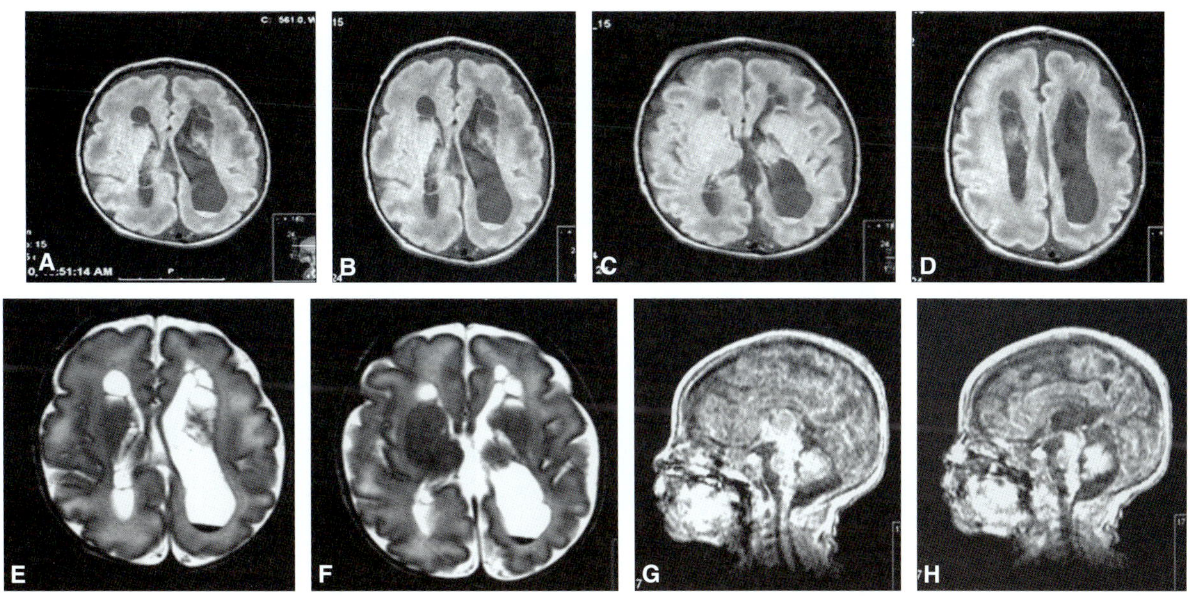


**Figure 10–28.** MRI of intraventricular hemorrhage grade II of the newborn (same case as in Figures 10–20, 10–21, 10–22, and 10–26). Showing areas of bleeding as well as some intracranial adhesions consistent with the fetal intracranial hemorrhage. **(A–F)** Axial sections. **(G, H)** Sagittal sections.

the vermis. In fetuses as in neonates, blood appears highly echogenic, and the echogenicity is comparable to that of the normal choroid plexus.

### Differential Diagnosis

Cerebellar tumor

### Prognosis

The prognosis for the fetus with a significant cerebellar hemorrhage is considered dismal. In the case reported by Jennette et al,[80] the infant died at age 46 hours despite supportive treatment, and in the case reported by Hadi et al,[94] the infant died at age 18 hours. On the other hand, Ghi and colleagues[61] reviewed a case of cerebellar hemorrhage causing progressive cerebellar hypoplasia with no apparent neurologic or clinical compromise in follow-up at 1 year of age.

### Obstetric Management

A detailed anatomical survey, as well as a targeted brain scan, is suggested. Consultations with neonatology, pediatric neurology, pediatric neurosurgery, and maternal-fetal medicine should be included. MRI may be helpful in further evaluating the extent of the hemorrhage. Given the poor prognosis associated with cerebellar hemorrhage, termination of pregnancy should be offered to the patient. At present, there are no established guidelines regarding the delivery route for fetuses with a cerebellar hemorrhage. However, in cases in which the lesions are severe and are associated with a poor neonatal outcome, conservative management may be offered.

## SUBDURAL HEMORRHAGE

### Definition

Intracranial bleeding confined to the subdural space.

### Synonyms

None

### Incidence

In fetuses, a subdural hemorrhage is a rare condition with an unknown incidence, although improvement in imaging has helped prenatal diagnosis by sonography. In preterm neonates, the incidence of subdural hemorrhage

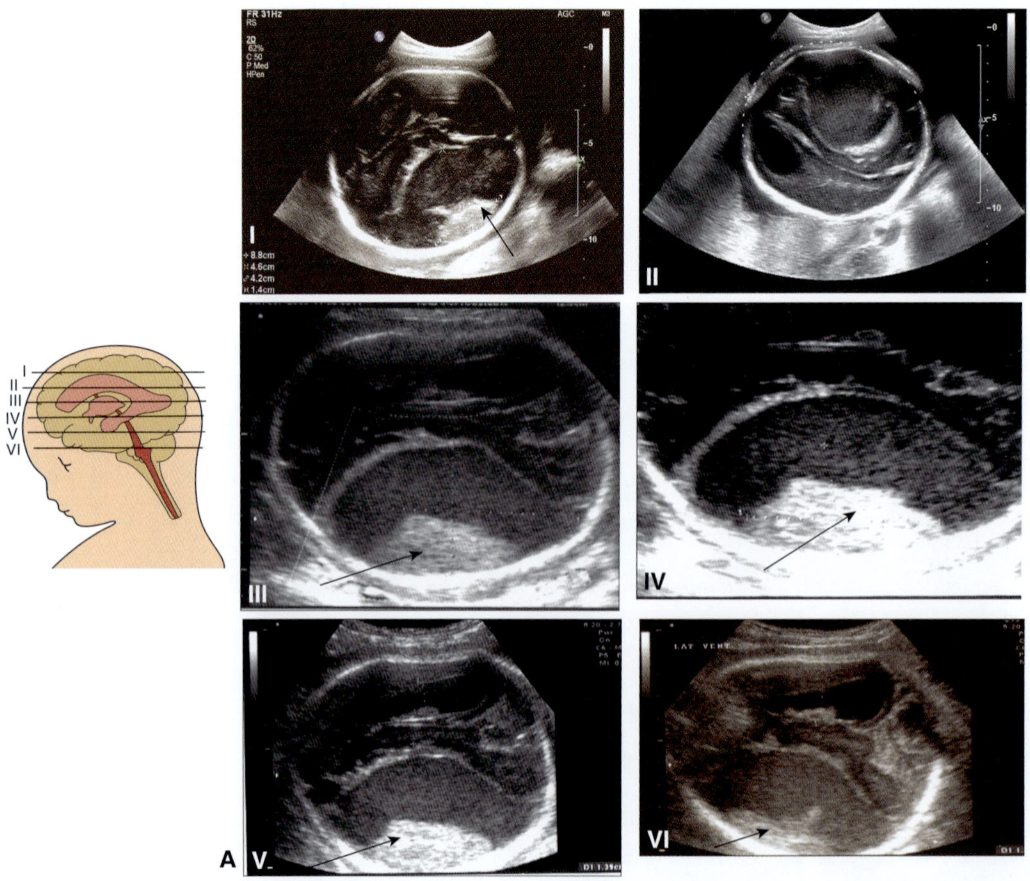


**Figure 10–29.** Fetal subdural hematoma. **(A)** Serial axial sections of a subdural hematoma from top **(I)** toward the base of the skull. The far hemisphere is severely compressed and displaced toward the midline, which is shifted. The arrows point to the clot (**III**, cerebellum). The hematoma is 8.8 × 4.6 cm. The clot is 4.2 × 1.4 cm.

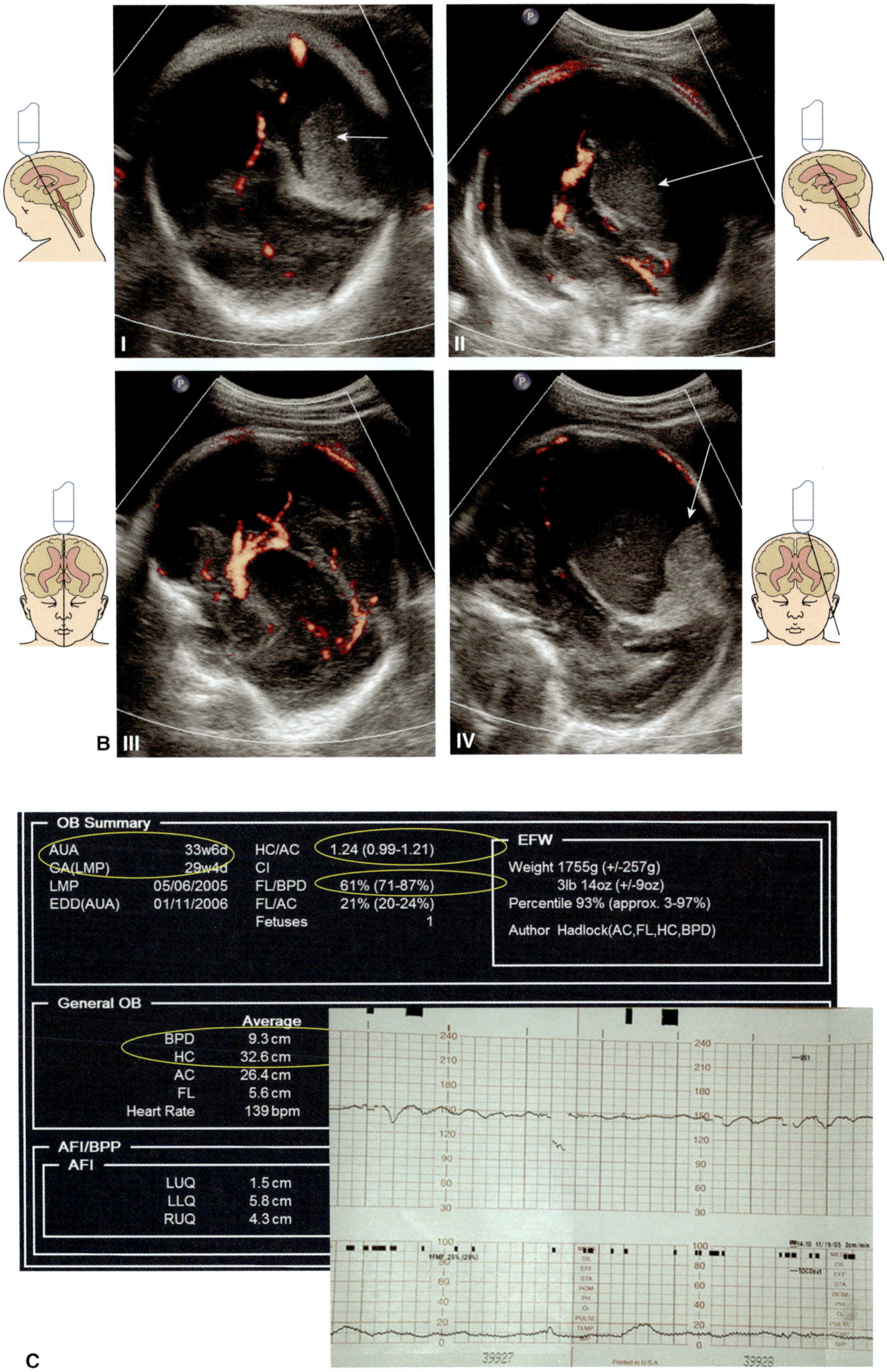


**Figure 10–29.** *(continued)* **(B)** Power Doppler imaging of **I** left-sided temporoparietal subdural hematoma: (**I** and **II**) coronal sections (**III**) and (**IV**) are median and left parasagittal, respectively. The arrow points to the hematoma and the hyperechoic clot distorting the course of the vessels. **(C)** Biometry of the fetus. Note the enlarged fetal head measurements. Inlay: Electronic monitoring demonstrates decreased short-term fetal heart rate variability and a sinusoidal pattern.

ranges from 3% to 18%. Most of these subdural hematomas in neonates are related to trauma during the perinatal period.[99]

### Etiology

Fetal subdural hematomas have been reported to occur as a result of trauma (the result of a motor vehicle accident or abdominal trauma),[70,100] maternal drug ingestion (warfarin),[101] maternal medical complication of pregnancy (pancreatitis), acoagulation factor deficiency (factor X),[102] or spontaneous subdural hemorrhage with unknown etiology.[103–105]

### Pathogenesis

The subdural hematoma is venous in nature, either secondary to shearing forces along the subdural perforating venous channels or a predisposing coagulopathic factor.

### Associated Anomalies

Other sonographic findings described with fetal subdural hematoma are hydrocephaly, polyhydramnios, and fetal hydrops.

### Risk of Recurrence

The recurrence risk for spontaneous subdural hematoma is unknown. The risk of fetal subdural bleeding secondary to maternal predisposing factor could be modifiable depending on the etiology.

### Sonographic Diagnosis

The sonographic appearance is that of extracerebral fluid collection with compression of the cortical surfaces (Figure 10–29). Ben-Chetrit et al[99] performed Doppler velocimetry studies on a patient with a fetal subdural hematoma and found that the MCA had a high resistance pattern with reverse diastolic flow. In utero subdural hematomas are usually located over the cerebral hemisphere rather than infratentorially.[103]

### Differential Diagnosis

There are reports of subarachnoid[106] and extradural fetal hemorrhages,[107] which would warrant differentiation. A large subdural hematoma could be mistaken for significant intracranial or intraventricular bleeding.[103]

### Prognosis

The outcomes for neonates with an in utero diagnosis of subdural hematoma have ranged from in utero fetal death to survival with no gross neurodevelopmental abnormalities.[99,104,108–110] The prognosis of subdural hemorrhage also depends on the location and extent of the subdural hemorrhage. A large posterior fossa hemorrhage could cause brainstem compression and result in in utero shock and death. There is also a report of spontaneous resolution of prenatally diagnosed bilateral subdural hematoma.[111]

### Obstetric Management

A detailed neurosonogram and anatomical survey to evaluate other anomalies are indicated. Antenatal evaluation to rule out maternal coagulopathy is suggested. Consultations with neonatology, pediatric neurology, pediatric neurosurgery, and maternal-fetal medicine should be included. MRI may be helpful in further evaluating the extent of the hemorrhage. Given the poor prognosis associated with subdural hemorrhage, termination of pregnancy should be offered to the patient. At present, there are no established guidelines regarding the delivery route for fetuses with a subdural hemorrhage. However, in cases in which the lesions are severe and are associated with a poor neonatal outcome, conservative management may be offered. In cases in which the pregnancy will be continued, MRI, as well as serial follow-up US evaluation, could help in monitoring the size of the hematoma.

## REFERENCES

1. Govaert P. Prenatal stroke. *Semin Fetal Neonatal Med.* 2009;14:250–266.
2. Govaert P, Ramenghi L, Taal R, de Vries L, Deveber G. Diagnosis of perinatal stroke I: Definitions, differential diagnosis and registration. *Acta Paediatr.* 2009;98:1556–1567.
3. Volpe JJ. *Neurology of the Newborn.* Philadelphia: Saunders/Elsevier; 2008.
4. Cheong JL, Cowan FM. Neonatal arterial ischaemic stroke: Obstetric issues. *Semin Fetal Neonatal Med.* 2009;14:267–271.
5. Raju TN, Nelson KB, Ferriero D, Lynch JK. Ischemic perinatal stroke: Summary of a workshop sponsored by the National Institute of Child Health and Human Development and the National Institute of Neurological Disorders and Stroke. *Pediatrics.* 2007;120:609–616.
6. Benders MJ, Groenendaal F, de Vries LS. Preterm arterial ischemic stroke. *Semin Fetal Neonatal Med.* 2009;14:272–277.
7. Simchen MJ, Goldstein G, Lubetsky A, Strauss T, Schiff E, Kenet G. Factor V Leiden and antiphospholipid antibodies in either mothers or infants increase the risk for perinatal arterial ischemic stroke. *Stroke.* 2009;40:65–70.
8. Gul A, Gungorduk K, Yildirim G, Gedikbasi A, Ceylan Y. Prenatal diagnosis of porencephaly secondary to maternal carbon monoxide poisoning. *Arch Gynecol Obstet.* 2009;279:697–700.
9. Simonazzi G, Pilu G, Palareti G, Bernardi B, Rizzo N. Foetal cerebral hemispheric atrophy and porencephaly after intrauterine exposure to maternal warfarin for mechanical prosthetic heart valve. *Prenat Diagn.* 2008;28:157–159.
10. Eller KM, Kuller JA. Porencephaly secondary to fetal trauma during amniocentesis. *Obstet Gynecol.* 1995;85:865–867.
11. Sensi A, Cerruti S, Calzolari E, Vesce F. Familial porencephaly. *Clin Genet.* 1990;38:396–397.
12. Shastri NJ, Bharani SA, Modi UJ, Trivedi C. Familial porencephaly. *Indian J Pediatr.* 1993;60:459–463.
13. Vilain C, Van Regemorter N, Verloes A, David P, Van Bogaert P. Neuroimaging fails to identify asymptomatic carriers of familial porencephaly. *Am J Med Genet.* 2002;112:198–202.
14. Zonana J, Adornato BT, Glass ST, Webb MJ. Familial porencephaly and congenital hemiplegia. *J Pediatr.* 1986;109:671–674.
15. Lynch JK, Han CJ, Nee LE, Nelson KB. Prothrombotic factors in children with stroke or porencephaly. *Pediatrics.* 2005;116:447–453.
16. Lynch JK. Epidemiology and classification of perinatal stroke. *Semin Fetal Neonatal Med.* 2009;14:245–249.
17. Alamowitch S, Plaisier E, Favrole P, et al. Cerebrovascular disease related to COL4A1 mutations in HANAC syndrome. *Neurology.* 2009;73:1873–1882.
18. Filly R. Ultrasound evaluation of the fetal neural axis. In: Callen P, ed. *Ultrasonography in Obstetrics and Gynecology.* Philadelphia: W.B. Saunders; 1994;189–234.

19. Sonographic examination of the fetal central nervous system: Guidelines for performing the basic examination and the fetal neurosonogram. *Ultrasound Obstet Gynecol.* 2007;29:109–116.
20. Kirton A, deVeber G. Advances in perinatal ischemic stroke. *Pediatr Neurol.* 2009;40:205–214.
21. Bussel J. Diagnosis and management of the fetus and neonate with alloimmune thrombocytopenia. *J Thromb Haemost.* 2009;7(Suppl 1): 253–257.
22. Ward MJ, Pauliny J, Lipper EG, Bussel JB. Long-term effects of fetal and neonatal alloimmune thrombocytopenia and its antenatal treatment on the medical and developmental outcomes of affected children. *Am J Perinatol.* 2006;23:487–492.
23. Berkowitz RL, Bussel JB, McFarland JG. Alloimmune thrombocytopenia: State of the art 2006. *Am J Obstet Gynecol.* 2006;195: 907–913.
24. Hehr U, Pineda-Alvarez DE, Uyanik G, et al. Heterozygous mutations in SIX3 and SHH are associated with schizencephaly and further expand the clinical spectrum of holoprosencephaly. *Hum Genet.* 2010;127:555–561.
25. Yakovlev PI, Wadsworth, RC Schizencephalies: A study of the congenital clefts in the cerebral mantle. 1. Clefts with fused lips. *J Neuropath Exp Neurol.* 1946:116–130.
26. Szabo N, Gyurgyinka G, Kobor J, Bereg E, Turi S, Sztriha L. Epidemiology and clinical spectrum of schizencephaly in South-Eastern Hungary. *J Child Neurol.* 2010;25(11):1335–1339.
27. Curry CJ, Lammer EJ, Nelson V, Shaw GM. Schizencephaly: Heterogeneous etiologies in a population of 4 million California births. *Am J Med Genet A.* 2005;137:181–189.
28. Sener RN. Schizencephaly and congenital cytomegalovirus infection. *J Neuroradiol.* 1998;25:151–152.
29. Huang WM, Monteagudo A, Bennett GL, Fowkes ME, Timor-Tritsch IE. Schizencephaly in a dysgenetic fetal brain: Prenatal sonographic, magnetic resonance imaging, and postmortem correlation. *J Ultrasound Med.* 2006;25:551–554.
30. Oh KY, Kennedy AM, Frias AE, Jr., Byrne JL. Fetal schizencephaly: Pre- and postnatal imaging with a review of the clinical manifestations. *Radiographics.* 2005;25:647–657.
31. Martin Fernandez-Mayoralas D, Fernandez-Jaen A, Jimenez-de-la-Pena M, Recio-Rodriguez M, Munoz-Jareno N, Arroyo-Gonzalez R. Schizencephaly: Pre- and postnatal magnetic resonance imaging. *J Child Neurol.*
32. Goez H, Zelnik N. Schizencephaly in infants with thrombophilia. *J Child Neurol.* 2009;24:421–424.
33. Laurichesse-Delmas H, Beaufrere AM, Martin A, Kaemmerlen AG, Dechelotte P, Lemery D. First-trimester features of Fowler syndrome (hydrocephaly-hydranencephaly proliferative vasculopathy). *Ultrasound Obstet Gynecol.* 2002;20:612–625.
34. Lam YH, Tang MH. Serial sonographic features of a fetus with hydranencephaly from 11 weeks to term. *Ultrasound Obstet Gynecol.* 2000;16:77–79.
35. McAbee GN, Chan A, Erde EL. Prolonged survival with hydranencephaly: Report of two patients and literature review. *Pediatr Neurol.* 2000;23:80–84.
36. Ozduman K, Pober BR, Barnes P, et al. Fetal stroke. *Pediatr Neurol.* 2004;30:151–162.
37. Edmondson SR, Hallak M, Carpenter RJ, Jr., Cotton DB. Evolution of hydranencephaly following intracerebral hemorrhage. *Obstet Gynecol.* 1992;79:870–871.
38. Greene MF, Benacerraf B, Crawford JM. Hydranencephaly: US appearance during in utero evolution. *Radiology.* 1985;156: 779–780.
39. Belfar HL, Kuller JA, Hill LM, Kislak S. Evolving fetal hydranencephaly mimicking intracranial neoplasm. *J Ultrasound Med.* 1991; 10:231–233.
40. Bae JS, Jang MU, Park SS. Prolonged survival to adulthood of an individual with hydranencephaly. *Clin Neurol Neurosurg.* 2008;110: 307–309.
41. Saracco P, Parodi E, Fabris C, Cecinati V, Molinari AC, Giordano P. Management and investigation of neonatal thromboembolic events: Genetic and acquired risk factors. *Thromb Res.* 2009;123:805–809.
42. deVeber G, Andrew M, Adams C, et al. Cerebral sinovenous thrombosis in children. *N Engl J Med.* 2001;345:417–423.
43. Carletti A, Colleoni GG, Perolo A, et al. Prenatal diagnosis of cerebral lesions acquired in utero and with a late appearance. *Prenat Diagn.* 2009;29:389–395.
44. Laurichesse Delmas H, Winer N, Gallot D, et al. Prenatal diagnosis of thrombosis of the dural sinuses: Report of six cases, review of the literature and suggested management. *Ultrasound Obstet Gynecol.* 2008;32:188–198.
45. Spampinato MV, Hardin V, Davis M, Chang E, Rumboldt Z. Thrombosed fetal dural sinus malformation diagnosed with magnetic resonance imaging. *Obstet Gynecol.* 2008;111:569–572.
46. McInnes M, Fong K, Grin A, et al. Malformations of the fetal dural sinuses. *Can J Neurol Sci.* 2009;36:72–77.
47. Grange G, LeTohic A, Merzoug V, Adamsbaum C. Prenatal demonstration of afferent vessels and progressive thrombosis in a torcular malformation. *Prenat Diagn.* 2007;27:670–673.
48. Schwartz N, Monteagudo A, Bornstein E, Timor-Tritsch IE, Zagzag D, Kudla M. Thrombosis of an ectatic torcular herophili: Anatomic localization using fetal neurosonography. *J Ultrasound Med.* 2008; 27:989–991.
49. Barbosa MG, Mahadevan J, Weon YC, et al. Dural sinus malformations (DSM) with giant lakes, in neonates and infants: Review of 30 consecutive cases. *Interven Neuroradiol.* 2003:407–424.
50. Merzoug V, Flunker S, Drissi C, et al. Dural sinus malformation (DSM) in fetuses: Diagnostic value of prenatal MRI and follow-up. *Eur Radiol.* 2008;18:692–699.
51. Grigoriadis S, Cohen JE, Gomori JM. Prenatal thrombosis of torcular herophili with spontaneous resolution and normal outcome. *J Neuroimaging.* 2008;18:177–179.
52. Rossi A, DeBiasio P, Scarso E, et al. Prenatal MR imaging of dural sinus malformation: A case report. *Prenat Diagn.* 2006;26:11–16.
53. Komiyama M, Ishiguro T, Kitano S, Sakamoto H, Nakamura H. Serial antenatal sonographic observation of cerebral dural sinus malformation. *AJNR Am J Neuroradiol.* 2004;25:1446–1448.
54. Visentin A, Falco P, Pilu G, et al. Prenatal diagnosis of thrombosis of the dural sinuses with real-time and color Doppler ultrasound. *Ultrasound Obstet Gynecol.* 2001;17:322–325.
55. Lasjaunias P, Magufis G, Goulao A, Suthipongchai S, Rodesch R, Alvarez H. Anatomoclinical aspects of dural arteriovenous shunts in children: Review of 29 cases. *Interven Neuroradiol.* 1996:179–191.
56. Jackson JC, Blumhagen JD. Congenital hydrocephalus due to prenatal intracranial hemorrhage. *Pediatrics.* 1983;72:344–346.
57. Achiron R, Pinchas OH, Reichman B, et al. Fetal intracranial haemorrhage: Clinical significance of in utero ultrasonographic diagnosis. *Br J Obstet Gynaecol.* 1993;100:995–959.
58. Canapicchi R, Cioni G, Strigini FA, Abbruzzese A, Bartalena L, Lencioni G. Prenatal diagnosis of periventricular hemorrhage by fetal brain magnetic resonance imaging. *Childs Nerv Syst.* 1998;14: 689–692.
59. Elchalal U, Yagel S, Gomori JM, et al. Fetal intracranial hemorrhage (fetal stroke): Does grade matter? *Ultrasound Obstet Gynecol.* 2005;26:233–343.
60. Folkerth RD, McLaughlin ME, Levine D. Organizing posterior fossa hematomas simulating developmental cysts on prenatal imaging: Report of 3 cases. *J Ultrasound Med.* 2001;20:1233–1240.
61. Ghi T, Simonazzi G, Perolo A, et al. Outcome of antenatally diagnosed intracranial hemorrhage: Case series and review of the literature. *Ultrasound Obstet Gynecol.* 2003;22:121–130.
62. Guerriero S, Ajossa S, Mais V, et al. Color Doppler energy imaging in the diagnosis of fetal intracranial hemorrhage in the second trimester. *Ultrasound Obstet Gynecol.* 1997;10:205–208.
63. McGahan JP, Haesslein HC, Meyers M, Ford KB. Sonographic recognition of in utero intraventricular hemorrhage. *AJR Am J Roentgenol.* 1984;142:171–173.
64. Meagher SE, Walker SP, Choong S. Mid-trimester fetal subdural hemorrhage: Prenatal diagnosis. *Ultrasound Obstet Gynecol.* 2002;20:296–298.
65. Portman MA, Brouillette RT. Fatal intracranial hemorrhage complicating amniocentesis. *Am J Obstet Gynecol.* 1982;144:731–733.
66. Strigini FA, Cioni G, Canapicchi R, Nardini V, Capriello P, Carmignani A. Fetal intracranial hemorrhage: Is minor maternal trauma a possible pathogenetic factor? *Ultrasound Obstet Gynecol.* 2001;18:335–342.
67. Strigini FA, Nardini V, Carmignani A, Valleriani AM. Second-trimester diagnosis of intracranial vascular anomalies in a fetus with subdural hemorrhage. *Prenat Diagn.* 2004;24:31–34.
68. Vergani P, Strobelt N, Locatelli A, et al. Clinical significance of fetal intracranial hemorrhage. *Am J Obstet Gynecol.* 1996;175: 536–543.

69. Yuksel A, Batukan C. Fetal cerebellar hemorrhage in a severely growth-restricted fetus: natural history and differential diagnosis from Dandy-Walker malformation. *Ultrasound Obstet Gynecol.* 2003;22:178–181.
70. de Spirlet M, Goffinet F, Philippe HJ, Bailly M, Couderc S, Nisand I. Prenatal diagnosis of a subdural hematoma associated with reverse flow in the middle cerebral artery: Case report and literature review. *Ultrasound Obstet Gynecol.* 2000;16:72–76.
71. Brouwer MJ, de Vries LS, Pistorius L, Rademaker KJ, Groenendaal F, Benders MJ. Ultrasound measurements of the lateral ventricles in neonates: Why, how and when? A systematic review. *Acta Paediatr.* 2010;99(9):1298–1306.
72. Larroque B, Marret S, Ancel PY, et al. White matter damage and intraventricular hemorrhage in very preterm infants: The EPIPAGE study. *J Pediatr.* 2003;143:477–483.
73. Fanaroff AA, Wright LL, Stevenson DK, et al. Very-low-birth-weight outcomes of the National Institute of Child Health and Human Development Neonatal Research Network, May 1991 through December 1992. *Am J Obstet Gynecol.* 1995;173:1423–1431.
74. Morioka T, Hashiguchi K, Nagata S, et al. Fetal germinal matrix and intraventricular hemorrhage. *Pediatr Neurosurg.* 2006;42: 354–361.
75. Grant EG. Pathophysiology of germinal matrix-related hemorrhage and ischemia. In: Grant EG, ed. *Neurosonography of the Pre-term Neonate.* New York, Springer-Verlag;1986:25–32.
76. Volpe JJ. Brain injury in the premature infant—from pathogenesis to prevention. *Brain Dev.* 1997;19:519–534.
77. Volpe JJ. Edward B. Neuhauser lecture: Current concepts of brain injury in the premature infant. *AJR Am J Roentgenol.* 1989;153: 243–251.
78. Burrows RF, Caco CC, Kelton JG. Neonatal alloimmune thrombocytopenia: Spontaneous in utero intracranial hemorrhage. *Am J Hematol.* 1988;28:98–102.
79. Fogarty K, Cohen HL, Haller JO. Sonography of fetal intracranial hemorrhage: Unusual causes and a review of the literature. *J Clin Ultrasound.* 1989;17:366–370.
80. Jennett RJ, Daily WJ, Tarby TJ, Manwaring KH. Prenatal diagnosis of intracerebellar hemorrhage: Case report. *Am J Obstet Gynecol.* 1990;162:1472–1474, discussion 1474–1475.
81. Knuppel RA, Salvatore DL, Agarwal R, Leiman S, Sikka A. Documented fetal brain damage resulting from a motor vehicle accident. *J Ultrasound Med.* 1994;13:402–404.
82. Lustig-Gillman I, Young BK, Silverman F, et al. Fetal intraventricular hemorrhage: sonographic diagnosis and clinical implications. *J Clin Ultrasound.* 1983;11:277–280.
83. Zalneraitis EL, Young RS, Krishnamoorthy KS. Intracranial hemorrhage in utero as a complication of isoimmune thrombocytopenia. *J Pediatr.* 1979;95:611–614.
84. Crespin M, Alhenc-Gelas M, Grange G, Fallet-Bianco C, Fontenay M. Fetal intracerebral hemorrhage in familial thrombophilia. *Pediatr Neurol.* 2009;41:291–293.
85. Ramenghi LA, Fumagalli M, Righini A, Triulzi F, Kustermann A, Mosca F. Thrombophilia and fetal germinal matrix-intraventricular hemorrhage: Does it matter? *Ultrasound Obstet Gynecol.* 2005; 26:574–576.
86. Coulson CC, Kuller JA, Sweeney WJ. Nonimmune hydrops and hydrocephalus secondary to fetal intracranial hemorrhage. *Am J Perinatol.* 1994;11:253–254.
87. Serrarens-Janssen VM, Semmekrot BA, Novotny VM, et al. Fetal/neonatal allo-immune thrombocytopenia (FNAIT): Past, present, and future. *Obstet Gynecol Surv.* 2008;63:239–252.
88. Huang YF, Chen WC, Tseng JJ, Ho ES, Chou MM. Fetal intracranial hemorrhage (fetal stroke): Report of four antenatally diagnosed cases and review of the literature. *Taiwan J Obstet Gynecol.* 2006;45:135–141.
89. Grant EG. Neurosonography: Germinal matrix-related hemorrhage. In: Grant EG, ed. *Neurosonography of the Pre-term Neonate.* New York, Springer-Verlag;1986:85–90.
90. Rutherford MA. Magnetic resonance imaging of the fetal brain. *Curr Opin Obstet Gynecol.* 2009;21:180–186.
91. Glenn OA. MR imaging of the fetal brain. *Pediatr Radiol.* 2010;40:68–81.
92. Papile LA, Burstein J, Burstein R, Koffler H. Incidence and evolution of subependymal and intraventricular hemorrhage: A study of infants with birth weights less than 1,500 gm. *J Pediatr.* 1978;92:529–534.
93. Sarkar S, Bhagat I, Dechert R, Schumacher RE, Donn SM. Severe intraventricular hemorrhage in preterm infants: Comparison of risk factors and short-term neonatal morbidities between grade 3 and grade 4 intraventricular hemorrhage. *Am J Perinatol.* 2009;26: 419–424.
94. Hadi HA, Finley J, Mallette JQ, Strickland D. Prenatal diagnosis of cerebellar hemorrhage: Medicolegal implications. *Am J Obstet Gynecol.* 1994;170:1392–1395.
95. Lerner A, Gilboa Y, Gerad L, Malinger G, Kidron D, Achiron R. Sonographic detection of fetal cerebellar cavernous hemangioma with in-utero hemorrhage leading to cerebellar hemihypoplasia. *Ultrasound Obstet Gynecol.* 2006;28:968–971.
96. Hiller LT, McGahan JP, Bijan B, Melendres G, Towner D. Sonographic detection of in utero isolated cerebellar hemorrhage. *J Ultrasound Med.* 2003;22:649–652.
97. Limperopoulos C, Benson CB, Bassan H, et al. Cerebellar hemorrhage in the preterm infant: Ultrasonographic findings and risk factors. *Pediatrics.* 2005;116:717–724.
98. Martin R, Roessmann U, Fanaroff A. Massive intracerebellar hemorrhage in low-birth-weight infants. *J Pediatr.* 1976;89:290–293.
99. Ben-Chetrit A, Anteby E, Lavy Y, Zacut D, Yagel S. Increased middle cerebral artery blood flow impedance in fetal subdural hematoma. *Ultrasound Obstet Gynecol.* 1991;1:357–358.
100. Piastra M, Pietrini D, Massimi L, et al. Severe subdural hemorrhage due to minimal prenatal trauma. *J Neurosurg Pediatr.* 2009;4: 543–546.
101. Robinson MJ, Cameron MD, Smith MF, Ayers AB. Fetal subdural haemorrhages presenting as hydrocephalus. *Br Med J.* 1980;281:35.
102. de Sousa C, Clark T, Bradshaw A. Antenatally diagnosed subdural haemorrhage in congenital factor X deficiency. *Arch Dis Child.* 1988;63:1168–1170.
103. Akman CI, Cracco J. Intrauterine subdural hemorrhage. *Dev Med Child Neurol.* 2000;42:843–846.
104. Gunn TR, Mok PM, Becroft DM. Subdural hemorrhage in utero. *Pediatrics.* 1985;76:605–610.
105. Nogueira GJ. Chronic subdural hematoma in utero: Report of a case with survival after treatment. *Childs Nerv Syst.* 1992;8:462–464.
106. Kiryabwire J, Chaseling R, Lang EW. Extensive in utero traumatic subarachnoid haemorrhage and abruptio placentae. *J Trauma.* 2005; 59:236–238.
107. Bonnefoy O, Maugey-Laulom B, Diris B, Dallay D, Diard F. Fetal extradural hematoma: Prenatal diagnosis and postmortem examination. *Fetal Diagn Ther.* 2005;20:262–265.
108. Demir RH, Gleicher N, Myers SA. Atraumatic antepartum subdural hematoma causing fetal death. *Am J Obstet Gynecol.* 1989;160: 619–620.
109. Hanigan WC, Ali MB, Cusack TJ, Miller TC, Shah JJ. Diagnosis of subdural hemorrhage in utero: Case report. *J Neurosurg.* 1985;63: 977–979.
110. Kawabata I, Imai A, Tamaya T. Antenatal subdural hemorrhage causing fetal death before labor. *Int J Gynaecol Obstet.* 1993;43: 57–60.
111. Barozzino T, Sgro M, Toi A, et al. Fetal bilateral subdural haemorrhages: Prenatal diagnosis and spontaneous resolution by time of delivery. *Prenat Diagn.* 1998;18:496–503.

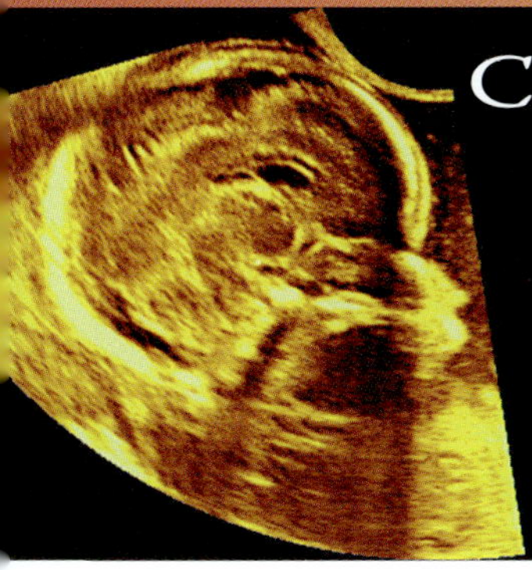

# Chapter 11

# INTRACRANIAL CYSTS

*Eran Bornstein • Ana Monteagudo • Ilan E. Timor-Tritsch*

**KEY POINTS**

1. One of the most common and usually benign fetal brain tetralogy pathology.
2. Easily detected due to its obvious anechoic appearance at places that should not be located present.
3. Larger cysts may exert pressure on adjacent organs causing displacement of structures or obstruct the flow of cerebrospinal fluid.
4. Although mostly isolated, they can be associated with other pathologies, therefore targeted neuroscan and anatomy scan is warranted.

Intracranial cysts are relatively common findings encountered in the prenatal sonographic assessment of the fetal brain. The vast majority of these fluid collections (arachnoid and choroid plexus cysts) are of a benign nature, remain clinically silent, do not evolve, and regress spontaneously. When these lesions are not associated with other fetal anomalies, they are compatible with normal life regardless of whether they require postnatal treatment or not.[1,2] Nevertheless, due to the numerous differential diagnostic entities, as well as the associated parental anxiety, clinically, these findings present a dilemma in need of appropriate diagnosis and counseling.

The differential diagnoses of intracranial cysts encompass multiple etiologic and pathologic processes. Advancements in imaging techniques, especially in fetal sonography, have facilitated the workup of such cysts by depicting their exact location, size, relationship to the ventricular system, and midline structures. Additionally, fetal sonography allows for evaluation of the presence of solid components seen in cases of brain tumors or blood clots and for performance of Doppler studies of blood flow patterns in cases of vascular malformations, such as an aneurysm of the vein of Galen. Nevertheless, imaging studies may come short of distinguishing between some of these lesions, which require histologic examination of the cyst wall to establish the correct diagnosis.[3] In this chapter, we classify intracranial cysts based on the location of their origin into one of three groups: extra-axial, intraventricular, and intraparenchymal (Table 11–1).

## CLASSIFICATION OF INTRACRANIAL CYSTS

### CYSTS OF EXTRA-AXIAL ORIGIN

This group of lesions consists of arachnoid cysts, glioependymal cysts, endodermal cysts, cystic teratomas, and dural separation due to dural sinus thrombosis.

#### Arachnoid Cysts

Arachnoid cysts are by far the most common lesion in this group, and our review will focus on them.

#### Synonyms

None

#### Definition

Arachnoid cysts were first described by Bright in 1831[3] as "serous cysts forming in connection with the arachnoid and apparently lying between its layers." Like other intracranial cysts, arachnoid cysts are collections of cerebrospinal fluid (CSF) on the brain surface bordered by a cyst wall.

#### Incidence

Arachnoid cysts account for 1% of all intracranial masses in children.[2–4] They usually occur in a sporadic fashion as an isolated single lesion. Multiple and bilateral arachnoid cysts are unusual; familial occurrence has been reported in only a few cases. The left side of the brain is affected more commonly, and a male predominance with a 2:1 male-to-female ratio has been shown.[5–8]

#### Pathogenesis

The exact pathogenesis is not clear, but it is thought to develop mostly in the second and third trimesters. Arachnoid cysts are usually benign, congenital, space-occupying lesions with a cavity that is entirely surrounded by a transparent arachnoid membrane. These collections of CSF are located within the layers of the arachnoid membranes and

**Table 11–1. CLASSIFICATION OF INTRACRANIAL CYSTS**

| Extra-axial Cyst | Intraventricular Cyst | Intraparenchymal Cyst |
|---|---|---|
| Arachnoid cyst | Choroid plexus cyst | Periventricular pseudocyst |
| Glioependymal cyst | Choroid plexus hemorrhage | Cystic periventricular leukomalacia |
| Endodermal cyst | | Porencephalic cyst |
| Dural separation | | Cystic brain tumor |
| Cystic tumors (teratoma) | | Holoprosencephaly |
| Vascular malformations | | Schizencephaly |

may or may not communicate with the subarachnoid space. Postnatally, they usually are the result of head trauma, which provokes a proliferation of fibroblasts that form a loculated cyst within the leptomeninges. These can enlarge because the fluid within (CSF) is trapped and can only increase. As a congenital lesion, the cause is less certain, but the prevailing theory is that an arachnoid cyst is a disturbance of the mesencephalic neural crest, the origin of the meninges, which forms a splitting of the primordial membrane into which fluid accumulates and becomes loculated, analogous to a dissecting aneurysm. Whereas a cleft may form during this period, it does not necessarily fill with fluid to separate the two leaves until later in gestation or even postnatally; hence, it is plausible that it would not be identified in the second trimester by neuroimaging, because it may be detectable only microscopically at that time.

## Etiology

An arachnoid cyst may present as a primary or an acquired lesion. Primary cysts commonly arise from an abnormal developmental process of the leptomeningeal formation, whereas acquired arachnoid cysts (secondary cysts) generally result from entrapment of CSF within arachnoid adhesions following in utero hemorrhage, infection, or trauma.[9–13]

## Pathology

On histologic examination, the cyst wall is lined with collagen and cells of the arachnoid matter (meningothelial cells). Electron microscopic findings confirm that the origin of these cysts is arachnoid cells and not epithelial cells.[14] Immunohistochemical markers have also been used to differentiate arachnoid cysts from epithelial cysts. The cells lining the arachnoid cyst are not ciliated and do not stain with antibodies against glial fibrillary acidic protein (GFAP), S-100, transthyretin, and carcinoembryonic antigen (CEA).[15]

## Associated Anomalies

Arachnoid cysts usually present as isolated lesions. Several central nervous system (CNS) anomalies have been described in association with them. These include agenesis of the corpus callosum, absent septum pellucidum, deficient cerebellar lobulation, Arnold-Chiari type I malformation, malformations of cortical development, and arteriovenous malformation.[16] We believe interhemispheric cysts that present in fetuses with commissural anomalies are probably not true arachnoid cysts but rather cystic processes that develop from an abnormal meninx that cause by themselves the defect, as they block the pathway of the axonal fibers through the midline. Non-CNS malformations associated with arachnoid cysts are tetralogy of Fallot, sacrococcygeal tumor, and neurofibromatosis type I.[11,12,17–19] In addition, a few case reports point to the possible association of arachnoid cysts with nonchromosomal syndromes, such as distichiasis-lymphedema and Mohr syndrome, as well as trisomy 12q24.31.[20–22] However, the strength of this association is questionable and may suffer from publication bias due to the limited number of case reports.

## Risk of Recurrence

Generally, the finding of an arachnoid cyst is not thought to represent an increased risk for future pregnancies. However, arachnoid cyst is associated with a few hereditary conditions that confer increased risk of recurrence mostly in an autosomal recessive or an X-linked pattern. Aicardi syndrome, for example, is a rare X-linked dominant syndrome that includes agenesis of the corpus callosum, interhemispheric cyst, choroidal anomalies, and infantile seizures (Figure 11–1A).

## Sonographic Diagnosis

Most of the arachnoid cysts are sonographically detectable in the second or third trimester, which is consistent with the belief that these lesions only develop around this time. Prenatal diagnosis before 20 weeks' gestation is uncommon. In one of the largest series evaluating fetuses with arachnoid cysts, there were no cases diagnosed prior to 20 postmenstrual weeks. Moreover, in this series 55% of the arachnoid cysts were diagnosed between 20 and 30 postmenstrual weeks and 45% only after the 30th week despite an earlier scan.[2] Nevertheless, first trimester sonographic diagnosis coupled with histologic

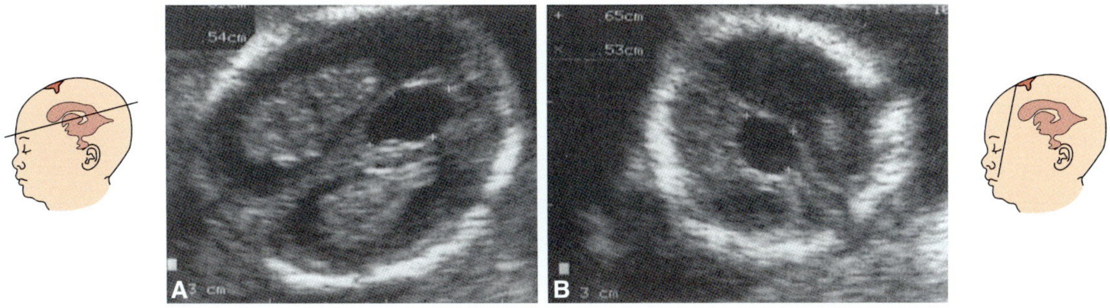

**Figure 11–1.** Arachnoid cyst at 16 postmenstrual weeks. **(A)** Axial plane showing the 0.7 × 0.54 cm cystic structure between the frontal lobes of the hemispheres. **(B)** A midcoronal section localizes the cyst between the hemispheres in the longitudinal sulcus. The exact localization of this arachnoid cyst was in the suprachiasmatic area. In spite of the favorable counseling, the patient elected for termination of the pregnancy. (Courtesy of Leibovitz Zvi Haifa, Israel.)

confirmation of an arachnoid cyst has been described (Figure 11–1).[1,23]

The characteristic sonographic appearance is that of a sonolucent cystic mass with a thin, smooth wall (Figures 11–2 to 11–9). Arachnoid cysts do not communicate with the lateral ventricles (unlike some of the intraparenchymal cysts or lesions, such as porencephaly, dorsal cysts of holoprosencephaly, and schizencephaly).[9,10] In severe cases, secondary hydrocephaly may be the result of an obstruction in the flow of CSF due to the mass effect. Most arachnoid cysts are supratentorial, with ~50% to 65% located in the middle cranial fossa, 5% to 10% in the suprasellar cistern, 5% to 10% in the quadrigeminal cistern, 5% spread along the convexities, and only 5% to 10% in the posterior fossa at the level of the cerebellopontine angle and the cisterna magna. Pierre-Kahn and Sonigo[2] published the largest series including 54 patients with arachnoid cysts. Based on their experience, 63% of the cysts were supratentorial, mostly intrahemispheric (25%), with few in the base, suprasellar, or interventricular area. They found 22.2% of the cysts to be located at the infratentorial area.[2]

## Differential Diagnosis

The differential diagnosis of an arachnoid cyst includes other extra-axial lesions, as well as intraparenchymal or intraventricular cystic lesions, as displayed in Table 11–1. With the exception of brain cystic tumors, which may be heterogeneous and contain solid components, all other lesions are sonolucent fluid cystlike masses that can be associated with secondary hydrocephaly due to a mass effect. In experienced hands, ultrasound (US) can distinguish between the different groups of intracranial cysts. For example, porencephalic cysts can be seen in the brain parenchyma and communicate with the ventricles and subarachnoid space.

Malformations of the vein of Galen have turbulent flow, which becomes evident using two- (2D) or three-dimensional (3D) color or power angiography.[24–27] The sonolucent structure of the dilated vein of Galen does

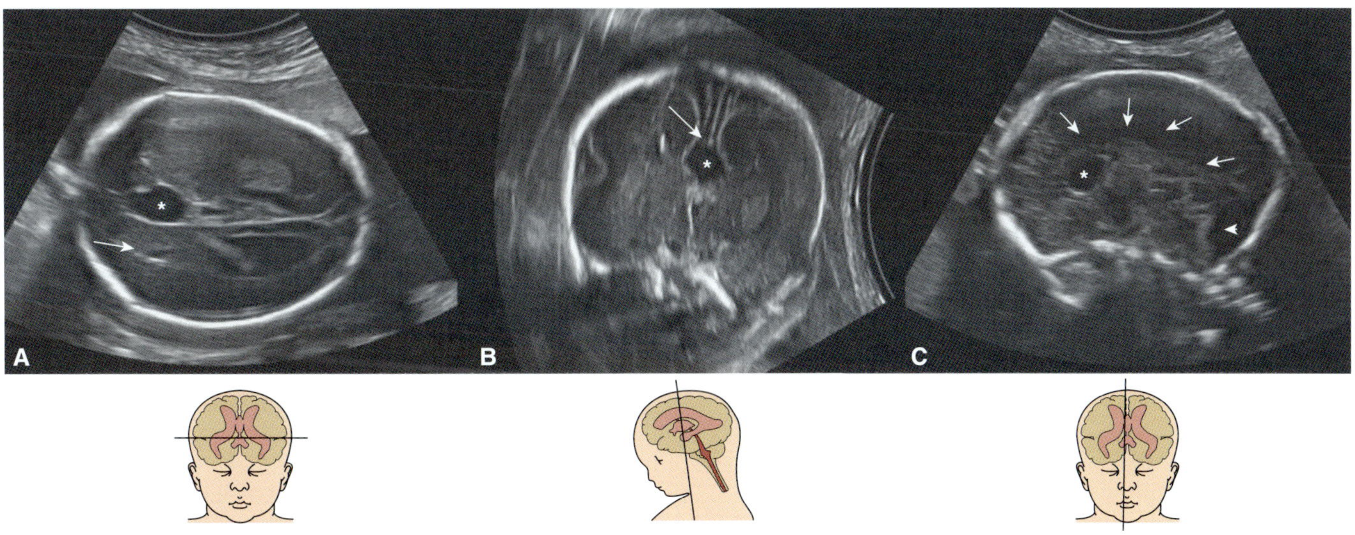

**Figure 11–2.** Interhemispheric arachnoid cyst (*) associated with agenesis of the corpus callosum in a fetus at 22 weeks of gestation. **(A)** Axial view showing typical ventricular colpocephaly with a sharp shape of the anterior horn (*arrow*). **(B)** Coronal view. The interhemispheric fissure is continuous with the arachnoid cyst due to agenesis of the corpus callosum. **(C)** Median plane fails to show the corpus callosum (*arrows*); note also the presence of a severely dysgenetic vermis (*arrowhead*).

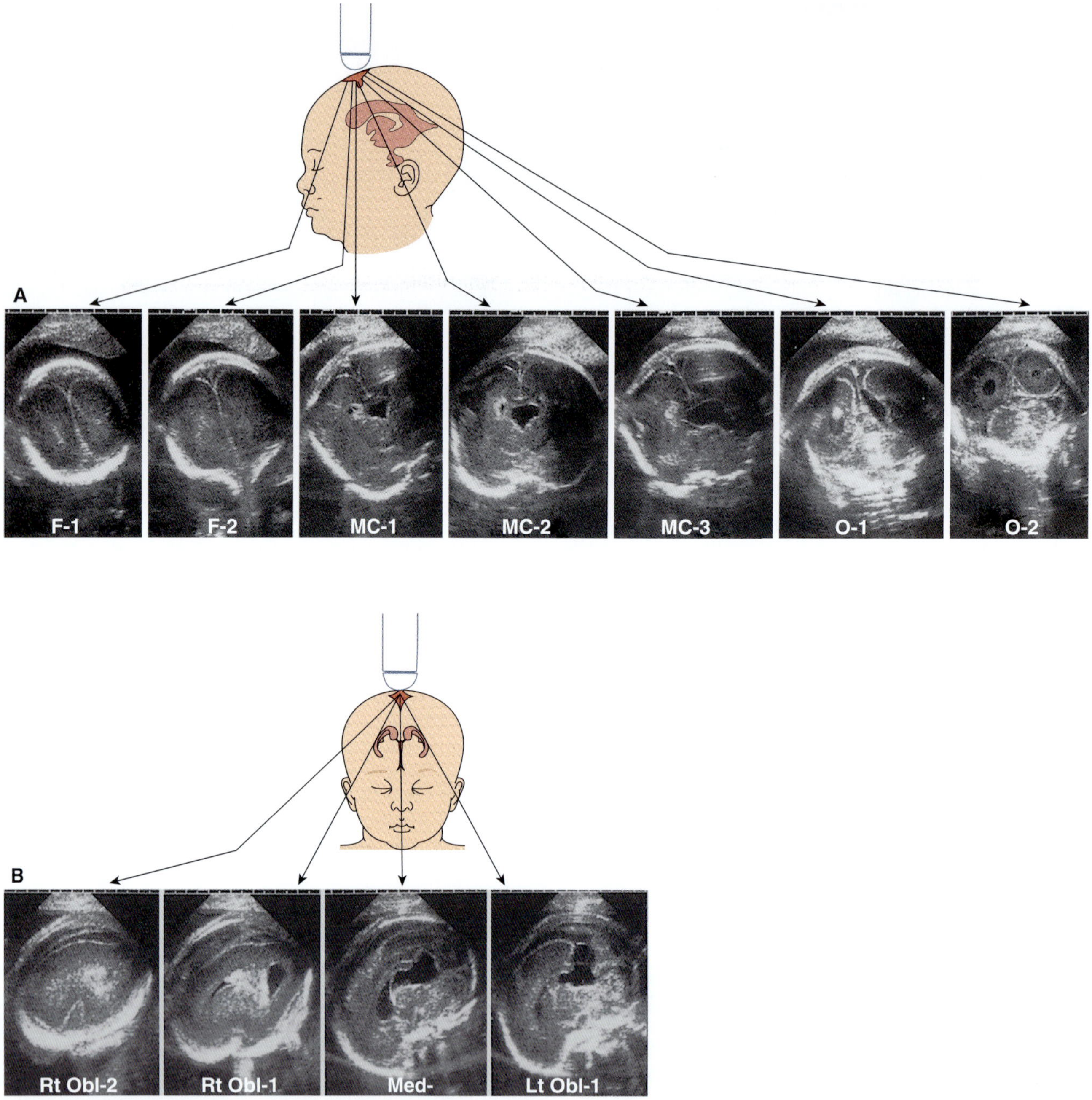


**Figure 11–3.** Transvaginal brain study of a fetus at 25 postmenstrual weeks showing a quadrigeminal cistern arachnoid cyst. **(A)** Serial coronal sections from frontal–1 to occipital–2 (F-1 to O-2), with F-1 and frontal–2 (F-2) section showing the parenchyma of the frontal lobes. Midcoronal–1 (MC-1) to midcoronal–3 (MC-3) shows the midline anechoic cyst. In occipital–1 (O-1), the cyst can be seen slightly impinging on the posterior lobe of the brain. **(B)** Median (Med) and right and left oblique (Rt. and Lt. Obl) sections showing the extended and exact location of the cyst. Right oblique–1 and –2 (Rt. Obl-1 and -2) show the normal right cerebral hemispheres. Note that there is no dilation of lateral ventricles. On the median section, the arachnoid cyst is seen below the tail of the corpus callosum extending almost to the cranial bone. On left oblique–1 (Lt. Obl-1), more of the cyst is seen extending all the way to the outer surface of the brain. This fetus has a normal corpus callosum; therefore, the prognosis is good.

not communicate with the ventricles or the subarachnoid space and is located in the area of the quadrigeminal plate cistern (Figures 11–10 and 11–11). The aneurysm probably represents a remnant of the embryonic median prosencephalic vein. The diagnosis is generally made postnatally, and the clinical signs include cyanosis, systolic murmur, cardiomegaly, and increased pressure with hydrocephaly due to obstruction of the sylvian aqueduct by the dilated aneurysm. In severe cases, nonimmune hydrops fetalis may result from severe high-output congestive heart failure. Gerards and colleagues[28] described their experience with two cases of aneurysm of the vein of Galen. Their experience suggests that Doppler studies, 3D sonography, and magnetic resonance imaging (MRI) may be used to evaluate for prognostic factors, such as drainage and secondary damage.

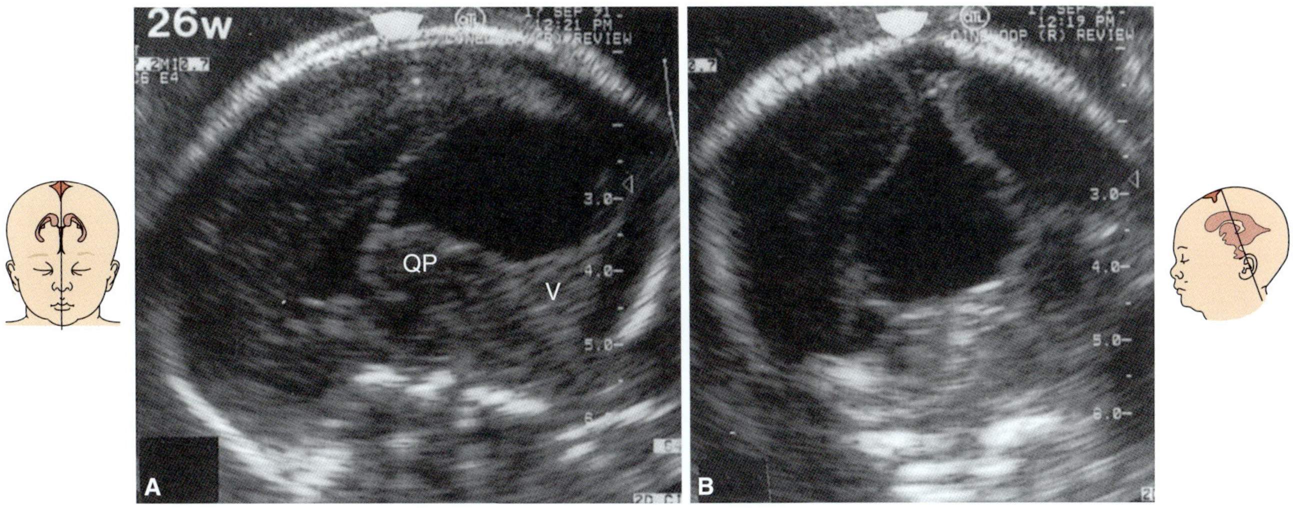


**Figure 11–4.** Images of a large quadrigeminal plate arachnoid cyst at 26 postmenstrual weeks. **(A)** Median section showing the displacement of a quadrigeminal plate (QP) and the vermis of the cerebellum (V). **(B)** Midcoronal section showing the symmetrical position of the cyst displacing the hemispheres.

Fetal brain tumors are extremely rare, have a heterogeneous pattern, are usually within the brain parenchyma, and may communicate with the ventricles.[11] Teratomas are probably the only tumor that may appear as a completely cystic intracranial extra-axial neoplasm. Cassart et al[29] published their experience with US and MRI of fetal intracranial tumors. Of 13 teratomas in their series, 12 had a significant cystic component, and few were completely cystic. These cystic components correspond to necrotic lesions and were extremely uncommon in other types of tumors. In a different series of fetal brain tumors, the authors diagnosed seven cases of brain tumors, of which six were confirmed postnatally. One case of a supratentorial arachnoid cyst was mistaken for a teratoma with cystic components. Out of the six cases of suspected teratomas, one was revealed to be a glioblastoma, one an arachnoid cyst, and one a primitive neuroectodermal tumor. The authors concluded that prenatal ultrasonography is a useful tool to identify any intracranial space-occupying lesion >10 mm, with 86% specificity. As expected, the accuracy of US in diagnosing the tumor's histologic type was limited (57%).[30] For a more detailed discussion and images of fetal CNS tumors, see Chapter 13.

Other extra-axial cysts, such as glioependymal and endodermal cysts, are extremely rare and cannot be distinguished sonographically from arachnoid cysts. Glioependymal cysts, also called ependymal cysts, choroidal epithelial cysts, neuroepithelial cysts, and epithelial cysts, have a glioependymal lining that distinguishes them from arachnoid cysts histologically. They may be located both extra-axially and intraparenchymally and have been reported to be detected in association with agenesis of the corpus callosum.[31] This lesion is thought to arise from displaced neuroectodermal tissue most closely resembling the area forming the tela choroidea and may also have a heterogeneous sonographic appearance. Like arachnoid cysts, these lesions can grow and reach significant proportions.[31] Several reports describe the detection of glioependymal cysts in fetuses undergoing neurosonographic evaluation or brain MRI for the evaluation of ventriculomegaly.[32,33] The authors stressed the importance of considering this entity in the differential diagnosis of fetal cystic brain lesions, especially when callosal abnormalities coexist. Endodermal cysts are extremely uncommon congenital lesions that are rarely diagnosed prenatally. Most cases are located in the spinal canal, and of the intracranial ones, most are located in the posterior fossa.[34]

Dural separation is a benign, mostly isolated finding that may appear as a "cystlike" structure in the extra-axial space of the brain.

Thrombosis of the dural sinus and thrombosis of the torcular herophili following a thrombotic event are rare events that are thought to result from trauma, dural sinus malformation, or a genetic thrombophilia. The diagnosis and management may be difficult, as this lesion may mimic an intracranial tumor and display both solid and cystic components. In utero resolution of the lesion was reported in a few cases that had favorable outcome (after an 18-month follow-up).[35,36] Laurichesse Delmas and colleagues[37] reported their experience based on six cases of dural sinus thrombosis. They found that sonographic evidence of brain damage, cardiac failure, increased size of the thrombus, and secondary brain ischemic damage were associated with a poor outcome, whereas findings of either partial or total regression, as well as the absence of fetal decompensation, are considered good prognostic factors associated with a favorable outcome. They further concluded that based on the limited data available, the outcome in cases in which the thrombus did not decrease in size and there was no fetal decompensation or brain anomaly could not be predicted. Our group had evaluated three cases in which thrombus of the torcular herophili was diagnosed on prenatal US. Separation of the dura with

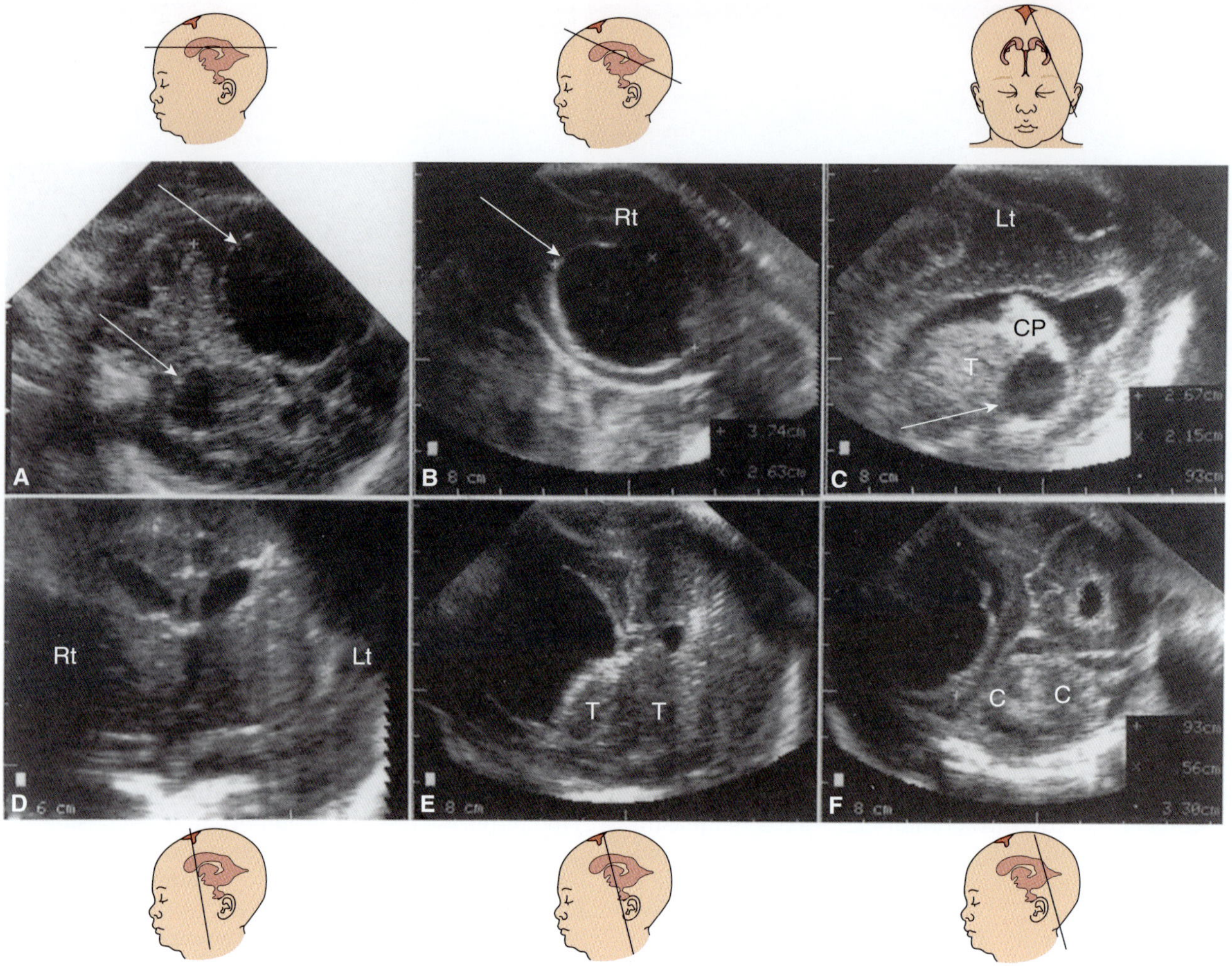


**Figure 11–5.** Bilateral cysts at 32 postmenstrual weeks. The working diagnosis based on the sonographic evaluation was bilateral choroid plexus cysts. **(A)** "Horizontal"" section. The cysts are marked by arrows; the right is larger than the left. **(B)** Posterior angled "horizontal" section. The arrow points to the larger right–sided cyst. **(C)** Left oblique–1 section. Note the slightly dilated posterior horn and the smaller cyst (*arrow*) below the choroid plexus. **(D)** Midcoronal–1 section. Note that the anterior horns are slightly dilated. **(E)** Midcoronal–2 section. The cyst on the right side is shown. T, thalamus. **(F)** Occipital–1 section. The larger right-sided cyst is seen extending posteriorly even on this section. C, cerebellum. The neonate was born at term. The MRI images suggested the diagnosis of arachnoid cyst rather than cyst arising from the choroid plexus.

a cystlike area at the level of the torcular herophili containing a focus of clotted blood could be detected on a detailed sonographic evaluation. These findings were supported by a fetal MRI and further confirmed on the post mortem examination.[38] For an illustrative case of thrombosis of the torcular herophili, see Chapter 10, Figures 10–12, 10–13, 10–14, 10–16, and 10–18.

It is extremely hard to differentiate arachnoid cysts that are located in the posterior fossa from megacisterna magna (MCM) or Dandy-Walker malformation. Nevertheless, an attempt to distinguish between them is important because of the significant difference in the outcomes of these conditions. The hallmark of this lesion is a cyst compressing the cerebellum against the brainstem (Figure 11–12), with the vermis remaining intact, whereas in MCM, there are no signs of compression, and in Dandy-Walker malformation, the vermis is either absent or hypoplastic. The distinction between these conditions can be established by identifying the normally formed fourth ventricle and the presence of the complete cerebellar vermis. In these cases, we recommend visualizing the median plane (either by transvaginal US or by 3D reconstruction) in order to evaluate the size of the cerebellar vermis, which may be displaced by the cyst resembling a Dandy-Walker malformation. Hogge and colleagues[22] reported a case of an infratentorial posterior fossa arachnoid cyst that was associated with an unbalanced X;9 translocation. In one of our cases (Figure 11–13), the first US at 15½ postmenstrual weeks was completely normal; however, at 28 postmenstrual weeks, a cyst of the posterior fossa was imaged, and at 31 postmenstrual weeks, it appeared like a Dandy-Walker malformation. Postnatal MRI and computed tomography (CT) scan confirmed the diagnosis of a posterior fossa arachnoid cyst.

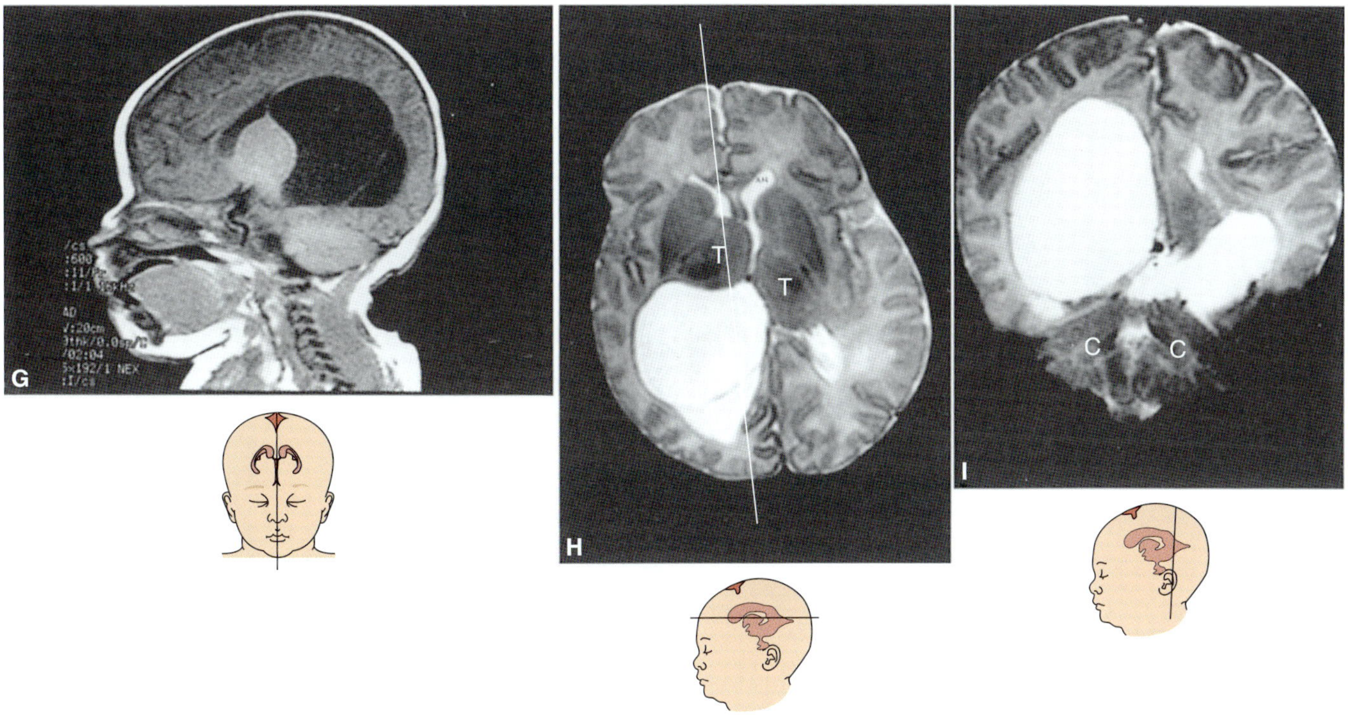


**Figure 11–5.** *(continued)* **(G)** Slightly right paramedian section notes the thin wall of the cysts in the right lateral ventricle. This plane was obtained along the white line transecting the brain in Figure 11–5H. **(H)** "Horizontal" section. Note that the anterior horns (AH) are not dilated and that the right thalamus (T) is pushed slightly forward. **(I)** Coronal section through the two cystic structures and the cerebellum (C).

## Implications for Targeted Examination

When managing a fetus with an arachnoid cyst, the exact location and the effect on the brain structures in its immediate vicinity should be determined. Our practice is to perform a targeted detailed neurosonographic examination, preferably using a high-frequency transvaginal probe to scrutinize the brain. The focus is on the exact location and size, the relationship to the ventricles, and the presence of any associated intracranial malformations or secondary anomalies. We also follow up these cases longitudinally with US and consider a brain MRI, which may be valuable in detecting additional anomalies (specifically, migrational disorders in places distant to the cyst),[16] as well as providing further reassurance. We obtain a detailed fetal scan looking for extracranial anomalies, a fetal echocardiogram, genetic counseling, and possibly genetic testing for women who are diagnosed with fetal extra-axial cyst.

## Prognosis

The clinical manifestations are directly related to the size of the cyst and its location within the brain. Small cysts

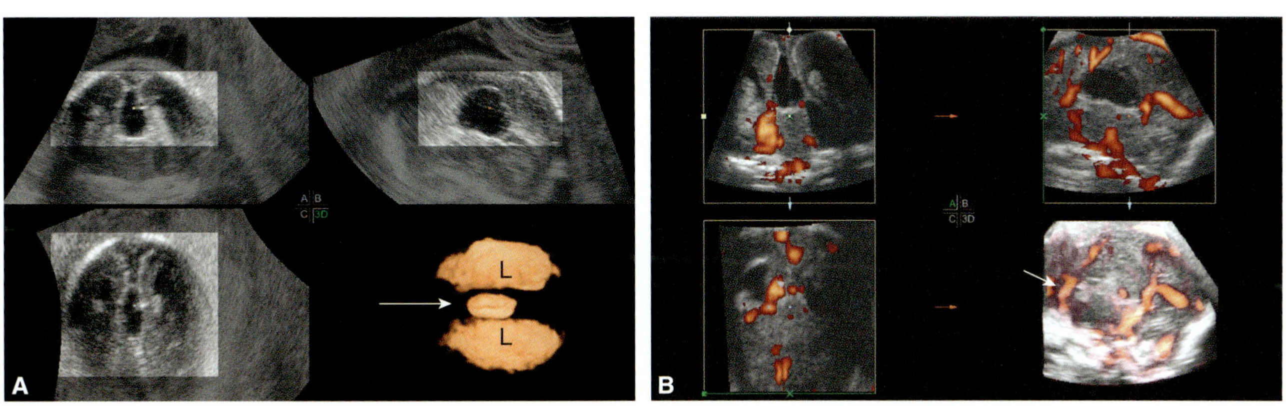


**Figure 11–6.** Interhemispheric arachnoid cyst at 21 postmenstrual weeks affecting the corpus callosum. **(A)** Three-dimensional (3D) orthogonal planes: coronal (box A), sagittal (box B), axial (box C). Box D displays inversion rendering of the lateral ventricles (L) and the arachnoid cyst (*arrow*). **(B)** 3D power Doppler study. The planes are the same as in Figure 11–6A. Box D displays the short pericallosal artery (*arrow*).

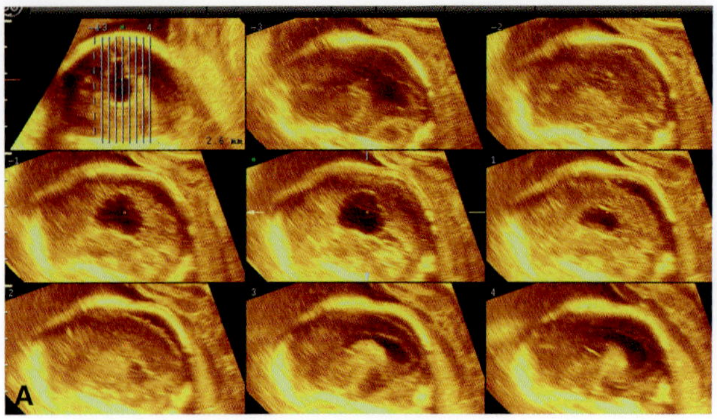

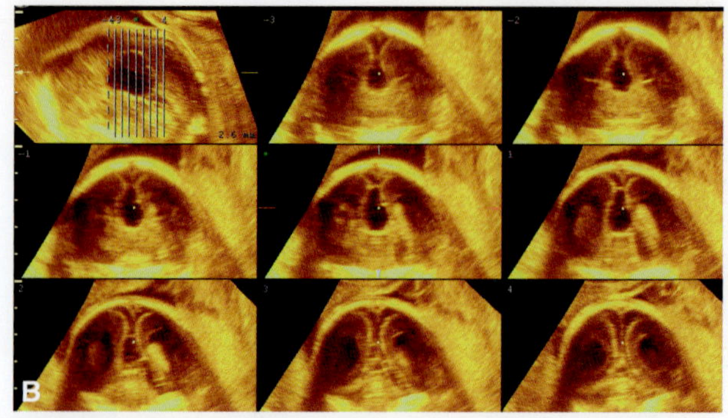

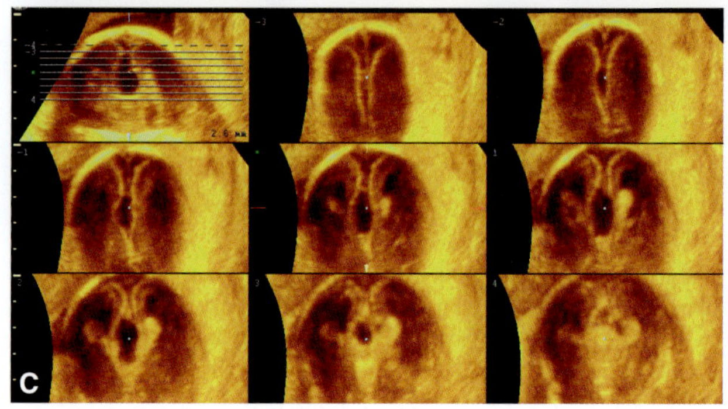

**Figure 11–7.** 3D tomographic representation of the interhemispheric arachnoid cyst. Same case as in Figure 11–6. **(A)** Sagittal planes along the lines seen in the first box. **(B)** Coronal planes along the lines seen in the first box. **(C)** Axial planes along the lines seen in the first box.

generally present as incidental findings, whereas larger cysts may come to attention during a workup of seizures, headache, hydrocephaly, or focal neurologic signs, which are caused by the mass effect.[39] Approximately 60% to 80% of arachnoid cysts are a symptomatic. Even a large cyst producing pressure on brain structures may remain asympomatic.[1] In infants there may be increased head circumference and calvarial asymmetry in severe cases of hydrocephaly.[7]

The prognosis of fetuses with arachnoid cysts is mostly dependent on the presence of associated congenital or chromosomal anomalies. As mentioned before, the prognosis is generally good even in those cases requiring drainage of a hydrocephaly in the neonatal or infancy period.[40–43] Vergani and colleagues[3] published their experience distinguishing between interhemispheric cystic lesions that are related to physiologic median brain structures and cysts from pathologic fluid collections. In their sonographic evaluation, they used an evaluation of the cyst's location, size, and change in size over time, as well as associated anomalies. They detected 12 fetuses with interhemispheric cysts that were related to median structures (enlargement of the cavum septi pellucidi [3 fetuses] or of the cavum Vergae [2 fetuses] and cysts of the velum interpositum [7 fetuses]). These cysts were unilocular, ranging from 10 to 30 mm, and were not associated with overt fetal anomalies. Moreover, the cysts resolved in five cases, remained stable in the rest, and all had normal pediatric follow-up. In contrast, seven cases that were diagnosed as "pathologic lesions" were significantly larger, ranging from 10 to 80 mm, and grew over time. In five of these cases, associated intracranial anomalies, such as partial or total agenesis of the corpus callosum and overt hydrocephaly, were present. The neonatal outcome in these cases was also significantly worse and included one elective termination of pregnancy, one infant death at 4 months of age, two neonates with neurodevelopmental delay, and three that appeared to be neurologically intact at a mean follow-up of 43 months. Cyst shunting was necessary in five of six cases.[3] In a different report, five fetuses who were diagnosed with isolated cyst of the cavum veli interpositi had a normal neurologic and neurosonographic follow-up.[44] Other investigators reached similar findings, supporting the conclusion that isolated, "benign-appearing" cysts of the median structures carry a favorable neonatal outcome.

## Obstetric Management and Prognosis

Management includes the workup that we previously described. The mode of delivery should not be affected by the presence of an arachnoid cyst unless hydrocephaly does not permit vaginal delivery. Management of neonates with arachnoid cysts varies based on their symptoms and the degree of hydrocephaly. Most arachnoid cysts that are found incidentally can be managed expectantly and have favorable outcome. However, patients who are symptomatic should be regarded as surgical candidates. The surgical options for treatment include ventriculoperitoneal and cystoperitoneal shunting, open or endoscopic fenestration, and stereotactic aspiration.[41–45] Recent advances in neurosurgical techniques and neuroendoscopy continue

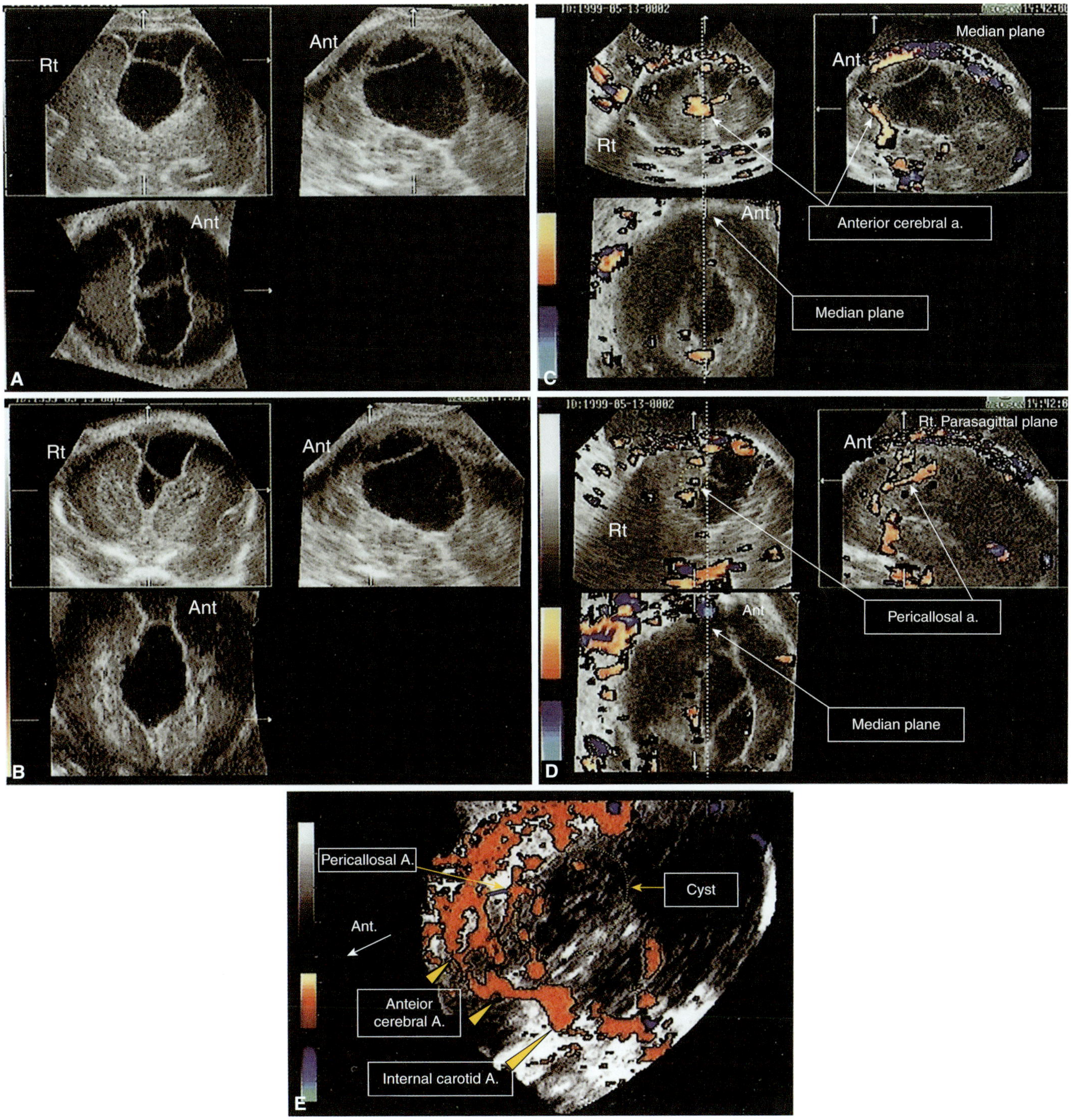


**Figure 11–8.** An arachnoid cyst originating from the quadrigeminal plate at 23 postmenstrual weeks. **(A)** The septated cyst displacing the falx to the right is shown by the coronal (box A), sagittal (box B), and axial (box C) planes. **(B)** Another set of orthogonal planes were selected to study the extent of the lesion. **(C)** Color Doppler study. The picture in the active box (box B) highlighted by the frame is generated in the median plane (*dotted vertical white line* through boxes A and C). Only the anterior cerebral artery, but not the pericallosal artery, is seen (the latter should be evident in this plane). **(D)** The plane is moved to the right. Now the active box (box B) is generated in the right parasagittal plane. In this plane, the pericallosal artery is clearly detected. This proves that the corpus callosum is not destroyed by the cyst. The dotted vertical white line was kept to mark the median plane. **(E)** A 3D color flow rendering of the anterior cerebral and pericallosal arteries. The approximate place of the arachnoid cyst is marked.

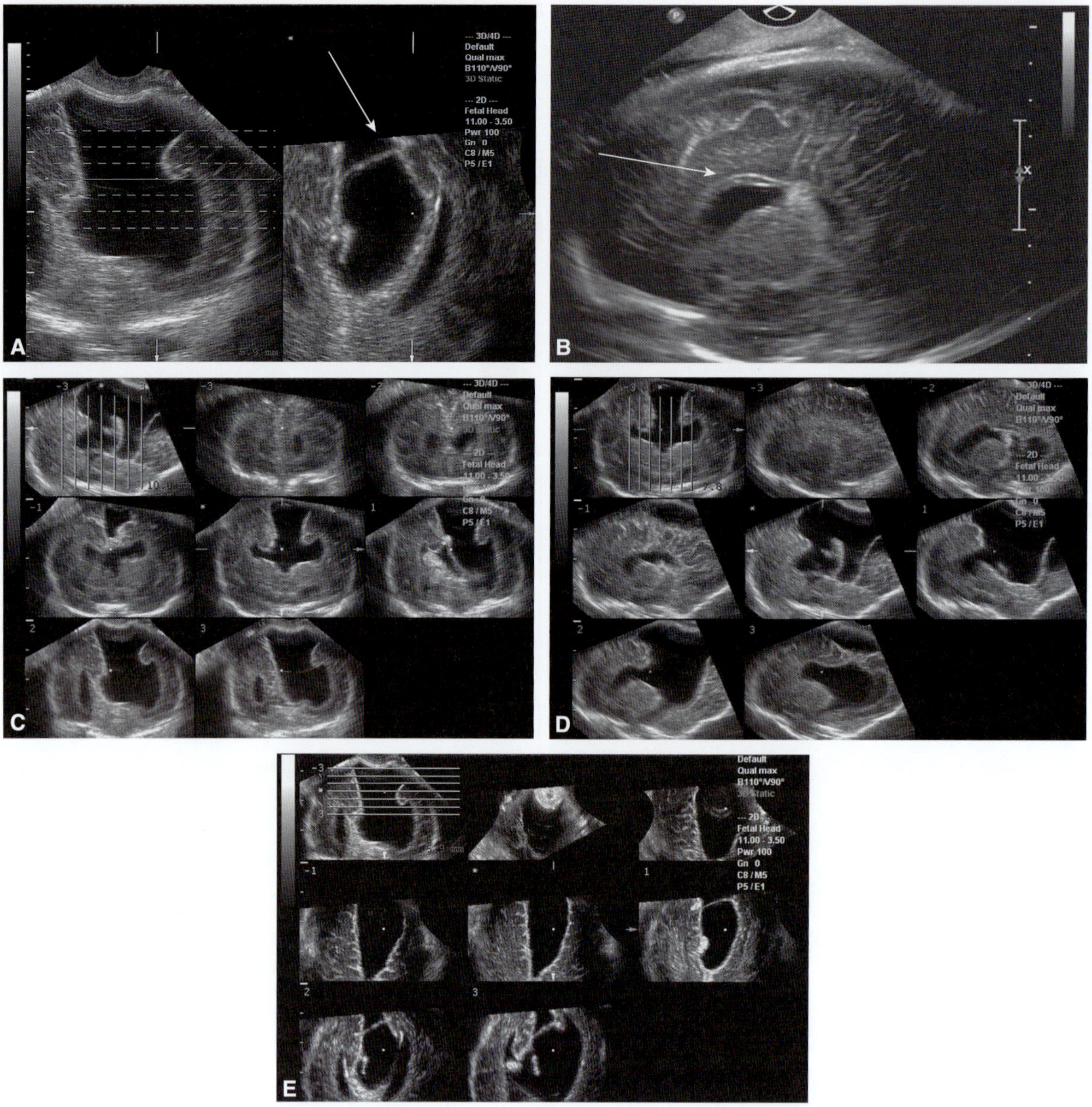

**Figure 11–9.** Interhemispheric arachnoid cyst. **(A)** Two side-by-side coronal views of the cyst. Note the thin cyst wall (*arrow*) that depicts the diagnosis. **(B)** Although some views raised the suspicion of agenesis of the corpus callosum, this parasagittal image (especially some radially oriented gyri) shows the presence of a laterally displaced but normal-appearing corpus callosum (*arrow*). **(C)** 3D coronal tomographic sequence of the cyst. **(D)** 3D sagittal tomographic sequence of the cyst. **(E)** 3D axial tomographic sequence of the cyst. In addition to the above mentioned possible differential diagnosis of a partial agenesis of the corpus callosum we also considered schizencephaly as an alternative diagnosis. A postnatal MRI confirmed the diagnosis of arachnoid cyst parting the two hemispheres.

to favor fenestration over shunt insertion as the method of choice for initial cyst decompression.[41] A recent retrospective review presented the outcomes of 42 infants who underwent craniotomy for fenestration of an arachnoid cyst prior to the age of 2 years.[40] Based on these authors' experience, they recommended that infants with arachnoid cyst and ventriculomegaly should have fenestration initially. Shunt placement may be necessary later in most cases. In infants who presented with nonspecific macrocephaly, initial fenestration was sufficient in 40%. These did not require subsequent shunting procedure. Only 10% of the patients who presented with other symptoms, such as seizures, headache, motor deficits, or developmental delay, required subsequent shunting procedure after fenestration.

The long-term prognosis of more than 60 children with arachnoid cysts showed that 64% had a complete recovery after treatment, 15% had a slight deficit, 13% had severe postoperative deterioration, and 8% died.[46] The outcome of these children was dependent on the location

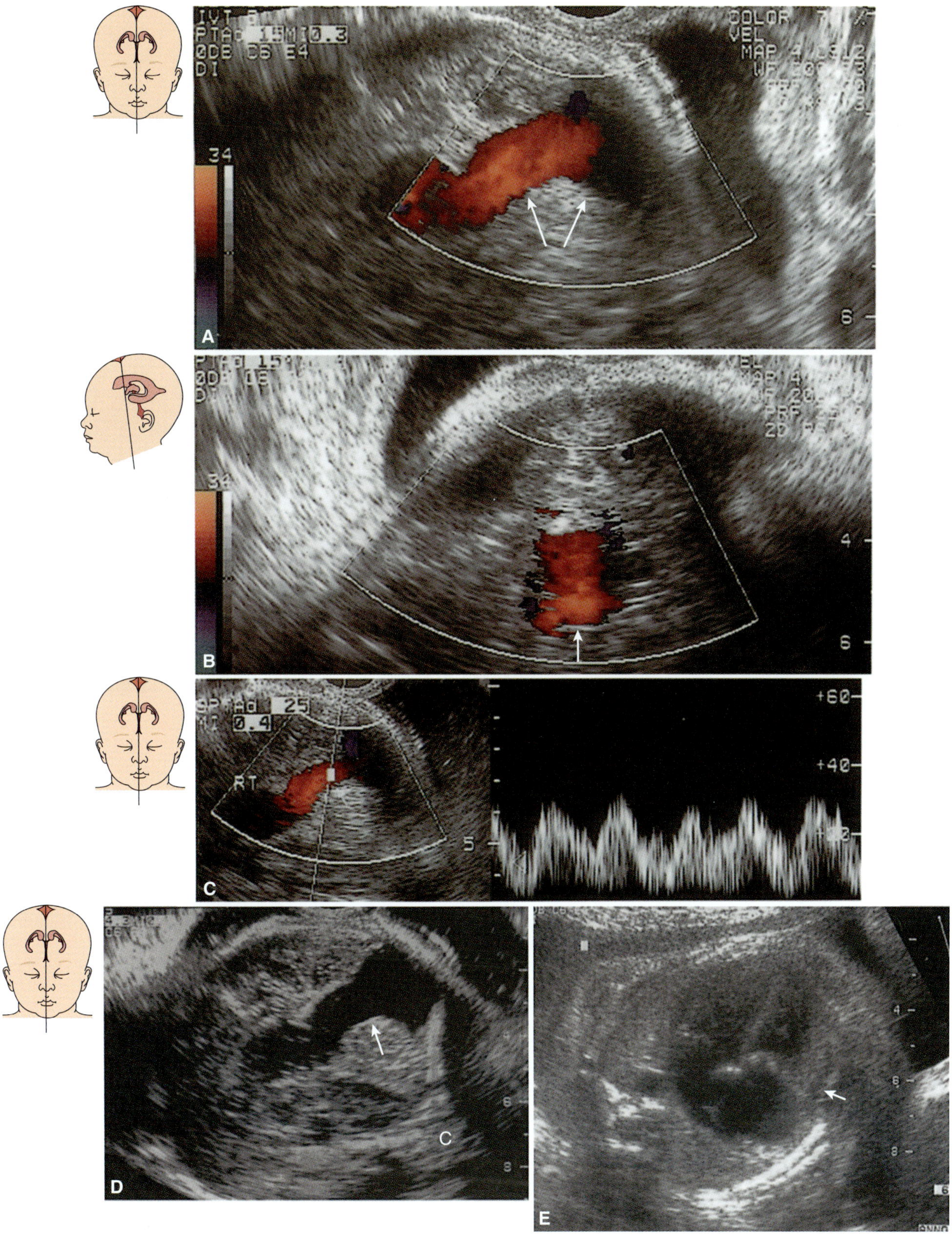


**Figure 11–10.** Aneurysm of the vein of Galen at 33 postmenstrual weeks. **A–C.** C-coded Doppler images of the lesion (*arrows*). **(A)** The median plane. **(B)** The midcoronal–1 plane. **(C)** In the median plane, note the wide (~1.2 cm) structure above the cerebellum (C) with flow toward the posterior pole of the brain. The Doppler evaluation showed a pulsating venous flow. **(D)** Grayscale image in the median plane. **(E)** Four-chamber view of the heart showing relative cardiomegaly; heart-to-chest diameter ratio: 0.65 (normal 0.45–0.5) and a very small amount of pericardial effusion (*arrow*). There was no atrioventricular valve regurgitation, but the heart had hyperdynamic motion consistent with a cerebral arteriovenous malformation. There was no dilation of the vessels in the neck of the fetus. Three attempts at embolization were performed after the delivery, but the neonate died during the last such attempt.

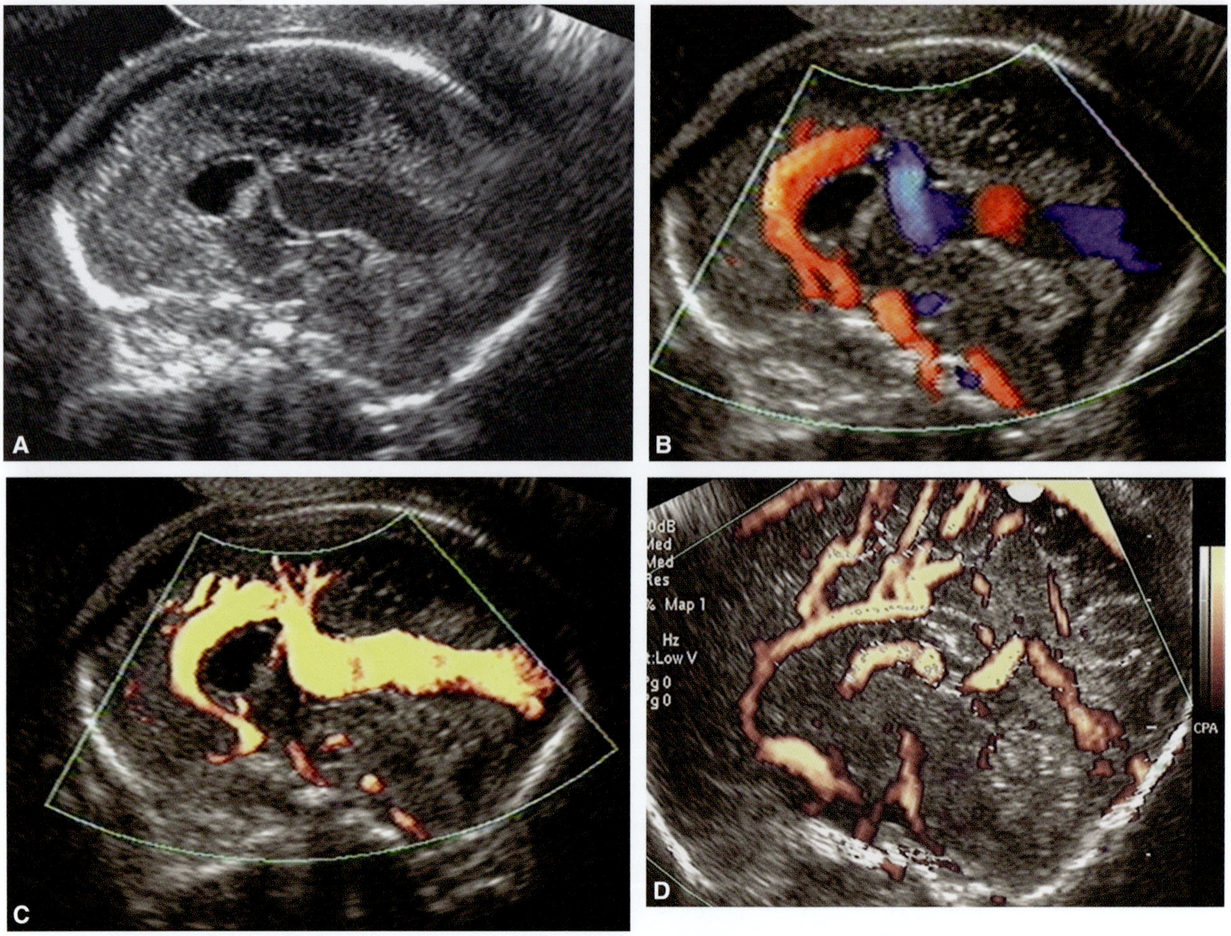


**Figure 11–11.** Aneurysm of the vein of Galen at 22 postmenstrual weeks. **(A)** Two-dimensional (2D) grayscale median plane. **(B)** 2D color Doppler median plane. **(C)** 2D power Doppler median plane. **(D)** 2D power Doppler median plane of a normal vascular pattern for comparison.

of the cyst; of those children with temporal cysts, 93% had full recovery or minimal deficit, and none died, versus 64% of patients with cysts in other locations did well, and 16% died.

## INTRAVENTRICULAR CYST

Choroid plexus cysts (CPCs) are the most common type of intraventricular cystic lesion.

### Synonyms

None

### Definition

This is a fluid-filled cystic space that accumulates within the choroid plexus.

### Incidence

CPC is a common finding during the second trimester of pregnancy, with a reported incidence of 0.95% (range 0.18–3.6%) of all fetuses scanned.[47–54] CPCs are usually not diagnosed before 17 to 18 postmenstrual weeks, and in the majority of cases, do resolve by 26 postmenstrual weeks.

### Pathogenesis

The choroid plexus is responsible for the production of CSF. CPCs are thought to result from filling of the neuroepithelial folds with CSF. At 6 to 7 postmenstrual weeks, the choroid plexus starts developing in the roof of the fourth ventricle, next in the lateral ventricle, and then in the third ventricle, as fingerlike projections of neuroepithelium into the ventricles, creating choroidal villi. The choroid plexus grows rapidly and by 9 postmenstrual weeks fills 75% of the cavity of the lateral ventricle. Portions of the epithelium are pinched off and become either tubules or cysts lined with neuroepithelium within the choroidal matrix. By the 20th week, the choroid plexus has achieved its adult appearance.[48–50] The choroid plexus cyst may be unilateral or bilateral and vary in size, although they tend to be < 10 mm in diameter. Resolution of the cysts is frequently seen regardless of the fetal karyotype.

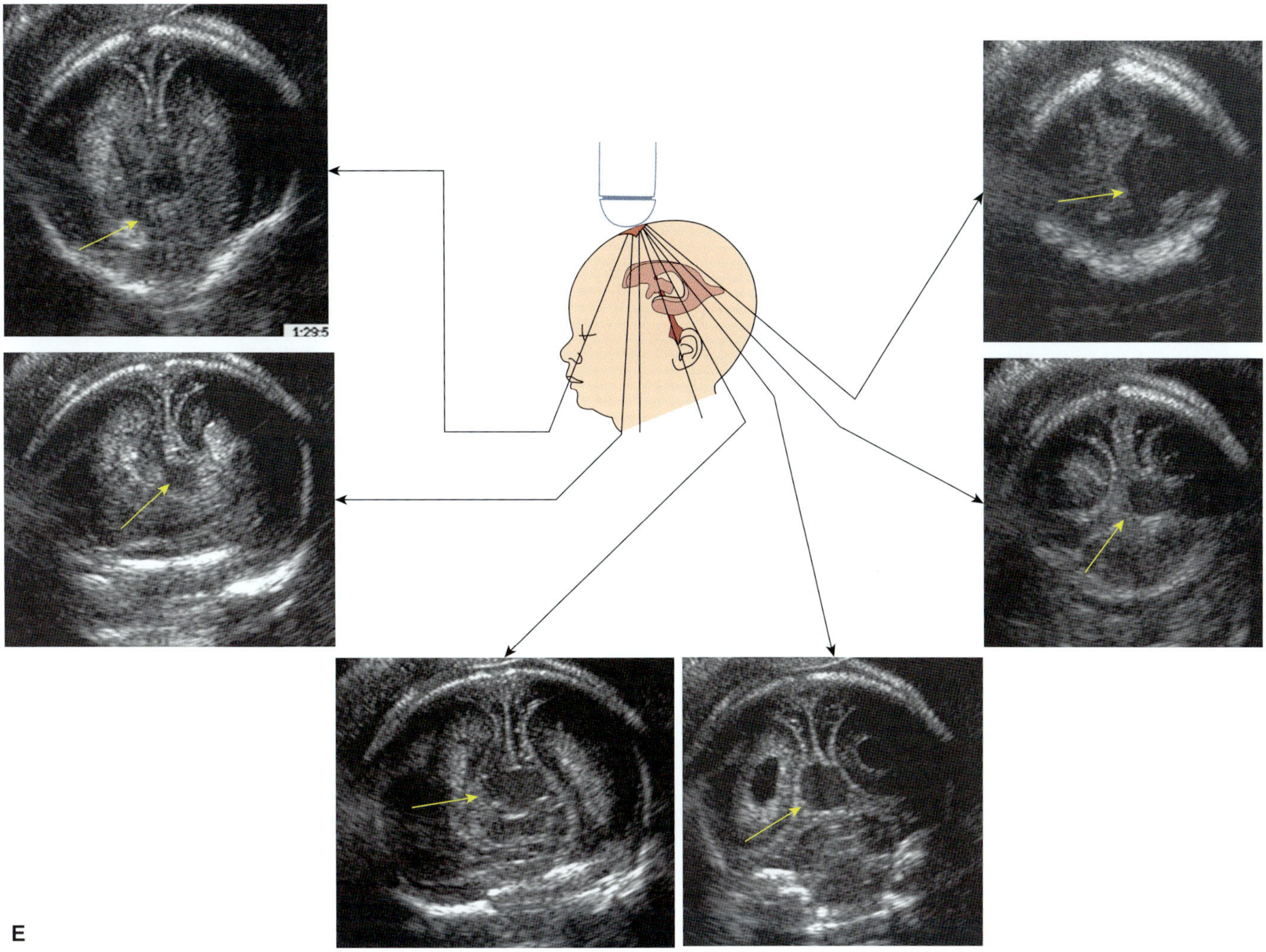


**Figure 11–11.** *(continued)* **(E)** Serial coronal 2D grayscale images of the pathology.

## Etiology

The etiology of CPC is not well understood, as most fetuses who have CPC do not have any other structural or chromosomal malformation. However, the presence of this finding, especially in conjunction with additional sonographic abnormalities, has been associated with trisomy 18; in fact, as many as 50% of the fetuses with trisomy 18 may have a choroid plexus cyst. In addition, choroid plexus cysts have been reported in association with cri du chat (5p-) syndrome and mosaic trisomy 9.[51–55] A possible association between CPC and trisomy 21 has been ruled out by almost all well-designed studies.[56]

## Pathology

Arachnoid cysts are generated by splitting of the arachnoid membrane which is then reinforced by a thick layer of collagen to result in a cyst. They are lined with a layer of meringothelial cells. They may be unilocular or multilocular.

## Associated Anomalies

Most CPCs are isolated findings in normal fetuses. Nevertheless, the detection of CPC mandates a meticulous targeted scan to look for other malformations, in particular those that are seen in fetuses with trisomy 18.[57] These anomalies include congenital heart malformations (more commonly ventricular septal defect, polyvalvular dysplasia, bicuspid aortic or pulmonary valves, and coarctation of the aorta), brain anomalies (eg, holoprosencephaly, meningomyelocele, Arnold-Chiari malformation, abnormal gyration, and hydrocephaly), facial anomalies (eg, low-set or malformed ears, micrognathia, and cleft palate), renal abnormalities (eg, horseshoe kidney, hydroureter, and hydronephrosis), skeletal anomalies (eg, overlapping fingers, rockerbottom feet, and clubfoot), nuchal thickening, cystic hygroma, and single umbilical artery.[54,58,59] Most investigators believe that cyst size or laterality is not an indication of an associated chromosomal anomaly and that all CPCs warrant similar investigation.

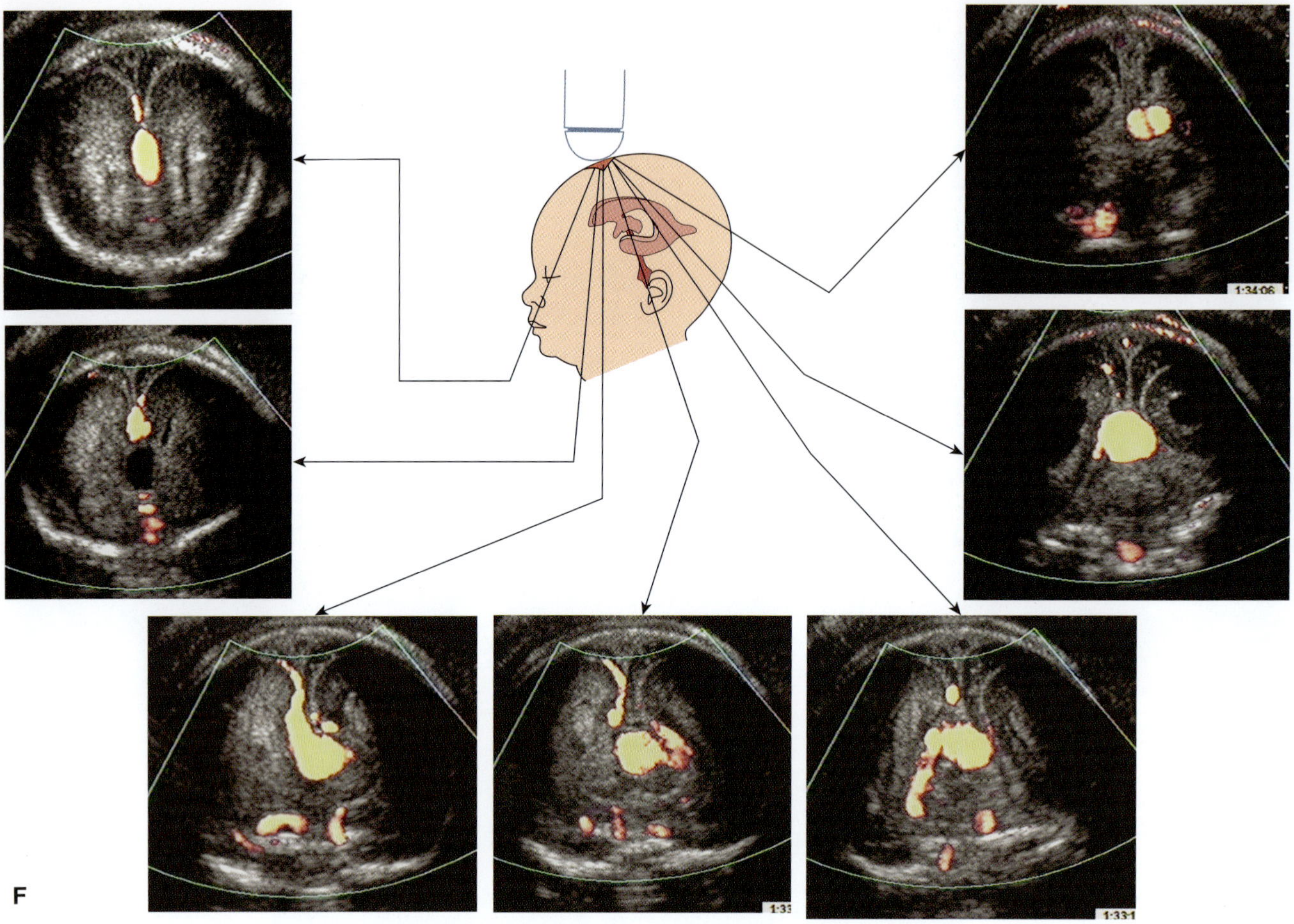


**Figure 11–11.** *(continued)* **(F)** Serial coronal 2D power Doppler images of the pathology.

## Risk of Recurrence

Most of these lesions resolve spontaneously and are not associated with an abnormal fetal condition and thus do not recur in subsequent pregnancies. Even in cases in which CPCs are associated with trisomy 18, they are mostly sporadic, and the risk of recurrence in subsequent gestations is not thought to be significantly higher. Trisomy 18 is generally a nonrecurrent chromosomal anomaly, and unlike trisomy 21, chromosome 18 is not acrosomal and thus is not frequently involved in unbalanced translocations. However, rare familial translocations have a higher recurrence risk, depending on the specific translocation.

## Sonographic Diagnosis

The sonographic appearance of a choroid plexus cyst is that of a sonolucent structure within the hyperechogenic choroid plexus. The CPCs are usually small, measuring <10 mm in size, with a range of 3 to 20 mm. Their borders are well delineated and are located within the choroid plexus; they may be unilateral or bilateral and contain debris or other small cystlike structures.[50,52,60–64] Several examples are presented in Figures 11–14, 11–15, and 11–16. Although most CPCs are isolated findings in normal fetuses, the detection of a CPC mandates a meticulous targeted scan to look for other malformations, as we previously described.

## Differential Diagnosis

The differential diagnosis of CPC includes: epidermoid cysts, colloid cysts, focal porencephaly and arachnoid cysts. Another entity that may results in an intraventricular cyst is choroid plexus hemorrhage, which has a hyperechogenic appearance in the first 72 hours, after which the cyst becomes less echogenic as the blood clot dissolves.[1] Choroid plexus papilloma can also present as a cystic structure in a choroid plexus.

## Implications for Targeted Examination

The detection of a choroid plexus cyst is an indication to perform a targeted detailed sonographic evaluation looking for other intracranial and extracranial anomalies, with particular attention to the systems involved in cases of trisomy 18. Follow-up until the CPC disappears

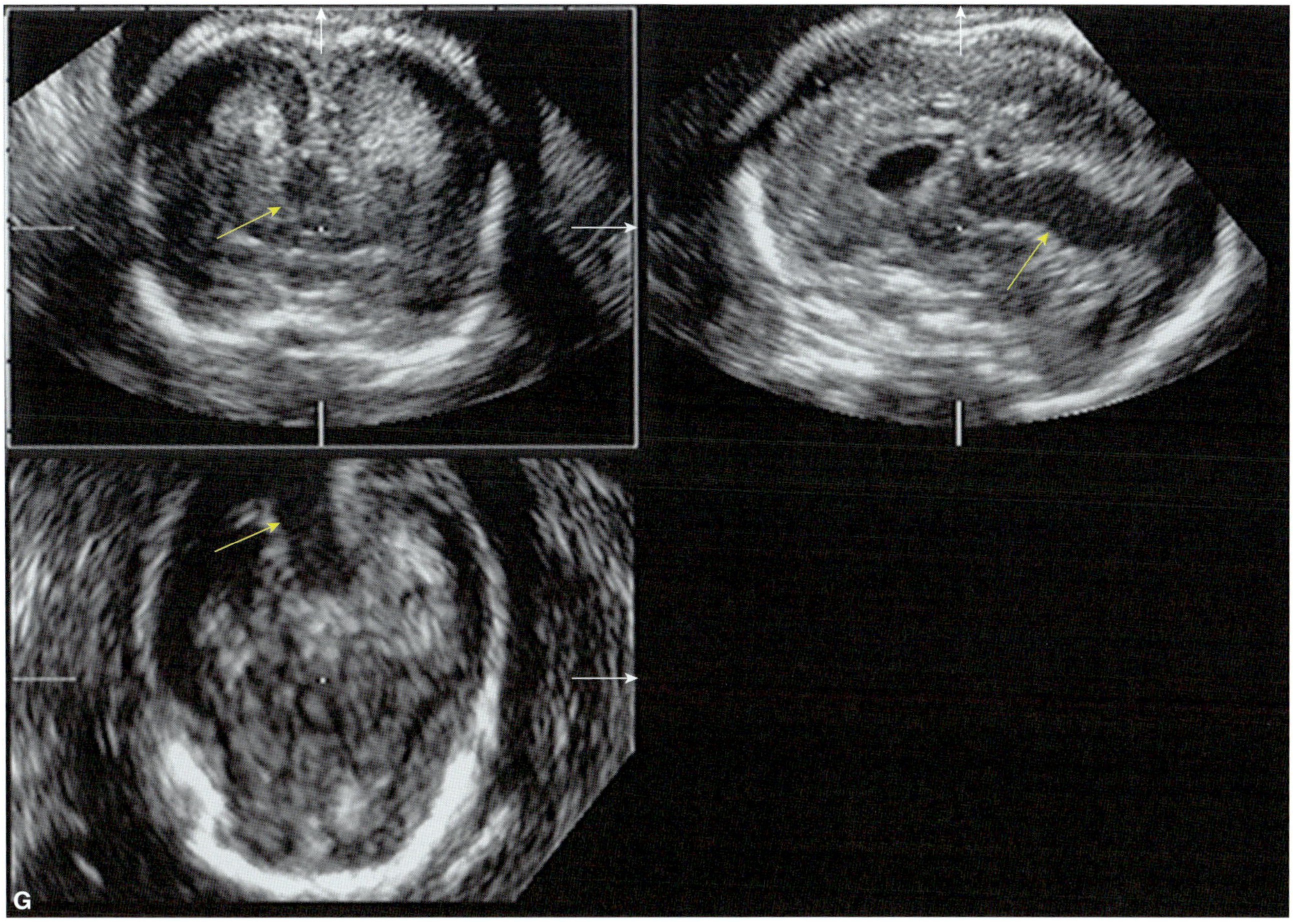


**Figure 11–11.** *(continued)* **(G)** 3D grayscale multiplanar views of the pathology. The arrows point to the dilated vein.

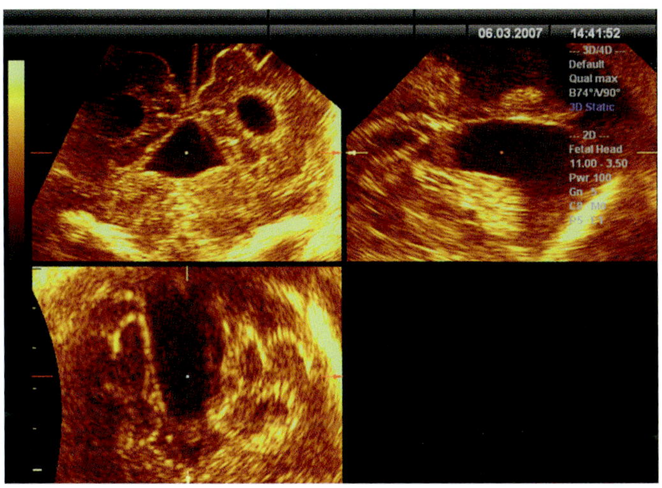


**Figure 11–12.** 3D orthogonal display of a posterior fossa arachnoid cyst in a fetus at 22 postmenstrual weeks. Note the misleading axial section (*lower image*) with the widely displaced cerebellar hemispheres. However, the median plane (*upper right image*) clearly demonstrates the intact but anteriorly displaced vermis and the pressure on the medulla.

may be indicated because of the rare possibility of an obstructive hydrocephaly.[65]

## Prognosis

These cysts are usually asymptomatic and benign. They commonly resolve by the midtrimester (26 weeks) and have been associated with both a normal and an abnormal fetal karyotype.[61,62,64,66–68] Similarly, the number of cysts, bilaterality, and size are not thought to be associated with an increased risk of chromosomal abnormality. Failure to resolve after 25 to 26 weeks' gestation does not alter the prognosis, but these patients should be followed because of the extremely rare possibility of ventricular obstruction with the development of ventriculomegaly due to obstruction of the foramen of Monro.

## Obstetric Management

Management of pregnancies with a choroid plexus cyst has been a subject of great controversy, with several studies with conflicting data regarding the association of isolated CPC and trisomy 18. Subsequently, a wide

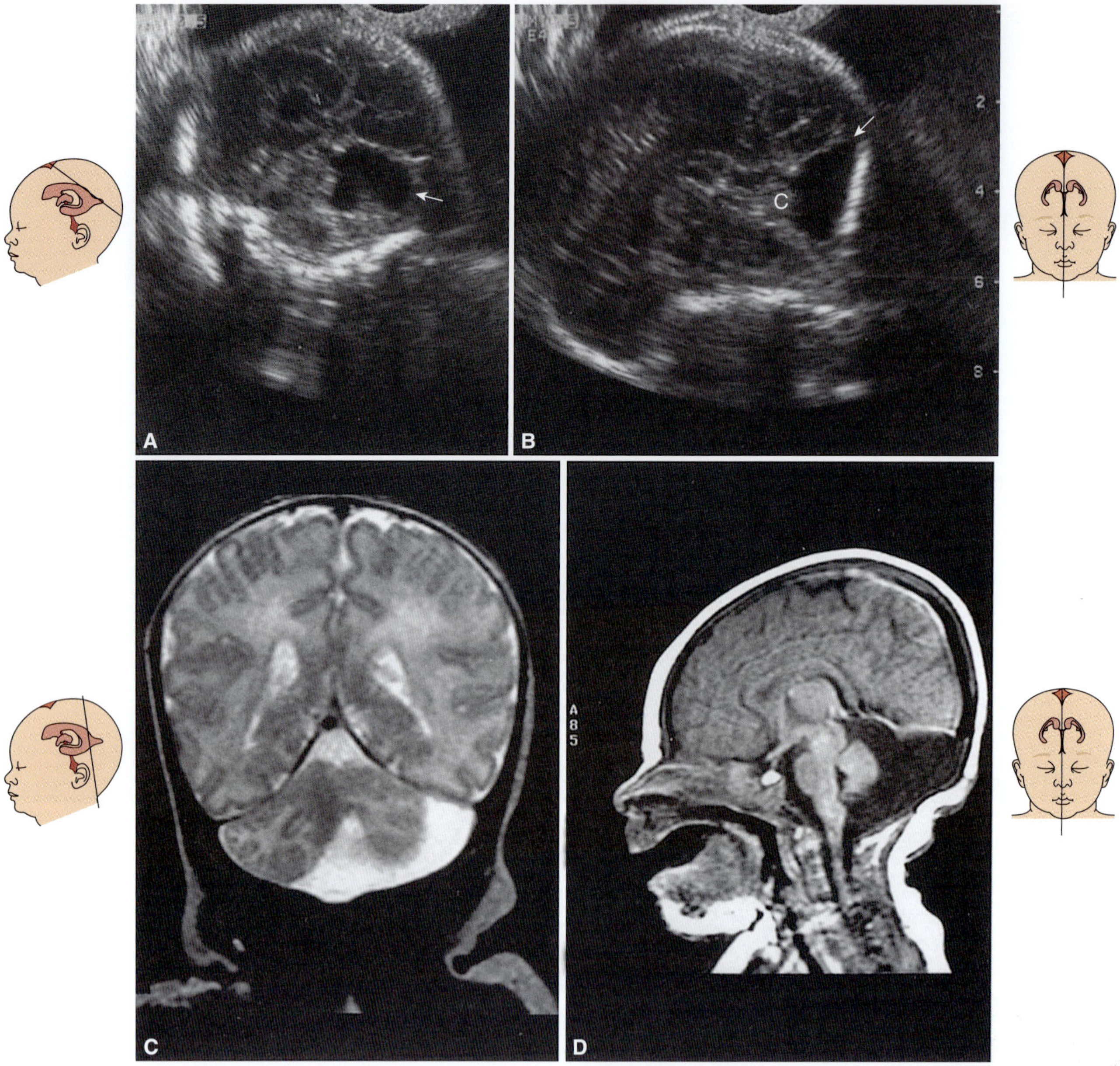


**Figure 11–13.** A large posterior fossa (mainly to the left) arachnoid cyst of a fetus at 28 postmenstrual weeks. **(A)** Occipital–1 section showing the cystic structure (*white arrow*). **(B)** Median section showing the normal-appearing midline structures, as well as the sonolucent structure (*white arrow*) displacing the cerebellum (C). The lesion was followed up until delivery occurred. **C, D.** MRI of the neonate. **(C)** Coronal image of the posterior fossa showing what appeared to be a cerebellar arachnoid cyst displacing both lobes of the cerebellum. **(D)** Median image of the brain clearly showing the cystic structure in the posterior fossa with displacement of the cerebellum and midbrain. The diagnosis of arachnoid cyst was arrived at because there was minimal deformity of the vermis, which is the mark of Dandy-Walker malformation. The fourth ventricle is of normal size but slightly pushed by the increasing cerebrospinal fluid (CSF) pressure. The lateral and third ventricles were of appropriate size. There was no evidence of hemorrhage.

range of clinical practices have emerged regarding the need to check the fetal karyotype or inform patients of such a finding when it is indeed isolated. When a fetus with CPC has other malformations or a soft sonographic marker, there is no doubt that genetic counseling is indicated, and genetic testing should be offered. The disagreement pertains to the need for genetic counseling and fetal karyotyping in cases in which the CPC is an isolated finding. Some authors recommend that all patients should be offered genetic testing because the experience, equipment, and/or ability of all sonographers or sonologists may not be equal, and some less experienced operators may miss an associated malformation.[47,50,58,64,67,69–72] Other authors believe that only in the presence of an associated congenital anomaly is genetic testing justified and that invasive testing is not indicated for isolated CPC.[54,59,61,73] Kupferminc et al[58] reported the risk of chromosomal abnormality in cases of isolated choroid plexus cyst to be 1:25. In their series of 98 cases of isolated CPC, 4 abnormal karyotypes were found among 75 women

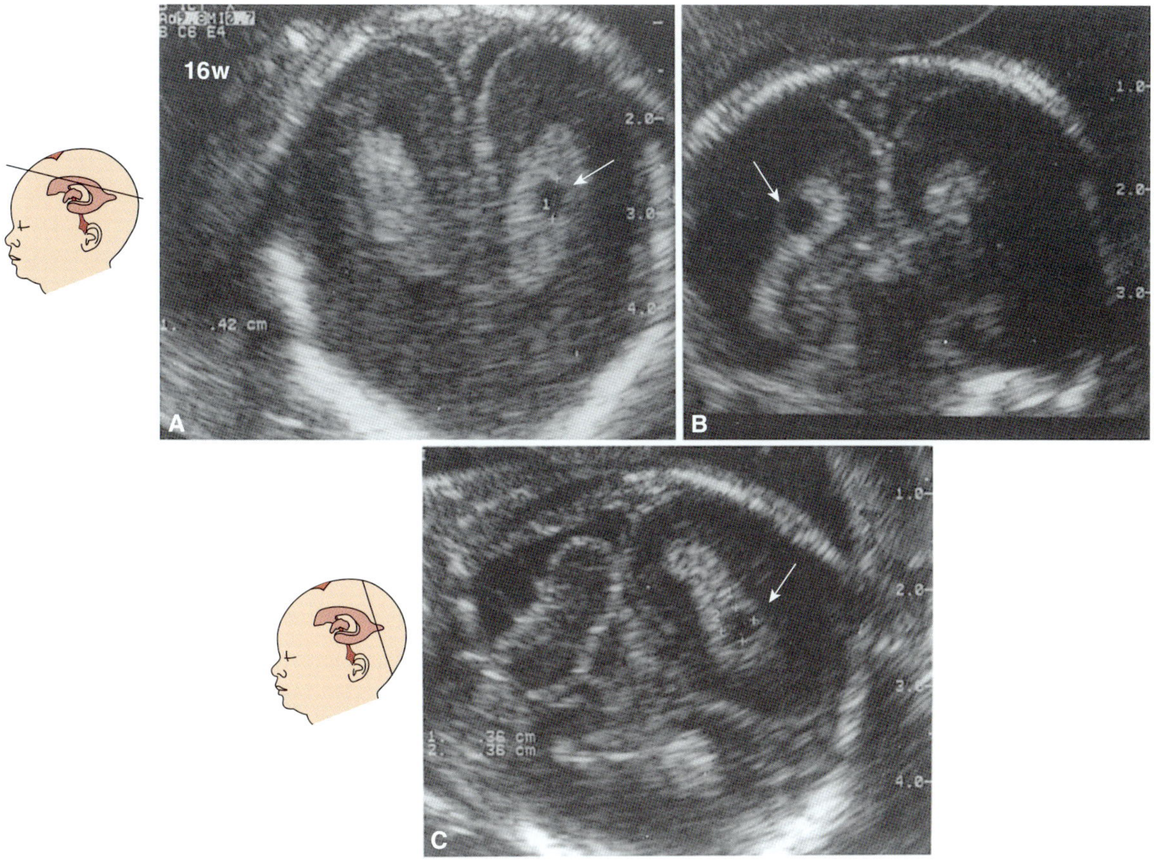


**Figure 11–14.** Routine structural evaluation at 16 postmenstrual weeks revealed a unilateral choroid plexus cyst measuring 0.4 × 0.36 × 0.36 cm. The white arrow points to the small choroid plexus cyst. **(A)** "Horizontal" section. **(B)** Midcoronal–3 section. **(C)** Occipital–1 section.

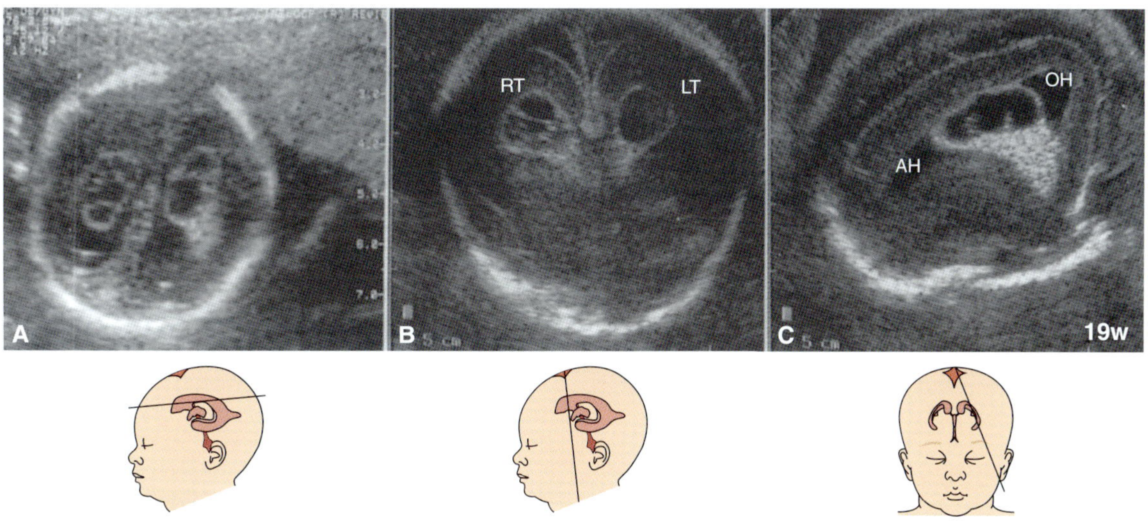


**Figure 11–15.** Three different views of bilateral and septated choroid plexus cysts at 19 postmenstrual weeks. **(A)** "Horizontal" section. **(B)** Midcoronal–1 section. **(C)** Oblique–1 section showing the normal anterior horn (AH) and posterior horn (OH). The neonate was normal.

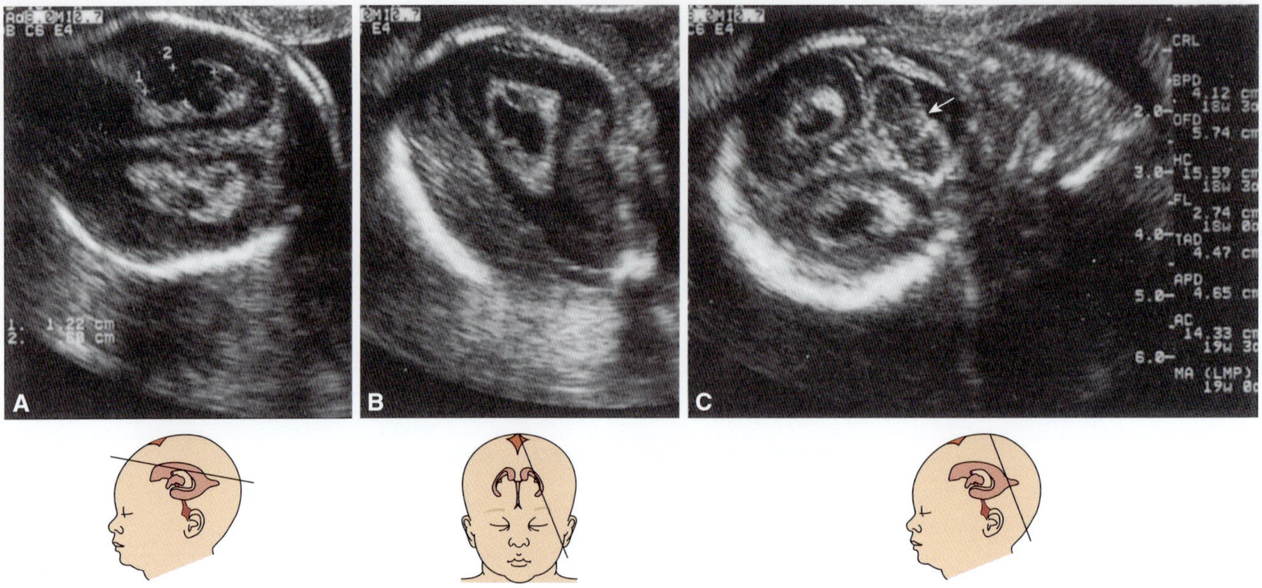


**Figure 11–16.** Three views of bilateral choroid plexus cysts at 19 postmenstrual weeks. **(A)** "Horizontal" section, with the largest cyst measuring 1.2 × 2.6 cm. **(B)** Occipital–2 section. **(C)** Occipital–1 section depicting both posterior horns and the cerebellum with the normal vermis (*white arrow*). At 24 postmenstrual weeks, the choroid plexus on the left side was no longer apparent, and all the lateral ventricle measurements were within the normal limits. At 29 postmenstrual weeks, the left choroid plexus cyst disappeared. A repeated scan at 33 postmenstrual weeks showed normal brain anatomy. The neonate was normal.

who elected to have amniocentesis. Of the four abnormal karyotypes, three were Down syndrome (trisomy 21) and one trisomy 18.[58] Gross et al[54] subsequently reported on the risk of trisomy 18 in cases of isolated choroid plexus cyst. Using a meta-analysis and their own cases, they were able to calculate a risk of trisomy 18 in cases of isolated choroid plexus to be 1:374.[54]

It is our practice to inform the patient of this finding and to incorporate it into our counseling, which is based on the patient's a priori risk of fetal trisomy. We do not recommend invasive testing for fetal karyotyping in cases of isolated CPC in which other fetal anomalies or soft sonographic markers were excluded and first and/or second trimester screening tests were normal.

## INTRAPARENCHYMAL CYST

Intraparenchymal cystic structures may result from different insults, such as hemorrhage, ischemia, infection, and tumor. The prognosis depends primarily on the etiology, location, and size of the lesion and the presence or absence of associated anomalies.

### Periventricular Pseudocyst

#### Definition

A small intraparenchymal periventricular cystic lesion that is not lined by epithelium and lacks a real cyst wall (i.e. periventricular pseudocyst).

#### Synonyms

Germinolysis, periventricular cyst.

#### Incidence

This finding is uncommon during the ultrasonographic evaluation of the fetus; however, the incidence is ~1% among newborns in the general population and as high as 3% in newborns admitted to the intensive care unit.[74–76]

#### Pathogenesis

The pathogenesis of periventricular pseudocysts is unclear, as well as the exact timing in which it occurs. The latter is probably related to the specific etiology or precipitating exposure. Pathologic examination of such lesions detected that the pseudocysts are lined with macrophages, suggesting the process of prior malacia, whereas others show positive staining for iron pigment, suggesting prior hemorrhage.

#### Etiology

Periventricular pseudocysts are thought to be the result of antenatal cystic matrix regression or germinolysis and are probably the outcome of hemorrhage or microinfarction of the germinal matrix. The most common etiology associated with these findings is infection with cytomegalovirus (CMV). Other, less common etiologies are other TORCH infections (toxoplasmosis, other infections, rubella, herpes simplex virus), cardiac malformations, chromosomal microdeletion (4p-), and metabolic or mitochondrial disorders.[1]

#### Associated Anomalies

Other anomalies or sonographic findings that can be detected in association with periventricular pseudocysts

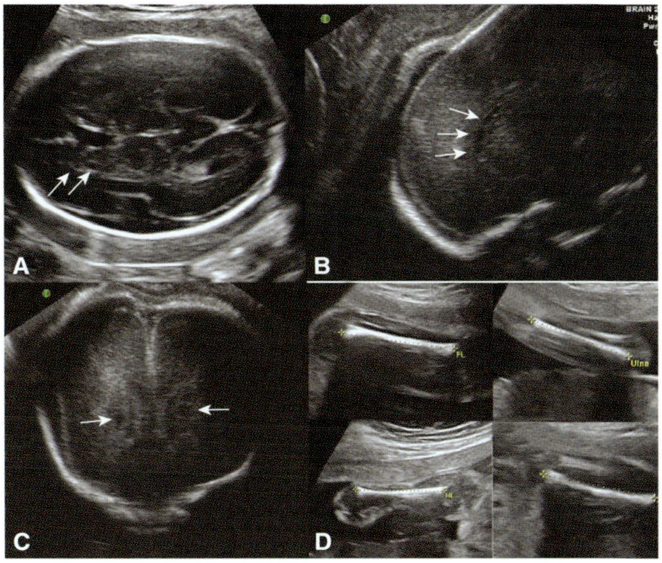


**Figure 11–17.** Periventricular pseudocysts (*arrows* in **A–C**) in a fetus with suspected skeletal dysplasia (**D**) at 24 weeks' gestation. Note that the cysts are difficult to visualize in the transabdominal axial image (**A**).

are those characteristic for CMV infection. These findings include intraparenchymal calcifications, ventriculomegaly, large cisterna magna, intraventricular adhesions, periventricular cysts, abnormal sulcation, hypoplastic corpus callosum, and liver calcifications.[77]

## Risk of Recurrence

Periventricular pseudocysts[78–85] are generally sporadic and do not recur in future pregnancies. Rare exceptions are cases associated with hereditary metabolic or mitochondrial disorders.

## Sonographic Diagnosis

The prenatal sonographic diagnosis of periventricular pseudocysts has been described by Malinger et al.[78] Based on their experience, these lesions could be suspected and at times detected using the traditional abdominal axial scanning planes (Figure 11–17). However, transvaginal, high-frequency scan of the fetal brain in the coronal and sagittal planes provided additional information and helped the authors to distinguish these lesions from periventricular leukomalacia (Figure 11–18).

Periventricular pseudocysts are usually located in the germinal matrix, in the caudothalamic groove, caudate nucleus, or lateral aspect of the frontal horns of the lateral ventricles[76] below the level of the roof of the lateral ventricles.[77] The cysts may be unilateral or bilateral, as well as unilocular or multilocular. Our experience shows that large cysts, even when isolated, may carry a poorer prognosis than smaller ones.[79]

The role of MRI in the diagnosis of periventricular pseudocyst is unclear. In one series describing five cases of periventricular pseudocysts that were confirmed by high-resolution transvaginal neurosonography by an experienced examiner, MRI did not diagnose the pseudocysts in two cases.[78] The authors hypothesized that this was due to the small size of the pseudocyst or the thin wall and its proximity to the ventricle. The benefit of doing MRI in such cases is its ability to better depict brain migrational anomalies that may coexist. Therefore, the authors concluded that an MRI should be performed in every case of periventricular pseudocyst in order to rule out additional pathologies and provide further reassurance.[78]

## Differential Diagnosis:

1. The complete differential diagnosis is displayed in Table 11–1; however, the most difficult sonographic distinction is between periventricular pseudocyst and periventricular leukomalacia, which carry a significantly worse prognosis (Figure 11–18). Periventricular

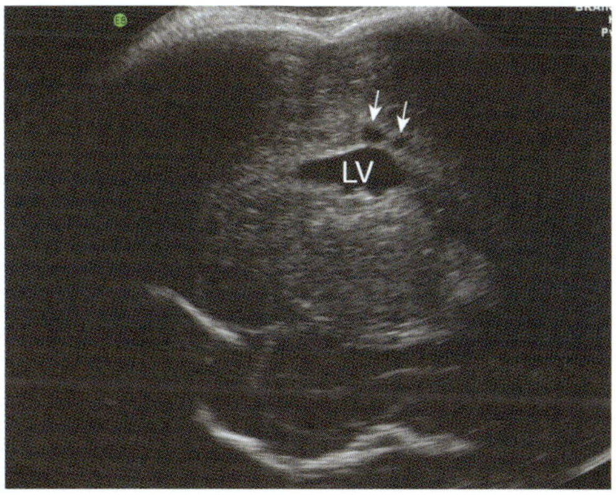


**Figure 11–18.** Periventricular leukomalacia (*arrows*) in a fetus at 31 weeks of gestation referred for evaluation because of mild asymmetric ventriculomegaly. The cysts are placed on the roof of the lateral ventricle instead of in the germinal matrix or caudate nuclei, as seen in patients with periventricular pseudocysts.

leukomalacia or white matter necrosis, is associated with prematurity and is detected mostly in preterm neonates, but it has also been detected in term neonates after a hypoxic-ischemic event. Its incidence is not clear and depends on the population that is studied. The pathogenesis is thought to be focal necrosis of the periventricular white matter, which, depending on its size, may appear as a cystlike structure. There is a softening in the hemispheric white matter. On pathologic evaluation, the lesion appears as a yellow-white spot or cavity with a chalky white border. It could be single or multiple, unilateral or bilateral, and measures several millimeters. The main etiologic factors associated with periventricular leukomalacia are prematurity and intra-amniotic infection. Maternal infection during pregnancy has been associated with this lesion and was also found to be associated with the development of cerebral palsy.[80] Moreover, histologic evidence of chorioamnionitis and congenital infection–related morbidity was more common among neonates with periventricular leukomalacia. Leukomalacia typically develops in the periventricular, unmyelinated white matter, especially in the corona radiata and centrum semiovale. Thus, neonates with these findings are at increased risk of developing cerebral palsy and visual disturbances. Leukomalacia commonly extends above the external angle of the lateral ventricle, characteristically located on top of the lateral ventricles, and not on their sides, as in the case of periventricular pseudocysts.[78] Soon after the insult, irregular zones of coagulative necrosis are surrounded by rings of intense eosinophilia. Later, fragmented and swollen axons are seen at the periphery of the lesion, with microglia, reactive astrocytes, and macrophages. Alternative appearances may include cavities surrounded by gliosis and mineralized axons and vessels, as well as gliotic or microcystic parenchyma with clusters of foamy macrophages.

2. An in-depth overview of most of the intraparenchymal cystic lesions is presented in Chapter 10.
3. *Holoprosencephaly*: This anomaly is covered in Chapter 6.
4. *Porencephalic cyst*: This anomaly is reviewed in Chapter 10.
5. *Brain tumors*: This subject is covered in Chapter 13.

## Implications for Targeted Examination

The detection of periventricular pseudocysts should prompt a meticulous workup. This should include detailed neurosonography, preferably using a transvaginal, high-resolution probe scrutinizing the brain in the coronal and sagittal planes. MRI should be performed during the third trimester. In addition, 3D ultrasound may be used to display successive thin slices through the brain, allowing for a detailed evaluation for even small intraparenchymal cysts. Investigation to rule out CMV infection is extremely important, as it is thought to be the etiologic factor in a large proportion of these cases. Other infectious causes should also be ruled out. In cases that are also growth restricted, amniocentesis with fluorescent in situ hybridization for 4p-deletions is indicated. Other rare conditions may be associated with periventricular pseudocysts (Table 11–2).

## Prognosis

It is thought that isolated periventricular pseudocysts generally carry a good prognosis and do not represent leukomalacia.[75,81] In the largest series of prenatally diagnosed periventricular pseudocysts, nine fetuses were detected, of which three underwent elective termination; there was also one stillbirth at 31 postmenstrual weeks, one neonatal death, and four fetuses who demonstrated normal development.[78] Further experience has shown that isolated large cysts may be associated with prenatally unrecognized or difficult to recognize pathologic conditions.[79]

**Table 11–2. PERIVENTRICULAR PSEUDOCYSTS: DIFFERENTIAL DIAGNOSIS AND EVALUATION**

| Etiology | Associated Findings | Diagnostic Procedures |
|---|---|---|
| Cytomegalovirus[82] | Calcifications, microcephaly | Amniocentesis: PCR-CMV |
| Wolf-Hirschhorn (-4p) syndrome[83] | IUGR, "Greek helmet" face, callosal anomalies, white matter disorders | Amniocentesis: FISH |
| Zellweger syndrome[84] | Ventriculomegaly, MCD, hypokinesia, renal hyperechogenicity | Amniocentesis: peroxisomal assays, molecular screening (defective *PEX* genes) |
| Glutaric aciduria[85] | Macrocephaly, increased extra-axial spaces | DNA analysis |
| Mitochondrial diseases[86] | None | Fetal muscle biopsy? |
| Idiopathic[78] | None | None |

CMV, cytomegalovirus; FISH, fluorescence in situ hybridization; IUGR, intrauterine growth retardation; MCD, malformation of cortical development; PCR, polymerase chain reaction.

## REFERENCES


1. Malinger G, Corral-Sereño E, Lerman-Sagie T. The differential diagnosis of fetal intracranial cystic lesions. *Ultrasound Clin.* 2008;3(4):553–558.
2. Pierre-Kahn A, Sonigo P. Malformative intracranial cysts: Diagnosis and outcome. *Childs Nerv Syst.* 2003;19(7–8):477–483.
3. Vergani P, Locatelli A, Piccoli MG, et al. Ultrasonographic differential diagnosis of fetal intracranial interhemispheric cysts. *Am J Obstet Gynecol.* 1999;180(2, Pt 1):423–428.
4. Bright R. Serous cysts in the arachnoid. In: Reese, Orme, Brown, Green, eds. *Diseases of the Brain and the Nervous System.* Vol 1. London: Longman;p 1831:437–439.
5. Galassi E, Tognetti F, Gaist G, Fagioli L, Frank F, Frank G. CT scan and metrizamide CT cisternography in arachnoid cysts of the middle cranial fossa: Classification and pathophysiological aspects. *Surg Neurol.* 1982;17(5):363–369.
6. Handa J, Okamoto K, Sato M. Arachnoid cyst of the middle cranial fossa: Report of bilateral cysts in siblings. *Surg Neurol.* 1981;16(2):127–130.
7. Naidich TP, McLone DG, Radkowski MA. Intracranial arachnoid cysts. *Pediatr Neurosci.* 1985;12(2):112–122.
8. Sato K, Shimoji T, Yaguchi K, Sumie H, Kuru Y, Ishii S. Middle fossa arachnoid cyst: clinical, neuroradiological, and surgical features. *Childs Brain.* 1983;10(5):301–316.
9. Banna M. Arachnoid cysts on computed tomography. *AJR Am J Roentgenol.* 1976;127(6):979–982.
10. Chuang S, Harwood-Nash D. Tumors and cysts. *Neuroradiology.* 1986;28(5–6):463–475.
11. Langer B, Haddad J, Favre R, Frigue V, Schlaeder G. Fetal arachnoid cyst: Report of two cases. *Ultrasound Obstet Gynecol.* 1994;4(1):68–72.
12. Menezes AH, Bell WE, Perret GE. Arachnoid cysts in children. *Arch Neurol.* 1980;37(3):168–172.
13. Robinson RG. Congenital cysts of the brain: arachnoid malformations. *Prog Neurol Surg.* 1971;4:133-174.
14. Hirano A, Hirano M. Benign cysts in the central nervous system: Neuropathological observations of the cyst walls. *Neuropathology.* 2004;24(1):1–7.
15. Inoue T, Matsushima T, Fukui M, Iwaki T, Takeshita I, Kuromatsu C. Immunohistochemical study of intracranial cysts. *Neurosurgery.* 1988;23(5):576–581.
16. Malinger G, Kidron D, Schreiber L, et al. Prenatal diagnosis of malformations of cortical development by dedicated neurosonography. *Ultrasound Obstet Gynecol.* 2007;29(2):178–191.
17. Galassi E, Tognetti F, Frank F, Fagioli L, Nasi MT, Gaist G. Infratentorial arachnoid cysts. *J Neurosurg.* 1985;63(2):210–217.
18. Jones RF, Warnock TH, Nayanar V, Gupta JM. Suprasellar arachnoid cysts: Management by cyst wall resection. *Neurosurgery.* 1989;25(4):554–561.
19. Pascual-Castroviejo I, Roche MC, Martinez Bermejo A, Arcas J, Garcia Blazquez M. Primary intracranial arachnoidal cysts: A study of 67 childhood cases. *Childs Nerv Syst.* 1991;7(5):257–263.
20. Elbers SE, Furness ME. Resolution of presumed arachnoid cyst in utero. *Ultrasound Obstet Gynecol.* 1999;14(5):353–355.
21. Pilu G, Falco P, Perolo A, et al. Differential diagnosis and outcome of fetal intracranial hypoechoic lesions: Report of 21 cases. *Ultrasound Obstet Gynecol.* 1997;9(4):229–236.
22. Hogge WA, Schnatterly P, Ferguson JE, II. Early prenatal diagnosis of an infratentorial arachnoid cyst: Association with an unbalanced translocation. *Prenat Diagn.* 1995;15(2):186–188.
23. Bretelle F, Senat MV, Bernard JP, Hillion Y, Ville Y. First-trimester diagnosis of fetal arachnoid cyst: prenatal implication. *Ultrasound Obstet Gynecol.* 2002;20(4):400–402.
24. Lee TH, Shih JC, Peng SS, Lee CN, Shyu MK, Hsieh FJ. Prenatal depiction of angioarchitecture of an aneurysm of the vein of Galen with three-dimensional color power angiography. *Ultrasound Obstet Gynecol.* 2000;15(4):337–340.
25. Heling KS, Chaoui R, Bollmann R. Prenatal diagnosis of an aneurysm of the vein of Galen with three-dimensional color power angiography. *Ultrasound Obstet Gynecol.* 2000;15(4):333–336.
26. Hirsch JH, Cyr D, Eberhardt H, Zunkel D. Ultrasonographic diagnosis of an aneurysm of the vein of Galen in utero by duplex scanning. *J Ultrasound Med.* 1983;2(5):231–233.
27. Sepulveda W, Platt CC, Fisk NM. Prenatal diagnosis of cerebral arteriovenous malformation using color Doppler ultrasonography: Case report and review of the literature. *Ultrasound Obstet Gynecol.* 1995;6(4):282–286.
28. Gerards FA, Engels MA, Barkhof F, van den Dungen FA, Vermeulen RJ, van Vugt JM. Prenatal diagnosis of aneurysms of the vein of Galen (vena magna cerebri) with conventional sonography, three-dimensional sonography, and magnetic resonance imaging: Report of 2 cases. *J Ultrasound Med.* 2003;22(12):1363–1368.
29. Cassart M, Bosson N, Garel C, Eurin D, Avni F. Fetal intracranial tumors: A review of 27 cases. *Eur Radiol.* 2008;18(10): 2060–2066.
30. D'Addario V, Pinto V, Meo F, Resta M. The specificity of ultrasound in the detection of fetal intracranial tumors. *J Perinat Med.* 1998;26(6):480–485.
31. Pelkey TJ, Ferguson JE, II, Veille JC, Alston SR. Giant glioependymal cyst resembling holoprosencephaly on prenatal ultrasound: Case report and review of the literature. *Ultrasound Obstet Gynecol.* 1997;9(3):200–203.
32. Muhler MR, Hartmann C, Werner W, Meyer O, Bollmann R, Klingebiel R. Fetal MRI demonstrates glioependymal cyst in a case of sonographic unilateral ventriculomegaly. *Pediatr Radiol.* 2007;37(4):391–395.
33. Hassan J, Sepulveda W, Teixeira J, Cox PM. Glioependymal and arachnoid cysts: unusual causes of early ventriculomegaly in utero. *Prenat Diagn.* 1996;16(8):729–733.
34. Chen PY, Wu CT, Lui TN, Jung SM. Endodermal cyst presenting as a prenatally diagnosed large intracranial cyst: Case report and review of the literature. *J Neurosurg.* 2007;106(6, Suppl):506–508.
35. Jung E, Won HS, Kim SK, et al. Spontaneous resolution of prenatally diagnosed dural sinus thrombosis: A case report. *Ultrasound Obstet Gynecol.* 2006;27(5):562–565.
36. Gicquel JM, Potier A, Sitruk S, Girard N. Normal outcome after prenatal diagnosis of thrombosis of the torcular herophili. *Prenat Diagn.* 2000;20(10):824–827.
37. Laurichesse Delmas H, Winer N, Gallot D, et al. Prenatal diagnosis of thrombosis of the dural sinuses: Report of six cases, review of the literature and suggested management. *Ultrasound Obstet Gynecol.* 2008;32(2):188–198.
38. Schwartz N, Monteagudo A, Bornstein E, Timor-Tritsch IE, Zagzag D, Kudla M. Thrombosis of an ectatic torcular herophili: Anatomic localization using fetal neurosonography. *J Ultrasound Med.* 2008;27(6):989–991.
39. Robertson SJ, Wolpert SM, Runge VM. MR imaging of middle cranial fossa arachnoid cysts: Temporal lobe agenesis syndrome revisited. *AJNR Am J Neuroradiol.* 1989;10(5):1007–1010.
40. Zada G, Krieger MD, McNatt SA, Bowen I, McComb JG. Pathogenesis and treatment of intracranial arachnoid cysts in pediatric patients younger than 2 years of age. *Neurosurg Focus.* 2007; 22(2):E1.
41. Pradilla G, Jallo G. Arachnoid cysts: Case series and review of the literature. *Neurosurg Focus.* 2007;22(2):E7.
42. Crimmins DW, Pierre-Kahn A, Sainte-Rose C, Zerah M. Treatment of suprasellar cysts and patient outcome. *J Neurosurg.* Aug 2006;105(2, Suppl):107–114.
43. Yang SH, Lee KS, Sung JH, Son BC, Jeun SS, Kang JK. Surgical decompression of supratentorial arachnoid cysts in pediatric patients younger than one year. *Pediatr Neurosurg.* 2008;44(6): 465–470.
44. D'Addario V, Pinto V, Rossi AC, Pintucci A, Di Cagno L. Cavum veli interpositi cyst: Prenatal diagnosis and postnatal outcome. *Ultrasound Obstet Gynecol.* 2009;34(1):52–54.
45. Marinov M, Undjian S, Wetzka P. An evaluation of the surgical treatment of intracranial arachnoid cysts in children. *Childs Nerv Syst.* 1989;5(3):177–183.
46. Richard KE, Dahl K, Sanker P. Long-term follow-up of children and juveniles with arachnoid cysts. *Childs Nerv Syst.* Jun 1989;5(3):184-187.
47. Achiron R, Barkai G, Katznelson MB, Mashiach S. Fetal lateral ventricle choroid plexus cysts: The dilemma of amniocentesis. *Obstet Gynecol.* 1991;78(5, Pt 1):815–818.
48. Chan L, Hixson JL, Laifer SA, Marchese SG, Martin JG, Hill LM. A sonographic and karyotypic study of second-trimester fetal choroid plexus cysts. *Obstet Gynecol.* 1989;73(5, Pt 1):703–706.

49. Chinn DH, Miller EI, Worthy LM, Towers CV. Sonographically detected fetal choroid plexus cysts: Frequency and association with aneuploidy [see comments]. *J Ultrasound Med.* 1991;10(5): 255–258.
50. Chitkara U, Cogswell C, Norton K, Wilkins IA, Mehalek K, Berkowitz RL. Choroid plexus cysts in the fetus: A benign anatomic variant or pathologic entity? Report of 41 cases and review of the literature. *Obstet Gynecol.* 1988;72(2):185–189.
51. Clark SL, DeVore GR, Sabey PL. Prenatal diagnosis of cysts of the fetal choroid plexus. *Obstet Gynecol.* 1988;72(4):585–587.
52. DeRoo TR, Harris RD, Sargent SK, Denholm TA, Crow HC. Fetal choroid plexus cysts: Prevalence, clinical significance, and sonographic appearance. *Am J Roentgenol.* 1988;151(6):1179–1181.
53. Gabrielli S, Reece EA, Pilu G, et al. The clinical significance of prenatally diagnosed choroid plexus cysts. *Am J Obstet Gynecol.* 1989;160(5, Pt 1):1207–1210.
54. Gross SJ, Shulman LP, Tolley EA, et al. Isolated fetal choroid plexus cysts and trisomy 18: A review and meta-analysis. *Am J Obstet Gynecol.* 1995;172(1, Pt 1):83–87.
55. Sarno AP, Jr., Polzin WJ, Kalish VB. Fetal choroid plexus cysts in association with cri du chat (5p-) syndrome. *Am J Obstet Gynecol.* 1993;169(6):1614–1615.
56. Bromley B, Lieberman R, Benacerraf BR. Choroid plexus cysts: Not associated with Down syndrome. *Ultrasound Obstet Gynecol.* 1996;8(4):232–235.
57. Snijders RJ, Shawa L, Nicolaides KH. Fetal choroid plexus cysts and trisomy 18: Assessment of risk based on ultrasound findings and maternal age. *Prenat Diagn.* 1994;14(12):1119–1127.
58. Kupferminc MJ, Tamura RK, Sabbagha RE, Parilla BV, Cohen LS, Pergament E. Isolated choroid plexus cyst(s): An indication for amniocentesis. *Am J Obstet Gynecol.* 1994;171(4):1068–1071.
59. Nadel AS, Bromley BS, Frigoletto FD, Jr., Estroff JA, Benacerraf BR. Isolated choroid plexus cysts in the second-trimester fetus: Is amniocentesis really indicated? *Radiology.* 1992;185(2):545–548.
60. Benacerraf BR. Asymptomatic cysts of the fetal choroid plexus in the second trimester. *J Ultrasound Med.* 1987;6(8):475–478.
61. Benacerraf BR, Harlow B, Frigoletto FD, Jr. Are choroid plexus cysts an indication for second-trimester amniocentesis? *Am J Obstet Gynecol.* 1990;162(4):1001–1006.
62. Benacerraf BR, Laboda LA. Cyst of the fetal choroid plexus: a normal variant? *American Journal of Obstetrics & Gynecology.* 1989;160(2):319–321.
63. Chudleigh P, Pearce JM, Campbell S. The prenatal diagnosis of transient cysts of the fetal choroid plexus. *Prenat Diagn.* 1984;4(2): 135–137.
64. Hertzberg BS, Kay HH, Bowie JD. Fetal choroid plexus lesions: Relationship of antenatal sonographic appearance to clinical outcome. *J Ultrasound Med.* 1989;8(2):77–82.
65. Nahed BV, Darbar A, Doiron R, Saad A, Robson CD, Smith ER. Acute hydrocephalus secondary to obstruction of the foramen of monro and cerebral aqueduct caused by a choroid plexus cyst in the lateral ventricle: Case report. *J Neurosurg.* 2007;107(3 Suppl):236–239.
66. Farhood AI, Morris JH, Bieber FR. Transient cysts of the fetal choroid plexus: Morphology and histogenesis. *Am J Med Genet.* 1987;27(4):977–982.
67. Fitzsimmons J, Wilson D, Pascoe-Mason J, Shaw CM, Cyr DR, Mack LA. Choroid plexus cysts in fetuses with trisomy 18. *Obstet Gynecol.* 1989;73(2):257–260.
68. Nicolaides KH, Rodeck CH, Gosden CM. Rapid karyotyping in nonlethal fetal malformations. *Lancet.* 1986;1(8476):283–287.
69. Gabrielli S, Reece EA, Pilu G, et al. The clinical significance of prenatally diagnosed choroid plexus cysts. *Am J Obstet Gynecol.* 1989;160(5, Pt 1):1207–1210.
70. Porto M, Murata Y, Warneke LA, Keegan KA, Jr. Fetal choroid plexus cysts: An independent risk factor for chromosomal anomalies. *J Clin Ultrasound.* 1993;21(2):103–108.
71. Perpignano MC, Cohen HL, Klein VR, et al. Fetal choroid plexus cysts: Beware the smaller cyst. *Radiology.* 1992;182(3):715–717.
72. Platt LD, Carlson DE, Medearis AL, Walla CA. Fetal choroid plexus cysts in the second trimester of pregnancy: A cause for concern. *Am J Obstet Gynecol.* 1991;164(6, Pt 1):1652–1655, discussion 1655–1656.
73. Ouzounian JG, Ludington C, Chan S. Isolated choroid plexus cyst or echogenic cardiac focus on prenatal ultrasound: Is genetic amniocentesis indicated? *Am J Obstet Gynecol.* 2007;196(6):e591–593.
74. Ramenghi LA, Domizio S, Quartulli L, Sabatino G. Prenatal pseudocysts of the germinal matrix in preterm infants. *J Clin Ultrasound.* 1997;25(4):169–173.
75. Larcos G, Gruenewald SM, Lui K. Neonatal subependymal cysts detected by sonography: Prevalence, sonographic findings, and clinical significance. *AJR Am J Roentgenol.* 1994;162(4):953–956.
76. Rademaker KJ, De Vries LS, Barth PG. Subependymal pseudocysts: Ultrasound diagnosis and findings at follow-up. *Acta Paediatr.* 1993;82(4):394–399.
77. Malinger G, Lev D, Zahalka N, et al. Fetal cytomegalovirus infection of the brain: The spectrum of sonographic findings. *AJNR Am J Neuroradiol.* 2003;24(1):28–32.
78. Malinger G, Lev D, Ben Sira L, Kidron D, Tamarkin M, Lerman-Sagie T. Congenital periventricular pseudocysts: Prenatal sonographic appearance and clinical implications. *Ultrasound Obstet Gynecol.* 2002;20(5):447–451.
79. Leshinsky-Silver E, Lev D, Malinger G, et al. Leigh disease presenting in utero due to a novel missense mutation in the mitochondrial DNA-ND3. *Mol Genet Metab.* 2010;100(1):65–70.
80. Bax M, Tydeman C, Flodmark O. Clinical and MRI correlates of cerebral palsy: The European Cerebral Palsy Study. *JAMA.* 2006;296(13):1602–1608.
81. Makhoul IR, Zmora O, Tamir A, Shahar E, Sujov P. Congenital subependymal pseudocysts: Own data and meta-analysis of the literature. *Isr Med Assoc J.* 2001;3(3):178–183.
82. Malinger G, Lev D, Lerman-Sagie T. Imaging of fetal cytomegalovirus infection. *Fetal Diagn Ther.* 2011;29(2)117–126.
83. Boog G, Le Vaillant C, Collet M, et al. Prenatal sonographic patterns in six cases of Wolf-Hirschhorn (4p-) syndrome. *Fetal Diagn Ther.* 2004;19(5):421–430.
84. Mochel F, Grebille AG, Benachi A, et al. Contribution of fetal MR imaging in the prenatal diagnosis of Zellweger syndrome. *AJNR Am J Neuroradiol.* 2006;27(2):333–336.
85. Twomey EL, Naughten ER, Donoghue VB, Ryan S. Neuroimaging findings in glutaric aciduria type 1. *Pediatr Radiol.* 2003;33(12): 823–830.
86. Leshinsky-Silver E, Malinger G, Ben-Sira L, Kidron D, Cohen S, Inbar S, Bezaleli T, Levine A, Vinkler C, Lev D, Lerman-Sagie T. A large homozygous deletion in the SAMHD1 gene causes atypical Aicardi-Goutieres syndrome associated with mtDNA deletions. *Eur J Hum Genet.* 2011;19(3):287–292.

Chapter 12

# METABOLIC DISORDERS

*Asuri N. Prasad • Gustavo Malinger • Tally Lerman-Sagie*

**KEY POINTS**

1. Inborn errors of metabolism (IEMs) are rare disorders, most of them only present after delivery.
2. Several IEMs may affect the fetus, producing congenital malformations and/or brain insults.
3. Prenatal diagnosis is usually possible following the birth of an affected child; in patients without a family history, even in the presence of severe malformations, a definitive diagnosis is usually only made after delivery.
4. Biochemical tests and molecular studies are indicated in selected cases.

## INBORN ERRORS OF METABOLISM AND FETAL BRAIN DEVELOPMENT

The in utero metabolic microenvironment during embryogenesis (fetal metabolome) profoundly influences the entire range of developmental processes underlying fetal organogenesis.

Inborn errors of metabolism (IEMs) are inherited disorders with mostly single gene defects resulting in the development of enzymatic blocks within biochemical pathways, often due to the deficiency of an enzyme or cofactor. There may be secondary accumulation or formation of toxic intermediaries, as well as deficiency of critical end products necessary for cell function. The resulting changes influence the internal and external cellular microenvironment, as well as cellular homeostatic mechanisms.[1] The association of IEMs with developmental malformations has long been recognized (Figure 12–1). Following initial reports of association of callosal dysgenesis with IEMs,[2] widespread developmental abnormalities in the morphogenesis of the brain have been described.[3] A logical extension of these observed associations is the exploration of the possibilities of detection and diagnosis during the prenatal period. A majority of these conditions are usually diagnosed in postnatal life in the index case. During subsequent pregnancies, early detection and diagnosis carry the potential for early therapeutic interventions in the fetus or carefully considered decisions to terminate the pregnancy in the event of the diagnosis of an incurable disorder with no hope for a meaningful quality of life.

A variety of interactions between the planes of genome–proteome and metabolome regulate developmental processes that ultimately influence the formation and maturation of all organ systems, including the fetal brain. In early fetal life, interference with formation of the telencephalic vesicles (holoprosencephaly), dysgenesis of the corpus callosum, absence of the septi pellucidi, cerebellar dysgenesis, and abnormalities in ventricular shape (colpocephaly and single ventricle) may be visualized through targeted neurosonography. As the brain grows in complexity, abnormalities may extend to involve the gray matter (atrophy of the cortical ribbon and basal ganglia), white matter (thinning out or loss of volume, demyelination, or dysmyelination of white matter), encephaloclastic lesions (porencephalic cysts), and neuronal migration defects (pachygyria) and can be identified with the aid of high-resolution fetal magnetic resonance imaging (MRI). Neuronal loss or cell death (neurotoxic or apoptotic) is followed by wallerian (secondary axonal) degeneration, leading to atrophy and volume loss in the gray and white matter. These changes result in ventriculomegaly and a prominence of the extra-axial fluid spaces. Porencephalic cysts are seen secondary to ischemic injury following vascular occlusion and focal neuronal necrosis. Secondary processes such as failure or interference with myelination by glial cells will result in demyelination or dysmyelination.[4]

IEMs involve different biochemical/metabolic pathways, substrates, intermediary compounds, and end products. There is a large body of literature usually in the form of case reports linking individual disorders to the malformations of the nervous system during embryogenesis. For instance, disorders involving folic acid metabolism and folate deficiency states result in neural tube defects, and defects in the glycine cleavage pathway have a well-documented association with agenesis of the corpus callosum. Defects in cholesterol metabolism interfere with the development of telencephalic vesicles and appear to lead to holoprosencephaly and its variants. The cerebellum appears to be peculiarly vulnerable to the effects of metabolic perturbations. Defects of cerebellar development

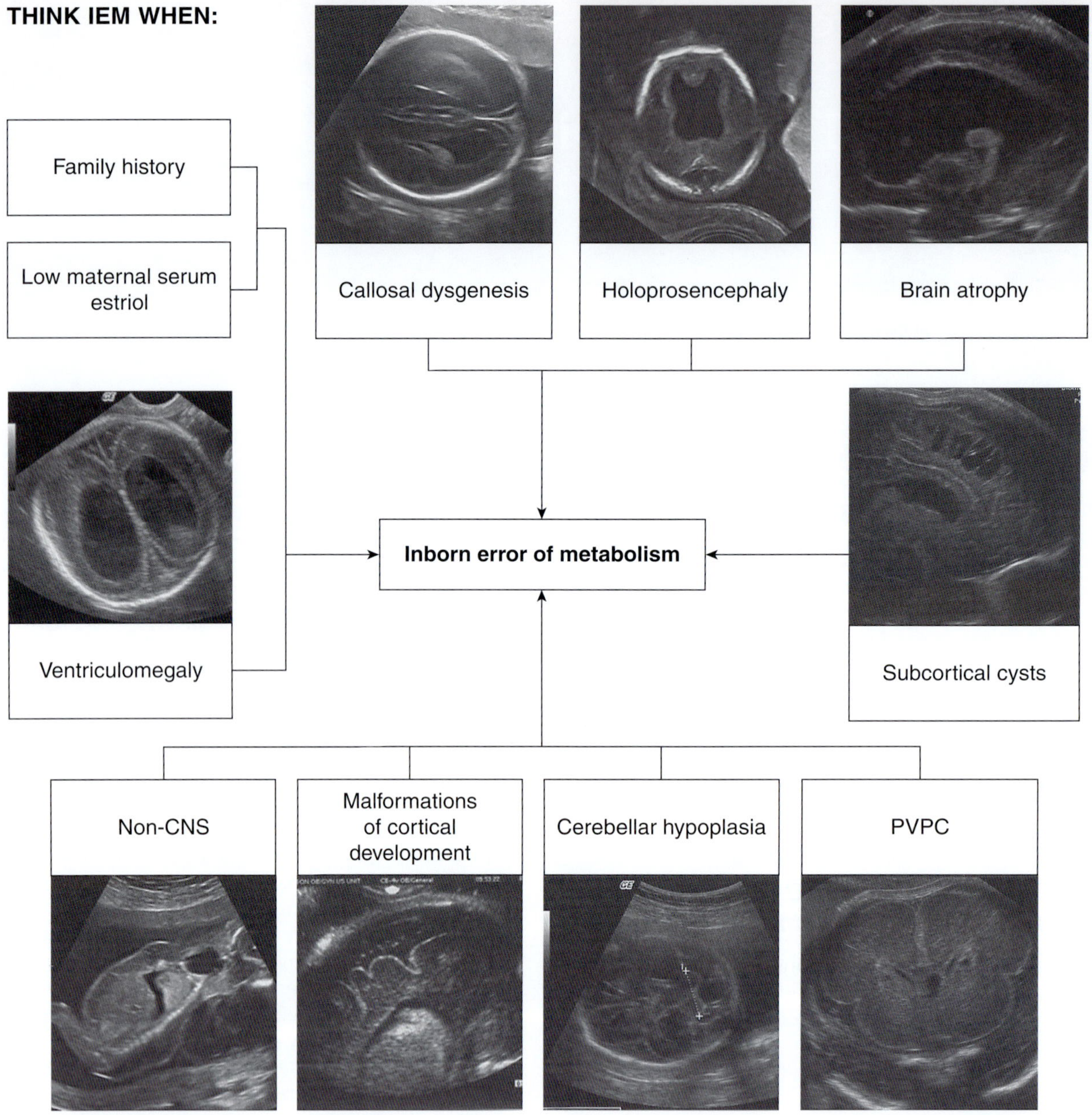


**Figure 12–1.** Markers of IEM's on fetal ultrasonography.

are associated with a variety of IEMs, such as congenital lactic acidosis, mitochondrial disorders, and disorders of glycosylation.[3]

Current technological advances in fetal ultrasonography and MRI permit visualization of the fetal brain in considerably greater detail than previously possible and enable detection of developmental malformations. Furthermore, these techniques permit a noninvasive tool to monitor serial changes over time. Recognition of specific patterns and associations with inborn errors of metabolism guide the neurologist and the metabolic specialist in targeting appropriate investigations, critical for diagnosis, treatment, and counseling.

When dealing with rare and infrequently diagnosed diseases, fetal imaging has two different goals. In families at risk, the examination should be conducted with the goal of identification of specific, predefined patterns; the examiner should be familiar with these patterns prior to the evaluation in order to target the examination accurately (Tables 12–1 and 12–2). When technical problems impair full visualization, it should be included in the report and a follow-up examination scheduled.

When one of the findings characteristic of IEMs is diagnosed during an ultrasound (US) or MRI examination, a differential diagnosis of the diseases known to be associated with this particular finding should be offered,

**Table 12–1. PATTERNS OF NERVOUS SYSTEM MALFORMATIONS IN INBORN ERRORS OF METABOLISM (IEM)**

| Inborn Error of Metabolism | Neural Tube Defects | Holoprosencephaly | Cerebellar Malformations | Hypoplastic Temporal Lobes |
|---|---|---|---|---|
| **Energy metabolism** | | | | |
| Respiratory chain enzyme deficiency | | | + | |
| Fatty acid oxidation | | | | |
| Glutaric acidemia 2 | | | + | + |
| **Folic acid metabolism** | | | | |
| Methylenetetrahydrofolate reductase deficiency | + | | | |
| **Organic aciduria** | | | | |
| Glutaric aciduria 1 | | | | + |
| Ethylmalonic aciduria | + | | | |
| **Cholesterol metabolism** | | | | |
| Smith-Lemli-Opitz | | + | | |
| **Glycoprotein metabolism** | | | | |
| Congenital disorder of glycosylation type 1a | | | + | |
| **Trace element metabolism** | | | | |
| Menkes kinky hair | | | + | |

followed by a repeat examination in search of other common anomalies known to be potentially present in the different entities (Table 12–3).

## PYRUVATE DEHYROGENASE DEFICIENCY

### Synonyms

Pyruvate dehydrogenase alpha 1 (PDHA1), pyruvate dehydrogenase complex E1 alpha (PDHCE1A), OMIM *608769.

### Definition

Pyruvate dehydrogenase alpha 1 deficiency is one of the most commont causes of congenital lactic acidosis. Mutations in genes coding for proteins involving the pyruvate dehydrogenase (PDH) complex (OMIM *300502 E1; EC 4.1.1.1) are associated with primary lactic acidosis presenting in the infantile period. The enzyme is a multienzyme complex with three components: pyruvate dehydrogenase (E1), dihydrolipoamide acetyltransferase (E2), and lipoamide dehydrogenase (E3).

The disorder is known to be associated with central nervous system (CNS) malformations in the prenatal period.[5,6]

### Etiology

The PDHCE1A complex catalyzes the first step involved in the conversion of pyruvate to acetyl coenzyme A (CoA). Mutations (occur de novo) in the gene coding for the alpha subunit of the PDHE1 component lead to an X-linked form of PDH deficiency.[7–11]

### Pathology

Infants present with either a metabolic form with severe lactic acidosis and encephalopathy at birth or in a neurologic form that may be detected prenatally on account of the associated anomalies. The phenotypic severity is linked to the underlying mutation and residual enzyme activity. Severe mutations tend to be lethal in male infants, whereas females present with brain abnormalities with minimal to no lactic acidosis. Milder mutations in males present with lactic acidosis and a neurologic phenotype, whereas females may be asymptomatic, often leading to a delay in diagnosis. The neuropathologic features associated include cerebral atrophy, cavitating lesions in the white matter and deep gray nuclei, callosal dysgenesis of varying severity, absence of the pyramids, heterotopias of the olivary complex, and abnormalities of the dentate nuclei.[12]

**Table 12–2. PATTERNS OF CEREBRAL MALFORMATIONS ASSOCIATED WITH SPECIFIC IEM**

| Inborn Error of Metabolism | Pachygyria | Polymicrogyria | Cortical Heterotopia | Cerebellar Dysplasia | Olivary Nuclei Dysplasia | Dysgenetic Corpus Callosum |
|---|---|---|---|---|---|---|
| **Peroxisomal disorders** | | | | | | |
| Zellweger | + | + | + | + | + | + |
| Infantile Refsum | | | | + | | + |
| Pseudoneonatal adrenoleukodystrophy | | | | + | + | + |
| Bifunctional enzyme deficiency | + | + | + | + | + | |
| Chondrodysplasia punctata | | | | | + | |
| **Energy metabolism** | | | | | | |
| Pyruvate dehydrogenase deficiency | + | | + | + | + | + |
| Fumarase deficiency | | + | + | + | | + |
| Fatty acid oxidation defects | | | | | | |
| Carnitine palmitoyl transferase 2 | | | + | | | |
| Glutaric acidemia 2 | + | | + | | | + |
| **Aminoacidurias** | | | | | | |
| Maternal phenylketonuria | | | | | | + |
| Nonketotic hyperglycinemia | + | | | | | + |
| Organic aciduria | | | | | | |
| 3-Hydroxyisobutyric aciduria | + | | | | | + |
| **Cholesterol metabolism** | | | | | | |
| Smith-Lemli-Opitz | + | + | + | + | | + |
| Trace elements | | | | | | |
| Menkes kinky hair syndrome | | | + | + | | + |
| **Glycoprotein metabolism** | | | | | | |
| Congenital disorder of glycosylation 1a | | | | | | + |

**Table 12–3. SPECIFIC ULTRASONOGRAPHIC MARKERS FLAGGING DISTINCT IEM DISORDERS**

| Fetal Ultrasonographic Features | Comments on Significance in Relationship to Inborn Errors of Metabolism |
|---|---|
| Intrauterine growth retardation | Nonspecific, wide differential, represents global effects of metabolic perturbation on the fetus |
| Fetal akinesia/hypokinesia | Indicative of hypotonia, weakness in utero |
| Anomalies in head size: microcephaly and macrocephaly | Indicates poor cerebral growth, can be severe in Amish microcephaly, macrocrania a feature of glutaric aciduria type I |
| Forebrain development differentiation, midline anomalies | Holoprosencephaly is a feature of Smith-Lemli-Opitz syndrome |
| Ventriculomegaly | Nonspecific feature indicates raised intracranial pressure, volume loss in the white matter |
| Callosal abnormalities | Callosal dysgenesis is a marker for several IEMs (eg, NKH, PDH deficiency) |
| Post fossa abnormalities | Cerebellar atrophy that is progressive is a feature of defects in energy metabolism, cerebellar hypoplasia is associated with CDG type 1a |
| Neural tube segmentation | Disorders of folate metabolism |
| Cerebral atrophy and calcifications | Nonspecific, indicates progressive disease as a consequence of neuronal loss/drop out, seen in mitochondrial disorders |
| Intracranial hemorrhage, effusions | Subdural hemorrhages and effusions associated with organic acidemias (eg, GA1) |
| Stroke/encephaloclastic lesions (porencephaly), | Nonspecific association with defects in energy metabolism, sulfite oxidase deficiency |
| Schizencephalic clefts lissencephaly/ pachygyria | These are more difficult to detect on US alone, may need fetal MRI, and follow-up postnatal imaging studies |

CDG, carbohydrate-deficient glycoprotein; IEM, inborn error of metabolism; MRI, magnetic resonance imaging; NKH, nonketotic hyperglycinemia; PDH, pyruvate dehydrogenase; US, ultrasound

## Recurrence Risk

PDHCE1A is inherited as a mendelian X-linked condition. Both males and heterozygous females carrying one copy of the defective gene tend to be symptomatic.

## Diagnosis

Prenatal US examination could be useful in identification of ventriculomegaly, callosal dysgenesis, and posterior fossa abnormalities usually recognized in the newborn (Figure 12–2). MRI may bring a higher level of resolution to the abnormalities involving the brainstem and cerebellum (Figure 12–3). Lactate elevation in the brain can be demonstrated on magnetic resonance spectroscopy.[13] Although enzyme activity in cultured fibroblasts is typically low, activity levels may be normal in heterozygous females; hence a reliable diagnosis requires a search for mutations in the gene coding for the PDHE1alpha subunit and should include DNA sequencing.[14]

## Differential Diagnosis

The principal differential diagnoses include mitochondrial disorders of the respiratory chain, which can also present with congenital lactic acidosis. With PDHCE1A deficiency, lactate/pyruvate ratios are normal in the cerebrospinal fluid (CSF), a distinctive feature in comparison to disorders of the respiratory chain.

### Implications for Targeted Examination

When there is a history of a previous child with a neonatal presentation of PDH deficiency, a targeted exam should be obtained from 18 weeks' gestation to monitor the development of the corpus callosum. Sonograms should be obtained every 2 to 3 weeks to monitor development of ventriculomegaly or periventricular cysts.

### Implications for Sonographic Screening

The changes in the brain in the form of ventriculomegaly and brain atrophy can be detected as early as 28 postmenstrual weeks.[15] The occurrence of structural brain anomalies is influenced by gender and the severity of the mutation. Ultrasonography may be useful in the detection of structural anomalies by the end of the second trimester.

## MRI Diagnosis

MRI of a fetus whose mother had a history of two prior infants affected with pyruvate dehydrogenase deficiency demonstrated ventriculomegaly, increased extra-axial CSF, and posterior fossa abnormalities (Figure 12–4). Magnetic

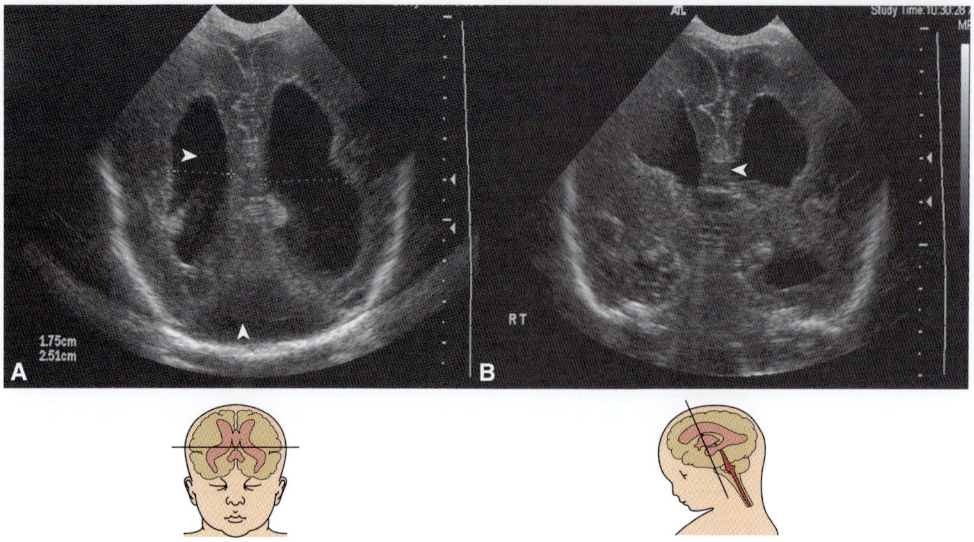

**Figure 12–2.** Axial sections on cranial ultrasound (US) in an infant with pyruvate dehydrogenase deficiency on day 1 of life. **(A)** Ventriculomegaly and posterior fossa cyst (*arrowheads*) can be identified. **(B)** Callosal dysgenesis (*arrowhead*) and unusual shape of the frontal horns are also identified. Note the abnormal sulcation in both figures.

resonance spectroscopy was normal. The diagnosis of PDH deficiency was made after delivery with the detection of severe lactic acidosis in the immediate neonatal period.[16]

## Obstetric Management

Management of a high-risk pregnancy should be made in coordination with a metabolic geneticist. Following delivery, the infant will need to be placed on a ketogenic diet, with symptomatic treatment for the management of lactic acidosis and seizures. In the absence of curative treatments, when brain malformations and/or extensive destructive lesions are identified, in utero termination of pregnancy, when legally possible, can be considered.

## Prognosis

Some forms of the PDH deficiency are thiamine responsive, and thiamine supplements are helpful; lactic acidosis may be treated with the introduction of a ketogenic diet and the concomitant use of dichloroacetate. The ketogenic diet has been used successfully in the rescue of a zebrafish model for PDH deficiency.[17] When there is established involvement of the prenatal brain, the prognosis is poor,

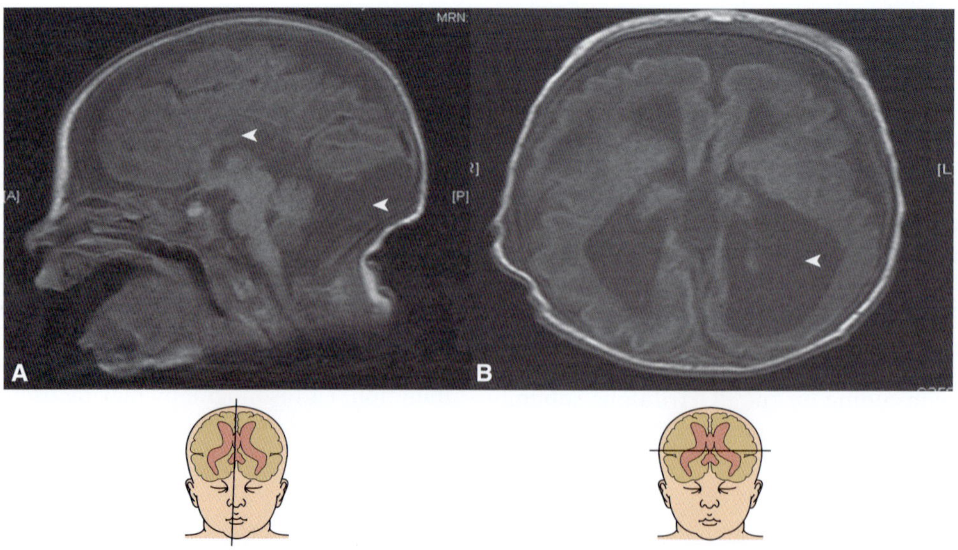

**Figure 12–3.** MRI T1-weighted images of the same infant as in Figure 12–2 on day 1 of life. **(A)** Median section confirms callosal and posterior fossa abnormalities (*arrowheads*) with large extra-axial spaces due to a reduction in brain mass. **(B)** Axial section shows bilateral ventriculomegaly (*arrowhead*). Note the presence of diffuse white matter abnormalities and pachygyria.

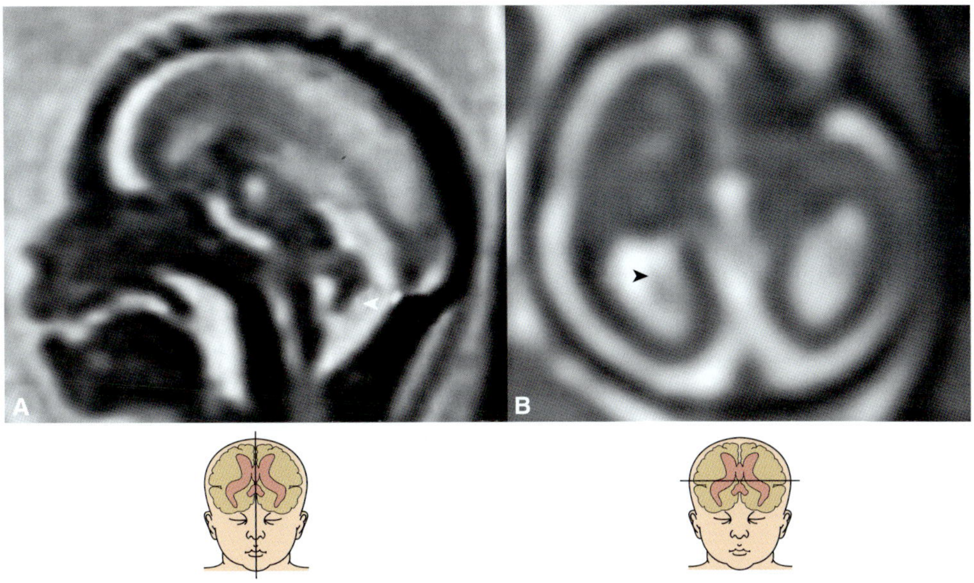


**Figure 12–4.** Single shot fast spin echo (SSFSE) fetal magnetic resonance imaging (MRI) during the third trimester of a patient with pyruvate dehydrogenase deficiency. **(A)** Sagittal section shows callosal and pontocerebellar abnormalities (*arrowhead*). **(B)** Axial section shows ventriculomegaly, particularly of the posterior horns (*arrowhead*).

and the children either die of fulminant lactic acidosis or are left with severe brain damage.

## SMITH-LEMLI-OPITZ SYNDROME

### Synonyms

SLO syndrome, RSH syndrome, Rutledge lethal multiple congenital anomaly syndrome, polydactyly, sex reversal, renal hypoplasia, unilobar lung, lethal acrodysgenital syndrome, OMIM 270400

### Definition

Smith-Lemli-Opitz (SLO) syndrome is a common birth defect (1:20,000–1:40,000) associated with malformations within multiple systems, craniofacial dysmorphic features, limb defects, and abnormalities of the heart, lungs, kidney, and genitalia[18–20] (Figure 12–5).

### Pathology

Although two forms of the disorder are described, a severe form with neonatal presentation and a milder form, these likely represent two ends of a pathologic spectrum. The CNS involvement is highly variable, with microcephaly, hypoplasia of the frontal lobes, holoprosencephaly, callosal dysgenesis, and cerebellar hypoplasia typical of the severe forms of the disorder. However, considerable clinical heterogeneity exists, and milder forms can be more difficult to diagnose in the prenatal period on the basis of CNS features alone.[21]

### Associated Anomalies

The occurrence of multiple malformations involving the face, limbs (polydactyly and syndactyly), genital abnormalities (hypospadias, ambiguous genitalia, micropenis, hypoplastic scrotum, and bifid scrotum), and renal anomalies (agenesis, renal cysts, and hydronephrosis), along with CNS abnormalities, are well recognized features of SLO syndrome.

### Etiology

This condition is caused by a defect in the enzyme 7-dehydrocholesterol reductase (DHCR7; OMIM *602858, EC 1.3.1.21), involved in the pathway for cholesterol

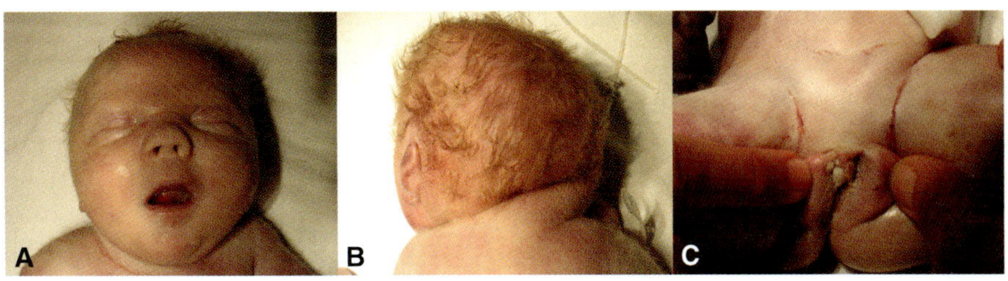


**Figure 12–5.** Smith-Lemli-Opitz syndrome in a deceased newborn delivered at 36 weeks of pregnancy. **(A)** Characteristic dysmorphism, including facial edema, hypertelorism, and anteverted nares. **(B)** Short, webbed neck. **(C)** Ambiguous genitalia in a genotypic male newborn.

biosynthesis. The DHCR7 gene maps to 11q12-q13 locus. Plasma cholesterol levels are typically low, whereas the levels of the precursor 7-dehydrocholesterol are elevated.[22]

## Recurrence Risk

The disorder is autosomal recessive in its inheritance. Each sibling of an affected individual has a 25% chance of being affected, a 50% chance of being an asymptomatic carrier, and a 25% chance of being unaffected and not a carrier.

## Diagnosis

Maternal serum and urinary dihydroxysteroid ratios in combination with fetal anomalies detectable on US greatly enhance the likelihood of establishing a prenatal diagnosis.[23,24] Identification of mutations in the gene encoding the enzyme sterol delta-7-reductase are diagnostic; common mutations can currently be identified through a polymerase chain reaction (PCR) assay.[25,26]

## Differential Diagnosis

The findings of SLO syndrome can be mimicked by other conditions, both genetic and metabolic; however, rarely is the combination of more than two of the above described anomalies and the biochemical defect replicated in other conditions. Other genetic considerations are trisomies 13 and 18, Meckel syndrome, and Simpson-Golabi syndrome. Metabolic conditions that can be considered with similar sterol synthesis defects include β-sitosterolemia (abnormal sterol biosynthesis, normal to elevated cholesterol levels, episodic hemolysis, tuberous xanthomatosis, and early atherosclerosis), CHILD syndrome (congenital hemidysplasia, ichthyosiform nevus, and limb defects), desmosterolosis (macrocephaly, hypoplastic nasal bridge, thick alveolar ridges, gingival nodules, cleft palate, total anomalous pulmonary venous drainage, ambiguous genitalia, short limbs, and generalized osteosclerosis), mevalonic aciduria (normal to slightly reduced cholesterol levels, developmental delay, dysmorphic facial features, central cataracts, anemia, and hepatosplenomegaly), and X-linked dominant chondrodysplasia punctata (alopecia, cataracts, ichthyosis, punctate calcification of bones, and rhizomelic limb shortening).

### Implications for Targeted Examination

A confirmed diagnosis of SLO syndrome in one child would suggest that the biological parents are likely carriers; consequently, future pregnancies carry a definite risk of recurrence. In such situations, the subsequent pregnancies should be followed from the first trimester so that abnormalities in the cleavage of the forebrain are not missed.

### Implications for Sonographic Screening

There is marked phenotypic variability in the presentation of SLO syndrome. A few reports have emphasized the clinical significance of the association of intrauterine growth retardation and nuchal edema detected on US examinations prenatally to be highly suggestive of SLO syndrome; however, milder cases may be missed despite the use of biochemical screening and prenatal ultrasonography.[21,24] In a single large series examining the antenatal expression of the disorder, intrauterine growth retardation was the only consistent feature, often in combination with other anomalies such as nuchal edema and cerebral, renal, or limb malformations. A considerable proportion (~15%) of the prenatal US studies were reported as normal; an early diagnosis of multiple malformations was possible in only 10%[23] (Figure 12–6). A combination of biochemical sterol analysis in the amniotic fluid and ultrasonographic examinations may be more helpful in milder cases.

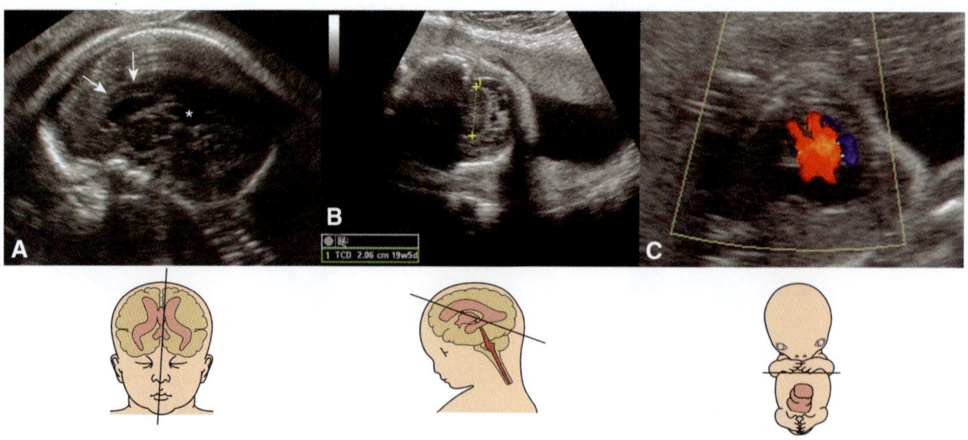


**Figure 12–6.** Prenatal US images of the same patient as in Figure 12–5 at 25 weeks of pregnancy. **(A)** Dysgenesis of the corpus callosum; the corpus callosum is thick and short (*arrows*), the splenium is missing and replaced by a cyst of the cavum interpositum (*asterisk*). **(B)** Cerebellar hypoplasia; the transverse cerebellar diameter is unusually small (2.06 mm = 19 weeks, 5 days). **(C)** Color Doppler of the heart showing atrioventricular canal. Other findings, not shown, included intrauterine growth retardation, microcephaly, pulmonic stenosis, and cleft palate.

### Obstetric Management

When severe, SLO syndrome is identified in utero; where legally possible, medical termination of pregnancy can be considered as an option.

### Prognosis

The prognosis is variable, with severe malformations resulting in a shortened life span, whereas milder cases may be compatible with a normal life span. Dietary cholesterol supplementation, as well as the use of simvastatin, a 3-hydroxy-3-methylglutaryl (HMG) CoA inhibitor, improves the biochemical profile,[27] but the effects on behavior remain unclear.

## GLUTARIC ACIDURIA TYPE I

### Synonyms

Glutaric acidemia type I, glutaryl CoA dehydrogenase deficiency, OMIM 231670

### Definition

Glutaric aciduria type I is an autosomal recessive disorder resulting from an inherited defect in the glutaryl-CoA dehydrogenase enzyme (GCDH; enzyme commission number, EC 1.3.99.7; OMIM*231670). The disorder causes an acute devastating neurologic syndrome in infants that is characterized by sudden-onset hypotonia, dystonia, and encephalopathy often in conjunction with a febrile illness. Survivors often have dystonic movements, seizures, and developmental delay.

### Pathology

Neuropathologic features are fairly characteristic for this disorder: macrocrania and increased brain size and weight, subdural effusions and hematomas, a pattern of frontotemporal hypoplasia associated with incomplete opercularization, and atrophy of the caudate and putamina bilaterally.[28]

### Associated Anomaly

Pathologic changes are confined to the nervous system; macrocephaly at birth is usually a marker.

### Pathogenesis

In a majority of patients, the principal pathologic changes follow the occurrence of encephalopathic crises often in postnatal life. A combination of the neurotoxic effects of intracerebral accumulation of intermediaries such as glutaric acid and 3-hydroxyglutaric acid and intrinsic vulnerability of striatal medium-sized γ-amino butyric acid neurons to neurotoxins and metabolic stress underlie the pathogenic effects.

### Etiology

GCDH is involved in the degradative pathway of the amino acids L-tryptophan, L-lysine, and L-hydroxylysine. The metabolic block results in accumulation of toxic intermediaries (glutaric acid [GA], 3-hydroxyglutaric acid [3-OH-GA], and glutaconic acid) in blood and to a lesser extent CSF. In the brain, de novo synthesis of these intermediaries and subsequent trapping due to poor efflux from the neuron account for abnormally high levels of accumulation. Urine organic acid analysis shows excretion of variable amounts of GA and 3-OH-GA and can be categorized into two groups, high and low excreters. Mutations in the gene at the GCDH locus (19p13.2) are diagnostic. There is considerable locus heterogeneity as well as a lack of genotype–phenotype correlation in this disorder.

### Recurrence Risk

Because the disorder is inherited in an autosomal recessive manner, a 25% recurrence risk is to be expected. There is strong evidence for intra- and interfamilial phenotypic variability.

### Diagnosis

Biochemical confirmation through assays of glutarylcarnitine in dried blood spots from the newborn using tandem mass spectrometry is an alternative.[29] Molecular genetic studies are available to identify GCDH mutations using DNA from chorionic villous biopsy or cultured amniocytes, enabling prenatal diagnosis if the mutation in the index case is already known.[30]

### Differential Diagnosis

GA1 must be distinguished from other organic acidurias presenting in early life, such as propionic acidemia, methylmalonic acidemia, and isovaleric acidemia. This distinction can be performed on the basis of biochemical analysis of body fluids using tandem mass spectrometry.[31]

#### Implications for Targeted Examination

In families at risk of carrying a fetus with GA1 following the diagnosis of the disease in a sibling, a targeted exam should be obtained in the third trimester.

#### Implications for Sonographic Screening

Although the typical neuropathologic findings are easily detected in the postnatal period on MRI, during the prenatal period, ultrasonographic studies seem to suggest that the combination of macrocrania, abnormal opercularization of the sylvian fissure, ventriculomegaly, and subdural effusions may be highly suggestive.[32–34] GA1 should also be considered in the differential diagnosis of periventricular pseudocysts (Figure 12–7), particularly when associated with macrocephaly or other CNS anomalies. After delivery, imaging findings can be confirmed through postnatal scans, biochemical confirmation through newborn screening of blood spots, and molecular DNA diagnostic tests.

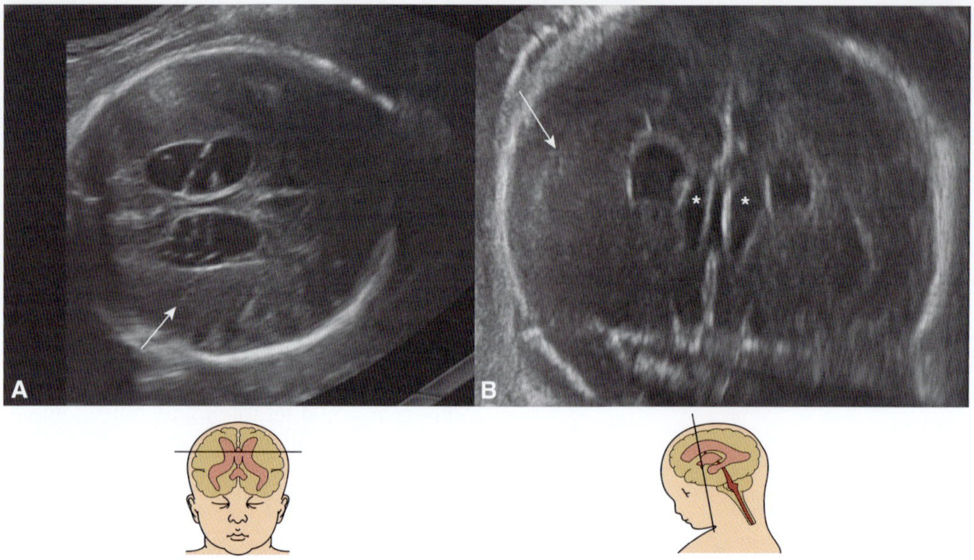


**Figure 12–7.** Prenatal appearance of glutaric aciduria in a 37-week fetus. **(A)** Axial plane showing huge bilateral periventricular pseudocyst (PVPC); note the abnormal echogenicity of the brain tissue, probably due to edema (*arrowhead*). **(B)** Axial plane at the level of the caudate nuclei shows bilateral, large PVPC. Note also in this section the almost complete lack of sulcation (*arrowhead*). The lateral ventricles are marked with an asterisk (*). (Courtesy of Dr. Waldo Sepulveda, Santiago, Chile.)

### Prognosis

Early diagnosis carries a significant impact on both survival and timely interventions to prevent and mitigate complications of the acute encephalopathic crisis.[35] Prognosis is variable, with improved outcome through supportive and prompt interventions during acute symptomatic crises reported for some groups, whereas the outcome remains poor in other populations.[36]

### Obstetric Management

Routine. Usually there are no perinatal sequelae directly attributable to delivery. However, postnatal follow-up, early diagnosis, and supportive interventions are critical to outcome.

## CONGENITAL DISORDERS OF GLYCOSYLATION

### Synonyms

Carbohydrate-deficient glycoprotein syndrome, CDG, OMIM 212065

### Definition

This is a group of recessively inherited disorders resulting from enzyme defects in the glycosylation pathways (pre-Golgi, endoplasmic reticulum, and Golgi complex). These disorders present with multisystem involvement, particularly the central and peripheral nervous system and coagulation and endocrine systems.[37,38]

There are two types of glycosylation reactions: N-glycosylation and O-glycosylation. The first disorder in the glycosylation pathway was first described in 1980 and was named the carbohydrate-deficient glycoprotein syndrome. The past decade has seen an explosion of interest resulting in the identification of several subtypes, and the original syndromic term has been replaced by disorders of glycosylation. Of the more than 10 subtypes known currently, CDG type Ia is the most frequently encountered and is the one with severe enough manifestations involving fetal brain malformations that can be detected by prenatal US.[39] We will restrict our discussion to this subtype.

### Pathology

Cerebellar hypoplasia is a consistently noted feature in this disorder. There is considerable heterogeneity in the presentation of this condition; therefore, it is likely that prenatal US may only be useful if the abnormalities are severe and above the threshold sensitivity for detection.

### Associated Anomalies

The initial descriptions of this condition included facial dysmorphic features, inverted nipples, and abnormal distribution of fat pads.[37]

### Pathogenesis

Deficient glycosylation of proteins results in improper trafficking and functioning of secretory and membranous glycoproteins, as well as lysosomal enzymes. This leads to widespread and multisystem effects of varying severity.

## Etiology

CDGIa results from mutations in the *PMM2* gene coding for the enzyme phosphomannomutase (OMIM 601785, EC 5.4.2.8). The resulting deficiency leads to reduced availability of guanosine diphosphate (GDP)–mannose required for the assembly of the dolicholpyrophosphate-linked oligosaccharide in the endoplasmic reticulum.[39]

## Recurrence Risk

A 25% recurrence risk is to be expected in this recessively inherited condition.

## Diagnosis

The diagnosis relies on demonstration of hypoglycosylation of serum proteins, particularly transferrins, using isoelectric focusing, which will show a cathodal shift in the presence of partial sialyl groups in transferrin.[40] Although the enzyme assay can be performed on cultured fibroblasts and amniocytes, the results are not considered uniformly reliable, as low values have been reported in the presence of a normal genotype. A molecular diagnostic study leading to prenatal diagnosis is possible in the presence of an affected proband.[39]

## Differential Diagnosis

In the postnatal period, the differential diagnosis is very wide, considering that infants present with central hypotonia. However, the combination of clinical features of inverted nipples, abnormal fat pads, and cerebellar hypoplasia is often considered highly suggestive of the diagnosis. There is considerable phenotypic variability, with milder cases diagnosed during adult life.

### Implications for Targeted Examination

In families at risk of having a fetus with CDG1a following the diagnosis of the disease in a sibling, targeted exam should be obtained from the second trimester to look for abnormal cerebellar development and hydrops fetalis.

### Implications for Sonographic Screening

Current neurosonographic techniques are sophisticated enough to permit detection of posterior fossa abnormalities in the right hands on serial imaging. However, there are diagnostic pitfalls that need to be considered that have been described in detail.[41] If the combination of cerebellar hypoplasia and fetal akinesia is detected, in our opinion, CDG1a should be a consideration. Other features, such as presentation with nonimmune hydrops fetalis, hyperechoic kidneys, and cardiomyopathy, have also been detected in prenatal studies leading to a diagnosis of CDG1a.[42–44]

## Prognosis

The outcome is variable; most infants demonstrate developmental delay, mental retardation, and failure to thrive. Symptomatic treatment measures and supportive care are all that can be offered, as there is no treatment currently available for this disorder.

## Obstetric Management

Routine management when termination of pregnancy is not an option

# NONKETOTIC HYPERGLYCINEMIA

## Synonyms

NKH, OMIM 605899, glycine encephalopathy

## Etiology

Nonketotic hyperglycinemia (NKH) is an inborn error of glycine metabolism in which large quantities of glycine accumulate in all body tissues, including the brain. It is caused by a defect in the glycine cleavage system (EC 2.1.2.10), which is confined to the mitochondria and composed of four protein components: P protein (a pyridoxal phosphate–dependent glycine decarboxylase), H protein (a lipoic acid–containing protein), T protein (a tetrahydrofolate-requiring enzyme), and L protein (a lipoamide dehydrogenase). NKH may be due to a defect in any one of these enzymes.

## Associated Anomaly

Only affects the CNS

## Pathogenesis

The placental circulation cannot lower the plasma glycine level sufficiently to lower the CSF/brain glycine level to the normal range. The intracellular accumulation of metabolites such as glycine can produce direct neurotoxic effects. Elevated glycine affects the developing fetal brain from early pregnancy. The first sign is agenesis of the corpus callosum.

## Risk of Recurrence

Autosomal recessive disorder with a recurrence rate of 25%

## Sonographic Diagnosis

Agenesis of the corpus callosum is a pathognomonic feature.

## MRI Diagnosis

MRI demonstrates agenesis or thinning of the corpus callosum, dysmyelination, and gyral abnormalities.[45–48]

### Implications for Targeted Examination

In families at risk of having a fetus with NKH following the diagnosis of the disease in a sibling, targeted exam should be obtained from the second trimester to look for abnormal callosal development.

The differential diagnosis upon prenatal diagnosis of agenesis of the corpus callosum with or without associated cortical malformations should include NKH.

**Implications for Sonographic Screening, Including Earliest Recognition**

Paupe et al[49] reported the prenatal diagnosis at 22 postmenstrual weeks of hypoplasia of the corpus callosum in a fetus that was diagnosed with NKH.

Prenatal diagnosis for pregnancies at increased risk is possible by analysis of DNA extracted from fetal cells obtained by amniocentesis. Prenatal testing using measurement of amniotic fluid glycine concentration and the glycine/serine ratio are unreliable because normal and affected values overlap.

### Prognosis

Death may occur in the neonatal period. Long-term survival may occur, usually with minimal mental development, but surprisingly little gross brain destruction.

### Obstetric Management

When legally possible, termination of pregnancy should be offered.

## MITOCHONDRIAL DISORDERS

### Synonyms

Disorders of energy metabolism, respiratory chain disorders, oxidative phosphorylation disorders

### Pathology

Mitochondrial disorders are disorders of the respiratory chain that cause defective oxidative phosphorylation resulting in energy deficiency of any organ or tissue. The decrease in energy supply may manifest any time, from prenatal to postnatal life. The most affected organs are those that require the largest amount of energy (brain, muscle, and heart).

The mitochondrial respiratory chain (RC) catalyzes the oxidation of fuel molecules and the concomitant energy transduction into adenosine triphosphate (ATP) via five complexes, which are embedded in the inner mitochondrial membrane. Complex I (nicotinamide adenine dinucleotide [NADH] coenzyme Q [CoQ] reductase) carries reducing equivalents from NADH to CoQ (ubiquinone) and consists of 40 different polypeptides. Complex II (succinate-CoQ reductase) carries reducing equivalents from 5,10-methylenetetrahydrofolate reductase (FADH2) to CoQ and contains four polypeptides, including the FAD-dependent succinate dehydrogenase and iron-sulfur proteins. Complex III (reduced CoQ–cytochrome c reductase) carries electrons from CoQ to cytochrome c; it contains 11 subunits. Complex IV (cytochrome c oxidase [COX]), the terminal oxidase of the RC, catalyzes the transfer of reducing equivalents from cytochrome c to molecular oxygen. It is composed of 2 cytochromes (cytochromes a and a3), 2 copper atoms, and 13 different protein subunits. During the oxidation process, electrons are transferred to oxygen via the energy-transducing complexes of the RC. The free energy generated from the redox reactions is converted into a transmembrane proton gradient. Complex V (ATP synthase) allows protons to flow back into the mitochondrial matrix and uses the released energy to synthesize ATP. Three ATP molecules are produced for each NADH molecule oxidized.[50]

The mitochondrial RC is composed of approximately 100 different proteins. Only 13 of the proteins are encoded by mitochondrial genes; the others are encoded by nuclear genes. All complexes of the RC except complex II have a double genetic origin.

### Associated Anomalies

Von Kleist-Retzow et al[51] reviewed 300 cases of proven respiratory chain enzyme deficiency for fetal development. Twenty patients had an antenatal presentation, the most common being intrauterine growth retardation and multiple anomalies of organs sharing no common function or embryologic origin.

### Pathogenesis

Mitochondrial disorders can present at any age and affect all organs; however, they rarely present in utero. Aerobic metabolism in the brain tends to increase during periods of rapid neuronal proliferation, differentiation, and neuronal migration. Therefore, disorders of the respiratory chain are associated with multiple developmental defects in the nervous system.

### Risk of Recurrence

Disorders of the respiratory chain may be inherited in all modes of inheritance: maternal, autosomal recessive, autosomal dominant, and X-linked. Large-scale deletions in the mitochondrial DNA (mtDNA) may occur de novo. The risk of recurrence depends on the specific genetic defect.

### Sonographic Diagnosis

Fetal brain involvement that can be depicted by US includes ventriculomegaly, porencephalic cysts, Dandy-Walker malformation, cerebellar hypoplasia, pontocerebellar hypoplasia, and agenesis of corpus callosum.[51,52,53] In one reported case, ventriculomegaly and porencephalic germinal matrix cysts were found at 22 weeks' gestation and later resolved.[51] We have also found periventricular pseudocysts in a fetus that later developed a Leigh disease presentation (Figure 12–8).

Samson et al[54] described ventriculomegaly and intracerebral calcifications in two fetuses with a familial mitochondrial encephalopathy. An autopsy showed extensive encephalopathy with cavitation and calcification in the cerebral hemispheres, polymicrogyria, multiple neuronal heterotopia, partial callosal dysgenesis, and severe Leigh syndrome. We have also observed white matter

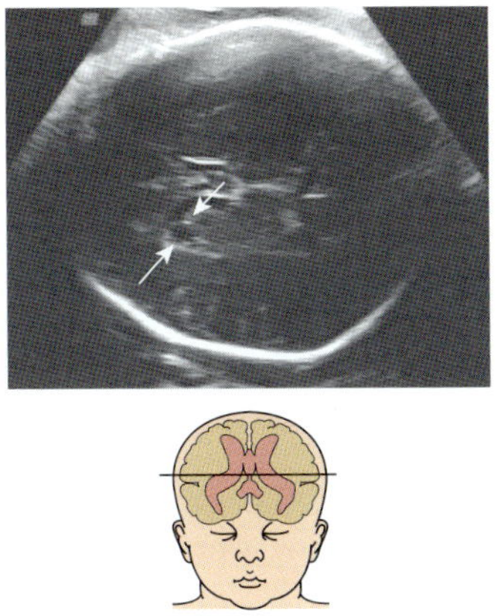

**Figure 12–8.** Periventricular pseudocysts in a fetus at 38 weeks' gestation diagnosed postnatally as suffering from Leigh syndrome.

calcifications in two consecutive pregnancies of fetuses with multiple mtDNA deletions (Figure 12–9).

## MRI Diagnosis

Gire at al[55] described the neuroradiological features of six neonates with mitochondrial disorders. Five had antenatal involvement. A prenatal MRI in one demonstrated ventricular and parenchymal hemorrhages.

### Implications for Targeted Examination

When a previous child with a diagnosed mitochondrial disorder shows fetal brain involvement, US should be obtained from the second trimester to look for ventriculomegaly, periventricular cysts, calcifications, and cerebellar abnormalities.

### Implications for Sonographic Screening

Abnormalities of the respiratory chain may cause both brain dysplasia and disruption. There is a continuum of early and late brain involvement that can be identified by US at different stages of gestation. The US may identify agenesis of the corpus callosum as early as midpregnancy, and later in the third trimester identify cerebellar hypoplasia and malformations of cortical development.[56] Ventriculomegaly and periventricular pseudocysts may prove to be a relatively common presentation of in utero energy deficiency.

When a fetus presents with an association of multiorgan malformations without a common embryologic origin, intrauterine growth retardation, and brain dysplasia/

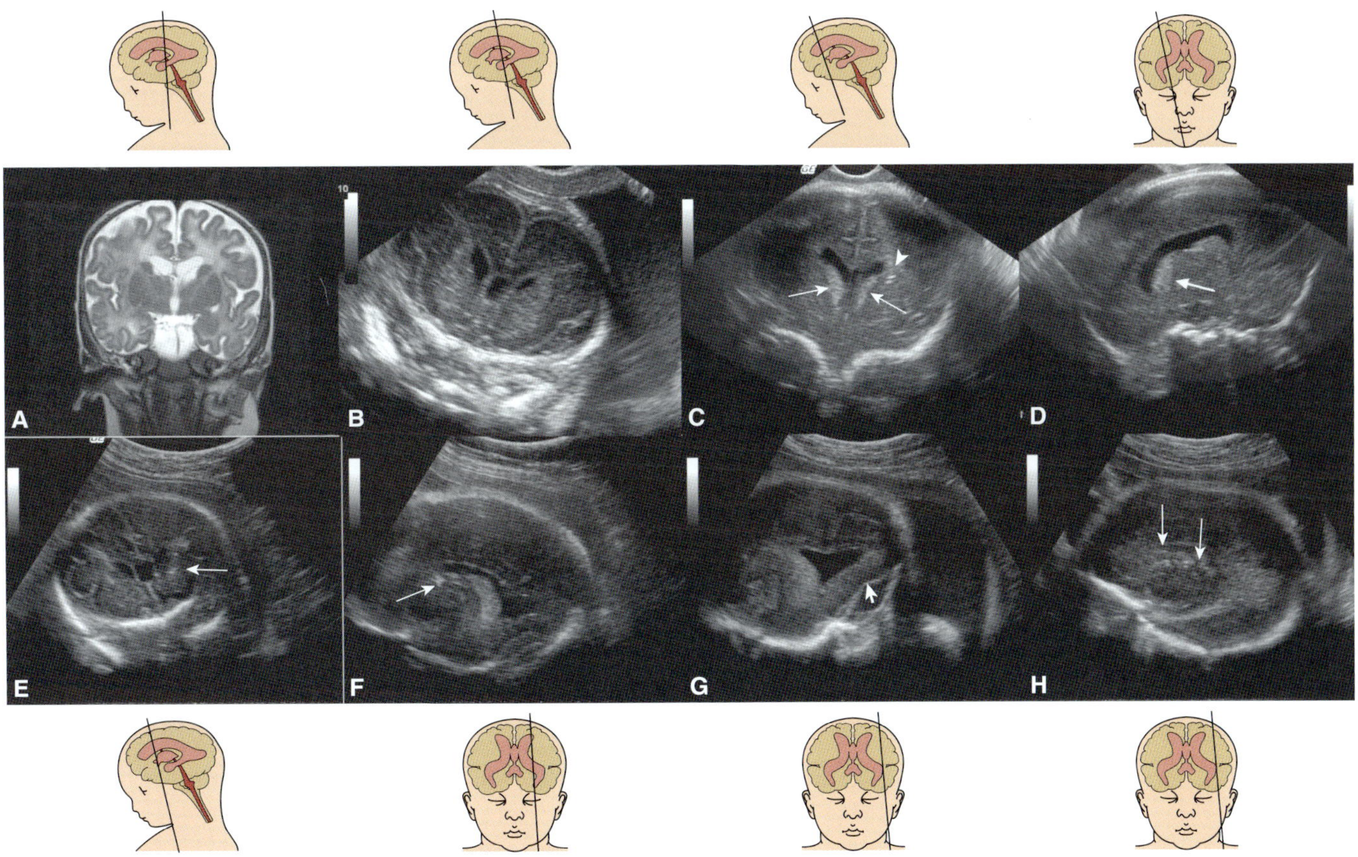


**Figure 12–9.** Siblings with autosomal recessive multiple mitochondrial DNA (mtDNA) deletions. **(A)** T2-weighted brain MRI of the propositus at 3 years of age shows diffuse white matter involvement and caudate nuclei cystic formations. **(B)** Coronal transvaginal sonography (TVS) of the first fetus at 24 weeks is normal. **(C)**. **(D)** Abnormal US findings diagnosed at 33 weeks' gestation in the same fetus as in B showing hyperechogenic caudate nuclei (*arrows*) and small calcification foci (arrowhead). Coronal **(E)** and sagittal **(F–H)** images of the second fetus at 34 weeks' gestation show caudothalamic calcifications (*arrows*) and abnormal occipital white matter with abnormal sulcation (*arrowhead*).

disruption, a mitochondrial disorder should be suspected. However, when there is no family history, prenatal diagnosis cannot be offered.

## Prognosis

When mitochondrial disorders present in utero, the postnatal presentation is usually early (neonatal period to infancy), and the course is frequently fatal.[51] The presentation may be fulminant, with lactic acidosis and multiorgan failure culminating in early demise.

## Obstetric Management

When the disease-causing mutation in the nuclear DNA is known, prenatal diagnosis is available. However, when the mutation is in the mtDNA, very little information is available, because the ratio of mutant versus wild-type mtDNA (heteroplasmy) in fetal DNA is considered to be a poor indicator of postnatal outcome. Nevertheless, prenatal diagnosis has been attempted in MELAS (myopathy, encephalopathy, lactic acidosis, and strokelike syndrome) due to the 3243 mtDNA[57] mutation, and in maternally related Leigh syndrome due to the 8993 mtDNA mutation.[58]

Assessment of the respiratory chain in amniotic cells is not reliable because the abnormal enzyme activity may be tissue specific and not involve amniotic cells, and the expression of respiratory chain deficiency during fetal life is time dependent due to differential expression or regulation of the mutant proteins.[59]

# MATERNAL PHENYLKETONURIA

## Synonym

Maternal PKU

## Definition

The maternal phenylketonuria (PKU) syndrome refers to the teratogenic effects of phenylalanine during pregnancy. These effects include mental retardation, microcephaly, congenital heart disease, and intrauterine growth retardation.[60]

## Pathology

Phenylketonuria (OMIM 261600) is an autosomal recessive IEM resulting from a deficiency of phenylalanine hydroxylase (PAH; EC 1.14.16.1), an enzyme that catalyzes the hydroxylation of phenylalanine to tyrosine, the rate-limiting step in phenylalanine catabolism.

## Associated Anomaly

Congenital heart disease in 15%

## Pathogenesis

When the mother has classic PKU with a blood phenylalanine level > 1200 μM (20 mg/dL), there is a high frequency of teratogenicity in the offspring, with microcephaly and mental retardation in 75% to 90%. There is a dose-response relationship with progressively lower frequencies of these abnormalities at lower phenylalanine levels.

The pathogenesis may be related to inhibition by phenylalanine of large neutral amino acid transport across the placenta or to direct toxicity of phenylalanine, a phenylalanine metabolite, or both in certain fetal organs. Although phenylalanine hydroxylase is expressed in the fetus as early as the sixth week of gestation, the large load of toxic phenylalanine from the mother overwhelms the limited hydroxylating capacity of the fetus.[61] The oligodendroglia switch to a nonmyelinating phenotype that expresses an astrocyte marker, glial fibrillary acidic protein. The impairment of intrauterine myelination can explain the hypoplastic corpus callosum.

## Risk of Recurrence

The teratogenic effects of phenylalanine can recur in every pregnancy if the mother does not keep a strict low-phenylalanine diet.

## Sonographic Diagnosis

Dysgenesis of the corpus callosum associated with progressive microcephaly is pathognomonic of maternal PKU.

## MRI Diagnosis

Brain MRI may demonstrate a dysgenetic corpus callosum and delayed myelination.[61]

### Implications for Targeted Examination

When the mother has PKU, she should be monitored for phenylalanine levels even before conception, and her diet should be strictly adjusted. A fetal US should be obtained serially throughout pregnancy. It can demonstrate progressive microcephaly and dysgenesis of the corpus callosum associated with a congenital heart defect.

### Implications for Sonographic Screening, Including Earliest Recognition

Dysgenesis of the corpus callosum can be recognized by US as early as 22 weeks, whereas progressive microcephaly can only be diagnosed in the third trimester.

## Prognosis

Because the fetus does not have PKU, the effect of the increased phenylalanine levels in utero is nonprogressive. The child may be born microcephalic with a congenital heart defect and then show a picture of static developmental delay.

## Obstetric Management

The treatment of maternal PKU consists of biochemical control through a phenylalanine-restricted diet during pregnancy. The best results are obtained with diet initiation before conception or no later than the earliest weeks of pregnancy.

## PEROXISOMAL BIOGENESIS DISORDERS

### Synonyms

PBD; OMIM 601539

### Definition

The peroxisomal biogenesis disorders (PBDs) are autosomal recessive disorders of peroxisome assembly that lead to deficiency of multiple peroxisomal enzymes. They have overlapping phenotypic features and various genetic causes (defects in over 25 *PEX* genes). Due to their heterogeneity, PBDs had been divided into four groups: Zellweger syndrome (ZS; MIM 214100), neonatal adrenoleukodystrophy (NALD; MIM 202370), infantile Refsum disease (IRD; MIM 266510), and rhizomelic chondrodysplasia punctata (RCDP; MIM 215100).[62]

### Pathology

Peroxisomes are organelles present in almost all eukaryotic cells. They are essential for the metabolism of branched chain and very long chain fatty acids (VLCFAs), ether lipids, polyamines, amino acids, and glyoxylate. During some of these metabolic processes, peroxisomes generate and subsequently inactivate reactive oxygen species.[62] It has been estimated that at least 85 proteins are associated with peroxisome structure and function in humans. Peroxisome matrix proteins are synthesized in the cytosol prior to import into the peroxisome. Peroxins, encoded by a family of *PEX* genes, are involved in peroxisome biogenesis, with functions ranging from membrane synthesis and matrix protein import to organelle division.[62]

Biochemical studies performed in blood and urine are used to screen for PBD. They include elevated plasma, VLCFAs, bile acids, and phytanic, pristanic, and pipecolic acids contrasting with low plasma plasmalogens. Impaired enzymatic activity of dihydroacetone-phosphate acyltransferase deficiency can be detected in fibroblasts.

### Associated Anomalies

Zellweger syndrome, also known as cerebrohepatorenal syndrome, is the classic and most severe peroxisomal biogenesis disorder. Associated anomalies are prominent forehead, large anterior fontanelle, hypoplastic supraorbital ridges, broad nasal bridge, hypertelorism and deformed earlobes, limb anomalies, hepatomegaly, cataracts, stippled epiphyses, and renal cysts.

### Pathogenesis

Accumulation of phytanic acid, VLCFAs, pipecolic acid, and abnormal bile acids in multiple organs are thought to be the underlying mechanism of this fatal condition.

### Risk of Recurrence

Inheritance is autosomal recessive. The risk of recurrence is 25%.

### Sonographic Diagnosis

Migration anomalies can be diagnosed in utero by ultrasonography based on the presence of specific deviations from the normal pattern of development as early as the 18th postmenstrual week.[56] The ultrasonographic findings leading to the diagnosis of malformations of cortical development are abnormally overdeveloped gyri and sulci for gestational age, delay in sulcation, abnormally thin cortex, and abnormally wide and broad sulci.

### MRI Diagnosis

Migration anomalies are well documented in peroxisomal disorders. In the Zellweger syndrome spectrum, these anomalies consist of lissencephaly, perirolandic and occipital pachygyria, frontal and perisylvian polymicrogyria (Figure 12–10), periventricular heterotopias, band heterotopias, hypoplastic corpus callosum, abnormal layering of the cerebellum, and dysplasia of the inferior olivary nuclei and olfactory bulb.[63–72] Mochel et al[73] described the fetal MRI features in two fetuses with Zellweger syndrome. One depicted asymmetric ventriculomegaly, abnormally small cerebral convolutions, mostly in the frontal and in the perisylvian cortex, periventricular leukodystrophy predominating in the frontal area, and germinolytic cysts in the subependymal areas; the other depicted bilateral ventricular enlargement associated with a large cavum, abnormal gyration pattern mostly in the frontal and perisylvian cortex, and periventricular leukodystrophy, mainly in the frontal area and irregular ventricular walls revealing bilateral subependymal pseudocysts. The combination of cortical malformations of the perisylvian and perirolandic regions, hypomyelination, and germinolytic cysts seems specific for Zellweger syndrome.

#### Implications for Targeted Examination

When there is a history of a previously affected child, specific deviations from the normal pattern of cortical development should be evaluated by US every 2 to 3 weeks starting at 22 weeks' gestation.

#### Implications for Sonographic Screening

The first sign of fetal Zellweger syndrome is increased nuchal translucency.[74] Later, suspicion would be raised in a fetus with hypokinesia, cerebral ventricular enlargement, renal hyperechogenicity, and hepatosplenomegaly. Prenatal US supplemented with MRI can identify abnormal cortical development in the third trimester.

### Prognosis

There is a clinical overlap between Zellweger syndrome, neonatal adrenoleukodystrophy, and infantile Refsum disease. Affected individuals can be recognized at birth

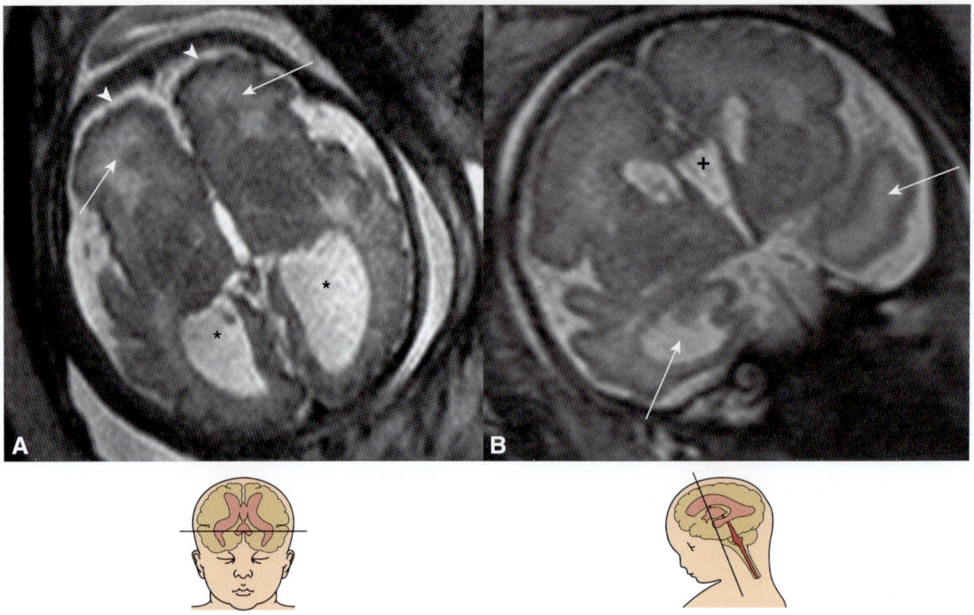


**Figure 12–10.** Zellweger syndrome. Brain MRI T2-weighted images in fetus at 35 weeks' gestation. Axial **(A)** and coronal **(B)** sections show bilateral frontal polymicrogyria (*arrowheads*) and abnormally high signal intensity of the frontal and temporoparietal white matter (*arrows*) consistent with abnormal white matter maturation. Note the presence of asymmetric ventriculomegaly (*) and a large cavum septi pellucidi (+). (Courtesy of Dr. Gregor Kasparian and Daniela Prayer, Vienna, Austria.)

because of prominent hypotonia, hyporeflexia, seizures, craniofacial dysmorphism, limb abnomalities, liver dysfunction, optic atrophy, glaucoma, cataract, failure to thrive, renal cysts, stippled epiphyses, and prominent mental retardation. Death usually occurs within the first year of life in Zellweger syndrome.

### Obstetric Management

When there is a family history, and both disease-causing alleles of the affected family member have been identified, a molecular diagnosis can be made. However, when the suspicion is raised because of the association of the typical brain anomalies with kidney and liver abnormalities, the prenatal diagnosis can be made by VLCFA content and plasmalogen synthesis measured in cultured chorionic villus sampling (CVS) or amniocytes.[75]

## MOLYBDENUM COFACTOR DEFICIENCY

### Synonyms

MOCOD, OMIM 252150, combined deficiency of sulfite oxidase, xanthine dehydrogenase, and aldehyde oxidase, molybdenum cofactor deficiency, complementation group A, molybdenum cofactor deficiency, complementation group B, molybdenum cofactor deficiency, complementation group C

### Definition

Molybdenum is a trace element that, in its complex form molybdopterin, is essential for the function of three enzymes: sulfite oxidase, xanthine dehydrogenase, and aldehyde oxidase. Molybdenum cofactor deficiency (MoCD) is a rare autosomal recessive disorder that may be mistaken for ischemic encephalopathy.

### Pathology

MoCD can be caused by mutations at either of two separate steps in the formation of molybdenum cofactor. MOCS1 (603707) encodes two enzymes for synthesis of the precursor. The conversion of the precursor into the organic moiety of molybdenum cofactor is catalyzed by molybdopterin synthase (MOCS2; 603708), which encodes the small and large subunits of this heteromeric enzyme. MOCS1 is defective in patients with complementation group A deficiency. MOCS2 is defective in patients with complementation group B deficiency. The phenotype is identical in both complementation groups. In addition, a third type of MoCD, complementation group C, is caused by mutation in the gephyrin gene (GEPH; 603930). The diagnosis is established by the presence of low blood uric acid levels, positive urine sulfite reaction, and MoCD gene analysis.[76]

### Associated Anomalies

MoCD mainly affects the CNS, but renal stones and dislocated lens may be associated anomalies.

### Pathogenesis

Disruption of mitochondrial energy production by sulfite accumulation inhibits glutamate dehydrogenase. Sulfur-containing compounds that are formed as a result of

MoCD cause excitotoxic neuronal injury in the presence of excess magnesium. Pockets of neuronal cell death or focal ischemia may lead to encephaloclastic lesions, such as porencephalic cysts.[77–80] These lesions may develop at the end of pregnancy.

## Risk of Recurrence

Autosomal recessive inheritance, 25% risk of recurrence

## Sonographic Diagnosis

Encephaloclastic white matter cysts associated with cerebellar hypoplasia are pathognomonic of MoCD[81] and may sometimes be identified in utero (Figure 12–11).

## MRI Diagnosis

The MRI demonstrates shortly after birth atrophy of the cerebral hemispheres in association with multiple cystic cavities resembling multicystic encephalomalacia located in the subcortical region. The cerebellum is hypoplastic. There may be bilateral subacute subdural hematoma.[82–86]

### Implications for Targeted Examination

Following the birth of an affected child, the pregnancy should be monitored for abnormal cerebellar development and ischemic lesions toward the end of pregnancy.

### Implications for Sonographic Screening, Including Earliest Recognition

It is not clear how often brain involvement is manifested prenatally. In some cases, there is documentation that the first US/MRI was normal[81,86] and that the lesions developed in the neonatal period. It seems obvious that the ischemic like brain cysts develop either at the very end of pregnancy or shortly after delivery.

## Prognosis

The prognosis is poor. Most of the infants die in the first days or weeks of their lives, and effective therapy is not available for this rare disease. Presentation is usually in the newborn period or early infancy with intractable seizures, metabolic acidosis, intracranial hemorrhage, feeding difficulties, exaggerated startle reactions, dysmorphic facial features, profound mental retardation, alterations in muscle tone, microcephaly, lens dislocation, and renal stones.[87]

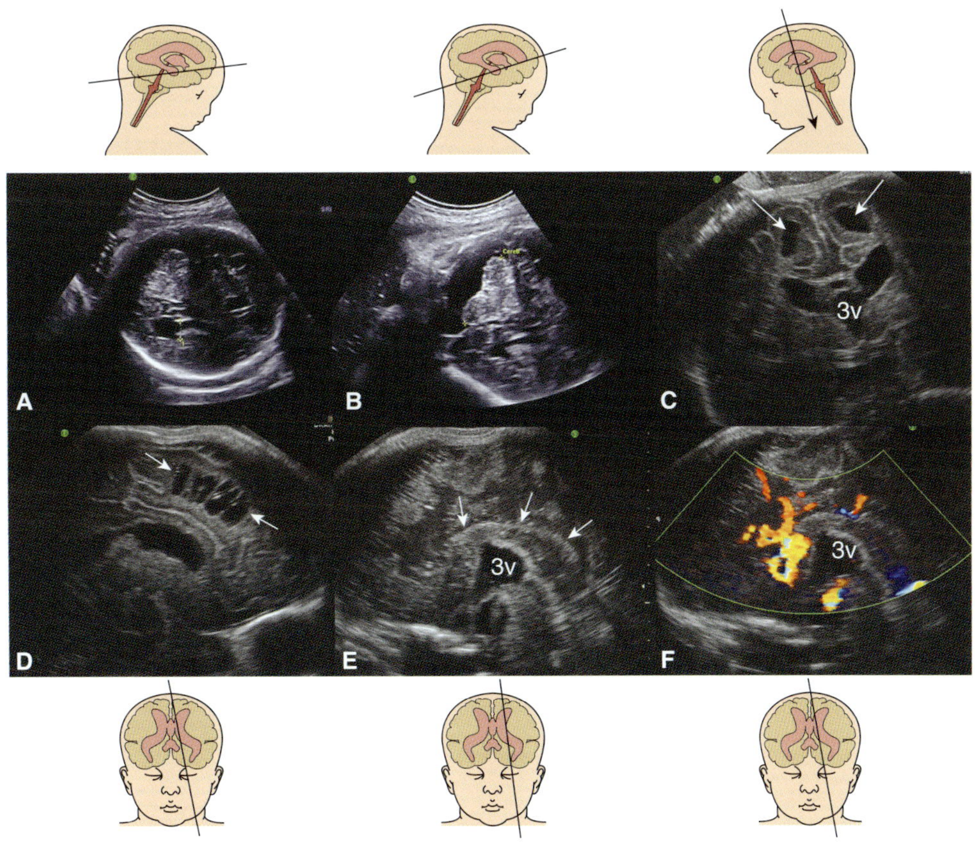


**Figure 12–11.** Prenatal appearance of molybdenum cofactor deficiency in fetus at 35 weeks' gestation. **(A)** Transabdominal axial plane shows only mild ventriculomegaly (lateral ventricle width (LVW) 10.2 mm). **(B)** Transabdominal axial plane shows cerebellar hypoplasia with mega cisterna magna. **(C)** Transvaginal coronal plane at the level of the third ventricle shows lateral and third ventricle dilation; the subcortical white matter has been replaced by multiple encephaloclastic lesions. **(D)** Transvaginal paramedian plane shows the multiple, multilocular pattern of the cysts. **(E, F)** Paramedian planes show severe dysgenesis of the corpus callosum with abnormal vasculature particularly from vessels originating from the aberrant anterior cerebral artery.

## Obstetric Management

When multiple porencephalic cysts are diagnosed in pregnancy, termination should be suggested when legally possible. The deficiencies can be diagnosed prenatally by monitoring sulfite oxidase activity in CVS. In those families in which the specific defects have been identified, diagnosis can be achieved by mutation analysis or linkage studies directed at affected genes.[88]

## REFERENCES


1. Graf W. Cerebral dysgenesis secondary to metabolic diseases in fetal life. In: Aminoff MJ, Boller F, Swaab DF, ed. *Handbook of Clinical Neurology.* Amsterdam: Elsevier; 2008;459–476.
2. Bamforth F, Bamforth S, Poskitt K, Applegarth D, Hall J. Abnormalities of corpus callosum in patients with inherited metabolic diseases. *Lancet.* 1988;2(8608):451.
3. Nissenkorn A, Michelson M, Ben-Zeev B, Lerman-Sagie T. Inborn errors of metabolism: a cause of abnormal brain development. *Neurology.* 2001;56(10):1265–1272.
4. Siu VM, Ratko S, Prasad AN, Prasad C, Rupar CA. Amish microcephaly: long-term survival and biochemical characterization. *Am J Med Genet A.* 2010;152A(7):1747–1751.
5. Israels S, Haworth JC, Dunn HG, Applegarth DA. Lactic acidosis in childhood. *Adv Pediatr.* 1976;22:267–303.
6. Aleck KA, Kaplan AM, Sherwood WG, Robinson BH. In utero central nervous system damage in pyruvate dehydrogenase deficiency. *Arch Neurol.* 1988;45(9):987–989.
7. de Meirleir LJ, Lissens W, Vamos E, Liebaers I. Pyruvate dehydrogenase deficiency due to a mutation of the E1 alpha subunit. *J Inherit Metab Dis.* 1991;14(3):301–304.
8. De Meirleir L, Lissens W, Vamos E, Liebaers I. Pyruvate dehydrogenase (PDH) deficiency caused by a 21-base pair insertion mutation in the E1 alpha subunit. *Hum Genet.* 1992;88(6):649–652.
9. Chun K, MacKay N, Petrova-Benedict R, Robinson BH. Mutations in the X-linked E1 alpha subunit of pyruvate dehydrogenase leading to deficiency of the pyruvate dehydrogenase complex. *Hum Mol Genet.* 1993;2(4):449–454.
10. Hansen LL, Brown GK, Brown RM, Dahl HH. Pyruvate dehydrogenase deficiency caused by a 5 base pair duplication in the E1 alpha subunit. *Hum Mol Genet.* 1993;2(6):805–807.
11. Otero LJ, Brown RM, Brown GK. Arginine 302 mutations in the pyruvate dehydrogenase E1alpha subunit gene: Identification of further patients and in vitro demonstration of pathogenicity. *Hum Mutat.* 1998;12(2):114–121.
12. Chow CW, Anderson RM, Kenny GC. Neuropathology in cerebral lactic acidosis. *Acta Neuropathol (Berl).* 1987;74(4):393–396.
13. Zand DJ, Simon EM, Pulitzer SB, et al. In vivo pyruvate detected by MR spectroscopy in neonatal pyruvate dehydrogenase deficiency. *AJNR Am J Neuroradiol.* 2003;24(7):1471–1474.
14. Brown RM, Brown GK. Prenatal diagnosis of pyruvate dehydrogenase E1 alpha subunit deficiency. *Prenat Diagn.* 1994;14(6):435–441.
15. Wada N, Matsuishi T, Nonaka M, Naito E, Yoshino M. Pyruvate dehydrogenase E1alpha subunit deficiency in a female patient: Evidence of antenatal origin of brain damage and possible etiology of infantile spasms. *Brain Dev.* 2004;26(1):57–60.
16. Robinson JN, Norwitz ER, Mulkern R, Brown SA, Rybicki F, Tempany CM. Prenatal diagnosis of pyruvate dehydrogenase deficiency using magnetic resonance imaging. *Prenat Diagn.* 2001;21(12):1053–1056.
17. Taylor MR, Hurley JB, Van Epps HA, Brockerhoff SE. A zebrafish model for pyruvate dehydrogenase deficiency: Rescue of neurological dysfunction and embryonic lethality using a ketogenic diet. *Proc Natl Acad Sci U S A.* 2004 30;101(13):4584–4589.
18. Opitz JM, Penchaszadeh VB, Holt MC, Spano LM. Smith-Lemli-Opitz (RSH) syndrome bibliography. *Am J Med Genet.* 1987;28(3):745–750.
19. Penchaszadeh VB. The nosology of the Smith-Lemli-Opitz Syndrome. *Am J Med Genet.* 1987;28(3):719–721.
20. Porter FD. Smith-Lemli-Opitz syndrome: Pathogenesis, diagnosis and management. *Eur J Hum Genet.* 2008;16(5):535–541.
21. Nowaczyk MJ, Heshka T, Kratz LE, Kelley RE. Difficult prenatal diagnosis in mild Smith-Lemli-Opitz syndrome. *Am J Med Genet.* 200011;95(4):396–398.
22. Irons M, Elias ER, Tint GS, et al. Abnormal cholesterol metabolism in the Smith-Lemli-Opitz syndrome: Report of clinical and biochemical findings in four patients and treatment in one patient. *Am J Med Genet.* 1994;50(4):347–352.
23. Goldenberg A, Wolf C, Chevy F, et al. Antenatal manifestations of Smith-Lemli-Opitz (RSH) syndrome: A retrospective survey of 30 cases. *Am J Med Genet A.* 2004;124A(4):423–426.
24. Shinawi M, Szabo S, Popek E, Wassif CA, Porter FD, Potocki L. Recognition of Smith-Lemli-Opitz syndrome (RSH) in the fetus: Utility of ultrasonography and biochemical analysis in pregnancies with low maternal serum estriol. *Am J Med Genet A.* 2005;138(1):56–60.
25. Battaile KP, Maslen CL, Wassif CA, Krakowiak P, Porter FD, Steiner RD. A simple PCR-based assay allows detection of a common mutation, IVS8-1G→C, in DHCR7 in Smith-Lemli-Opitz syndrome. *Genet Test.* 1999;3(4):361–363.
26. Wassif CA, Maslen C, Kachilele-Linjewile S, et al. Mutations in the human sterol delta7-reductase gene at 11q12-13 cause Smith-Lemli-Opitz syndrome. *Am J Hum Genet.* 1998;63(1):55–62.
27. Haas D, Garbade SF, Vohwinkel C, et al. Effects of cholesterol and simvastatin treatment in patients with Smith-Lemli-Opitz syndrome (SLOS). *J Inherit Metab Dis.* 2007;30(3):375–387.
28. Funk CB, Prasad AN, Frosk P, et al. Neuropathological, biochemical and molecular findings in a glutaric acidemia type 1 cohort. *Brain.* 2005;128(Pt 4):711–722.
29. Baric I, Zschocke J, Christensen E, et al. Diagnosis and management of glutaric aciduria type I. *J Inherit Metab Dis.* 1998;21(4):326–340.
30. Busquets C, Coll MJ, Merinero B, et al. Prenatal molecular diagnosis of glutaric aciduria type I by direct mutation analysis. *Prenat Diagn.* 2000;20(9):761–764.
31. Shigematsu Y, Hata I, Nakai A, et al. Prenatal diagnosis of organic acidemias based on amniotic fluid levels of acylcarnitines. *Pediatr Res.* 1996;39(4, Pt 1):680–684.
32. Forstner R, Hoffmann GF, Gassner I, et al. Glutaric aciduria type I: Ultrasonographic demonstration of early signs. *Pediatr Radiol.* 1999;29(2):138–143.
33. Lin SK, Hsu SG, Ho ES, et al. Glutaric aciduria (type I): Prenatal ultrasonographic findings. *Ultrasound Obstet Gynecol.* 2002;20(3):305–307.
34. Lin SK, Hsu SG, Ho ES, et al. Novel mutation and prenatal sonographic findings of glutaric aciduria (type I) in two Taiwanese families. *Prenat Diagn.* 2002;22(8):725–729.
35. Superti-Furga A, Hoffmann GF. Glutaric aciduria type 1 (glutaryl-CoA-dehydrogenase deficiency): Advances and unanswered questions. Report from an international meeting. *Eur J Pediatr.* 1997;156(11):821–828.
36. Kolker S, Christensen E, Leonard JV, et al. Guideline for the diagnosis and management of glutaryl-CoA dehydrogenase deficiency (glutaric aciduria type I). *J Inherit Metab Dis.* 2007;30(1):5–22.
37. Jaeken J, Carchon H. The carbohydrate-deficient glycoprotein syndromes: An overview. *J Inherit Metab Dis.* 1993;16(5):813–820.
38. Krasnewich D, Gahl WA. Carbohydrate-deficient glycoprotein syndrome. *Adv Pediatr.* 1997;44:109–40.
39. Matthijs G, Schollen E, Van Schaftingen E. The prenatal diagnosis of congenital disorders of glycosylation (CDG). *Prenat Diagn.* 2004;24(2):114–116.
40. Jaeken J, Carchon H, Stibler H. The carbohydrate-deficient glycoprotein syndromes: Pre-Golgi and Golgi disorders? *Glycobiology.* 1993;3(5):423–428.
41. Malinger G, Lev D, Lerman-Sagie T. The fetal cerebellum: Pitfalls in diagnosis and management. *Prenat Diagn.* 2009;29(4):372–380.
42. Hertz-Pannier L, Dechaux M, Sinico M, et al. Congenital disorders of glycosylation type I: A rare but new cause of hyperechoic kidneys in infants and children due to early microcystic changes. *Pediatr Radiol.* 2006;36(2):108–114.
43. Malhotra A, Pateman A, Chalmers R, Coman D, Menahem S. Prenatal cardiac ultrasound finding in congenital disorder of glycosylation type 1a. *Fetal Diagn Ther.* 2009;25(1):54–57.
44. van de Kamp JM, Lefeber DJ, Ruijter GJ, et al. Congenital disorder of glycosylation type Ia presenting with hydrops fetalis. *J Med Genet.* 2007;44(4):277–280.

45. Press G, Barshop BA, Haas RH, et al. Abnormalities of the brain in nonketotic hyperglycinemia: MR manifestations. *AJNR Am J Neuroradiol.* 1989;10:315–321.
46. Fletcher JM, Bye AME, Naynar V, et al. Non-ketotic hyperglycinemia presenting as pachygyria. *J Inher Metab Dis.* 1995;18:665–668.
47. Alejo J, Rincon P, Vaquerizo J, et al. Transient non-ketotic hyperglycinemia: Ultrasound, CT and MRI. Case report. *Neuroradiology.* 1997;39:658–660.
48. Scher MS, Bergman I. Neurophysiological and anatomical correlations in neonatal nonketotic hyperglycinemia. *Neuropediatrics.* 1986;17:137–143.
49. Paupe A, Bidat L, Sonigo P, et al. Prenatal diagnosis of hypoplasia of the corpus callosum in association with non-ketotic hyperglycinemia. *Ultrasound Obstet Gynecol.* 2002;20(6):616–619.
50. Rötig A, Munnich A. Genetic features of mitochondrial respiratory chain disorders. *J Am Soc Nephrol.* 2003;14(12):2995–3007.
51. von Kleist-Retzow JC, Cormier-Daire V, Viot G, et al. Antenatal manifestations of mitochondrial respiratory chain deficiency. *J Pediatr.* 2003;143(2):208–212.
52. Lincke CR, van den Bogert C, Nijtmans LG, et al. Cerebellar hypoplasia in respiratory chain dysfunction. *Neuropediatrics.* 1996;27: 216–218.
53. de Koning TJ, de Vries LS, Groenendaal F, et al. Pontocerebellar hypoplasia associated with respiratory-chain defects. *Neuropediatrics.* 1999;30(2):93–95.
54. Samson JF, Barth PG, de Vries JI, et al. Familial mitochondrial encephalopathy with fetal ultrasonographic ventriculomegaly and intracerebral calcifications. *Eur J Pediatr.* 1994;153(7):510–516.
55. Gire C, Girard N, Nicaise C, Einaudi MA, Montfort MF, Dejode JM. Clinical features and neuroradiological findings of mitochondrial pathology in six neonates. *Childs Nerv Syst.* 2002;18(11): 621–628.
56. Malinger G, Kidron D, Schreiber L, et al. Prenatal diagnosis of malformations of cortical development by dedicated neurosonography. *Ultrasound Obstet Gynecol.* 2007;29(2):178–191.
57. Bouchet C, Steffann J, Corcos J, et al. Prenatal diagnosis of myopathy, encephalopathy, lactic acidosis, and stroke-like syndrome: Contribution to understanding mitochondrial DNA segregation during human embryofetal development. *J Med Genet.* 2006;43(10):788–792.
58. Dahl HH, Thorburn DR, White SL. Towards reliable prenatal diagnosis of mtDNA point mutations: Studies of nt8993mutations in oocytes, fetal tissues, children and adults. *Hum Reprod.* 2000;15(Suppl 2):246–255.
59. Minai L, Martinovic J, Chretien D, et al. Mitochondrial respiratory chain complex assembly and function during human fetal development. *Mol Genet Metab.* 2008;94(1):120–126.
60. Levy HL, Ghavami M. Maternal phenylketonuria: A metabolic teratogen. *Teratology.* 1996;53(3):176–184.
61. Levy HL, Lobbregt D, Barnes PD, et al. Maternal phenylketonuria: Magnetic resonance imaging in offspring. *J Pediatr.* 1996;128(6): 770–775.
62. Yik WY, Steinberg SJ, Moser AB, et al. Identification of novel mutations and sequence variation in the Zellweger syndrome spectrum of peroxisome biogenesis disorders. *Hum Mutat.* 2009;30(3): E467–480.
63. Volpe JJ, Adams RD. Cerebro-hepato-renal syndrome of Zellweger: An inherited disorder of neuronal migration. *Acta Neuropathol.* 1972;20:175–198.
64. Liu MH, Bangaru BS, Kidd J, et al. Neuropathological considerations in cerebro-hepato-renal syndrome (Zellweger's syndrome). *Acta Neuropathol.* 1976;34:115–123.
65. Gichrist KW, Gilbert EF, Goldfarb S, et al. Studies of malformation syndromes of Man XIB: The cerebro-hepato-renal syndrome of Zellweger. Comparative pathology. *Eur J Pediatr.* 1976;121: 99–118.
66. Evrard P, Caviness VS, Prats-Vinas J, et al. The mechanism of arrest of neuronal migration in the Zellweger malformation: An hypothesis based upon cytoarchitectonic analysis. *Acta Neuropathol.* 1978; 41:109–117.
67. Sarnat HB, Treven CL, Darwish HS. Ependymal abnormalities in cerebro-hepato-renal disease of Zellweger. *Brain Dev.* 1993;15: 270–277.
68. Van der Knaap MS, Valk J. The MR spectrum of peroxisomal disorders. *Neuroradiol.* 1991;33:30–37.
69. Barkovich AJ, Peck WW. MR of Zellweger syndrome. *AJNR Am J Neuroradiol.* 1997;18:1163–1170.
70. Torvik A, Torp S, Kase BF, et al. Infantile Refsum disease: A generalized peroxisomal disorder. Case report with postmortem examination. *J Neurol Sci.* 1988;85:39–53.
71. Kyllerman M, Blomstrand S, Mansson JE, et al. Central nervous system malformations and white matter changes in pseudo-neonatal adrenoleukodystrophy. *Neuropediatrics.* 1990;21:199–201.
72. Young S, Rabi Y, Lodha AK. Band heterotopia in Zellweger syndrome (cerebro-hepato-renal syndrome). *Neurol India.* 2007;55(1):93.
73. Mochel F, Grébille AG, Benachi A, et al. Contribution of fetal MR imaging in the prenatal diagnosis of Zellweger syndrome. *AJNR Am J Neuroradiol.* 2006;27(2):333–336.
74. Johnson JM, Babul-Hirji R, Chitayat D. First-trimester increased nuchal translucency and fetal hypokinesia associated with Zellweger syndrome. *Ultrasound Obstet Gynecol.* 2001;17:344–346.
75. Steinberg SJ, Dodt G, Raymond GV, et al. Peroxisome biogenesis disorders. *Biochim Biophys Acta.* 2006;1763(12):1733–1748.
76. Schwarz G. Molybdenum cofactor biosynthesis and deficiency. *Cell Mol Life Sci.* 2005;62(23):2792–2810.
77. Zhang X, Vincent AS, Halliwell B, et al. A mechanism of sulfite neurotoxicity: Direct inhibition of glutamate dehydrogenase. *JBiolog Chem.* 2004;279(41):43035–43045.
78. Schiaffino MC, Fantasia AR, Minniti G, et al. Isolated sulphite oxidase deficiency: clinical and biochemical features in an Italian patient. *J Inherit Metab Dis.* 2004;27(1):101–102.
79. Rupar CA, Gillett J, Gordon BA, et al. Isolated sulfite oxidase deficiency. *Neuropediatrics.* 1996;27(6):299–304.
80. Roth A, Nogues C, Monnet JP, et al. Anatomo-pathological findings in a case of combined deficiency of sulphite oxidase and xanthine oxidase with a defect of molybdenum cofactor. *Virchows Arch A Pathol Anat Histopathol.* 1985;405(3):379–386.
81. Serrano M, Lizarraga I, Reiss J, et al. Cranial ultrasound and chronological changes in molybdenum cofactor deficiency. *Pediatr Radiol.* 2007;37(10):1043–1046.
82. Per H, Gümüş H, Ichida K, Cağlayan O, Kumandaş S. Molybdenum cofactor deficiency: clinical features in a Turkish patient. *Brain Dev.* 2007;29(6):365–368.
83. Arslanoglu S, Yalaz M, Gökşen D, et al. Molybdenum cofactor deficiency associated with Dandy-Walker complex. *Brain Dev.* 2001;23(8):815–818.
84. Topcu M, Coskun T, Haliloglu G, Saatci I. Molybdenum cofactor deficiency: Report of three cases presenting as hypoxic-ischemic encephalopathy. *J Child Neurol.* 2001;16(4):264–270.
85. Appignani BA, Kaye EM, Wolpert SM. CT and MR appearance of the brain in two children with molybdenum cofactor deficiency. *AJNR Am J Neuroradiol.* 1996;17(2):317–320.
86. Schuierer G, Kurlemann G, Bick U, Stephani U. Molybdenum-cofactor deficiency: CT and MR findings. *Neuropediatrics.* 1995;26(1):51–54.
87. Mize C, Johnson JL, Rajagopalan KV. Defective molybdopterin biosynthesis: Clinical heterogeneity associated with molybdenum cofactor deficiency. *J Inherit Metab Dis.* 1995;18(3):283–290.
88. Reiss J, Christensen E, Dorche C. Molybdenum cofactor deficiency: First prenatal genetic analysis. *Prenatal Diag.* 1999;19: 386–388.

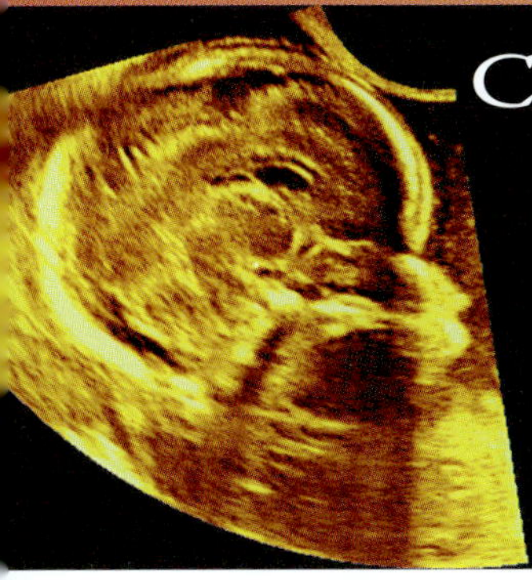

# Chapter 13

# TUMORS OF THE BRAIN

*Israel Meizner*

**KEY POINTS**

1. Fetal brain tumors are rare and usually diagnosed only in the 3rd trimester of pregnancy or even only after delivery.
2. Most types have a poor prognosis lipomas and choroid plexus papillomas are the exception having a better prognosis.

## CONGENITAL CENTRAL NERVOUS SYSTEM TUMORS

### Definition

Congenital central nervous system (CNS) tumors represent a distinct group of tumors that differs from familial and genetic CNS tumors. It is accepted that these tumors include those present at birth or diagnosed during the first year of life.

### Incidence/Prevalence

Congenital CNS tumors have been reported to represent between 0.5% and 1.5% of all pediatric brain tumors.[1] The fact that many of the congenital CNS tumors often result in intrauterine fetal demise makes the accurate assessment of the true incidence difficult.

The incidence in the United States as reported in the Third National Cancer Survey in 1971 was 14 CNS tumors per 1 million live births per year.[2] A similar study from Germany showed an incidence much higher (3.6 per 100,000 births).[3]

### Pathogenesis

We still have no knowledge or means to identify the cause or causes of malignancies that occur in early life. Fetal and/or maternal exposure to exogenous factors, including ionizing irradiation, drugs, and viruses, may start the biological mechanisms responsible for tumor formation.[4] Developmental errors during embryonic and fetal maturation may result in congenital tumors.[5] More than 100 years ago, Durante[6] and Cohnheim[7] proposed the "cell rest" theory that may be adapted to embryonic tumors. These authors believed that more cells are produced than required for the formation of an organ or tissue and that the origins of embryonic tumors rest in developmental errors in these surplus embryonic rudiments. Embryonic tumors developing after infancy are explained by the persistence of cell rests or developmental vestiges.[8] Developmentally anomalous tissues (ie, hamartomas and dysgenic gonads) are a source of neoplasms in older children and adults. When any of these developmentally abnormal tissues are present at birth, it is inferred that the cells failed to mature, migrate, or differentiate properly during intrauterine life.

A genetic model of carcinogenesis has been introduced in an attempt to clarify the pathogenesis and behavioral peculiarities of certain embryonic tumors.[9] According to this hypothesis, embryonic neoplasms arise as a result of two mutational events in the genome. The first mutation is prezygotic in familial cases and postzygotic in nonfamilial; the second mutation is always postzygotic.

The concept that teratogenesis and oncogenesis have shared mechanisms has been well documented by numerous examples. There is probably simultaneous or sequential cellular and tissue reaction to specific injurious agents. The degree of cytodifferentiation, the metabolic or immunological state of the embryo or fetus, and the length of time of exposure to the agent will determine whether the effect is teratogenic, oncogenic, both, or neither. Many biological, chemical, and physical agents known to be teratogenic to the fetus or embryo are carcinogenic postnatally.[10] Alternatively, a teratogenic event during intrauterine life may predispose the fetus to an oncogenic event later in life. This would explain neoplastic transformation occurring in hamartomas, developmental vestiges, heterotopias, and dysgenetic tissues. It is postulated that the anomalous tissues harbor latent oncogenes that, under certain environmental conditions, are activated, resulting in malignant transformation of a tumor.

## Cytogenetics

The type of chromosomal abnormalities appearing in the pediatric brain tumors differs from that found in adult brain tumors. Genetic abnormalities detected at the chromosomal and molecular level have been observed in several fetal brain tumors.[11,12] The most common abnormality in medulloblastoma is the partial or total loss of chromosome 17, a monosomy of (17q), which is observed in ~50% of tumors.[13] Chromosome 1 deletions (del 1q) have been reported in childhood astrocytomas.[14] Studies conducted on fetal brain teratomas have found that a normal 46XY or 46XX karyotype exists for both the patient and tumor.[15]

An interesting association between monosomy 22, the most frequent chromosomal abnormality in pediatric and adult meningiomas, has been described with primitive neuroectodermal tumor.[16] Also, the gene for neurofibromatosis has been mapped to the long arm of chromosome 22. It may be possible to suspect a possible association between neurofibromatosis and CNS tumors sharing a common pathogenetic mechanism in tumorigenesis.[17]

## Pathology

Large studies on fetal intracranial tumors have provided data about the different histologic subtypes.[18–21] Interestingly, the distribution of the various types of perinatal brain tumors varies in different countries and medical centers. Astrocytoma, medulloblastoma, and choroid plexus papilloma are the major neuroglial perinatal tumors, and teratoma is the leading nonneuroglial tumor. The teratomas are responsible for the largest number of stillbirths, accounting for over one-third to one-half of cases.

Incorporation of electron microscopy and immunohistochemistry techniques is mandatory for identification and classification of brain tumors. The immunohistochemical markers specifically used for evaluation of CNS neoplasms include the glial fibrillary acidic protein (GFAP) and the neurofilament protein (NFP) antibodies.[22,23] The GFAP is helpful in distinguishing between glial and nonglial neoplasms and in identifying astrocytic elements. Monoclonal antibodies directed against neuroectoderm-associated antigens include neuron-specific enolase (NSE) and the S-100 protein, which cross-reacts with many types of tissues, both neural and nonneural.[24] Tumors such as neuroblastoma, medulloblastoma, and primitive neuroectodermal tumor (PNET) generally exhibit NSE positivity and are focally positive to S-100 protein. Synaptophysin has been found to be a useful marker for identifying these tumors. Alphafetoprotein (AFP) and human chorionic gonadotropin (hCG) immunoperoxidase antibodies also aid in the diagnosis of intracranial germ tumors, yolk sac tumor, and choriocarcinoma. For tumors posing a severe diagnostic challenge, one may use electron microscopy.[22] Karyotyping is increasingly becoming an aid in detecting certain brain tumors. We will present the pathologic hallmarks of the most common fetal brain tumors.

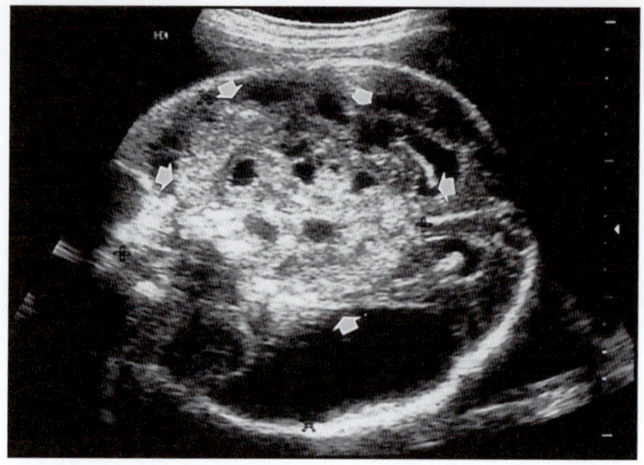

**Figure 13–1.** Brain teratoma. Note the huge echogenic solid tumor mass (*arrowheads*) replacing a large volume of the normal brain tissue.

### Intracranial Teratoma

Intracranial teratoma is the most common intracranial neoplasm diagnosed during the first year of life and the leading cause of tumor-related fetal death.[18,19,21] Perinatal intracranial teratomas consist of mature and immature tissues of various types. Most of them arise from midline supratentorial locations, such as the pineal body and third ventricle and suprasellar regions, but occasionally they originate in the cerebral hemispheres or brainstem.[25] In ~50% of cases, the teratoma reaches gigantic size, effacing normal brain tissue elements; thus, it destroys any identifiable clue for site of origin.

A classification of intracranial teratomas into three subtypes has been proposed:[26]

- Teratomas replacing the brain tissue (Figure 13–1)
- Smaller tumors usually not causing hydrocephaly (Figures 13–2, 13–3, and 13–4)
- Teratomas with local extension into the face (Figures 13–5 and 13–6)

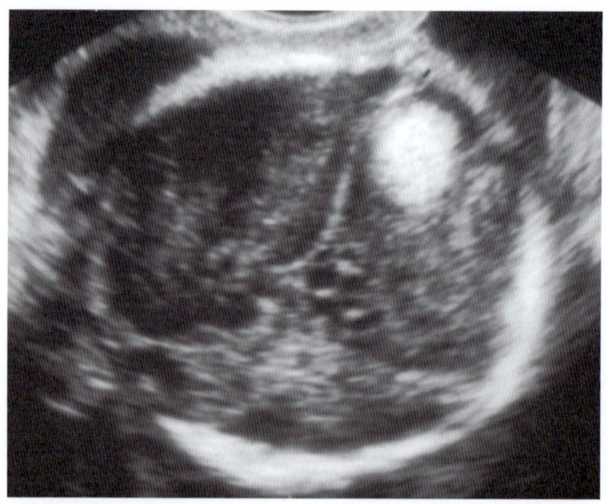

**Figure 13–2.** Brain teratoma. Note the tumor mass (T) without aparent dilated lateral ventricles.

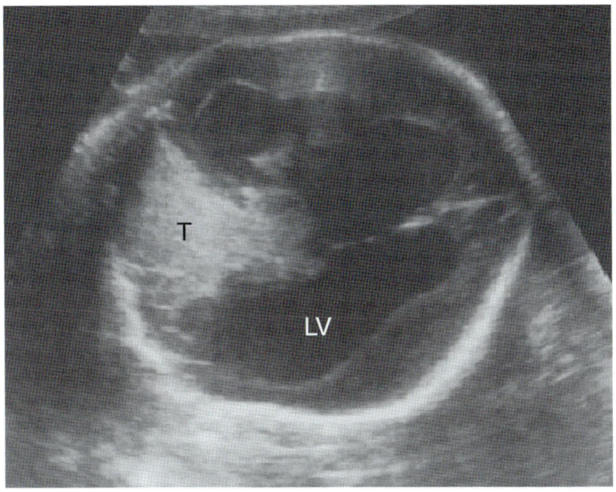


**Figure 13–3.** Small echogenic brain teratoma (T). LV, lateral ventricle.

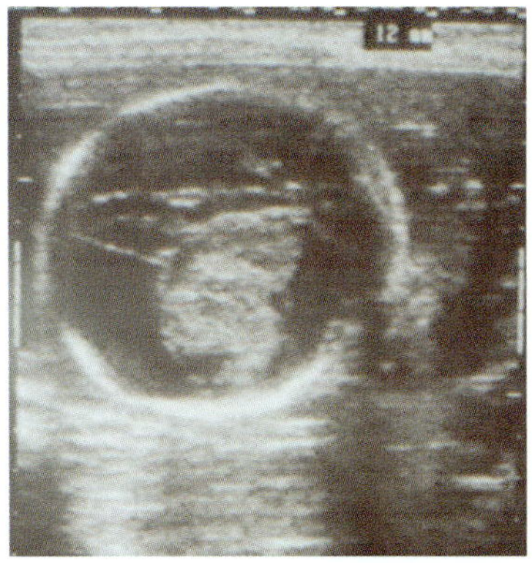

**Figure 13–5.** Brain teratoma. Note the absence of normal brain architecture. Solid areas surrounded by septated liquified areas are present. (Courtesy of Ron Rabinovitz, MD, Jerusalem, Israel.)

Hydrocephaly may be the initial finding. In several cases it has been reported that hydrocephaly has progressed rapidly on serial scans prior to the detection of a huge teratoma.[15] This observation suggests that early obstruction to the flow of cerebrospinal fluid (CSF) by the midline location of the tumor is followed by effacement of the brain by continued tumor growth. Neonates, having small lesions, may show evidence of hydrocephaly after birth caused by aqueductal stenosis.

Despite recent advances in diagnosis and therapy, with fetal and neonatal intracranial teratomas, stillbirth or perinatal death occurs in most cases.[27–29] In some cases, dystocia may happen.[30]

### Fetus in Fetu

An extremely rare congenital condition, fetus in fetu has been described as presenting as a mass. The mass may be present intracranially (Figure 13–7), intra-abdominally, retroperitoneally, or in the scrotum. The exact relationship between teratoma and fetus in fetu is controversial.[31–36] Some feel that this might in fact be two edges of the same entity, namely, a teratoma.[32] However, it has been stated that to distinguish between fetus in fetu and teratoma, the vertebral column must be present.[37]

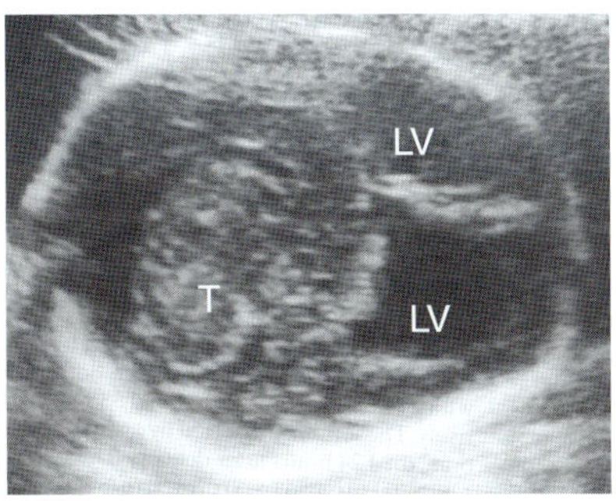


**Figure 13–4.** Brain teratoma causing hydrocephaly. T, tumor mass; LV, lateral ventricles.

### Astrocytoma

Astrocytoma is the leading neuroglial tumor of infancy. In the fetus, it is usually supratentorial. The cerebral hemisphere is the most common primary site (two-thirds of cases). Those arising from the cerebral hemispheres are frequently large, may involve more than one lobe, and occupy an extensive part of the brain (Figure 13–8). Hydrocephaly is the main presenting feature in both fetus and neonate, regardless of site of origin. Almost half of perinatal astrocytomas are malignant, and some have been called anaplastic astrocytomas.

### Glioblastoma multiforme

Originating from the glia, glioblastoma multiforme (GBM) this is an extremely rare tumor in the fetal brain. Its prenatal diagnosis is possible and was reported to occur usually after 25 weeks.[38] Fetal glioblastomas are characteristically fast-growing intracranial tumors presenting as polyhydramnios and hydrocephaly and a fast-growing echogenic, vascularized brain lesion (see

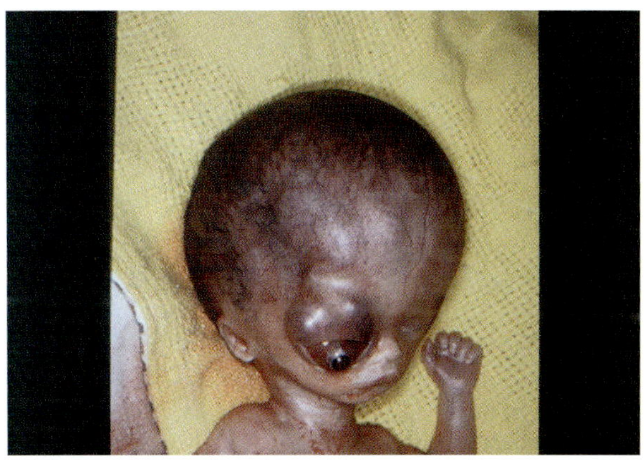

**Figure 13–6.** Post mortem picture of the fetus in Figure 13–5. Note the macrocephaly and eye protrusion due to extension of the tumor into the orbit. (Courtesy of Ron Rabinovitz, MD, Jerusalem, Israel.)

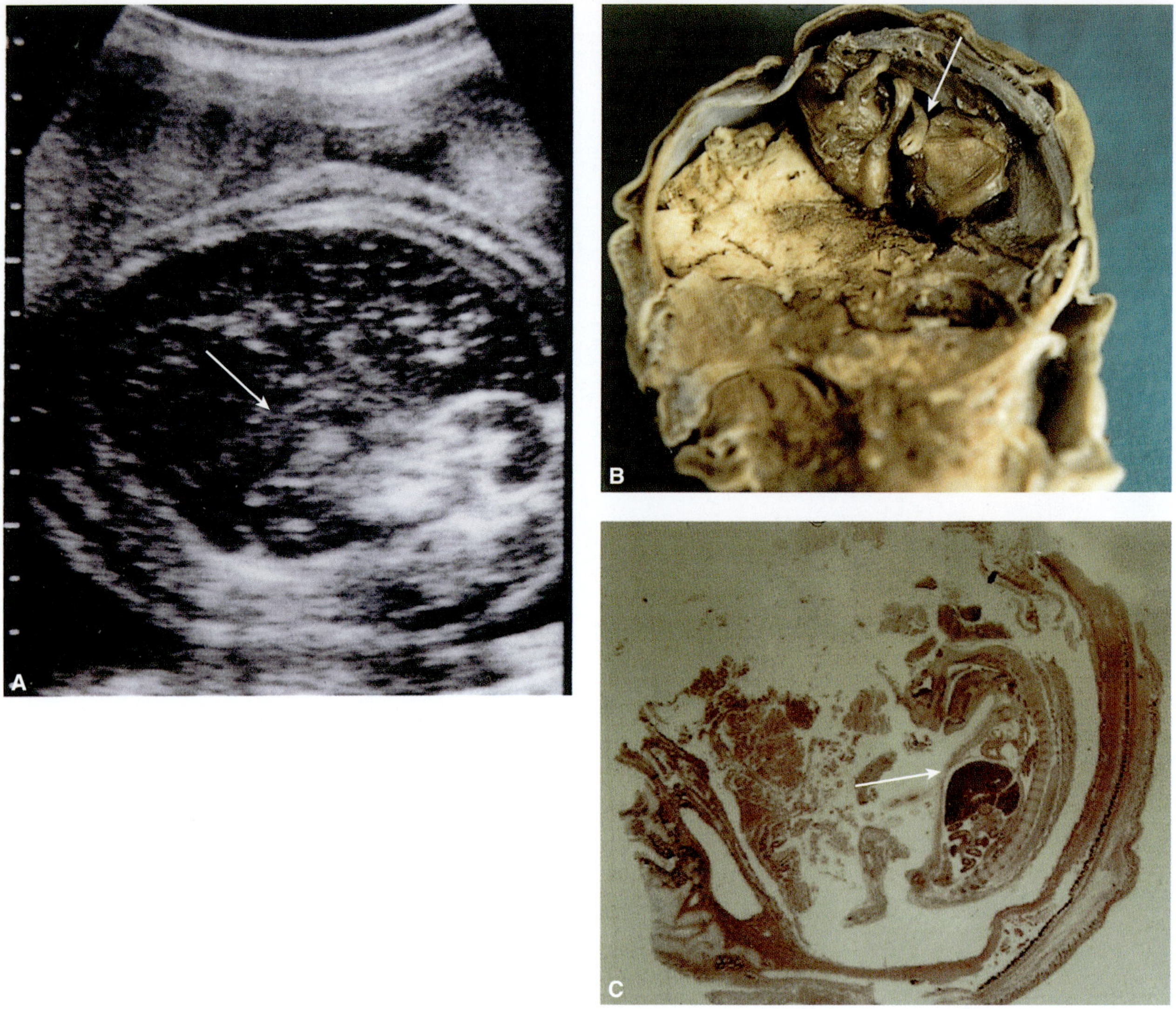


**Figure 13–7.** A very rare case of a true intracranial fetus-in-fetu that presented at 17 weeks with an intracranial mass. Upon closer inspection, the mass had the sonographic appearance of a fetus. **(A)** Transabdominal scan at 17 weeks showing intracranial mass (*arrow*). Patient elected to terminate the pregnancy. **(B)** Picture of the gross specimen showing the well-formed fetus (*arrow*) within the cranial cavity pushing the brain to one side. **(C)** Histology demonstated a well-formed fetal vertebral column. (Courtesy of Prof. A. lanniruberto, Italy.)

Figure 13–8). Most cases of GBM occur supratentorially. The prognosis is almost uniformly grim. All neonates in the published literature succumbed at birth or shortly thereafter.[39–45]

### Primitive Neuroectodermal Tumor

PNET occurs in several locations, including the cerebellum, cerebral hemispheres, pineal body, brainstem, spinal cord, olfactory nerve, and retina[24] (Figure 13–9). Microscopically, PNETs are represented by groups of small, poorly differentiated, darkly stained cells. They occur primarily in the pediatric age group and are characterized by very aggressive behavior, regardless of their primary site or histologic components. This type of tumor metastasizes widely within the CSF pathways and seeds the meninges of the brain and spinal cord.[22]

### Medulloblastoma

Medulloblastoma, also called PNET of the cerebellum, is the leading infratentorial tumor. It is associated with a high frequency of stillbirth, hydrocephaly, and congenital defects.[46] Anomalies described to appear in conjunction with this tumor include cleft palate, omphalocele, malrotation of the intestine, imperforate anus, and bladder exstrophy.[46] A tendency toward a familial occurrence of this tumor has been reported.[47] An association with rhabdoid tumor of the kidney has also been reported, suggesting that the neural crest is the common denominator.[48]

### Choroid Plexus Papilloma

Choroid plexus papilloma is a benign tumor composed of epithelial cells that line the ventricular choroid plexuses.[49]

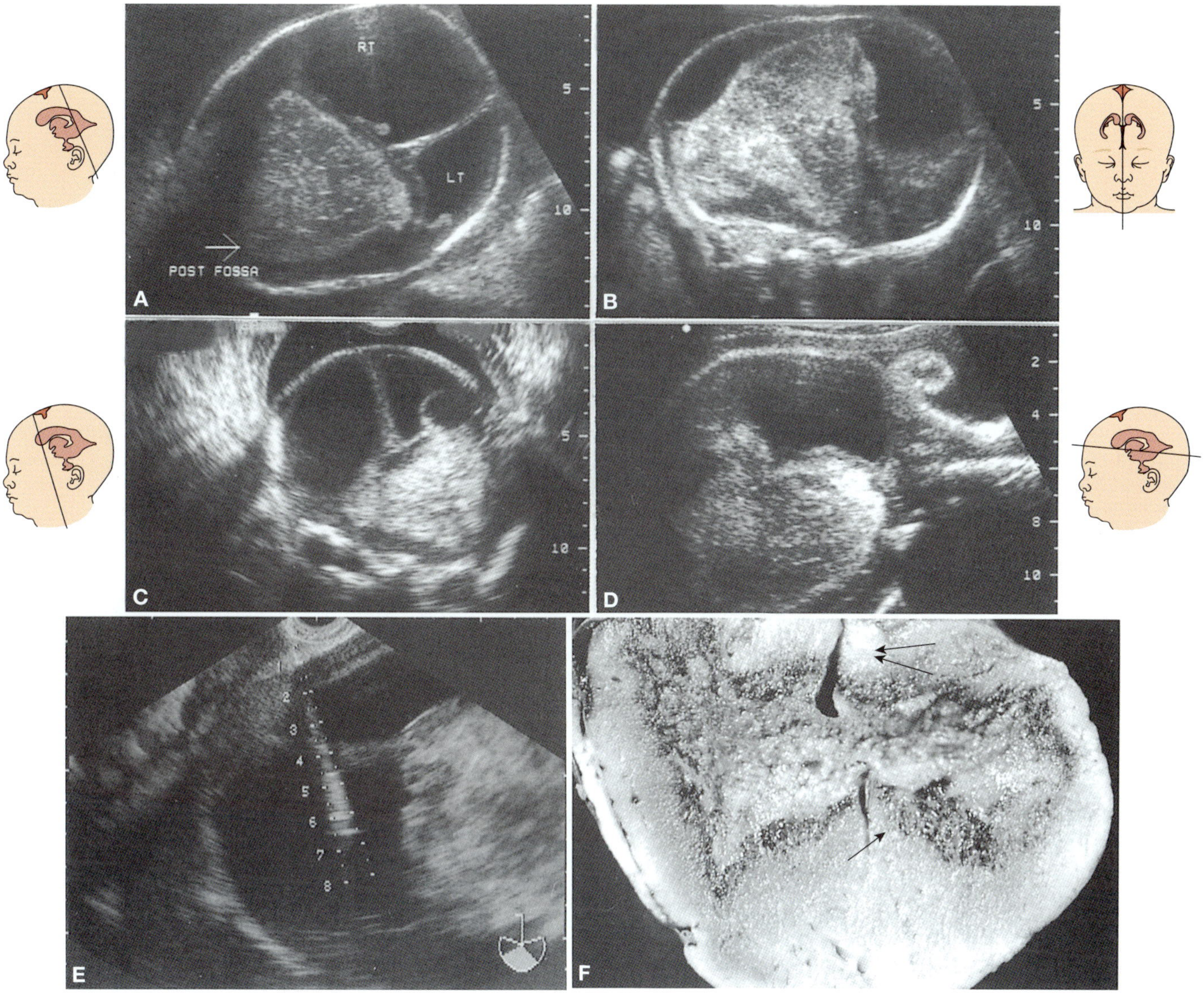


**Figure 13–8.** Four views of the brain of a fetus at 34 postmenstrual weeks having a tumor of the brain. **(A)** Midcoronal–3, almost occipital–1, section showing the dilated right and left lateral ventricles, the thin and dangling hyperechoic choroid plexus, and the extremely thin posterior fossa (*arrow*). **(B)** Median section showing the extent of the tumor in the midline, above and behind which the dilated ventricles are seen. **(C)** Midcoronal–1 section. **(D)** Horizontal section. After the diagnosis of the space-occupying lesion in the brain, causing severe obstructive hydrocephaly, it was decided that the patient's labor would be induced. Cephalocentesis, to decrease the size of the head by draining cerebrospinal fluid (csf), was performed. **(E)** The needle is seen in the fluid at a depth of 6.5 cm. The head circumference decreased from 40 cm to enable vaginal birth, which was achieved after inducing labor. **(F)** The stillborn neonate was examined by the pathologist. The arrow indicates the third ventricle, and the double arrow indicates the longitudinal sulcus. Histologic examination of the tumor revealed a glioblastoma. (Courtesy of Susan M. Staugaitis, MD, PhD; Departments of Neurosciences and Anatomic Pathology, Cleveland Clinic.)

The incidence is inversely correlated with age, and ~50% of cases in patients in the pediatric age group are detected during the first year of life.[50] These neoplasms rank third in frequency of congenital CNS tumors. The main presentation is rapidly developing hydrocephaly caused by the growing papilloma into the lateral ventricles, sometimes into the third or fourth ventricle. This overgrowth produces a large, space-occupying nodular lesion that is readily observed on imaging studies (Figure 13–10). The tumor may produce large amounts of CSF, causing hydrocephaly. The prognosis of patients having choroid plexus papilloma is comparatively good and is the most favorable of all newborn brain tumors.[51] It is important to diagnose choroid plexus papilloma preoperatively, as surgical removal is usually curative.

## PERICALLOSAL LIPOMA

Pericallosal lipoma is caused by the abnormal resorption of the meninx primitive and its differentiation into lipomatous tissue. Two different groups have been described: curvilinear and tubulonodular. In the curvilinear type, the lipomatous tissue extends in a regular pattern into the

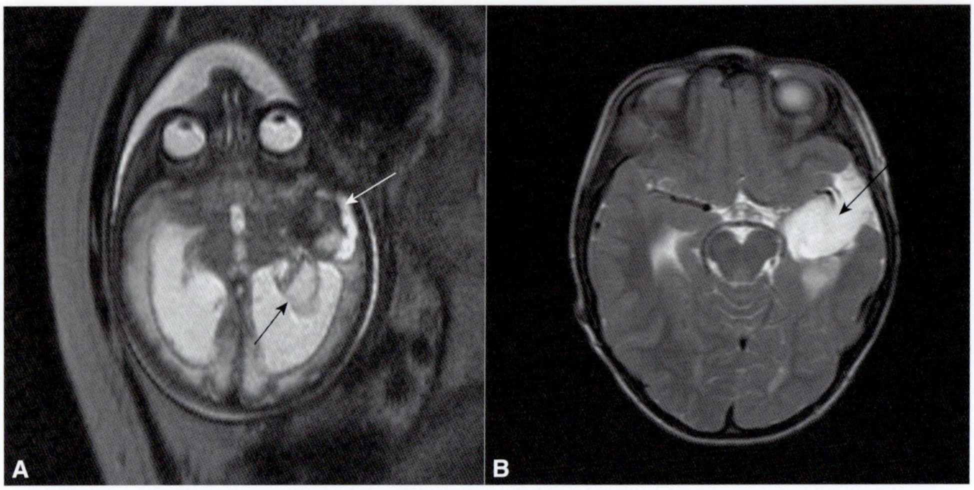


**Figure 13–9.** Primitive neuroectodermal tumor. **(A)** Fetal brain MRI at 34 weeks of gestation shows the mass involving the brain parenchyma (*white arrow*) and extending into the lateral ventricle (*black arrow*). Note the presence of marked ventriculomegaly. **(B)** Brain MRI at 5 years of age shows complete remission following surgery. (Courtesy of Daniela Prayer, Vienna, Austria.)

callosal sulcus, covering the upper aspect of the corpus callosum (Figure 13–11). In the tubulonodular type, the tumor is usually anteriorly situated and round or cylinder-shaped. These lipomas are generally > 2 cm in diameter (Figure 13–12) and have a high incidence of corpus callosum dysgenesis, frontal lobe anomalies, and frontal encephaloceles.[52] The tumor mass may extend to the region of the lateral ventricle choroid plexus in the caudothalamic groove (25%). Bilateral ventriculomegaly may accompany the lesion.

## Clinical Aspects

The clinical features of congenital CNS tumors are entirely different from those found in older children or adults. Hydrocephaly and macrocephaly are the main presenting signs in the fetus and neonate, as opposed to the older child, in whom signs of lateralization are common (hyperreflexia, ataxia, cranial nerve palsy, hemiparesis, and seizures) (Figure 13–13). Brain tumors in the fetus and newborn may appear as intracranial hemorrhage, subdural hematoma, unexplained hydrocephaly, distortion of the cranium, and bony defects[54] (Figure 13–14). As suggested by Volpe,[53] the clinical findings of fetal and neonatal brain tumors can be classified into four main groups of presentations. The first is characterized by tumors that are huge, producing severe macrocephaly leading to cephalopelvic disproportion, dystocia, stillbirth, and preterm birth associated with severe obstetrical complications. The second is characterized by the appearance of a large cranium and bulging fontanelles secondary to hydrocephaly. The third includes all specific neurologic findings related to the type and site of occurrence of the lesion and is typical for postnatal tumors. The fourth is characterized by a sudden onset of intracranial hemorrhage, which appears in 8% to 18% of neonates with brain tumors.

The remarkable ability of the skull to expand causes some tumors of the brain to expand enormously in utero. This may lead to dystocia and stillbirth. Large tumors are responsible for fetal hydrops or may necessitate decompression of the cranium to permit vaginal delivery.[29,30] The best example for such a tumor is intracranial teratoma. Hydrocephaly is caused by either compression of the ventricular system or intracranial hemorrhage from the tumor.

About two-thirds of congenital brain tumors of the fetus are supratentorial, and the rest are infratentorial.[55] Thus, the location of the tumors is completely different from that seen in the older child and adolescent. Primary intracranial tumors appearing in the older child and adolescent are infratentorial in the vast majority of cases and are found within the posterior fossa (brainstem and cerebellum). The majority of tumors appearing in the fetus and neonate are located above the tentorium.

As reported, congenital brain teratomas, primitive neuroectodermal tumors, and pineoblastomas appear in the midline, the pineal area, and the area of the third ventricle. The astrocytic tumors are located in close relationship with the dura mater in the cerebral cortex.[24,25] Tumors arising from the choroid plexus are found in the lateral ventricles, less frequently in the third ventricle.[25] Primary congenital astrocytomas arising in the spinal cord may affect the entire cord (holocord) or just a segment. It should be stressed that most spinal cord neoplasms are within the substance of the cord (intramedullary) but may be extramedullary and intradural or extradural.

## Differential Diagnosis

Congenital CNS tumor can mimic other CNS pathologies, such as ventriculomegaly, intracranial bleeding (subdural hematoma), intracranial cysts, vascular malformations (vein of Galen aneurysm), and intracranial abscesses. One should remember, however, that the leading cause of congenital hydrocephaly is not a tumor but rather obstruction of the subarachnoid space or aqueduct following infection or hemorrhage. The differential diagnosis should include the Arnold-Chiari malformation.[47]

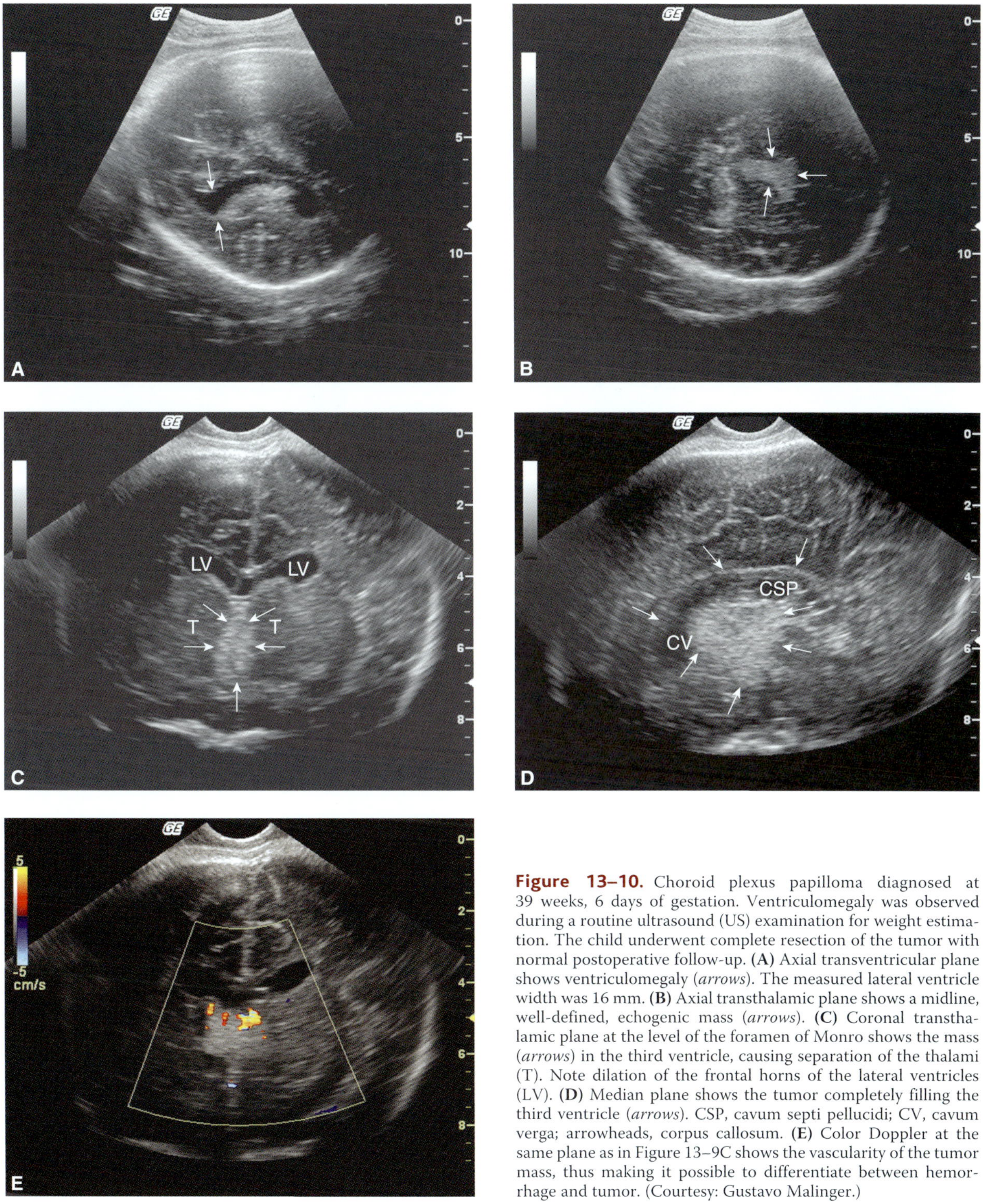


**Figure 13–10.** Choroid plexus papilloma diagnosed at 39 weeks, 6 days of gestation. Ventriculomegaly was observed during a routine ultrasound (US) examination for weight estimation. The child underwent complete resection of the tumor with normal postoperative follow-up. **(A)** Axial transventricular plane shows ventriculomegaly (*arrows*). The measured lateral ventricle width was 16 mm. **(B)** Axial transthalamic plane shows a midline, well-defined, echogenic mass (*arrows*). **(C)** Coronal transthalamic plane at the level of the foramen of Monro shows the mass (*arrows*) in the third ventricle, causing separation of the thalami (T). Note dilation of the frontal horns of the lateral ventricles (LV). **(D)** Median plane shows the tumor completely filling the third ventricle (*arrows*). CSP, cavum septi pellucidi; CV, cavum verga; arrowheads, corpus callosum. **(E)** Color Doppler at the same plane as in Figure 13–9C shows the vascularity of the tumor mass, thus making it possible to differentiate between hemorrhage and tumor. (Courtesy: Gustavo Malinger.)

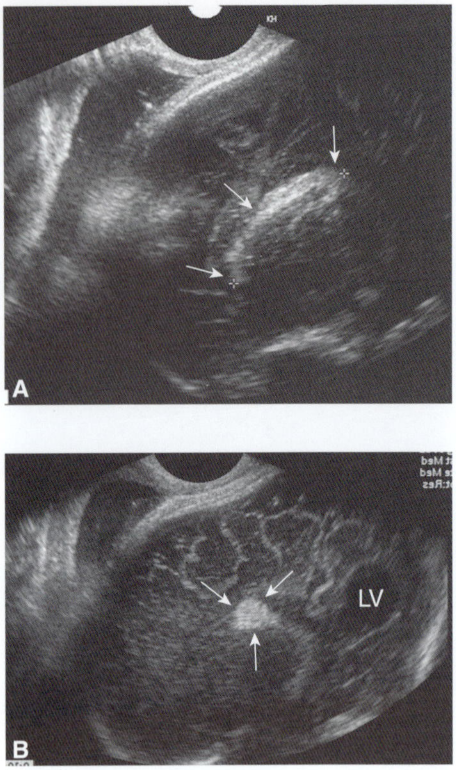


**Figure 13–11.** Pericallosal curvilinear lipoma diagnosed at 34 weeks of gestation. **(A)** Median plane shows the echogenic lipoma (*arrows*). The corpus callosum, which is positioned below the lipoma, is less echogenic and thus difficult to visualize. **(B)** Paramedian plane shows extension of the lipomatous mass into the choroid plexus (*arrows*). LV, lateral ventricle. (Courtesy of Gustavo Malinger.)

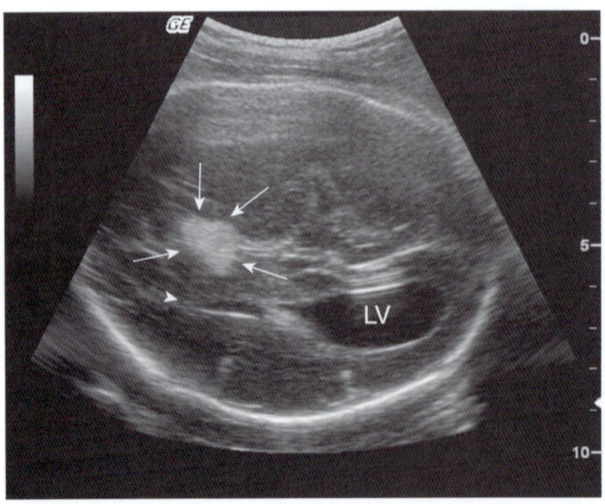


**Figure 13–12.** Pericallosal tubulonodular lipoma diagnosed at 30 weeks of gestation. Axial transventricular plane shows the nodular mass positioned anteriorly (*arrows*). Note the presence of associated colpocephaly with an abnormally shaped frontal horn (*arrowhead*). LV, lateral ventricle. (Courtesy of Gustavo Malinger.)

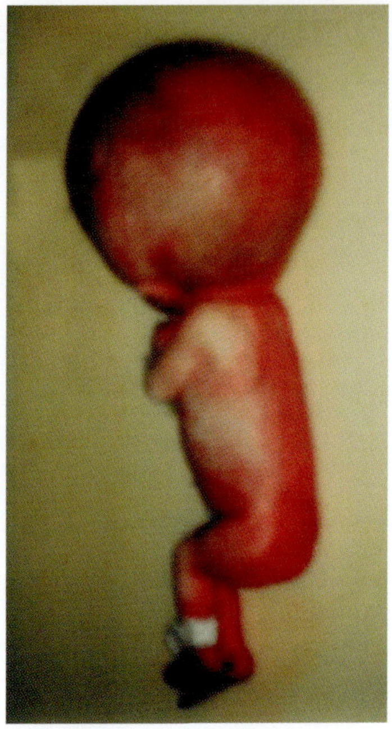

**Figure 13–13.** Abortus with huge intracranial teratoma. Note the extremely large size of the head.

## Risk of Recurrence

Congenital CNS tumors are usually sporadic and not associated with other malformations. A rare exception is the hypothalamic hamartoblastoma characteristic of the Pallister-Hall syndrome.[56] A definite association has been documented between neurofibromatosis type I and tuberous sclerosis,[24] choroid plexus papilloma and Aicardi syndrome,[57] and hemangioblastoma and von Hippel-Lindau disease.[58]

## Sonographic and Magnetic Resonance Imaging Diagnosis

With the widespread use of imaging modalities, namely, ultrasound (US) and magnetic resonance imaging (MRI), the ability to detect fetal tumors prenatally has improved dramatically. There are many case reports as well as

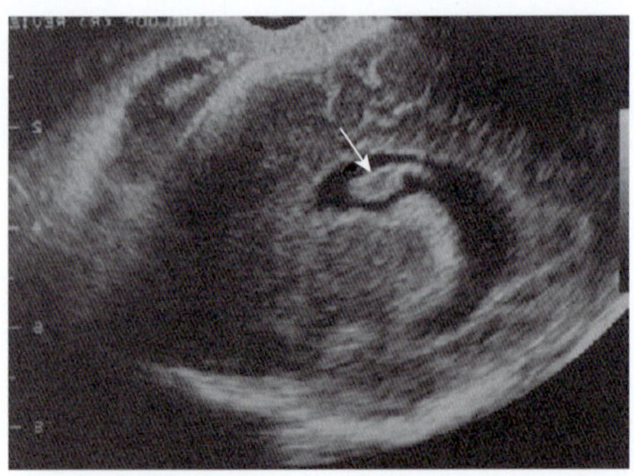

**Figure 13–14.** Paramedian plane in a fetus with a brain teratoma shows ventriculomegaly and intraventricular hemorrhage (*arrow*).

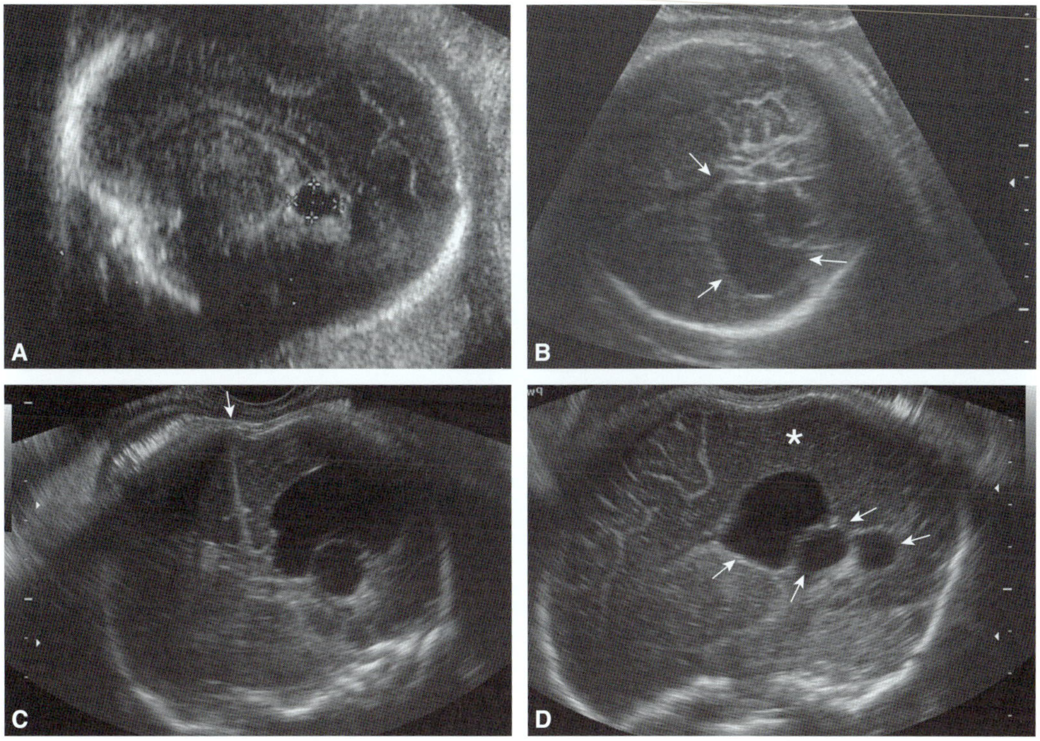


**Figure 13–15.** Rapid development of choroid plexus papilloma of the lateral ventricle. **(A)** Paramedian plane at 28 weeks of gestation shows a small cystic formation within the choroid plexus. This finding was not present at 23 weeks of gestation. **(B)** Axial plane at 35 weeks of gestation shows a much larger multicystic mass. **(C)** Coronal plane at the level of the occipital lobe shows displacement of the falx from the midline. **(D)** Parasagittal plane shows the lack of normal sulcation in the brain parenchyma around the mass (*asterisk*). (Courtesy of Zeev Efrat and Gustavo Malinger.)

some review studies of fetal brain tumors diagnosed in utero.[27,59–62] All these studies are helpful in establishing guidelines for correct prenatal diagnosis of such lesions. Furthermore, imaging studies can be helpful in identifying and distinguishing potentially curable tumors, such as choroid plexus papillomas, from rapidly fatal ones, such as teratomas and PNETs.

Ultrasonography is the main method used to establish a correct diagnosis in utero, once a solid, cystic, or calcified lesion has been observed. It is also the best modality for evaluating fetal macrocrania.[62] Most brain tumors show a similar sonographic image represented by disorganized structures within the fetal brain accompanied by areas of calcification and cysts. Polyhydramnios is a common finding due to inhibition of swallowing caused by the tumor. The head circumference measurement will show a huge head size, far beyond what is expected for gestational age. One should bear in mind that intracranial hemorrhage can cause echogenic areas that may mimic intracranial calcifications. According to Isaacs,[21] the most prevalent clinical signs of intracranial fetal tumor are macrocephaly, hydrocephaly, intracranial mass, polyhydramnios, breech presentation, hydrops, stillbirth, dystocia, and enlarged uterus.

According to Garel,[64] the contribution of MRI is relatively limited but may help in determining the remaining brain structures and the exact localization of the tumor, as well as in differentiating between tumor and hemorrhage. Recently, Cassart et al[61] studied 27 fetuses with intracranial tumors; in 24 an MRI was also performed. The authors found that the heterogeneous pattern characteristic of teratoma was better depicted by MRI. In addition, in two patients with teratoma, MRI helped in the assessment of tumor extension.[61] We find MRI very useful in counseling families with operable tumors regarding the apparent lack of associated findings and the relatively good prognosis expected following conservative management or surgery.

We should remember that fetal intracranial tumors have consistently been diagnosed relatively late in pregnancy, during the late second trimester, third trimester, or even at birth.[65] This may be due to the fact that they may grow very rapidly[66] (Figure 13–15), they are of similar echogenicity as the surrounding structures (Figure 13–16) or to changes in echogenicity occurring during pregnancy (Figure 13–17).

### Teratoma

Around 100 reports on the prenatal diagnosis of fetal intracranial teratomas have been published since the first US description by Hoff and Mackay in 1980.[67] The sonographic and MRI appearance of the fetal intracranial teratoma is usually that of an irregular solid mass, in some cases with cystic and/or calcified components, distorting brain anatomy[68] (see Figures 13–1 to 13–5). Intratumoral vascularization as demonstrated by color Doppler may be useful in the differential diagnosis between teratoma and

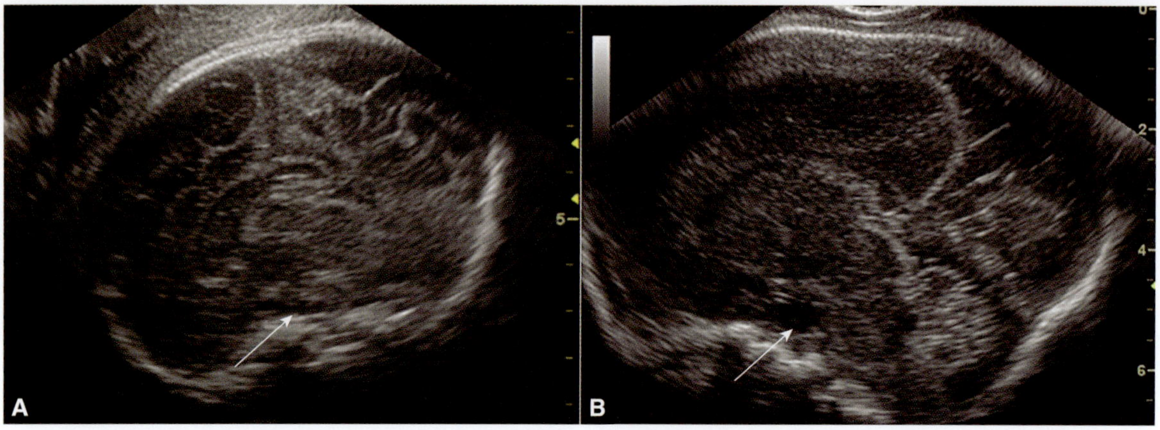

**Figure 13–16.** **(A)** Median plane in a fetus at 31 weeks of gestation diagnosed at 6 months of age as suffering from Pallister-Hall syndrome. The arrow points to the basal cistern filled with a mass of similar echogenicity as the surrounding brain, later on proved to represent a hypothalamic hamartoblastoma. **(B)** Normal basal cistern (*arrow*) in a fetus at the same gestational age. (Courtesy of Gustavo Malinger.)

hemorrhage (Figure 13-9).[69] Although in most cases teratomas have been described relatively late in pregnancy, there are isolated reports of first or early second trimester diagnosis.[70] Associated findings may include hydrocephaly[71,72] (see Figures 13–3 to 13–5, 13–10, and 13–14), macrocephaly,[56,58] brain atrophy or destruction[74] (see Figures 13–1 and 13–7), facial involvement[27,75] (see Figure 13–6), polyhydramnios,[76] and fetal hydrops with cardiac failure.[77]

### Astrocytoma

Although second in frequency, fetal astrocytomas have been described to less extent than teratomas.[78] By prenatal imaging, it seems difficult to differentiate between them[66,79,80] (see Figure 13–8). A possible clue in the differential diagnosis may be the presence of intratumoral hemorrhage.[81,82]

### Primitive Neuroectodermal Tumor

Prenatal diagnosis of PNET is extremely rare and less than 10 cases have been described.[83] In one recent case, an echogenic mass was visualized by US and MRI at 24 weeks' gestation causing severe ventriculomegaly; the diagnosis was made only at autopsy.[60] In postnatal cases, the tumor is usually solid, but in some cases, it may be composed of solid and cystic structures (Figure 13–8).

### Medulloblastoma

Medulloblastomas are characteristically infratentorial tumors. To the best of our knowledge, they have never been diagnosed during the prenatal period. A description of a 13-day-old girl with hydrocephaly starting at 22 weeks' gestation has been published.[84]

### Choroid Plexus Papilloma

Choroid plexus papillomas (CPPs) have been reported occasionally during the prenatal period. In 1989 Romero and colleagues[85] described CPP of the lateral ventricle in a fetus presenting with hydrocephaly at 30 weeks of gestation. They found that a comparison between the size of the choroid plexus and the presence of an echogenic mass

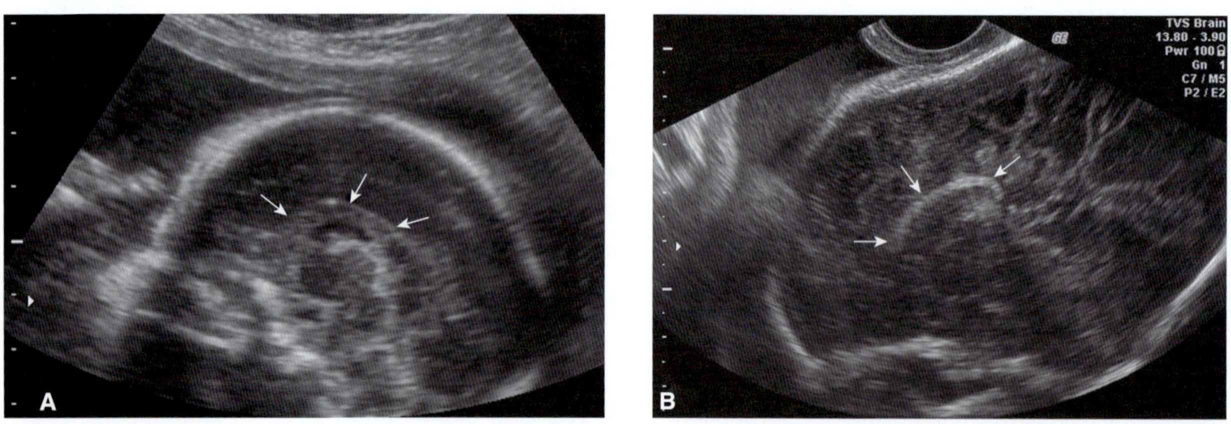

**Figure 13–17.** Pericallosal curvilinear lipoma. **(A)** Median plane at 23 weeks of gestation. The corpus callosum, although present, is not clearly visualized (*arrows*). **(B)** At 32 weeks of pregnancy in the same plane, the hyperechogenic lipoma is clearly depicted (*arrows*). The diagnosis was confirmed postnatally (Courtesy of Gustavo Malinger).

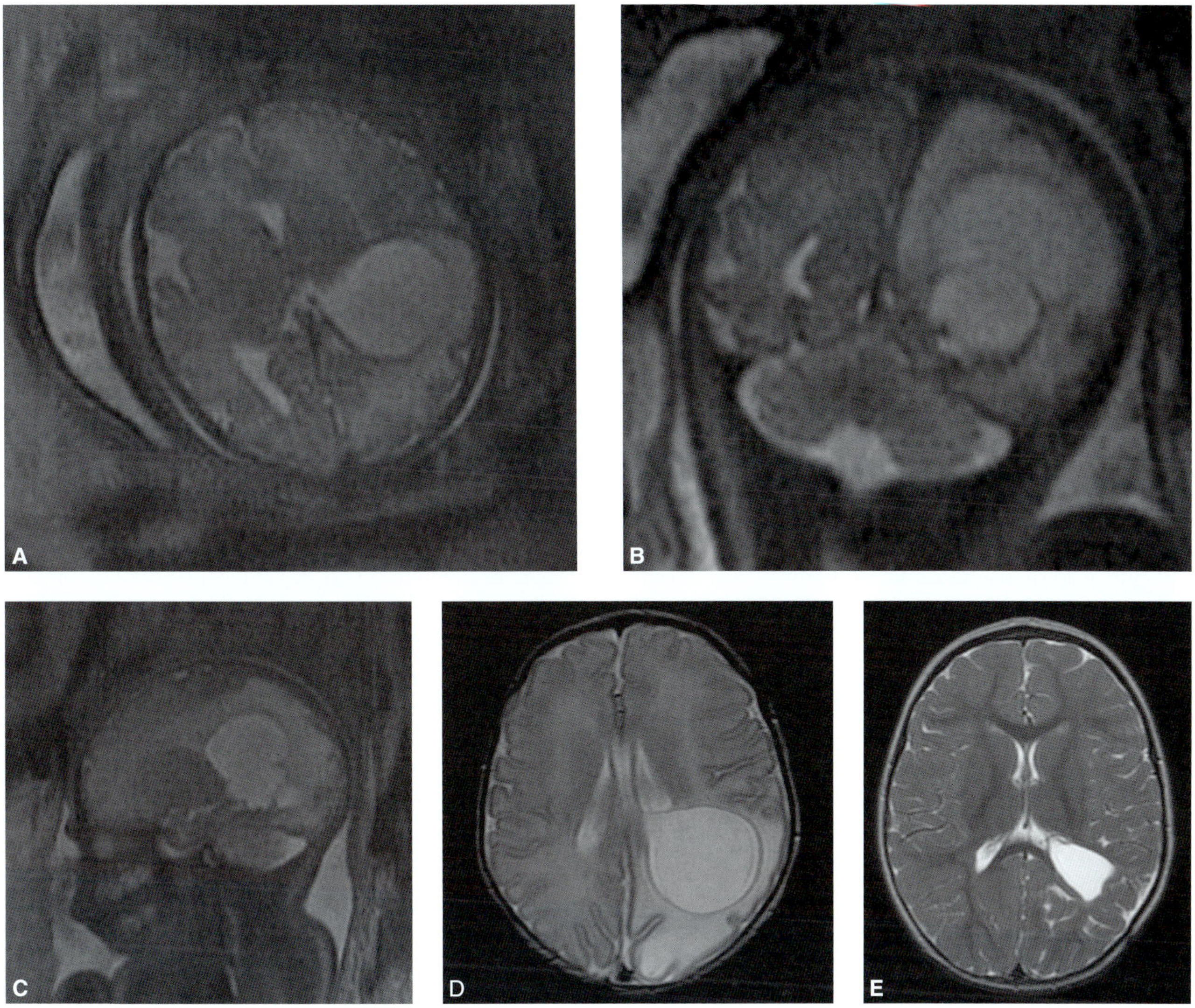


**Figure 13–18.** Prenatal and postnatal magnetic resonance imaging (MRI) in a patient with lateral ventricle choroid plexus papilloma (CPP; same patient as in Figure 13–14). Axial **(A),** coronal **(B),** and paramedian **(C)** planes at 36 weeks of gestation show the large, predominantly cystic tumor and the abnormal surrounding brain parenchyma. **(D)** Axial plane at the age of 9 days. **(E)** Same plane at 15 months of age following surgical resection of the tumor. Normal neurologic and developmental follow-up was done at 3 years of age. (Courtesy of Liat Ben Sira, MD, Tel Aviv, Israel.)

in the side where the choroid plexus seems larger may be helpful hints for diagnosis.[85]

CPPs may develop in the lateral ventricle (see Figures 13–15 and 13–18), third ventricle (see Figures 13–10 and 13–19), and fourth ventricle. Characteristically, they are diagnosed during the third trimester and are always associated with unilateral or bilateral ventriculomegaly. In our own experience with two cases, the second-trimester examinations were normal, but in one fetus, a repeated US examination at 28 weeks detected what appeared to be a small choroid plexus cyst; only follow-up examination at 35 weeks depicted the fully developed CPP. US and MRI depicted in this case the abnormal adjacent parenchyma (see Figures 13–15 and 13–18). In the other patient with a third ventricle CPP diagnosed at 39 weeks, color Doppler showing a very vascularized mass was more useful than MRI in differentiating between hemorrhage and CPP (see Figure 13–10 and 13–19).

### Lipoma

Pericallosal lipomas occasionally have been diagnosed using US and MRI. A literature review found fewer than 25 reported diagnoses. Mulligan and Meier[86] and Jeanty and colleagues[87] published the first prenatal descriptions in fetuses with agenesis of the corpus callosum and Goldenhar syndrome, respectively. The only published series described the US and MRI findings in seven fetuses. The lipomas were visible by US in all the patients, but in one of them it was wrongly considered a hemorrhage; in six patients the diagnosis was made during the third trimester and in one at 23 weeks' gestation.[88] In the same study, MRI enabled better characterization of the anomalies of the corpus callosum. The very rare Pai syndrome (midline cleft of the upper lip, facial skin polyps, and CNS lipomas) should be considered when a pericallosal lipoma is diagnosed.[89]

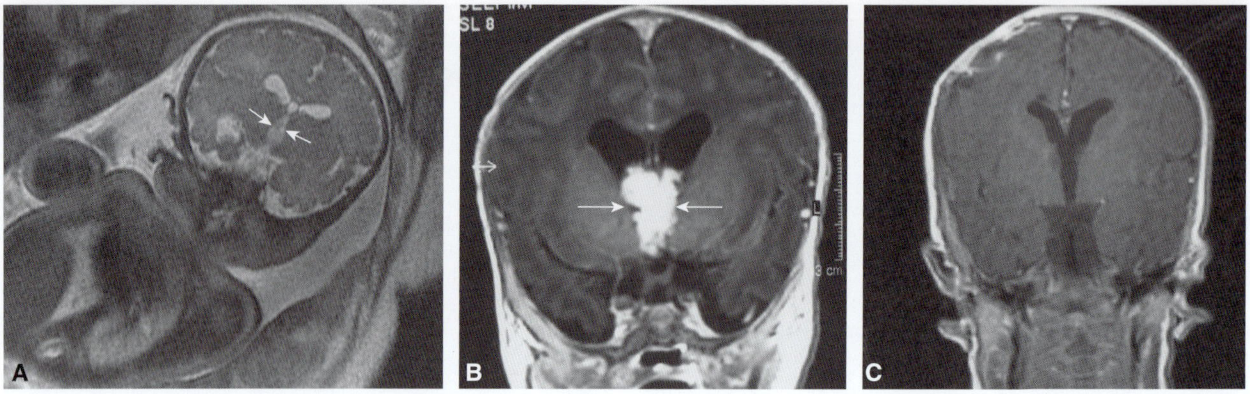


**Figure 13–19.** Prenatal and postnatal MRI in a patient with third ventricle CPP (same patient as in Figure 13–9). **(A)** Prenatal MRI at 40 weeks of gestation shows the CCP causing dilation of the third ventricle (*arrows*). **(B)** Postnatal MRI confirms the diagnosis (*arrows*). Note that the mass extends into the lateral ventricles. **(C)** Same plane at 10 months of age following surgical resection of the tumor. Normal neurologic and developmental follow-up was done at 4 years of age.

In our experience pericallosal lipomas are usually diagnosed during the third trimester following apparently normal second-trimester examinations or following US examinations in which callosal dysgenesis was suspected (see Figures 13–11, 13–12, and 13–17). Extension to the choroid plexus is frequent and seems not to alter the generally good prognosis (Figure 13–10).

In some patients, T2-weighted MRI sequences may fail to depict the lipoma.[90]

## Prognosis

With the exception of CPP and lipomas, the prognosis of prenatally diagnosed fetal tumors is poor.[54,91] The overall survival rates have improved somewhat with newer imaging and neurosurgical techniques. Survival figures and degrees of neurologic deficits are variable and are related to the patient's age and the size, location, and histology of the tumor. Although surgery remains the treatment of choice, there is a high rate of mortality, and it is not indicated in cases of neonates with enormous tumors that replace the entire brain tissue.[54] Radiotherapy is not recommended as a therapeutic option, as there is a deleterious effect of this type of treatment on the immature, developing brain.[92] The same applies for radiation therapy under 2 years of age. Chemotherapy usage is highly controversial; however, some investigators try to combine it with surgery for malignant tumors only (eg, PNET and astrocytomas).[93]

Prenatal diagnosed and apparently isolated pericallosal lipomas have a good prognosis. Ickowits et al[88] reported on six children without associated malformations that were delivered; their follow-up was considered normal at a mean age of 3 years.

## Obstetric Management

Obstetrical management should not be modified in patients with suspected apparently isolated CPPs or lipomas. When other intracranial tumors are suspected, particularly those causing brain destruction, the option for termination of pregnancy should be offered if legally possible. In patients with severe hydrocephaly and/or macrocephaly, the possibility of dystocia should be contemplated and cephalocentesis considered for maternal reasons.

## REFERENCES

1. Stiller CA, Bunch KJ. Brain tumors in children aged under two years: Incidence and survival in Britain, 1971-85. *Br J Cancer.* 1992;66(Suppl 18):S50–S53.
2. Bader JL, Miller RW. U.S. cancer incidence and mortality in the first year of life. *Am J Dis Child.* 1989;133:157–159.
3. Janisch W. Zur epidemiologie der primaren Geschwulste des zentralnervensystems im ersten lebensjahr. *Arch Geschwulstforsch.* 1985;55:489–494.
4. Court Brown WM, Doll R, Hill RB. Incidence of leukaemia after exposure to diagnostic radiation in utero. *Br Med J.* 1960;2(5212):1539–1545.
5. Becker LE. Central neuronal tumors in childhood: Relationship to dysplasia. *J Neurooncol.* 1995;24(1):13–19.
6. Durante F. Nesso fisio-patologico tra la struttura dei nei materni e la genesi di alcuni tumori maligni. *Arch Memor Observ Chir Prat.* 1874;11:217.
7. Cohnheim J. *Lecture on General Pathology.* Vol 2. London: The New Syndenham Society; 1889.
8. Bolande R. *Cellular Aspects of Developmental Pathology.* Philadelphia: Lea & Fabriger; 1967.
9. Knudson AG, Jr. Mutagenesis and embryonal carcinogenesis. *Natl Cancer Inst Monogr.* 1979;51:19–24.
10. Bolande RP. Benignity of neonatal tumors and concept of cancer repression in early life. *Am J Dis Child.* 1971;122(1):12–14.
11. Leon SP, Zhu J, Black PM. Genetic aberrations in human brain tumors. *Neurosurgery.* 1994;34(4):708–722.
12. Fujii Y, Hongo T, Hayashi Y. Chromosome analysis of brain tumors in childhood. *Genes Chromosomes Cancer.* 1994;11(4):205–215.
13. Bigner SH, McLendon RE, Fuchs H, et al. Chromosomal characteristics of childhood brain tumors. *Cancer Genet Cytogenet.* 1997;97(2):125–134.
14. Vagner-Capodano AM, Gentet DC, Gambarelli D, et al. Cytogenetic studies in 45 pediatric brain tumors. *Pediatr Hematol Oncol.* 1992;9(3):223–235.
15. Odell JM, Allen JK, Badura RJ, et al. Massive congenital intracranial teratoma: A report of two cases. *Pediatr Pathol.* 1987;7(3):333–340.
16. Hansson CM, Buckley PG, Grigelloniene G, et al. Comprehensive genetic and epigenetic analysis of sporadic meningioma for

macro-mutations on 22q and micro-mutations within the NF2 locus. *BMC Genomics.* 2007;8:16.
17. Biegel JA, Rorke LB, Packer RJ, et al. Monosomy 22 in rhabdoid or atypical tumors of the brain. *J Neurosurg.* 1990;73(5): 710–714.
18. Wakai S, Arai T, Nagai M. Congenital brain tumors. *Surg Neurol.* 1984;21(6):597–609.
19. Raisanen JM, Davis RL. Congenital brain tumors. *Pathology (Phila).* 1993;2(1):103–116.
20. Shamji MF, Vassilydi M, Lam CH, et al. Congenital tumors of the central nervous system: The MCH experience. *Pediatr Neurosurg.* 2009;45(5):368–374.
21. Isaacs H, Jr. Perinatal brain tumors: A review of 250 cases. *Pediatr Neurol.* 2002;27(4):249–261.
22. Becker LE, Halliday WC. Central nervous system tumors of childhood. *Perspect Pediatr Pathol.* 1987;10:86–134.
23. Rickert CH, Paulus W. Prognosis-related histomorphological and immunohistochemical markers in central nervous system tumors of childhood and adolescence. *Acta Neuropathol.* 2005;109(1): 69–92.
24. Heideman RJ, Packer RJ, Albrigh LA. Tumors of the central nervous system. In: Pizzo PA, Poplack GP, eds. *Principles and Practice of Pediatric Oncology.* Philadelphia: Lippincott; 1993.
25. Mazewski CM, Hudgins RJ, Reisner A, et al. Neonatal brain tumors: A review. *Semin Perinatol.* 1999;23:286–298.
26. Parham DM, Jenkins JJ III. Pathology of selected pediatric embryonal neoplasms. *Mod Pathol.* 1994;7:501–509.
27. Alagappan A, Shattuck KE, Rowe T, et al. Massive intracranial immature teratoma with extracranial extension into oral cavity, nose, and neck. *Fetal Diagn Ther.* 1998;13(5):321–324.
28. Arslan E, Usul H, Baykal S, et al. Massive congenital intracranial immature teratoma of the lateral ventricle with retro-orbital extension: A case report and review of the literature. *Pediatr Neurosurg.* 2007;43(4):338–342.
29. Bolat F, Kayaselicuk F, Tarim E, et al. Congenital intracranial teratoma with massive macrocephaly and skull rupture. *Fetal Diagn Ther.* 2008;23(1):1–4.
30. Vibert-Guigue C, Gousale SM, Gouellet N, et al. Vaginal delivery using cranioclasia following prenatal diagnosis of a giant fetal intracranial teratoma. *Fetal Diagn Ther.* 2008;23(3):222–227.
31. Afshar F, King TT, Berry CL. Intraventricular fetus-in-fetu: Case report. *J Neurosurg.* 1982;56:845–849.
32. Goldstein I, Jackobi P, Groisman G, Itskovitz-Eldor J. Intracranial fetus-in-fetu. *Am J Obstet Gynecol.* 1996;175:1389–1390.
33. Hung CF, Lam MS. Intracranial fetus in fetu: Report of a case. *J Formos Med Assoc.* 1993;92:920–922.
34. Wakai S. On the origin of intracranial teratomas. *No To Shinkei.* 1989;41:947–953.
35. Yang ST, Leow SW. Intracranial fetus-in-fetu: CT diagnosis. *AJNR Am J Neuroradiol.* 1992;13:1326–1329.
36. Yasuda Y, Mitomori T, Matsuura A, Tanimura T. Fetus-in-fetu: Report of a case. *Teratology.* 1985;31:337–344.
37. Willis RA. *The Borderline of Embryology and Pathology.* London: Butterworth; 1985:147.
38. Riboni G, De Simoni M, Leopardi O, Molla R. Ultrasound appearance of a glioblastoma in a 33 week fetus in utero. *J Clin Ultrasound.* 1985;13:345–346.
39. McConachie NS, Twining P, Lamb MP. Case report: Antenatal diagnosis of congenital glioblastoma. *Clin Radiol.* 1991;44: 121–122.
40. Morof DF, Levine D, Stringer KF, Grable I, Folkerth R. Congenital glioblastoma multiforme: Prenatal diagnosis on the basis of sonography and magnetic resonance imaging. *J Ultrasound Med.* 2001;20: 1369–1375.
41. Brown K, Mapstone TB, Oakes WJ. A modern analysis of intracranial tumors of infancy. *Pediatr Neurosurg.* 1997;26:25–32.
42. Kamitoma M, Sameshima H, Uetsuhara K, et al. Fetal glioblastoma: Rapid growth during the third trimester. *Fetal Diagn Ther.* 1998;13:339–342.
43. Doug-Yeob L, Yeon-Mee K, Shi-Joon Y, et al. Congenital glioblastoma diagnosed by fetal sonography. *Childs Nervous Syst.* 1999;15:197–201.
44. Geraghty AV, Knott PD, Hanna HM. Prenatal diagnosis of fetal glioblastoma multiforme. *Prenatal Diagnosis.* 2005;9:613–616.
45. Kasliwal MK, Gupta DK, Mahapatra AK, Sharma MC. Congenital glioblastoma multiforme: A case report and review of literature. *J Pediatr Neurosci.* 2007;2:69–71.
46. Werb P, Scurry J, Ostor A, et al. Survey of congenital tumors in perinatal necropsies. *Pathology.* 1992;24(4):247–253.
47. Ciara E, Piekutowska-Abramczuk D, Popowska E, et al. Heterozygous germ-line mutations in the NBN gene predispose to medulloblastoma in pediatric patients. *Acta Neuropathol.* 2010;119(3): 325–334.
48. Bonnin JM, Rubenstein LG, Palmer NF, et al. The association of embryonal tumors originating in the kidney and in the brain. A report of seven cases. *Cancer.* 1984;54(10):2137–2146.
49. Wolburg H, Paulus W. Choroid plexus: Biology and pathology. *Acta Neuropathol.* 2010;119(1):75–88.
50. Galassi E, Conado V, Cavallo M, et al. Intracranial tumors during the 1st year of life. *Childs Nerv Syst.* 1989;5(5):288–298.
51. McEvoy AW, Harding BM, Phipps KP, et al. Management of choroid plexus tumours in children: 20 years experience at a single neurosurgical centre. *Pediatr Neurosurg.* 2000;32(4):192–199.
52. Demaerel P, Van de Gaer P, Wilms G, et al. Interhemispheric lipoma with variable callosal dysgenesis: relationship between embryology, morphology, and symptomatology. *Eur Radiol.* 1996;6(6): 904–909.
53. Buetow PC, Smirniotopoulos JG, Done S. Congenital brain tumors: A review of 45 cases. *AJNR Am J Neuroradiol.* 1990;11(4):793–799.
54. Volpe JJ. Brain tumors and vein of Galen malformation. In: *Neurology of the Newborn.* Philadelphia: WB Saunders; 2008:989–1006.
55. Isaacs H, Jr. Perinatal brain tumors: a review of 250 cases. *Pediatr Neurol.* 2002;27(5):333–342.
56. Graham JM, Saunders R, Fratkin J. A cluster of Pallister-Hall syndrome cases (congenital hypothalamic hamartoblastoma syndrome). *Am J Med Genet Med.* 1986;2(Suppl):53–63.
57. Frye RE, Polling JS, Ma LC. Choroid plexus papilloma expansion over 7 years in Aicardi syndrome. *J Child Neurol.* 2007;22(4):484–487.
58. Diguet A, Laquerriere A, Eurin D, et al. Fetal capillary haemangioblastoma: An exceptional tumour. A review of the literature. *Prenat Diagn.* 2002;22(11): p. 979-983.
59. Alvarez M, Chitakara U, Lynch L, et al. Prenatal diagnosis of fetal brain tumors. *Fetal Ther.* 1987;2(4):203–208.
60. Sahin FK, Koken G, Casar E, et al. A prenatal diagnosed case of primitive neuroectodermal tumor. *Fetal Diagn Ther.* 2008;23(4): 267–270.
61. Cassart M, Bosson M, Garec C, et al. Fetal intracranial tumors: A review of 27 cases. *Eur Radiol.* 2008;18(10):2060–2066.
62. D'Addario V, Pinto V, Meo F, et al. The specificity of ultrasound in the detection of fetal intracranial tumors. *J Perinat Med.* 1998;26(6):480–485.
63. Weyerts LK, Katangarite V, Jones MC, et al. Prenatal diagnosis of a giant intracranial teratoma associated with pulmonary hypoplasia. *J Med Genet.* 1993;30(10):880–882.
64. Garel C. *MRI of the Fetal Brain: Normal Development and Cerebral Pathologies.* Berlin: Springer; 2004:267.
65. Isaacs H. Fetal brain tumors: A review of 154 cases. *Am J Perinatol.* 2009;26(6):453–466.
66. Sylvestre G, Sherer DM. Prenatal sonographic findings associated with malignant astrocytoma following normal early third-trimester ultrasonography. *Am J Perinatol.* 1998;15(10):581–584.
67. Hoff NR, Mackay IM. Prenatal ultrasound diagnosis of intracranial teratoma. *J Clin Ultrasound.* 1980;8(3):247–249.
68. Chien YH, Tsao PN, Lee WT, et al. Congenital intracranial teratoma. *Pediatr Neurol.* 2000;22(1):72–74.
69. Saada J, Enza-Razavi F, Delahaye S, et al. Early second-trimester diagnosis of intracranial teratoma. *Ultrasound Obstet Gynecol.* 2009;33(1):109–111.
70. Horton D, Pilling DW. Early antenatal ultrasound diagnosis of fetal intracranial teratoma. *Br J Radiol.* 1997;70(840):1299–1301.
71. Bare JB, Abramowsky CR, Denton TD, et al. Congenital immature teratoma of the central nervous system: Three case reports with literature review. *Fetal Pediatr Pathol.* 2007;26(3):109–118.
72. Koken G, Yilmazer E, Sahin FK, et al. Prenatal diagnosis of a fetal intracranial immature teratoma. *Fetal Diagn Ther.* 2008;24(4): 368–371.
73. Uysal A, Oztekin O, Oztekin D, et al. Prenatal diagnosis of a fetal intracranial tumor. *Arch Gynecol Obstet.* 2005;272(1):87–89.

74. Muhonen MG, Bierma JS, Hussain NS, et al. Giant intracranial teratoma and lack of cortical development in a fetus. Case report. *J Neurosurg.* 2005;103(2 Suppl);180–183.
75. Kuller JA, Laifer SA, Martin JD, et al. Unusual presentations of fetal teratoma. *J Perinatol.* 1991;11(3):294–296.
76. Sherer DM, Onyeije CI. Prenatal ultrasonographic diagnosis of fetal intracranial tumors: A review. *Am J Perinatol.* 1998;15(5):319–328.
77. Sherer DM, Abramowicz JS, Eggers PC, et al. Prenatal ultrasonographic diagnosis of intracranial teratoma and massive craniomegaly with associated high-output cardiac failure. *Am J Obstet Gynecol.* 1993;168(1, Pt 1):97–99.
78. Phi JH, Park SH, Chae JH, et al. Congenital subependymal giant cell astrocytoma: clinical considerations and expression of radial glial cell markers in giant cells. *Childs Nerv Syst.* 2008;24(12):1499–1503.
79. Mirkin LD, Ey EH, Chaparro M. Congenital subependymal giant-cell astrocytoma: Case report with prenatal ultrasonogram. *Pediatr Radiol.* 1999;29(10):776–780.
80. Lee DY, Kim YM, Soo SJ, et al. Congenital glioblastoma diagnosed by fetal sonography. *Childs Nerv Syst.* 1999;15(4):197–201.
81. Seker A, Ozek MM. Congenital glioblastoma multiforme: Case report and review of the literature. *J Neurosurg.* 2006;105(6 Suppl): 473–479.
82. Sell M, Huber-Schumacher S, van Landeghem FK. Congenital glioblastoma multiforme with abnormal vascularity presenting as intracranial hemorrhage in prenatal ultrasound. *Childs Nerv Syst.* 2006;22(7):729–733.
83. Nejat F, Kazmi SS, Ardakani SB. Congenital brain tumors in a series of seven patients. *Pediatr Neurosurg.* 2008;44(1):1–8.
84. Komatsu F, Tsugu H, Nonako M, et al. Congenital medulloblastoma with atypical MRI appearance. *Pediatr Neurosurg.* 2008;44(2): 165–168.
85. Romero R, Pilu G, Jeanty P, et al., eds. Choroid plexus papilloma. In: *Prenatal Diagnosis of Congenital Anomalies.* Norwalk, CT: Appleton & Lange; 1989:34–36.
86. Mulligan G, Meier P. Lipoma and agenesis of the corpus callosum with associated choroid plexus lipomas: In utero diagnosis. *J Ultrasound Med.* 1989;8(10):583–588.
87. Jeanty P, Zaleski W, Fleischer AC. Prenatal sonographic diagnosis of lipoma of the corpus callosum in a fetus with Goldenhar syndrome. *Am J Perinatol.* 1991;8(2):89–90.
88. Ickowitz V, Eurin D, Rypens F, et al. Prenatal diagnosis and postnatal follow-up of pericallosal lipoma: report of seven new cases. *AJNR Am J Neuroradiol.* 2001;22(4):767–772.
89. Choustan A, Ville D, James I, et al. Pericallosal lipoma associated with Pai syndrome: prenatal imaging findings. *Ultrasound Obstet Gynecol.* 2008;32(5):708–710.
90. Malinger G, Ben-Sira L, Lev D, et al. Fetal brain imaging: a comparison between magnetic resonance imaging and dedicated neurosonography. *Ultrasound Obstet Gynecol.* 2004;23(4):333–340.
91. Cavalheiro S, Moron AF, Hisaba W, et al. Fetal brain tumors. *Childs Nerv Syst.* 2003;19(7–8):529–536.
92. Jooma R, Kendall B, Hayward R. Intracranial tumors in neonates: A report of seventeen cases. *Surg Neurol.* 1984;21:165–175.
93. Haddad SF, Menezes AH, Bell WE, et al. Brain tumors occurring before 1 year of age: A retrospective reviews of 22 cases in an 11-year period (1977–1987). *Neurosurgery.* 1991;29(1):8–13.

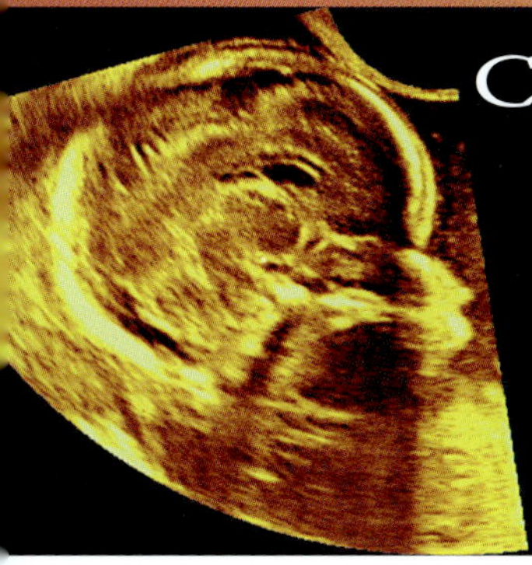

Chapter 14

# THE FETAL EYE

*Zeev Blumenfeld • Moshe Bronshtein*

## KEY POINTS

1. A fetal neuroscan is not complete without a thorough examination of the orbits, the eyes, and their surroundings.
2. Malformations of the eyes can be solitary or in association with other anomalies. Therefore, a search for those should be undertaken.
3. Any alteration in the shape or size of the orbits, the interorbital distances should be evaluated as a possible sign of other anomalies.
4. Whenever fetal position enables, transvaginal sonography should be used.

The ultrasonographic examination of the eyes is an important and integral part of the fetal face survey. This chapter describes the methodology of the orbit and eye evaluation, the ultrasonic landmarks of the normal eye, and the features of congenital abnormalities that may be detected in the fetus. The presented data are a summary of the English literature on this topic, as well as the authors' experience.

## EPIDEMIOLOGY OF CONGENITAL BLINDNESS

Congenital blindness is a common disorder in developing countries in contrast to Western countries.[1–4] Robinson and coworkers[1] reported a prevalence of 3 per 10,000 births for eye malformations in British Columbia. Stoll and associates[4] found congenital eye malformations in 7.5 per 10,000 births in France. Studies in Great Britain[5,6] have shown that about half of the cases of childhood blindness are genetically determined. Twenty percent of all cases were autosomal dominant, 17% autosomal recessive, 5% X-linked, and 8% were thought to be multifactorial.[5] Intrauterine infections such as rubella and toxoplasmosis are also regarded as major factors contributing to eye malformations. More recently, fetal alcohol syndrome has become well recognized as a cause of ocular abnormalities, particularly of optic nerve hypoplasia.[5,7]

The most commonly described ocular abnormalities were cataract (30%), microphthalmia (24%), coloboma (9%), and anophthalmia (4%).[1,4–5] Robinson et al[1] and Phillips et al[6] also reported that cataract was the most common eye abnormality associated with congenital blindness.

As extending the previous study performed in France, Stoll et al,[7] reporting on 212,479 deliveries, found a slightly lower prevalence of congenital eye malformations of 6.8 per 10,000. In this study, the prevalence of cataract was 2.7/10,000; of microphthalmia, 1.7/10,000;[7] of anophthalmia, 0.23/10,000; and of coloboma, 1.4/10,000.[5] Associated fetal anomalies included clubfeet, microcephaly, hydrocephaly, cleft lip and palate, and facial dysmorphism.[7] The affected neonates were smaller, weighed less, had smaller head circumference and lower placental weight, and were more often complicated by threatened abortion or oligo- or polyhydramnios than controls.[7] Their mothers more often used drugs during pregnancy, and their fathers were more often exposed to occupational hazards than fathers of controls.[7] Eye malformations were associated with parental consanguinity.[7] The recurrence risk for first-degree relatives of probands was 8.9%;[7] this risk was more than 3 times that for additional, nonocular malformations.[7]

Genetic counseling of the affected families is of utmost importance. The genetics of several congenital malformations with eye abnormalities is known (eg, cataract Coppock-like, Lowe syndrome, Norrie disease, X-linked retinitis pigmentosa, chorioderemia, and retinoblastoma).[1,8,9] In these cases, early prenatal diagnosis is therefore possible.

The importance of ultrasound (US) in the prenatal detection of eye abnormalities is discussed later in this chapter.

## DEVELOPMENT OF THE FETAL EYE

Figure 14–1 depicts the developmental process of the embryonic and fetal eye. Ages here are given as postconceptional days and weeks, for the first few weeks, then later on as postmenstrual weeks. The eyes first appear in the 22-day-old embryo as a pair of lateral grooves that

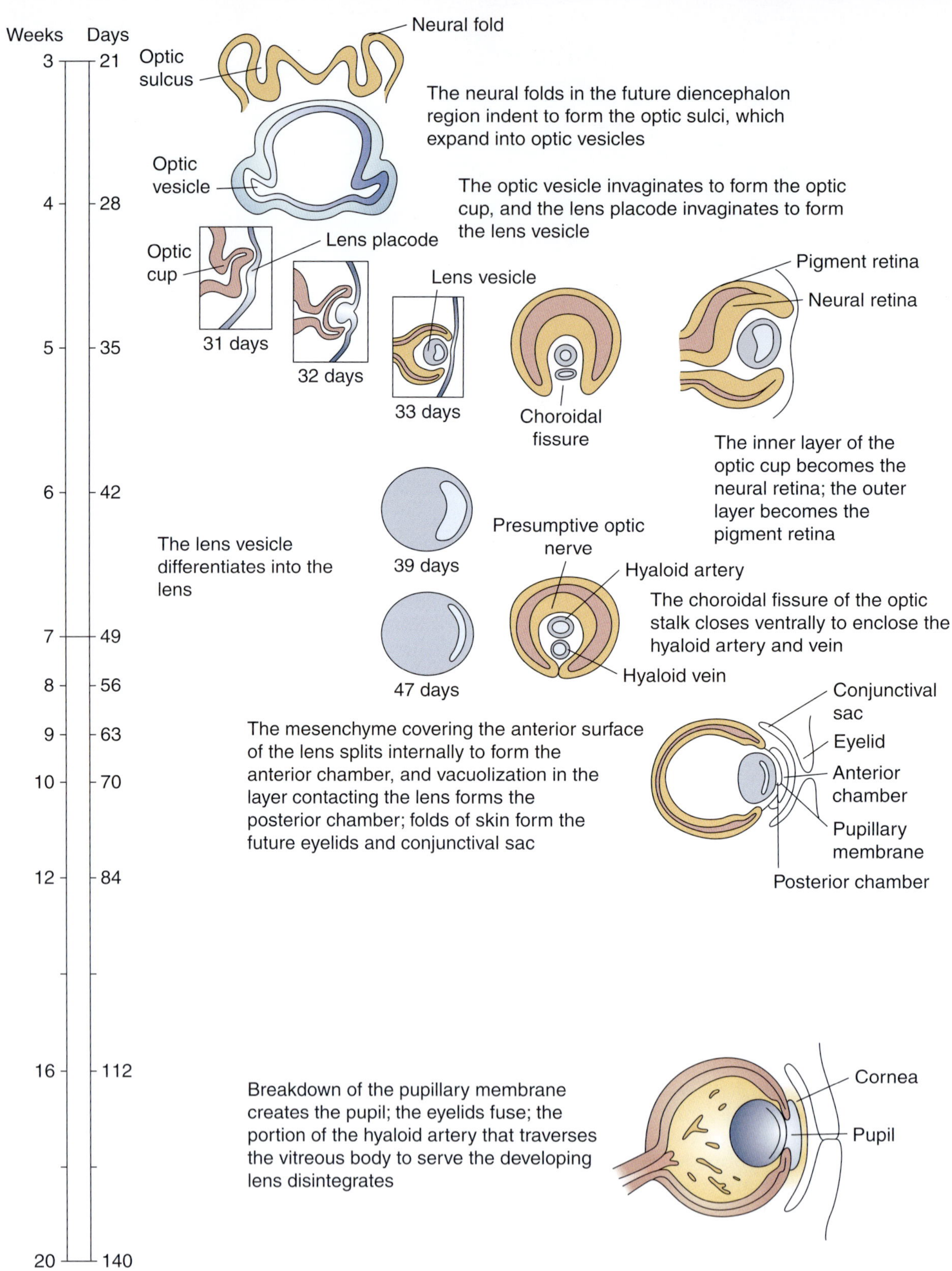


**Figure 14–1.** Development of the eye from day 21 to day 40 (postconception). (From Larsen, 2001,[11] with permission.)

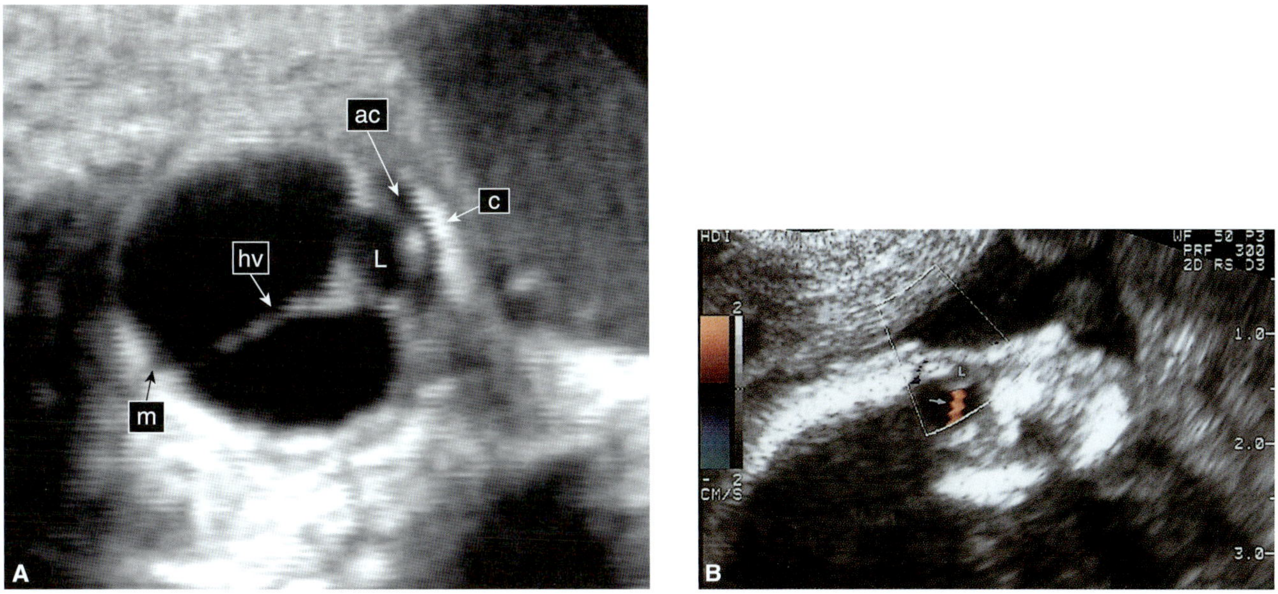


**Figure 14–2.** The normal fetal eye **(A)** Normal fetal eye at 27 weeks, visualized by transvaginal sonography (TVS). ac, anterior chamber; c, cornea; hv, hyaloid vessels; L, lens; m, macula. **(B)** Color-flow imaging reveals the active arterial flow in the hyaloid artery (*arrow*) toward the lens (L).

originate from the neural fold of the forebrain and form the optic vesicles.[10,11] Subsequently, the optic vesicles invaginate and form the optic cup.

The lens vesicle originates from the surface ectoderm at 33 days and subsequently differentiates into the lens at 39 to 47 days. Both the developing lens and the retina are vascularized by the hyaloid artery.

The optic cup is connected to the brain by the optic stalk. The nerve fibers that emerge from the retina are connected with the brain through the optic stalk, which develops into the optic nerve during gestational week 8. At the end of the fifth week, the optic capsule is completely surrounded by a loose mesenchyme. This tissue differentiates into an inner layer comparable to the pia mater of the brain and an outer layer comparable to the dura mater. At 6 to 7 postmenstrual weeks, the choroid originates from the inner layer, and the outer layer develops into the sclera. The anterior chamber of the eye comes from the mesenchyme that overlies the lens. At 8 postmenstrual weeks, the cornea differentiates from the external layer of the anterior chamber. The eyelids are mesodermal folds lined with ectoderm that meet in front of the cornea by the eighth week.[10,11]

The hyaloid artery originates from the ophthalmic artery. It runs through the center of the eye and terminates at the posterior surface of the lens (Figure 14–2).[10–12] Its primary function is to nourish the developing lens. There is a normal process of regression of the hyaloid vessels toward the end of pregnancy.[10–13] A delay in the process of regression is associated with fetal abnormalities mainly of the central nervous system (CNS).[13] The flow in the hyaloid artery can be seen using color Doppler sonography. Figure 14–2B depicts hyaloid arterial flow at 16 weeks.

Ocular growth during fetal life was studied in products of spontaneous and induced abortions.[14,15] The development of the diameter and circumference of the eyeball showed an almost linear increase during gestation. The horizontal diameter of the eyeball was longer than the sagittal, and the vertical diameter was the shortest one. The average diameters of the eye in male fetuses were longer than in female fetuses.[14] At birth, the various dimensions of the eyeball were approximately one-third of the adult size.

When eyeball measurements were compared with gestational age, weight, height, head circumference, and abdominal circumference, it was found that the fetal head circumference correlated best with ocular growth.[15,16]

## ULTRASONOGRAPHIC EVALUATION OF THE FETAL EYE

### Technique

A detailed ultrasonic examination of the fetal eye was first reported by Birnholz[16] and de Elejalde and Elejalde.[17] The eyes were analyzed in both axial and coronal planes. In the axial plane, scanning is done from the top of the skull across the fetal face. In the coronal plane, the scanning focus was moved from the tip of the nose to the posterior aspect of the eye.[16,17] In both studies, the eyelids, lens, cornea, sclera, irises, hyaloid artery, retina, and optic nerve were depicted. However, such a detailed examination is not always possible, and sonologists are advised to refer to these studies in order to better understand the ultrasonic features of the different parts of the fetal eye.[16,17] For practical purposes, most sonologists examine qualitatively the size and location of the orbits, eyelids, hyaloid artery, and lens (Figures 14–2, 14–3, 14–4, 14–5, 14–6, and 14–7). Whenever an ocular malformation is suspected and the fetus is in the vertex presentation, the use of transvaginal sonography (TVS) may in some cases provide better visualization of the different eye structures. The use of

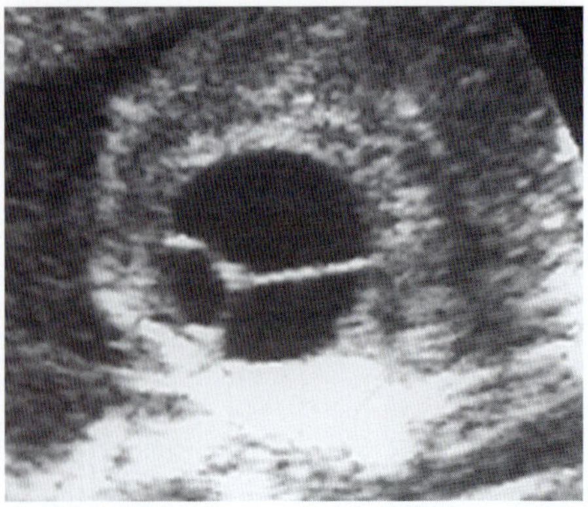

**Figure 14–3.** Normal fetal eye at 22 postmenstrual weeks, imaged by TVS. The straight hyaloid vessel is clearly demonstrated approaching the lens.

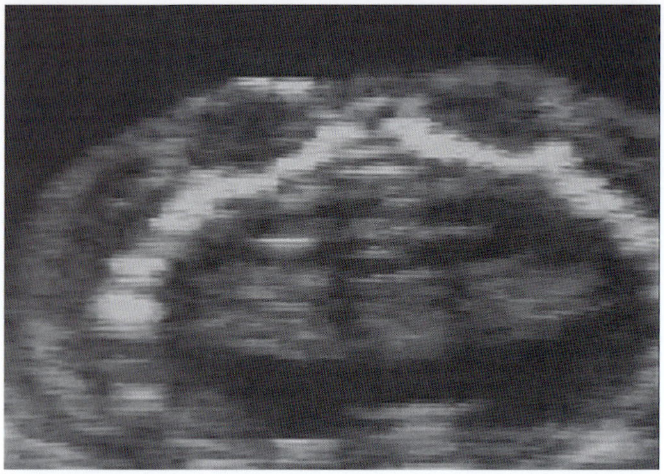

**Figure 14–5.** Fetal cataract diagnosed by lack of visualization of the lens at 14 postmenstrual weeks. Termination of pregnancy (TOP) at 15 weeks demonstrated the cataracts.

high-resolution abdominal probes enables good visualization of these structures.

## Biometric Measurements

Nomograms have been constructed providing data on fetal axial eye length, interocular distance, binocular distance, lens diameter, and a timetable for hyaloid artery regression and flow cessation.[18–24] Use of these nomograms may be helpful in the detection of fetal hypo- or hypertelorism, as well as other fetal eye and face malformations (Tables 14–1 and 14–2). (See also Chapter 3.)

Although the nomograms are useful and important, we do not routinely measure the ocular biometry in low-risk pregnancies, but instead use a qualitative approach comparing the two orbits and eyes in the same plane. When a facial anomaly is suspected, as well as in patients with a familiar history of malformations involving the eyes, we recommend a more extensive investigation that includes measurements and comparison with nomograms.

# PATHOLOGY OF THE LENS

The normal lens appears on the coronal ultrasonic facial view as a smooth, hyperechogenic circular line with a hypoechogenic content (Figures 14–4 and 14–5). In the axial view of the fetal head and orbits, the lenses are visualized as a pair of small dotted echoes originating from their near and far margins (Figure 14–2).

## Cataracts

Cataracts are opacities of the lens that cause visual impairment. The mechanism of cataract formation is denaturation of lens protein and formation of an opaque insoluble precipitate that causes loss of lens translucency.[25] This may be unilateral or bilateral. It has been estimated that this anomaly accounts for ~10% of the cases of blindness in preschool children.[25,26] Approximately one-third of cataract cases are idiopathic, and many of these are familial. Both autosomal dominant and autosomal recessive inheritance have been reported.[26,27] Other possible etiologies are intrauterine infections, chromosomal disorders, and systemic syndromes.[25–28]

Cataracts may produce different US imaging patterns. Thick, irregular, or crenate hyperechogenic borders, clusters of hypoechogenic material, or homogeneous opacities may be observed (Figures 14–8, 14–9, 14–10, 14–11, and 14–12).[29–37] In some cases of cataracts, we failed to demonstrate the hyaloid artery. It is possible that the opacity

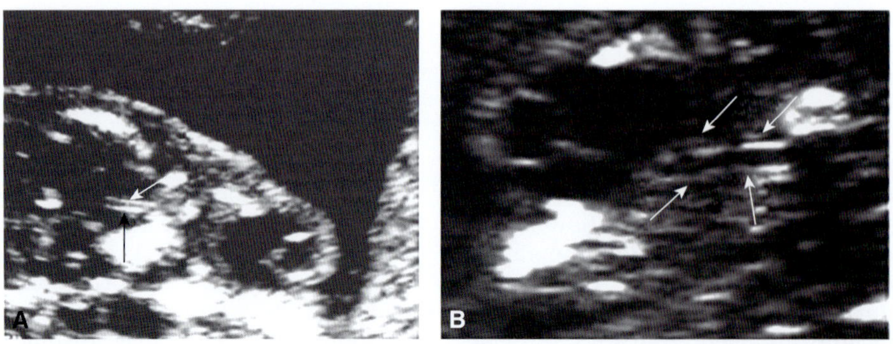


**Figure 14–4.** The fetal optic nerve **(A)**, **(B)** Visualization of the normal fetal optic nerve as two parallel lines (*arrows*) at 15 postmenstrual weeks by TVS.

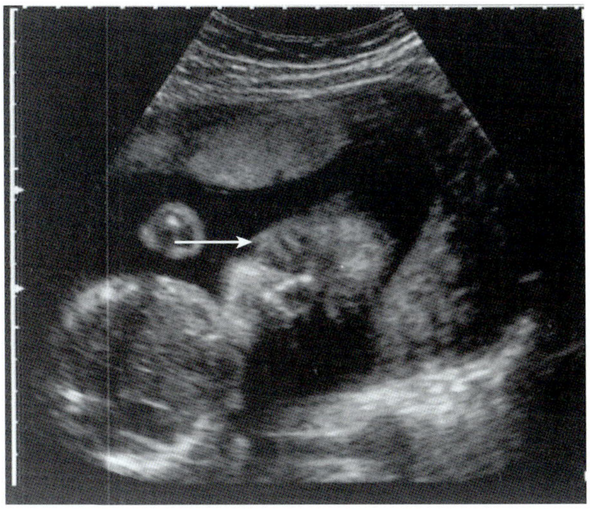

**Figure 14–6.** The eyelids are visualized in a cross section of the fetal face (*arrow*).

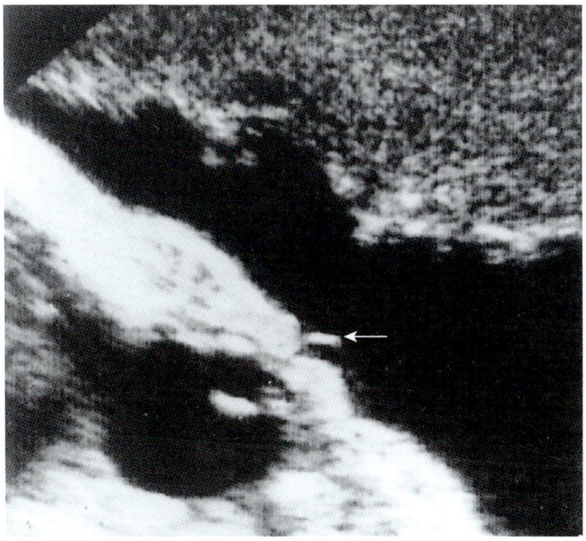

**Figure 14–7.** Eyelashes (*arrow*) observed in front of the fetal eye.

of the lens interfered with the visualization of this vessel. It can also be speculated that there is an association between congenital cataract and pathologies of the hyaloid artery.[38]

It should be noted that demonstration of apparently normal lenses on US does not exclude the presence of cataract. Additionally, the transparency of the lens on clinical examination is due to the free passage of light, whereas sonolucency refers to free passage of US waves through the lens. We have failed to diagnose some cases of mild cataract.[31] Therefore, it is understandable and can be summarized that at present the threshold for the ultrasonic identification of cataract is still uncertain, and mild to moderate or even severe cases might not be sufficiently abnormal for sonographic detection and recognition.[32,33] As for the earliest possible detection of congenital cataracts, Monteagudo et al[33] reported an early diagnosis using transvaginal scan at 14 weeks of gestation.

## PATHOLOGY OF THE EYELIDS

Because the normal eyelid and its opening and closure can be detected, it is expected that a thorough, targeted examination of the eyelids can potentially detect abnormalities. Figure 14–11A depicts a fetus with fixed, partially open eyelids detected during ultrasonography. Examination of the stillborn fetus confirmed this finding. The detected syndrome was the Neu-Laxova syndrome (Figure 14–11B); similar findings have been reported by Shapiro and associates.[30]

## PATHOLOGY OF THE EYEBALL

### Microphthalmia and Anophthalmia

Congenital microphthalmia can be sporadic or hereditary.[38–46] Some sporadic cases are secondary to exogenous factors, such as infections (eg, rubella, toxoplasma, and syphilis). Sutcliffe and colleagues[41] reported two cases of bilateral severe microphthalmia and one case of anophthalmia associated with treatment of carbamazepine during pregnancy.

Microphthalmia may present as an isolated anomaly or may be a component of multiple malformation syndromes. All patterns of mendelian inheritance have been reported.[44–46] Right and left eyes alone or together are about equally affected.[44] When bilateral, these patients are blind or have poor vision due to disorganization of the ocular globe as a whole or of one or more of its constituent parts. Common associated anomalies are cataract, corneal scarring or vascularity, and colobomas of the iris or choroid. The possibility of Fraser and Walker-Warburg syndromes should be considered.[40–44]

Anophthalmia, or the complete absence of ocular primordial structure is considered the most extreme form of microphthalmia. Clinical distinction between severe microphthalmia and anophthalmia may be difficult or even impossible in utero, and the accurate diagnosis can be done only after pathologic examination.[42,43]

The sonographic diagnosis of microphthalmia should be suggested in cases of a small orbital diameter falling below the accepted nomograms of orbital growth (Figures 14–10, 14–13, 14–14, 14–15, and 14–16). The prenatal diagnosis of microphthalmia has been reported by several investigators.[38–46] Both isolated cases and microphthalmia in multiple malformation syndromes have been identified. The earliest gestational age of detection was reported by Porges and collaborators,[44] who found the anomaly in a fetus at 11 weeks of gestation.

Sonographic diagnosis of anophthalmia also has been reported.[46,48,49] However, sonographers should be cautious because fetal head position, especially in the cephalic prone position with the head deep inside the pelvis, may preclude visualization of the eyes. In such cases, vaginal sonography may be of significant value even in the advanced pregnancy. The sonographic diagnosis of anophthalmia should therefore be suggested in

**Table 14–1. GROWTH OF THE OCULAR PARAMETERS**

| | Binocular Distance (mm) | | | Interocular Distance (mm) | | | Ocular Diameter (mm) | | |
|---|---|---|---|---|---|---|---|---|---|
| Age (postmenstrual weeks) | 5th | 50th | 95th | 5th | 50th | 95th | 5th | 50th | 95th |
| 11 | 5 | 13 | 20 | — | — | — | — | — | — |
| 12 | 8 | 15 | 23 | 4 | 9 | 13 | 1 | 3 | 6 |
| 13 | 10 | 18 | 25 | 5 | 9 | 14 | 2 | 4 | 7 |
| 14 | 13 | 20 | 28 | 5 | 10 | 14 | 3 | 5 | 8 |
| 15 | 15 | 22 | 30 | 6 | 10 | 14 | 4 | 6 | 9 |
| 16 | 17 | 25 | 32 | 6 | 10 | 15 | 5 | 7 | 9 |
| 17 | 19 | 27 | 34 | 6 | 11 | 15 | 5 | 8 | 10 |
| 18 | 22 | 29 | 37 | 7 | 11 | 16 | 6 | 9 | 11 |
| 19 | 24 | 31 | 39 | 7 | 12 | 16 | 7 | 9 | 12 |
| 20 | 26 | 33 | 41 | 8 | 12 | 17 | 8 | 10 | 13 |
| 21 | 28 | 35 | 43 | 8 | 13 | 17 | 8 | 11 | 13 |
| 22 | 30 | 37 | 44 | 9 | 13 | 18 | 9 | 12 | 14 |
| 23 | 31 | 39 | 46 | 9 | 14 | 18 | 10 | 12 | 15 |
| 24 | 33 | 41 | 48 | 10 | 14 | 19 | 10 | 13 | 15 |
| 25 | 35 | 42 | 50 | 10 | 15 | 19 | 11 | 13 | 16 |
| 26 | 36 | 44 | 51 | 11 | 15 | 20 | 12 | 14 | 16 |
| 27 | 38 | 45 | 53 | 11 | 16 | 20 | 12 | 14 | 17 |
| 28 | 39 | 47 | 54 | 12 | 16 | 21 | 13 | 15 | 17 |
| 29 | 41 | 48 | 56 | 12 | 17 | 21 | 13 | 15 | 18 |
| 30 | 42 | 50 | 57 | 13 | 17 | 22 | 14 | 16 | 18 |
| 31 | 43 | 51 | 58 | 13 | 18 | 22 | 14 | 16 | 19 |
| 32 | 45 | 52 | 60 | 14 | 18 | 23 | 14 | 17 | 19 |
| 33 | 46 | 53 | 61 | 14 | 19 | 23 | 15 | 17 | 19 |
| 34 | 47 | 54 | 62 | 15 | 19 | 24 | 15 | 17 | 20 |
| 35 | 48 | 55 | 63 | 15 | 20 | 24 | 15 | 18 | 20 |
| 36 | 49 | 56 | 64 | 16 | 20 | 25 | 16 | 18 | 20 |
| 37 | 50 | 57 | 65 | 16 | 21 | 25 | 16 | 18 | 21 |
| 38 | 50 | 58 | 65 | 17 | 21 | 26 | 16 | 18 | 21 |
| 39 | 51 | 59 | 66 | 17 | 22 | 26 | 16 | 19 | 21 |
| 40 | 52 | 59 | 67 | 18 | 22 | 26 | 16 | 19 | 21 |

From Romero and colleagues, 1988,[56] with permission.

**Table 14–2. THE DIAMETER OF THE FETAL LENS (MM)**

| | | | Centiles | | | | |
|---|---|---|---|---|---|---|---|
| GA (postmenstrual weeks) | Mean | 95% CI | 10 | 25 | 50 | 75 | 90 |
| 14 | 2.5 | 2.3–2.7 | 2.1 | 2.4 | 2.5 | 2.7 | 2.9 |
| 15 | 2.9 | 2.9–3.0 | 2.7 | 2.8 | 2.9 | 3.1 | 3.2 |
| 16 | 2.9 | 2.8–3.0 | 2.7 | 2.8 | 2.9 | 3.1 | 3.2 |
| 17–18 | 3.3 | 3.0–3.6 | 2.8 | 2.9 | 3 | 3.3 | 5 |
| 19–20 | 4.1 | 4.0–4.3 | 3.6 | 4 | 4 | 4.3 | 5 |
| 21 | 4.4 | 4.1–4.6 | 3.7 | 3.9 | 4 | 5 | 5 |
| 22 | 4.4 | 4.2–4.7 | 3.9 | 4 | 4.3 | 5 | 5 |
| 23 | 4.6 | 4.3–4.8 | 3.8 | 4 | 5 | 5 | 5 |
| 24 | 4.6 | 4.4–4.8 | 4 | 4.3 | 4.6 | 5 | 5 |
| 25 | 4.8 | 4.6–5.0 | 4.2 | 4.6 | 5 | 5.1 | 5.2 |
| 26 | 5 | 4.8–5.2 | 4.4 | 4.8 | 5.1 | 5.2 | 5.5 |
| 27 | 5 | 4.8–5.2 | 4.4 | 4.8 | 5.1 | 5.2 | 5.5 |
| 28 | 5.1 | 5.0.5.2 | 4.5 | 5 | 5.2 | 5.2 | 5.5 |
| 29 | 5.3 | 5.1–5.5 | 4.6 | 5.2 | 5.2 | 5.5 | 5.9 |
| 30–31 | 5.3 | 5.2–5.5 | 4.8 | 5.1 | 5.5 | 5.5 | 5.7 |
| 32–33 | 5.6 | 5.4–5.8 | 4.8 | 5.2 | 5.5 | 5.9 | 6.2 |
| 34–36 | 5.8 | 5.6–6.0 | 5.4 | 5.5 | 5.7 | 6 | 6.5 |

CI, confidence interval; Ga, gestational age.

From Goldstein and colleagues, 1998,[20] with permission.

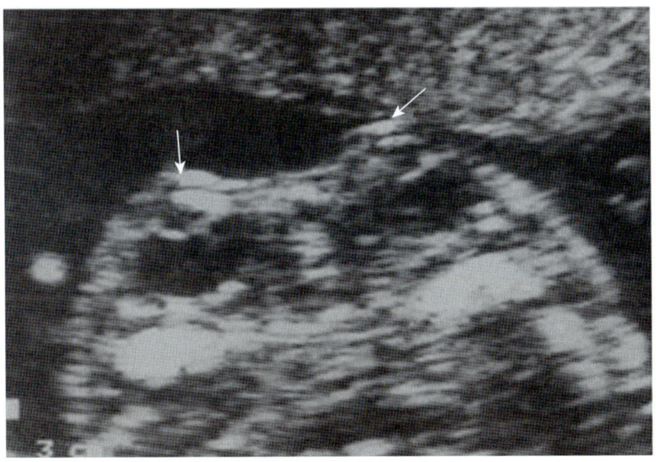

**Figure 14–8.** One of the suggestive findings of possible future development of fetal cataract: edema of the fetal eyes (15 weeks, *arrows*).

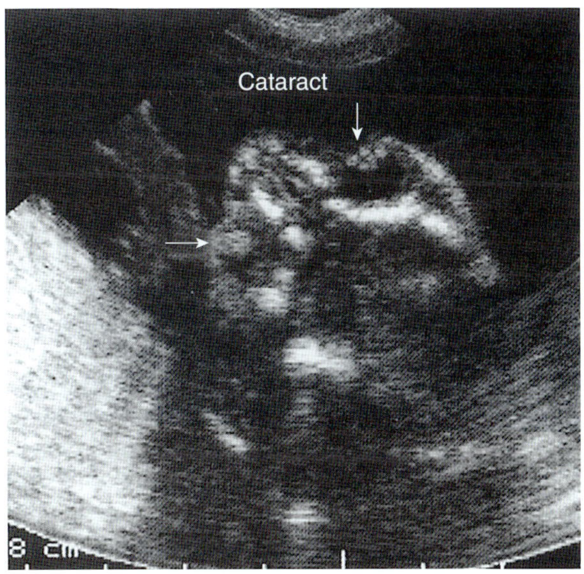


**Figure 14–9.** Homogeneous hyperechogenicity of the right lens and clusters of hypoechogenic material in the left eye (cataract). (From Zimmer et al, 1993,[26] with permission.)

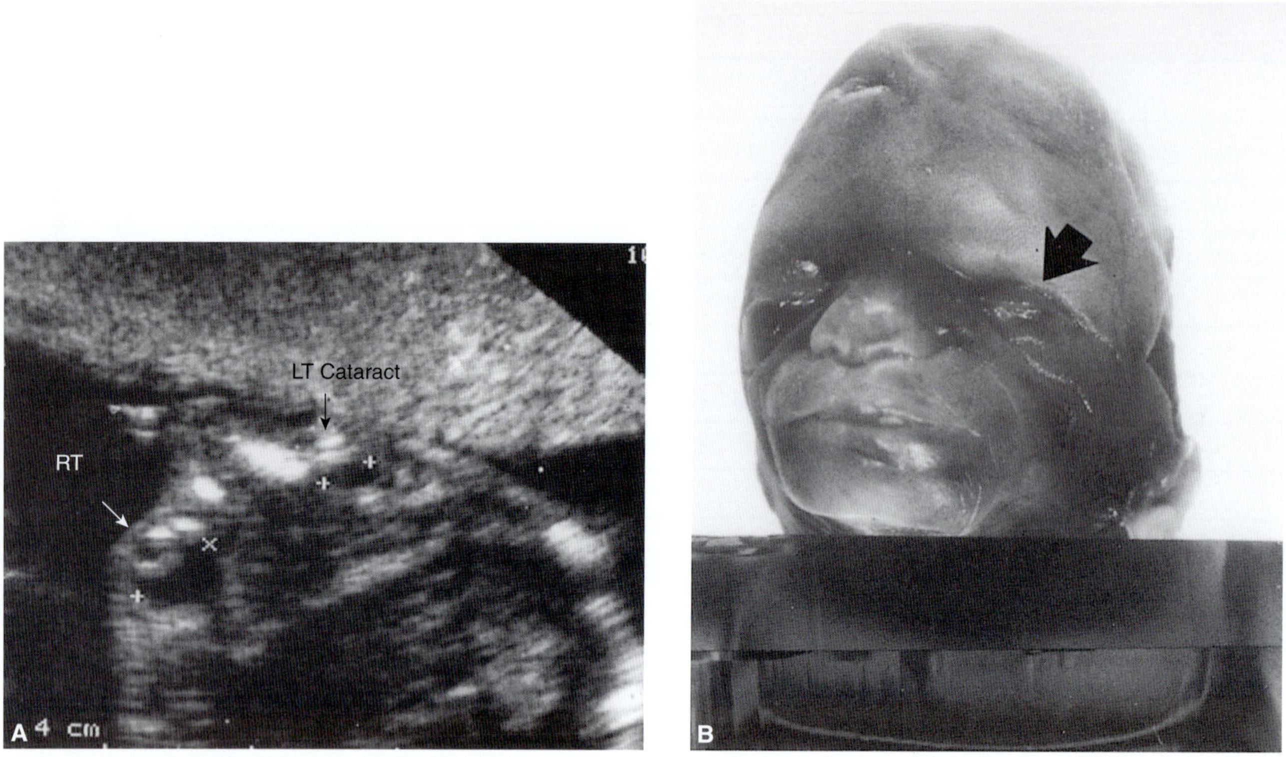


**Figure 14–10.** Microphthalmia in utero and in the aborted specimen **(A)** Microphthalmia with cataract. A normal orbit and lens are imaged on the right side (RT). On the left side, the orbit is small, and the lens contains hypoechogenic material. **(B)** An aborted fetus with microphthalmia.

cases in which a complete view of the fetal face failed to demonstrate one or both orbits. However, we are aware of two cases in which, although normal orbits were observed during early pregnancy, the newborns suffered from anophthalmia. The reason for this unexpected sequence of events is still unclear. In one of these cases, we diagnosed bilateral anophthalmia at 15 weeks of pregnancy (Figure 14–15), and the newborn had congenital anophthalmia and a cardiac malformation. One of the patient's sisters was followed in two successive pregnancies. The first resulted in a normal newborn; however, her next pregnancy resulted in a fetus with unilateral microphthalmia that underwent termination of pregnancy. The autopsy confirmed the diagnosis in both cases (Figures 14–15 and 14–16).

In cases of early microphthalmia, a high incidence of associated anomalies, mainly cerebral, facial, and chromosomal disorders, are usually diagnosed by TVS.[43–45] It

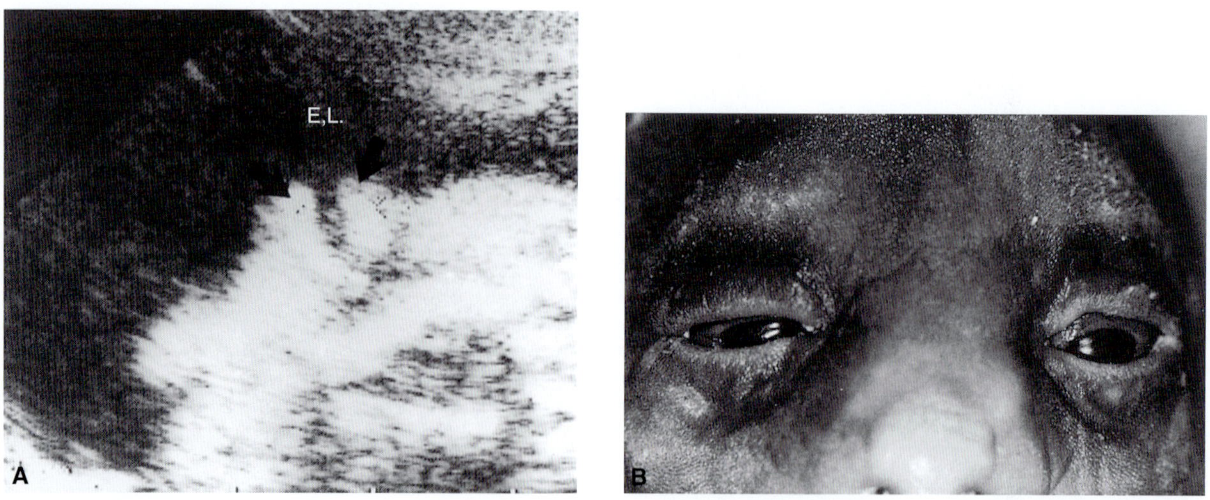


**Figure 14–11.** Atrophy of the eyelids **(A)** Eyelids (EL). The upper and lower eyelids (*arrow*) were small and open throughout the ultrasound (US) examination. Partial atrophy was therefore suggested. **(B)** The aborted fetus with Neu-Laxova syndrome. There is partial atrophy of the eyelids, as well as cataract.

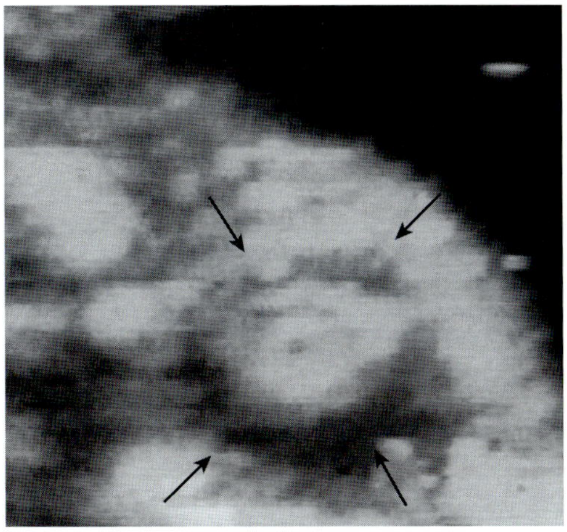

**Figure 14–12.** Fetal cataract at 16 postmenstrual weeks, appearing as concentric opacities (*arrows*), like "onion rings."

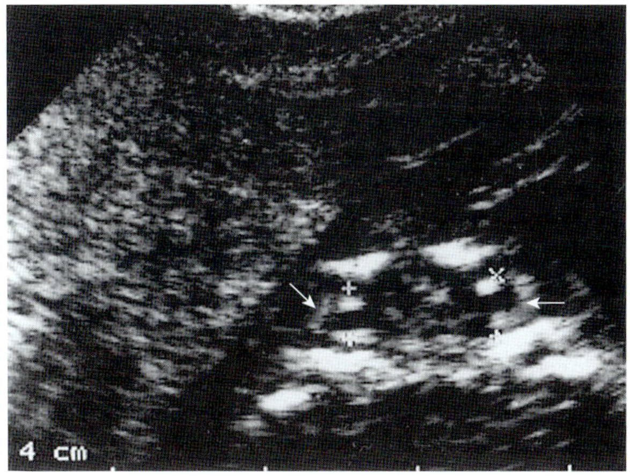


**Figure 14–13.** Bilateral microphthalmia at 15 postmenstrual weeks. The orbits are marked by an arrow and crosses.

should be noted, however, that normal measurements of the fetal eyes in early and midpregnancy do not exclude the possibility of subsequent development of microphthalmia. The precise underlying causes for late-onset microphthalmia are not yet established.

## Late-Onset Microphthalmia

Severe cataract and microphthalmia may be correctly diagnosed by sonography.[31,43,45] However, TVS failed to detect moderate cataract in a case of repeat cataract in a subsequent gestation.[45] Also, anophthalmia may sometimes be secondary to a degenerative process in middle and late pregnancy. In a retrospective group of late-onset microphthalmia, we confirmed the normal eye measurements performed in early and midpregnancy.[45] Like late-appearing microcephalus, there may be a late arrest of eye development, bringing about normal fetal screening at 15 and even 22 to 23 postmenstrual weeks, as well as later development of microphthalmia.

## Exophthalmos

Prominent eyes, or exophthalmia, are the result of shallow orbits or large eyeballs. The ultrasonographic diagnosis is done by imaging the protrusion of the eye on the axial section, usually used for interorbital and binocular biometry (Figure 14–17). Exophthalmos may appear with various fetal abnormalities. Prenatal sonographic diagnosis of exophtalmos has been reported in cases of holoprosencephaly,[43] Saethre-Chotzen syndrome,[49] Crouzon syndrome,[50] Roberts syndrome,[51] and akinesia-hypokinesia sequence.[52]

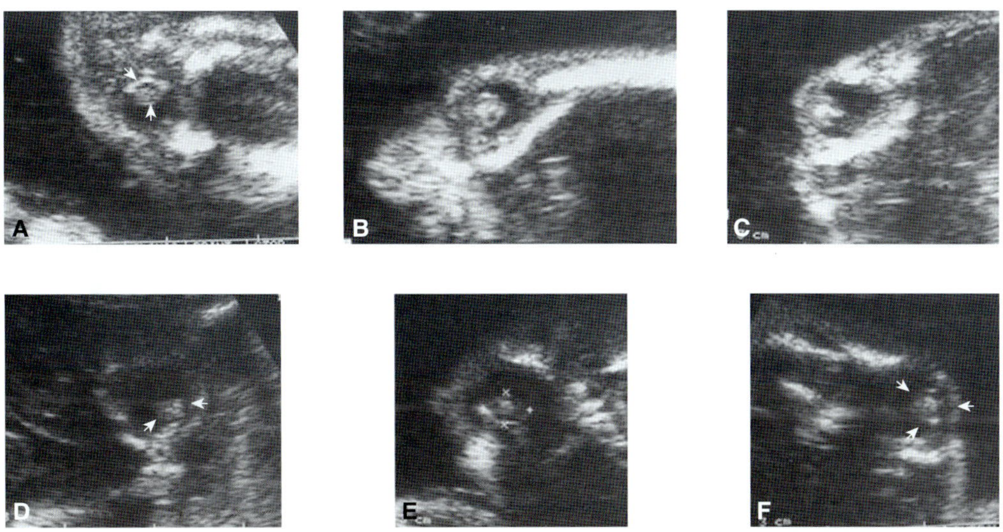


**Figure 14–14.** Autosomal familial dominant cataract that affected the father and grandmother diagnosed at 15 postmenstrual weeks' gestation as a central homogeneous echogenicity of the fetal lens **(A)–(C)** and at 18 postmenstrual weeks **(D)–(F)** (*arrows*). Neonatal cataract was confirmed at delivery as the only isolated neonatal malformation.

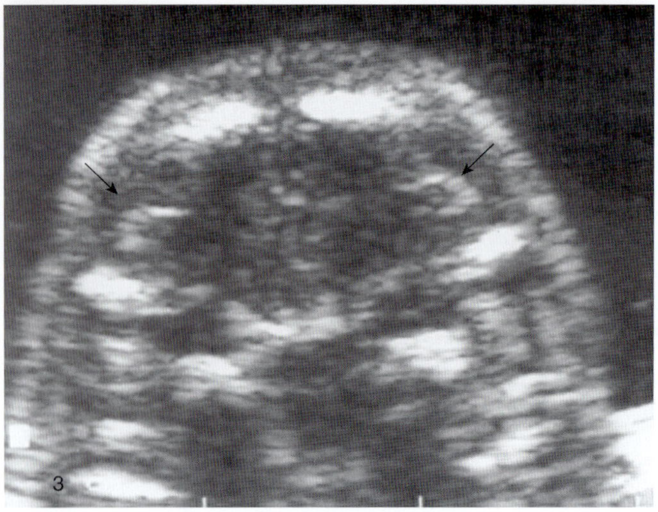


**Figure 14–15.** Bilateral familial anophthalmia at 15 postmenstrual weeks. The patient's sister was delivered of a neonate with congenital anophthalmia and cardiac malformation. The next pregnancy in the same patient was normal. However, the third pregnancy generated a fetus with unilateral microphthalmia and was subsequently terminated. The postmortem examinations validated the intrauterine-diagnosed anophthalmia.

## ABNORMALITIES OF HYALOID VASCULATURE

During early gestation, a conic net of blood vessels emerges from the posterior portion of the eye to the anterior lens, through the vitreous body, forming the primary vitreous body. From the 7th through the 32nd week of gestation, an apoptotic process causes this abundant blood vessel network to degenerate, generating a bloodless vitreous body, the secondary vitreous body (Figure 14–18). Using TVS, only the central part of the abundant blood vessels network is visualized, as the hyaloid artery. Complete or partial inhibition of the apoptotic process leading to the degeneration of the vascular network may cause late sequelae. Incomplete disruption of the vascular vessels in the anterior end of the vitreous results in the formation of the Mittendorf dot, whereas incomplete disruption of the vascular vessels at its posterior end results in the formation of the Bergmeister papillae. Both formations are compatible with normal vision. Mittendorf dot, also called the hyaloid body, is the embryonic remnant of the hyaloid artery as it joins the tunica vasculosa lentis.[53] Although Mittendorf dot is present in normal eyes, representing the remains of the anterior portion of the hyaloid artery, it may be associated with posterior lenticonus and produce a posterior polar cataract, through extension of the fetal vasculature through a gap in the lens.[53] This may be the pathophysiology of at least some forms of prenatal and neonatal cataract.[54,55] The hyaloid artery does not always appear as a straight line connecting the retina to the lens, but instead may have several normal variants (Figures 14–19 and 14–20).

### Persistent Hyperplastic Primary Vitreous

Persistent hyperplastic primary vitreous (PHPV) is an infrequent developmental malformation of the eye characterized by the presence of a vascular membrane behind the lens. The prevalence of this very rare fetal malformation in our population is about 1 in 60,000, occurring when the hyaloid artery and the associated abundant vitreous vessels fail to degenerate by 32 weeks' gestation, resulting in the development of cataract and microphthalmia. This anomaly is usually sporadic and unilateral, but when bilateral, trisomies 13 and 18 should be ruled out. Only one case report has been published in which the diagnosis was made at 23 weeks.[54] The accurate diagnosis in this case report[54] is equivocal, as PHPV can be diagnosed

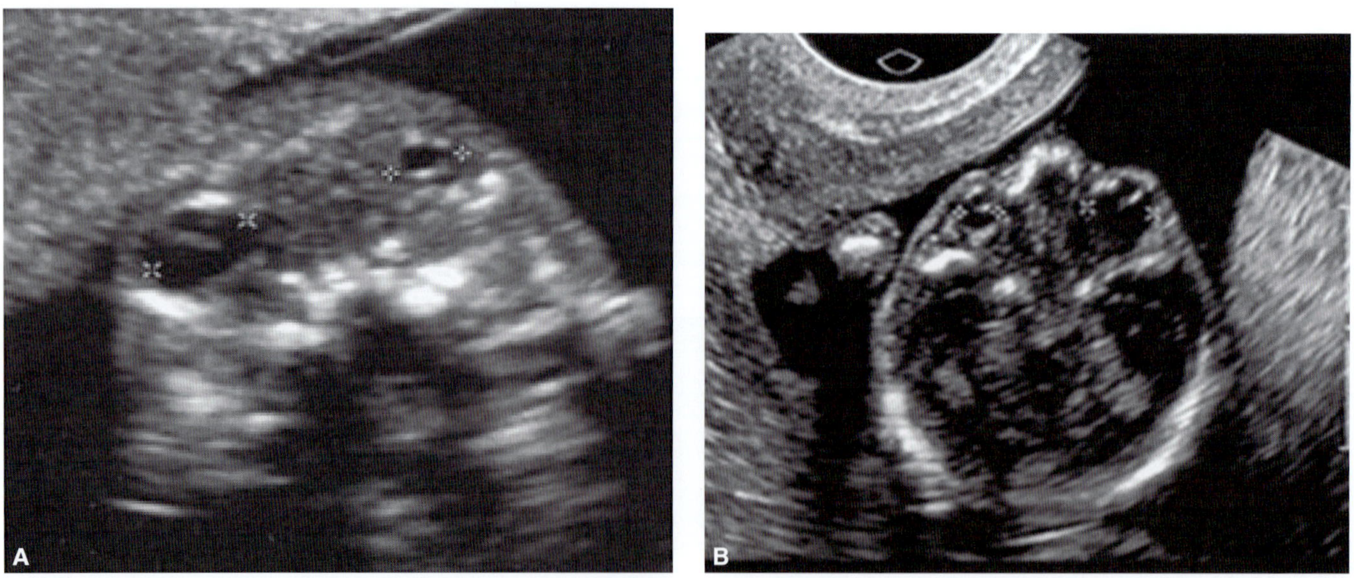


**Figure 14–16.** Unilateral microphthalmia: **(A)**, **(B)** Unilateral microphthalmia at 15 postmenopausal weeks. One of these two fetuses is from the third pregnancy of the patient described in **Figure 14–15.**

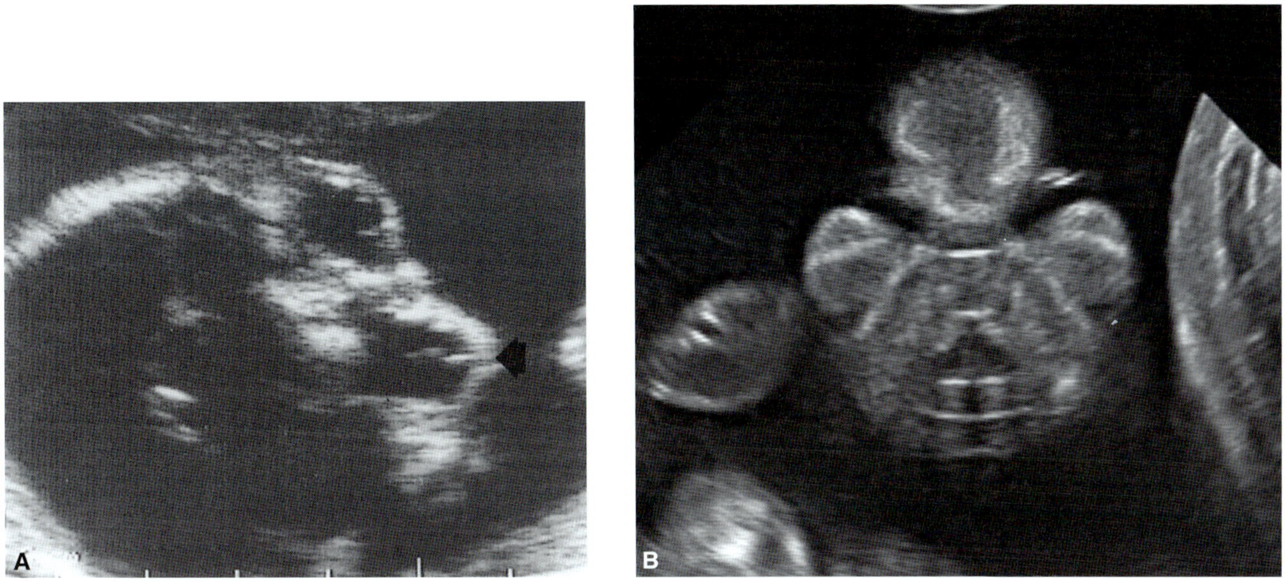


**Figure 14–17.** (**A**) Exophthalmos of the right eye in a fetus at 19 postmenstrual weeks. (**B**) Bilateral exophthalmos in a fetus with Raine syndrome at 21 postmenstrual weeks.

only during the third trimester, when physiologically, the apoptotic regression of the vitreous blood vessels is completed. In contrast to this case report, Figure 14–21 describes a true case of PHPV at 34 weeks, with bilateral cataract and microphthalmia associated with trisomy 13 (see also Figure 14–22).

## PATHOLOGY OF THE INTERORBITAL DISTANCES

### Hypotelorism

Hypotelorism is defined as a decreased interorbital distance (Figure 14–23) (see Chapter 2). It is usually associated with other fetal abnormalities, mainly holoprosencephaly (arhinencephaly).[55,56] Cyclopia represents the most severe form of the spectrum and is usually associated with midline deficiencies in facial development and incomplete morphogenesis of the forebrain. There is a single eye or partially divided eye in a single orbit and arhinia with proboscis. In most cases, other malformations are present.[57–65] Of the various karyotypes associated with cyclopia, trisomy D has been described with the greatest frequency.[62–64]

Environmental factors such as viremia and salicylates have been suggested as a possible cause of this abnormality.[65] In ethmocephaly, there is extreme hypotelorism but separate orbits, as well as arhinia with proboscis. In cebocephaly, hypotelorism is associated with a proboscis-like nose or a single-nostril nose, but there is no median or cleft lip.[49,55,56,66] An accurate sonographic diagnosis of these three different types of orbital anomalies is not easy. It may be difficult to differentiate between a single orbital cavity and very close or fused orbits. Furthermore, in some cases the observers failed to identify the orbits, and the diagnosis relied on the demonstration of a proboscis in a fetus with a brain anomaly.[58,60] Three-dimensional (3D) US may be useful in detecting cyclopia and proboscis, as demonstrated in a fetus at 13 weeks' gestation.[67]

Hypotelorism has been described in fetuses with microcephaly, oculu-dento-digital dysplasia and medical syndrome.[56]

### Hypertelorism

Hypertelorism is a craniofacial defect that consists of abnormally spaced orbits. The sonographic diagnosis therefore relies on the measurement of an abnormally large interorbital distance. Hypertelorism may be isolated or associated with many malformation syndromes. Romero and colleagues[56] summarized nearly 150 fetal syndromes with hypertelorism.

Prenatal diagnosis was reported by several investigators in fetuses with diverse associated malformations.[42,56,68,69–74] Recently, mycophenolate mofetil (CellCept), an immunosuppressant drug used by young women with autoimmune diseases, such as systemic lupus erythematosus, has been found to be teratogenic and capable of producing hypertelorism.[72]

### Retinal Disorders

Prenatal sonographic diagnosis of retinal detachment and dysplasia is extremely rare and has been reported in only a few cases, (Figure 14–24) most of them associated with Walker-Warburg syndrome.[73–76] In some cases of Walker-Warburg syndrome, recurrence can be suspected as early as the first trimester, but the diagnosis cannot be excluded on the basis of normal appearance on US until later in pregnancy.[73–76] This syndrome is characterized by the presence of cobblestone lissencephaly with other brain malformations, eye anomalies, and muscular

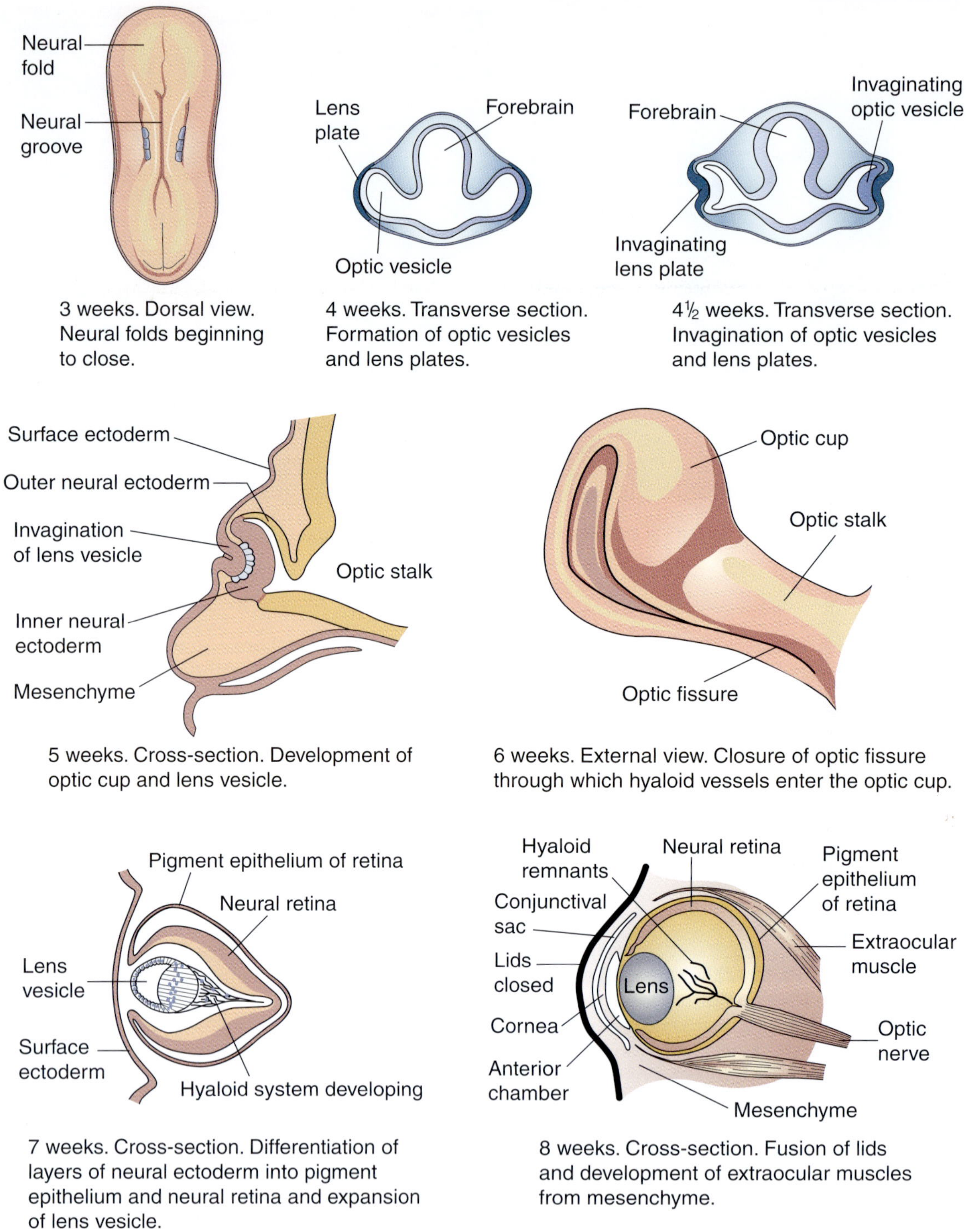


**Figure 14–18.** The apoptotic degeneration of the conic vascular network in the primary vitreous, in the seventh and ninth weeks (left), to the "blood vessel–free" secondary vitreous body, after the seventh month of gestation (right). (Reproduced with permission from Riordan-Eva P, Whitcher JP. Vaughan & Asbury's General Ophthalmology 17th ed. New York: McGraw-Hill, 2008. Fig. 1–28.)

dystrophy. Ultrasound of the fetal eye reveals a conical structure within the globe with its base toward the lens and its apex pointing posteriorly toward the optic nerve. In one case,[73] this ultrasonic image was obtained in one eye only. However, at the time of autopsy, the anomaly was identified in both eyes. Monteagudo et al[74] described this syndrome at 34 postmenstrual weeks in a fetus presenting with hydrocephaly and retinal detachment. (See also Chapter 16.)

In another case,[77] a similar conical structure was seen on US of the fetal orbits; examination of the newborn showed disorganized fibrous structures within the vitreous

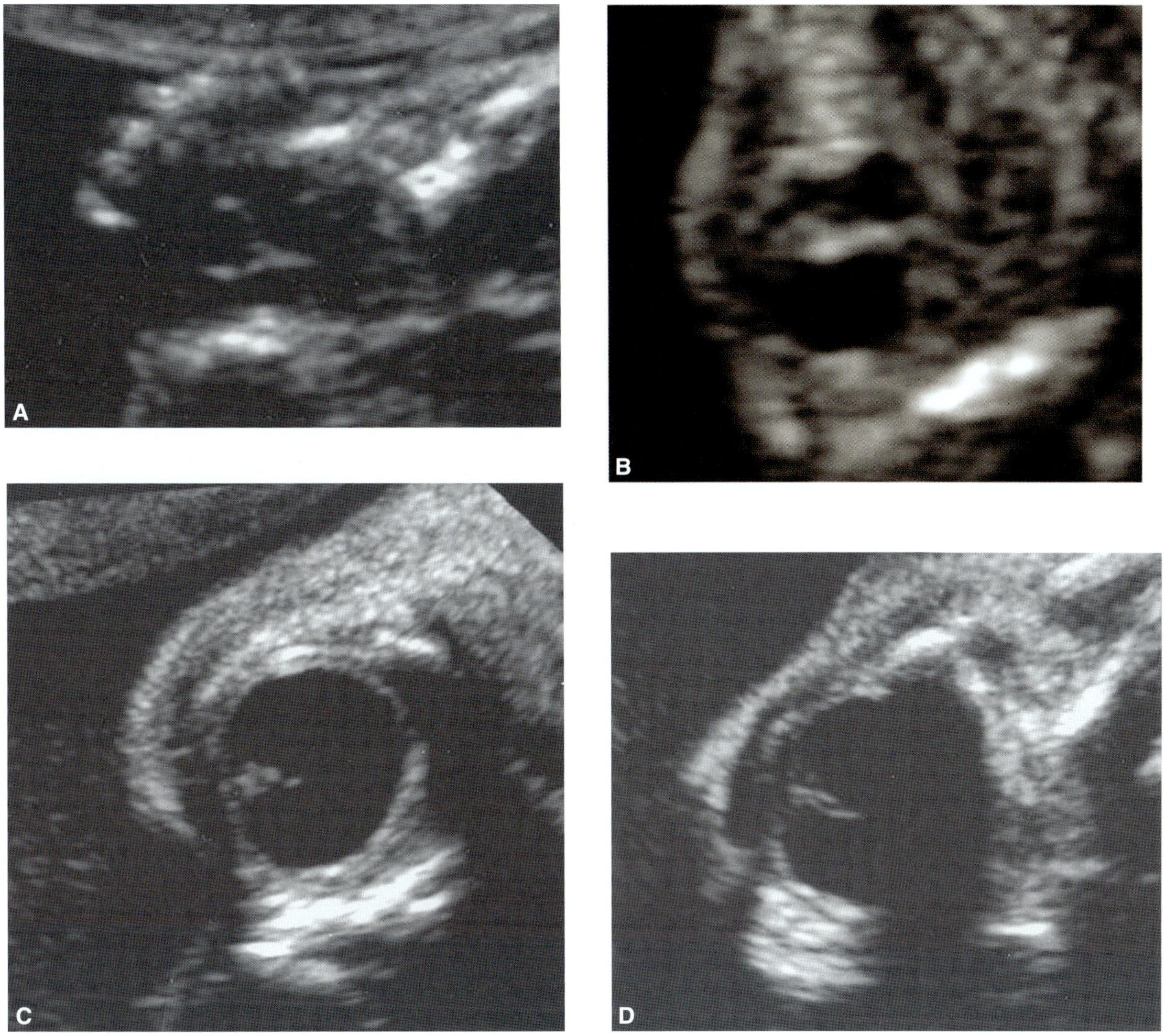


**Figure 14–19.** Variants of a hyaloid artery. **(A), (B)** Wide bifurcated hyaloid artery at 15 postmenstrual weeks' gestation. **(C), (D)** Threadlike structured hyaloid artery at 23 weeks' gestation.

cavity. On physical examination, absence of the irises and pupils was noted.

Bilateral retinal detachment was also imaged by US in a fetus with Norrie disease.[78] The principal feature of this disease is retinal dysplasia with resultant retinal detachment (Figure 14–24).

Maat-Kievit and colleagues[79] reported on the detection of a large retinoblastoma in a fetus at 21 postmenstrual weeks' gestation. The oval-shaped tumor protruded from the right side of the fetal face. The right orbit, as well as the fetal nose and mouth, could not be imaged, and a deformity of the normal anatomy of the facial bones was noted. Another case of fetal ocular neoplasm, rhabdomyosarcoma, is shown in Figure 14–25. Retinoblastoma is a very rare tumor, with an estimated annual incidence of between 1 in 15,000 and 1 in 34,000 in childhood, and about 1 in 30,000 prenatal incidence.[79,80]

Recent studies[81,82] have reported on the use of molecular techniques to screen prenatally for retinoblastoma, and others have reported on the first newborn delivered following preimplantation genetic exclusion of retinoblastoma.[83] Prenatal diagnosis of other rare disorders has been reported, including orbital heterotopic brain tissue[84,85] and orbital teratoma.[86]

## CONGENITAL NASOLACRIMAL DUCT CYST

The presence of fetal periorbital cystic structures raises the possibility of dacrocystocele;[87] this condition is usually apparent only in late pregnancy. Congenital nasolacrimal obstruction occurs in 1.75% to 6% of newborns.[88–95] The abnormality may be unilateral or bilateral. Epiphora is the only clinical sign in most cases, and spontaneous resolution occurs during infancy. However, in some cases, cysts

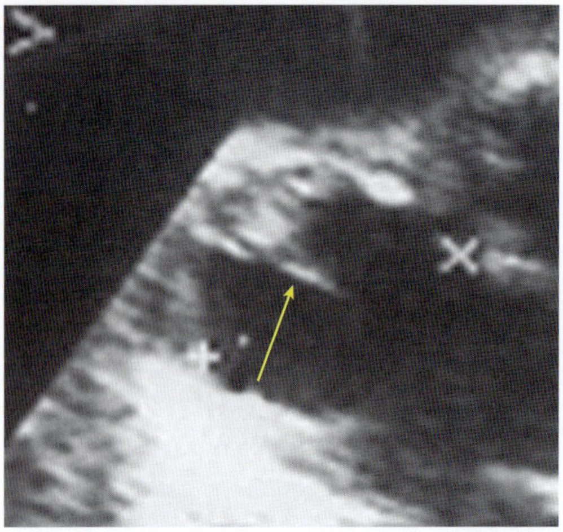

**Figure 14–20.** Hyaloid artery bifurcation associated with fetal cataract detection in utero.

are formed because of mucus accumulation. Complete obstruction may lead to an increased respiratory effort or even respiratory distress. In such cases, probing of the duct or silicone intubation is indicated.[89,90,92]

Although congenital dacryocystoceles may resolve without surgical intervention, some become infected and require systemic antibiotic treatment and even surgical drainage.[88] Prenatal sonographic diagnosis should be suggested if a cystic mass is visualized adjacent to the orbit and the base of the nose.[89–96] The differential diagnosis includes other anomalies in this region, such as encephalocele or hemangioma. Bilateral dacrocystocele has been detected in utero (Figure 14–26). Other periorbital findings are an epidermoid cyst that was detected in our patient at 29 weeks' gestation (Figure 14–27) and retinal coloboma diagnosed prenatally by Bault and Quarello[97] (Figure 14–28).

## TRAUMA OF THE EYE DURING AMNIOCENTESIS

The possible association between amniocentesis and fetal damage is well known. However, there are only a few cases reported on ophthalmologic complications;[98–103] in these case reports, cystic lesions, perforations, and scars were noted in the different parts of the eye. In some of the reports, the damage was corrected by surgery; but in others, the damage was severe, leading to hemianopia, gaze palsy,[101] microphthalmia, and total blindness.[99]

Ultrasound-guided amniocentesis has now become the standard of care. It is expected that this technique will reduce to a minimum the incidence of fetal trauma during the procedure.

## PHYSIOLOGIC ASPECTS OF THE FETAL EYE

### Fetal Eye Movements

Fetal eye movements are best evaluated by ultrasonographic observation of positional changes of the lenses. The pattern of fetal eye movements was studied and correlated with the emergence of fetal behavior states.

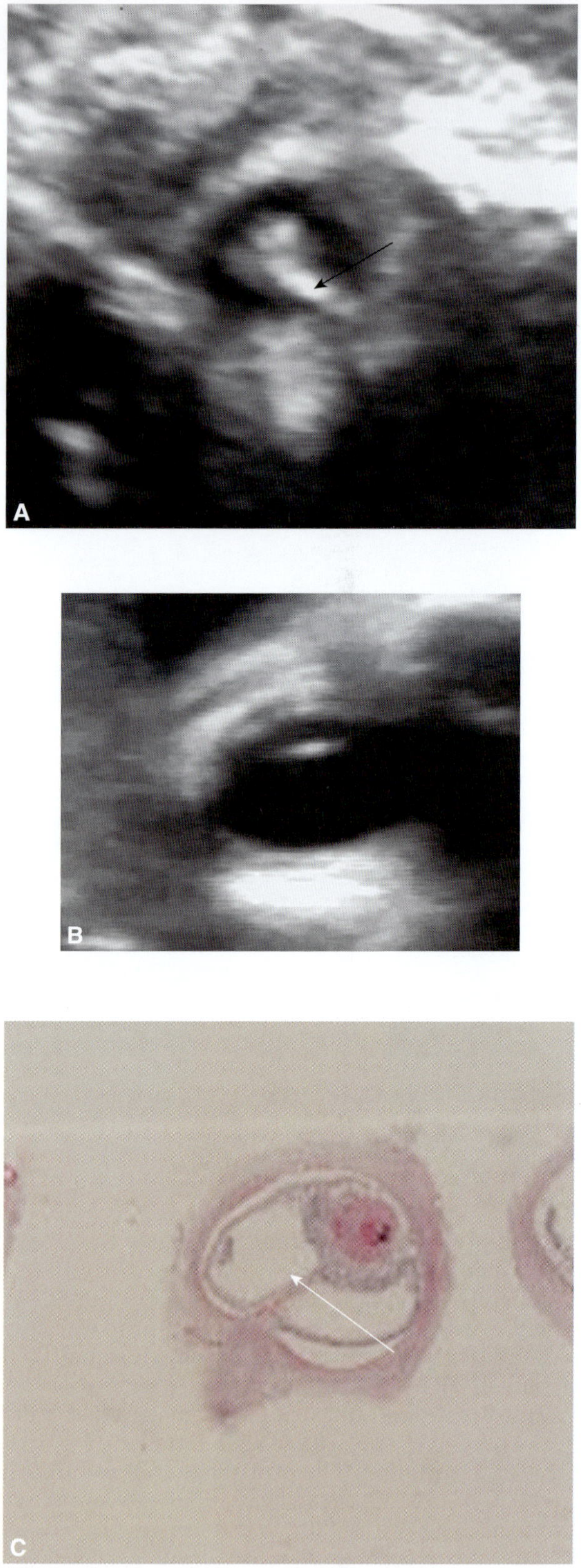

**Figure 14–21.** Persistent hyaloid vessels **(A)** Persistent hyperplastic primary vitreous (PHPV) at 34 postmenstrual weeks in a fetus with trisomy 13. The hyaloid aretery (HA) is fibrotic, going from the retina to the opaque lens, the ocular globe is small, and the lens is horizontal. **(B)** A normal eye with sonolucent lens, and no hyaloid artery visualized at 34 postmenstrual weeks. **(C)** Histology of the fetal eye demonstrating the persistent hyaloid vessels defining the PHPV. (Courtesy of Dr Y. Ben-Arieh.)

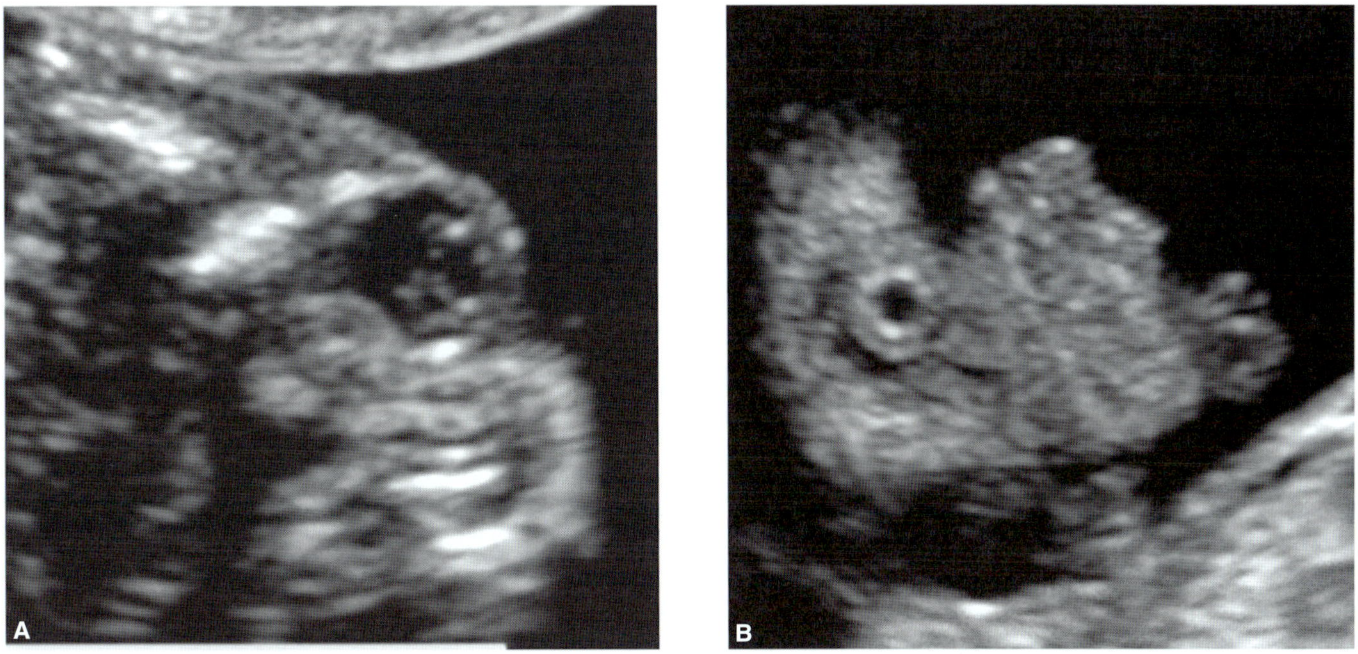


**Figure 14–22.** The problematic diagnosis of PHPV before 32 weeks is demonstrated by the following cases. **(A)** At 15 postmenopausal weeks, the hyaloid vessels are congested and hyperplastic in a fetus with trisomy 18, which is associated with PHPV. **(B)** The congested hyaloid vessels form a concentric double halo around the fetal lens at 15 postmenstrual weeks. This anomaly disappeared by 32 weeks, and the pregnancy generated a completely normal neonate.

Birnholz[104] described four types of eye movements:

1. Type I: single transient linear deviation, usually from midposition to a lower, outer orbital margin, followed by a slightly slower return to the initial position
2. Type II: prolonged but single deviation to a medial or lateral position
3. Type III: complex sequence of deviations, including rotatory components without apparent spatial or temporal periodicity (these movements are typically brisk and jerky)
4. Type IV: repetitive or nystagmoid deviations

Birnholz regarded types I and II as slow eye movements, and types III and IV as rapid eye movements. Arduini and coworkers[105] considered as rapid eye movements rapid nystagmus-like movements with a frequency >6/min. Eye movements with a frequency <6/min were defined as slow eye movements.[105]

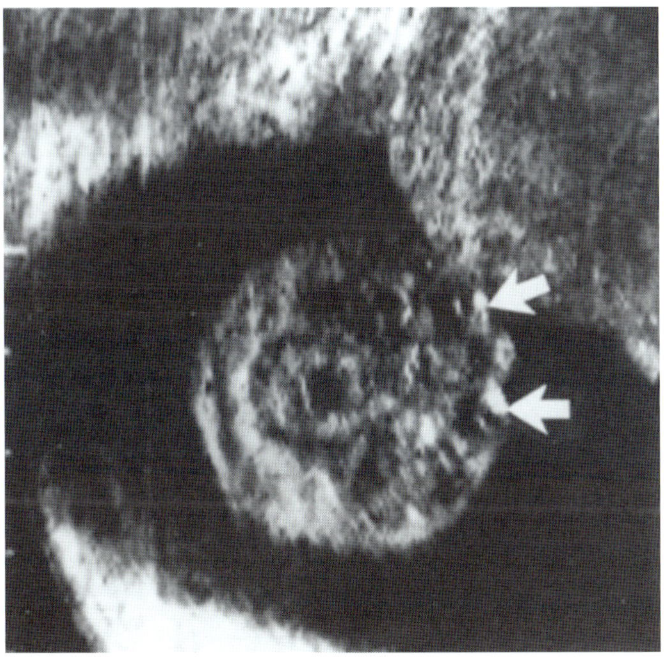

**Figure 14–23.** Hypotelorism. The orbits (*arrows*) of this fetus at 15 postmenstrual weeks are very close to each other.

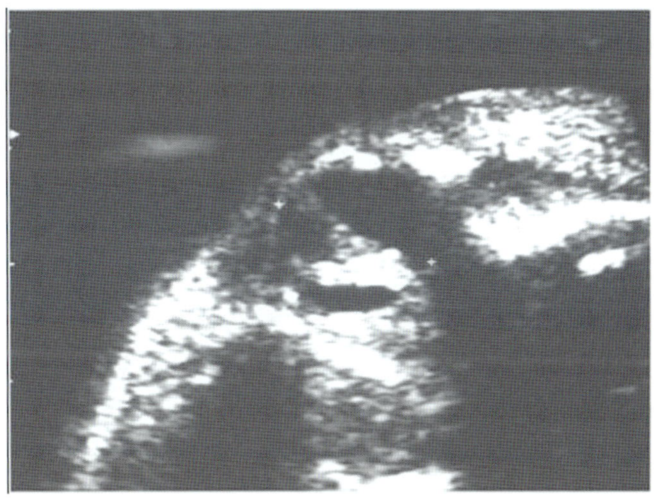

**Figure 14–24.** Retinal detachment diagnosis in a fetus at 26 postmenstrual weeks. (From Blin G, et al,[77] with permission.)

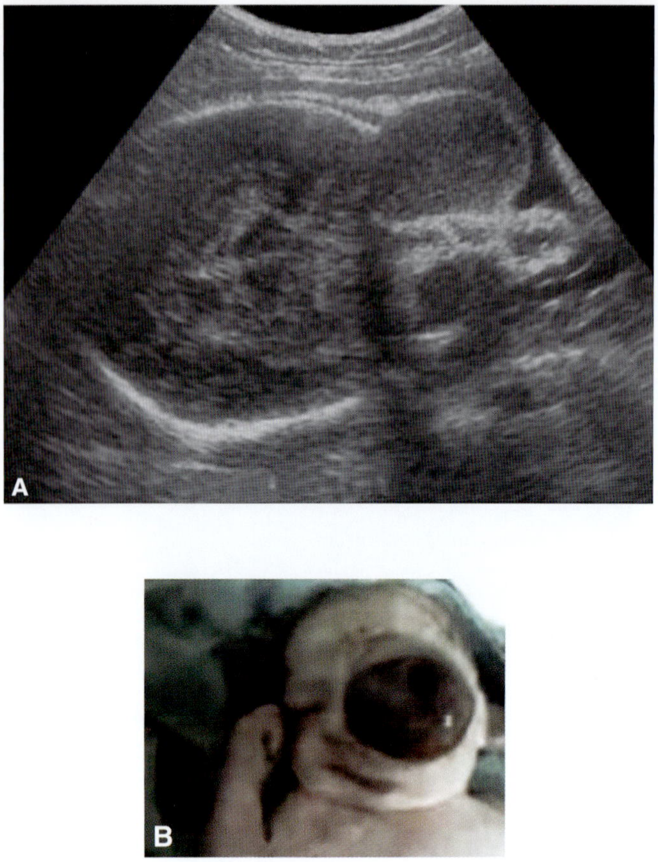


**Figure 14–25.** A case of ocular rhabdomyosarcoma at 35 postmenstrual weeks. Transverse section through the fetal skull showing an enlarged left ocular bulb protruding out of the orbit **(A)** and after delivery **(B)** in the neonate. (Courtesy of Bajram H. Syla. Reproduced, with permission, from www.thefetus.net.)

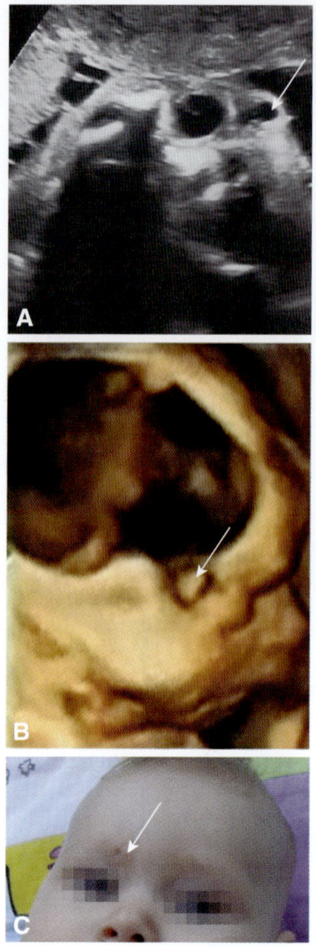


**Figure 14–27.** A case of epidermoid cyst detected at 29 postmenstrual weeks by two-dimentional US **(A)**, three-dimentional US **(B)**, and after delivery, in the neonate **(C)**.

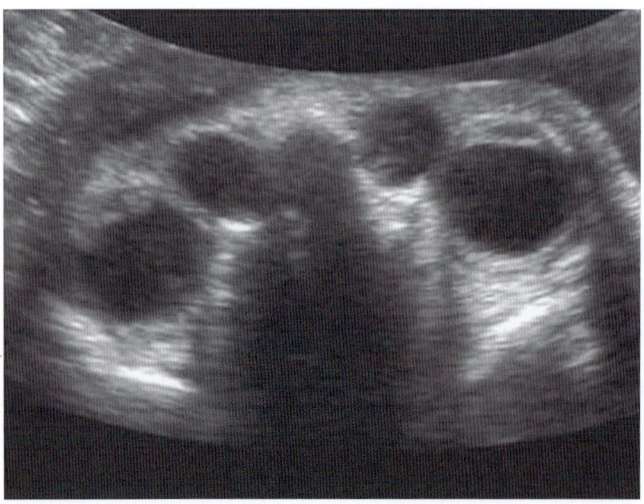

**Figure 14–26.** A case of bilateral dacrocystocele detected in utero at 30 postmenstrual weeks. (Courtesy of Yinon Gilboa. Reproduced, with permission, from www.thefetus.net.)

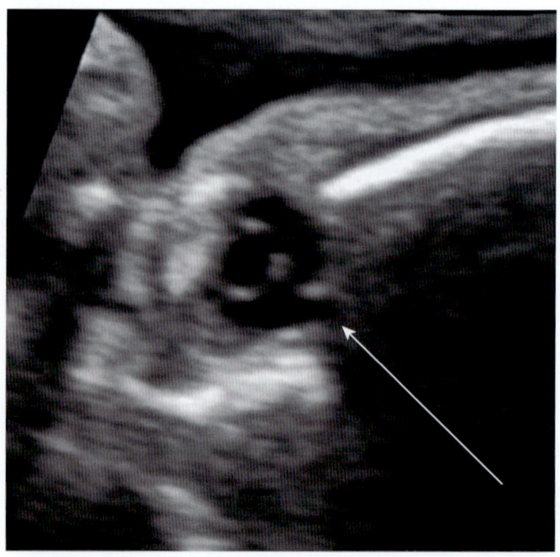

**Figure 14–28.** A case of fetal retinal coloboma (*arrow*) detected at 16 weeks.

Horimoto and associates[106] noted two types of eye movements. Those with duration of 0.07 up to 0.6 to 0.8 second were regarded as rapid eye movements. The others with duration of 0.6 to 0.8 up to 4 to 5 seconds were considered slow eye movements.[106] Differences in gestational age distribution of the various types of eye movements have been observed. Birnholz[104] reported that type I movements were apparent between 16 and 26 postmenstrual weeks' gestation, whereas type IV movements were recognized only after 32 postmenstrual weeks.

The patterns of eye movements, as well as the periodicity of absent eye movements, are important in the definition of fetal behavioral states. Nijuis and collaborators[107] defined four types of fetal behavior at 36 to 40 postmenstrual weeks. According to their classification, there is absence of fetal eye movements in state 1F. In the other three states, 2F, 3F, and 4F, both slow and rapid eye movements are continually present.[107]

Arduini's group[105] reported that during quiet phases of fetal behavior, slow eye movements, as well as absence of eye movement, was recorded. Rapid eye movements were never observed at this phase of fetal activity. On the other hand, during the active phases of fetal activity, both slow and rapid eye movements, as well as the absence of eye movement, could be noted. However, after 36 postmenstrual weeks, a significant prevalence of rapid eye movements during the active phases and absence of eye movement during the quiet phases were observed.[105]

A change in fetal eye movements (blinking response) may be induced by vibroacoustic stimulation. This is part of the startle response and change in fetal behavior state occurring in healthy fetuses following stimulation.[107]

Horimoto and colleagues[109] evaluated changes in pupillary diameters in relation to fetal eye movements. Pupillary diameters were found to be differentiated with statistical significance into two groups: 9.7% for the dilated pupil (range 2.1–3.4 mm) and 90.3% for the constricted pupil (range 1.4–1.9 mm). The percentage of dilated pupils during eye movement period (14.3%) was significantly greater than that during no eye movement period (2.3%).[109] This relation between papillary diameter and eye movement is in agreement with data from adults.

## COLOBOMA

Congenital optic coloboma represents an important cause of childhood visual impairment and blindness; it can be either isolated or, more often, associated with several syndromes. Coloboma is a rare malformation consisting of a wedge malformation in the ocular bulb. Although not included in any screening protocol, it may be prenatally diagnosed, at least in some cases, by US (Figure 14–28). Retinal coloboma can be diagnosed in utero using a new technique, the so-called virtual fetal eyeground.[97] However, in our experience the traditional B mode is also accurate for the detection of coloboma. We also believe that in cases where a satisfactory sonographic evaluation of the fetal eyes is possible and accessible, high-resolution US may be more accurate and informative than magnetic resonance imaging.[110]

## REFERENCES


1. Robinson GC, Jan JE, Kinnis C. Congenital ocular blindness in children, 1945 to 1984. *Am J Dis Child.* 1987;141:1321–1324.
2. Goggin M, O'Keefe M. Childhood blindness in the Republic of Ireland: A national survey. *Br J Opthalmol.* 1991;75:425–429.
3. Foster A. Gilbert C. Epidemiology of childhood blindness. *Eye.* 1992;6:173–176.
4. Stoll C, Alembik Y, Dott B, Roth MP. Epidemiology of congenial eye malformations in 131,760 consecutive births. *Opthalmic Pediatr Genet.* 1992;13:179–186.
5. Jay B. Causes of blindness in school children. *Br Med J.* 1987;294: 1183–1184.
6. Phillips CI, Levy AM, Newton M, Stokoe NL. Blindness in school children: Importance of heredity, congenial cataract and prematurity. *Br J Opthalmol.* 1987;71:578–584.
7. Stoll C, Alembik Y, Dott B, Roth MP. Congenital eye malformations in 212,479 consecutive births. *Ann Genet.* 1997;40:122–128.
8. Nicolaides KH, Salversen DR, Sijders RJM, Gosdes CM. Fetal facial defects: Associated malformations and chromosomal abnormalities. *Fetal Diagn Ther.* 1993;8:1–9.
9. Wilkie AOM, Amberger JS, McKusick VA. The gene map of congenital malformations. *J Med Genet.* 1994;31:507–517.
10. Sadler TW, ed. Eye. In: *Langsman's Medical Embryology.* 6th ed. Baltimore: Williams & Wilkins; 1990:338–346.
11. Larsen WJ, ed. Development of the eyes. In: *Human Embryology.* 4th ed. Churchill Livingstone; Philadelphia. 2001:379–389.
12. Ko M-K, Chi JG, Chang B-L. Hyaloid vascular pattern in the human fetus. *J Pediatr Opthalmol Strabismus.* 1985;22:188–193.
13. Birnholz JC, Farrell EE. Fetal hyaloid artery: Timing of regression with US. *Radiology.* 1988;166:781–783.
14. Harayama K, Amemiya T, Nishimura H. Development of the eyeball during fetal life. *J Pediatr Ophthalmol Strabismus.* 1981;18:37–40.
15. Denis D, Righini M, Scheiner C, et al. Ocular growth in the fetus: 1. Comparative study of axial length and biometric parameters in the fetus. *Ophthalmologica.* 1993;207:117–124.
16. Birnholz JC. Ultrasonic fetal ophthalmology. *Early Hum Dev.* 1985;12:199–209.
17. de Elejalde MM, Elejalde BR. Ultrasonographic visualization of the fetal eye. *J Craniofac Genet Dev Biol.* 1985;5:319–326.
18. Jeanty P, Dramaix-Wilmet M, Van Gansbeke D, Van Regemorter N, Rodesch F, Fetal ocular biometry by ultrasound. *Radiology.* 1982;143:513–516.
19. Mayden KL, Tortora M, Berkowitz RL, Bracken M, Hobbins JC. Orbital diameters: A new parameter for prenatal diagnosis and dating. *Am J Obstet Gynecol.* 1982;144:289–297.
20. Goldstein I, Tamir A, Zimmer EZ, Itskovitz-Eldor J. Growth of the fetal orbit and lens in normal pregnancies. *Ultrasound Obstet Gynecol.* 1998;12:175–179.
21. Dilmen G, Köktener A, Turhan NO, Tez S. Growth of the fetal lens and orbit. *Int J Gynaecol Obstet.* 2002;76(3):267–271.
22. Sukonpan K, Phupong V. Fetal ocular distance in normal pregnancies. *J Med Assoc Thai.* 2008;91:1318–1322.
23. Achiron R, Gottlieb Z, Yaron Y, et al. The development of the fetal eye: In utero ultrasonographic measurements of the vitreous and lens. *Prenat Diagn.* 1995;15:155–160.
24. Achiron R, Kreiser D, Achiron A. Axial growth of the fetal eye and evaluation of the hyaloid artery: In utero ultrasonographic study. *Prenat Diagn.* 2000;20:894–899.
25. Nelson LB. Diagnosis and management of cataracts in infancy and childhood. *Ophthalmic Surg.* 1984;15:688–697.
26. Kohn BA. The differential diagnosis of cataracts in infancy and childhood. *Am J Dis Child.* 1976;130:184–192.
27. Merin S, Crawford JS. The etiology of congenital cataracts: a survey of 386 cases. *Can J Ophthalmol.* 1971;6:178–182.
28. Taylor D. Congenital cataract: The history, the nature and the practice. *Eye.* 1998;12:9–36.
29. Walton DS. Eye evaluation in the newborn. In: Oski FA, DeAngelis CD, Feigin RD, Warshaw JB, eds. *Principles and Practice of Pediatrics.* Philadelphia: Lippincott Williams & Wilkins' 1990:468–470.
30. Shapiro I, Borochowitz Z, Degani S, Dar H, Ibschitz I, Sharf M. Neu-Laxova syndrome: Prenatal ultrasonographic diagnosis, clinical and pathological studies and new manifestations. *Am J Med Genet.* 1992;43:602–605.

31. Zimmer EZ, Bronshtein M, Ophir E, et al. Sonographic diagnosis of fetal congenital cataracts. *Prenat Diagn.* 1993;13:503–511.
32. Gaary EA, Rawnsley E, Marin-Padilla JM, Morse CL, Crow HC. In utero detection of fetal cataracts. *J Ultrasound Med.* 1993;12: 234–236.
33. Monteagudo A, Timor-Tritsch IE, Friedman AH, Santos R. Autosomal dominant cataracts of the fetus: Early detection by transvaginal ultrasound. *Ultrasound Obstet Gynecol.* 1996;8:104–108.
34. Drysdale K, Kyle PM, Sepulveda W. Prenatal detection of congenital inherited cataracts. *Ultrasound Obstet Gynecol.* 1997;9:62–63.
35. Romain M, Awoust J, Dugauquier C, van Maldergem L. Prenatal ultrasound detection of congenital cataract in trisomy 21. *Prenat Diagn.* 1999;19:780–782.
36. Pedreira DAL, Diniz EMA, Schultz R, Faro LB, Zugaib M. Fetal cataract in congenital toxoplasmosis. *Ultrasound Obstet Gynecol.* 1999;13:266–267.
37. Müllner-Eidenböck A, Amon M, Moser E, Klebermass N. Persistent fetal vasculature and minimal fetal vascular remnants: A frequent cause of unilateral congenital cataracts. *Ophthalmology.* 2004;111:906–913.
38. Zeiter HJ. Congenital microphthalmus. *Am J Ophthalmol.* 1963;55:910–922.
39. Duke-Elder S, Cooke C. Microphthalmos: Congenital deformities. In: Duke-Elder S, ed. *System of Ophthalmology.* Vol 3. St. Louis, MO: CV Mosby; 1964:488–495.
40. Warburg M. Genetics of microphthalmos. *Int Ophthalmol.* 1981;4:45–65.
41. Sutcliffe AG, Jones RB, Woodruff G. Eye malformations associated with treatment with carbamazepine during pregnancy. *Ophthalmic Genet.* 1998;19:59–62.
42. Schauer GM, Dunn LK, Godmilow L, Eagle RC, Knisely AS. Prenatal diagnosis of Fraser syndrome at 18.5 weeks gestation, with autopsy finding at 19 weeks. *Am J Med Genet.* 1990;37:583–591.
43. Bronshtein M, Zimmer EZ, Gershoni-Baruch R, Yoffe N, Meyer H, Blumenfeld Z. First and second trimester diagnosis of fetal ocular defects and associated anomalies: Report of eight cases. *Obstet Gynecol.* 1991;77:443–449.
44. Porges Y, Gershoni-Baruch R, Leibu R, et al. Hereditary microphthalmia with colobomatous cyst. *Am J Ophthalmol.* 1992;114:30–34.
45. Blazer S, Zimmer EZ, Mezer E, Bronshtein M. Early and late onset fetal microphthalmia. *Am J Obstet Gynecol.* 2006;194:1354–1359.
46. Shulman LP, Gordon PL, Emerson DS, Wilroy RS, Elias S. Prenatal diagnosis of isolated bilateral microphthalmia with confirmation by evaluation of products of conception obtained by dilation and evacuation. *Prenat Diagn.* 1993;13:403–409.
47. Schneider A, Bardakjian TM, Zhou J, et al. Familial recurrence of SOX2 anophthalmia syndrome: Phenotypically normal mother with two affected daughters. *Am J Med Genet A.* 2008;146A:2794–2798.
48. Vutova K, Peicheva Z, Popova A, Markova V, Mincheva N, Todorov T. Congenital toxoplasmosis: Eye manifestations in infants and children. *Ann Trop Paediatr.* 2002;22:213–218.
49. Turner GM, Twining P. The facial profile in the diagnosis of fetal abnormalities. *Clin Radiol.* 1993;47:389–395.
50. Menashe Y, Ben Baruch G, Rabinovitch O, Shalev Y, Katznelson MBM, Shalev E. Exophthalmus—Prenatal ultrasonic features for diagnosis of Crouzon syndrome. *Prenat Diagn.* 1989;9:805–808.
51. Gershoni-Baruch R, Drugan A, Bronshtein M, Zimmer EZ. Roberts syndrome or "X linked Amelia"? *Am J Med Genet.* 1990;37: 569–572.
52. Bocino CA, Platt LD, Garber A, et al. Fetal akinesia hypokinesia sequence: Prenatal diagnosis and intrafamilial variability. *Prenat Diagn.* 1993;13:1011–1019.
53. Amaya L, Taylor D, Russell-Eggitt I, Nischal KK, Lengyel D. The morphology and natural history of childhood cataracts [review]. *Surv Ophthalmol.* 2003;48:125–144.
54. Katorza E, Rosner M, Zalel Y, Gilboa Y, Achiron R. Prenatal ultrasonographic diagnosis of persistent hyperplastic primary vitreous. *Ultrasound Obstet Gynecol.* 2008;32:226–228.
55. DeMyer W, Zeman W, Palmer CG. The face predicts the brain: Diagnostic significance of median facial anomalies for holoprosencephaly (arhinencephaly). *Pediatrics.* 1964;34:256–263.
56. Romero R, Pilu G, Jeanty P, Chidini A, Hobbins JC, eds. The face. In: *Prenatal Diagnosis of Congenital Anomalies.* East Norwalk, CT: Appleton & Lange; 1988:81–113.
57. Khudr G, Olding L. Cyclopia. *Am J Dis Child.* 1973;125:120–122.
58. Elejalde Br, de Elejalde MM, Hamilton PR, Christenson R, Broekhuizen F. Prenatal diagnosis of cyclopia. *Am J Med Genet.* 1983;14:15–19.
59. Toth Z, Csecsei K, Szeifert G, Papp Z. Early prenatal diagnosis of cyclopia associated with holoprosencephaly. *J Clin Ultrasound.* 1986;14:550–553.
60. Meizner I, Drawall D, Mazor M, Katz. Sonographic findings in a rare case of fetal cyclopia. *Isr J Med Sci.* 1987;23:910–912.
61. Van Allen MI, Ritchie S, Toi A, Fong K, Winsor E. Trisomy 4 in a fetus with cyclopia and other anomalies. *Am J Med Genet.* 1993;46:193–197.
62. Arakaki DT, Waxman SH. Trisomy D in a cyclops. *J Pediatr.* 1969;74:620–622.
63. Jaschevatzky OE, Goldman B, Georghiou P, Grunstein S, Pevzner S. Trisomy D in a cyclops with cardiovascular defects. *Acta Obstet Gynecol Scand.* 1976;55:73–76.
64. Taysi K, Tinaztepe K. Trisomy D and the cyclops malformation. *Am J Dis Child.* 1972;124:710–713.
65. Mollica F, Pavone L, Nuciforo G, Gorge G. A case of cyclopia: Role of environmental factors. *Clin Genet.* 1979;16:69–71.
66. Rolland M, Sarramon MF, Bloom MC. Astomia-agnathia-holoprosencephaly association: Prenatal diagnosis of a new case. *Prenat Diagn.* 1991;11:199–203.
67. Cho FN, Kan YY, Chen SN, Lee TC, Hsu TJ, Hsu PH. Prenatal diagnosis of cyclopia and proboscis in a fetus with normal chromosome at 13 weeks of gestation by three-dimensional transabdominal sonography. *Prenat Diagn.* 2005;25:1059–1060.
68. Pilu G, Reece EA, Romero R, Bovicelli L, Hobbins JC. Prenatal diagnosis of craniofacial malformations with ultrasonography. *Am J Obstet Gynecol.* 1986;155:45–50.
69. Chervenak FA, Tortora M, Mayden K, et al. Antenatal diagnosis of median cleft face syndrome: Sonographic demonstration of cleft lip and hypertelorism. *Am J Obstet Gynecol.* 1984;149:94–97.
70. Shever DM, Shah YG, Wang N, Metlay LA, Wood JR, Jr. Prenatal diagnosis and subsequent management of a fetus with a 46 XYr (4) (p15-q35) karyotype. *Am J Perinatol.* 1991;8:53–55.
71. Trout T, Budorick NE, Pretorius DH, McGahan JP. Significance of orbital measurements in the fetus. *J Ultrasound Med.* 1994;13: 937–943.
72. Anderka MT, Lin AE, Abuelo DN, Mitchell AA, Rasmussen SA. Reviewing the evidence for mycophenolate mofetil as a new teratogen: Case report and review of the literature. *Am J Med Genet A.* 2009;149A:1241–1248.
73. Farrel SA, Leadman TML, Davidson RG, Caco C. Prenatal diagnosis of retinal detachment in Walker-Warburg syndrome. *Am J Med Genet.* 1987;28:619–624.
74. Monteagudo A, Ayalon A, Mayberry P. Walker-Warburg syndrome: Case report and review of the literature. *J Ultrasound Med.* 2001;20:419–426.
75. Vohra N, Ghidini A, Alvarez M, Lockwood C. Walker–Warburg syndrome: Prenatal ultrasound findings. *Prenat Diagn.* 1993;13: 575–579.
76. Chitayat D, Toi A, Babul R, et al. Prenatal diagnosis of retinal nonattachment in the Walker-Warburg syndrome. *Am J Med Genet.* 1995;56:351–358.
77. Blin G, Rabbé A, Ansquer Y, Meghdiche S, Floch-Tudal C, Mandelbrot L. First-trimester ultrasound diagnosis in a recurrent case of Walker-Warburg syndrome. *Ultrasound Obstet Gynecol.* 2005;26:297–299.
78. Redmond RM, Vaughan JI, Jay M, Jay B. In utero diagnosis of Norrie disease by unltrasonography. *Ophthalmol Pediatr Genet.* 1993;14: 1–3.
79. Maat-Kievit JA, Oepkes D, Hartwig NG, Vermeij-Keers C, Van Kamp IL, Van De Kamp JJP. A large retinoblastoma detected in a fetus at 21 weeks of gestation. *Prenat Diagn.* 1993;13:377–384.
80. Salim A, Wiknjosastro GH, Danukusumo D, Barnas B, Zalud I. Fetal retinoblastoma. *J Ultrasound Med.* 1998;17:717–720.
81. Singh AD, Black SH, Shields CL, Shields JA. Prenatal diagnosis of retinoblastoma. *J Pediatr Ophthalmol Strabismus.* 2003;40:2 22–224.
82. Lau CS, Choy KW, Fan DS, et al. Prenatal screening for retinoblastoma in Hong Kong. *Hong Kong Med J.* 2008;14(5):391–394.
83. Xu K, Rosenwaks Z, Beaverson K, Cholst I, Veeck L, Abramson DH. Preimplantation genetic diagnosis for retinoblastoma: The first reported liveborn. *Am J Ophthalmol.* 2004;137:18–23.

84. Sueters M, Peek AM, Ball LM, et al. Prenatal detection of orbital rhabdomyosarcoma. *Arch Ophthalmol.* 2005;123:276–279.
85. Hingorani M, Mannor G, Vardy SJ, et al. Prenatal diagnosis of orbital heterotopic brain tissue. *J Pediatr Surg.* 1997;32:1348–1350.
86. Moon YJ, Hwang HS, Kim YR, Park YW, Kim YH. Prenatally detected congenital orbital teratoma. *Ultrasound Obstet Gynecol.* 2008;31:107–109.
87. Abbasi AH, Haj N, Nseir T, Garzozi HJ. Prenatal diagnosis of dacryocystocele. *Eye.* 2007;21:1537–1538.
88. Wong RK, VanderVeen DK. Presentation and management of congenital dacryocystocele. *Pediatrics.* 2008;122:e1108–1112.
89. Yen MT, Tse DT. Congenital orbital cyst detected and monitored by prenatal ultrasonography. *Ophthal Plast Reconstr Surg.* 2001;17:443–446.
90. Kushner BJ. Congenital nasolacrimal system obstruction. *Arch Ophthalmol.* 1982;100:597–600.
91. Harris GJ, DiClementi D. Congenital dacryocystocele. *Arch Ophthalmol.* 1982;100:1763–1765.
92. Paul TO, Shepard R. Congenital nasolacrimal duct obstruction: Natural history and the timing of the optimal intervention. *J Pediatr Opthalmol Strabismus.* 1994;31:362–367.
93. Davis WK, Mahoney BS, Carroll BA, Bowie JD. Antenatal sonographic detection of benign dacrocystoceles (lacrimal duct cysts). *J Ultrsound Med.* 1987;6:461–465.
94. Alper CM, Chan KH, Hill LM, Chenevey P. Antenatal diagnosis of congenital nasolacrimal duct cyst by ultrasonography: A case report. *Prenat Diagn.* 1994;14:623–626.
95. Walsh G. Dubbins PA. Antenatal sonographic diagnosis of dacryocystocele. *J Ultrasound Med.* 1994;22:457–460.
96. Sharony R, Raz J, Aviram R, Cohen I, Beyth Y, Tepper R. Prenatal diagnosis of dacryocystocele: A possible marker for syndromes. *Ultrasound Obstet Gynecol.* 1999;14:71–73.
97. Bault JP, Quarello E. Retinal coloboma: Prenatal diagnosis using a new technique, the "virtual fetal eyeground." *Ultrasound Obstet Gynecol.* 2009;33:495–496.
98. Cross HE, Maumenee AE. Ocular trauma during amniocentesis. *Arch Ophthalmol.* 1973;90:303–304.
99. Merin S, Beyth Y. Uniocular congenital blindness as a complication of midtrimester amniocentesis. *Am J Ophthalmol.* 1980;89: 299–301.
100. Isenberg SJ, Heckenlively JR. Traumatized eye with retinal damage from amniocentesis. *J Pediatr Ophthalmol Strabismus.* 1985;22: 65–67.
101. Admoni MM, Ben Ezra D. Ocular trauma following amniocentesis as a cause of leukocoria. *J Pediatr Ophthalmol Strabismus.* 1988;25:196–197.
102. Naylor G, Roper JG, Willshaw HE. Ophthalmic complications of amniocentesis. *Eye.* 1990;4:845–849.
103. Rummelt V, Rummelt C, Naumann GOH. Congenital nonpigmented epithelial iris cyst after amniocentesis: Clinicopathologic report on two children. *Ophthalmology.* 1993;100:776–781.
104. Birnholz JC. The development of human fetal eye movement patterns. *Science.* 1981;213:679–681.
105. Arduini D, Rizzo G, Giorlandino C, Valensise H, Dellacqua S, Romanini C. The development of fetal behavioral states: A longitudinal study. *Prenat Diagn.* 1986;6:117–124.
106. Horimoto N, Koyanagi T, Satoh S, Yoshizato T, Nakano H. Fetal eye movement assessed with real time ultrasonography: Are these rapid and slow eye movements? *Am J Obstet Gynecol.* 1990;163: 1480–1484.
107. Nijhuis JG, Prechtl HFR, Martin BR, Jr, Bates RSGM. Are there behavioral states in the human fetus? *Early Hum Develop.* 1982;6:177–195.
108. Birnholz JC, Benacerraf BR. The development of human fetal hearing. *Science.* 1983;222:516–518.
109. Horimoto N, Koyanagi T, Takashima T, Akazawa K, Nakano H. Changes in pupillary diameter in relation to eye movement and no eye movement periods in the human fetus at term. *Am J Obstet Gynecol.* 1992;167:1465–1469.
110. Righini A, Avagliano L, Doneda C, et al. Prenatal magnetic resonance imaging of optic nerve head coloboma. *Prenat Diagn.* 2008;28:242–246.

Chapter 15

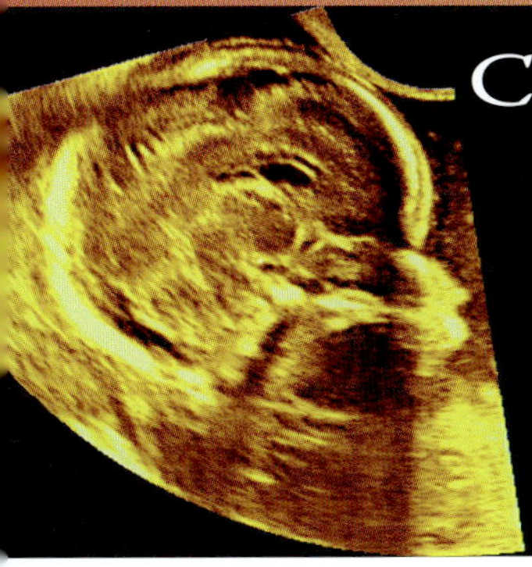

# FETAL CEREBRAL CIRCULATION

*Ritsuko K. Pooh • Shimon Degani*

## KEY POINTS

1. Data collected from Doppler velocity recordings using both spectral and color Doppler mode confirm the fundamental aspects of the fetoplacental circulation. Changes in placental vascular resistance, cardiac contractibility, vessel compliance, and blood viscosity alter the normal dynamics of fetal cerebral circulation.
2. Reference values have been established for the main cerebral vessels. During the last trimester of normal pregnancies, the values of Doppler waveform indices decrease in all main cerebral vessels. After birth, vascular resistance decreases, and later stabilizes. Cerebral autoregulation persists from fetal to postnatal life, with low waveform indices in cerebral vessels of growth-retarded fetuses and neonates. The low indices indicate decreased cerebrovascular resistance, representing the redistribution of flow, or the brain-sparing effect.
3. Combined parameters recorded from different vascular beds may provide support for the diagnosis of significant hemodynamic changes and are of prognostic value in predicting fetal outcome such as fetal IUFGR and Rh disease.
4. As far as imaging of the vascularization (arterial and venous) of the prenatal brain, it should be clear that no brain scan should be considered complete without looking at its main vessels or at least at the pericallosal artery on a median section. Should such a protocol be too complicated to achieve in all anomaly scans, it is important to scrutinize brain vascularization in each and every case of suspected brain anomaly.
5. Three-dimensional power Doppler US technology, especially combined with high-frequency TVS, as described in this and other chapters, is the most preferable noninvasive and reproducible imaging method to be used. The accurate information about deviant brain vascularity may help to render proper obstetric, neurologic, and neurosurgical management.

Recent sonographic advances have contributed to accurate and reliable visualization of intrauterine vascularity. The first breakthrough in the assessment of fetal circulation was the Doppler system. Technical developments in Doppler ultrasound (US) equipment, especially highly sensitive color Doppler, power Doppler, and bidirectional power Doppler imaging techniques, have made it possible to study the fetal circulatory system, including cerebral vascularization. Early fetal circulation has been demonstrated by conventional two-dimensional (2D) color Doppler since the 1990s.[1] Fine vessels inside the choroid plexus were depicted and assessed in 1994.[2,3] Two-dimensional color/power Doppler combined with transvaginal sonography (TVS) became a powerful tool to demonstrate early fetal vascularization.[4,5] Embryonal/fetal development is amazingly rapid, and the structure of the brain changes throughout pregnancy. Introduction of three-dimensional (3D) power Doppler technology in the late 1990s enabled visualization of intracranial vessels. This assessment, combined with TVS, has provided 3D sonoangiographic images, and adds useful information in the prenatal evaluation of normal brain development, vascular malformation, and tumoral vascularity.[6,7]

## DEVELOPMENT OF EMBRYONAL CEREBRAL CIRCULATION

Vascular endothelial cells cover the entire inner surface of blood vessels and are influenced by vascular endothelial growth factor (VEGF), which is a potent angiogenic factor working as an endothelial cell-specific mitogen and exerting a trophic effect on neurons and glial cells. Both of these activities are essential during central nervous system (CNS) vascularization, development, and repair. In these cells, VEGF expression developmentally regulates and is correlated with angiogenesis, which in turn responds to the high metabolic demands of the developing fetal brain.[8]

From the beginning of cardiac development, the cranial parts of the truncus arteriosus enlarge and transform into the aortic sac, which later gives rise to the aortic branches. After splitting of the truncus arteriosus by the aorticopulmonal septum, the primoridal aortic sac becomes part of the ventral aorta, while a pair of the dorsal aortae develop independently of the cardiac tube. During later development, extensive changes occur, leading to loss of the symmetrical state of these primitive vessels. In brief, the common aortic artery, along with the first part of the internal carotid artery (ICA), arises from the third aortic branch, while the rest of the vessels develop from the cranial part of the dorsal aorta. The external carotid artery develops as a cranial part of the third aortic branch, while the vertebral arteries emerge from the dorsal aorta. In the development of cerebral fetal veins, the upper cardinal veins play the most important role, draining the blood from the cranial part of the embryo.

During fetal development (approximately 35 gestational days), the craniocerebral circulation is characterized by temporary connections between the primitive carotid and the paired dorsal longitudinal neural arteries (precursors of the vertebrobasilar system). They include persistent trigeminal, ottic, hypoglossal, and proatlantic intersegmental arteries. Normal embryonic development underwrites the regression of all these vessels totally. Sometimes the regression does not occur, resulting in a persistent trigeminal artery, which is the most frequent reason (85% of cases) of primitive carotid-to-basilar artery anastomoses.[9]

## NORMAL VASCULARIZATION OF THE FETAL CENTRAL NERVOUS SYSTEM

It should be said at the outset that the best way to study fetal circulation during its development is by employing 2D as well as 3D color and power Doppler technologies. Due to their physical limitations, transabdominal transducers cannot achieve high enough resolution to accurately display fine vessel anatomy. Therefore, high-frequency transvaginal probes have to be used for the best results.

Also the use of color and power Doppler should be used judiciously and sparingly during the first trimester according to the ALARA (as low as reasonably achievable) radiation safety suggestion (Title 10, Section 20.103 of the Code of Federal Regulators (USFNR).

Assessment of cerebral vascularization becomes possible from the seventh postmenstrual week of gestation, capturing low-velocity flow signals with an obvious absence of diastolic flow, from the periphery (walls) of the rhombencephalic cavity.[3] At that stage the lateral ventricles are small evaginations located laterally and rostrally from the cavity of the diencephalon directly contiguous with the mesencephalon (Figure 15–1). The isthmus rhombencephali represents the connection to the rhombencephalic cavity and the future fourth ventricle. At this time of the evolution, the cavity of the rhombencephalon is the largest brain cavity visible in the embryonic head, as shown in Figure 15–1. From 8 postmenstrual weeks of gestation, it is possible to detect blood flow signals from the ICA and vertebral artery. At this stage, the rhombencephalic cavity (future fourth ventricle) decreases in size and moves toward the occipital part. Upon reaching the brain, the two ICAs turn dorsally and course alongside the diencephalon, giving off their branches. The ICA and its branches—the anterior cerebral artery (ACA), the middle cerebral artery (MCA), and the posterior communicating artery—form a polygonal-shaped communicating vessel called the circulus arteriosus, or the circle of Willis. The vessels arising from the circle of Willis supply the blood flow to the entire brain. Other vessels that form the circle are the vertebral arteries running between the transverse processes of C2 to C6 and giving a branch called the basilar artery and the posterior cerebral artery (PCA). The main components of the circulus arteriosus are present at Carnegie stage 16 (crown-rump [C-R] length of 10 mm, or 38 days postconception), and the circle is complete with Carnegie stage 16 (see Chapter 1). Arteries originating from the vertebral arteries are important for the supply of the cerebellum and brainstem. Within the symmetrical cerebellar hemispheres, it is possible to visualize the intracerebellar arteries. Blood flow signals from the intracerebellar arteries can be obtained from the ninth postmenstrual week of gestation,

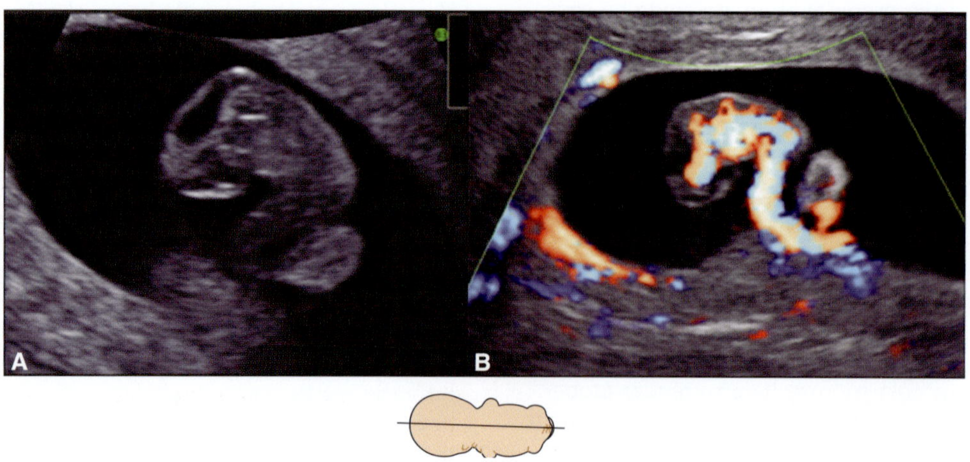


**Figure 15–1.** Early embryonal vascularity at 7 postmenstrual weeks. **(A)** Sagittal sonographic image of the embryo. **(B)** Bidirectional power Doppler image on the same section.

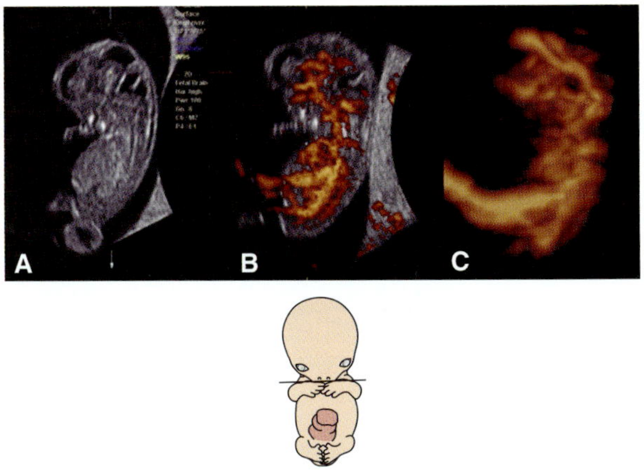


**Figure 15–2.** Early embryonal vascularity at 9 postmenstrual weeks. **(A)** Sagittal sonographic image of the fetus. **(B)** Three-dimensional (3D) power Doppler image of fetal vascularity with surface display mode. **(C)** 3D power Doppler angiographic image of the vascular system.

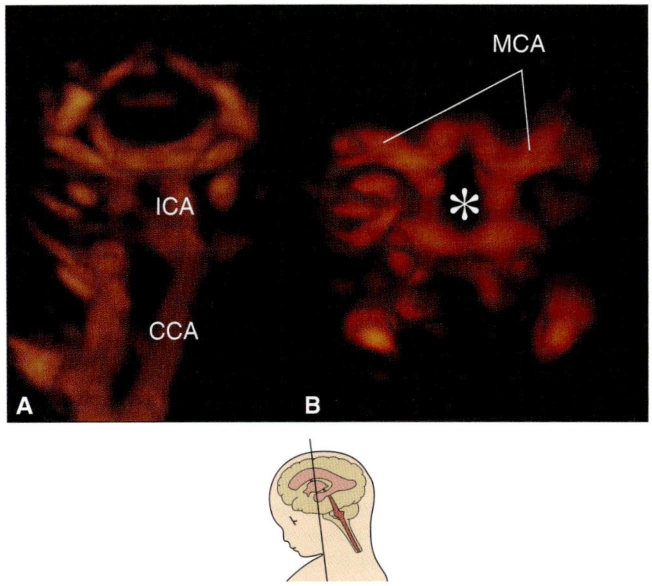


**Figure 15–3.** Vascular structure of normal 12 postmenstrual week brain by 3D power Doppler angiographic rendering. **(A)** Coronal power Doppler image of common carotid arteries (CCA), internal carotid arteries (ICA), and their branches. **(B)** Axial or horizontal 3D power Doppler angiographic image obtained from the parietal direction. The circle of Willis (asterisk) is clearly visualized. MCA, middle cerebral arteries.

as shown in Figure 15–2. After the ninth postmenstrual week, the cerebellar superior, anteroinferior, and posterior arteries can be detected and separated from other cerebral arteries. These arteries are characterized by low to moderate impedance to blood flow. Three-dimensional power Doppler imaging presents the early vascular anatomy at the base of the skull with branches evolving laterally to the mesencephalon and cephalic flexure.[10]

With advancing gestational age, a progressive increase in blood flow velocity is noted for all cerebral arteries. Between the 9th and 10th postmenstrual weeks, the diastolic velocity component begins to emerge, but it is inconsistently present. From the 11th postmenstrual week, the end-diastolic blood-flow component of the velocity waveform begins to be consistently present. The posterior lateral choroidal artery derives from the PCA, whereas the lateral choroidal artery derives from the MCA and the ICA. Blood flow signals from the choroid plexus are obtained during the 9th and 10th postmenstrual weeks of gestation as subtle color and pulsed Doppler signals at the inner edge of the choroid plexus of the lateral ventricle. This developmental period is also the time of active neurogenesis. Choroid plexus vascularity during weeks 9 and 10 has two typical features: the presence of prominent venous blood flow signals and the absence of diastolic flow.[2,11] In parallel, at this early age the cranial venous system, important for brain drainage, develops gradually. The venous circulation drains the blood into the dural sinuses, which meet in the confluence of the sinuses (torcular herophili) at the occipital pole of the skull, from where the blood flow drains into the jugular veins. As stated before, color/power Doppler and pulsed Doppler enable imaging and evaluation of the carotid artery[8] and cerebral arterial blood flows. The MCA has been of particular interest to clinicians and clinical researchers alike and is therefore the objective of Doppler measurements and studies as the most important representative blood vessel of the brain. This interest is evident even at present, as measurements of blood flow profiles have stayed in daily clinical practice. The MCA is the largest branch of the ICA, supplying ~80% of the cerebral hemisphere. In middle and late pregnancy, the greater wings of the sphenoid bone, between the anterior and middle fossae, are good reference points for locating the MCA. It runs laterally in the sylvian fissure as a continuation of the intracranial carotid artery. This vessel consists of four segments—M1, M2, M3, and M4—and sends branches to the corpus striatum, the internal capsule, and the leuticulostriate nucleus. The preferable site for Doppler assessment is the M1 segment, as it maintains a more constant diameter. It then continues to cruise posteriorly over the surface of the insula and the inferior frontal gyrus.

In Figure 15–3, the bilateral common carotid arteries, the ICA and the basilar arteries, were imaged in the coronal plane, as seen on the left side of the figure, while the circle of Willis and two MCAs were demonstrated from the parietal view using 3D power Doppler reconstructed imaging, seen on the right of Figure 15–3, at 12 postmenstrual weeks' gestation. The ACA and its branches can be demonstrated using the sagittal plane from the late first trimester. From the late first or early second trimester, the MCA, ACA, and their branches can be demonstrated by transvaginal 3D power Doppler (Figure 15–4). In the second trimester, the MCA is also easy visible, and its peak systolic velocity (PSV) values increase from the 22nd to 38th postmenstrual week.[12] Figure 15–5 shows the median 2D/3D bidirectional power Doppler images by TVS/transfontanelle sonography of the ACA, callosomarginal artery, and their branches. Figure 15–6 shows serial, consecutive tomographic US images of coronal and sagittal sections of the above arteries. If a more accentuated impression of the brain vessels is sought, 3D rendering

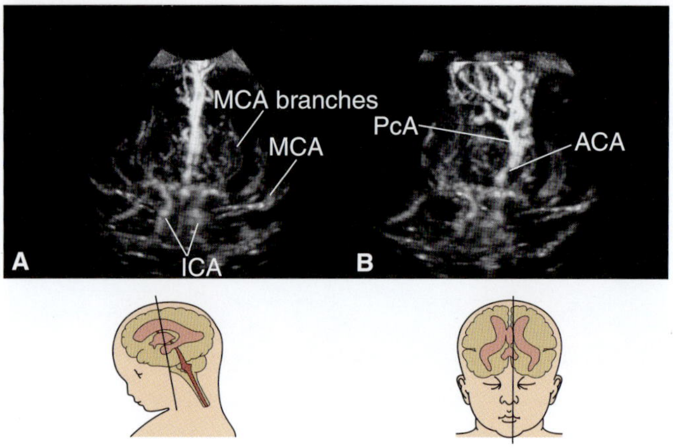


**Figure 15–4.** Conventional 3D power Doppler image of fetal brain circulation. **(A)** Cranial view. The bilateral internal carotid arteries (ICA) and middle cerebral arteries (MCA), as well as the branches of MCA, are demonstrated. **(B)** Anterior oblique view. The anterior cerebral artery (ACA) and the pericallosal artery (PcA) are demonstrated.

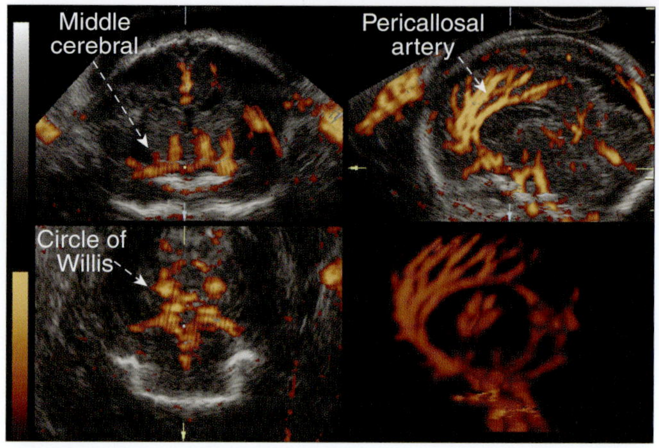


**Figure 15–5.** Fetal brain vascularity at 20 postmenstrual weeks. **(A)** Coronal lane. **(B)** Median plane. **(C)** Axial/horizontal plane. **(D)** 3D angiographic rendering. ACA, anterior cerebral artery; PCA, pericallosal artery. (Courtesy of Timor-Tritsch et al.)

will provide those images. These are excellent teaching materials. Figure 15–7 shows such reconstructed 3D angiography of normal cerebral circulation at 31 postmenstrual weeks.

Tomographic US imaging is useful for obtaining orientation of cerebral vessels. High-frequency TVS employing a 6 to 12 MHz transducer (Voluson E8, GE Healthcare, Waukesha, Wisconsin) has enabled the demonstration of vessels on the cerebral pial surface, as shown in Figures 15–8 and 15–9. Furthermore, the author (RKP) succeeded in demonstrating the fine medullary vessels running from the pial surface toward the subependymal area by bidirectional power Doppler with 3D angiostructural imaging,[7,13] as shown in Figure 15–10. As seen on these images, 3D imaging technology with high-frequency TVS and 3D power Doppler allows the images to be assessed on the orthogonal display as well as on the rendered planes. Conventional 3D power Doppler technology could not depict small-caliber blood vessels; however, recent advances in 3D technology using bidirectional power Doppler allows tiny blood vessels to be depicted.

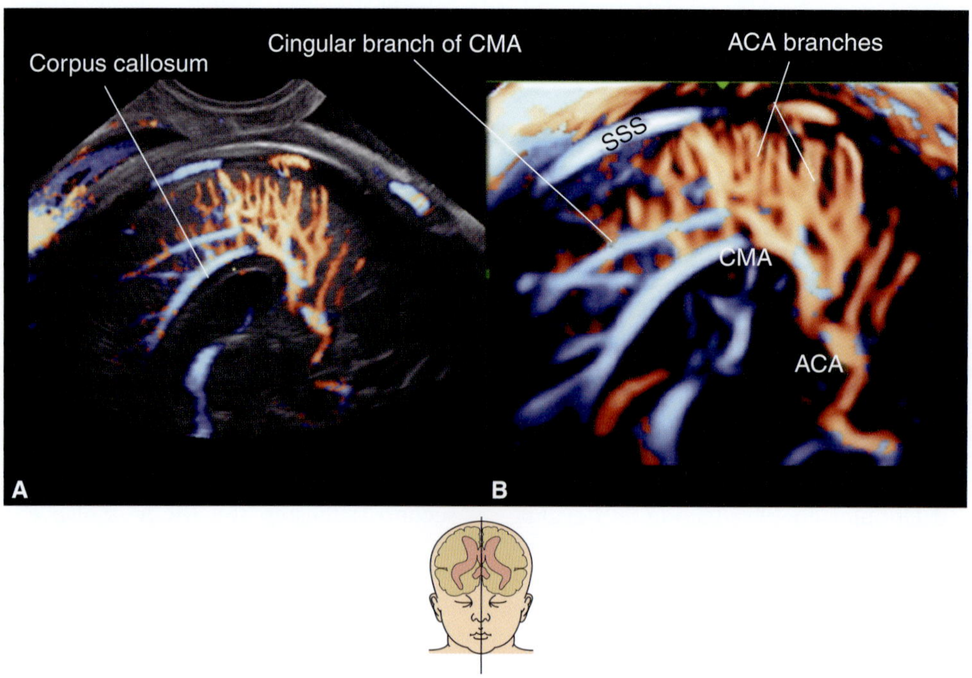


**Figure 15–6.** Anterior cerebral artery and its branches in a 24 postmenstrual weeks' normal brain (median view). **(A)** Two-dimensional (2D) power Doppler image by B-mode demonstrates the corpus callosum (CC). **(B)** 3D reconstructed angiographic image. ACA, anterior cerebral artery; CMA, callosomarginal artery; SSS, superior sagittal sinus. The cingular branch of the CMA runs along the cingulate gyrus.

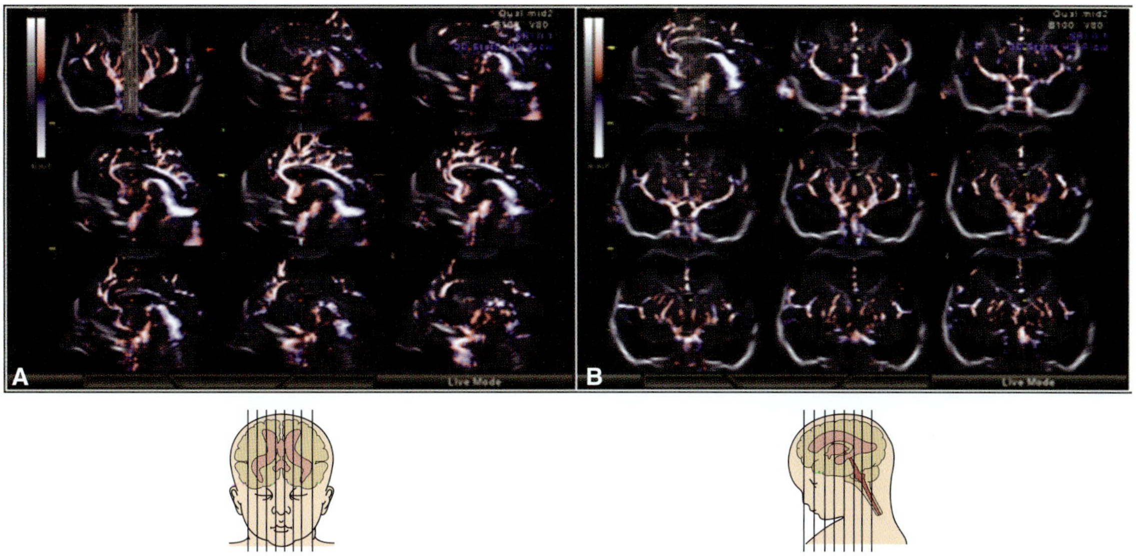

**Figure 15–7.** 3D tomographic ultrasound (US) image of brain circulation at 31 postmenstrual weeks. **(A)** Tomographic power Doppler imaging of serial sagittal sections on which the anterior cerebral arteries and their branches are seen. The image at the center represents the perfect median section. **(B)** Successive and serial coronal sections. The middle cerebral arteries and their branches are seen on these sections.

Using this technique, medullary vessels are detectable from the early second trimester developing into numerous "showerlike" vessels. Before 20 weeks, as seen in Figure 15–9, the medullary veins are demonstrated as red color or red/blue colors by bidirectional power Doppler, and thereafter remarkably rapid development is seen in the previously mentioned showerlike vessels (Figure 15–11). In the fetal brain, the medullary vessels within the deeper cerebral white matter are more developed than the subcortical veins located within the subcortical white matter.[14] The maldevelopment of medullary vessels may indicate developmental abnormalities and may predict subsequent hydrocephaly and postnatal neurologic deficit. At this time we have no scientific proof of the clinical importance of this fascinating display of the fine details of fetal brain circulation. The author (RKP) has been investigating the assessment of medullary veins in normal and abnormal brain structure. It is expected that the investigation will be one of the clues in evaluation of the relations between the fetal brain development and postnatal neurologic findings.

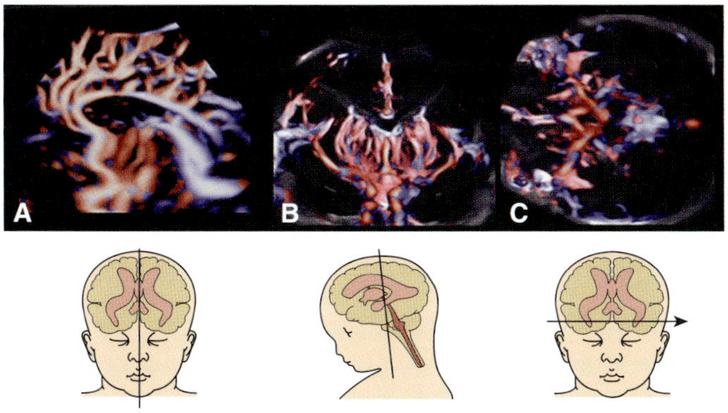

**Figure 15–8.** Reconstructed 3D angiography of normal cerebral circulation at 31 postmenstrual weeks. 3D bidirectional power Doppler angiograms of sagittal (**A**), coronal (**B**), and axial (**C**) sections.

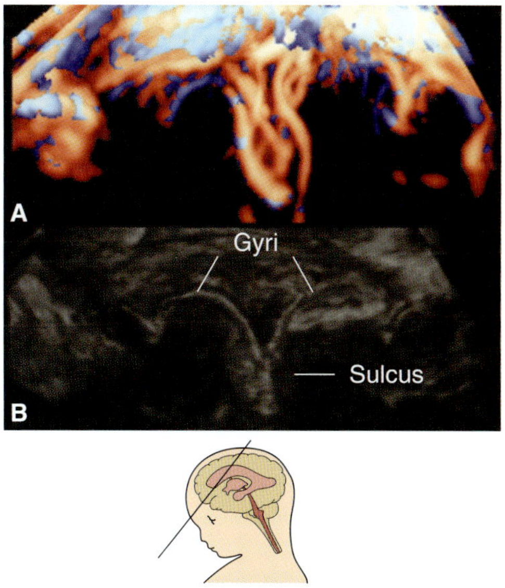


**Figure 15–9.** Coronal view of pial vascularity along the cerebral sulci and gyri by 3D bidirectional power Doppler angiography at 33 postmenstrual weeks of gestation. **(A)** 3D bidirectional power Doppler angiogram of pial vessels along the gyri and sulci. **(B)** 3D reconstructed image of the cerebral by surface y gray scale. Protrusion of the brain surface due to gyral formation is demonstrated.

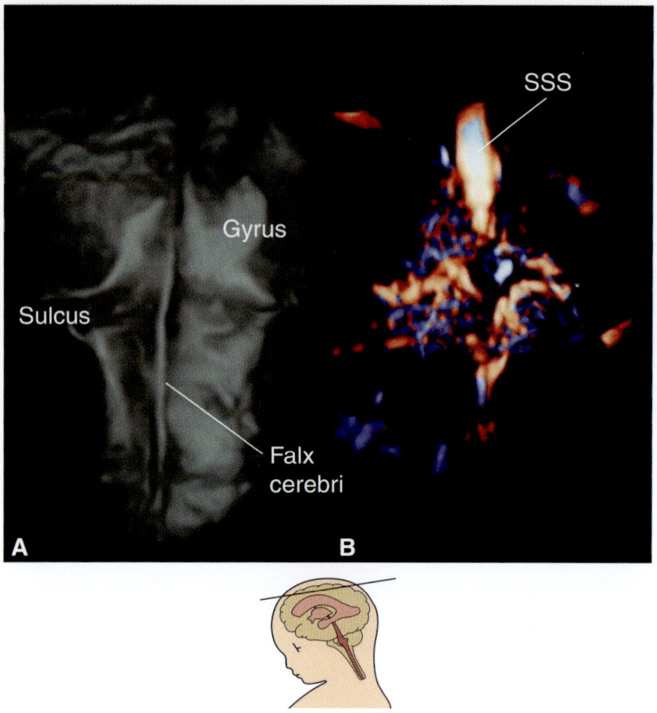


**Figure 15–10.** Parietal/tangential view of pial vascularity along cerebral sulci and gyri by 3D bidirectional power Doppler at 30 weeks of gestation. **(A)** 3D reconstructed gray scale image of the cerebral surface. Falx cerebri and gyral formation are well demonstrated. **(B)** 3D bidirectional power Doppler sonoangiogram of superficial vascularity and pial vessels along the gyri and sulci. SSS, superior sagittal sinus.

## TECHNICAL CONSIDERATIONS AND DOPPLER CRITERIA

For studying the MCA according to anatomical data, Mari and collaborators[15] suggested a plane more caudal to the cerebral peduncles in the section containing the pons and the medulla oblongata and greater paired wings of the sphenoid. It can also be visualized at the level of the cerebral peduncles at its anterolateral border, running anterolaterally toward the lateral edge of the orbit.

The base of the skull at the level of the temporal and sphenoidal bones is the preferred plane for recording Doppler signals from the ACA and PCA. The ACA flow-velocity waveforms can be obtained close to the midline, anterior to the pulsating ICA, and half the distance from the midbrain to the frontal bone. The PCA recordings are done at the level of the transverse cerebral fissure on the side of the midbrain.

Using the transabdominal route, a prerequisite for recording cerebral Doppler signals is that the head is not too deeply engaged in the maternal pelvis.[16] Transvaginal scanning of cerebral vessels was recommended by Lewinsky et al.[17] The coronal section obtained by this approach showed separate and easily distinguishable images of these arteries, because the ICAs are located medially and inferiorly to the corresponding MCAs. With the use of a transfontanelle approach in the newborn, detection of flow is easily obtained from the ACA, where it curves around the corpus callosum.[18] In most studies of the fetal cerebral circulation, Doppler-derived data

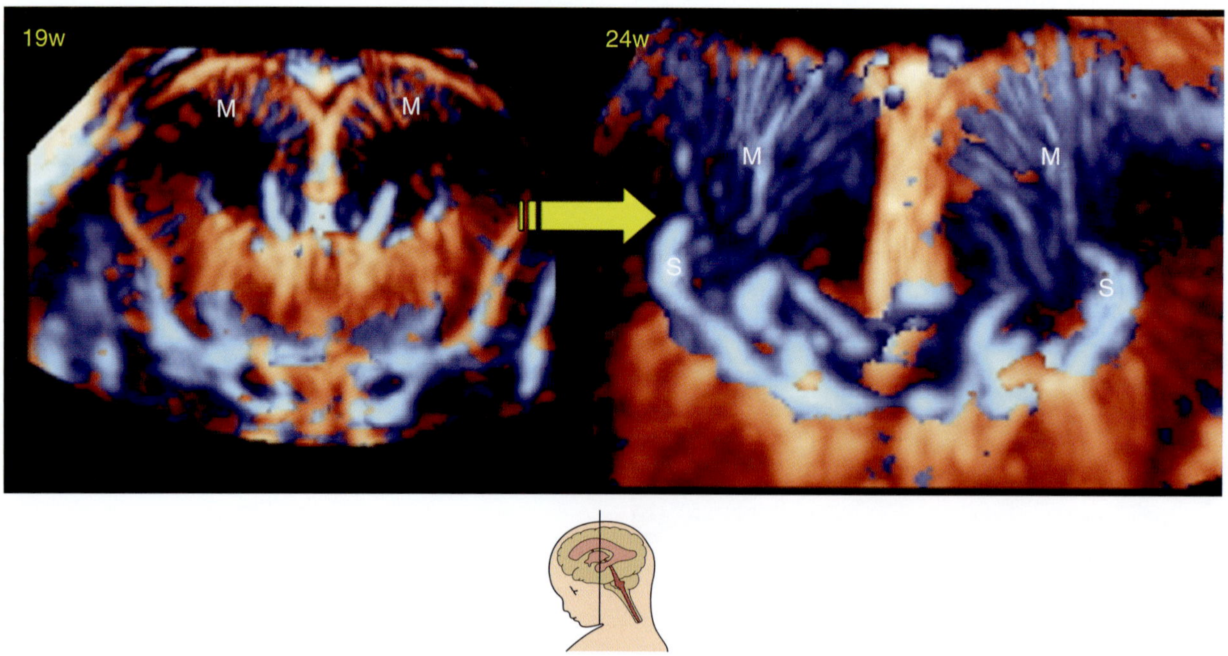


**Figure 15–11.** Development of medullary vessels with advanced gestational age. 3D reconstructed coronal power Doppler images from the same fetus at 19 postmenstrual weeks of gestation **(A)** and 24 postmenstrual weeks **(B)**. At 19 postmenstrual weeks, medullary vessels (M) are immature, and most of the veins run toward the pia mater. With advancing gestational weeks, medullary vessels (M) mature and increase in numbers. The vessels run in the central direction from the cerebral cortex toward the longitudinal caudate vein of Schlesinger (S).

are gained from the MCA and ICA due to the ease of obtaining recordings. Few studies have reported on data collected from other cerebral vessels (ie, the ACA and PCA).[19–21] To correlate fetal with neonatal cerebral flow data, the same vessels should be studied.[22,23]

Detection of vessels is based on visualization of pulsatile flow-velocity waveforms with duplex systems or by using color flow imaging.[24] Transducers with carrier frequencies of 2.5, 3.5, and 5 MHz are usually used, the sample gate not exceeding 3 to 4 mm. This allows clear flow-velocity signals without interference from other nearby vessels. A high-pass filter of 50 to 150 Hz is applied to remove signals originating from slow-moving tissues in the path of the Doppler beam. The angle of insonation is kept as small as possible, and the low-power output mode should be used throughout the study. For standard conditions, all samples are taken with subjects in the semi-recumbent position and during fetal apnea, as high-amplitude fetal breathing modulates the blood flow.[25]

For calculation of qualitative Doppler indices, velocity waveforms are recorded, and peak velocity, end-diastolic velocity, and mean maximum velocity are measured. Three to five consecutive waveforms are analysed, and the results are averaged. Using these Doppler variables, the pulsatility index (PI), defined as the difference between the PSV and end-diastolic value divided by the mean maximum flow velocity,[26] may be calculated. Substantial interobserver agreement and intraobserver repeatability were found for cerebral vessels studied.[27,28]

Other qualitative parameters may be determined but are less frequently used: the ratio of peak systolic to maximum end-diastolic velocity (S/D ratio), the resistance index (RI) (the difference between peak systolic and end-diastolic velocities divided by the PSV), and the cerebral index (PSV minus S/D ratio).[29] Ratios of qualitative parameters in other fetal vessels are also in use: the ratio of RI in the fetal common carotid artery to the RI in the umbilical artery, as described by Arabin et al,[30] or the ratio between the cerebral RI and the placental RI, as described by Arbeille and colleagues.[21] The use of color flow imaging enables accurate measurement of the angle of vessel insonation to determine absolute mean blood flow velocity values in intracranial vessels.[31]

The venous circulation of the fetal brain can be identified by color Doppler. Recently, the US-anatomical correlates were established for the venous blood flow in the fetal brain, and the reference values for flow-velocity waveforms in the transverse sinus were documented.[32]

Power Doppler improves the sensitivity of detection of the presence of flow, when compared with conventional color Doppler velocity imaging. Fetal intracerebral arteries and veins that could not have been imaged by the transabdominal approach were demonstrated using a combination of TVS and power Doppler flow mapping.[4]

## Normal Fetuses

The intracranial circulation becomes visible as early as the 8th week of pregnancy, when arterial pulsation can be detected on an axial view of the embryonic skull. In a study by Kurjak and coworkers[33] using transvaginal US, the visualization rate of pulsation on the base of the skull increased from 50% at the 8th gestational week to 83% at the 10th week. From the 11th week onward, it became a constant finding. It is very difficult to distinguish blood flow between the various cerebral arteries because the distances are in a range of a few millimeters or even less. The waveform signal profile at this gestational age is characterized by the absence of an end-diastolic component.

During the third trimester, continuous flow is present throughout the cardiac cycle in the ICA, confirming the existence of low peripheral vascular resistance in the fetal brain.[34] Flow-velocity waveforms from the fetal MCA are highly pulsatile, and the presence of end-diastolic frequencies becomes more common with advancing gestation.[31] Thus, end-diastolic frequencies were present in 75% of fetuses at 18 to 25 weeks and in all fetuses examined after 34 weeks' gestation.[31]

The PI of the MCA was found to be higher than that for either the ICA or the proximal ACA.[15] Hata et al[35] found the RI of the PCA to be lower than that of the MCA and ACA.

These differences emphasize the need for an exact definition of the vessel that is being insonated and could be caused by different resistances in various portions of the cerebral circulation. In vitro examination of the contractile properties of the common carotid artery in the fetal lamb has shown that this vessel has less dilating capacity in response to hypoxia than do the intracranial arteries.[36] However, in cross-sectional studies, mean blood flow velocities in the common carotid artery increased throughout pregnancy in contrast to aortic velocities, which tend to decrease toward the end of pregnancy. The PI in the aorta remains constant, whereas in the common carotid artery, it falls steeply after 32 postmenstrual weeks.[37] A significant decrease in the PI was also observed in the MCA, especially after 36 weeks (Table 15–1)[38–40]. These results suggest that with advancing gestation there is redistribution of the fetal circulation, with decreased impedance to flow to the fetal brain, presumably to compensate for the progressive decrease in fetal blood $PO_2$. In studies of the MCA in the second trimester,[41–43] an increasing PI was found until the late second trimester, followed by a decline in the third trimester. Mari and Deter[43] attributed the low PI values at the beginning and end of pregnancy to increased metabolic requirements and therefore lower cerebral vascular impedance to blood flow.

Studies of waveforms recorded from the fetal ICA demonstrated that the PI remains fairly constant during the last trimester of pregnancy, and only during the last 4 weeks does there seem to be a slight decrease.[31] Reference RIs of the fetal MCA were established in a large and minimally selected population attending a single clinic.[44] Cerebral vascular resistance decreases constantly up to gestational week 42.[44]

In a longitudinal study,[22] fetal and neonatal cerebral blood flow velocities were assessed in the MCA in 40 uncomplicated pregnancies during the third

**Table 15–1. PULSATILITY INDEX OF THE MIDDLE CEREBRAL ARTERY IN NORMAL FETUSES AS A FUNCTION OF GESTATIONAL AGE: REGRESSION EQUATIONS**

| Authors | Regression Equation | $r^2$ | References |
|---|---|---|---|
| Van den Wijngaard and colleagues | PI = −3.44 + 0.36 × GA − 0.006 × GA$^2$ | — | 51 |
| Arstrom and colleagues | PI = 5.13 − 0.09 × GA | 0.52 | 173 |
| Arduini and Rizzo | PI = 0.006 + 0.144 × GA − 0.003 × GA$^2$ | 0.52 | 41 |
| Mari and Deter | PI = 1.97 + 0.327 × GA − 0.006 × GA$^2$ | 0.45 | 43 |

PI, pulsatility index; GA, gestational age; $r^2$, coefficient of determination.

Reproduced from Marsal and colleagues, 1994,[71] with permission.

trimester and in 22 neonates born from these pregnancies (Table 15–2). PSV, temporal mean, and end-diastolic flow velocities increased during the third trimester and were significantly higher from 36 weeks' gestation on, as compared with values obtained at 28 postmenstrual weeks, suggesting an increase in actual blood flow. The PI and RI of the MCA did not differ significantly during this period. Immediately after birth, flow velocities decreased significantly and remained lower during the first 5 postnatal days compared with fetal values. The PI and RI of the MCA tended to decrease during the first postnatal day but stabilized afterward. These alterations in cerebral blood flow in the transition from the fetal to the neonatal state are explained by local rather than central cardiovascular changes, mainly the local effect of oxygen on peripheral vessels.[45]

Doppler flow studies in twins without growth retardation or discordance demonstrated changes throughout pregnancy similar to those in singletons.[46,47]

## PHYSIOLOGIC VARIABLES AFFECTING CEREBRAL BLOOD FLOW IN NORMAL PREGNANCY

The physiologic changes to cerebral blood flow in normal pregnancy are summarized in Table 15–3.

### Fetal Heart Rate

An inverse correlation was found between fetal heart rate and PI in the MCA of fetuses with heart rate decelerations[48] and with tachycardia secondary to ritodrine infusion.[49] Within the normal range of fetal heart rate, Doppler indices did not alter significantly.

### Fetal Breathing Movements

High-amplitude fetal breathing movements modulate flow-velocity waveforms in the fetal ICA.[50] This is similar to

**Table 15–2. REFERENCE VALUES FOR DOPPLER INDICES OF CEREBRAL VESSELS IN THE THIRD TRIMESTER OF PREGNANCY**

| Vascular Index | 26 to 27 Weeks* | 40 Weeks* | References |
|---|---|---|---|
| Common carotid artery pulsatility index | 2.13 ± 0.11 | 1.89 ± 0.07 | 37 |
| Internal carotid artery pulsatility index | 1.63 ± 0.35 | 1.31 ± 0.41 | 33 |
| Middle cerebral artery | | | |
| Pulsatility index | 2.30 ± 0.48 | 1.82 ± 0.38 | 31 |
| Systolic/diastolic ratio | 6.89 ± 1.48 | 4.23 ± 0.67 | 68 |
| Resistance index | 0.93 ± 0.049 | 0.68 ± 0.087 | 35 |
| Mean velocity (cm/sec) | 5.3 ± 2.3 | 11.3 ± 3.1 | 31 |
| Anterior cerebral artery resistance index | 0.83 ± 0.05 | 0.79 ± 0.04 | 172 |
| Posterior cerebral artery resistance index | 0.73 ± 0.05 | 0.70 ± 0.06 | 118 |

*Postmenstrual weeks.

Reproduced from Degani and colleagues, 1988,[118] with permission.

**Table 15–3. CHANGES IN IMPEDANCE CRITERIA (PULSATILITY AND RESISTANCE INDICES) IN FETAL CEREBRAL ARTERIAL VASCULATURE SECONDARY TO VARIOUS PHYSIOLOGICAL AND NONPHYSIOLOGICAL STATES IN PREGNANCY**

| State | Impedance | | | | Mean Blood Velocity | References |
|---|---|---|---|---|---|---|
| | Internal Carotid Artery | Middle Cerebral Artery | Anterior Cerebral Artery | Posterior Cerebral Artery | | |
| Gestational age | ↓ | N/↓ | ↓ | ↓↓ | ↑ | 31, 33, 37, 39, 46, 47 |
| ↑ Fetal heart rate | ↓ | — | — | — | — | 49 |
| ↓ Fetal heart rate | ↑ | — | — | — | — | 48, 49 |
| Fetal breathing movement | ↑/↓ | — | — | — | — | 50 |
| Fetal behavior stage 2F | ↓ | — | — | — | — | 52 |
| Plasma glucose concentration | ↑ | ↓/↑[a] | — | — | — | 53, 54, 56 |
| Fetal head compression | ↑ | ↑ | — | — | — | 57 |
| Uterine contractions | ↑/N | ↑/↓ | — | — | — | 60–62 |
| Fetal anemia | ↑/N | ↑/N | — | — | ↑ | 64, 65 |
| Oilgohydramnios | ↑ | ↑ | — | — | — | 58, 90–94 |
| Growth retardation | ↓↓ | ↓↓/↓ | ↓ | ↓ | ↑ | 15, 17, 21, 29, 31, 43, 68, 69 |
| Fetal hydrocephaly | ↑ | ↑/N/↓ | — | — | — | 118–120 |
| Arteriovenous malformation | — | ↓ | — | — | — | 156–157 |
| ↑ $P_{CO_2}$ | ↓ | ↓ | — | — | — | 133, 134 |
| ↓ $P_{CO_2}$ | ↓ | ↓ | — | — | ↑ | 31, 69 |

↑, Increased; ↓, decreased; N, normal.
[a]Depending on fetal behavior stage.
Reproduced from Degani, and colleagues, 1988,[118] with permission.

findings in the umbilical artery and vein and fetal descending aorta, where changes in PI ranging from −25% to +30% have been observed.[25] It is recommended, therefore, that cerebral flow-velocity waveforms be recorded under a standardized condition (eg, a period of fetal apnea).

## Fetal Behavioral States

Nijhuis et al[50] described behavioral states in the human fetus from 36 weeks on. Based on changes in fetal heart rate patterns, body movements, and eye movements, four states were defined. Doppler flow-velocity waveforms recorded from the fetal ICA in normal pregnancies at 37 to 38 weeks' gestation during fetal behavioral states 1F (quiet sleep) and 2F (active sleep) demonstrated a significant reduction of the PI in state 2F compared with that in state 1F.[52] This reduction of PI was not related to heart rate only and could be demonstrated at standardized heart rate. Increased oxygen demand during fetal activity is followed by increased cerebral blood flow, reflecting autoregulation. It is suggested that fetal neurologic development expressed by the emergence of fetal behavior is associated with specific hemodynamic adaptation.

## Plasma Glucose Concentration

We found a significant positive correlation between maternal plasma glucose concentration and the PI of the ICA.[53] Similar changes were demonstrated in the fetal MCA after a glucose challenge test.[54] In preterm infants, hypoglycemia was found to be associated with an increase in cerebral blood flow.[55] This may be a compensatory mechanism to maintain glucose supply to the brain.

An indirect effect, mediated through induced changes in behavioral state, was suggested by others.[56]

### Fetal Head Compression

The increase in the PI of flow-velocity waveforms from the MCA was found to be associated with maternal abdominal pressure, even from the US transducer,[57] olighydramnios,[58] polyhydramnios,[59] or uterine contractions during labor.[60] Fetal head compression was suggested as the underlying mechanism of these changes. End-diastolic flow velocities are reduced, and in some cases reverse diastolic flow is seen.

Transvaginal Doppler assessment of the fetal MCA could not confirm a change in peripheral resistance in the fetal cerebral vascular bed during the first stage of normal labor.[61,62] The growing list of internal and external variables affecting cerebral circulation emphasizes the need for strict standards in study design.

### Labor and Delivery

Fetal aortic blood flow was demonstrated to be increased with the progress of labor.[56] The umbilical circulation seems to remain unaffected by uterine contractions.[64,65] However, conflicting results are reported on changes in fetal cerebral vascular resistance during and between contractions. Yagel and collaborators[60] found a reduction of 40% in vascular resistance in the fetal MCA during labor. Their hypothesis suggests a protective mechanism to prevent fetal cerebral hypoxia.

During contractions, increased PI values were found in the fetal ICA,[60] but no difference was found in the ACA[66] and MCA.[61] The varying results may be related to other variables (eg, the intensity of the contractions, the fetal head position and station, or the degree of molding of the skull).

In pregnancies complicated by preterm labor with intact membranes, significantly reduced PI values from the MCA were recorded when compared with fetuses delivered later or normal reference limits for gestation.[67]

The mode of delivery does not seem to influence cerebral blood flow velocities in healthy term newborns.[70] Decompression of the fetal head during vaginal delivery may influence cerebral blood flow. Marsal et al[71] and Maesel et al[72] found a very high cerebral blood flow velocity and low resistance values at the moment of birth. Ipsiroglu and associates,[73] in a study of infants delivered by cesarean section, reported the highest blood velocities among infants after prolonged and difficult delivery of the head.

## PATHOLOGIC PREGNANCIES

### Fetal Anemia

In neonatal polycythemia, partial plasma-exchange transfusion improves cerebral hemodynamics; the exchange procedure results in significantly decreased hematocrit, viscosity, and PI.[18]

Vyas and colleagues[74] found mean blood flow velocity in the fetal MCA to be increased with anemia. The blood flow velocity in red cell–isoimmunized pregnancies was not related to fetal blood $PO_2$, and the relation of increased velocity to anemia was not affected by the PI; therefore, these authors suggest that the hyperdynamic circulation is a consequence of decreased blood viscosity.[75] Increased PSV in the MCA was found to be reliable in detecting anemia in pregnancies complicated by maternal blood group immunization.[76] Intravascular transfusion to correct anemia was not associated with a significant difference in the PI values of cerebral vessels when measured 1 day after the procedure.[40] In fact, the PI was reduced significantly immediately after transfusion but returned to pretransfusion levels by the following day.[18] These data suggest that the PI cannot be used as an indicator of fetal anemia. However, new data suggest that MCA PSV evaluation is now the investigation of choice for noninvasive diagnosis of fetal anemia due to Rh alloimmunization and has practically replaced amniocentesis for amniotic fluid $OD_{450}$ in centers well trained in assessment of MCA PSV. Originally described in the 1990s, MCA Doppler PSV has been studied extensively as a noninvasive method of detecting fetal anemia. Mari and colleagues[77] established MCA PSV above threshold of 1.5 multiples of the median (MoMs) as an effective tool of prenatal diagnosis of moderate to severe fetal anemia in patients with Rh alloimmunization. Before use of MCA Doppler evaluation, serial amniocentesis to determine the bilirubin level in amniotic fluid—by detecting change in optical density at wavelengths of 450 nm—was the mainstay of management of alloimmunization in pregnancy. In a multicenter prospective study, Oepkes et al[78] concluded that MCA PSV Doppler evaluation was more sensitive and accurate than amniotic fluid $OD_{450}$ in the diagnosis of severe fetal anemia, with MCA PSV sensitivity, specificity, and accuracy of 88%, 82%, and 85%, respectively as compared with 76%, 77%, and 76%, respectively, for amniotic fluid $OD_{450}$.

The MCA PSV is measured in the axial view of the fetal head with pulsed Doppler gate over the vessel close to its base at the circle of Willis for accurate measurement (Figures 15–12 and 15–13). Three measurements should be taken during the period of fetal apnea and absent fetal

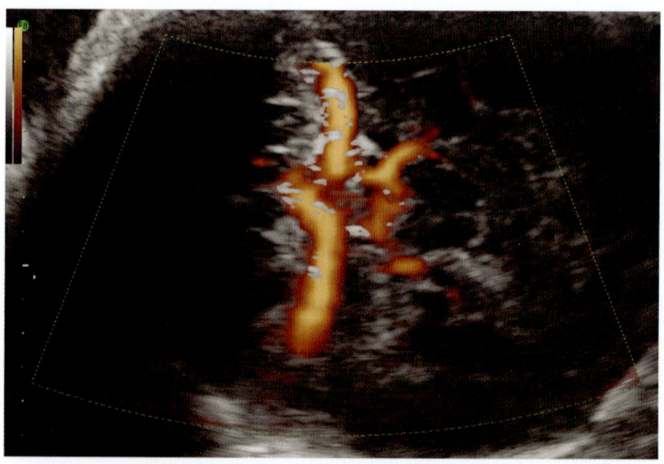

**Figure 15–12.** The technique for obtaining the correct positioning of the middle cerebral artery (MCA) for Doppler velocity measurements.

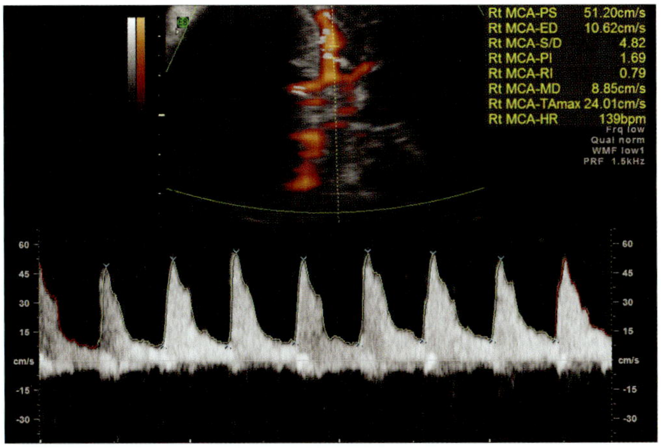


**Figure 15–13.** The technique for obtaining the correct measurement. The angle of insonation and the direction of the MCA is 0°. The measurements velocity and resistive indices are displayed on the right.

movement.[79,80] In pregnancies complicated by alloimmunization, MCA Doppler evaluation should be initiated in the second trimester and performed weekly, and intrauterine transfusion is indicated for severe anemia.

## Elevated Placental Resistance and Growth Retardation

The fetoplacental circulation is a low-resistance system in which downstream flow continues throughout the cardiac cycle. The effects of elevated placental resistance on diastolic blood flow in the main fetal arteries were studied by Fouron et al.[81] Placental resistance was mechanically increased in exteriorized lambs by tightening a string inserted into an exposed section of the umbilical cord around the vein. Doppler flow-velocity waveforms were measured over the cord through an acoustic bag. Compression of the umbilical vein continued until retrograde diastolic flow was observed in the umbilical artery.

The patterns of diastolic flow observed after compression were as follows: descending aorta and aortic arch, retrograde; ascending aorta, bidirectional; and cephalic aorta, forward. These were quite different from their respective baseline patterns. The appearance of reverse diastolic flow in the umbilical artery[82] indicates, first, that the lowest vascular resistance in the fetal circulatory network is no longer at the placental but at the cerebral level, and, second, that preplacental blood with low oxygen content from the descending aorta and pulmonary artery is being shifted toward the brain.

Loss of end-diastolic velocities in the fetal aorta and/or umbilical artery was observed by Arabin and collaborators[83] in 30 of 137 high-risk pregnancies, indicating a high downstream impedance. All the fetuses were growth-retarded, and the observations of absent end-diastolic velocities were made nearly 8 days before pathologic cardiotocographic findings. In nine cases, the ratio of the blood flow volume in the common carotid artery to that of the fetal aorta could be determined. The values were significantly increased compared with values of undisturbed pregnancies, demonstrating a redistribution of fetal blood flow in favor of the cerebral circulation.

Failure of the physiologic invasion of myometrial spiral arteries by cytotrophoblasts in the second trimester and the development of acute atherosis are phenomena associated with higher vascular resistance of the fetoplacental vasculature.[84]

Animal experiments have suggested that fetal growth retardation is associated with reduced umbilical and placental blood flow and increased distal resistance.[85,86] Under experimental conditions in animal models during hypoxia, the redistribution of cardiac output and increased peripheral vascular resistance, with the aim of maintaining cerebral blood flow, resulted in the "brain-sparing" effect.[45,87] This phenomenon (see Figures 15–2 and 15–3) has been suggested as the pathophysiologic mechanism for asymmetrical growth retardation in the human fetus and is characterized by relative sparing of the brain with respect to body weight. This reflex of centralization of the fetal circulation has already been established in fetal hypoxia.[31,88] Maximum reduction in PI was found when the fetal $PO_2$ was 2 to 4 standard deviations below the normal mean for gestation. When the oxygen deficit was greater, there was a tendency for the PI to rise, and this presumably reflected the development of brain edema.[31] Compensatory redistribution is regulated by more than one mechanism; hypoxemia, alone or with hypercapnia, is responsible for cerebral vascular responses.[89]

In growth-retarded pregnancies, pulsatility in all of the major intracranial arteries was significantly reduced compared with normal pregnancy, suggesting participation in a brain-sparing effect in the presence of chronic fetal hypo xia.[15,17,21,29,31,43,68,69,90–100] Antenatally raised ratios were found to be associated with poor obstetric outcome (ie, fetal death and severe growth retardation).[101] Therefore, the brain-sparing effect is suggested as a mechanism to prevent fetal brain hypoxia, rather than as a sign of impending brain damage.

Several studies have proposed Doppler criteria involving intracranial vessels to predict small-for- gestational-age (SGA) neonates. We analyzed published data concerning these criteria, for which sensitivity and specificity could be determined.[102] The predictive values were computed using Bayes theorem, based on an SGA prevalence rate of 10%. Intracranial vessels had positive predictive values ranging between 49% and 66%. The use of a lower prevalence rate in Bayes formula would decrease the positive predictive value of all parameters.

Conflicting findings preclude the clinical use of cerebral Doppler alone as a predictor of growth retardation. For example, McCown and Duggan[103] found in 28 SGA fetuses a highly significant association between an abnormal ICA waveform and a poor outcome; this was particularly pronounced at a gestational age of less than 34 weeks, when the sensitivity, specificity, and predictive values were all 100%. On the other hand, in a study of 44 cases of intrauterine growth retardation (IUGR) with eight perinatal deaths, Wladimiroff and colleagues[100] found no correlation between the indicators of fetal well-being (ie, Apgar score at 1 min, fetal heart rate [FHR] patterns, and umbilical arterial pH) and the ICA PI. This group[24] considered the end velocities in the ACA and MCA to be the most sensitive parameters discriminating between SGA fetuses and controls but found the umbilical artery PI to be the best indicator for the SGA fetuses.

Maternal hyperoxygenation has been suggested for treatment of growth-retarded and hypoxic fetuses.[104,105] No effect was observed on placental RIs, but flow waveforms were modified in cerebral arteries.[106] Such a positive response was found to be a good prognostic factor, in contrast to the poor prognosis associated with a negative test response, which may indicate gross placental failure such that fetal $PO_2$ cannot be improved.[107,108]

## Twin Discordance

The value of Doppler waveform analysis in the surveillance of twin fetuses was assessed by us in a prospective longitudinal study.[47] Measurements of indices from the ICA and umbilical artery gave an overall sensitivity in prediction of an SGS fetus of 58% and a positive predictive value of 71%. These data were not as sensitive and specific as our earlier data.[46] However, Doppler changes preceded US diagnosis of growth retardation by a mean interval of 3.7 weeks and demonstrated greater specificity and sensitivity. A combination of these parameters improved sensitivity to 84% and may complement real-time ultrasonography for the early diagnosis of abnormal growth in twin pregnancies. Rizzo et al[109] found different trends in Doppler serial recordings according to the underlying mechanism of growth defect. Gaziano and colleagues[110] studied fetal growth and blood flow distribution in diamniotic monochorionic compared with dizygotic (diamniotic dichorionic) twins. They found that diamniotic monochorionic twins from the lower-birth-weight group more often show blood flow redistribution compared with dizygotic twins of similar low birth weight. Placental vascular connections and the attendant hemodynamic changes in this group probably account for this difference. Brain sparing events occurred commonly without clinical twin transfusion syndrome.

Degani et al[108] studied the Doppler flow velocity changes in cerebral vessels of seven monochorionic twins with twin-to-twin transfusion syndrome (TTTS). These were compared with 8 monochorionic pairs and 11 dichorionic twin pairs. They found significant changes in Doppler flow velocity and indices, which suggest instability of cerebral blood flow with episodes of "hyperperfusion" in monochorionic twins with TTTS. Although interesting and to some extent logical, these data need to be correlated and applied to neonatal neurologic outcomes. The MCA PSVs in uncomplicated twin pregnancies were found to be comparable with published singleton norms with a median intertwine MCA PSV difference of ~5 cm/s.[109]

The role of MCA PSVs was studied by Klaritsch et al[110] in monochorionic diamniotic twins as a longitudinal study. This group's goal was to establish terms for calculating conditional reference intervals appropriate for individual serial measurements. Based on 824 observations in 100 fetuses, normative ranges of 15 to 37 weeks were comparable for those in singletons. Their conclusion was that between 18 and 37 weeks, reference ranges of singletons can be used to assess fetal anemia in monochorionic/diamniotic pregnancies. Prior to 18 weeks, the application of singleton references may lead to an increased number of false-positive diagnoses of presumed fetal anemia in such twin pregnancies.

Grazianno et al[111] studied Doppler velocimetry in twins with low-birth-weight groups. They evaluated Doppler velocimetry to determine redistribution of fetal blood flow and correlated growth restriction in diamniotic-monochorionic and dizygotic twins. They concluded that diamniotic-monochorionic twins from the lower-birth-weight groups more often showed blood flow redistribution compared with dizygotic twins of similar birth weights. Placental vascular connections and the attendant hemodynamic changes in fetuses of amniotic monochorionic twins probably account for this difference. Brain-sparing events occur commonly without clinical twin transfusion syndrome in this group.

### Ventriculomegaly and Increased Intracranial Pressure

In adults, the volume of blood, spinal fluid, and brain tissue in the cranium at any time must be relatively constant (Monro-Kellie doctrine).[104] During fetal life, the fontanelles and the open skull sutures enable better adaptation to increased intracranial volume. Hill and Volpe[113] found the ventriculomegaly to be a more critical factor than the intracranial pressure in the pathogenesis of the impaired flow in infantile hydrocephaly.

The effect of ventriculomegaly on cerebral pulsatile flow was studied by us in four hydrocephalic fetuses.[114] The PI in the ICA showed progressive elevation, proportional to the developing ventriculomegaly.

Van den Wijngaard et al[115] presented data on nine fetuses with bilateral symmetrical hydrocephaly and four with unilateral hydrocephaly. An elevated ICA PI was demonstrated in five cases. The fetal outcome was poor: Only one infant seemed to be developing normally at 1 year of age. However, in contrast to reports on elevated PI, according to Kirkinen and colleagues,[116] blood flow patterns seem to differ individually from case to case. Normal, increased, and decreased velocity waveform indices could be measured. The discrepancies in results may be related to different pathophysiologic mechanisms of hydrocephaly.

Posterior fossa subdural hematoma was diagnosed antenatally by Ben-Chetrit et al[119] in a fetus at 30 weeks' gestation. Doppler studies of the MCA showed an abnormally high resistance pattern with reverse end-diastolic flow, reflecting high intracranial pressure; associated quadriplegia was noted during US assessment. Color Doppler energy imaging (power Doppler) may help in the diagnosis of intracranial hemorrhage.[118] Another case of cerebral intraparenchymal hemorrhage[119] allowed the authors to analyze the evolution of cerebral Doppler abnormalities, but the modifications in Doppler velocimetry could not be predicted.

The underlying disorder and the presence of other malformations rather than cerebral blood flow measurements are of greater prognostic value regarding brain damage in fetuses with hydrocephaly.

### Arteriovenous Malformations

A cerebral cystic structure in the median plane with turbulent flow pattern in the lesion and decreased cerebral vascular resistance is typical of an arteriovenous malformation (AVM).[112–114] An aneurysm of the vein of Galen may lead to cardiac failure and nonimmune hydrops fetalis[113,115] (see Chapter 9). Fetuses without evidence of hydrocephaly or signs of cardiac insufficiency were followed and treated postnatally by embolization.[116–118] Very-high-volume blood flow in the draining prosencephalic vein was measured in two cases by Goelz and colleagues.[119] The huge shunting of blood flow in this vein was associated with the development of severe encephalomalacia and progressive heart failure of both fetuses.

## PHARMACOLOGICAL ASPECTS

Various drugs administered during pregnancy are reported to affect cerebral blood flow.

Ritodrin infusion for premature uterine contractions was associated with significantly decreased waveform indices in the MCA and renal artery. There was no change in the indices of the umbilical artery.[49]

Magnesium supplementation during pregnancy, particularly in cases of preterm labor, was found to be associated with a decrease in vascular resistance, both in the umbilical artery and in the fetal MCA.[118]

Indomethacin for preterm labor or polyhydramnios resulted in constriction of the ductus arteriosus in 11 of 13 fetuses within 48 hours of therapy.[119] In the fetuses that manifested both ductal constriction and tricuspid insufficiency, the PI of the MCA decreased significantly.[119] In another randomized controlled trial,[120] indomethacin did not significantly affect cerebral blood flow. If antenatal indomethacin in the preterm fetus increases the risk of intraventricular hemorrhage, it would appear to be by another mechanism.

Prostaglandin $E_2$ administered intracervically for preinduction cervical ripening was found to be associated with increased pulsatility in the cerebral artery.[121]

Nifedipine therapy for preterm labor had no influence on Doppler criteria of either fetal or uteroplacental circulation.[122]

Betamethasone administration causes a transient but considerable reduction in fetal body and breathing movements and in fetal heart rate variation. No significant changes occurred in the PI of uterine arteries, umbilical arteries, fetal aorta and renal artery, and fetal cerebral arteries, suggesting that the change is not mediated through fetal hypoxemia.[123]

Nicotine injections induced vasoconstriction on the umbilical and cerebral arteries of ovine fetuses and were associated with poor perinatal outcome.[124]

Extradural anesthesia (eg, with bupivacaine) had no detrimental effects on the uteroplacental and fetal circulation in the uncomplicated pregnancy when maternal hypotension was avoided with rapid prehydration.[125]

Oxygen administration to the mother was followed by an increase of maternal $PO_2$, which raised the pressure difference in $PO_2$ across the placenta.[101,102] Fetal $PO_2$ increased if it was below the normal range. Oxygen administration had no effect on placental RIs but modified the waveforms in cerebral arteries.[103] Maternal oxygenation results in velocity waveform changes that suggest an increase in cerebral vascular resistance and a redistribution of blood from the brain to the vascular beds supplied by the ascending aorta.[104,105] Absent or reversed end-diastolic velocity in the aortic isthmus appears to be an early sign of blood redistribution in SGA fetuses.[126]

Carbon dioxide is also an important determinant of cerebral blood flow. Inhalation of a prepared gas mixture with 2% to 3% carbon dioxide or increased $PCO_2$ in patients undergoing controlled hyperventilation selectively caused a decrease in resistance in the fetal cerebral circulation.[127,128]

Both maternal and fetal cerebral vascular resistances were decreased by 30% nitrous oxide inhalation.[129] No adverse effects to the mother or fetus have been demonstrated in clinical practice. However, preterm fetuses are susceptible to intracranial hemorrhage, and the cerebral hyperemia by nitrous oxide might increase the risk of hemorrhage in these fetuses. From animal experiments it is known that nitric oxide (NO) influences cerebral vascular tone both in the normal fetus and in the hypoxemic fetus.[130] Prostaglandins are important in facilitating the full expression of NO-induced vasodilation.

## FETAL DISTRESS

The significant alterations in cerebral flow velocity and PI in fetal hypoxemia and acidemia suggest the use of Doppler criteria to detect imminent fetal distress in complicated pregnancies. Combinations of Doppler parameters from various vessels may be used:

1. The cerebroumbilical Doppler ratio (the ratio between the PI of the MCA and the PI of the umbilical artery) is usually constant during the last 10 weeks of gestation.[131] Using a single cut-off value, it was found to provide a better predictor for adverse perinatal outcome than the PI of either artery alone. The predictive value of the ratio in diagnosing SGA newborns was 70%, compared with 54.4% for the MCA and 65.5% for the umbilical artery.
2. Serial measurement of mean velocity of the fetal descending thoracic aorta is the best fetal parameter identifying prolonged pregnancy at increased risk for perinatal complications,[132] but the velocity ratio of the fetal common carotid artery to the fetal descending thoracic aorta had the highest predictive capacity for the SGA pregnancy complicated by fetal distress.[84]

Arduini and colleagues[133] reported on Doppler studies from fetal vessels preceding the onset of late decelerations in growth-retarded fetuses. Maximum vasodilation in cerebral arteries was reached 2 weeks before the onset of antepartum late fetal heart rate deceleration, whereas significant changes in the peripheral and umbilical vessels occurred close to the onset of abnormal fetal heart rate patterns. Weiner et al[134] reported on abnormal fetal heart rate pattern in fetuses with absent end-diastolic velocity in the umbilical artery when the MCA begins to lose its compensatory dilation.

In another preliminary report, pathologic fetal heart rate changes were associated with changes in diastolic flux to the brain; in one case the change was biphasic, returning to basic levels, and was interpreted as possible loss of cerebrovascular autoregulation.[135] Hypoxemia at delivery appeared to be better recognized by the fetal velocity waveform of the MCA than by the fetal heart rate analysis.[136]

The responses of the ovine fetus to umbilical cord comprehension with variable-type heart rate deceleration were studied by Richardson and coworkers.[137] Although cerebral oxidative metabolism appeared to be well maintained during moderate to severe variable deceleration, the need to increase fractional oxygen extraction and the redistribution of blood flow from carcass tissue may contribute to an accumulation of lactic acid both within the brain and systemically when such an insult occurs repeatedly.

High perinatal mortality has been reported in association with the finding of absent end-diastolic flow velocity in the umbilical artery. In these cases, abnormal end-diastolic umbilical venous pulsation in the cord is a late and ominous sign of a severely compromised fetus,[138] whereas abnormal blood flow velocimetry in the MCA might be an earlier sign of fetal hypoxia, with a better prognosis. Visualization of the fetal coronary blood flow in severe uteroplacental insufficiency was suggested as a preterminal event.[139,140]

In prolonged pregnancy,[141,142] resistance in the MCA did not change abruptly when gestation exceeded 287 days. Doppler studies in pregnancies with preterm prelabor amniorhexis[143] demonstrated that microbial invasion of the amniotic cavity and fetal bacteremia are not associated with detectable changes in fetal circulation and oxygenation.

## FETAL DEATH

Reverse end-diastolic flow in the MCA may be an ominous sign and was suggested as one of the terminal hemodynamic events preceding fetal death.[144] In the majority of cases, the cause of the observed phenomenon remains unknown, but an increase in pressure in the right ventricle and possible tricuspid regurgitation should be considered.[145] Few reports on the terminal patterns of the fetal cerebral blood velocity have been published.[144–147] Two pregnant women with hypertension and early severe IUGR and one with lupus anticoagulants showed decreasing PI on follow-up examinations. Increased impedance to flow was found in Doppler measurements obtained close to fetal death. This pattern may reflect a phase of decompensation with loss of the brain-sparing phenomenon. Preterminal brain edema has been suggested as the underlying cause of this effect, which has been noted in studies on monkey fetuses deprived of oxygen.[2] Heart rate pattern with loss of long- and short-term variability with or without decelerations is suggestive of severe brain impairment and described after fetal decerebration.[148]

### Cerebral Vascular Abnormalities

If the principal pathologic causes of spontaneous intracranial malformations in the first year of life of neonates are aneurysms, AVMs, cavernous vascular malformations, and vascular tumors, these may also be the ones to be considered when such pathologies are suspected in the fetal brain.

Two- and 3D color/power Doppler sonoangiography is a powerful tool to detect the presence of abnormal intracranial vessels, their location, and the extent of damage they cause.

#### Arteriovenous Malformations: Vein of Galen Aneurysm

A cerebral cystic structure in the median plane with turbulent flow pattern within the lesion and decreased cerebral vascular resistance is typical of an AVM.[144–151] An aneurysm of the vein of Galen may lead to cardiac failure and nonimmune hydrops fetalis.[150–152] Fetuses without evidence of hydrocephaly or signs of cardiac insufficiency were followed and treated postnatally by embolization.[153–155] Very-high-volume blood flow in the draining prosencephalic vein was measured in two cases by Goelz and colleagues.[156] The huge shunting of blood flow in this vein was associated with the development of severe encephalomalacia and progressive heart failure of both fetuses.

These congenital malformations of the fetal brain are rare, with the incidence estimated at ~1 in 25,000 to 1 in 10,000 deliveries. The main structure is direct arteriovenous fistulas in which blood shunts from choroidal and/or quadrigeminal arteries into an overlying single median venous sac. These lead to progressive aneurysmal dilation of the vein, whose wall becomes thick and tough. A vein of Galen aneurysm is not a real aneurysm but an AVM. The vein of Galen aneurysmal malformation (VGAM) is a choroidal type of AVM involving the vein of Galen forerunner (see also Chapter 2). This is distinct from an AVM with venous drainage into a dilated but already formed vein of Galen[156] These anomalies can be associated with anomalies of other systems, such as cardiomegaly due to high cardiac output, secondary hydrocephaly, macrocrania, cerebral ischemia (intracranial steal phenomenon), and subarachnoid/cerebral/intraventricular hemorrhages. The detection of VGAM includes the visualization of vascular anomaly itself, as shown in Figure 15–14 (see Chapter 11). Differential diagnosis includes arachnoid cyst, porencephalic cyst, and intracranial teratoma. Color/power Doppler assessment is easily utilized for differentiation from those other abnormalities. The clinical

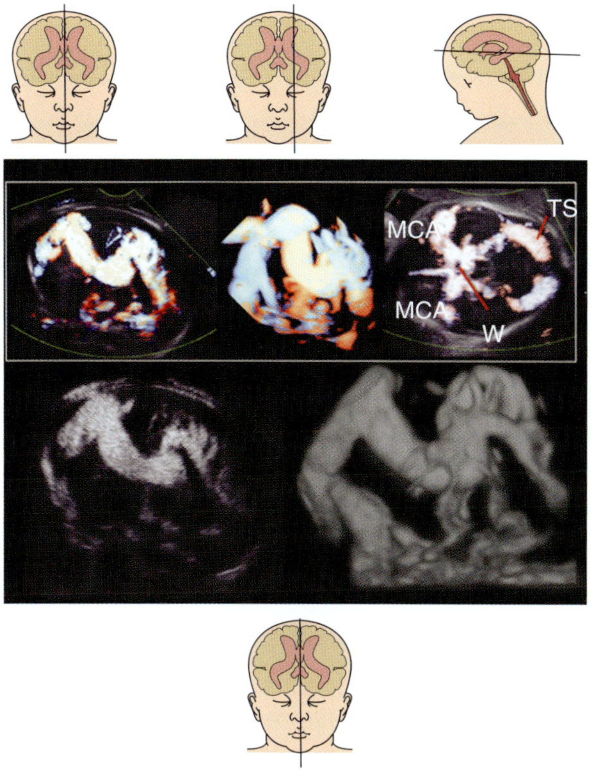


**Figure 15–14.** Vein of Galen aneurysmal malformation at 28 postmenstrual weeks. **(A)** Median section of 2D power Doppler image. The abnormally dilated vein of Galen is demonstrated (*left*). Lateral view of 3D reconstructed power Doppler image (*middle*). Axial section of 2D power Doppler image (*right*). The abnormally dilated middle cerebral arteries (MCA) and circle of Willis (W) are demonstrated. The transverse sinus (TS) is also dilated, and the blood flow direction is in the opposite direction. **(B)** Median section using 2D B-flow image. The abnormally dilated vein of Galen is demonstrated (*left*). Lateral view of 3D reconstructed B-flow image (*right*). This case is a choroidal type vein of Galen malformation with aplasia of the straight sinus. Many of the arteries directly enter into the dilated vein of Galen. This anomaly is considered an abnormal arteriovenous shunt.

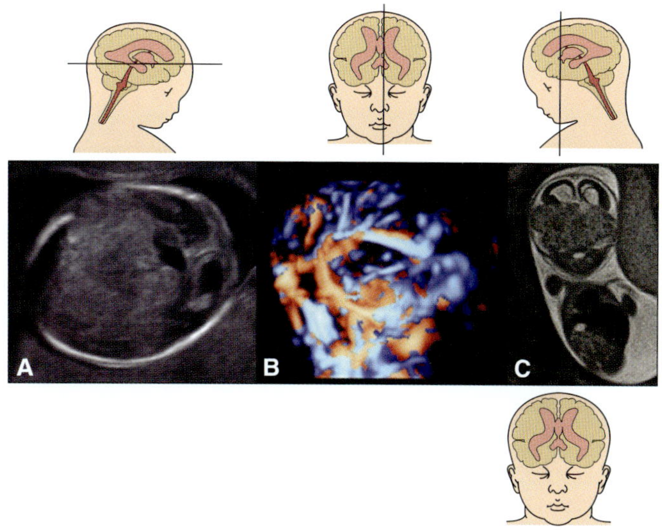


**Figure 15–15.** Brain tumor at 14 postmenstrual weeks of gestation. **(A)** 2D axial section. A large hyperechogenic mass occupies more than half of the cranial cavity. **(B)** Intratumoral vascularity demonstrated by 3D bidirectional power Doppler angiogram. **(C)** Fetal magnetic resonance imaging (MRI): coronal image. Bilaterally, the hemispheres are displaced above the tumor.

features differ with the age at presentation. Neonates can have progressive high-output cardiac failure seen within the first few hours after birth. Older children with this condition may be diagnosed in the course of an investigation of macrocephaly or headaches and/or subarachnoid hemorrhage in adolescence or adult life.

According to an earlier review, outcomes did not differ between treated and nontreated groups, and over 80% of neonates died.[157] However, recent advances in treatment have improved the outcome so that 60% to 100% survive,

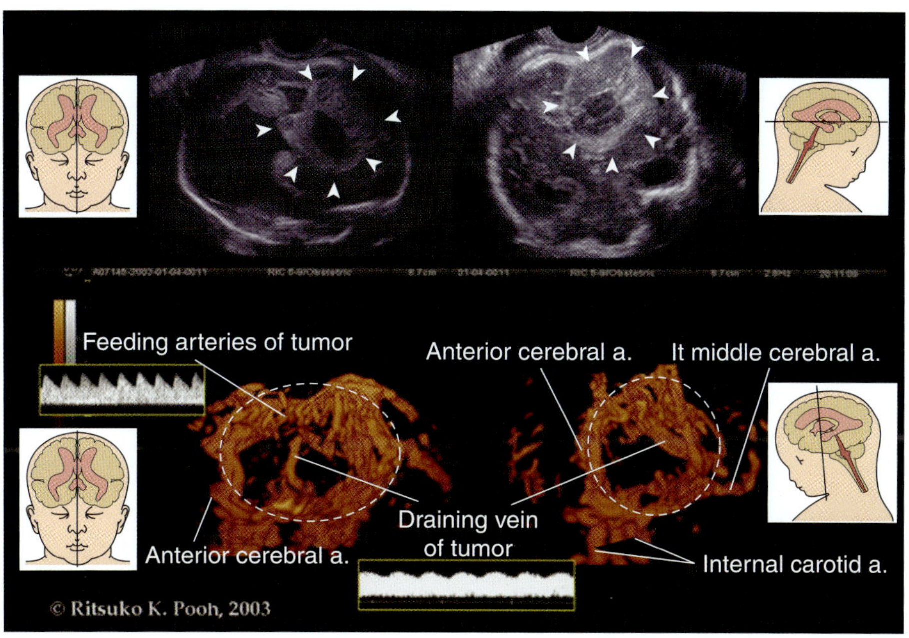


**Figure 15–16.** Intracranial tumor with interventricular hemorrhage at 35 postmenstrual weeks. **(A)** Sagittal and coronal US images. Large tumor (*arrowheads*) with hemorrhage within the tumor in the frontoparietal lobe, complicated with unilateral hydrocephaly with intraventricular hemorrhage. **(B)** Oblique sagittal view of 3D reconstructed power Doppler angiogram image depicted from the fetal left side (*left*). Oblique coronal view from the anterior. The tumor is fed by numerous feeding arteries from the anterior cerebral artery. Feeder arteries have low-resistant flow waveforms. One large vein that drains blood from the tumor is visible. The draining vein has pulsatile flow (*right*). (Reproduced, with permission, from Ritsuko K. Pooh.)

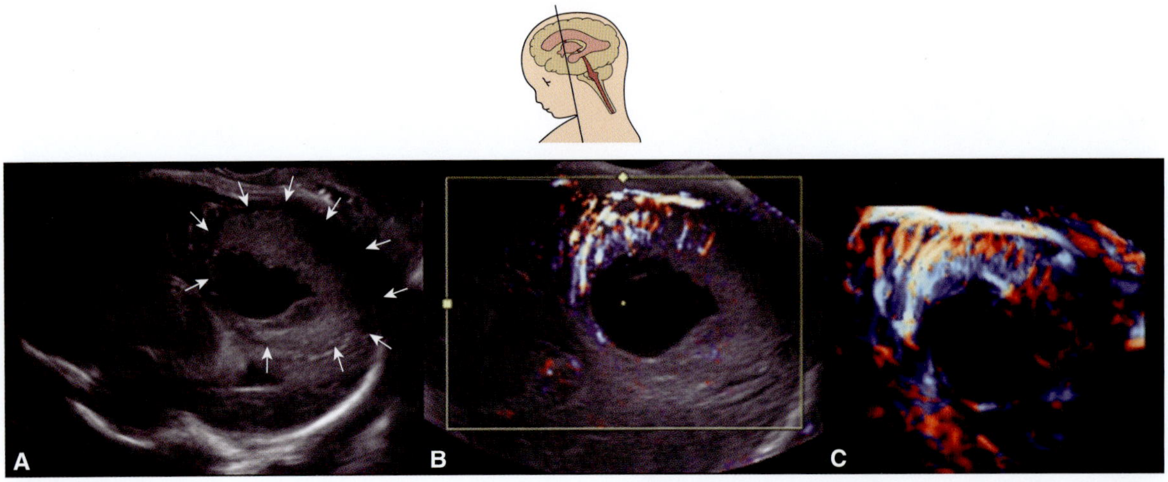


**Figure 15–17.** Brain tumor at 40 postmenstrual weeks of gestation. **(A)** 2D sagittal section. An echogenic mass (*arrows*) is demonstrated. **(B)** 2D power Doppler image demonstrating intratumoral vascularity. **(C)** 3D power Doppler reconstructed angiographic image.

and >60% have a good neurologic outcome.[156–159] The outcome of those cases diagnosed antenatally and actively treated postnatally is better than those diagnosed postnatally due to the opportunity to choose the mode and timing of delivery.

Evaluation of the fetal high-output cardiac state is necessary for the proper obstetric management. Transfer to a department having all the requisite skills in neonatal intensive care, pediatric interventional radiology, and neonatal anesthesia is required. Percutaneous embolization by microcoils is recent and constitutes the main postnatal treatment, remarkably improving outcome.

### Vascularization of Brain Tumors

Brain tumors during the fetal and neonatal period are extremely rare. Brain tumors are divided into teratomas and nonteratomatous tumors. Teratomas are most commonly reported and have a variety of histologic or cellular maturity. Nonteratomatous tumors include neuroepithelial tumors, such as medulloblastoma, astrocytoma, choroid plexus papilloma, choroid plexus carcinoma, ependymoma, ependymoblastoma, and mesenchymal tumors, such as craniopharyngioma, sarcoma, fibroma, hemangioblastoma, hemangioma, and meningioma, as well as lipoma of the corpus callosum and the subependymal giant-cell astrocytoma associated with tuberous sclerosis.[160,161]

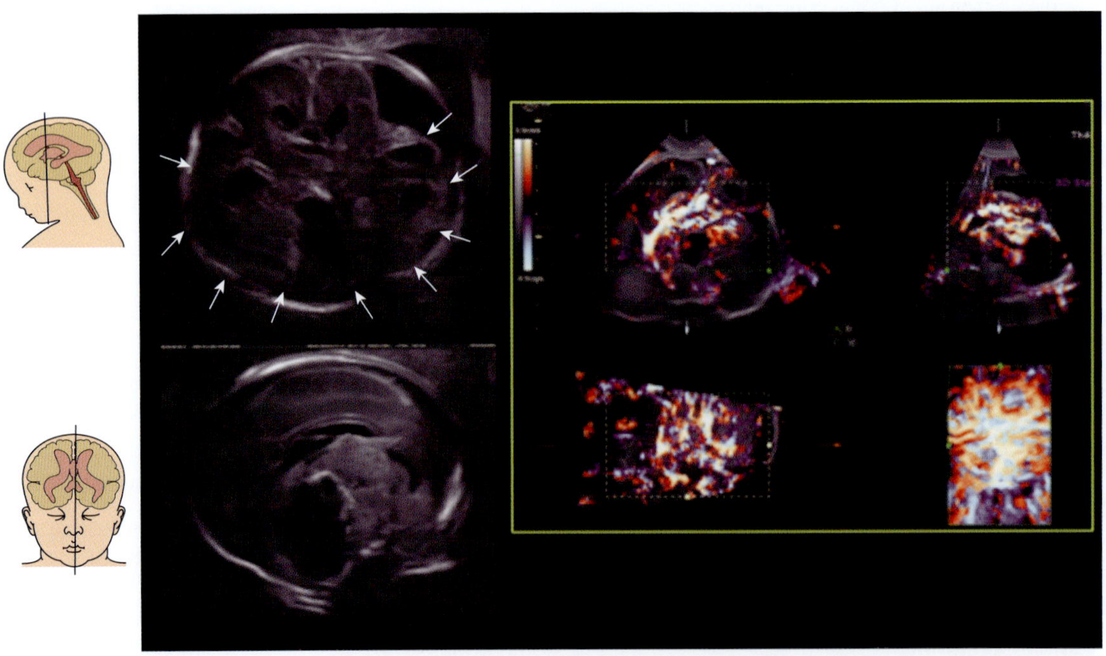

**Figure 15–18.** Brain tumor at 24 postmenstrual weeks of gestation. **(A)** 2D coronal section. A large mass (*arrows*) occupies the lower hemispheres. Between the cerebral hemispheres the tumor is not clearly defined. **(B)** 2D median section (*right*). The three orthogonal views and the reconstructed image of intratumoral vascularity by bidirectional power Doppler angiogram with the chaotic tumoral vessels are demonstrated.

Tumor vascularization by prenatal 2D/3D power Doppler sonoangiography is shown in Figures 15–15 to 15–18. As expected and like tumors in other organs, immature teratomas, nonteratomatous malignant tumors, and hemangiomas demonstrate intense vascularization by power Doppler and 3D angiography due to vascular neoangiogenesis. Recent advances of 3D power Doppler technology provide information not only about intratumoral vascular structure but also about the origin of their feeding arteries and/or location of their draining veins (Figure 15–15). The flow-velocity waveforms of intratumoral vessels often have abnormal patterns of resistance to flow,[162,163] as shown in Figure 15–15, as well as massive neovascularization with low resistance to flow. Indirectly, this may occasionally lead to predicting the degree of their invasive nature. Prenatal information of tumor vascularity may prove to be useful to plan the postnatal neurosurgical strategy.[7]

## REFERENCES


1. Kurjak A, Zudenigo D, Predanic M, Kupesic S. Recent advances in the Doppler study of early fetomaternal circulation. *J Perinat Med.* 1993;21:419–439.
2. Kurjak A, Schulman H, Predanic A, et al. Fetal choroid plexus vascularization assessed by color flow ultrasonography. *J Ultrasound Med.* 1994;13:841–844.
3. Kupesic S, Kurjak A, Babic M. New data on early cerebral circulation. *Prenat Neonat Med.* 1997;2:48–55.
4. Pooh RK, Aono T. Transvaginal power Doppler angiography of the fetal brain. *Ultrasound Obstet Gynecol.* 1996;8:417–421.
5. Pooh RK, Pooh KH, Nakagawa Y, Maeda K, Fukui R, Aono T. Transvaginal Doppler assessment of fetal intracranial venous flow. *Obstet Gynecol.* 1999;93:697–701.
6. Pooh RK, Pooh KH. Transvaginal 3D and Doppler ultrasonography of the fetal brain. *Semin Perinat.* 2001;25:38–43.
7. Pooh RK. Neuroscan of congenital brain abnormality. In: Pooh RK, Kurjak A, eds. *Fetal Neurology.* New Delhi: Jaypee Brothers Medical Publishers; 2009:59–139.
8. Risau W. Developing brain produces an angiogenesis factor. *Dev Biol.* 1986;83:3855–33859.
9. Virgintino D, Errede M, Robertson D, et al. VEGF expression is developmentally regulated during human brain angiogenesis. *Histochem Cell Biol.* 2003;119(3):227–232.
10. Osborn AG. The internal carotid artery: Cavernous, clinoid, ophthalmic and communicating segments. In: Osborn AG, Jacobs JM, eds. *Diagnostic Cerebral Angiography.* 2nd ed. Philadelphia: Lippincott Williams & Wilkins; 1999:91–93.
11. Kurjak A, Pooh RK, Merce LT, et al. Structural and functional early human development assessed by three-dimensional and four-dimensional sonography. *Fertil Steril.* 2005;84(5):1285–1299.
12. Gadelha-Costa A, Spara-Gadelha P, Mauad-Filho F, et al. The maximum systolic velocity increases in middle cerebral artery of normal fetus from 22nd to 38th week of gestation. *Acta Med Port.* 2006;19:105–108.
13. Pooh RK, Pooh KH. Fetal neuroimaging. *Fetal Matern Med Rev.* 2008;19:1–31.
14. Takashima S, Hirayama A, Okoshi Y, et al. Vascular, Axonal and glial pathogenesis of periventricular leukomalacia in fetuses and neonates. *Neuroembryology.* 2002;1:72–77.
15. Mari G, Moise, KJ, Deter RL, Kirshon B, Carpenter RJ, Huhta JC. Doppler assessment of the pulsatility index in cerebral circulation of the human fetus. *Am J Obstet Gynecol.* 1989;160:698–703.
16. Arbeille PH, Tranquart F, Benson M, Roncin A, Saliba E, Pomcelot I. Visualization of the fetal circle of Willis and intracerebral arteries by color-coded Doppler. *Eur J Obstet Gynecol Reprod Biol.* 1989; 32:195–198.
17. Lewinsky RM, Farine D, Ritchie JWK. Transvaginal Doppler assessment of the fetal cerebral circulation. *Obstet Gynecol.* 1991;78: 637–640.
18. Bada HS, Korones SB, Kolni HW, et al. Partial plasma-exchange transfusion improves cerebral hemodynamics in symptomatic neonatal polycythemia. *Am J Med Sci.* 1986;291,157–163.
19. Mari G, Moise KJ, Deter RL. Flow velocity waveforms of the umbilical and cerebral arteries before and after intravascular transfusion. *Obstet Gynecol.* 1990;75:584–589.
20. Mirro R, Gonzalez A. Perinatal anterior cerebral artery Doppler flow indexes: Methods and preliminary results. *Am J Obstet Gynecol.* 1987;156,1227–1231.
21. Arbeille P, Roncin A, Berson M, Patat D, Pourcelot L. Exploration of the fetal cerebral blood flow by duplex Doppler-linear assay system in normal and pathological pregnancies. *Ultrasound Med Biol.* 1987;13:329–337.
22. Meerman RJ, Van Bel F, Van Zuiten PH, Oepkes D, Deb-Ouden L. Fetal and neonatal cerebral blood velocity in the normal fetus and neonate. *Early Hum Dev.* 1990;24:209–217.
23. Raju TN. Cerebral Doppler studies in the fetus and newborn infant. *J Pediatr.* 1991;119:165–174.
24. Noordam MJ, Heydanus R, Hop WC, et al. Doppler color flow imaging of fetal intracerebral arteries and umbilical artery in the small for gestational age fetus. *Br J Obstet Gynaecol.* 1994;101: 504–508.
25. Marsal K, Lindblad A, Lingman G, et al. Blood flow in the fetal descending aorta: Intrinsic factors affecting fetal blow flow, i.e., fetal breathing movements and cardiac arrhythmia. *Ultrasound Med Biol.* 1984;10:339–349.
26. Gosling RG, King DH. Ultrasound angiology. In: Marcus AW, Adamson L, eds. *Arteries and Veins.* Edinburgh: Churchill-Livingstone;1975:61–75.
27. Fong K, Ryan ML, Cohen H, et al. Doppler velocimetry of the fetal middle cerebral and renal arteries: Interobserver reliability. *J Ultrasound Med.* 1996;15:317–321.
28. Alcazar JL. Intraobserver variability of pulsatility index measurements in three fetal vessels in the first trimester. *J Clin Ultrasound.* 1997;25:366–371.
29. Arbeiile P, Body G, Saliba E, et al. Fetal cerebral circulation assessment by Doppler ultrasound in normal and pathological pregnancies. *Eur J Obstet Gynecol Reprod Biol.* 1988;29:261–273.
30. Arabin B, Mohnhaupt A, Becker R, et al. Comparison of the prognostic value of pulsed Doppler blood flow parameters to predict SGA and fetal distress. *Ultrasound Obstet Gynecol.* 1992;2: 272–278.
31. Vyas S, Nicolaides KH, Bower S, et al. Middle cerebral artery flow velocity waveforms in fetal hypoxaemia. *Br J Obstet Gynaecol.* 1990;97:797–803.
32. Laurichesse-Delmass H, Grimaud O, Moscoso G, et al. Color Doppler study of the venous circulation in the fetal brain and hemodynamic study of the cerebral transverse sinus. *Ultrasound Obstet Gynecol.* 1999;13:34–42.
33. Kurjak A, Predonic M, Kupesic S, et al. Transvaginal color Doppler study of middle cerebral blood flow in early normal and abnormal pregnancy. *Ultrasound Obstet Gynecol.* 1992;2:424–428.
34. Wladimiroff JW, van den Wijngaard JAGW, Degani S, Noordam MJ, Van Eyck J, Tonge HM. Cerebral and umbilical arterial blood flow velocity waveforms in normal and growth-retarded pregnancies. *Obstet Gynecol.* 1987;69:705–709.
35. Hata K, Hata T, Makihara K, Aoki S, Takamiya O. Fetal intracranial arterial hemodynamics assessed by color and pulsed Doppler ultrasound. *Int J Gynecol Obstet.* 1991;35:139–145.
36. Gilbert RD, Pearce W, Ashwal S, Longo ID. Effects of hypoxia on contractility of isolated fetal cerebral arteries. *J Dev Physiol.* 1990;13:199–203.
37. Bilardo CM, Campbell S, Nicolaides KH. Mean blood velocities and flow impedance in the fetal descending thoracic aorta and common carotid artery in normal pregnancy. *Early Hum Dev.* 1988;18: 213–221.
38. Ferrazi E, Gementi P, Bellotti M, Rodolfi M, Gella Peruta S. Doppler velocimetry: Critical analysis of umbilical cerebral and aortic reference values. *Eur J Obstet Gynecol Reprod Biol.*1991;38:189–196.
39. Satoh S, Kojanagi T, Hara K, Shimokawa H, Nakamo J. Developmental characteristics of blood flow in the middle cerebral artery in the human fetus in utero, assessed using the linear assay-pulsed Doppler method. *Early Hum Dev.* 1988;17:195–203.

40. Veille JC, Hanson R, Tatum K. Longitudinal quantitation of middle cerebral artery blood flow in normal human fetuses. *Am J Obstet Gynecol.* 1994;169:1393–1398.
41. Arduini D, Rizzo G. Normal values of pulsatility index from fetal vessels: A cross sectional study on 1556 healthy fetuses. *J Perinat Med.* 1990;18:165–172.
42. van den Wijngaard JAGW, Groenenberg IAI, Wladimiroff JW, Hop WCJ. Cerebral Doppler ultrasound of the human fetus. *Br J Obstet Gynecol.* 1989;96:845–849.
43. Mari G, Deter RL. Middle cerebral artery flow velocity waveforms in normal and small-for-gestational-age fetuses. *Am J Obstet Gynecol.* 1992;166:1262–1270.
44. Jaeren H, Funk A, Goetz M, et al. Development of quantitative Doppler indices for uteroplacental and fetal blood flow during the third trimester. *Ultrasound Med Biol.* 1996;22:823–835.
45. Peeters LLH, Sheldon RE, Jones MD, Makowski EL, Neschin G. Blood flow to fetal organs as a function of arterial oxygen content. *Am J Obstet Gynecol.* 1979;135:637–646.
46. Degani S, Paltiel Y, Lewinsky R, Shapiro I, Sharf M. Fetal internal carotid artery flow velocity time waveforms in twin pregnancies. *J Perinat Med.* 1988;16:405–409.
47. Degani S, Gonen R, Shapiro I, Paltiel Y, Sharf M. Doppler flow velocity waveform analysis in fetal surveillance of twins: A prospective longitudinal study. *J Ultrasound Med.* 1992;11:537–541.
48. Mari S, Moise KJ, Jr, Deter RL, Carpenter RJ. Fetal heart rate influence on the pulsatility index in the middle cerebral artery. *J Clin Ultrasound.* 1991;19:149–153.
49. Rasanen J. The effect of ritrodrine infusion on fetal myocardial function and fetal hemodynamics. *Acta Obstet Gynecol Scand.* 1990;69:487–492.
50. Wladimiroff JW, Van Bel F. Fetal and neonatal cerebral blood flow. *Semin Perinatol.* 1987;11:335–346.
51. Nijhuis JG, Prechtl HFR, Martin CB, Jr. Are there behavioral states in the human fetus? *Early Hum Dev.* 1982;6:177–195.
52. Van Eyck J, Wladimiroff JW, van den Wijngaard JA, Noordam MJ, Prechtl HF. The blood flow velocity waveform in the fetal internal carotid and umbilical artery: Its relation to fetal behaviour in normal pregnancy at 37-38 weeks. *Br J Obstet Gynaecol.* 1987;94: 736–741.
53. Degani S, Paltiel Y, Gonen R, Sharf M. Fetal internal carotid artery pulsed Doppler velocity waveforms and maternal plasma glucose levels. *Obstet Gynecol.* 1991;7:379–381.
54. Pardo J, Orvieto N, Rabinerson D, et al. Fetal middle cerebral and umbilical artery flow assessment after glucose challenge test. *Int J Gynecol Obstet.* 1999;65:255–259.
55. Pryds O, Greisen G, Friis-Hansen B. Compensatory increase of CBF in preterm infants during hypoglycemia. *Acta Peadiatr Scand.* 1988;77:632–637.
56. Gillis S, Conners G, Potts P, Hunse C, Richardson B. The effect of glucose on Doppler flow velocity waveforms and heart rate pattern in the human fetus. *Early Hum Dev.* 1992; 30:1–10.
57. Vyas S, Campbell S, Bower S, Nicolaides KH. Maternal abdominal pressure alters fetal cerebral blood flow. *Br J Obstet Gynaecol.* 1990;97:740–742.
58. van den Wijngaard JAGW, Wladimiroff JW, Reuss A, Stewart PA. Oligohydramnios and fetal cerebral blood flow. *Br J Obstet Gynaecol.* 1988;95:1309–1311.
59. Mari G, Wasserstrum N, Kirshon B. Reduction in the middle cerebral artery pulsatility index after decompression of polyhydramnios in twin gestation. *Am J Perinatal.* 1992;9:381–384.
60. Fendel H, Funk A, Jorn J. Cerebral blood flow during labour. *Z Geburtsh Perinatol.* 1990;194:272–274.
61. Maesel A, Lingman G, Marsal K. Cerebral blood flow during labor. *Z Geburtsh Perinatol.* 1990;194:272–274.
62. Yagel S, Anteby E, Levy Y, et al. Fetal middle cerebral artery blood flow during normal active labour and in labour with variable decelerators. *Br J Obstet Gynaecol.* 1992;99:483–485.
63. Lindblad A, Berman J, Marsal K. Obstetric analgesia and fetal aortic blood flow during labour. *Br J Obstet Gynaecol.* 1987;94:306–311.
64. Fleischer A, Anyaegbumam AA, Schulman H, Farmakides G, Randolph G. Uterine and umbilical artery velocimetry during normal labor. *Am J Obstet Gynecol.* 1987;157:40–43.
65. Brar HS, Platt ID, De Vore GR, Horenstein J, Medearis AI. Qualitative assessment of maternal uterine and fetal umbilical artery blood flow and resistance in laboring patients by Doppler velocimetry. *Am J Obstet Gynecol.* 1988;158:952–956.
66. Mirro R, Gonzalez A. Perinatal anterior cerebral artery Doppler flow indexes: Methods and preliminary results. *Am J Obstet Gynecol.* 1987;156:1227–1231.
67. Rizzo G, Capponi A, Arduini D, et al. Uterine and fetal blood flows in pregnancies complicated by preterm labor. *Gynecol Obstet Invest.* 1996;42:163–166.
68. Woo JK, Liang ST, Lo RS, Chan FY. Middle cerebral artery Doppler flow velocity waveforms. *Obstet Gynecol.* 1987;70:613–616.
69. Wladimiroff JW, Tonge HM, Stewart PA. Doppler ultrasound assessment of cerebral blood flow in the human fetus. *Br J Obstet Gynaecol.* 1986;93:471–475.
70. Shuto H, Yashuhara A, Sugimoto T, Iwause S, Kobayaski Y, Nakamura M. Longitudinal determination of cerebral blood flow velocity in neonates with the Doppler technique. *Neuropediatrics.* 1988;18:218–221.
71. Marsal K, Gunmarsson G, Ley D, Maesel A, Laurini RN. Cerebral circulation in the perinatal period. In: Kurjak A, Chervenak FA, eds. *The Fetus as a Patient.* New York and London: Parthenon Publishing Group; 1994:4.
72. Maesel A, Sladkevicius P, Valentin L, et al. Fetal cerebral blood flow velocity during labor and the early neonatal period. *Ultrasound Obstet Gynecol.* 1995;4:372–376.
73. Ipsiroglu OS, Stockler S, Hausler MCH, et al. Cerebral blood flow velocities in the first minutes of life. *Eur J Pediatr.* 1993;152:269–271.
74. Vyas S, Nicolaides KH, Campbell S. Doppler examination of the middle cerebral artery in anemic fetuses. *Am J Obstet Gynecol.* 1990;162:1066–1068.
75. Mari G, Moise KJ, Jr, Deter RL, Kirshon B, Stefos T, Carpenter RJ, Jr. Flow velocity waveforms of the vascular system in the anemic fetus before and after intravascular transfusion for severe red blood cell alloimmunization. *Am J Obstet Gynecol.* 1990;162: 1060–1064.
76. Mari G, Adrignolo A, Abuhamed AZ, et al. Diagnosis of fetal anemia with Doppler ultrasound in the pregnancy complicated by maternal blood group immunization. *Ultrasound Obstet Gynecol.* 1995;5:400–405.
77. Mari G, Deter RL et al. Noninvasive diagnosis by Doppler ultrasonography of fetal anemia due to maternal red-cell alloimmunization. Collabrative group for Doppler assessmen of the blood velocityin anemic fetuses. N Engl J Med 2000;342:9-14.
78. Cosmi E, Segata M, Altaye M, et al. Doppler ultrasonography versus amniocentesis to predict fetal anemia. *N Engl J Med.* 2006;355:156–164.
79. Vandenbusshe FP, Windrion R, Kingdom J, et al. Middle cerebral artery peak systolic velocity: Technique and variability. *J Ultrasound Med.* 2005;24:425–430.
80. Moise KJ, Jr. The usefulness of middle cerebral artery Doppler assessment in the treatment of the fetus at risk for anemia. *Am J Obstet Gynecol.* 2008;198:161–164.
81. Fouron JC, Teyssier G, Maroto E, Lessard M, Marquette G. Diastolic circulatory dynamics in the presence of elevated placental resistance and retrograde diastolic flow in the umbilical artery: A Doppler echographic study in lambs. *Am J Obstet Gynecol.* 1991;164: 195–203.
82. Fouron JC, Teyssier G, Shalaby L, et al. Fetal central blood flow alterations in human fetus with umbilical artery reversed diastolic flow. *Am J Perinatol.* 1993;10:197–207.
83. Arabin B, Siebert M, Jimenez E, Saling, E. Obstetrical characteristics of a loss of end-diastolic velocities in the fetal aorta and/or umbilical artery using Doppler ultrasound. *Gynecol Obstet Invest.* 1988;25:173–180.
84. Khong TY, De Wolf F, Robertson WB, Brosens, L. Inadequate maternal vascular response to placentation in pregnancies complicated by small for gestational age infants. *Br J Obstet Gynaecol.* 1986;93:1049–1059.
85. Clap JF, Szeto HH, Larrow R, Hewitt J, Mann LI. Umbilical blood flow response to embolization of the uterine circulation. *Am J Obstet Gynecol.* 1980;138:60–67.
86. Creasy RK, Barret T, De Swiet M, Kahanna KV, Rudolph AM. Experimental intrauterine growth retardation in the sheep. *Am J Obstet Gynecol.* 1972;112:566–573.

87. Berman RE, Less MH, Peterson EN, DeLannoy CW. Distribution of the circulation in the normal and asphyxiated fetal primate. *Am J Obstet Gynecol.* 1970;108:956–969.
88. Bilardo CM, Nicolaides KH, Campbell S. Doppler measurements of fetal and uteroplacental circulations: Relationship with umbilical venous blood gases measured at cordocentesis. *Am J Obstet Gynecol.* 1990;162:115–120.
89. Akalin Sel T, Nicolaides KH, Peacock J, et al. Doppler dynamics and their complex interrelation with fetal oxygen pressure, carbon dioxide pressure and pH in growth retarded fetuses. *Obstet Gynecol.* 1994;84:439–444.
90. Kirkinen P, Muller R, Huch R, Huch A. Blood flow velocity waveforms in human fetal intracranial arteries. *Obstet Gynecol.* 1987;70:617–621.
91. Lingman G, Marsal K. Noninvasive assessment of cranial blood circulation in the fetus. *Biol Neonate.* 1989;56:129–135.
92. Veille JC, Cohen I. Middle cerebral artery blood flow in normal and growth-retarded fetuses. *Am J Obstet Gynecol.* 1990;162:391–396.
93. Degani S, Paltiel J, Lewinsky R, Shapiro I, Sharf, M. Fetal blood flow velocity waveforms in pregnancies complicated by intrauterine growth retardation. *Isr J Med Sci.* 1990;26:250–254.
94. Campbell S, Vyas S, Nicolaides KH. Doppler investigation of the fetal circulation. *J Perinat Med.* 1991;19:21–26.
95. Arbeille P. Fetal arterial Doppler-IUGR and hypoxia. *Eur J Obstet Gynecol Reprod Biol.* 1997;75:51–53.
96. Loy GL, Lin CC, Chien EK, et al. Cerebral and umbilical vascular resistance response to vibroacustic stimulation in growth restricted fetuses. *Obstet Gynecol.* 1997;90:947–952.
97. Yoshima S, Masuzaki H, Miura K, et al. Fetal blood flow redistribution in term intrauterine growth retardation and postnatal growth. *Int J Gynecol Obstet.* 1998;60:3–8.
98. Forouzan I, Tian ZY. Fetal middle cerebral artery blood flow velocities in pregnancies complicated by intrauterine growth restriction and extreme abnormality in umbilical artery Doppler velocity. *Am J Perinatol.* 1996;13:139–142.
99. Bahado-Singh RO, Kovanci E, Jeffres A, et al. The Doppler cerebroplacental ratios and perinatal outcome in intrauterine growth restriction. *Am J Obstet Gynecol.* 1999;180:750–756.
100. Harrington K, Carpenter RG, Nguyen M, et al. Changes observed in Doppler studies of the fetal circulation in pregnancies complicated by preeclampsia or the delivery of a SGA baby: 1. Cross-sectional analysis. *Ultrasound Obstet Gynecol.* 1995;6:19–28.
101. Scherjon SA, Smolders-de-Haas H, Kok JH, Zondervan HA. The "brain-sparing" effect: Antenatal cerebral Doppler findings in relation to neurologic outcome in very preterm infants. *Am J Obstet Gynecol.* 1993;169:169–175.
102. Degani S, Sharf M. Predictive values of Doppler criteria for intrauterine growth retardation in non-umbilical fetal vessels. *Isr J Obstet Gynecol.* 1991;2:138–142.
103. McCowan JME, Duggan PM. Abnormal internal carotid and umbilical artery Doppler in the small for gestational age fetus predicts an adverse outcome. *Early Hum Dev.* 1992;30:249–259.
104. Wladimiroff JW, Noordam MJ, van der Wijngaard JAGW, Hop WCJ. Fetal internal carotid and umbilical artery blood flow velocity waveforms as a measure of fetal well-being in intrauterine growth retardation. *Pediatr Res.* 1988;24:609–612.
105. Nicolaides KH, Campbell S, Bradley KJ, Bilardo CM, Soothill PW, Gibb D. Maternal oxygen therapy for intrauterine growth retardation. *Lancet.* 1987;1:942–945.
106. Arduini P, Rizzo G, Mancuso S, Romanini C. Short-term effects of maternal oxygen administration in blood flow velocity waveforms in healthy and growth-retarded fetuses. *Am J Obstet Gynecol.* 1988;159:1077–1080.
107. Arduini D, Rizzo G, Romanini C, Mancuso S. Fetal haemodynamic response to acute maternal hyperoxygenation as predictor of fetal distress in intra-uterine growth retardation. *Br Med J.* 1989;298:1561–1562.
108. de Rochambeau B, Poix P, Mellier G. Maternal hyperoxygenation: A fetal blood flow velocity prognosis test in small-for-gestational-age fetuses? *Ultrasound Obstet Gynecol.* 1992;2:279–282.
109. Caforio L, Caruso A, Testa AC, et al. Short term maternal oxygen administration in fetuses with absence or reversal of end diastolic velocity in umbilical artery: pathophysiological and clinical considerations. *Acta Obstet Gynecol Scand.* 1998;77:707–711.
110. Rizzo G, Arduini D, Romanini C. Cardiac and extracardiac flows in discordant twins. *Am J Obstet Gynecol.* 1994;170:1321–1327.
111. Gaziano E, Gaziano C, Brandt D, et al. Doppler velocimetry determined redistribution of fetal blood flow: Correlation with growth retardation in diamniotic monochorionic and dizygotic twins. *Am J Obstet Gynecol.* 1998;178:1359–1367.
112. Degani S, Leibovitz Z, Shapiro I, Gonen R, et al. Instability of Doppler cerebral blood flow in monochorionic twins. *J Ultrasound Med.* 2006;25:449–454.
113. Dashe JS, Ramus RM, Santos-Ramos R, McIntire DD, Twickler DM. Middle cerebral artery peak systolic velocity in monochorionic and dichorionic twin pregnancies. *J Ultrasound Med.* 2007;26: 195–200.
114. Klaritsch P, Deprest J, Van Mieghem T, et al. Reference ranges for middle cerebral artery peak systolic velocity monochorionic diamniotic twins in longitudinal study. *Ultrasound Obstet Gynecol.* 2009;34:149–154.
115. Gaziano E, Gaziano C, Brandt D. Doppler velocimetry determined redistribution of fetal blood flow: Correlation with growth restriction in diamniotic monochorionic and dizigotic twins. *Am J Obstet Gynecol.* 1998;178;1359–1367.
116. Adams RD, Victor M, eds. *Principles of Neurology.* 3rd ed. New York: McGraw-Hill; 1985:463.
117. Hill A, Volpe JJ. Decrease in pulsatile flow in the anterior cerebral arteries is infantile hydrocephalus. *Pediatrics.* 1982;69:4–7.
118. Degani S, Lewinsky R, Shapiro I, Sharf M. Decrease in pulsatile flow in the internal carotid artery in fetal hydrocephalus. *Br J Obstet Gynaecol.* 1988;95:138–141.
119. van den Wijngaard JAGW, Reuss A, Wladimiroff JW. The blood flow velocity waveform in the fetal internal carotid artery in the presence of hydrocephaly. *Early Hum Dev.* 1988;18:95–99.
120. Kirkinen P, Muller R, Baumann H, et al. Cerebral blood flow velocity waveforms in hydrocephalic fetuses. *J Clin Ultrasound.* 1988;16:493–498.
121. Ben-Chetrit A, Anteby E, Lavy Y, Zacut D, Yagel, S. Increased middle cerebral artery blood flow impedance is fetal subdural hematoma. *Ultrasound Obstet Gynecol.* 1991;1:357–358.
122. Guerriero S, Ajossa V, Mais A, et al. Color Doppler energy imaging in the diagnosis of fetal intracranial hemorrhage in the second trimester. *Ultrasound Obstet Gynecol.* 1997;10:205–208.
123. Sibony O, Fondacci C, Oury JF, et al. In utero fetal cerebral intraparenchymal hemorrhage associated with an abnormal cerebral Doppler. *Fetal Diagn Ther.* 1993;8:126–128.
124. Facchinetti, F., Battaglia, C., Benatti, R., Borella, P. and Genazzani, A.R. Oral magnesium supplementation improves fetal circulation. Magnesium Res., 1992;5:179–181
125. Mari G, Moise KJ, Jr, Deter RL, et al. Doppler assessment of the pulsatility index of the middle cerebral artery during constriction of the fetal ductus arteriosus after indomethacin therapy. *Am J Obstet.* 1989;161:1528–1531.
126. Parilla BV, Tamura RK, Cohen LS, et al. Lack of effect of antenatal indomethacin on fetal cerebral blood flow. *Am J Obstet Gynecol.* 1997;176:1166–1169.
127. Degani S, Gonen R, Lewinsky RM, et al. Intracervical prostaglandin $E_2$ is associated with increased pulsatility in fetal cerebral vessels. *J Matern Fetal Invest.* 1994;161:1514–1518.
128. Mari G, Kirshon B. Doppler assessment of the fetal and uteroplacental circulation during nifedipine therapy for preterm labor. *Am J Obstet Gynecol.* 1989;161:1514–1518.
129. Cohen BJ, Stiger RH, Derks JB, et al. Absence of significant hemodynamic changes in the fetus following maternal betamethasone administration. *Ultrasound Obstet Obstet Gynecol.* 1996;8: 252–255.
130. Arbeille P, Bose M, Vaillant MC, et al. Nicotine induced changes in the cerebral circulation in ovine fetuses. *Am J Perinatol.* 1992;9: 270–274.
131. Alahuhta S, Rasanen J, Jouppila P, et al. Ultraplacental and fetal haemodynamics during extradural anaesthesia for caesarean section. *Br J Anaesth.* 1991;66:319–323.
132. Brantberg A, Sonesson SE. Central arterial hemodynamics in small for gestational age fetuses before and during maternal hyperoxygenation: A Doppler velocimetric study with particular attention to the aortic isthmus. *Ultrasound Obstet Gynecol.* 1999; 14:237–243.

133. Potts P, Connors G, Gillis S, Hunse C, Richardson B. The effects of carbon dioxide on Doppler flow velocity waveforms in the human fetus. *J Dev Physiol.* 1992;17:119–123.
134. Veille JC, Penry M. Effects of maternal administration of 3% carbon dioxide on umbilical and fetal renal and middle cerebral artery Doppler waveforms. *Am J Obstet Gynecol.* 1992;167:1668–1671.
135. Polvi HJ, Pirhonen JP, Erkkola RV. Nitrous oxide inhalation: Effects on maternal and fetal circulation at term. *Obstet Gynecol.* 1996;87:1045–1048.
136. Van Bel F, Sola A, Roman C, et al. Perinatal regulation of the cerebral circulation: Role of nitric oxide and prostaglandins. *Pediatr Res.* 1997;42:299–304.
137. Gramellini D, Folli MC, Raboni S, Vadora E, Merialdi A. Cerebral umbilical Doppler ratio as a predictor of adverse perinatal outcome. *Obstet Gynecol.* 1992;79:416–420.
138. Battaglia C, Larocca E, Lanzani A, Coukos G, Genazzani AR. Doppler velocimetry in prolonged pregnancy. *Obstet Gynecol.* 1991;77:213–216.
139. Arduini D, Rizzo G, Romanini C. Changes of pulsatility index from fetal vessels preceding the onset of late decelerations in growth-retarded fetuses. *Obstet Gynecol.* 1992;79:605–610.
140. Weiner Z, Farmakides G, Schulman H, et al. Central and peripheral hemodynamic changes in fetuses with absent end-diastolic velocity in umbilical artery: correlation with computerized fetal heart rate pattern. *Am J Obstet Gynecol.* 1994;170:509–515.
141. Cynober E, Cabrol D, Uzan M. Fetal cerebral blood flow velocity during labor. *Fetal Diagn Ther.* 1992;7:93–101.
142. Chandran R, Serra-Serra V, Sellers SM, Redman CW. Fetal cerebral Doppler in the recognition of fetal compromise. *Br J Obstet Gynaecol.* 1993;100:139–144.
143. Richardson BS, Carmichael L, Homan L, et al. Fetal cerebral circulatory and metabolic responses during heart rate decelerations with umbilical cord compression. *Am J Obstet Gynecol.* 1996;175: 929–936.
144. Gudmundsson S, Tulzer G, Huhta JC, et al. Venous Doppler in the fetus with absent end-diastolic flow in the umbilical artery. *Ultrasound Obstet Gynecol.* 1996;7:262–267.
145. Gembruch U, Baschatt AA. Demonstration of fetal coronary blood flow by color coded and pulsed wave Doppler sonography: A possible indicator of severe compromise and impending demise in intrauterine growth retardation. *Ultrasound Obstet Gynecol.* 1996; 7:10–16.
146. Baschatt AA, Harman CR, Alger LS, et al. Fetal coronary and cerebral blood flow in acute fetomaternal hemorrhage. *Ultrasound Obstet Gynecol.* 1998;12:128–131.
147. Zimmerman P, Alback T, Koskinen J, et al. Doppler flow velocimetry of the umbilical artery, uteroplacental arteries and fetal middle cerebral artery in prolonged pregnancy. *Ultrasound Obstet Gynecol.* 1995;53:189–197.
148. Devine PA, Bracero LA, Lysikiewicz A, et al. Middle cerebral to umbilical artery Doppler ratio in post date pregnancies. *Obstet Gynecol.* 1994;84:856–860.
149. Carrol SG, Papaioannou S, Nicolaides KH. Doppler studies of the placental and fetal circulation in pregnancies with preterm prelabor amniorrhexis. *Ultrasound Obstet Gynecol.* 1995;5:184–188.
150. Sepulveda W, Shennan AH, Peek MJ. Reverse end-diastolic flow in the middle cerebral artery: An agonal pattern in the human fetus. *Am J Obstet Gynecol.* 1996;174:1645–1647.
151. Respondek M, Woch A, Kaczmarek P, et al. Reversal of diastolic flow in the middle cerebral artery of the fetus during the second half of pregnancy. *Ultrasound Obstet Gynecol.* 1997;9:324–329.
152. Mari G, Wasserstrum N. Fetal flow velocity waveforms of the fetal circulation preceding fetal death in a case of lupus anticoagulant. *Am J Obstet Gynecol.* 1991;164:776–778.
153. Chandran R, Serra W, Sellers SM, Redman CWG. Fetal middle cerebral artery flow velocity waveforms: A terminal pattern, case report. *Br J Obstet Gyneacol.* 1991;98:937–938.
154. Rizzo G, Capponi A, Pietropolli A, Bufalino LH, Arduini D, Romanini C. Fetal cardiac and extracardiac flows preceding intrauterine death. *Ultrasound Obstet Gynecol.* 1994;4:139–142.
155. Nijhuis JG, Crevels CAI, van Dongen PWI. Fetal brain death: The definition of a fetal heart pattern and its clinical consequences. *Obstet Gynecol Serv.* 1990;46:229–232.
156. Rizzo G, Arduini D, Colosimo C, Jr, Boccolini MR, Mancuso S. Abnormal fetal cerebral blood flow velocity waveforms as a sign of an aneurysm of the vein of Galen. *Fetal Ther.*1987;2:75–79.
157. Johnson W, Berry JM, Einzig S, Bass JL. Doppler findings in nonimmune hydrops fetalis and cerebral arteriovenous malformations. *Am Heart J.*1988;115:1138–1140.
158. Dan U, Shalev E, Greif M, et al. Prenatal diagnosis of fetal brain arteriovenous malformation: the use of color Doppler imaging. *J Clin Ultrasound.* 1992;20:149–151.
159. Jeanty, P, Kepple, D, Roussis, P, Shah, D. In utero detection of cardiac failure from an aneurysm of the vein of Galen. *Am J Obstet Gynecol.* 1990;163:50–51.
160. Dorn M, Tercanly S, Holzgreve W. Prenatal sonographic diagnosis of a vein of Galen aneurysm: Relevance of associated malformations for timing and mode of delivery. *Ultrasound Obstet Gynecol.* 1995;6:287–289.
161. Sepulveda W, Platt CC, Fisk NM. Prenatal diagnosis of arteriovenous malformation using color Doppler ultrasonography: Case report and review of the literature. *Ultrasound Obstet Gynecol.* 1995;6:282–286.
162. Mai R, Rempen A, Kirsten P. Prenatal diagnosis of a vein of Galen aneurysm assessed by pulsed and color Doppler sonography. *Ultrasound Obstet Gynecol.* 1996;7:228–230.
163. Goelz R, Mielke G, Gonser M, et al. Prenatal assessment of shunting blood flow in vein of Galen malformation. *Ultrasound Obstet Gynecol.* 1996;8:210–212.
164. Lasjaunias PL, Chng SM, Sachet M, et al. The management of vein of Galen aneurysmal malformations. *Neurosurgery.* 2006;59:184–194.
165. Hoffman HJ, Chuang S, Hendrick EB, et al. Aneurysms of the vein of Galen: Experience at the Hospital for Sick Children, Toronto. *J Neurosurg.* 1982;57:316–322.
166. Campi A, Rodesch G, Scotti G, et al. Aneurysmal malformation of the vein of Galen in three patients: Clinical and radiological follow-up. *Neuroradiology.* 1998;40:816–821.
167. Friedman DM, Verma R, Madrid M, et al. Recent improvement in outcome using transcatheter embolization techniques for neonatal aneurysmal malformations of the vein of Galen. *Pediatrics.* 1993;91:583–586.
168. Wakai S, Arai T, Nagai M, et al. Congenital brain tumors. *Surg Neurol.* 1984;21:597–609.
169. Volpe JJ. Brain tumors and vein of Galen malformation. In: Volpe JJ, ed. *Neurology of the Newborn.* 4th ed. Philadelphia: WB Saunders; 2001:841–856.
170. Pinto V, Meo F, Loiudice L, D'Addario V. Prenatal sonographic imaging of an immature intracranial teratoma. *Fetal Diagn Ther.* 1999;14:220–222.
171. Sherer DM, Anyaegbunam A, Onyeije C. Antepartum fetal intracranial hemorrhage, predisposing factors and prenatal sonography: A review. *Am J Perinatol.* 1998;15:431–441.
172. Perlman JM, Volpe JJ. Episodes of apnea and trachycardia in the preterm newborn: Impact on cerebral circulation. *Pediatrics.* 1985;76:333–338.
173. Orstrom K, Eliasson A, Horeide JH, Marsal K. Fetal blood velocity waveforms in normal pregnancies: A longitudinal study. *Acta Obstet Gynecol Scand.* 1989;68:171–178.

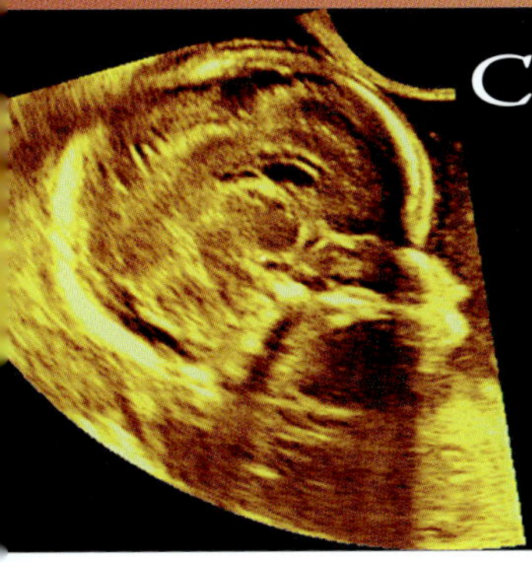

# Chapter 16

# CRANIOFACIAL ANOMALIES

*Gianluigi Pilu • Gustavo Malinger • Tullio Ghi*

## KEY POINTS

1. The most frequent craniofacial malformations are facial clefts. Different varieties exist. These conditions can be corrected surgically with good results. However, they are frequently associated with other malformations and syndromes that may have a major influence on the prognosis.
2. In expert hands, facial clefts can be accurately identified and categorized with sonography since early gestation. Three-dimensional (3D) ultrasound (US) may be helpful, and magnetic resonance imaging (MRI) can also be employed. However, the diagnosis is not simple, and indeed in standard sonographic examinations it is frequently missed.
3. In addition to facial clefts, other craniofacial anomalies can be identified sonographically. The list is long and includes ocular anomalies, such as microphthalmia, cataracts, micrognathia, and craniosynostosis. However, the diagnosis is generally difficult and is hampered by their progressive development.
4. Modern US equipment and 3D sonography in particular reveal many details of fetal craniofacial anatomy and may allow the diagnosis of even subtle dysmorphism. Evaluation of the fetal face is important in the assessment of fetuses with extracraniofacial anomalies because it may provide important clues to the diagnosis of syndromes.
5. Craniofacial anomalies are also discussed in Chapters 2 and 7.

Craniofacial anomalies include a wide spectrum of malformations. They may be clinically relevant as such, but they may also be associated with other congenital anomalies or be part of a syndrome. Evaluation of the face is indeed an important part of the clinical genetic examinations performed postnatally. Therefore, any time a fetal anomaly is identified during an antenatal US scan, the diagnostic workup should include a detailed examination of the fetal face. Apart from obvious malformations, a prenatal sonogram may also identify subtle dysmorphisms that may be crucial for a definitive diagnosis.

Prenatal sonographic diagnosis of craniofacial anomalies is possible in early gestation.[1–5] The diagnostic accuracy of referral centers in the investigation of selected patients at increased risk is quite high,[2–6] whereas the sensitivity of standard examinations of low-risk patients is low, in the range of 20% to -40%, with a general tendency to recognize facial malformations associated with other anomalies and to miss the isolated ones.[7–10] However, until a few years ago, most national guidelines for the standard examination of fetal anatomy suggested only demonstration of the orbits and the eyes. More recently, the recommendations include visualization of the nose, lips, and chin, with an expected positive impact on the detection of craniofacial anomalies.

## IMAGING OF THE FETAL FACE

With two-dimensional (2D) US, a combination of planes must be used to assess facial anomalies.[1,3,6] Midgestation is probably the most favorable time to evaluate the fetal face. However, many details of facial anatomy can be identified as early as 11 postmenstrual weeks. In the third trimester, the examination fails frequently because of intrauterine crowding and unfavorable fetal position. The median plane allows the visualization of the profile (Figure 16–1) with the forehead, nose, and jaw, which are readily appreciated in this view. Axial or coronal planes are used to assess the integrity of the eyes and lips. Nomograms for binocular distance, interocular distance, and ocular diameter are available (see Chapter 3). By moving the transducer caudally, the anterior lip and palate can be visualized. Further caudal shift of the probe will display the tongue inside the oral cavity and the mandible.

The advantages of 3D US over conventional 2D US include the visualization of a panoramic view of the face, as well as a clear visualization of sutures and fontanelles (Figure 16–2). The limitations of the technique are the same as for 2D sonograms. If the fetal face is not accessible, or if there is no pocket of amniotic fluid separating the face from the surrounding structures, 3D will be of

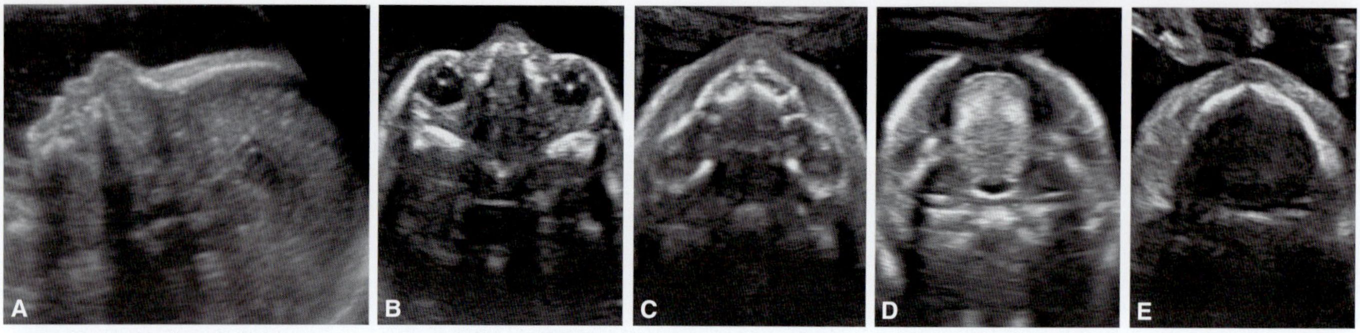


**Figure 16–1.** Two-dimensional (2D) sonographic evaluation of the fetal face at midgestation. **(A)** Median view demonstrating the fetal profile. **(B)–(E)** Axial scans demonstrating the eyes, the maxilla, the tongue within the oral cavity, and the mandible. (Reproduced, with permission, from *Visual Encyclopedia of Ultrasound in Obstetrics and Gynecology*, www.isuog.org.)

little help. However, in expert hands, a full and complete exam is possible in the majority of cases in the second to early third trimester. The relative value of 2D over 3D US has been debated.[4,6,11] In expert hands, 2D US is effective in identifying and categorizing craniofacial malformations. The authors have not found any significant diagnostic advantage over 3D US.[6] However, special 3D techniques may allow visualization of the posterior palate, which is seldom if ever possible with 2D US (Figures 16–3 and 16–4).[11–15] It has also been suggested that 3D US has other potential benefits, such as offering the parents an understandable image of the anomaly, and allowing better communication with and counseling by the specialists involved in the management of the neonate. Most of the experience with 3D US has been derived from referral centers. The impact of this technique in routine anatomy scans has yet to be assessed. In general, 3D US is complex and probably beyond the scope of a basic routine evaluation of fetal anatomy in low-risk pregnancies. It is possible that real-time 3D US (also referred to as 4D), which allows a continuous, rapid, and accurate visualization of the external surface of the fetus in motion, could prove useful for assessment of facial anatomy.

MRI has also been used in the diagnostic workup of craniofacial anomalies and may be helpful, particularly in the assessment of facial clefts.[16,17] The advantages of MRI include clear visualization of the posterior palate, which is imaged with great difficulty with US.

## FACIAL CLEFTS

Facial clefts are the most frequent craniofacial anomalies and the second most common congenital malformation, accounting for 13% of all anomalies. The incidence is ~1.4 cases per 1000 live births.[7,18] The anatomy and pathogenesis of these defects can be better understood in light of its embryological development. The fetal splanchnocranium derives from outgrowths of mesenchyma that surrounds the primitive oral cavity or stomodeum. These outgrowths (frontonasal prominence, maxillary prominence, and mandibular prominence) are separated by grooves that eventually undergo fusion and obliteration. The palate originates from the fusion of three palatine processes with the nasal septum, which divides the nasal cavities. The palate is commonly divided in three parts: the anterior or primary palate, the posterior or secondary palate, and the soft palate.

Most frequently, facial clefts derive from the persistence of the grooves between the frontonasal and maxillary prominences and involve the ideal line running between each nostril and the central part of the posterior palate. However, defects can occur in any part of the face. We will describe separately the typical cleft lip/palate, the

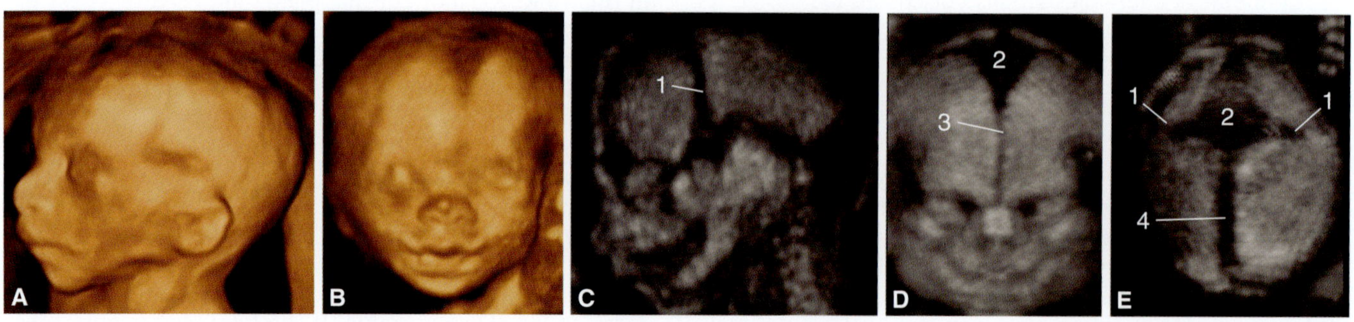


**Figure 16–2.** Three-dimensional (3D) sonographic examination of the fetal face at midgestation. **(A)**, **(B)** Surface rendering from a lateral and frontal perspective. **(C)–(E)** Maximum rendering demonstrating the skull and the sutures and fontanels interposed among the different bones (1, coronal suture; 2, bregmatic fontanelle; 3, metopic or frontal suture; 4, sagittal suture). (Reproduced, with permission, from Pilu G. *Atlas of Obstetric Ultrasound*, The Global Library of Women's Medicine, www.glowm.com.)

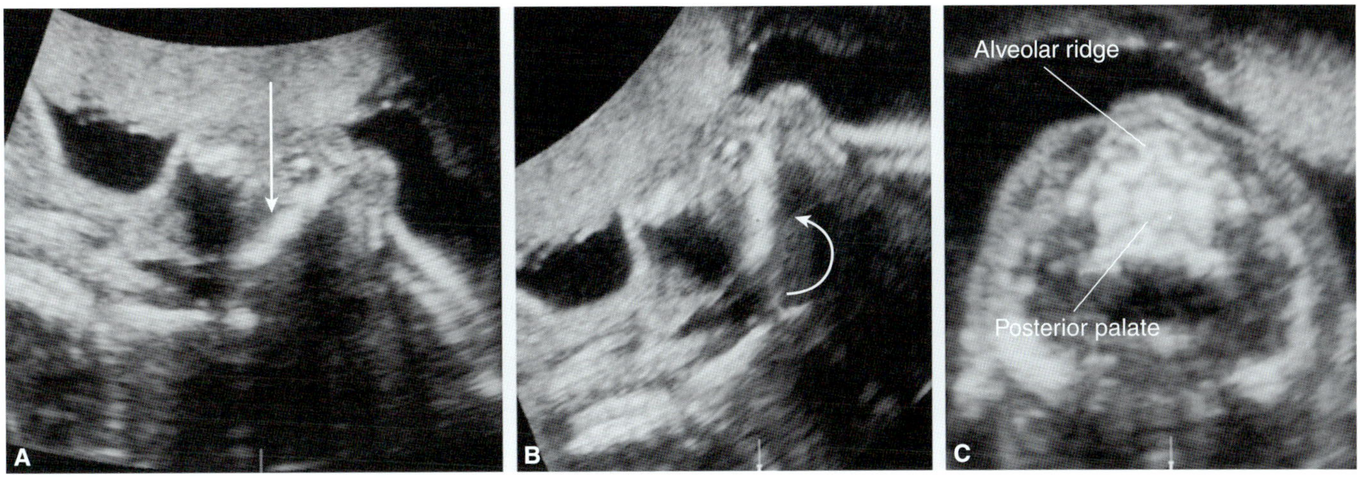


**Figure 16–3.** 3D sonographic evaluation of the posterior palate. **(A)** The palate is insonated with a 45° angle. **(B)** The volume that is obtained is rotated 45° counterclockwise to bring the palate in a vertical position. **(C)** The corresponding axial section effectively demonstrates the full length of the posterior palate; compare this image with the axial section that is obtained with a direct scan in Figure 16–1C. (Reproduced, with permission, from Pilu G, Segata M. A novel technique for visualization of the normal and cleft fetal secondary palate: angled insonation and three-dimensional ultrasound. *Ultrasound Obstet Gynecol* 2007;29[2]:166–169.)

cleft palate, and atypical facial clefts, as these categories differ in the etiology, clinical implications, and diagnostic approach.

## Typical Cleft Lip/Palate

The most frequent facial clefts are linear defects running between the ideal line connecting each nostril to the central portion of the palate. Roughly, in one-third of cases, there is an isolated defect of the lip (cleft lip). In the remaining two-thirds of cases, the opening extends variably into the palate (cleft lip/palate). The cleft may reach only the alveolar ridge, but in the majority of cases, it involves the secondary palate as well, reaching the floor of the nasal cavity or even the floor of the orbit. Cleft lip is bilateral in 20% of cases, whereas cleft lip/palate is bilateral in 25%.

In the vast majority of cases, cleft lip/palate has a multifactorial etiology. In some cases, however, it may be part of well-established genetic and nongenetic syndromes. The claimed risk associated with intake of diazepam and steroidal agents has not been confirmed in carefully controlled studies. Chromosomal abnormalities are rare in postnatal series but rather frequent in the prenatal ones.[2,6,19] The discrepancy may be due to a high rate of intrauterine

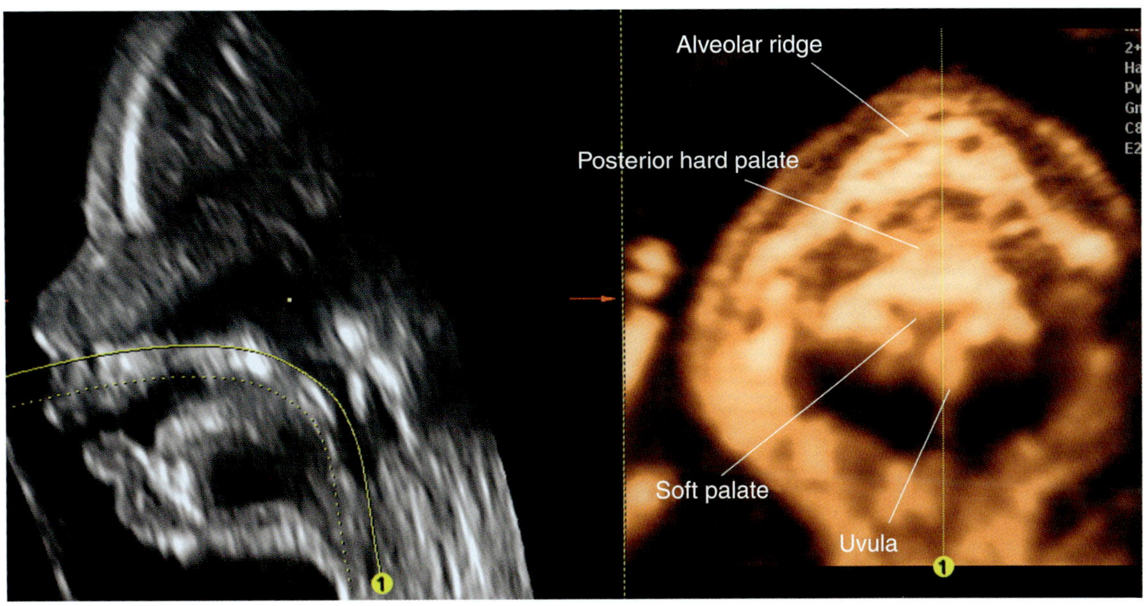


**Figure 16–4.** 3D sonography of the fetal palate. The mouth of the fetus is slightly open, and some fluid is found between the palate and the tongue. By using a curvilinear cut, it is possible to demonstrate both the hard and the soft palate, including the uvula. (Reproduced, with permission, from Pilu G. *Atlas of Obstetric Ultrasound,* The Global Library of Women's Medicine, www.glowm.com.)

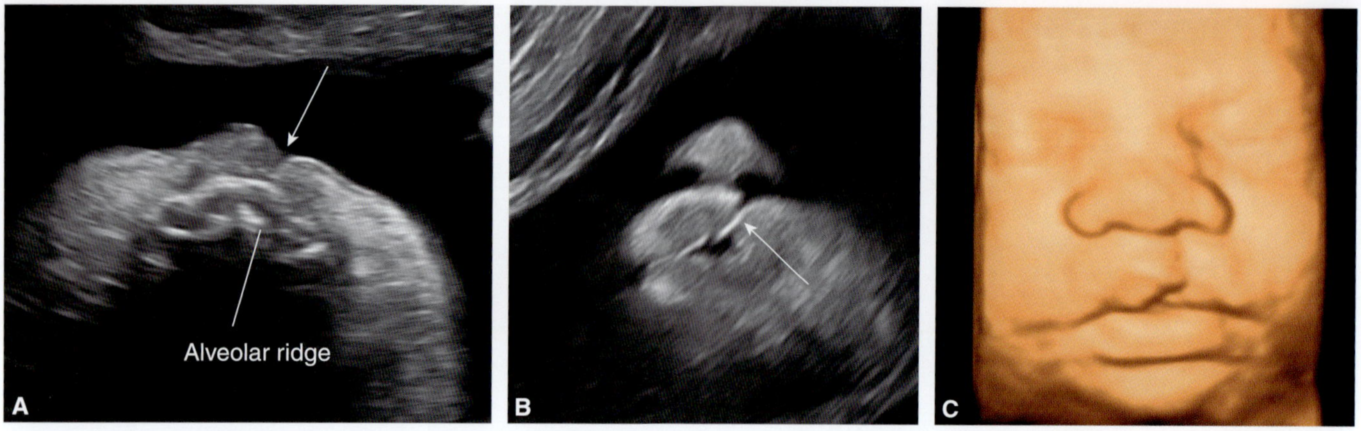


**Figure 16–5.** Unilateral cleft lip in the third trimester of gestation. **(A)** Axial section of the palate demonstrating a defect in the upper lip (*arrow*), while the alveolar ridge appears intact. **(B)** Coronal section of the face demonstrating the cleft extending between the nostril and the oral cavity (*arrow*). **(C)** 3D sonogram with surface rendering in the same fetus. (Reproduced, with permission, from *Visual Encyclopedia of Ultrasound in Obstetrics and Gynecology*, www.isuog.org.)

selection of aneuploid fetuses, as well as to the inclusion of an excess of atypical clefts.

Extrafacial anomalies are found in ~13% of infants with cleft lip/palate and up to 60% of fetuses with facial clefting.[2,3,19,20] A long list of genetic and nongenetic syndromes is associated with facial clefts. The most frequent malformations are nervous, skeletal, and cardiovascular anomalies.

The sonographic diagnosis of cleft lip/palate in the fetus depends on demonstration of a groove extending from one of the nostrils into the lip and possibly into the alveolar ridge. With standard 2D US, facial clefts can be recognized and categorized by a combination of coronal and axial scans (Figures 16–5, 16–6, 16–7, and 16–8). In our experience, cleft lip is best visualized in an anterior coronal plane demonstrating a linear defect extending from one nostril to the oral rim, usually associated with distortion of both the upper lip and nose (Figure 16–5). Extension of the defect into the palate is better demonstrated in an axial scan of the maxilla (Figure 16–7). By angling the transducer or using the 3D approaches for the previously described posterior palate, it is usually possible to evaluate the degree of extension of the defect, that is, to identify whether the lesion is limited to the most anterior part of the palate, the alveolar ridge, or continues into the posterior palate. Indirect sonographic findings can also be noted that correlate with the type of defect. In the typical form of bilateral cleft lip/palate, the axial and sagittal views demonstrate a protrusion of the central portion of the palate and lip that is commonly referred to as the "maxillary pseudomass"[2] (see Figure 16–8). We would like to emphasize that this maxillary pseudomass is generated by the "rolled up" tissue of the philtrum and appears as a hyperechoic protrusion pathognomonic on a median plane (profile) as well as a coronal or tangential plane of the upper lip. With bilateral cleft lip/palate there is a major distortion of facial anatomy and the pseudomass is a more obvious and reliable finding than the visualization of the clefts that is sometimes difficult. With unilateral cleft lip/palate or bilateral cleft lip the profile view is

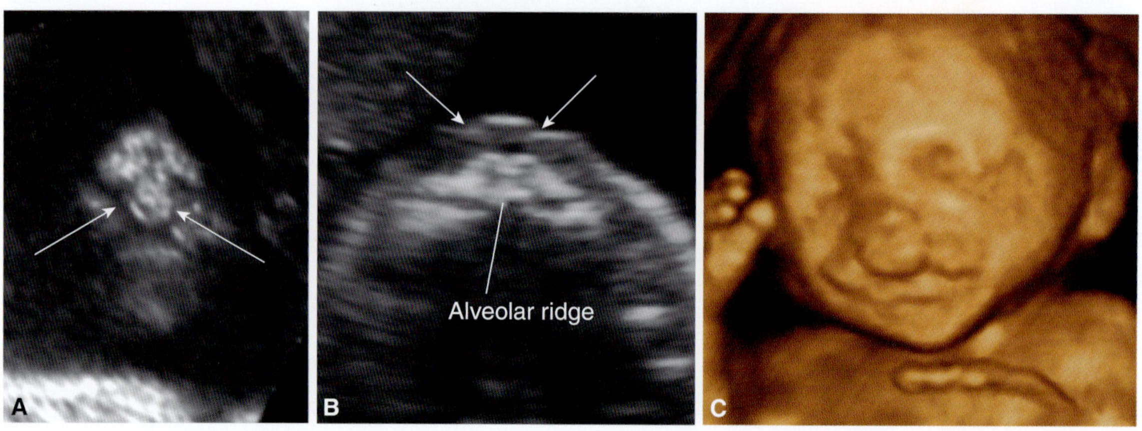


**Figure 16–6.** Bilateral cleft lip (*arrows*) in the second trimester. Coronal (**A**) and axial (**B**) 2D sonograms demonstrating the clefts in the upper lip and the intact alveolar ridge. **(C)** 3D sonogram with surface rendering in the same fetus. (Reproduced, with permission, from *Visual Encyclopedia of Ultrasound in Obstetrics and Gynecology*, www.isuog.org.)

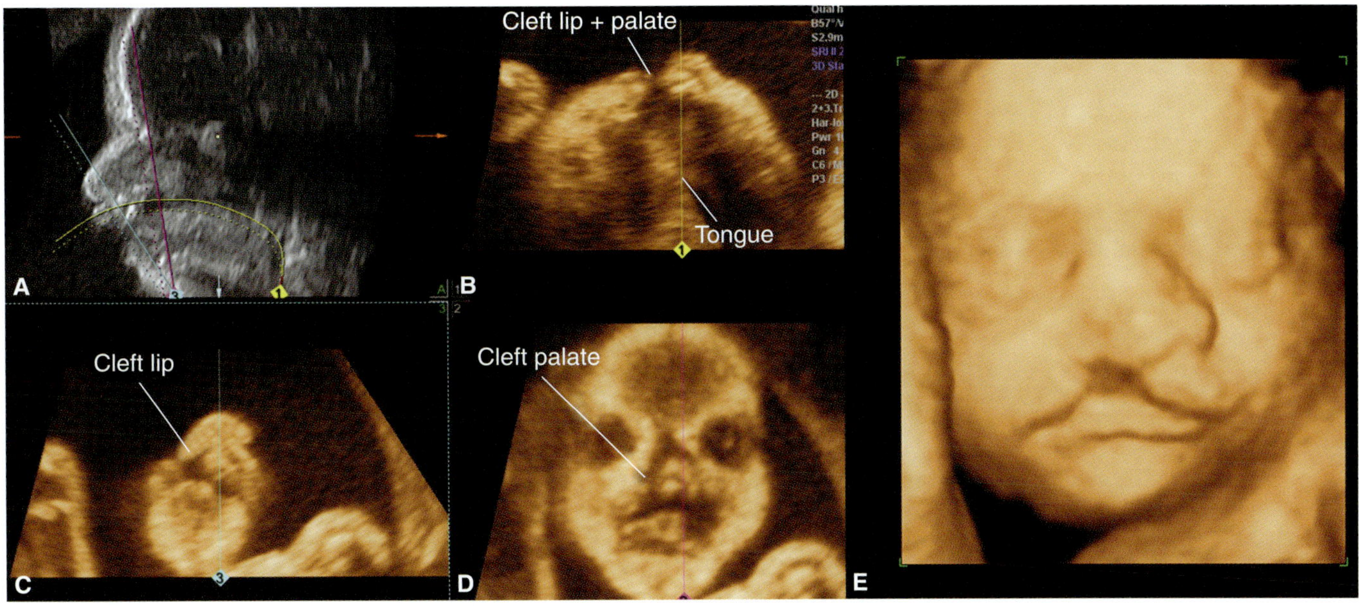


**Figure 16–7.** Unilateral cleft lip/palate: multisectional analysis of an ultrasound (US) volume. **(A–D)** and 3D sonogram with surface rendering **(E)** demonstrate a square-shaped defect in the upper lip and major distortion of the nose. (Reproduced, with permission, from Pilu G. *Atlas of Obstetric Ultrasound,* The Global Library of Women's Medicine, www.glowm.com.)

usually unremarkable. Unilateral cleft lip is always associated with some degree of asymmetry and distortion of the tip of the nose and nostrils, which is maximal with cleft lip/palate. A few cases of bilateral cleft lip/palate are not associated with a pseudomass but rather to flat facies with nasal hypoplasia.[21] This rare anomaly is probably closely related to median cleft lip, in that it is found with extreme flattening of the nose, usually in association with multiple anomalies and chromosomal aberrations, trisomy 18 in particular (Figure 16–9).

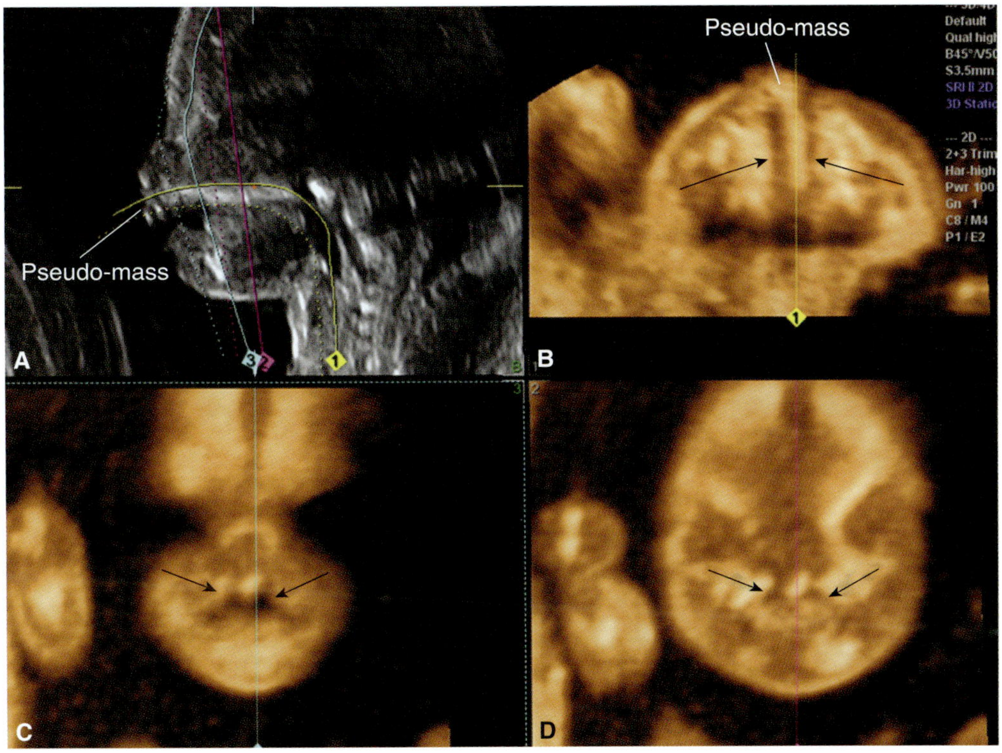


**Figure 16–8.** Bilateral cleft lip/palate (*arrows*) demonstrated with multisectional analysis of a US volume. The anterior protrusion of the central portion of the maxilla in the sagittal **(A)** and axial **(B)** views results in a typical premaxillary pseudomass. Coronal sections **(C–D)** reveal the clefts extending into the palate (Reproduced, with permission, from Pilu G. *Atlas of Obstetric Ultrasound,* The Global Library of Women's Medicine, www.glowm.com.)

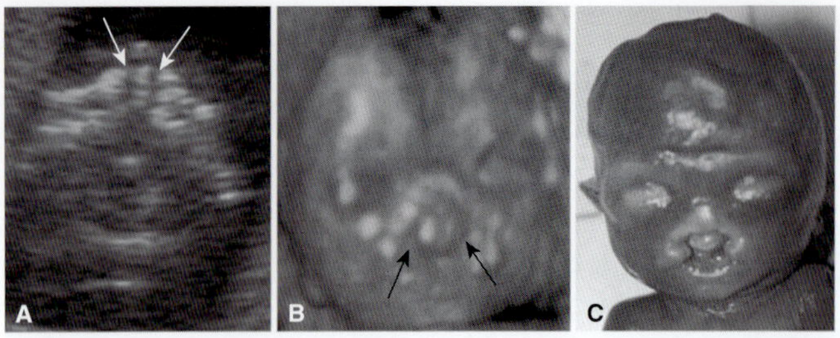


**Figure 16–9.** Bilateral cleft lip/palate (*arrows*) with flat face. **(A), (B)** Antenatal 2D and 3D sonograms. **(C)** Postnatal appearance. This fetus was affected by mosaic trisomy 8.

At times, evaluation of the palate is difficult with sonography, particularly in advanced gestation. MRI is usually quite effective in depicting the normal and abnormal palate and may be used in selected cases[16,17,22] (Figure 16–10).

The diagnosis of cleft lip/palate, mostly of the bilateral type, has been described even in early gestation, at 11 to 14 weeks, usually because of the demonstration of indirect signs of a premaxillary pseudomass or flat face.[21,23]

Prognosis depends primarily on the presence and type of associated anomalies. Mild clefts, such as lineal indentations of the lips or submucosal cleft of the soft palate, may not require surgical correction. Larger defects cause cosmetic, swallowing, and respiratory problems. Recent advances in surgical technique have produced good cosmetic and functional results. Cases that are associated with a defect in the posterior palate represent the greatest challenge for surgical correction, as the soft palate is involved in the process of swallowing and vocalizing. Furthermore, inner ear/tubal disorders may lead in time to acoustic problems and deafness.

## Cleft Palate

The term *cleft palate* refers to a defect of the posterior portion of the palate (secondary palate) in the presence of a normal upper lip and anterior (primary) palate. Cleft lip/palate and cleft palate are two different anomalies. With exceedingly rare exceptions, recurrences are type specific. If the index case has cleft lip/palate, there is no increased risk for cleft palate, and vice versa. Roughly, 25% of facial clefts are cleft lip, 50% cleft lip/palate, and 25% cleft palate. In the vast majority of cases, cleft palate has a multifactorial etiology. Cleft of the palate may include defects of the hard palate, the soft palate, or both or the submucosal tissue.

At present the US diagnosis of isolated cleft palate appears difficult. In general 2D US fails to demonstrate the condition.[3,6] Specific 3D US techniques have been described to overcome the physical limitations of US (Figure 16–11), but very few accurate diagnoses have been reported thus far.[24] Conversely, MRI does not suffer the physical limitations of US and is likely to be more effective than US (Figure 16–12).[16,17,24]

The prognosis of cleft palate depends primarily upon the presence of associated malformations. Surgical correction is frequently challenging as the soft palate is involved in the process of swallowing and vocalizing. Furthermore, tubal disorders may lead in time to acoustic problems and deafness.

## Atypical Facial Clefts

About 3% of clefts occur in portions of the face different from the line joining the nostrils to the posterior palate. Their prevalence was reported to be much higher in prenatal studies due to both the high intrauterine fatality rate that is associated with some of these conditions and probably the higher detection rate due to the frequency of associated malformations.

Tessier proposed a classification of these clefts that is demonstrated in Figure 16–13.[25,26] The median cleft, or Tessier cleft 0, is the type most frequently reported in prenatal studies. This is a quadrangular defect in the central portion of the upper lip and palate, usually associated with a flattened nose (Figure 16–14). It accounts for 0.2% to 0.7% of all cases of cleft lip. It is considered to represent the consequence of underdevelopment of the frontonasal prominence, which normally joins the two maxillary

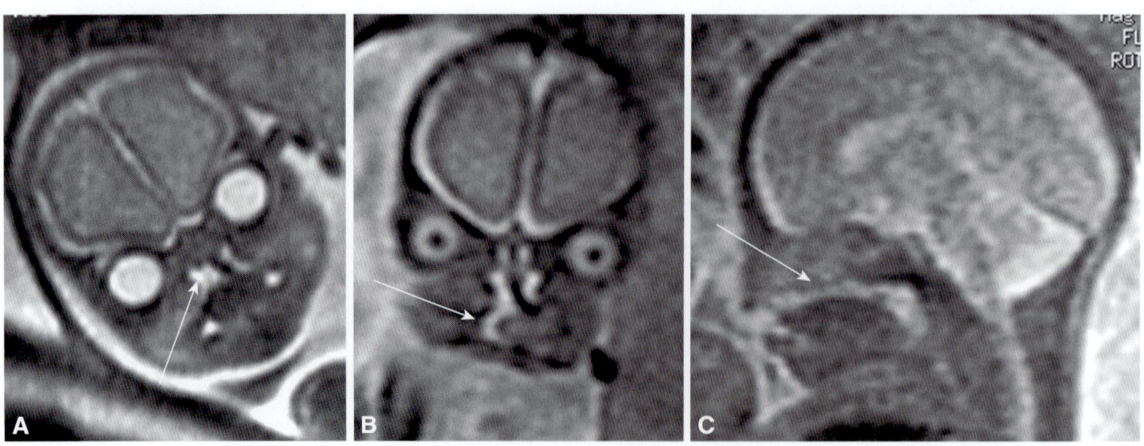


**Figure 16–10.** Magnetic resonance imaging (MRI) demonstrating a fetal facial cleft. **(A), (B)** Coronal sections. **(C)** Median section demonstrating the central absence of the posterior palate. (Reproduced, with permission, from Ghi T, Tani G, Savelli L, Colleoni GG, Pilu G, Bovicelli L. Prenatal imaging of facial clefts by magnetic resonance imaging with emphasis on the posterior palate. *Prenat Diagn.* 2003;23[12]:970–975.)

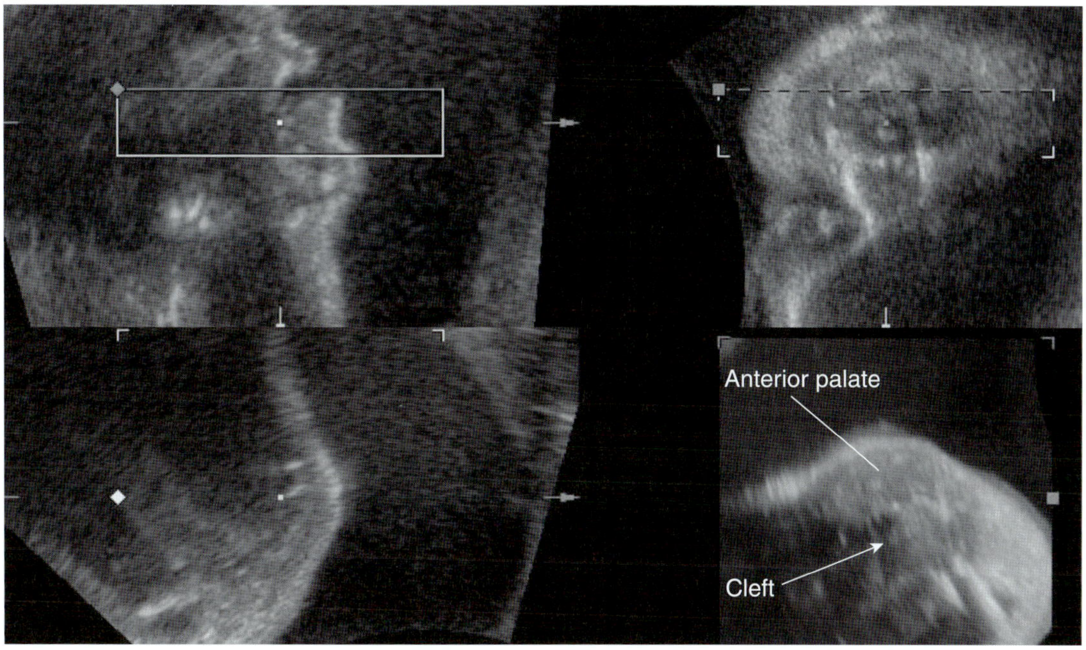


**Figure 16–11.** 3D sonographic diagnosis of cleft palate. (Reproduced, with permission, from Benacerraf BR, Sadow PM, Barnewolt CE, Estroff JA, Benson C. Cleft of the secondary palate without cleft lip diagnosed with three-dimensional ultrasound and magnetic resonance imaging in a fetus with Fryns' syndrome. *Ultrasound Obstet Gynecol.* 2006;27[5]:566–570.)

prominences creating the philtrum. Development of the midface is induced by the prechordal mesenchyma, which is also responsible for the differentiation of the midline structures of the brain. This explains the frequent association of median clefts with orbital anomalies (Figure 16–15) and cerebral malformations. There is a striking correlation between severe holoprosencephaly and craniofacial malformations, including mostly cyclopia, median cleft lip with hypotelorism, absence of the nose, and the presence of a proboscis[3,27,28] (Figure 16–16). Alobar and semilobar holoprosencephaly both have a very severe prognosis.[27]

Median cleft lip may also occur in association with hypertelorism (increased interorbital diatance), a

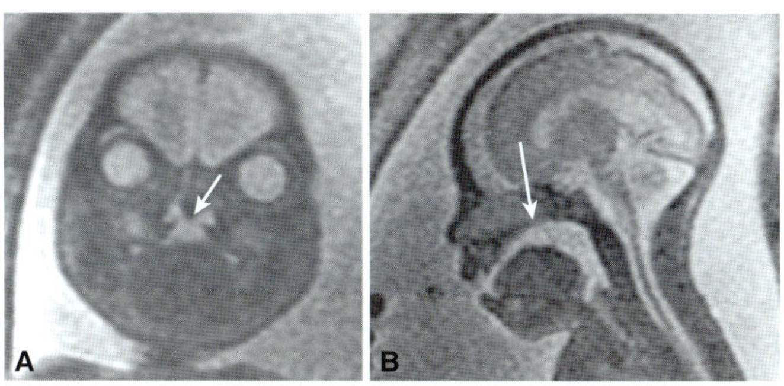


**Figure 16–12.** Same case as in Figure 16–11. MRI effectively confirms the central defect in the posterior palate (arrows) both in the coronal plane (**A**) as well as sagittal plane (**B**). (Reproduced, with permission, from Benacerraf BR, Sadow PM, Barnewolt CE, Estroff JA, Benson C. Cleft of the secondary palate without cleft lip diagnosed with three-dimensional ultrasound and magnetic resonance imaging in a fetus with Fryns' syndrome. *Ultrasound Obstet Gynecol.* 2006;27[5]:566–570.)

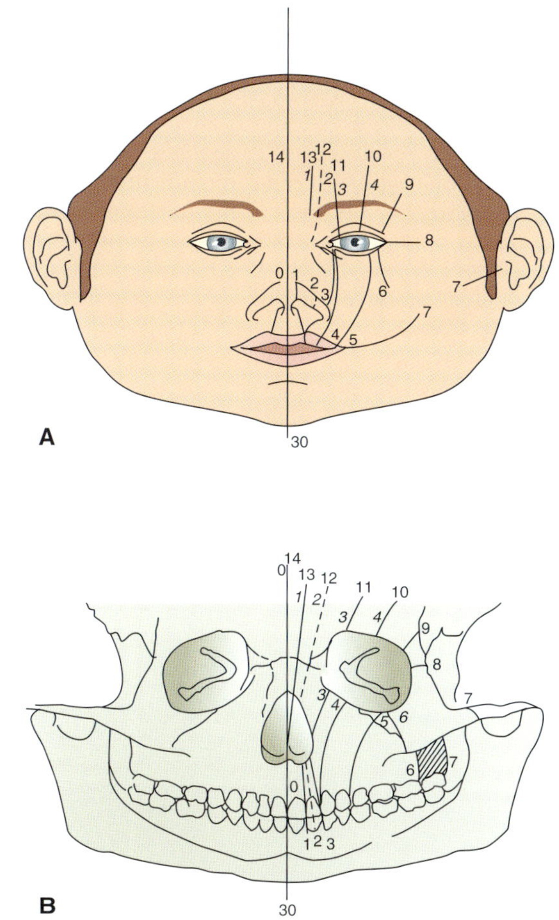


**Figure 16–13.** Tessier classification of craniofacial clefts (**A**) soft tissues, (**B**) skull.

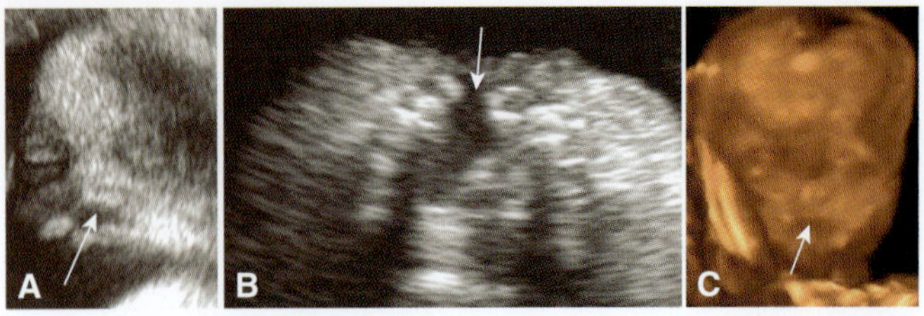

**Figure 16–14.** Median cleft lip (*arrows*). **(A), (B)** Coronal and axial 2D sonograms. **(C)** 3D sonogram with surface rendering. (Reproduced, with permission, from *Visual Encyclopedia of Ultrasound in Obstetrics and Gynecology*, www.isuog.org.)

combination that is pathognomonic of the median cleft face syndrome or frontonasal dysplasia.[29,30] The pathogenesis is much different in these cases. The premaxilla is present, as well as the nose, which is usually bifid; however, the brain is normal in most cases.

The prognosis of median cleft lip depends entirely on the association with other anomalies. Median cleft face syndrome is associated in 80% of cases with normal intelligence.[30] In such cases radical cosmetic surgery may be required. The most common atypical cleft found at birth is the lateral one (or Tessier 7), which has an estimated incidence of 1 in 3000 to 5600 live births and may be either unilateral (more frequently on the left side) or bilateral. It is probably due to defective development of the branchial arches and is characterized by a variable degree of widening of the oral commissure (macrostomia) associated with hypoplasia of the lateral skeleton of the face (maxilla, zygomatic bone, and ascending branch of the mandible) and external ear. A handful of cases have been diagnosed antenatally. Sonographic findings include unusual deepening of the corners of the mouth and asymmetry between the two sides of the face. 3D US is particularly valuable for recognizing lateral clefts. The central portion of the face, nose, lips, and alveolar ridge is well visualized with a standard 2D scan; however, the lateral part of the fetal face may not be easy. A panoramic view of the entire face using the surface mode of 3D US is certainly the best approach to establish the diagnosis (Figure 16–17).[25,26,31–33] Lateral clefts of the face are usually isolated malformations. Their surgical correction is possible but is extremely challenging due to the association with underlying skeletal abnormalities involving the mandible. Ear abnormalities are also frequent, further compounding the operative task.

## ORBITAL AND OCULAR DEFECTS

In early development, the eyes are placed laterally in the primitive face in a fashion similar to that of lower animals with panoramic vision. As gestation progresses, they migrate toward the midline, creating favorable conditions for the development of stereoscopic vision. Abnormalities of orbital diameters include hypotelorism (decreased interorbital distance) and hypertelorism (increased orbital distance) (Figure 16–15). Hypotelorism is almost always found in association with other severe anomalies, and in particular with holoprosencephaly.[3,28] The prognosis, which depends on the associated anomalies, is usually very poor. Hypertelorism can be either an isolated finding or associated with many clinical syndromes or malformations. Mild hypertelorism is a common variant. However, there is a high likelihood of mental retardation when either associated anomalies or an extreme degree of hypertelorism are found. The most common anomalies with hypertelorism are the "median cleft face syndrome," craniosynostoses such as Apert, Crouzon, and Pfeiffer syndromes, agenesis of the corpus callosum and anterior encephaloceles. Hypertelorism per se results only in cosmetic problems and possible impairment of stereoscopic binocular vision. For severe cases, a number of operative procedures, such as canthoplasty, orbitoplasty, surgical positioning of the eyebrows, and rhinoplasty, have been proposed.

Microphthalmia is defined as a decreased size of the eyeball, and anophthalmia refers to the absence of the eye; however, the term *anophthalmia* should be reserved for the pathologist, who must demonstrate not only absence of the eye but also of optic nerves, chiasma, and tracts. Microphthalmia/anophthalmia, which is either unilateral or bilateral, is frequently associated with genetic and nongenetic syndromes. Prenatal diagnosis of microphthalmia is based on the demonstration of decreased ocular diameter and careful examination of the intraorbital anatomy is indicated to identify lens, pupil, and optic nerve (Figure 16–18).[34,35] It has been reported that at least in some cases this anomaly may develop throughout gestation and early prenatal diagnosis may be impossible.[34] Congenital microphthalmia is frequently associated with visual disorders and with other anomalies. Goldenhar syndrome is characterized by hypoplasia of one half of the face (hemifacial microsomia) that often includes unilateral anophthalmia, ear, dental, and facial abnormalities.[36,37]

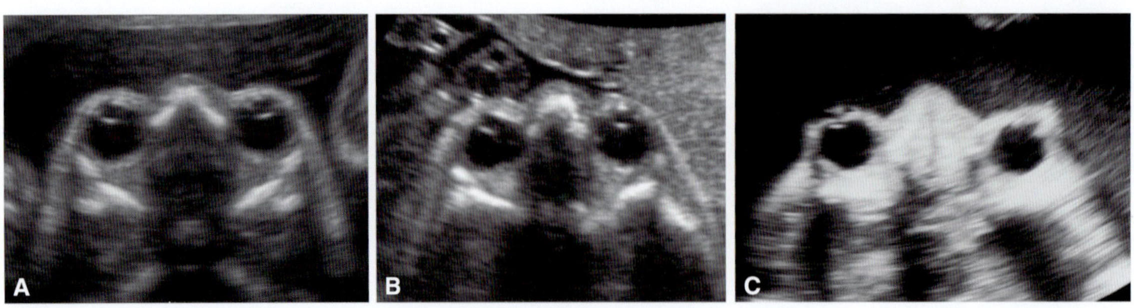


**Figure 16–15.** Abnormalities of interorbital distance. **(A)** Normal fetus. **(B)** Hypotelorism. **(C)** Hypertelorism. (Reproduced, with permission, from *Visual Encyclopedia of Ultrasound in Obstetrics and Gynecology*, www.isuog.org.)

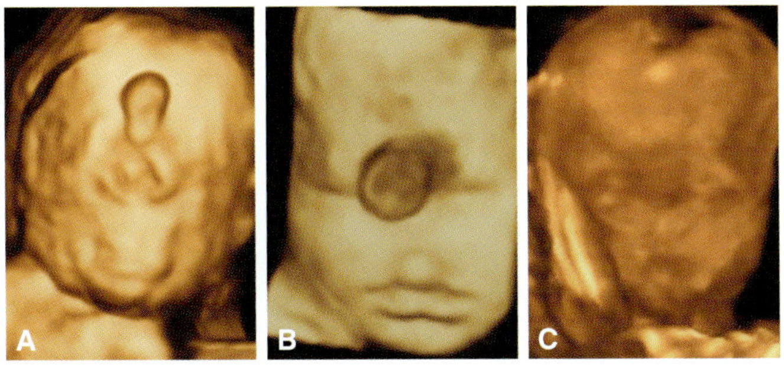


**Figure 16–16.** Craniofacial abnormalities associated with severe holoprosencephaly. **(A)** Cyclopia. **(B)** Ethmocephaly. **(C)** Median cleft lip with hypotelorism. (Courtesy of T. Esser, MD.)

A cataract is a clouding of the lens in the eye that affects vision. Most cataracts are related to aging. Cataracts are very common in older people. Rarely, this is found at birth, and in these cases the disease is usually bilateral. Sonographically, cataract is associated with an echogenic lens (see Figure 16–18). Prenatal diagnosis of cataracts have been reported.[38,39] In the majority of cases, they are a part of multiple anomalies and syndromes, or are associated with congenital infections. Congenital cataracts can be treated by removal of the lens. The prognosis however depends largely upon the associated anomalies.

Congenital obstruction of the nasolacrimal duct results in cystic dilatation of the proximal part of the duct, or dacrocystoceles. This has been identified prenatally as an anechoic mass medial and slightly inferior to the eye.[40,41] Although the differential diagnosis includes an anterior encephalocele, hemangioma, and a dermoid cyst, the sonographic appearance is typical (Figure 16–19). Postnatally, dacrocystoceles resolve spontaneously in ~90% of cases within the first 6 months of life.

A coloboma is a congenital gap in one of the structures of the eye. It may involve the iris, retina, choroid, or optic disc. The prenatal sonographic diagnosis of retinal coloboma has been described recently.[42] This appeared as an irregular extroflession of the posterior contour of the eye (Figure 16–20). Retinal colobomas are an important cause of visual impairment. The main interest in diagnosing this condition antenatally is, however, its association with syndromes including CHARGE and PHACE.[42]

## MICROGNATHIA AND RETROGNATHIA

The mandible arises from the merging of the two mandibular prominences that inferiorly delimit the stomodeum. The mandible forms the floor of the oral cavity and contains the tongue. If the mandible is severely hypoplastic (micrognathia) or posteriorly displaced (retrognathia) a typical sequence of malformations occurs: the tongue is displaced superiorly and posteriorly, leading to both abnormal closure of the palatine process, that results in either a cleft palate or a high arched palate, and glossoptosis that may cause suffocation at birth. This sequence is frequently referred to as the Robin anomalad, that may be a sporadic isolated finding (in ~40% of cases) or it may be associated with other anomalies or with recognized genetic and nongenetic syndromes. Micrognathia/retrognathia is frequently associated with genetic syndromes (eg, Treacher Collins, Robin, and Robert syndromes), chromosomal abnormalities (mainly trisomy 18 and triploidy) and teratogenic drugs (eg, methotrexate). Otocephaly is a rare, lethal, sporadic abnormality characterized by severe hypoplasia of the mandible (agnathia) and severe midline defects, including holoprosencephaly, anterior encephalocele, cyclopia, aglossia, microstomia, and midfacial location of the ears ("ear head").[43]

Micrognathia/retrognathia encompasses a wide spectrum of severity, and probably most mild cases cannot be recognized in utero. Conversely, severe forms can be identified since early gestation and different approaches have been suggested from time to time.[3,5,6,44–47] Probably, the simplest one is the profile view to demonstrate that the midportion of the mandible is not aligned with the maxilla.[47] In this view, the upper lip is usually very prominent and the chin is receding (Figure 16–21). This, however, is a subjective observation, and at times it is associated with many uncertainties. The index of suspicion increases when the tongue appears displaced posteriorly

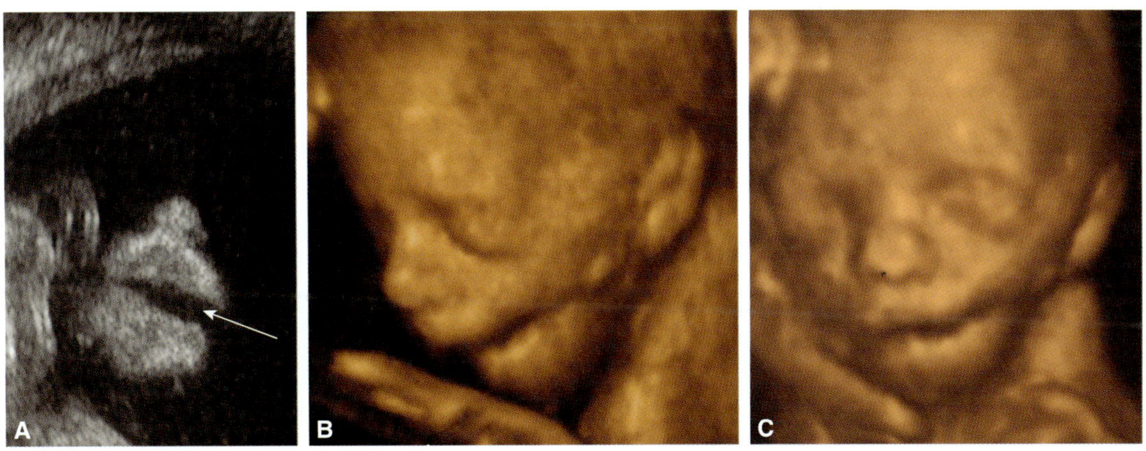


**Figure 16–17.** Lateral cleft of the face (Tessier type 7 cleft). **(A)** 2D coronal sonogram demonstrating asymmetry of the mouth (*arrow*). **(B), (C)** 3D sonograms. (Reproduced, with permission, from Pilu G, Visentin A, Ambrosini G, D'Antona D, Andrisani A. Three-dimensional sonography of unilateral Tessier number 7 cleft in a mid-trimester fetus. *Ultrasound Obstet Gynecol.* 2005;26[1]:98–99.)

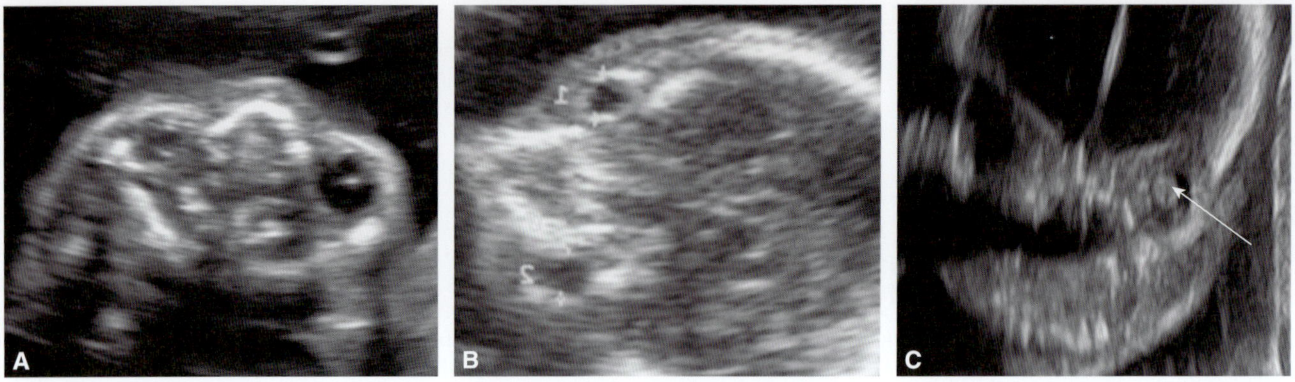


**Figure 16–18.** Ocular anomalies. **(A)** Unilateral microphthalmia. **(B)** Bilateral microphthalmia. **(C)** Cataract (*arrow*). (Reproduced, with permission, from *Visual Encyclopedia of Ultrasound in Obstetrics and Gynecology*, www.isuog.org.)

and superiorly[46] (Figure 16–22). Measurement of the mandible has also been proposed. Distinguishing micrognathia from retrognathia is not simple, and the two conditions frequently coexist. Intrauterine development of micrognathia, limiting early prenatal diagnosis has been suggested.[47] The use of 3D US has been suggested to increase the accuracy of 2D US diagnosis[45] (Figure 16–23).

Severe micrognathia can be a neonatal emergency due to airway obstruction by the normal tongue in the small oral cavity. If prenatal diagnosis is made a pediatrician should be present in the delivery room and be prepared to intubate the infant.[48] The prognosis however depends mostly on the presence of associated anomalies. Probably, only the most severe cases and those with associated malformations are detected in utero, and this may explain the poor outcome of most neonatal series.[43]

## TUMORS OF THE FACE

Epignathus is a very rare teratoma arising from the oral cavity or pharynx. Most cases of epignathus arise from the sphenoid bone. Some arise from the hard and soft palate, the pharynx, the tongue, and jaw. From their sites of origin, the tumors grow into the oral or nasal cavity or intracranially. The tumors, which are usually benign, consist of tissues derived from any of the three germinal layers; most of them contain adipose tissue, cartilage, bone, and nervous tissue. Prenatal diagnosis in the first and second trimester was published demonstrating a solid tumor arising from the oral cavity; calcifications and cystic components may also be present[49–54] (Figure 16–24). Polyhydramnios (due to pharyngeal compression) is frequently found. A careful examination of the brain is important because the tumor may grow intracranially. The outcome depends on the size of the lesion and the involvement of vital structures. Lesions detected antenatally have been very large. Polyhydramnios has been associated with poor prognosis. The major cause of neonatal death is asphyxia due to airway obstruction. Surgical resection and normal postoperative course are possible. Figure 16–25 describes a case in which a growing epiguatus (epidic) was longitudinally watched from 22 to 39 postmenstrual weeks throughout the delivery.[57] 3D US and Doppler studies were performed to establish the diagnosis and develop management strategies.

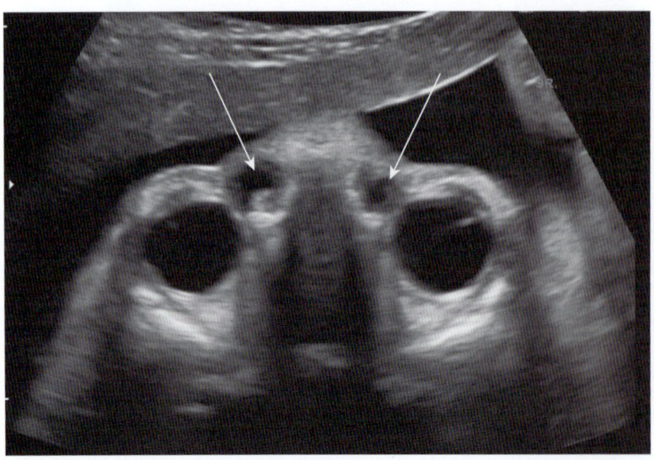

**Figure 16–19.** Dacrocystoceles (*arrows*). (Reproduced, with permission, from *Visual Encyclopedia of Ultrasound in Obstetrics and Gynecology*, www.isuog.org.)

Myoblastoma is a very rare benign tumor that usually arises from the oral cavity. The tumor occurs in females exclusively, and it may be the consequence of excessive production of estrogens by the fetal ovaries under human chorionic gonadotropin stimulation. The US features are those of a large solid mass protruding from the fetal mouth. Vascular connections between the tumor and the floor of the oral cavity may be demonstrated using color Doppler US. Polyhydramnios (due to pharyngeal compression) is common.

Intracranial teratoma, which is considered in detail elsewhere in this book (Chapter 13), may grow outside the skull, protruding from the orbits.

## FACIAL DYSMORPHISM

Modern high-resolution US allows detailed evaluation of the fetal face and an expert sonologist can now perform an anatomical examination on a living fetus in early gestation that in many ways is similar to clinical evaluations performed on live infants. Subtle facial dysmorphism is now amenable to antenatal detection and 3D US is certainly valuable in this setting. The detection of even the most subtle facial findings has been useful to diagnose or corroborate the diagnosis of

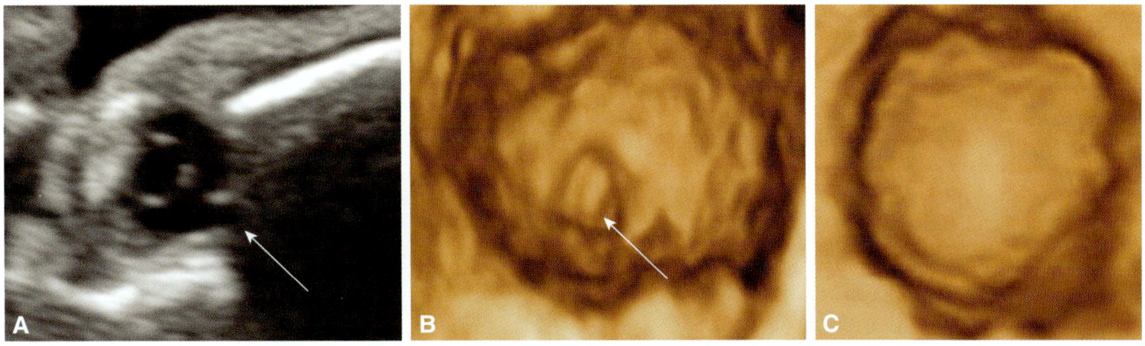


**Figure 16–20.** Retinal coloboma in a fetus at 27 postmenstrual weeks. **(A)** 2D US image of the left eye showing a small notch on the bottom of the eyeball (*arrow*). **(B)** Visualization of the fetal coloboma at the level of the papilla using 3D US (the virtual fetal eyeground). **(C)** A normal retina visualized using the technique at the same gestational age. (Reproduced, with permission, from Bault JP, Quarello E. Retinal coloboma: prenatal diagnosis using a new technique, the "virtual fetal eyeground." *Ultrasound Obstet Gynecol.* 2009;33[4]:495–496.)

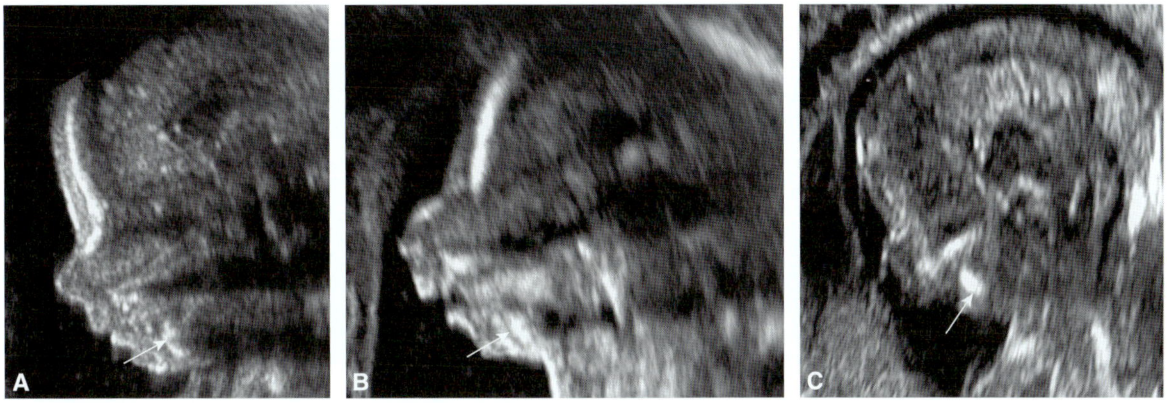


**Figure 16–21.** Median scan demonstrating the facial profile. **(A)** In a normal midtrimester fetus. **(B)** In a midtrimester fetus with multiple anomalies and severe micrognathia (*arrow*). **(C)** In a fetus with multiple anomalies and severe micrognathia at 12 postmenstrual weeks. (Reproduced, with permission, from *Visual Encyclopedia of Ultrasound in Obstetrics and Gynecology,* www.isuog.org.)

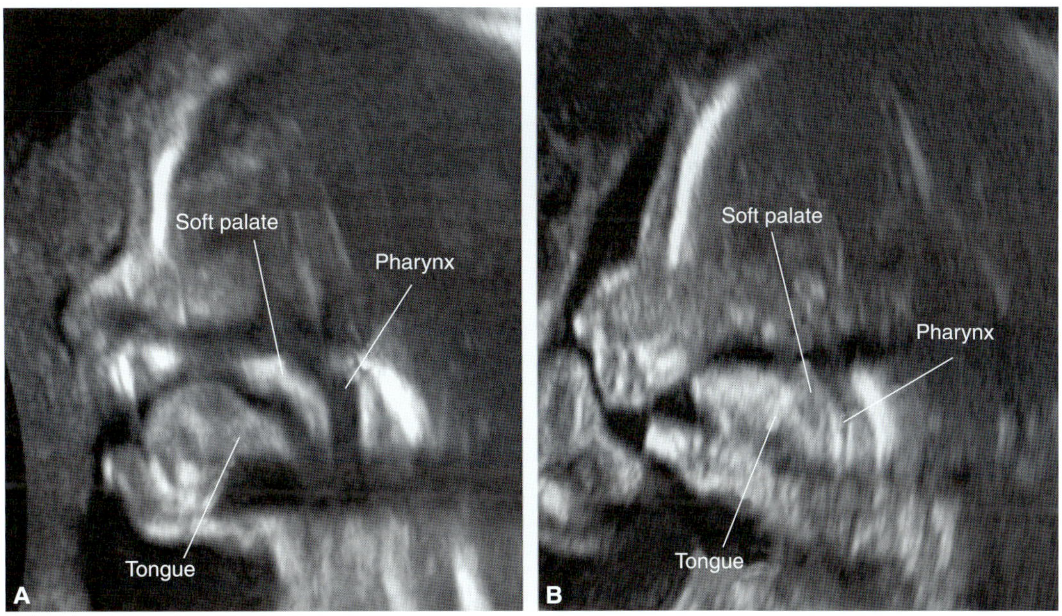


**Figure 16–22.** Median scans in demonstrating the oral cavity in midtrimster fetuses. **(A)** Normal anatomy. Note the tongue, soft palate, and open pharynx during swallowing. **(B)** Fetus with multiple anomalies and severe micrognathia. The floor of the oral cavity is small because of the diminutive mandible, and the tongue is displaced posteriorly, compressing the pharynx. When this pattern is persistent, it is highly suggestive of glossoptosis and carries a high risk of respiratory failure after delivery. (Reproduced, with permission, from *Visual Encyclopedia of Ultrasound in Obstetrics and Gynecology,* www.isuog.org.)

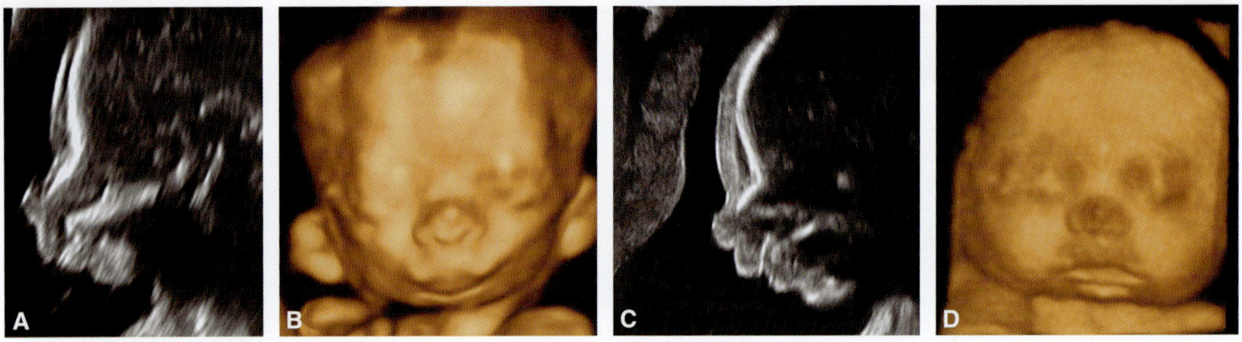


**Figure 16–23.** 3D US adds a further dimension to the diagnosis of micrognathia. In both cases, the 2D sonograms **(A), (C)** are less remarkable than the corresponding 3D images **(B), (D)**. (Reproduced, with permission, from *Visual Encyclopedia of Ultrasound in Obstetrics and Gynecology,* www.isuog.org.)

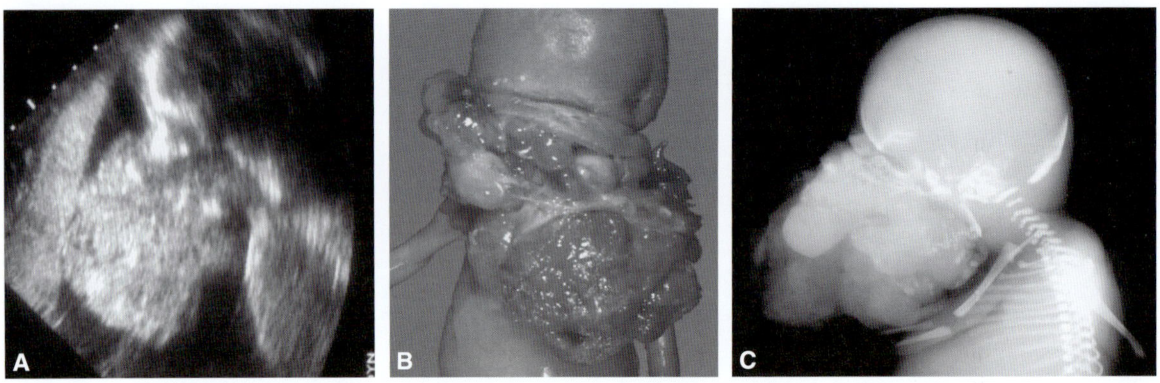


**Figure 16–24.** Epignathus. **(A)** Antenatal sonogram. **(B)** Postnatal image. **(C)** Postnatal radiogram. (B, C courtesy of Frank Chervenak, MD.)

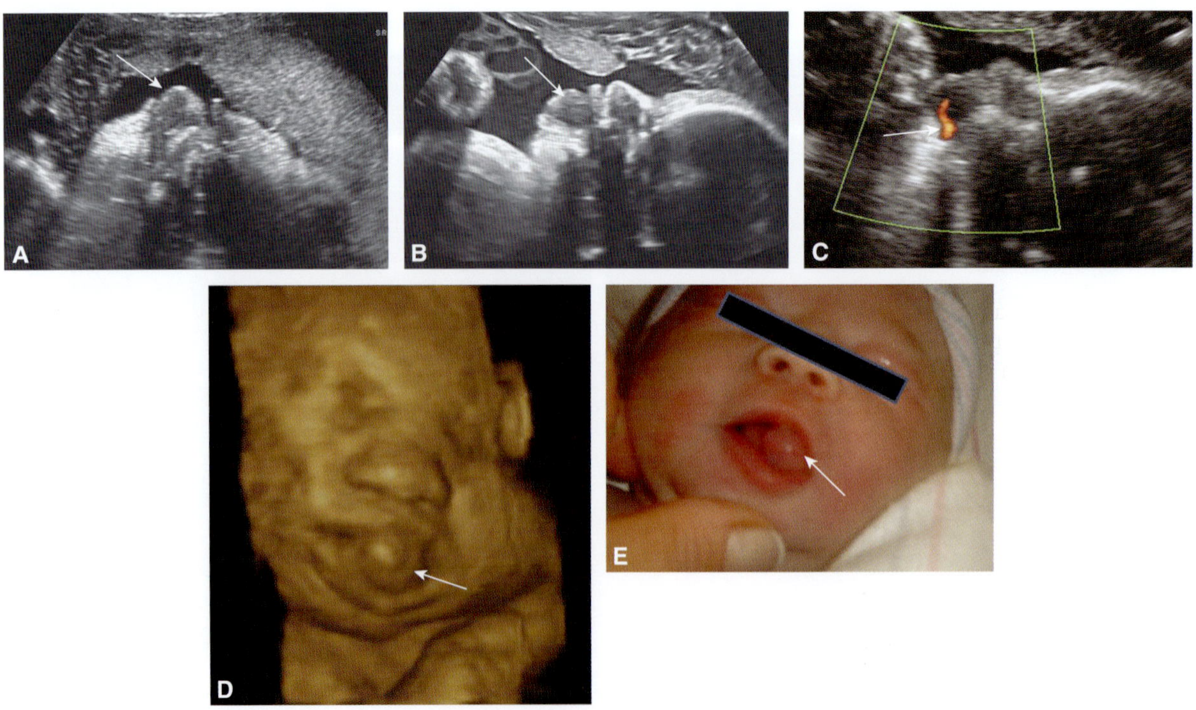


**Figure 16–25.** 2D and 3D evaluation of epignathus arising from the left lower lobular. Arrows show the mass. **(A)** Axial section. **(B)** Parasagittal section. **(C)** Vascular supply by power Doppler. **(D)** 3D surface rendering. **(E)** The neonate at birth (From Bornstein E, et al,[55] 2009, with permission).

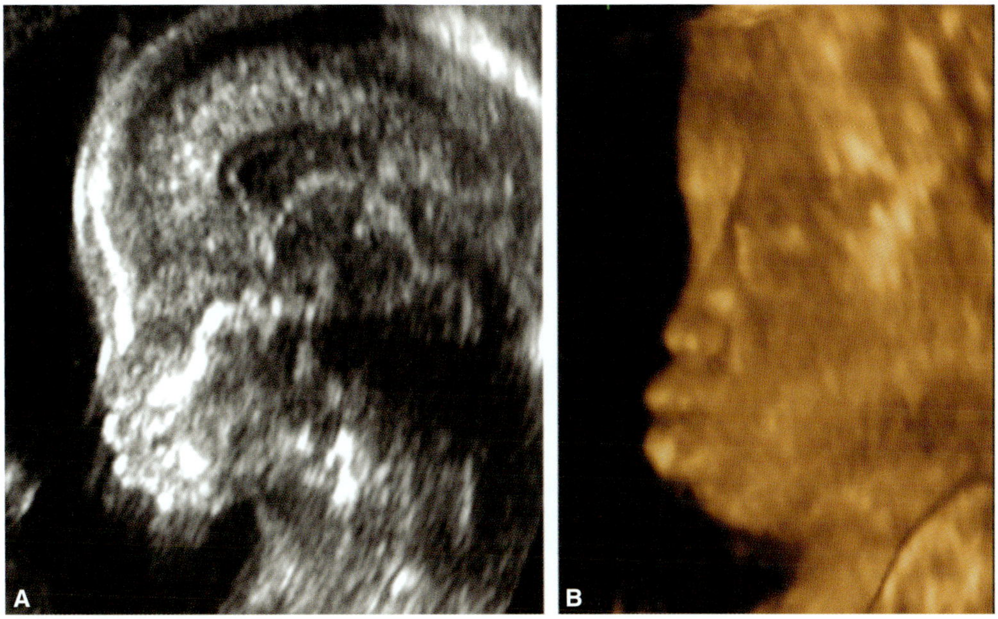


**Figure 16–26.** 2D (**A**) and 3D (**B**) sonograms of the profile of a midtrimester fetus demonstrating the pathognomonic findings of Binder syndrome: a small, flat nose that does not form an angle with the forehead; the maxilla and mandible are prominent. (Reproduced, with permission, from *Visual Encyclopedia of Ultrasound in Obstetrics and Gynecology*, www.isuog.org.)

syndromes in pregnancies at increased risk. However, some caution is necessary since facial features may demonstrate extreme variations even in normal individuals.

One of the conditions that can be reliably identified is Binder syndrome or "maxillonasal dysplasia" that is characterized by the association of an extremely small and flat nose, a convex upper lip, and malocclusion.[56] Prenatal diagnosis of this condition has been reported.[57,58] The profile view is particularly striking, with an extremely small and flat nose that does not form an angle with the forehead (Figure 16–26). This condition does not seem to affect neurological development and surgical treatment is available. An association with chondrodysplasia punctata has also been described.[56]

## CRANIOSYNOSTOSIS

Premature ossification and closure of the cranial sutures results in abnormal shape and size of the skull. In severe cases, this condition can also cause compression on cranial nerves and increased pressure on the growing brain. The final result depends upon the sutures that are involved and the time the closure takes place (Figure 16–27). Craniosynostosis (or craniostenosis) occurs in about 1 of 2100 to 2500 births.[59,60]

In most cases, only one suture is affected, and the condition is isolated and sporadic. However, in a minority of cases, closure of multiple sutures is possible, and associated anomalies are present. Craniosynostosis is part of many genetic syndromes. The genetic defect underlying some of these has been identified.[61] Most frequently, this is a mutation in the genes encoding the fibroblast growth factor receptors.[62]

The most frequent craniosynostosis is due to closure of the sagittal suture that is responsible for about half of the cases, resulting in an elongated head (scaphocephaly). The second most frequent type has changed over the years from coronal to metopic craniosynostosis;[63,64] the cause of this change is not yet clear.[65,66] In a recent study involving 629 patients with single-suture nonsyndromal craniosynostosis, closure of the sagittal suture was found

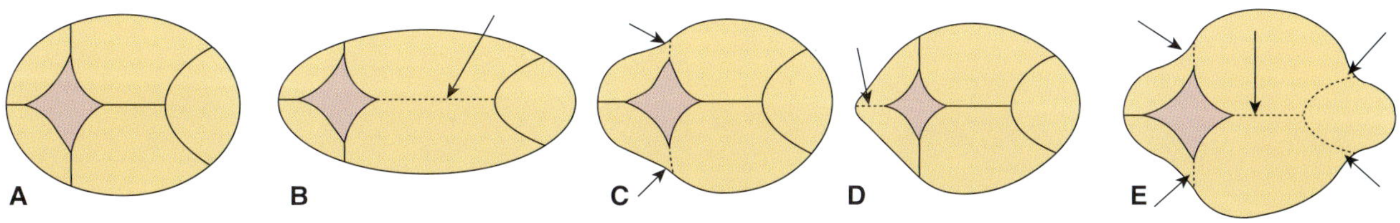


**Figure 16–27.** Schematic representation of the main types of craniosynostosis. (**A**) Normal head. (**B**) Premature closure of sagittal suture (*arrow*) or scaphocephaly. (**C**) Premature closure of both coronal sutures (*arrows*). (**D**) Premature closure of metopic suture (*arrow*) or trigonoscephaly. (**E**) Premature closure of multiple sutures (*arrows*) leading to cloverleaf skull. (Reproduced, with permission, from *Visual Encyclopedia of Ultrasound in Obstetrics and Gynecology*, www.isuog.org.)

in 45%, of the metopic in 28%, and of a single coronal suture in 24%.[66]

Crouzon and Apert syndromes are the most common of the craniosynostosis syndromes. Crouzon syndrome occurs in ~1 in 25,000 births. It may be transmitted as an autosomal dominant genetic condition or appear as a new mutation. In Crouzon syndrome craniosynostosis usually involves the coronal, sagittal, and lambdoid sutures. Other common features include hypertelorism, exophthalmos and external strabismus, parrot-beaked nose, short upper lip, hypoplastic maxilla, and a relative mandibular prognathism.[67] The phenotype of an infant with Crouzon syndrome can vary in severity from a mild presentation with subtle midface characteristics to severe forms with multiple cranial sutures fused and marked midface and ocular problems. The incidence of Apert syndrome is ~1 in 100,000 births, and most cases are fresh mutations. The general craniofacial features of a child with Apert syndrome are similar to those in Crouzon syndrome; however, there is not as much variability between cases, and the degree of presentation is more severe.[67]

Pfeiffer syndrome occurs in 1 in 100,000 births and is characterized by closure of all sutures with cloverleaf skull (also referred to as Kleeblattschädel syndrome), or by trigonocephaly, which is due to closure of the metopic suture resulting in a triangular forehead. Associated anomalies may include broad and deviated thumbs and big toes, partial syndactyly on hands and feet, hydrocephaly, severe ocular proptosis, ankylosed elbows, abnormal viscera, and slow development.[68] Shprintzen-Goldberg syndrome is even rarer and presents with anomalies involving the face, brain, bones, and heart.[69]

The experience with prenatal diagnosis of craniosynostosis is limited and consists mostly of case reports and small series of severe types. In general, suspicion arises because of an abnormal shape of the fetal head (Figure 16–28). Cloverleaf skull has a typical appearance, although this may appear only in late gestation: The head contour is polylobulated, with deep notches in the site of the coronal suture, the metopic suture is widened, and there is hypertelorism and exophthalmos (Figures 16–28 and 16–29).[6,70–73] Apert syndrome may be suspected early in pregnancy because of the characteristic "mittenlike" hand, but craniosynostosis is usually not detected until the second trimester[74] or even later on,[75] depending on its severity (Figure 16–30). Three-dimensional US is useful in these cases because the demonstration of a wide metopic suture with the maximum mode increases the index of suspicion (Figure 16–31). Crouzon syndrome has been demonstrated by the presence of cranial findings similar to those encountered with Apert syndrome: hypertelorism, exophthalmos, frontal bossing, notching at the level of the coronal sutures, and wide metopic suture.[6]

Miller et al[76] reviewed 109 cases of postnatally diagnosed craniosynostosis, but only 19 prenatal sonographic images were available for retrospective review; the authors were able to recognize abnormal findings in only 12 of them, including children with cloverleaf skull, Saethre-Chotzen syndrome, Crouzon syndrome, bilateral and unilateral coronal suture synostoses, and trigonocephaly.

Delahaye et al[77] reviewed retrospectively the US findings in 40 fetuses at risk of craniosynostosis; of these, 16 had a familiar history, and 24 had abnormal sonographic findings detected at a standard examination. Craniosynostosis was suspected when cranial deformation was present, but a definitive diagnosis was made only after direct visualization of a loss of normal hypoechogenicity of any suture.[77] In the group of patients with familiar history, recurrences occurred in five, and although all of them were diagnosed, the sutures were always open in the four fetuses examined in the second trimester. In the group of 24 patients referred because of suspicious findings (15 with dolichocephaly, 1 with brachycephaly, and 8 with facial dysmorphism), only 3 were affected by syndromic craniosynostosis, and 1 case was a false-positive.[77]

This experience suggests that the majority of cases are missed antenatally, and that there is potential for false-positive diagnoses. From our experience, we are aware of many infants who were diagnosed after birth with craniosynostosis and had completely unremarkable prenatal sonograms. This may be due to the conjunction of different factors: Craniosynostosis may develop late in pregnancy; fetuses with closure of the sagittal suture, the most frequent type of craniosynostosis, may present with dolichocephaly, a frequent finding during fetal life that is uneventful in the vast majority of cases; and imaging sonographically a seemingly open suture does not exclude premature closure at some other segment of the same suture.

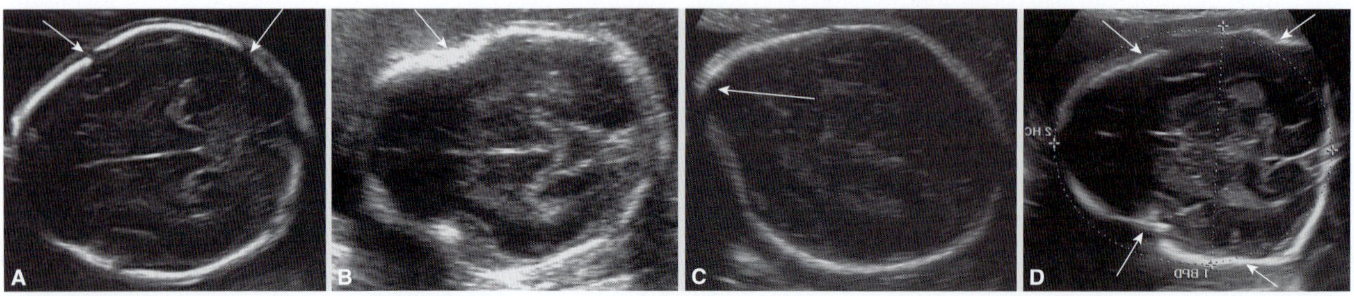


**Figure 16–28.** Sonography of normal fetal head and different types of craniosynostosis. **(A)** Normal fetus. The head has a regular ovular shape, and the coronal and lambdoid suture are well demonstrated as linear gaps in the ossified calvarium. **(B)** Bilateral coronal synostosis in a fetus with Crouzon syndrome. The coronal suture is not seen, and there is a notch in the contour of the head. **(C)** Trigonocephaly. The forehead is triangular. **(D)** Cloverleaf skull. Sutures are not seen, and the contour of the head is markedly irregular. (Reproduced, with permission, from *Visual Encyclopedia of Ultrasound in Obstetrics and Gynecology*, www.isuog.org.)

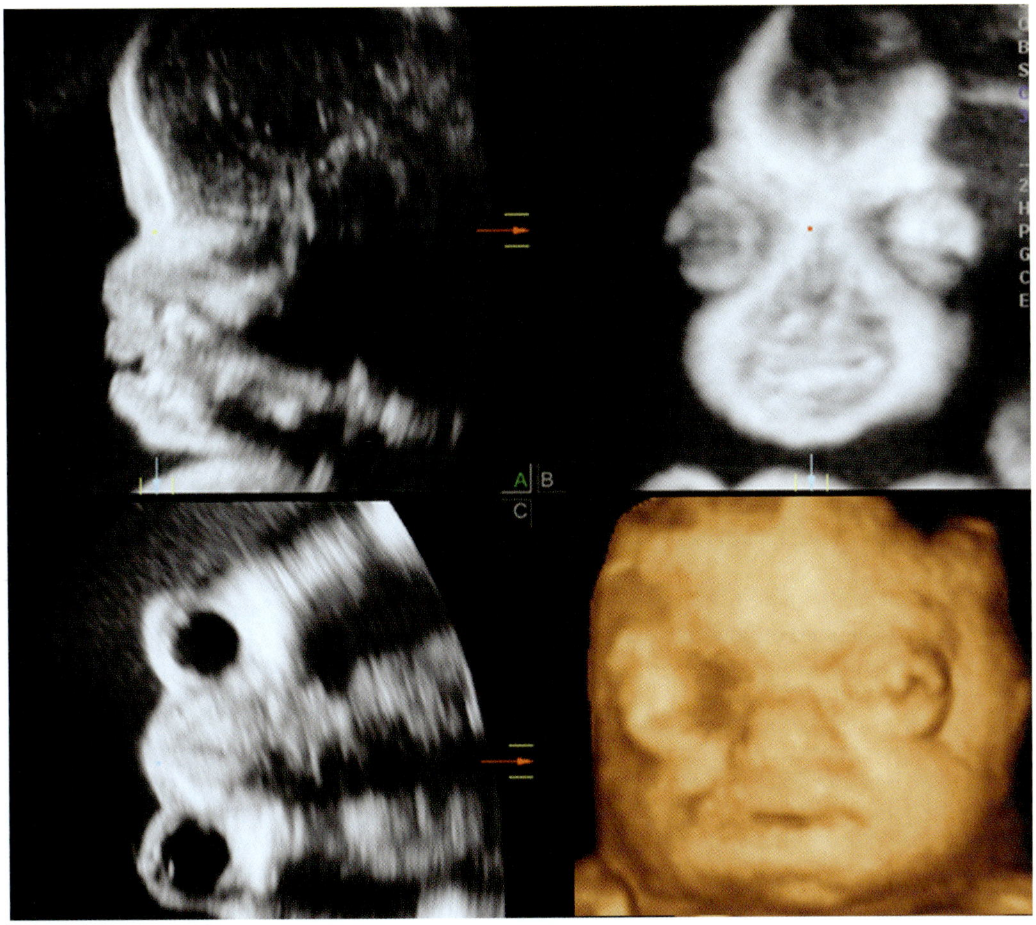


**Figure 16–29.** 3D US in a third-trimester fetus with severe Pfeiffer syndrome leading to neonatal death. Note the cloverleaf skull with frontal bossing and hypertelorism, Eeophthalmus with typically open eyelids, and prognatism. (Reproduced, with permission, from *Visual Encyclopedia of Ultrasound in Obstetrics and Gynecology*, www.isuog.org.)

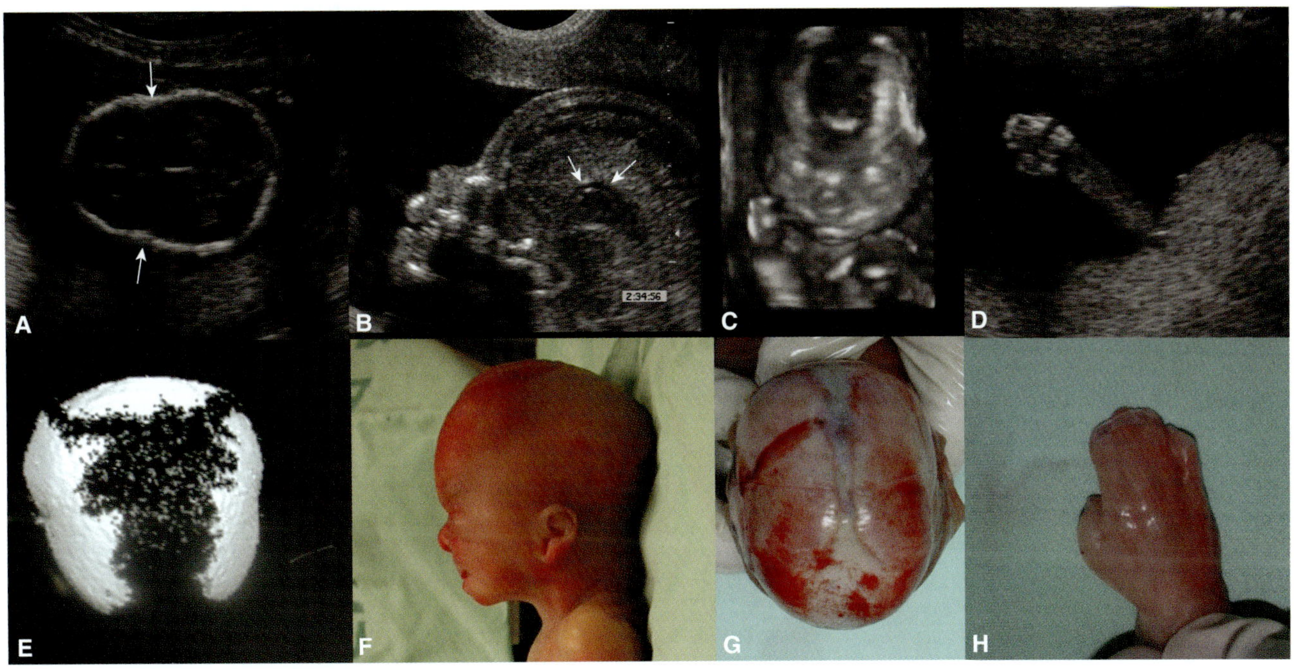


**Figure 16–30.** Apert syndrome diagnosed at 22 weeks of gestation. **(A)** Axial US shows the abnormal shape of the cranium due to synostosis of the coronal sutures (*arrows*), also shown in the post abortion CT **(E)**. **(B)** Median US shows frontal bossing, confirmed following delivery **(F)** and hypogenesis of the corpus callosum (arrows). **(C)** 3D US reconstruction shows the wide opening of the metopic suture and anterior fontanel; this finding was confirmed by post abortion CT **(E)** and autopsy **(G)**. Ultrasound **(D)** and autopsy specimen **(H)** demonstration of the "mitten-like" hand characteristic of Apert syndrome.

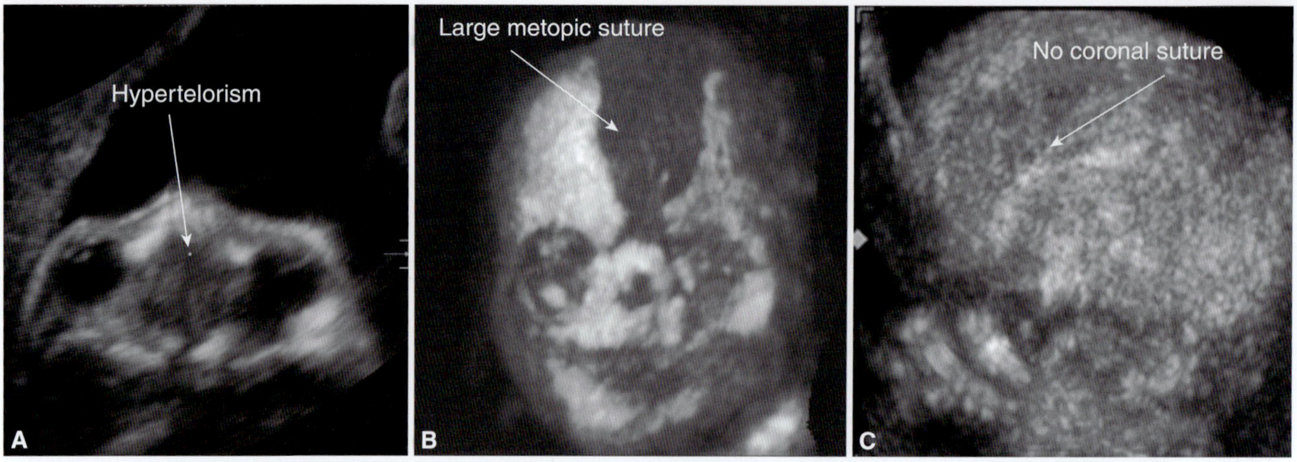


**Figure 16–31.** Cranial findings in a midtrimester fetus with Apert syndrome. **(A)** 2D US demonstrating hypertelorism. **(B), (C)** 3D US with maximum mode rendering demonstrating a wide metopic suture and no demonstrable coronal suture. (Reproduced, with permission, from *Visual Encyclopedia of Ultrasound in Obstetrics and Gynecology,* www.isuog.org.)

Even severe forms may be associated only with subtle findings, particularly in early gestation.

As suggested by Delahaye et al,[77] in high-risk patients or when the diagnosis of craniosynostosis is suspected, the initial analysis of the US images should include examination for overall head size, including circumference and cranial index; symmetry and continuity of the calvarium; size and shape of the orbits; brain anatomy; and detailed fetal examination. Following these steps, each suture should be assessed separately, searching for the loss of their characteristic hypoechogenic pattern and apparent overriding of the sutures (Figures 16–31 and 16–32). We have found that in patients with sagittal craniosynostosis, difficulty in the visualization of the median plane may be the first, and sometimes the only, sign of suture closure (Figure 16–33). Recently, reports on 3D US have described the normal appearance of the cranial sutures and fontanelles throughout pregnancy,[78,79] and it has been suggested that this technique may be valuable in the diagnosis of craniosynostosis.[79–81] Apart from the demonstration of panoramic views of the cranium using the standard surface mode, the transparent or maximum mode allows better visualization of the sutures, which is particularly useful for demonstrating the abnormal compensatory opening of the patent sutures that occurs when there is craniostenosis[82] (Figures 16–31 to 16–35).

The use of MRI in the diagnosis of fetal craniosynostosis has been proposed; published reports showed the abnormal shape of the head (Figure 16–36) and in some cases the presence of associated anomalies, but until now direct demonstration of abnormal sutures has not been described.[83–85] Genetic analysis may also be helpful in uncertain cases.[86]

The neurodevelopmental prognosis of individuals with craniosynostosis depends fundamentally on the etiology of the disease. Although syndromic cases and those with associated malformations have more sequelae than those with isolated, single-suture synostosis, the latter are at increased risk as well.[87] In a recent study, Chieffo et al[88] found that, even when treated early in life, children with

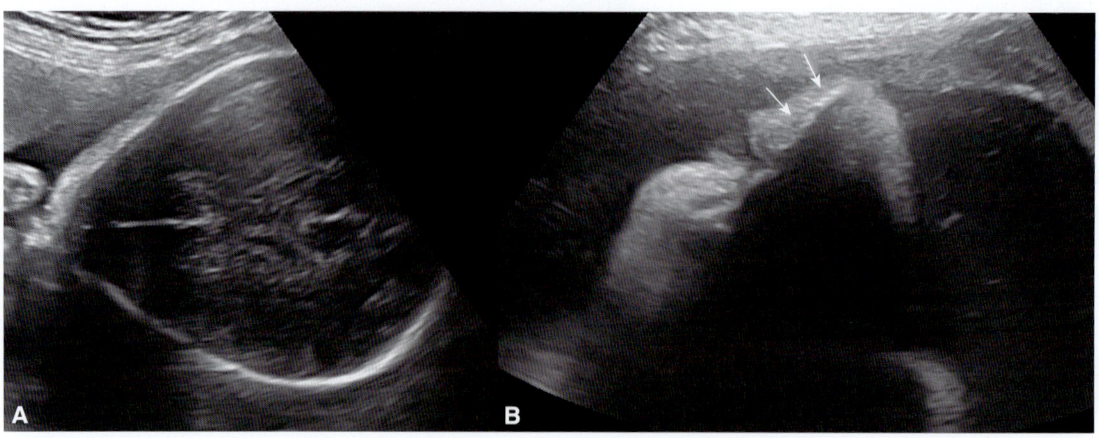


**Figure 16–32.** Isolated metopic craniosynostosis at 32 postmenstrual weeks. **(A)** The shape of the frontal bones raises the suspicion of early closure of the metopic suture. **(B)** Metopic craniosynostosis is demonstrated by the presence of a hyperechogenic frontal ridge (*arrows*).

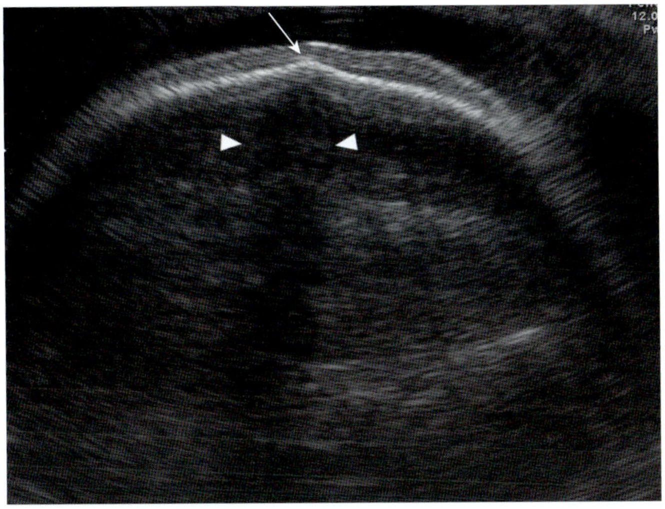

**Figure 16–33.** Autosomal dominant sagittal craniosynostosis at 27 postmenstrual weeks. The anterior portion of the brain appears normal, but visualization is sharply impaired for the posterior portion of the brain (*arrows*). This phenomenon is due to the fact that the anterior fontanelle is open, but the sagittal suture is closed.

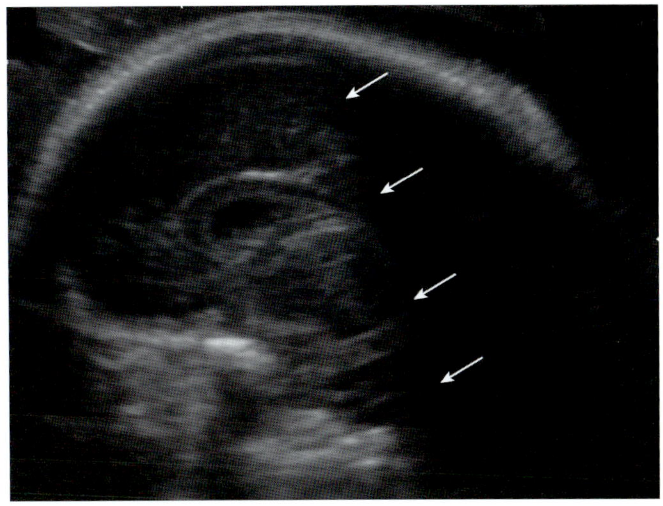

**Figure 16–34.** Isolated sagittal craniosynostosis at 27 postmenstrual weeks. The parietal bones are continuous; the hypechogenic suture is not demonstrated (*arrow*). Note the acoustic shadow produced by the synostosis (*arrowheads*).

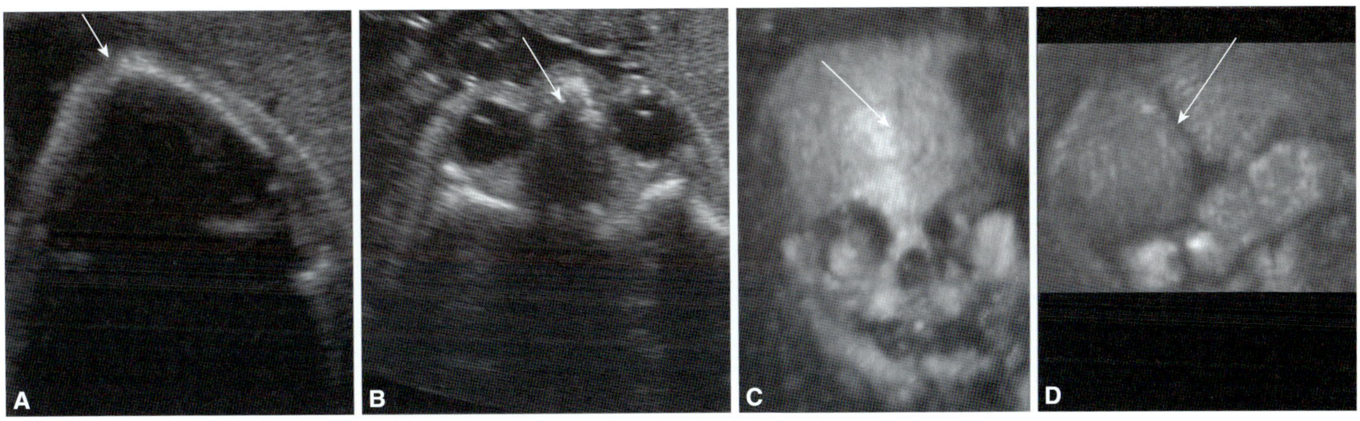


**Figure 16–35.** Trigonocephaly in a second-trimester fetus. **(A), (B)** 2D US demonstrating triangular forehead without evidence of central metopic suture and mild hypotelorism (*arrows*). **(C)** 3D US in maximum rendering mode of the skull confirming mild hypotelorism and no evidence of metopic suture (*arrow*). **(D)** 3D maximum mode rendering of the skull in a lateral projection demonstrating a patent coronal suture (*arrow*). (Reproduced, with permission, from *Visual Encyclopedia of Ultrasound in Obstetrics and Gynecology*, www.isuog.org.)

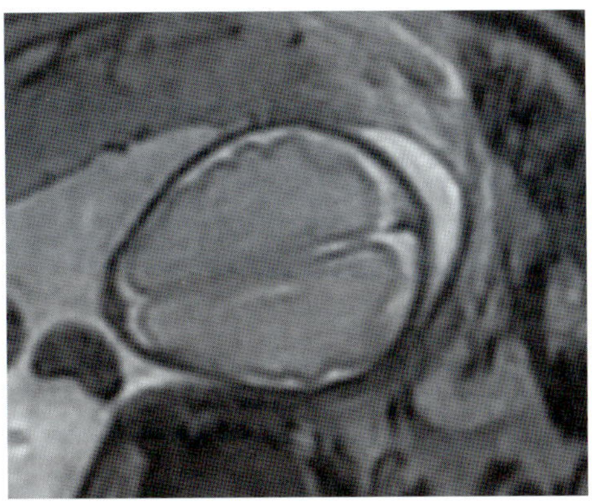

**Figure 16–36.** Fetal MRI at 30 postmenstrual weeks in a fetus with isolated metopic craniosynostosis.

sagittal or unilateral coronal craniosynostosis have neurodevelopmental deficits: 7% of those with sagittal craniosynostosis demonstrated visuospatial and constructional ability defects with associated visual memory recall deficits, 17% also exhibited selective and sustained attention deficits, and approximately one-third (30%) of the children with anterior plagiocephaly had processing and planning speech deficits. Children with metopic craniosynostosis appear to have a better prognosis.[89]

## REFERENCES


1. Benacerraf BR, Frigoletto FD, Jr., Bieber FR. The fetal face: Ultrasound examination. *Radiology.* 1984;153(2):495–497.
2. Nyberg DA, Sickler GK, Hegge FN, Kramer DJ, Kropp RJ. Fetal cleft lip with and without cleft palate: US classification and correlation with outcome. *Radiology.* 1995;195(3):677–684.
3. Pilu G, Reece EA, Romero R, Bovicelli L, Hobbins JC. Prenatal diagnosis of craniofacial malformations with ultrasonography. *Am J Obstet Gynecol.* 1986;155(1):45–50.
4. Rotten D, Levaillant JM. Two- and three-dimensional sonographic assessment of the fetal face: 2. Analysis of cleft lip, alveolus and palate. *Ultrasound Obstet Gynecol.* 2004;24(4):402–411.
5. Rotten D, Levaillant JM, Martinez H, Ducou le Pointe H, Vicaut E. The fetal mandible: A 2D and 3D sonographic approach to the diagnosis of retrognathia and micrognathia. *Ultrasound Obstet Gynecol.* 2002;19(2):122–130.
6. Ghi T, Perolo A, Banzi C, Contratti G, et al. Two-dimensional ultrasound is accurate in the diagnosis of fetal craniofacial malformation. *Ultrasound Obstet Gynecol.* 2002;19(6):543–551.
7. Jones MC. Prenatal diagnosis of cleft lip and palate: Detection rates, accuracy of ultrasonography, associated anomalies, and strategies for counseling. *Cleft Palate Craniofac J.* 2002;39(2): 169–173.
8. Sohan K, Freer M, Mercer N, Soothill P, Kyle P. Prenatal detection of facial clefts. *Fetal Diagn Ther.* 2001;16(4):196–199.
9. Stoll C, Dott B, Alembik Y, Roth M. Evaluation of prenatal diagnosis of cleft lip/palate by foetal ultrasonographic examination. *Ann Genet.* 2000;43(1):11–14.
10. Wayne C, Cook K, Sairam S, Hollis B, Thilaganathan B. Sensitivity and accuracy of routine antenatal ultrasound screening for isolated facial clefts. *Br J Radiol.* 2002;75(895):584–589.
11. Campbell S, Lees C, Moscoso G, Hall P. Ultrasound antenatal diagnosis of cleft palate by a new technique: The 3D "reverse face" view. *Ultrasound Obstet Gynecol.* 2005;25(1):12–18.
12. Campbell S, Lees CC. The three-dimensional reverse face (3D RF) view for the diagnosis of cleft palate. *Ultrasound Obstet Gynecol.* 2003;22(5):552–554.
13. Pilu G, Segata M. A novel technique for visualization of the normal and cleft fetal secondary palate: Angled insonation and three-dimensional ultrasound. *Ultrasound Obstet Gynecol.* 2007;29(2):166–169.
14. Platt LD, Devore GR, Pretorius DH. Improving cleft palate/cleft lip antenatal diagnosis by 3-dimensional sonography: The "flipped face" view. *J Ultrasound Med.* 2006;25(11):1423–1430.
15. Ten PM, Pedregosa JP, Santacruz B, Adiego B, Barron E, Sepulveda W. Three-dimensional ultrasound diagnosis of cleft palate: Reverse face, flipped face or oblique face—which method is best? Ultrasound Obstet Gynecol. 2009;33(4):399–406.
16. Ghi T, Tani G, Savelli L, Colleoni GG, Pilu G, Bovicelli L. Prenatal imaging of facial clefts by magnetic resonance imaging with emphasis on the posterior palate. *Prenat Diagn.* 200315;23(12): 970–975.
17. Kazan-Tannus JF, Levine D, McKenzie C, et al. Real-time magnetic resonance imaging aids prenatal diagnosis of isolated cleft palate. *J Ultrasound Med.* 2005;24(11):1533–1540.
18. Bellis TH, Wohlgemuth B. The incidence of cleft lip and palate deformities in the south-east of Scotland (1971–1990). *Br J Orthod.* 1999;26(2):121–125.
19. Berge SJ, Plath H, Van de Vondel PT, et al. Fetal cleft lip and palate: Sonographic diagnosis, chromosomal abnormalities, associated anomalies and postnatal outcome in 70 fetuses. *Ultrasound Obstet Gynecol.* 2001;18(5):422–431.
20. Nicolaides KH, Salvesen DR, Snijders RJ, Gosden CM. Fetal facial defects: Associated malformations and chromosomal abnormalities. *Fetal Diagn Ther.* 1993;8(1):1–9.
21. Gabrielli S, Piva M, Ghi T, et al. Bilateral cleft lip and palate without premaxillary protrusion is associated with lethal aneuploidies. *Ultrasound Obstet Gynecol.* 2009;34(4):416–418.
22. Mailath-Pokorny M, Worda C, Krampl-Bettelheim E, Watzinger F, Brugger PC, Prayer D. What does magnetic resonance imaging add to the prenatal ultrasound diagnosis of facial clefts? *Ultrasound Obstet Gynecol.* 2010;36(4):445–451.
23. Sepulveda W, Wong AE, Martinez-Ten P, Perez-Pedregosa J. Retronasal triangle: A sonographic landmark for the screening of cleft palate in the first trimester. *Ultrasound Obstet Gynecol.* 2010;35(1):7–13.
24. Benacerraf BR, Sadow PM, Barnewolt CE, Estroff JA, Benson C. Cleft of the secondary palate without cleft lip diagnosed with three-dimensional ultrasound and magnetic resonance imaging in a fetus with Fryns syndrome. *Ultrasound Obstet Gynecol.* 2006;27(5): 566–570.
25. David DJ, Moore MH, Cooter RD. Tessier clefts revisited with a third dimension. *Cleft Palate J.* 1989;26(3):163–184, discussion 84–85.
26. Kawamoto HK, Jr. The kaleidoscopic world of rare craniofacial clefts: Order out of chaos (Tessier classification). *Clin Plast Surg.* 1976;3(4):529–572.
27. Blaas HG, Eriksson AG, Salvesen KA, et al. Brains and faces in holoprosencephaly: Pre- and postnatal description of 30 cases. *Ultrasound Obstet Gynecol.* 2002;19(1):24–38.
28. Pilu G, Romero R, Rizzo N, Jeanty P, Bovicelli L, Hobbins JC. Criteria for the prenatal diagnosis of holoprosencephaly. *Am J Perinatol.* 1987;4(1):41–49.
29. Chervenak FA, Tortora M, Mayden K, et al. Antenatal diagnosis of median cleft face syndrome: Sonographic demonstration of cleft lip and hypertelorism. *Am J Obstet Gynecol.* 1984; 149(1):94–97.
30. DeMyer W. The median cleft face syndrome: Differential diagnosis of cranium bifidum occultum, hypertelorism, and median cleft nose, lip, and palate. *Neurology.* 1967;17(10):961–971.
31. Asai S, Tanaka M, Miyakoshi K, et al. A case of Tessier number 7 cleft with severe micrognathia: Prenatal sonographic and three-dimensional helical computed tomographic images. *Prenat Diagn.* 2010;30(2): 159–161.
32. Pilu G, Visentin A, Ambrosini G, D'Antona D, Andrisani A. Three-dimensional sonography of unilateral Tessier number 7 cleft in a mid-trimester fetus. *Ultrasound Obstet Gynecol.* 2005;26(1):98–99.
33. Presti F, Celentano C, Marcazzo L, Dolcetta G, Prefumo F. Ultrasound prenatal diagnosis of a lateral facial cleft (Tessier number 7). *Ultrasound Obstet Gynecol.* 2004;23(6):606–608.
34. Blazer S, Zimmer EZ, Mezer E, Bronshtein M. Early and late onset fetal microphthalmia. *Am J Obstet Gynecol.* 2006;194(5): 1354–1359.
35. Bronshtein M, Zimmer E, Gershoni-Baruch R, Yoffe N, Meyer H, Blumenfeld Z. First- and second-trimester diagnosis of fetal ocular defects and associated anomalies: Report of eight cases. *Obstet Gynecol.* 1991;77(3):443–449.
36. Ghi T, Contro E, Carletti A, et al. Prenatal sonographic imaging of Goldenhar syndrome associated with cystic eye. *Prenat Diagn.* 2008;28(4):362–363.
37. Tamas DE, Mahony BS, Bowie JD, Woodruff WW III, Kay HH. Prenatal sonographic diagnosis of hemifacial microsomia (Goldenhar-Gorlin syndrome). *J Ultrasound Med.* 1986;5(8):461–463.
38. Rosner M, Bronshtein M, Leikomovitz P, Berkenstat M, Barkai G, Barishak RY. Transvaginal sonographic diagnosis of cataract in a fetus. *Eur J Ophthalmol.* 1996;6(1):90–93.
39. Monteagudo A, Timor-Tritsch IE, Friedman AH, Santos R. Autosomal dominant cataracts of the fetus: Early detection by transvaginal ultrasound. *Ultrasound Obstet Gynecol.* 1996;8(2):104–108.
40. Davis WK, Mahony BS, Carroll BA, Bowie JD. Antenatal sonographic detection of benign dacrocystoceles (lacrimal duct cysts). *J Ultrasound Med.* 1987;6(8):461–465.
41. Goldberg H, Sebire NJ, Holwell D, Hill S. Prenatal diagnosis of bilateral dacrocystoceles. *Ultrasound Obstet Gynecol.* 2000;15(5): 448–489.

42. Bault JP, Quarello E. Retinal coloboma: Prenatal diagnosis using a new technique, the "virtual fetal eyeground." *Ultrasound Obstet Gynecol.* 2009;33(4):495–496.
43. Paladini D. Fetal micrognathia: Almost always an ominous finding. *Ultrasound Obstet Gynecol.* 2012;35(4):377–384.
44. Hsieh YY, Chang CC, Tsai HD, Yang TC, Lee CC, Tsai CH. The prenatal diagnosis of Pierre-Robin sequence. *Prenat Diagn.* 1999;19(6):567–569.
45. Lee W, McNie B, Chaiworapongsa T, et al. Three-dimensional ultrasonographic presentation of micrognathia. *J Ultrasound Med.* 2002;21(7):775–781.
46. Paladini D, Morra T, Teodoro A, Lamberti A, Tremolaterra F, Martinelli P. Objective diagnosis of micrognathia in the fetus: The jaw index. *Obstet Gynecol.* 1999;93(3):382–386.
47. Pilu G, Romero R, Reece EA, Jeanty P, Hobbins JC. The prenatal diagnosis of Robin anomalad. *Am J Obstet Gynecol.* 1986;154(3): 630–632.
48. Vettraino IM, Lee W, Bronsteen RA, Harper CE, Aughton D, Comstock CH. Clinical outcome of fetuses with sonographic diagnosis of isolated micrognathia. *Obstet Gynecol.* 2003;102(4):801–805.
49. Chervenak FA, Tortora M, Moya FR, Hobbins JC. Antenatal sonographic diagnosis of epignathus. *J Ultrasound Med.* 1984;3(5): 235–237.
50. Gull I, Wolman I, Har-Toov J, et al. Antenatal sonographic diagnosis of epignathus at 15 weeks of pregnancy. *Ultrasound Obstet Gynecol.* 1999;13(4):271–273.
51. Chen CP, Shih JC, Huang JK, et al. Two- and three-dimensional ultrasound demonstration of a giant epignathus. *Ultrasound Obstet Gynecol.* 2003;21(4):407–409.
52. Dar P, Rosenthal J, Factor S, Dubiosso R, Murthy AS. First-trimester diagnosis of fetal epignathus with 2- and 3-dimensional sonography. *J Ultrasound Med.* 2009;28(12):1743–1746.
53. Ruano R, Benachi A, Aubry MC, Parat S, Dommergues M, Manach Y. The impact of 3-dimensional ultrasonography on perinatal management of a large epignathus teratoma without ex utero intrapartum treatment. *J Pediatr Surg.* 2005;40(11):e31–e34.
54. Sherer DM, Zigalo A, Abulafia O. Prenatal 3-dimensional sonographic diagnosis of a massive fetal epignathus occluding the oral orifice and both nostrils at 35 weeks' gestation. *J Ultrasound Med.* 2006;25(11):1503–1505.
55. Bornstein E, Boozarjomehri F, Monteagudo A, Santos R, Milla SS, Timor-Tritsch IE. Diagnostic and prognostic aspects in the sonographic evaluation of a fetus with an oral mass. *J Ultrasound Med.* 2009;28(5):689–693.
56. Munro IR, Sinclair WJ, Rudd NL. Maxillonasal dysplasia (Binder's syndrome). *Plast Reconstr Surg.* 1979;63(5):657–663.
57. Cook K, Prefumo F, Presti F, Homfray T, Campbell S. The prenatal diagnosis of Binder syndrome before 24 weeks of gestation: Case report. *Ultrasound Obstet Gynecol.* 2000;16(6):578–581.
58. Cuillier F, Cartault F, Lemaire P, Alessandri JL. Maxillo-nasal dysplasia (Binder syndrome): Antenatal discovery and implications. *Fetal Diagn Ther.* 2005;20(4):301–305.
59. Lajeunie E, Le Merrer M, Bonaiti-Pellie C, Marchac D, Renier D. Genetic study of nonsyndromic coronal craniosynostosis. *Am J Med Genet.* 1995;55(4):500–504.
60. Boulet SL, Rasmussen SA, Honein MA. A population-based study of craniosynostosis in metropolitan Atlanta, 1989–2003. *Am J Med Genet A.* 2008;146A(8):984–991.
61. Wilkie AO, Byren JC, Hurst JA, et al. Prevalence and complications of single-gene and chromosomal disorders in craniosynostosis. *Pediatrics.* 2010;126(2):e391–e400.
62. Robin NH, Falk MJ, Haldeman-Englert CR. *FGFR-related Craniosynostosis Syndromes.* Seattle: University of Washington; 1998.
63. Anderson FM, Geiger L. Craniosynostosis: A survey of 204 cases. *J Neurosurg.* 1965;22:229–240.
64. Shillito J, Jr, Matson DD. Craniosynostosis: A review of 519 surgical patients. *Pediatrics.* 1968;41(4):829–853.
65. van der Meulen J, van der Hulst R, van Adrichem L, Arnaud E, Chin-Shong D, Duncan C, et al. The increase of metopic synostosis: A pan-European observation. *J Craniofac Surg.* 2009;20(2):283–286.
66. Kolar JC. An epidemiological study of nonsyndromal craniosynostoses. *J Craniofac Surg.* 2011;22(1):47–49.
67. Carinci F, Pezzetti F, Locci P, et al. Apert and Crouzon syndromes: Clinical findings, genes and extracellular matrix. *J Craniofac Surg.* 2005;16(3):361–368.
68. Vogels A, Fryns JP. Pfeiffer syndrome. *Orphanet J Rare Dis.* 2006;1:19.
69. Greally M. *Shprintzen-Goldberg Syndrome.* Seattle: University of Washington; 2006.
70. Brahman S, Jenna R, Wittenauer HJ. Sonographic in utero appearance of Kleeblattschadel syndrome. *J Clin Ultrasound.* 1979;7(6): 481–484.
71. Salvo AF. In utero diagnosis of Kleeblattschadel (cloverleaf skull). *Prenat Diagn.* 1981;1(2):141–145.
72. Benacerraf BR, Spiro R, Mitchell AG. Using three-dimensional ultrasound to detect craniosynostosis in a fetus with Pfeiffer syndrome. *Ultrasound Obstet Gynecol.* 2000;16(4):391–394.
73. Saal HM, Bulas DI, Allen JF, Vezina LG, Walton D, Rosenbaum KN. Patient with craniosynostosis and marfanoid phenotype (Shprintzen-Goldberg syndrome) and cloverleaf skull. *Am J Med Genet.* 1995;57(4):573–578.
74. Skidmore DL, Pai AP, Toi A, Steele L, Chitayat D. Prenatal diagnosis of Apert syndrome: Report of two cases. *Prenat Diagn.* 2003;23(12):1009–1013.
75. Filkins K, Russo JF, Boehmer S, et al. Prenatal ultrasonographic and molecular diagnosis of Apert syndrome. *Prenat Diagn.* 1997;17(11):1081–1084.
76. Miller C, Losken HW, Towbin R, et al. Ultrasound diagnosis of craniosynostosis. *Cleft Palate Craniofac J.* 2002;39(1):73–80.
77. Delahaye S, Bernard JP, Renier D, Ville Y. Prenatal ultrasound diagnosis of fetal craniosynostosis. *Ultrasound Obstet Gynecol.* 2003;21(4):347–53.
78. Ginath S, Debby A, Malinger G. Demonstration of cranial sutures and fontanelles at 15 to 16 weeks of gestation: A comparison between two-dimensional and three-dimensional ultrasonography. *Prenat Diagn.* 2004;24(10):812–815.
79. Chaoui R, Levaillant JM, Benoit B, Faro C, Wegrzyn P, Nicolaides KH. Three-dimensional sonographic description of abnormal metopic suture in second- and third-trimester fetuses. *Ultrasound Obstet Gynecol.* 2005;26(7):761–764.
80. Esser T, Rogalla P, Bamberg C, Kalache KD. Application of the three-dimensional maximum mode in prenatal diagnosis of Apert syndrome. *Am J Obstet Gynecol.* 2005;193(5):1743–1745.
81. Lam H, Lo TK, Lau E, Chin R, Tang L. The use of 2- and 3-dimensional sonographic scans in the evaluation of cranial sutures: Prenatal diagnosis of Apert syndrome. *J Ultrasound Med.* 2006;25(11): 1481–1484.
82. Faro C, Chaoui R, Wegrzyn P, Levaillant JM, Benoit B, Nicolaides KH. Metopic suture in fetuses with Apert syndrome at 22–27 weeks of gestation. *Ultrasound Obstet Gynecol.* 2006; 27(1):28–33.
83. Itoh S, Nojima M, Yoshida K. Usefulness of magnetic resonance imaging for accurate diagnosis of Pfeiffer syndrome type II in utero. *Fetal Diagn Ther.* 2006;21(2):168–171.
84. Fjortoft MI, Sevely A, Boetto S, Kessler S, Sarramon MF, Rolland M. Prenatal diagnosis of craniosynostosis: Value of MR imaging. *Neuroradiology.* 2007;49(6):515–521.
85. Weber B, Schwabegger AH, Vodopiutz J, Janecke AR, Forstner R, Steiner H. Prenatal diagnosis of Apert syndrome with cloverleaf skull deformity using ultrasound, fetal magnetic resonance imaging and genetic analysis. *Fetal Diagn Ther.* 2010;27(1):51–56.
86. Nazzaro A, Della Monica M, Lonardo F, et al. Prenatal ultrasound diagnosis of a case of Pfeiffer syndrome without cloverleaf skull and review of the literature. *Prenat Diagn.* 2004;24(11): 918–922.
87. Kapp-Simon KA, Speltz ML, Cunningham ML, Patel PK, Tomita T. Neurodevelopment of children with single suture craniosynostosis: A review. *Childs Nerv Syst.* 2007;23(3):269–281.
88. Chieffo D, Tamburrini G, Massimi L, et al. Long-term neuropsychological development in single-suture craniosynostosis treated early. *J Neurosurg Pediatr.* 2010;5(3):232–237.
89. Warschausky S, Angobaldo J, Kewman D, Buchman S, Muraszko KM, Azengart A. Early development of infants with untreated metopic craniosynostosis. *Plast Reconstr Surg.* 2005;115(6): 1518–1523.

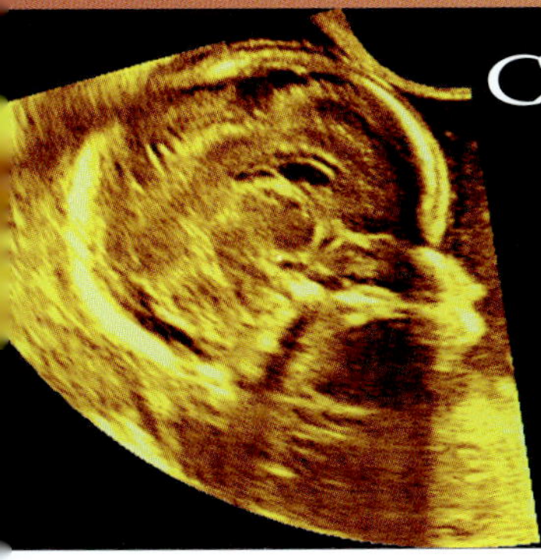

Chapter 17

# VERTEBRAL ANOMALIES

*Yinon Gilboa • Eldad Katorza • Reuven Achiron*

**KEY POINTS**

1. Sonographic evaluation of the vertebral column and the spine is a requirement of almost all governing bodies.
2. Starting the 13th postmenstrual weeks it is possible to ascertain a normal spine as well as a number of its anomalies.
3. 3D ultrasound is increasingly used and became instrumental in imaging the vertebral column in the three orthogonal planes using the X-ray or maximum mode rendering.
4. MRI may at times be necessary to complete the workup.

The assessment of the fetal vertebral column by transabdominal ultrasound (US) is an essential part of the second-trimester anatomical scan. The possibility of evaluating the spine at as early as 13 weeks of gestation by transvaginal high-resolution US has greatly improve its diagnostic capabilities and enabled the diagnosis of some of the common vertebral anomalies at this stage of pregnancy. Because not all spinal anomalies may be diagnosed during the late first or early second trimester, transabdominal US continues to be the "everyday" tool in the diagnosis of spinal and spinal cord malformations.[1] One example of this is the tethered cord that may be visible, in some but not all the cases, from the the midsecond trimester as the terminal spinal cord becomes more clearly defined.

The introduction of volume US with minimum intensity projection, or radiograph mode, contributes to projecting and locating the exact level of the malformation.[2] The additional value of this technology is still controversial, and the projection of a three-dimensional (3D) acquisition of the spine is not always reassuring, as it may miss small lesions in the lower spine.[3]

Magnetic resonance imaging (MRI) has been proposed as an additional tool in the diagnosis and counseling of patients with spinal cord anomalies, particularly regarding the evaluation of the spinal canal and its contents. So far this technology has not been widely used, but initial reports appear promising.[4,5] In this chapter, the terms *spine, spinal column,* and *vertebral column* are used interchangeably.

## DEVELOPMENT OF THE SPINE AND SPINAL CORD

The vertebrae develop during the sixth postmenstrual week of gestation, when chondrification centers appear for each mesenchymal vertebra. Each vertebral body has two primary ossification centers, one dorsal and one ventral. These centers fuse to form the centrum, which creates three primary ossification loci by the end of embryonic development; one develops in the vertebral body and the other two on each half of the vertebral arch.[6] According to US studies, by 16 postmenstrual weeks, S1 and S2 ossification centers are almost all visualized in coronal planes, but S3 is present in only about half of these fetuses; the nucleus of S4 develops slightly later and is observed in all fetuses at 21 weeks.[7] The posterior arch synchondrosis is not ossified in fetuses.

Closure of the neural tube seems to begin separately at several different levels. Progressive folding and closure of the neural structures and separation from ectoderm proceed both cranially and caudally from the point of initial closure, closing the neural tube in both directions. The most caudal end of the neural tube closes by 27 days of gestation. By 38 days, the lowest segment eventually becomes the most caudal portion of the conus medullaris, filum terminale, and ventriculus terminalis (focal dilation of the central canal in the conus medullaris).[8]

Because development and growth of the spinal cord are different from that of the vertebrae, the position of the conus medullaris in relation to the vertebral column is variable throughout pregnancy. On sagittal images, between 13 and 18 postmenstrual weeks, the conus medullaris is located below or at the level of L4 in all fetuses.[9] Then it undergoes progressive ascent until term, when it is always located above the level of L2–L3 (Figure 17–1).[10]

## ULTRASONOGRAPHIC EVALUATION OF THE FETAL SPINE

### Technique and Normal Anatomy

Whenever possible, US should be performed, when the fetal spine is positioned close to the transducer. Manipulation of the fetal body to correctly position the fetus is usually

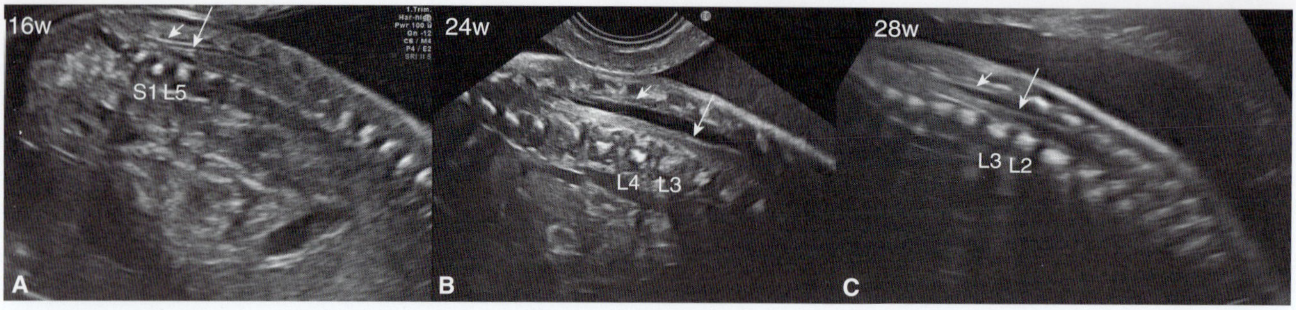


**Figure 17–1.** Normal anatomy of the spine and the spinal cord in fetuses at 16 **(A)**, 24 **(B)**, and 28 **(C)** postmenstrual weeks in the sagittal section. Conus medullaris (*large arrow*); dura mater (*small arrow*). Note the progressive displacement of the position of the conus medullaris from L5 at 16 postmenstrual. Weeks to L2–L3 at 28 postmenstrual weeks.

relatively easy during the late first and early second trimesters. Closer to term it may be more difficult and in some cases impossible due to fetal size and the relatively lower amount of amniotic fluid. If possible, one should minimize the applied pressure to the transducer to leave amniotic fluid between the proximal uterine wall and the spine, to serve as an acoustic window. It is important to remember that the quality of US images is highly influenced by maternal habitus and fetal position, therefore in some cases optimal visualization of the fetal spine may be difficult or even impossible. Two-dimensional (2D) US evaluation of the spine is adequately covered in most US textbooks. We would like to discuss here the somewhat less employed but highly diagnostic yield of 3D US imaging the vertebrae.

The spine may be evaluated using three planes: sagittal, coronal, and axial (Figure 17–2). Usually only two of these planes may be obtained by 2D US. Sonographic evaluation of the fetal spine is possible due to the presence of the previously mentioned ossification centers within the fetal vertebrae.[1,11]

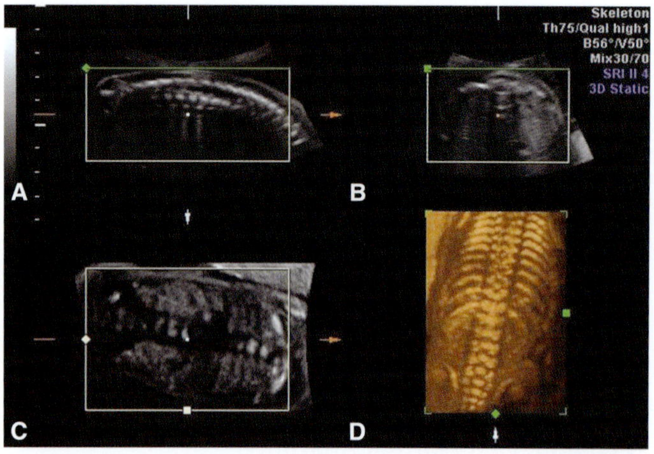


**Figure 17–2.** Three-dimensional (3D) multiplanar imaging of the spine shows the sagittal **(A)**, axial **(B)**, and coronal **(C)** planes. 3D reconstruction **(D)** enables evaluation mot only of individual vertebrae but also of ribs and iliac crests.

The sagittal planes enable visualization of the lateral ossification centers and each vertebral body. This is done by tilting the transducer from the midline (where the vertebral bodies are depicted) by about 15° to the right or left to reveal the lateral ossification centers. Fetal kyphosis may be identified in this plane. The skin, represented by an echogenic contour, should be meticulously evaluated to rule out the presence of skin-covered spinal dysraphism, which may be difficult or even impossible to detect, particularly before the third trimester. The curvature of the sacrum should be evaluated to include the normal anatomy of the rump to exclude sacral agenesis or sacrococcygeal teratoma. The spinal cord and meninges may be clearly visualized in these planes. Cord visualization is optimal in the fetus during the first and second trimesters due to partial bone mineralization and the small amount of soft tissue at the dorsum, creating a better sonolucent region than in the third trimester (see Figure 17–2).

The spinal cord is recognized as a hypoechoic tubular structure bordered by two echogenic lines, each line formed by the juxtaposed arachnoid and pia mater, with a hyperechoic central line representing the neural canal or the anterior median fissure.[12] As pregnancy advances, the conus medullaris, which is the lower end of the spinal cord, ascends. A significant ascent of the conus medullaris is detected between 13 and 40 postmenstrual weeks from the level of L4 or below (between 13 and 18 weeks) to a level above L2 at term[9] (see Figure 17–1). The visualization of a low-reaching conus medullaris during pregnancy should raise the suspicion of tethering.

The filum terminale, a delicate strand of fibrous tissue, appears as an echogenic midline string extending caudally from the conus medullaris through the coccyx.[12] Abnormal thickening of the filum terminale has been reported in postnatal cases of tethered cord.[13]

The coronal planes display paired parallel ossification centers of the spine and help in the evaluation of the degree of scoliosis.[1] Visualization of vertebral asymmetry raises the suspicion of hemivertebra (Figure 17–3).

The axial planes are produced by a dynamic shift starting either at the level of the head or from the sacrum cephalad and on the way demonstrate three ossification centers for each vertebra (see Figure 17–3). This plane is commonly used to exclude spinal defects and evaluate

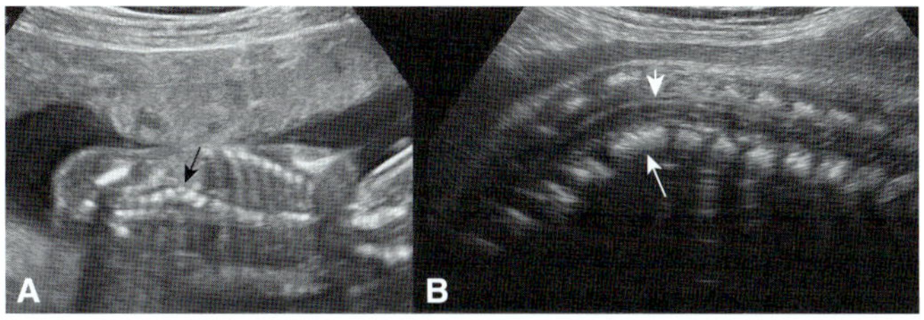


**Figure 17–3.** Hemivertebra with scoliosis. **(A)** At 14 postmenstrual weeks, the hemivertebra (*black arrow*) is clearly demonstrated in the coronal plane. **(B)** At 23 postmenstrual weeks, fusion of a normal vertebra and a hemivertebra is depicted as a large ossification center (*white arrow*) causing compression of the anterior and posterior borders of the cord (*arrowhead*).

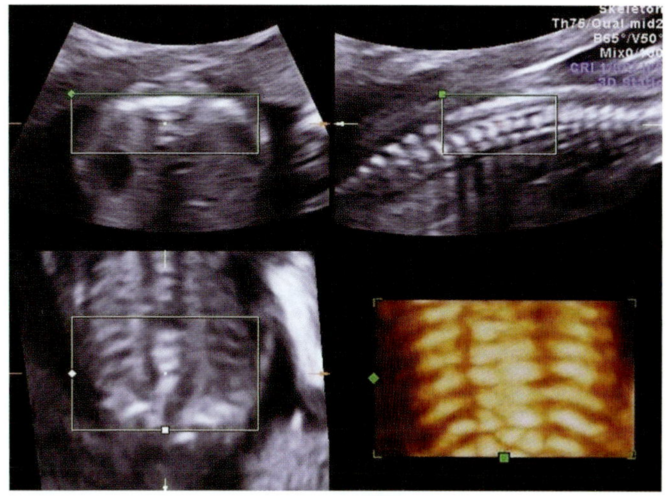

**Figure 17–4.** Multiplanar 3D ultrasound (US) helps to detect the level of the hemivertebra and demonstrates the severity of kyphoscoliosis.

the overlying soft tissues.[14] Chapter 5 contains additional, mostly 3D volume scans, with orthogonal displays and 3D renderings of the vertebral column.

## HEMIVERTEBRA

Hemivertebra is a relatively common congenital anomaly of the spine in which only one-half of the vertebral body develops. The reported incidence of hemivertebra is 0.5 to 1.0 per 1000 births,[15] with a male/female ratio of 0.31 for multiple vertebral anomalies and 0.68 for solitary vertebral anomalies.[16] In this malformation, a portion of the vertebra does not develop, producing a wedge-shaped vertebra. Depending on which ossification center fails to develop, the hemivertebra may be lateral or dorsal.[17] The main prenatal sonographic feature of hemivertebra is disruption of the normal spine alignment that leads to congenital scoliosis. When the suspicion of hemivertebra is raised, US is usually accurate in predicting the level and type of it. Usually the coronal plane allows the diagnosis by the display of the wedge-shaped hemivertebra and scoliosis (see Figure 17–3). By using the 3D multiplanar display with the volume acquisition in the midsagittal plane, the malformation may be projected forward, allowing observation of the exact level of the hemivertebra (Figure 17–4).

The diagnosis of isolated hemivertebra usually has a favorable outcome,[18–20] but hemivertebra is frequently associated with other congenital anomalies, and a meticulous anatomical scan should follow its diagnosis. The whole spine, ribs, pelvis, and limbs should be scanned, as hemivertebra may be part of syndromes involving other skeletal anomalies.[21] Extraskeletal anomalies, particularly cardiac and genitourinary tract anomalies, have been reported. They may be part of genetic syndromes, including Jarcho-Levin, Klippel-Feil, and VATER association (vertebral defects, imperforate anus, tracheoesophageal fistula, and radial and renal dysplasia).[22]

Wax et al[23] described a series of 19 fetuses with hemivertebra diagnosed during a period of 10 years. The diagnosis was made at a mean gestational age of 20.5 weeks; 14 (73.7%) fetuses had additional anomalies, of which 5 (35.7%) were syndromic (4 with cloacal exstrophy and omphaloceles and 1 with Jarcho-Levin syndrome). Fourteen (73.7%) neonates were live born, 2 (14.3%) of these neonates died; both had cloacal exstrophy and large omphaloceles. The remaining pregnancies were terminated or had a fetal death.[23]

From our experience, the progression of isolated cases cannot be predicted accurately, as demonstrated in Figure 17–5; in this case, the angle of scoliosis improved throughout pregnancy.

## DIASTEMATOMYELIA

Diastematomyelia, or split cord malformation (SCM), is a rare form of spinal dysraphism characterized by the presence of a sagittal cleft in the spinal cord. This condition is the result of the presence of an osseous or fibrocartilaginous septum producing a complete or incomplete sagittal division of the spinal cord into two hemicords. It may be isolated or associated with other segmental anomalies of the vertebral bodies.[24,25]

Splitting of the spinal cord may be partial or complete and can result in symmetrical or asymmetrical hemicords, which usually reunite caudally. Each segment has a central canal and dorsal as well as ventral nerve roots. Pang et al[24] proposed a classification for diastematomyelia. Type I SCM consists of two hemicords, each contained in a separate dural tube and separated by an osseocartilaginous septum. Type II SCM consists of a single dural sac containing both hemicords, the two hemicords being separated by a nonrigid fibrous septum. Type I split cords are technically more difficult to correct and are associated with more surgical morbidity than type II, especially if there is an oblique septum dividing the cords asymmetrically.[25]

Ultrasound in the axial plane may identify the hemicords and also the spur, which is usually echogenic (Figure 17–6). Diastematomyelia occurs most commonly

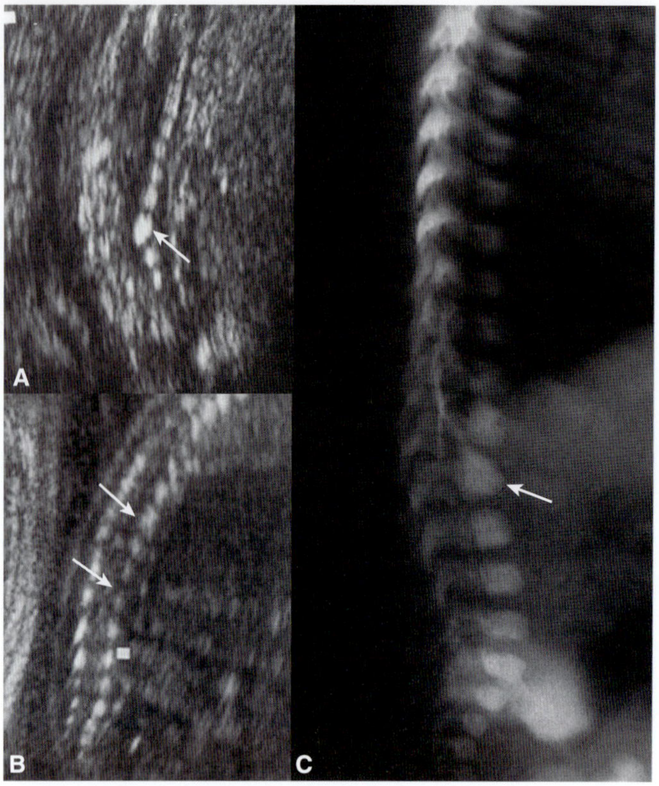


**Figure 17–5.** Hemivertebra diagnosed at 15 postmenstrual weeks (*arrow* in **A**), with improvement of scoliosis at 23 postmenstrual weeks (*arrows* in **B**). Normal clinical examination after delivery but a nonsegmented, fused vertebra was diagnosed by radiograph (*arrow* in **C**). (Courtesy of Bronshtein Moshe, MD, Haifa, Israel.)

in the thoracolumbar region; 50% to 75% of patients have cutaneous stigmata at the site of diastematomyelia.[26]

Diastematomyelia is commonly associated with tethering of the spinal cord ~75% of patients and syringohydromyelia in ~50% of patients. Both these abnormalities must therefore be looked for and excluded in the presence of diastematomyelia.[27]

Cutaneous signs of occult spinal dysraphism are frequently associated with SCM. Hypertrichosis (hairy patch) is the most common manifestation (56%); capillary hemangioma (26%), dermal sinuses (22%), and subcutaneous lipomas (11%) are also identified with increasing frequency.[28]

In a review of the literature, Has et al[29] found 26 reported patients; in 12 the malformation was isolated, and all of them had a good prognosis.

The use of MRI has been reported and will probably add information regarding the presence of associated spinal malformations that may be difficult to recognize by US alone.[30]

## TETHERED CORD

During the embryonic period, the spinal cord is positioned very low in the spinal canal; however, because of the accelerated growth of the bones of the vertebrae compared with the slower growth of the spinal cord, the cord "ascends" progressively until term to reach the level of L1–L2.[9,31] In the fetus, it is possible to localize the exact position of the conus medullaris using sagittal planes (see Figure 17–1). When the conus medullaris is positioned lower than expected, spinal dysraphism should be considered. Tethered cord syndrome (TCS) is a neurologic disorder caused by the fixation of the caudal portion of the cord by a tight and/or fatty infiltrated terminal filum. This results in a tight pull or stretching on the lower portion of the spinal cord and can lead to neurologic compromise. The true incidence of primary TCS is not known. Unlike open neural tube defects, closed defects such as TCS are usually diagnosed with the onset of symptoms or found incidentally during workup of unrelated problems.[31] Because of the continuous growth of the spinal column, the onset of symptoms may differ at different ages.[32] The syndrome is characterized by progressive neurologic, urologic, and/or orthopedic deterioration. Early diagnosis and treatment can prevent cord ischemia and functional deterioration. In some cases, prenatal diagnosis is possible by the demonstration of the conus medullaris in a position below the expected level for gestational age. Neurosurgical consultation followed by early neonatal surgery is expected to reduce the risks of neurologic damage and its sequelae, but it is important to remember that release of prenatally undiagnosed tethered cord is symptomatic children is adequate in maintaining neurologic, urologic, and orthopedic functioning.[33]

Tethered cord may be isolated or associated with other pathologies, including lipomata, lipomyelomeningocele, SCM (diastematomyelia), dermal sinus tract, fatty or tight filum, myelomeningocele (spina bifida or open spine), and caudal regression.[31]

Prenatal diagnosis has been rarely reported. Sohaey et al[34] reviewed the literature and presented their own cases, all of them with associated malformations, including fetuses with vertebral segmentation anomalies, VACTERL (vertebral, anal, cardiac, tracheal, esophageal, renal, and limb) association, myelocystocele, fetal tail, and open neural tube defect. We were able to reach a diagnosis during the second trimester in an otherwise normal fetus (Figure 17–7).

Recently, Sepulveda et al[35] described a case that remained unrecognized during first- and second-trimester US examinations.

## CAUDAL REGRESSION SYNDROME

Caudal regression syndrome (CRS) synonyms: sacral agenesis, sacral hypoplasia, sacral regression, corresponds to a spectrum of anomalies of the caudal end of the trunk. Malformations vary from isolated partial agenesis of the sacrococcygeal spine to severe malformations, such as dorsolumbosacral agenesis[36] and sirenomelia.[37–39] Associated malformations are imperforate anus, genitourinary anomalies, and renal dysplasia. The frequency of caudal regression syndrome is 1 in 7500 births, with no gender predominance but with an association with a

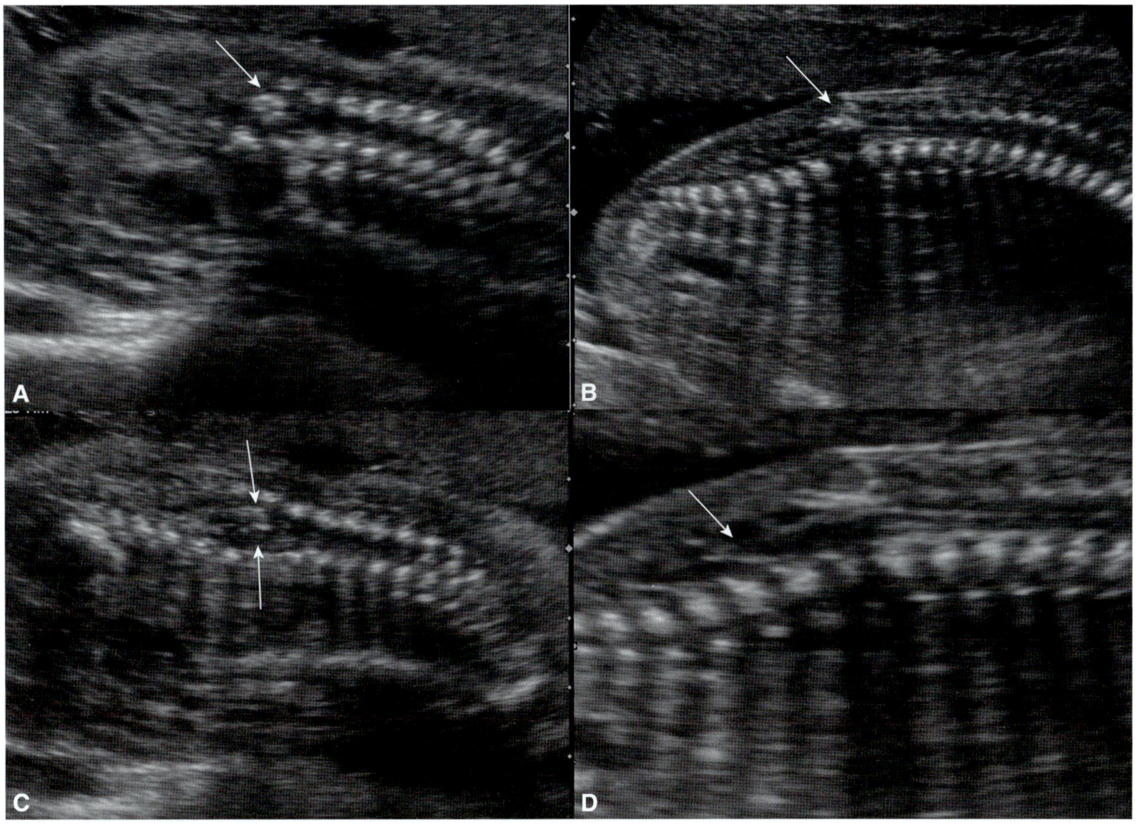


**Figure 17–6.** Diastematomyelia in a fetus at 23 postmenstrual weeks. Demonstration of the echogenic bone spur (*arrows*) in the coronal **(A)** and sagittal **(B)** planes is considered pathognomonic of this condition. In a more dorsal coronal plane **(C)**, the hemicords are observed (*arrows*). Tethered cord is commonly present.The arrow in **(D)** shows a low and dorsally positioned conus medullaris. (Courtesy of Dr. M. Teresa Higueras Sanz, Hospital Vall d'Hebron, Barcelona, Spain.)

diabetic mother. CRS is due to abnormal retrogressive differentiation of the developing spine and spinal cord, as well as disturbance of the caudal mesoderm, with failed development of the lumbar and sacral spine.[40–44] It is more common in infants of mothers with poorly controlled diabetes mellitus. Hyperglycemia is the most commonly recognized teratogen involved in this syndrome. In a patient with pregestational diabetes, caudal regression was diagnosed using transvaginal US.[41] At 9 postmenstrual weeks, shortening of the crown rump length and a protuberance at the lower spine (Figure 17–8A) suggested CRS. By 14 postmenstrual weeks, the diagnosis was certain (Figure 17–8B). Termination of the pregnancy was performed. The specimen was examined and confirmed the diagnosis (Figure 17–8C,D).

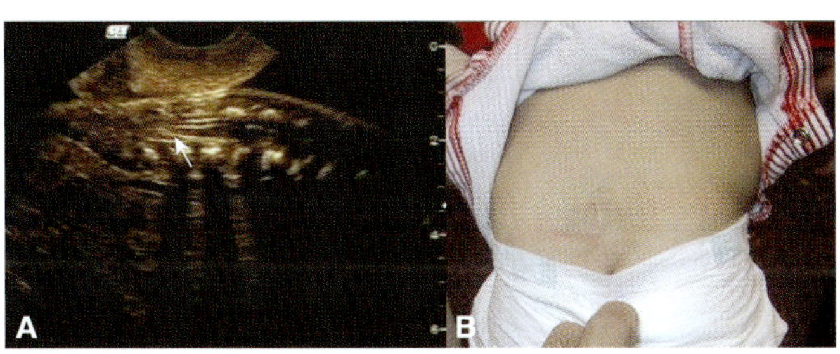


**Figure 17–7.** Tethered cord. **(A)** Image obtained from a video recording of a fetus at 23 postmenstrual weeks showing a conus medullaris positioned very low at the level of L5 (*arrow*). **(B)** The back of the child following successful tethered cord release; clinical follow-up showed no neurologic deficit.

The clinical presentation demonstrates a wide spectrum of abnormalities. Sacral agenesis is always associated with narrowing of the hips, hypoplastic gluteal muscles, and a flat intergluteal cleft. Orthopedic problems range from isolated deformities of the feet (eg, clubfoot) to complex deformities of the lower extremities. We can sonographically distinguish between partial sacral agenesis (Figure 17–9A) and complete sacral agenesis (Figure 17–9B). In patients with sirenomelia, complete lumbosacral agenesis and fused lower extremities are present.[37,38] Figures 17–10, 17–11, and 17–12 demonstrate two cases of early detection of sirenomelia at 11 postmenstrual weeks and 4 days (Figure 17–10) and 12 completed postmenstrual weeks (Figures 17–11 and 17–12), respectively. In these cases, color and power Doppler evaluation of the blood vessels in the lower limb and 3D surface rendering were instrumental. Not only was the

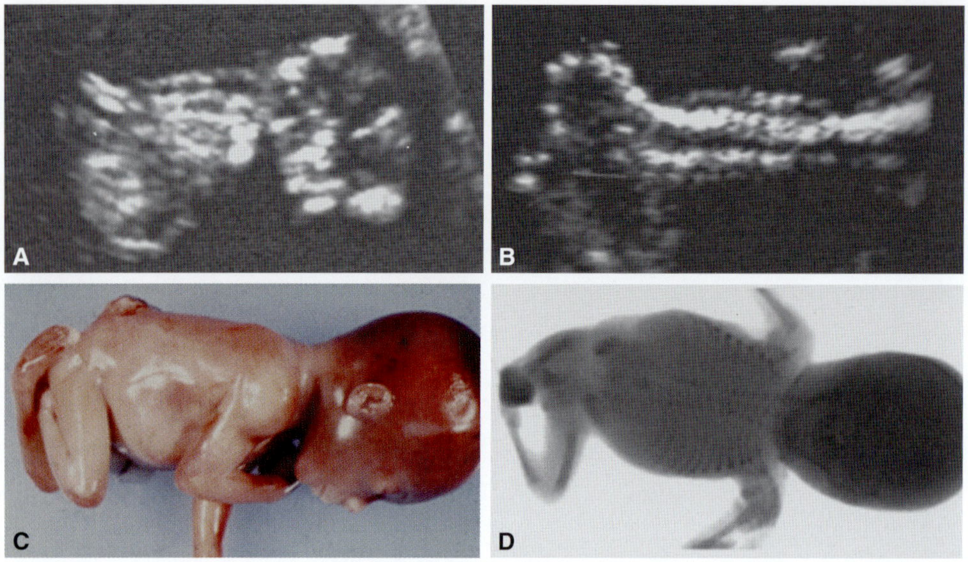

**Figure 17–8.** Caudal regression syndrome: early sonographic diagnosis. **(A)** At 9 postmenstrual weeks, the diagnosis was strongly suspected. **(B)** At 14 postmenstrual weeks, a firm diagnosis was made. **(C)** The specimen obtained by termination of the pregnancy revealed the deformity of the sacrum and the fixed, frog leg position of the lower limbs. **(D)** Radiographic study confirmed the lypoplastic sacrum, bones, and hip joints (Reproduced, with permission, from Baxi L et al, 1990[41]).

diagnosis made easier by the 3D rendering, but it contributed to the meaningful counseling of the couple. Different, extraskeletal anomalies are often associated with CRS. Genitourinary deformities include kidney malformations (agenesis or hydronephrosis) and various forms of duplication of the müllerian ducts. Neurologic deficiencies such as sensorimotor paresis or urinary bladder dysfunction can occur.

Various imaging methods allow differentiation of two groups of patients with caudal regression syndrome according to the configuration and level of the conus medullaris.[40] In group 1, spinal US demonstrates a blunt, deformed conus medullaris that terminates above the normal level of L1 and is sometimes associated with a dilated central canal or a cerebrospinal fluid–filled cyst at the lower end of the conus. In group 2, the conus medullaris is elongated

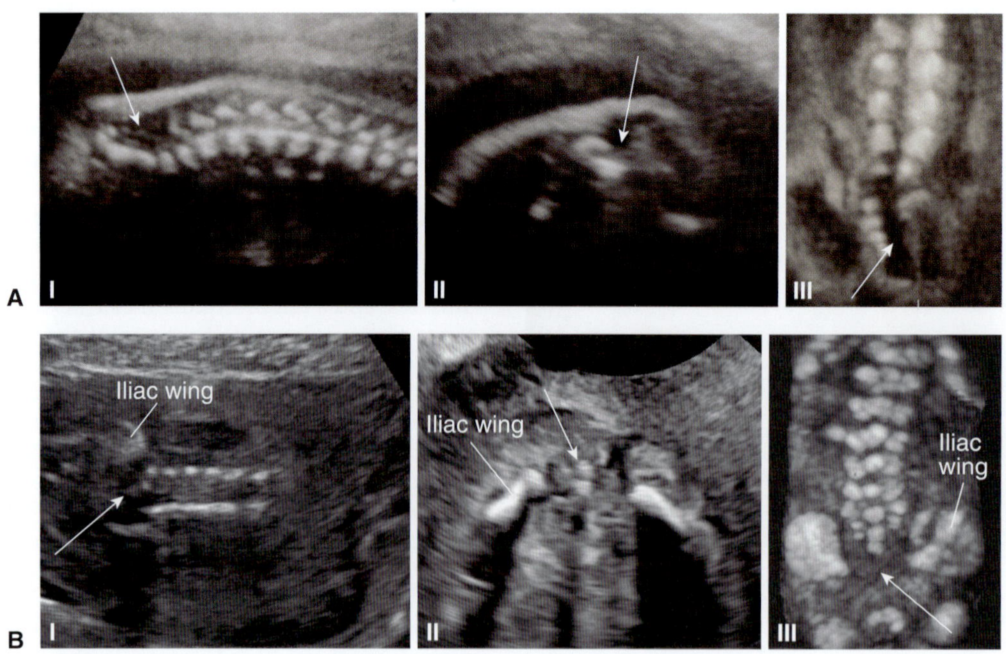


**Figure 17–9.** Types of sacral agenesis. **(A)** Partial: I. sagittal; II. axial; III. coronal. **(B)** Complete: I. coronal; II. axial; III. coronal (The white arrows point to the area of missing structures).

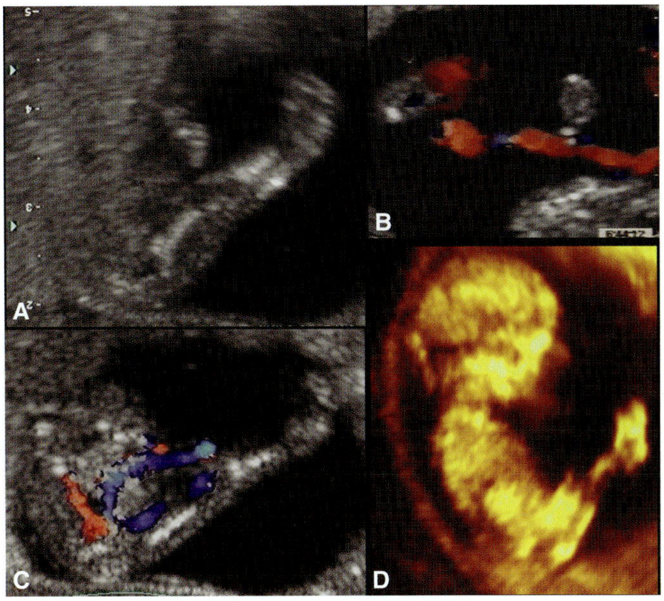

**Figure 17–10.** Sirenomelia in a fetus at 11 postmenstrual weeks. **(A)** One femur and two bones in the lower part of the leg are seen. **(B)** A two-vessel cord was detected. **(C)** One large artery is seen in the fused lips. **(D)** 3D renderings of the fetus. (Courtesy of Dr. Ana Monteagudo.)

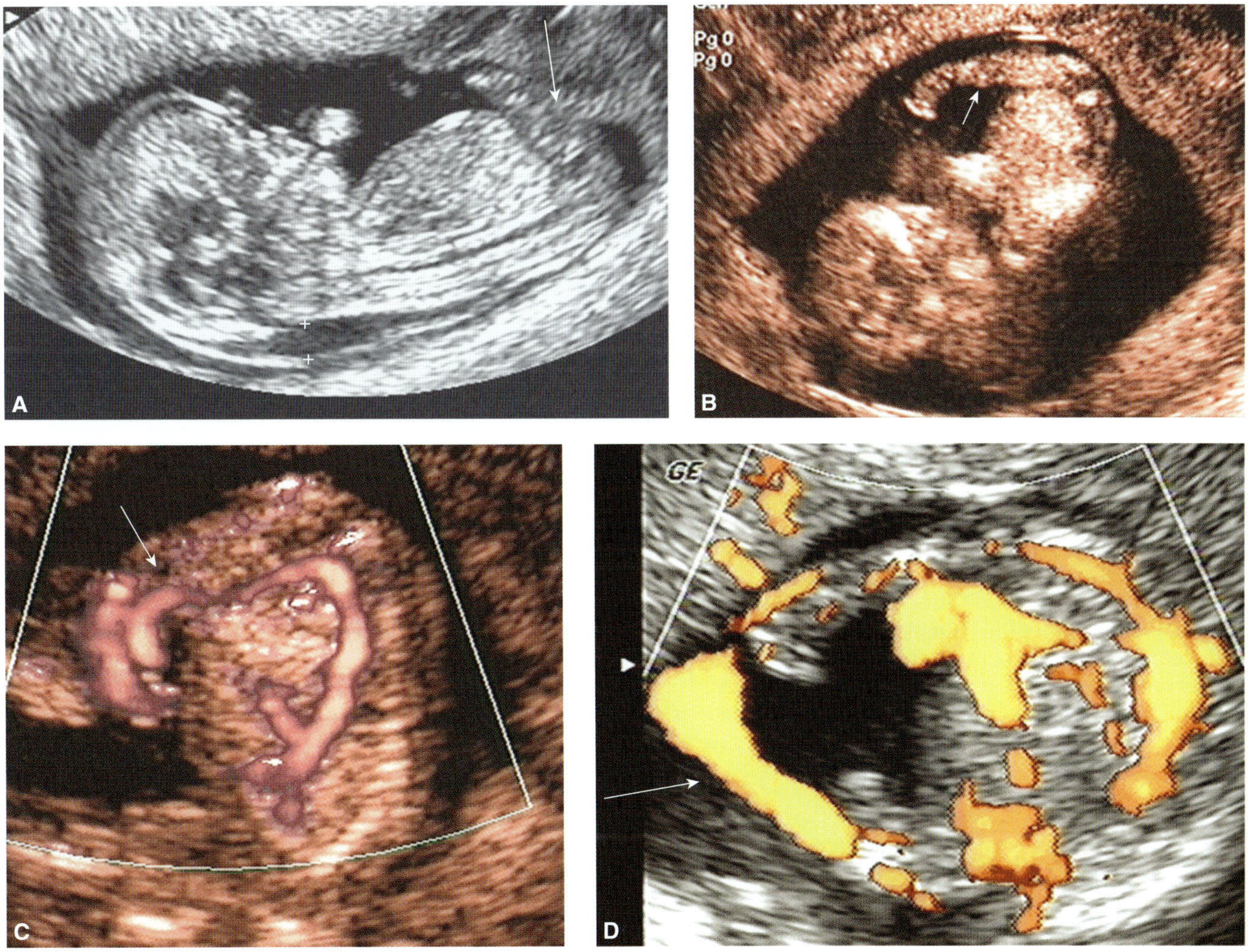

**Figure 17–11.** Anatomy scan at 11 postmenstrual weeks, 4 days at the time of the first trimester screening. **(A)** The nuchal translucency measures 8 mm. **(B), (C)** 3D "thick slice" rendering demonstrating the fused lower limb. **(D)** One single artery feeds the fused limb. **(E), (F)** 3D surface rendering of the feet with the toes. The white arrows point to the fused limb. (Courtesy of Dr. Ana Monteagudo)

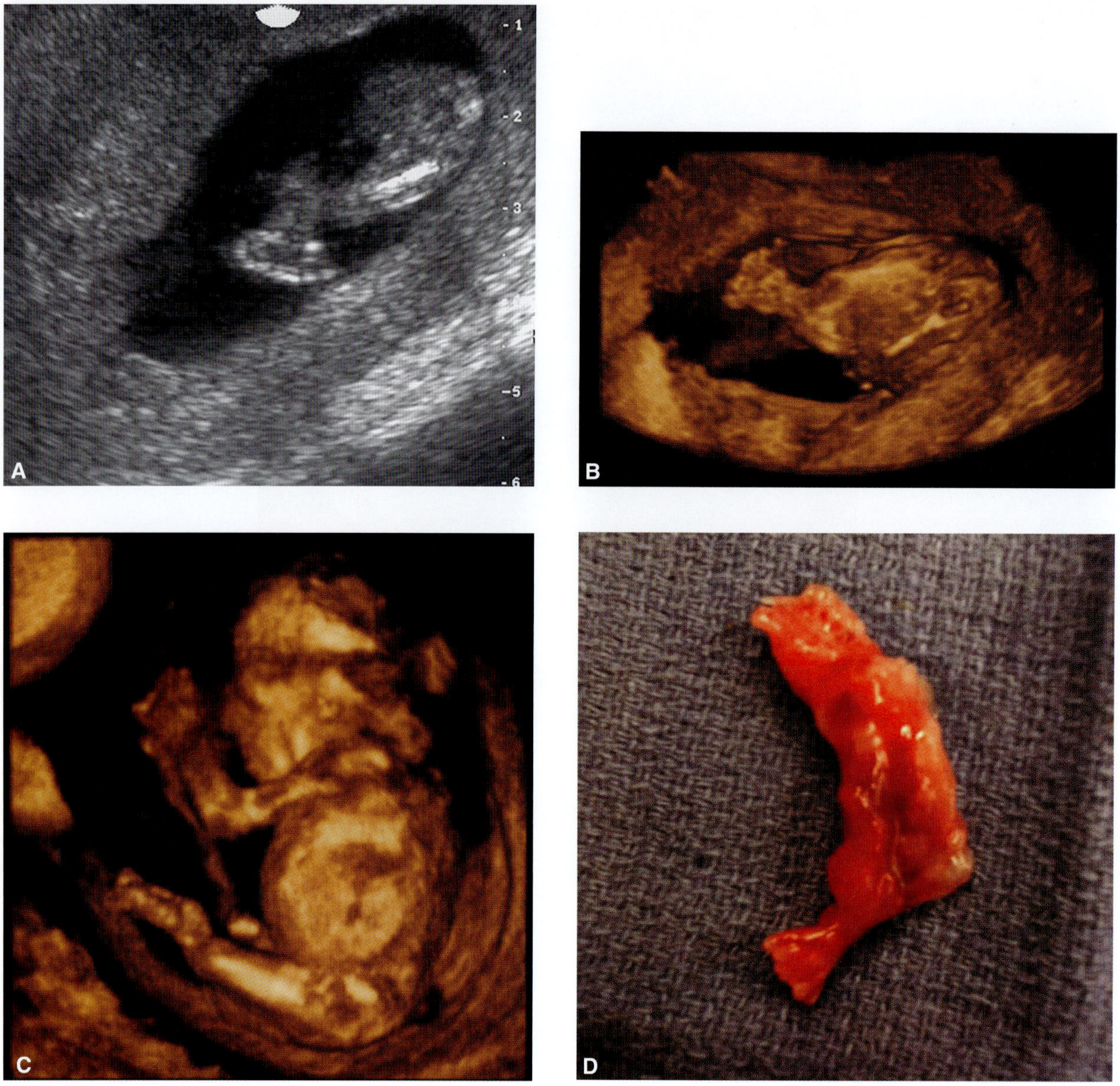

**Figure 17–12.** Sirenomelia in a fetus at 12 postmenstrual weeks. The pathology was detected at the time of the first trimester screening. **(A)** 2D gray-scale image. **(B)** 3D "thick slice" rendering. **(C)** 3D surface rendering of the fetus. At termination of the pregnancy, only the lower part of the body could be "salvaged" showing the pathology **(D)**. (Courtesy of Dr. Ilan Timor-Tritsch.)

and tethered by a thickened filum terminale or intraspinal lipoma and ends below L1. Patients in group 1 have major sacral deformities, whereas neurologic disturbances are more severe in group 2.[40]

Prenatal diagnosis is possible, even during the late first or early second trimester, by failing to demonstrate the caudal portion of the spine (see Figure 17–8).[36,43,44]

## REFERENCES

1. ISUOG. Sonographic examination of the fetal central nervous system: guidelines for performing the basic examination and the fetal neurosonogram *Ultrasound Obstet Gynecol.* 2007;29(1):109–116.
2. Lee W, Chaiworapongsa T, Romero R, et al. A diagnostic approach for the evaluation of spina bifida by three-dimensional ultrasonography. *J Ultrasound Med.* 2002;21(6):619–626.
3. Pilu G, Ghi T, Carletti A, Segata M, Perolo A, Rizzo N. Three-dimensional ultrasound examination of the fetal central nervous system. *Ultrasound Obstet Gynecol.* 2007;30(2):233–245.
4. von Koch CS, Glenn OA, Goldstein RB, Barkovich AJ. Fetal magnetic resonance imaging enhances detection of spinal cord anomalies in patients with sonographically detected bony anomalies of the spine. *J Ultrasound Med.* 2005;24(6):781–789.
5. Blaicher W, Mittermayer C, Messerschmidt A, Deutinger J, Bernaschek G, Prayer D. Fetal skeletal deformities:The diagnostic accuracy of prenatal ultrasonography and fetal magnetic resonance imaging. *Ultraschall Med.* 2004;25(3):195–199.
6. Barkovich J. Normal development of the neonatal and infant brain, skull and spine. In: Barkovich J, ed. *Pediatric Neuroimaging.* 4th ed. Philadelphia: Lippincott Williams & Wilkins; 2005: 17–75.
7. De Biasio P, Ginocchio G, Aicardi G, Ravera G, Venturini PL, Vignolo M. Ossification timing of sacral vertebrae by ultrasound in the mid-second trimester of pregnancy. *Prenat Diagn.* 2003;23(13): 1056–1059.

8. Barkovich J. Congenital anomalies of the spine. In: Barkovich J, ed. *Pediatric Neuroimaging.* Philadelphia: Lippincott Williams & Wilkins; 2005:704–772.
9. Zalel Y, Lehavi O, Aizenstein O, Achiron R. Development of the fetal spinal cord: time of ascendance of the normal conus medullaris as detected by sonography. *J Ultrasound Med.* Nov 2006;25(11): 1397–1401; quiz 1402–1393.
10. Unsinn KM, Geley T, Freund MC, Gassner I. US of the spinal cord in newborns: Spectrum of normal findings, variants, congenital anomalies, and acquired diseases. *Radiographics.* 2000;20(4): 923–938.
11. Budorick NE, Pretorius DH, Nelson TR. Sonography of the fetal spine: Technique, imaging findings, and clinical implications. *AJR Am J Roentgenol.* 1995;164(2):421–428.
12. Kirpekar M, Cohen HL. Ultrasonography of the normal spine. In: Timor-Tritsch I, Monteagudo A, Cohen HL, eds. *Ultrasonography of the Prenatal and Neonatal Brain.* New-York: McGraw-Hill; 2001:454–465.
13. Selden NR, Nixon RR, Skoog SR, Lashley DB. Minimal tethered cord syndrome associated with thickening of the terminal filum. *J Neurosurg.* 2006;105(3, Suppl):214–218.
14. Gray DL, Crane JP, Rudloff MA. Prenatal diagnosis of neural tube defects: Origin of midtrimester vertebral ossification centers as determined by sonographic water-bath studies. *J Ultrasound Med.* 1988;7(8):421–427.
15. Goldstein I, Makhoul IR, Weissman A, Drugan A. Hemivertebra: Prenatal diagnosis, incidence and characteristics. *Fetal Diagn Ther.* 2005;20(2):121–126.
16. Wynne-Davies R. Congenital vertebral anomalies: Aetiology and relationship to spina bifida cystica. *J Med Genet.* 1975;12:280–288.
17. Jeanty P, Valero G. Hemivertebra. www.thefetus.net. 2000.
18. Harrison LA, Pretorius DH, Budorick NE. Abnormal spinal curvature in the fetus. *J Ultrasound Med.* 1992;11(9):473–479.
19. Zelop CM, Pretorius DH, Benacerraf BR. Fetal hemivertebrae: Associated anomalies, significance, and outcome. *Obstet Gynecol.* 1993;81(3):412–416.
20. Weisz B, Achiron R, Schindler A, Eisenberg VH, Lipitz S, Zalel Y. Prenatal sonographic diagnosis of hemivertebra. *J Ultrasound Med.* 2004;23(6):853–857.
21. Lyngdoh TS, Mahalik S, Naredi B, Samujh R, Khanna S. Lumbocostovertebral syndrome with associated VACTERL anomaly. *J Pediatr Surg.* 2010;45(9):e15–e17.
22. Lazebnik N, Bornstein E, Timor-Tritsch I. The utility of volume sonography for the detection of fetal spine abnormalities. *Ultrasound Clin.* 2008;3(4):529–539.
23. Wax JR, Watson WJ, Miller RC, et al. Prenatal sonographic diagnosis of hemivertebrae: Associations and outcomes. *J Ultrasound Med.* 2008;27(7):1023–1027.
24. Pang D, Dias MS, Ahab-Barmada M. Split cord malformation: 1. A unified theory of embryogenesis for double spinal cord malformations. *Neurosurgery.* 1992;31(3):451–480.
25. Pang D. Split cord malformation: 2. Clinical syndrome. *Neurosurgery.* 1992;31(3):481–500.
26. Egelhoff JC. MR imaging of congenital anomalies of the pediatric spine. *Magn Reson Imaging Clin N Am.* Aug 1999;7(3):459–479.
27. Dick EA, Patel K, Owens CM, De Bruyn R. Spinal ultrasound in infants. *Br J Radiol.* 2002;75(892):384–392.
28. Winter RK, McKnight L, Byrne RA, Wright CH. Diastematomyelia: Prenatal ultrasonic appearances. *Clin Radiol.* 1989;40(3):291–294.
29. Has R, Yuksel A, Buyukkurt S, Kalelioglu I, Tatli B. Prenatal diagnosis of diastematomyelia: Presentation of eight cases and review of the literature. *Ultrasound Obstet Gynecol.* 2007;30(6):845–849.
30. Kulkarni M, Ruparel M, Redkar R. Fetal diastematomyelia: MR imaging. A case report. *Indian J Radiol Imaging.* 2009;19(1): 78–80.
31. Bui CJ, Tubbs RS, Oakes WJ. Tethered cord syndrome in children: A review. *Neurosurg Focus.* 2007;23(2):1–9.
32. Yamada S, Won DJ, Pezeshkpour G, et al. Pathophysiology of tethered cord syndrome and similar complex disorders. *Neurosurg Focus.* 2007;23(2):1–10.
33. Bowman RM, Mohan A, Ito J, Seibly JM, McLone DG. Tethered cord release: A long-term study in 114 patients. *J Neurosurg Pediatr.* 2009;3(3):181–187.
34. Sohaey R, Oh KY, Kennedy AM, Ameli JR, Selden NR. Prenatal diagnosis of tethered spinal cord. *Ultrasound Q.* 2009;25(2):83–87, quiz 93–95.
35. Sepulveda W, Wong AE, Fauchon DE. Fetal spinal anomalies in a first-trimester sonographic screening program for aneuploidy. *Prenat Diagn.* 2011;31(1):107–114.
36. Nagy GR, Csapo Z, Barakonyi E, Nagy B, Rigo J, Jr. Prenatal diagnosis and fetopathological investigation of dorsolumbosacral agenesis. *Pathol Res Pract.* 2009;205(7):490–493.
37. Malinger G, Treschan O, Rosen N, Zakut H. Sirenomelia in a twelve weeks abortus. *Early Hum Dev.* 1987;15(4):217–220.
38. Monteagudo A, Mayberry P, Rebarber A, Paidas M, Timor-Tritsch IE. Sirenomelia sequence: First trimester diagnosis with both two and three dimensional sonography. *J Ultrasound Med.* 2002;21: 915–920.
39. Pang D. Sacral agenesis and caudal spinal cord malformations. *Neurosurgery.* 1993;32(5):755–778, discussion 778–779.
40. Subtila D, Cossondo M, Houffina V, Valata AS, Puccha F. Early detection of caudal regression syndrome specific interest and findings in three cases. *Obstet Gynecol.* 1998;80:109–112.
41. Baxi L, Warren W, Collins MH, Timor-Tritsch IE. Early detection of caudal regression syndrome with transvaginal scanning. *Obstet Gynecol.* 1990;75:486–489.
42. Naidich TP, Zimmerman RA, McLone DG, Raybaud CA, Altman NR, Braffman BH. Congenital anomalies of the spine and spinal cord. In: Atlas SW, ed. *Magnetic Resonance Imaging of the Brain and Spine.* 2nd ed. New York: Lippincott-Raven; 1996:1265–1338.
43. Bashiri A, Sheizaf B, Burstein E, Landau D, Hershkovitz R, Mazor M. Three dimensional ultrasound diagnosis of caudal regression syndrome at 14 gestational weeks. *Arch Gynecol Obstet.* 2009;280(3):505–507.
44. Gonzalez-Quintero VH, Tolaymat L, Martin D, Romaguera RL, Rodriguez MM, Izquierdo LA. Sonographic diagnosis of caudal regression in the first trimester of pregnancy. *J Ultrasound Med.* 2002;21(10):1175–1178.

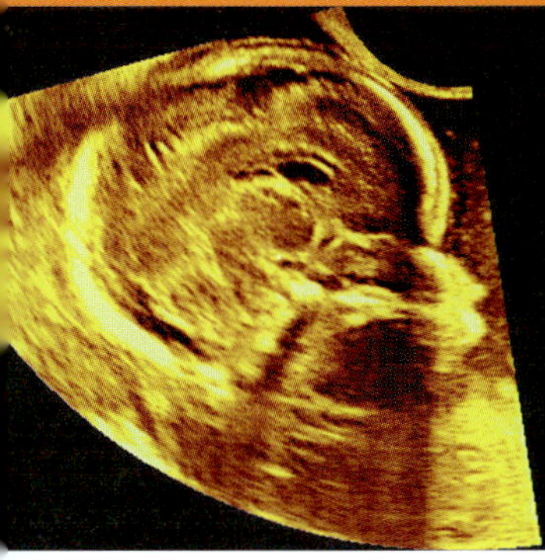

# INDEX

Page numbers followed by *f* or *t* indicate figures or tables, respectively.